BC Cancer Agency
Fraser Valley – Library
13750 96th Avenue
Surrey, BC Canada
V3V 1Z2

Interventional
Pain Management

Interventional Pain Management

SECOND EDITION

Steven D. Waldman, MD, JD
Director, The Pain Consortium of Greater Kansas City
Leawood, Kansas
Clinical Professor of Anesthesiology
University of Missouri at Kansas City
School of Medicine
Kansas City, Missouri

W.B. SAUNDERS COMPANY
An Imprint of Elsevier Science
Philadelphia London New York St. Louis Sydney Toronto

W. B. SAUNDERS COMPANY
An Imprint of Elsevier Science
The Curtis Center
Independence Square West
Philadelphia, PA 19106

Library of Congress Cataloging-in-Publication Data

Interventional pain management / editor, Steven D. Waldman.—2nd ed.

p. ; cm.

Includes bibliographical references and index.

ISBN 0-7216-8748-2

1. Analgesia. 2. Nerve block. 3. Pain—Treatment. I. Waldman, Steven D.
[DNLM: 1. Pain—therapy. 2. Analgesics—therapeutic use. 3. Nerve Block. 4. Neurosurgical Procedures. 5. Pain Measurement. WL 704 I619 2001]

RB127 .I59 2001

616′.0472—dc21 00-059487

Editor-in-Chief: Richard Lampert
Acquisitions Editor: Allan Ross
Developmental Editor: Ann Ruzycka
Project Manager: Tina Rebane
Production Manager: Pete Faber
Illustration Specialist: Walt Verbitski

INTERVENTIONAL PAIN MANAGEMENT ISBN 0-7216-8748-2

Copyright © 2001, 1996 by W.B. Saunders Company.

All rights reserved. No part of this publication may be reproduced or transmitted in any form or by any means, electronic or mechanical, including photocopy, recording, or any information storage and retrieval system, without permission in writing from the publisher.

Printed in the United States of America.

Last digit is the print number: 9 8 7 6 5 4 3 2

To
Drs. William and Marjorie Sirridge,
Marvin Bordy,
and
Alon Winnie,

whose dedication to teaching, the patient,
and love of medicine showed me
how it should be.

SDW

CONTRIBUTORS

Bernard M. Abrams, MD
Clinical Professor of Neurology, University of Missouri–Kansas City, Kansas City, Missouri; Neurologist, Menorah Medical Center, Overland Park, Kansas
Radiologic Testing in the Evaluation of the Patient in Pain

Susan R. Anderson, MD
Assistant Professor, Pain Clinic, Department of Anesthesiology, Texas Tech University Health Sciences Center, Lubbock, Texas
Atlantooccipital and Atlantoaxial Injections in the Treatment of Headache and Neck Pain; Stellate Ganglion Block; Continuous Regional Analgesia; Peripheral Neurolysis in the Management of Pain

Zahid H. Bajwa, MD
Assistant Professor of Anesthesia and Neurology, Harvard Medical School; Director, Pain Fellowship Program and Clinical Research, Beth Israel Deaconess Medical Center, Boston, Massachusetts
Facet Block and Neurolysis

Solomon Batnitzky, MD
Professor of Radiology and Surgery (Neurosurgery), and Chairman, Department of Radiology, University of Kansas School of Medicine; Radiologist in Chief, Kansas University Hospital, Kansas City, Kansas
Radiologic Testing in the Evaluation of the Patient in Pain

Marshall D. Bedder, MD, FRCP(C)
Medical Director, Advanced Pain Management Group, Inc., Portland, Oregon
Implantation Techniques for Spinal Cord Stimulation

David L. Brown, MD
Professor, Department of Anesthesiology, University of Iowa College of Medicine; Head, Department of Anesthesia, University of Iowa Health Care, Iowa City, Iowa
Occipital Nerve Block

Kenneth D. Candido, MD
Assistant Professor, Department of Anesthesiology, Rush Medical College; Chief, Section of Trauma Anesthesia, Department of Anesthesiology and Pain Management, Cook County Hospital, Chicago, Illinois
Differential Neural Blockade for the Diagnosis of Pain; Subarachnoid Neurolytic Blocks

Miles Day, MD
Assistant Professor, Pain Management/Anesthesiology, Texas Tech University Health Sciences Center, Lubbock, Texas
Sphenopalatine Ganglion Blockade

Meredith Dickens, MD
Neurological Pain Management, Department of Neurosurgery, The University of Texas M.D. Anderson Cancer Center, Houston, Texas
Receptors at the Spinal Cord Level: The Clinical Target

Charles D. Donohoe, MD
Associate Clinical Professor of Neurology, Kansas University Medical Center and University of Missouri at Kansas City, School of Medicine, Kansas City; President, Midwest Neuroscience, D.C., Independence, Missouri
Targeted History and Physical Examination; Rational Use of Laboratory Tests in the Evaluation of Pain

Anna Du Pen, ARNP, MN
Research Scientist, Cynergy Group, Bainbridge Island, Washington
Tunneled Epidural Catheters: Practical Considerations and Implantation Techniques

Stuart L. Du Pen, MD
Associate Director for Pain Research, Swedish Pain Management Group, Swedish Hospital; Clinical Associate Professor, Department of Anesthesiology, University of Washington School of Medicine, Seattle, Washington
Tunneled Epidural Catheters: Practical Considerations and Implantation Techniques

Donald A. Eckard, MD
Associate Professor of Radiology, and Chief, Division of Neuroradiology, University of Kansas School of Medicine, Kansas City, Kansas
Radiologic Testing in the Evaluation of the Patient in Pain

Valerie R. Eckard, MD
Senior Resident, Department of Radiology, University of Kansas School of Medicine, Kansas City, Kansas
Radiologic Testing in the Evaluation of the Patient in Pain

Philip M. Finch, FFP MANZCA
Perth Pain Management Centre, South Perth, Western Australia
Functional Anatomy of the Spine

Jason E. Garber, MD
Resident, Department of Neurosurgery, The University of Texas M.D. Anderson Cancer Center, Houston, Texas
Spinal Administration of Nonopiate Analgesics for Pain Management

Dan P. Gray, MD
Assistant Clinical Professor, Department of Anesthesia, Faculty of Medicine, University of Alberta; Staff Anesthesiologist, University of Alberta Hospital, Edmonton, Alberta, Canada
Facet Block and Neurolysis

Mark A. Greenfield, MD
Associate Director, Pain Consortium of Greater Kansas City, Leawood, Kansas
Phrenic Nerve Block

Rakesh Gupta, MD
Anesthesiologist, Virtua Memorial Hospital, Mt. Holly, New Jersey
Neurolytic Agents in Clinical Practice

Samuel J. Hassenbusch III, MD, PhD
Associate Professor and Associate Surgeon, Neurological Pain Management, Department of Neurosurgery, The University of Texas M.D. Anderson Cancer Center, Houston, Texas
Receptors at the Spinal Cord Level: The Clinical Target; Spinal Administration of Nonopiate Analgesics for Pain Management; Implantable Technology for Pain Control: Identification and Management of Problems and Complications

James E. Heavner, DVM, PhD
Professor, Departments of Anesthesiology and Physiology, and Director, Anesthesia Research, Texas Tech University Health Sciences Center, Lubbock, Texas
Percutaneous Epidural Neuroplasty; Peripheral Nerve Stimulation: Current Concepts

Donald W. Hinnant, PhD
Independent Practice, Behavioral Associates, Charleston, South Carolina
Psychological Evaluation of the Patient in Pain

Subhash Jain, MD
Associate Professor of Clinical Anesthesiology, Weill Medical College of Cornell University; Chief, Pain Service, Memorial Sloan-Kettering Cancer Center, New York, New York
Neurolytic Agents in Clinical Practice

Rudolph H. de Jong, MD
Professor (Hon) of Anesthesiology, Jefferson Medical College, Philadelphia, Pennsylvania
Local Anesthetics in Clinical Practice

Divakara Kedlaya, MD
Assistant Professor, Department of Physical Medicine and Rehabilitation, Loma Linda University School of Medicine, Loma Linda, California
Ilioinguinal-Iliohypogastric and Genitofemoral Nerve Blocks; Lateral Femoral Cutaneous Nerve Block; Spinal Administration of Opioids for Pain of Malignant Origin

Matthew T. Kline, MD
Private Practice in Interventional Pain Management, Philadelphia, Pennsylvania
Radiofrequency Techniques in Clinical Practice

Dan J. Kopacz, MD
Clinical Associate Professor, Department of Anesthesiology, University of Washington; Staff Anesthesiologist, Department of Anesthesiology, Virginia Mason Medical Center, Seattle, Washington
Intercostal Nerve Block

Elliot S. Krames, MD
Medical Director, Pacific Pain Treatment Centers, San Francisco, California
Mechanisms of Action of Spinal Cord Stimulation; Spinal Cord Stimulation and Intractable Pain: Patient Selection; When All Else Fails: A Role for Implantable Pain Management Devices; Intraspinal Analgesia for Nonmalignant Pain; Implantation Techniques for Totally Implantable Drug Administration Systems

Leland Lou, MD, MPH
Assistant Professor, Pain Service, Department of Anesthesiology, Texas Tech University Health Sciences Center, Lubbock, Texas
Percutaneous Epidural Neuroplasty

Ronald Melzack, PhD
Professor, Department of Psychology, McGill University; Research Director, Pain Centre, Montreal General Hospital, Montreal, Quebec, Canada
Toward a New Concept of Pain for the New Millennium

Michael Munz, MD, FRCS-C
Assistant Professor, Department of Neurosurgery, Temple University School of Medicine, Philadelphia, Pennsylvania
The Role of Neurosurgery in the Management of Intractable Pain

David P. Myers, MD, MBA
Assistant Professor of Clinical Anesthesiology, State University of New York at Buffalo School of Medicine and Biomedical Sciences; Staff Anesthesiologist, Roswell Park Cancer Institute, Buffalo, New York
Interpleural Catheters: Indications and Techniques

Kathleen A. O'Leary, MD
Assistant Professor of Clinical Anesthesiology, State University of New York at Buffalo School of Medicine and Biomedical Sciences; Chief of Surgical Anesthesia, Roswell Park Cancer Institute, Buffalo, New York
Interpleural Catheters: Indications and Techniques

John L. Pappas, MD
Department of Anesthesiology and Pain Management, William Beaumont Hospital, Royal Oak, Michigan
Cervical Plexus Blockade

Richard B. Patt, MD
President and Chief Medical Officer, The Patt Center for Cancer Pain and Wellness, Houston, Texas
Pharmacologic Management and Its Limitations; Celiac Plexus and Splanchnic Nerve Block; Superior Hypogastric Plexus Block: A New Therapeutic Approach for Pelvic Pain; Implantable Technology for Pain Control: Identification and Management of Problems and Complications

Valerie Phelps, PT
Faculty and Director, International Academy of Orthedic Medicine/US, Tucson, Arizona
Atlantooccipital and Atlantoaxial Injections in the Treatment of Headache and Neck Pain

Ricardo Plancarte, MD
Chief, Pain Clinic, National Cancer Institute, Mexico City, Mexico
Superior Hypogastric Plexus Block: A New Therapeutic Approach for Pelvic Pain

Gabor B. Racz, MD
Professor and Chair Emeritus, Department of Anesthesiology, and Director of Pain Services, Texas Tech University Health Sciences Center, and University Medical Center and Southwest Surgery Center, Lubbock, Texas
Atlantooccipital and Atlantoaxial Injections in the Treatment of Headache and Neck Pain; Sphenopalatine Ganglion Blockade; Percutaneous Epidural Neuroplasty; Peripheral Nerve Stimulation: Current Concepts

P. Prithvi Raj, MD
Professor of Anesthesiology, and Co-Director of Pain Services, Texas Tech University Health Sciences Center, Lubbock, Texas
Stellate Ganglion Block; Continuous Regional Analgesia; Peripheral Neurolysis in the Management of Pain; Peripheral Nerve Stimulation: Current Concepts

Somayaji Ramamurthy, MD
Professor, Department of Anesthesiology, University of Texas Health Science Center at San Antonio; Chief of University Pain Management Center, University Hospital, San Antonio, Texas
Thoracic Epidural Nerve Block; Obturator Nerve Block

Lowell Reynolds, MD
Assistant Professor of Anesthesiology, Loma Linda University, and Medical Director, Loma Linda University Center for Pain Management, Loma Linda, California
Ilioinguinal-Iliohypogastric and Genitofemoral Nerve Blocks; Lateral Femoral Cutaneous Nerve Block; Spinal Administration of Opioids for Pain of Malignant Origin

Steven M. Rosen, MD
Fox Chase Pain Management Associates, Jenkintown, Pennsylvania
Percutaneous Cordotomy

Lloyd R. Saberski, MD
Medical Staff, Yale New Haven Hospital, New Haven, Connecticut
Spinal Endoscopy: Current Concepts; Cryoneurolysis in Clinical Practice

Steven Simon, RPh, MD
Assistant Clinical Professor, Department of Physical Medicine and Rehabilitation, University of Kansas School of Medicine, Kansas City; Medical Director, MD America Rehabilitation Hospital, Overland Park, Kansas
Sacroiliac Joint Injection and Low Back Pain

Sunil K. Singh, MD
Interventional Neurology, Headache and Pain Relief Center, Minimally Invasive Surgery Center, Linwood, New Jersey
Percutaneous Laser Discectomy; Percutaneous Vertebroplasty; Chymopapain Chemonucleolysis

Steven M. Siwek, MD
Director, Intervention Pain Management Pain Consortium of Greater Kansas City, Leawood, Kansas
Interventional Pain Management: Programming for Success; Discography in Clinical Practice; Intradiscal Electrothermal Annuloplasty

Phillip S. Sizer, Jr, MEd, PT
Assistant Professor, Physical Therapy Program, Texas Tech University Health Sciences Center, Lubbock, Texas; Faculty, International Academy of Orthopedic Medicine/US, Tucson, Arizona
Atlantooccipital and Atlantoaxial Injections in the Treatment of Headache and Neck Pain

Michael Stanton-Hicks, MB, BS, MRCGPA, Dr Med (FFARCS, FRCA), AABM, FRCS, FRCA
Vice Chairman, Division of Anesthesiology, Pain Management, and Research, Cleveland Clinic Foundation, Cleveland, Ohio, and Professor, Johann Gutenberg University, Mainz, Germany
Lumbar Sympathetic Nerve Block and Neurolysis

James R. Taylor, Jr, MD, PhD, FAFRM
Adjunct Professor, Curtin University, and Visiting Professor, Australian Neuromuscular Research Institute, Perth, Western Australia
Functional Anatomy of the Spine

Gale E. Thompson, MD
Clinical Professor, Department of Anesthesiology, University of Washington; Staff Anesthesiologist, Department of Anesthesiology, Virginia Mason Medical Center, Seattle, Washington
Intercostal Nerve Block

C. David Tollison, PhD
Associate Clinical Professor, Department of Anesthesiology, Medical College of Georgia, Augusta, Georgia; Visiting Professor, Clemson University, Clemson, South Carolina
Psychological Evaluation of the Patient in Pain

Howard J. Waldman, MD, DO
Medical Director, Rehabilitation Physicians and Associates, Leawood; Director, Electrodiagnostic Medicine Laboratory and Pain Consortium, Kansas City, Kansas
Neurophysiologic Testing in the Evaluation of the Patient in Pain

Katherine A. Waldman, OTR, MBA
Director of Patient Services, Pain Consortium of Greater Kansas City, Leawood, Kansas
Interventional Pain Management: Programming for Success; Intradiscal Electrothermal Annuloplasty

Steven D. Waldman, MD, JD
Director, Pain Management Center of Greater Kansas, Leawood; Clinical Professor of Anesthesiology, University of Missouri at Kansas City School of Medicine, Kansas City, Missouri
Interventional Pain Management: Programming for Success; Discography in Clinical Practice; Blockade of the Gasserian Ganglion; Blockade of the Trigeminal Nerve and Its Branches; Glossopharyngeal Nerve Block; Vagus Nerve Block; Spinal Accessory Nerve Block; Cervical Epidural Nerve Block; Brachial Plexus Block; Suprascapular Nerve Block; Thoracic Paravertebral Block; Thoracic Sympathetic Ganglion Block; Lumbar Epidural Nerve Block; Celiac Plexus and Splanchnic Nerve Block; Caudal Epidural Nerve Block; Neuroadenolysis of the Pituitary: Indications and Technique; Intradiscal Electrothermal Annuloplasty

Carol A. Warfield, MD
Professor of Anesthesia, Harvard Medical School; Chairman, Department of Anesthesia, Beth Israel Deaconess Medical Center, Boston, Massachusetts
Cervical Plexus Blockade; Facet Block and Neurolysis

K. Dean Willis, MD
Associate Professor, University of Alabama in Huntsville, Vice President, American Neuromodulation Society, Huntsville, Alabama
Avoiding Difficulties in Spinal Cord Stimulation

Alon P. Winnie, MD, DABA, FACA, FFARCS(Eng), FFARACS, DABA Pain
Professor, Department of Anesthesiology, Rush Medical College; Chairman, Department of Anesthesiology and Pain Management, Cook County Hospital, Chicago, Illinois
Differential Neural Blockade for the Diagnosis of Pain; Subarachnoid Neurolytic Blocks

Gilbert Y. Wong, MD
Assistant Professor, Mayo Medical School; Consultant, Department of Anesthesiology, and Director of Psychosocial Program, Mayo Clinic Cancer Center, Mayo Clinic, Rochester, Minnesota
Occipital Nerve Block

Tony L. Yaksh, PhD
Professor and Vice Chair for Research, Department of Anesthesiology, and Professor of Pharmacology, University of California, San Diego, La Jolla, California
Anatomy of the Pain-Processing System; Pharmacology of the Pain-Processing System

Anthony T. Yarussi, MD
Assistant Professor of Clinical Anesthesiology, State University of New York at Buffalo, School of Medicine and Biomedical Sciences; Staff Anesthesiologist, Roswell Park Cancer Institute, Buffalo, New York
Interpleural Catheters: Indications and Techniques

Way Yin, MD
Medical Director, Interventional Medical Associates of Billingham, P.C., Billingham, Washington
Radiofrequency Techniques in Clinical Practice

Michael S. Yoon, MD
Resident, Department of Neurosurgery, Temple University Hospital, Philadelphia, Pennsylvania
The Role of Neurosurgery in the Management of Intractable Pain

PREFACE TO THE SECOND EDITION

It is hard to believe that over eight years have passed since the subspecialty of pain management devoted primarily to the provision of invasive procedures to treat pain was conceived. Its birth was the result of a request by Dr. Alon Winnie to put together a program to be sponsored by the Dannemiller Memorial Educational Foundation to be held in Nice, France, in conjunction with the International Association for the Study of Pain World Congress. The result was a program entitled Interventional Pain Management. When I presented the proposed program to Alon for his comments, he asked "What in the world is interventional pain management?" I explained I had coined the term interventional pain management (which I had liberally borrowed from our radiology colleagues) in an effort to recognize and distinguish the increasing number of pain management physicians who devoted their efforts to help patients in pain by the use of interventional pain management techniques as opposed to limiting their efforts to pharmacologic approaches. Hence, the subspecialty of pain management was born. The meeting was well received and it seemed logical that a text devoted to the same subject matter would be of value to pain management physicians. The result was the text *Interventional Pain Management*, published by W.B. Saunders Company. Little did either of us know that *Interventional Pain Management* would ultimately become the largest selling specialty pain management text in the world.

Since its initial publication in 1995 and through its four subsequent printings, the first edition of *Interventional Pain Management* has become a standard reference text for pain management physicians worldwide and has helped spur the growth of the subspecialty of interventional pain management. Just as the subspecialty has grown, so has the number of interventional techniques available to help our patients in pain. Thus, the need for an updated and expanded second edition of *Interventional Pain Management.* The current edition continues the conceptual emphasis on "how-to-do-it" started in the first edition and so popular with pain management physicians. This "how-to-do-it" approach is particularly evident in each of the eighteen new chapters of the second edition as well as in the completely revised old ones. New chapters include "rediscovered" old interventional techniques that have found new applications in pain management (e.g., brachial plexus block in the treatment of reflex sympathetic dystrophy), as well as reviews and descriptions of new techniques that did not exist when the first text was written (e.g., intradiscal electrothermal coagulation [IDET] and vertebroplasty). Throughout this edition of *Interventional Pain Management* the reader will find each chapter liberally illustrated with over 100 new or redrawn figures to help explain each procedure.

I want to thank each of the contributing authors who have given generously of their time and expertise to help make this edition of *Interventional Pain Management* a text we can all be proud of. Also, a special note of thanks to Allan Ross, Senior Medical Editor, and the other talented professionals at W.B. Saunders Company who helped make this text a reality. I hope you will find *Interventional Pain Management* meets your every expectation and helps you to better care for your patients in pain.

Steven D. Waldman, MD, JD

NOTICE

Anesthesiology is an ever-changing field. Standard safety precautions must be followed, but as new research and clinical experience broaden our knowledge, changes in treatment and drug therapy become necessary or appropriate. Readers are advised to check the product information currently provided by the manufacturer of each drug to be administered to verify the recommended dose, the method and duration of administration, and the contraindications. It is the responsibility of the treating physician, relying on experience and knowledge of the patient, to determine dosages and the best treatment for each individual patient. Neither the publisher nor the editor assumes any responsibility for any injury and/or damage to persons or property arising from this publication.

THE PUBLISHER

CONTENTS

PART V

Spinal Administration of Opioids and Other Analgesic Compounds

PART VI

Neurosurgical Techniques in the Management of Pain

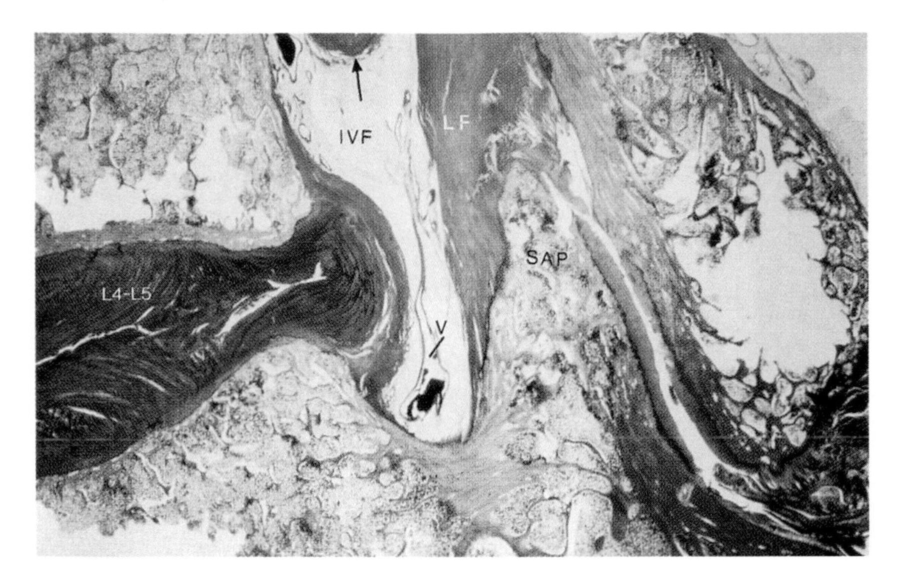

FIGURE 5–6 *Sagittal section of the posterior half of an L4-5 intervertebral disc from an elderly subject shows fissuring of the disc and posterior bulging of the annulus. The intervertebral foramen (*IVF*) behind the disc is empty apart from a segmental vein (*V*). The* arrow *indicates the spinal nerve in the upper part of the intervertebral foramen above the disc and facets.* LF, *ligamentum flavum;* SAP, *superior articular process of the facet joint.*

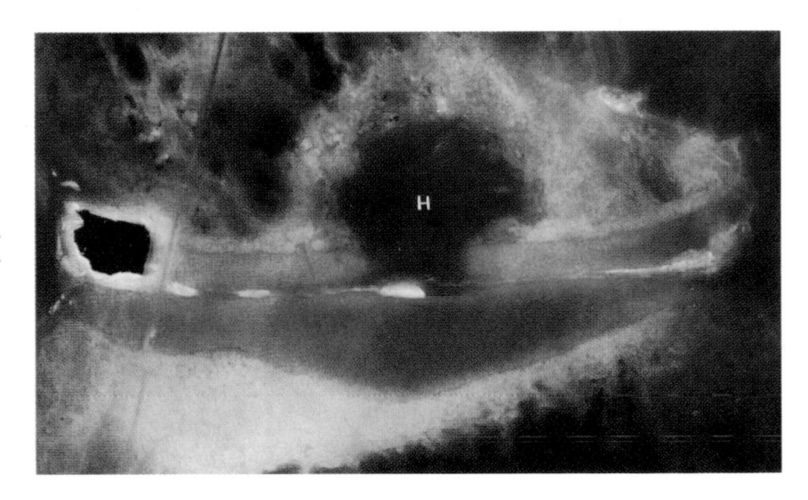

FIGURE 5–11 *A trauma-induced hemarthrosis in a lumbar facet joint of a 53-year-old woman.* H, *hematoma in subchondral bone.*

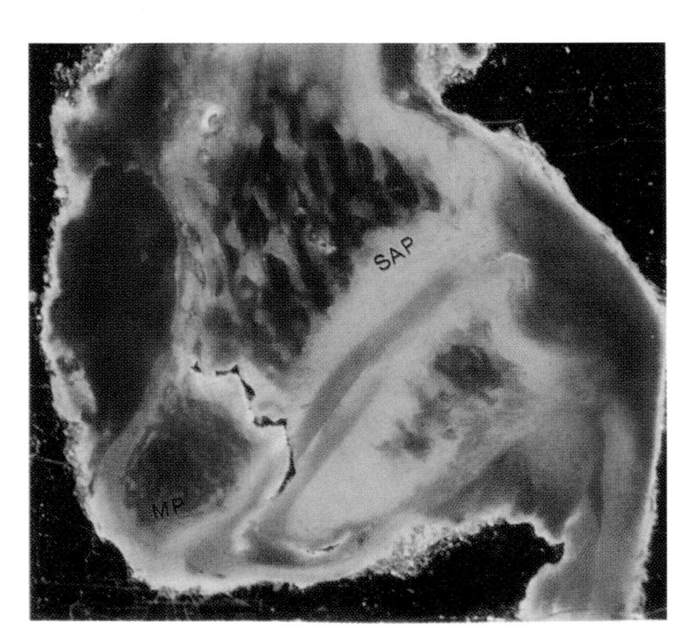

FIGURE 5–12 *A fracture of the mamillary process (*MP*) from the superior articular process (*SAP*) of L5 in a victim of a fatal traffic accident.*

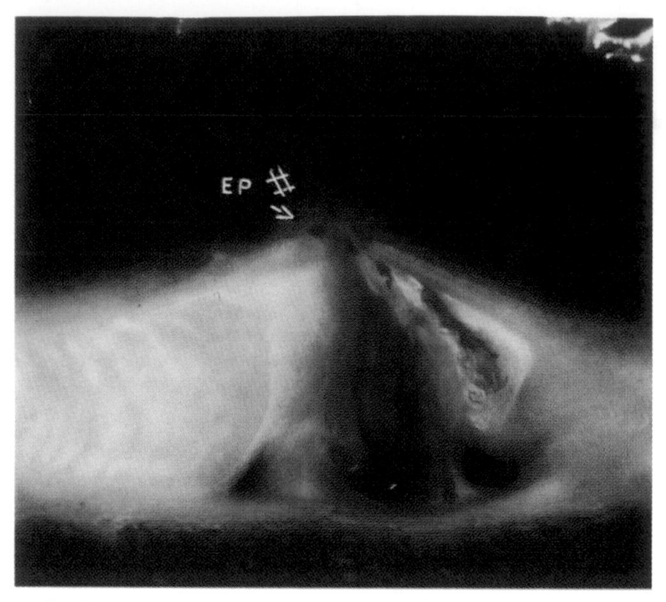

FIGURE 5–13 A fracture of the vertebral end plate of T9 (EP#) with bleeding into the disc in an 18-year-old man killed in a traffic accident.

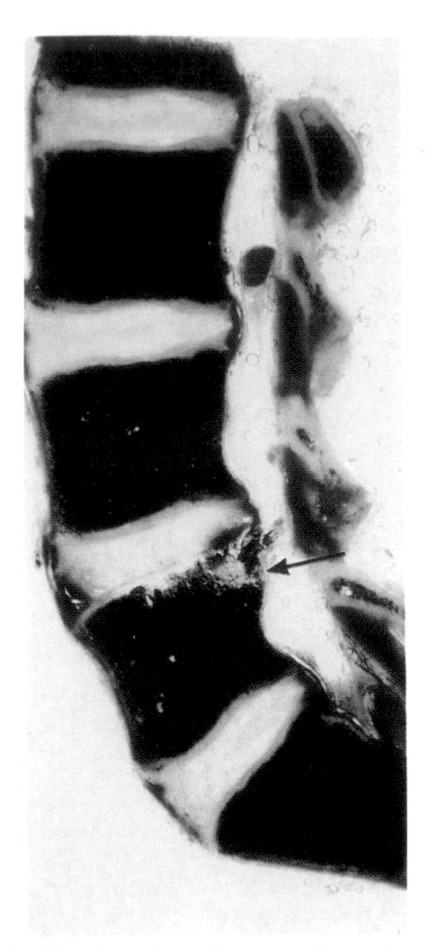

FIGURE 5–14 An unstained 2-mm sagittal section of the lumbar spine (L2 to sacrum) from a 19-year-old man who died after a traffic accident. Note the fracture of the upper posterior end plate of L5 with bleeding into the posterior annulus (arrow). There is also bleeding into the anterior annulus of L4-5 and, to a lesser degree, bleeding in the peripheral annuli of the other lumbar discs.

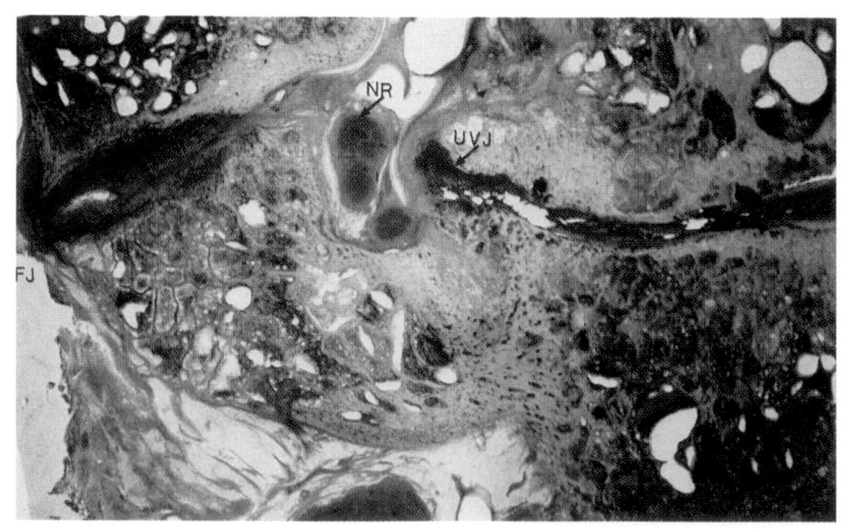

FIGURE 5–19 A 100-μm coronal section of a C6-7 motion segment, stained by hematoxylin and light green, from a 78-year-old woman, shows narrowing of the intervertebral foramen by disc resorption with laterally bulging uncovertebral osteophytes. There is an increase in the fibrous (green-stained) elements of the nerve roots (NR). UVJ, uncovertebral joint; FJ, facet joint.

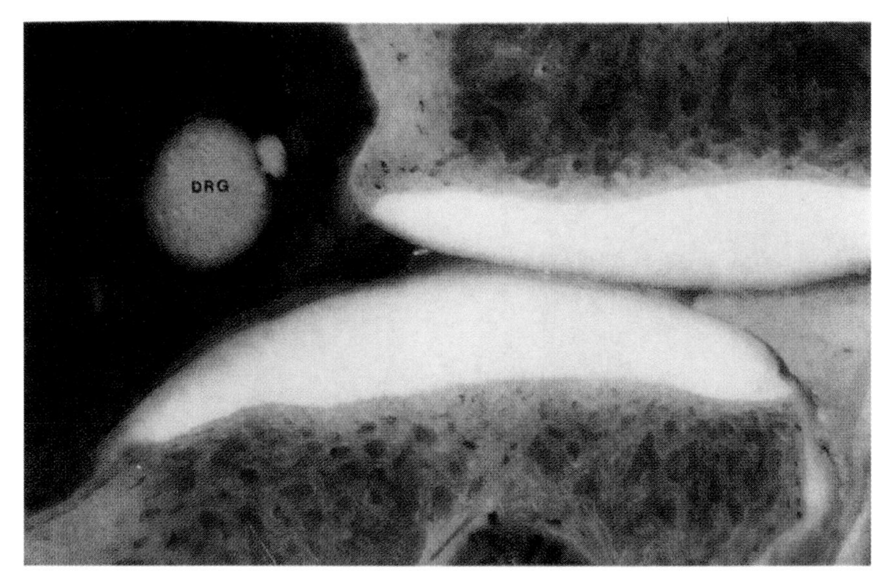

FIGURE 5–20 *A 2-mm, unstained sagittal section of an injured lateral atlantoaxial joint from a 13-year-old boy shows a large hematoma behind the joint (*left*) and in the posterior synovial fold of the joint. The dorsal root ganglion (*DRG*) is surrounded by the hematoma.*

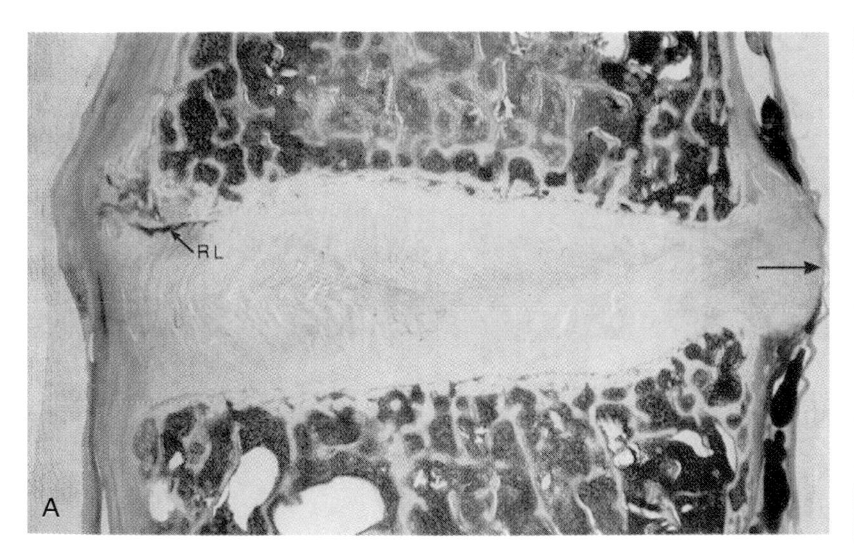

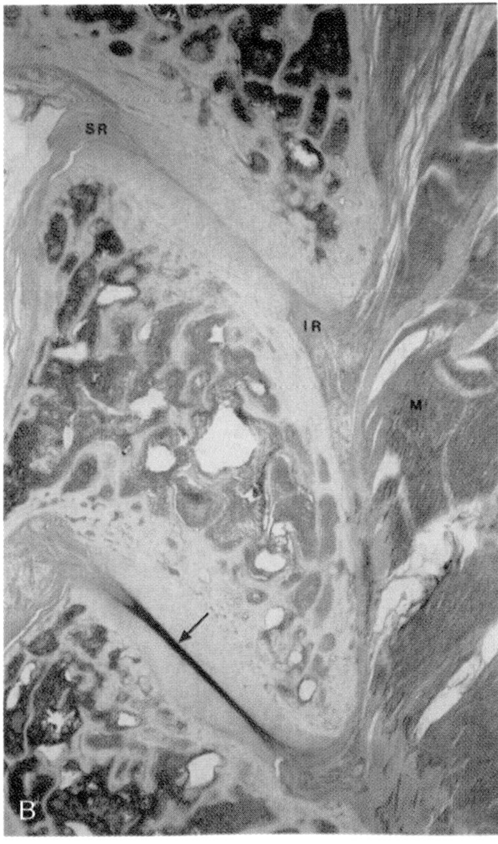

FIGURE 5–23 A, *This 100-μm section of the C6-7 disc from a 32-year-old man killed in a traffic accident shows an anterior rim lesion (*RL *and* arrow*) and a posterior traumatic disc herniation (*large arrow*) contained by a stretched but intact posterior longitudinal ligament.* B, *A 100-μm sagittal section of two facet joints from the same accident victim shows a normal joint above, with vascular synovial folds projecting into the superior recess (*SR*) and inferior recess (*IR*), which is enclosed by the multifidus muscle (*M*). The lower joint shows a traumatic hemarthrosis.*

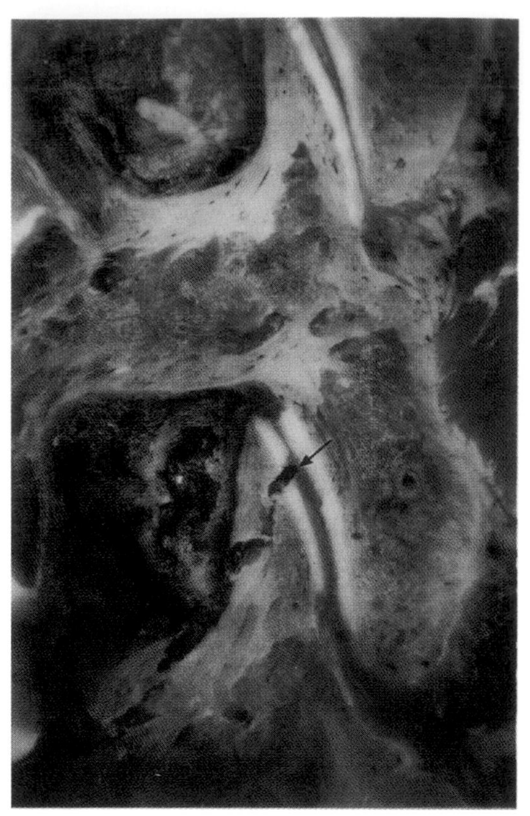

FIGURE 5–24 *A 2-mm unstained sagittal section of two lower cervical facet joints from a 16-year-old youth killed by a blow behind the vertex of the skull from a baseball bat. The axial compression injury has fractured the tip of the upper facet of T1* (arrow) *and the pedicle.*

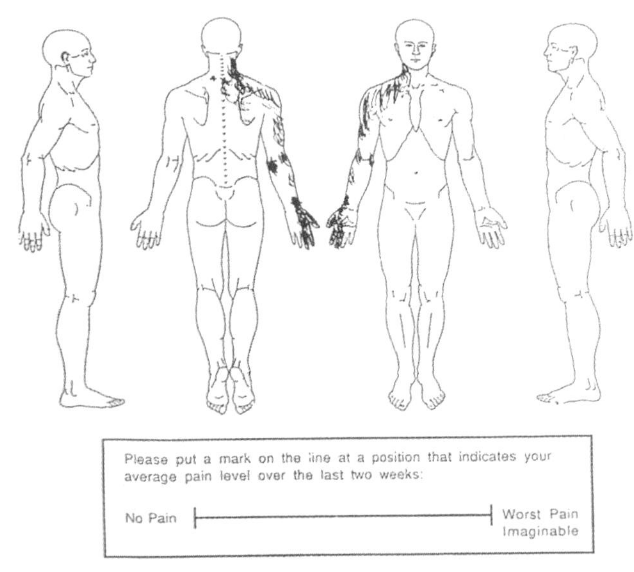

FIGURE 5–26 *Markings on this somatic pain diagram were supplied by the patient to represent pain. The diagram suggests involvement of the C6 nerve root.*

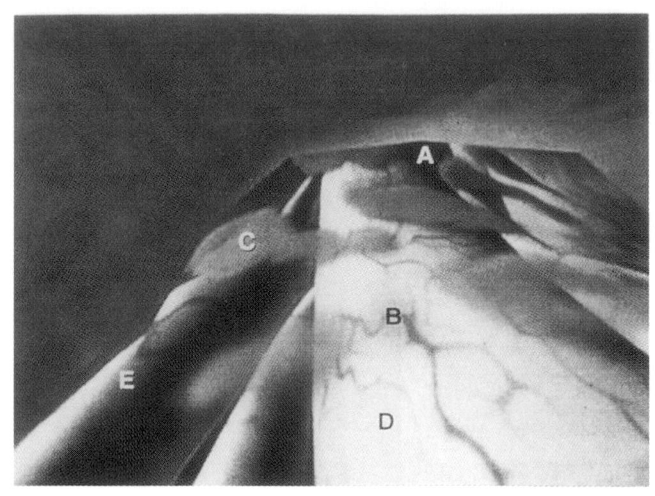

FIGURE 12–9 *Artist's rendering of the contents of the lower lumbar epidural space.* A, *Epidural space.* B, *Blood vessel.* C, *Epidural fat.* D, *Dura mater.* E, *Nerve root.*

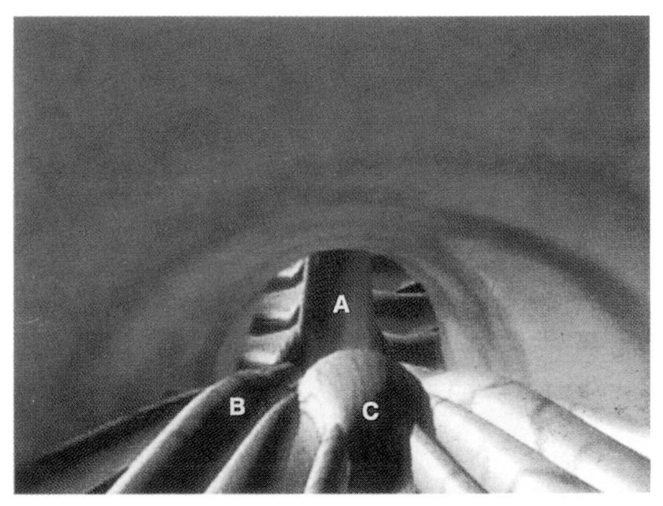

FIGURE 12–10 *Artist's rendering of the contents of the epidural space at the level of the conus medullaris (L1).* A, *Epidural space.* B, *Nerve root.* C, *Conus medullaris.*

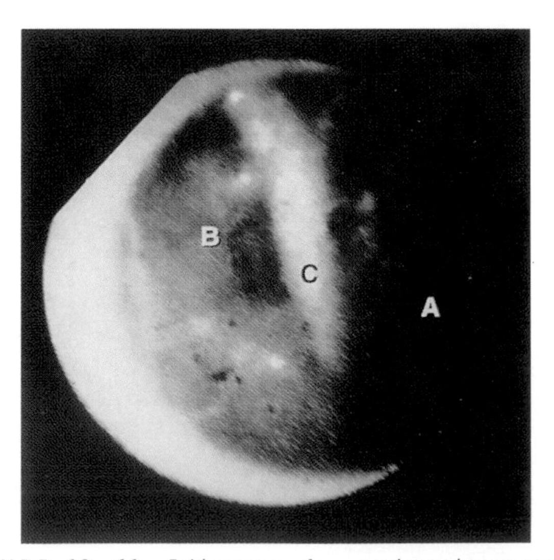

FIGURE 12–11 *Epiduroscopy of a normal sacral nerve root. The fiberoptic scope, introduced from the sacral hiatus, is on the right side, looking left toward a normal nerve root.* A, *Epidural space.* B, *Dura mater.* C, *Sacral nerve root.*

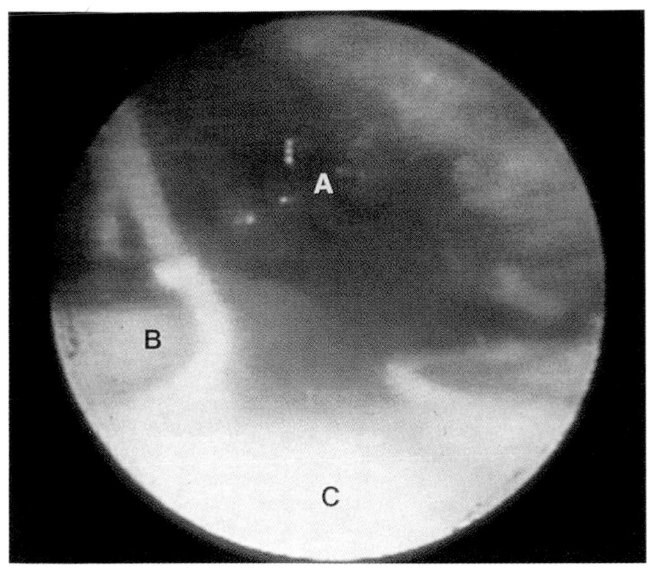

FIGURE 12–12 *Photograph of the lumbar epidural space caudad to the conus.* A, *Epidural space.* B, *Nerve root.* C, *Dura mater. See Figure 12–13 for an artist's rendering.*

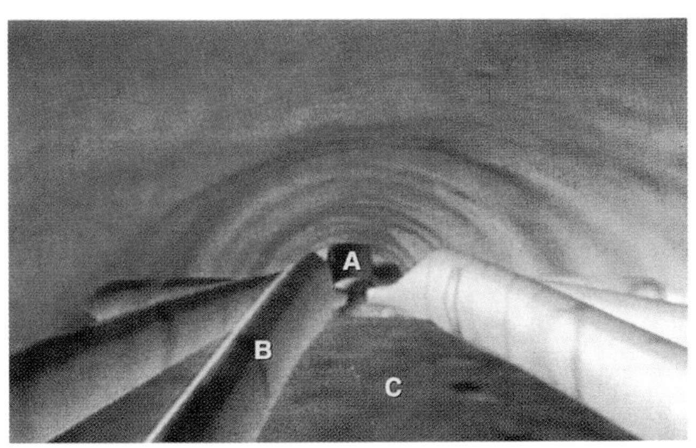

FIGURE 12–13 *Artist's rendering of the lumbar epidural space caudad to the conus shown in Figure 12–12.* A, *Epidural space.* B, *Nerve root.* C, *Dura mater.*

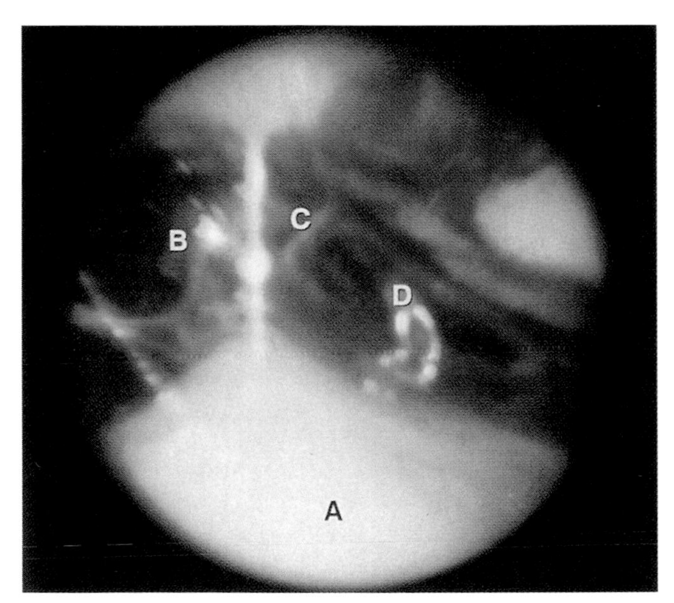

FIGURE 12–15 *Tuohy needle placed into the epidural space.* A, *Dura mater.* B, *Epidural space.* C, *Connective tissue band.* D, *Ligamentum flavum. (From Blomberg R, Olsson O: The lumbar epidural space in patients examined with epiduroscopy. Anesth Analg 68:157–160, 1989.)*

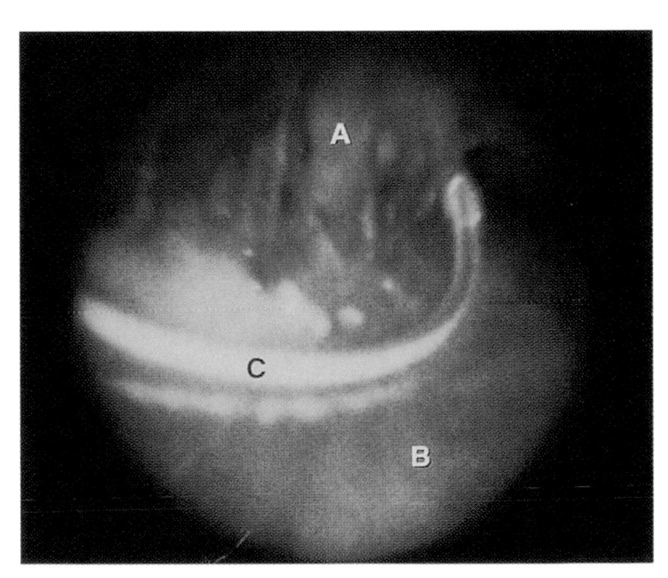

FIGURE 12–16 *Catheter passing into the epidural space from the Tuohy needle.* A, *Ligamentum flavum.* B, *Dura mater.* C, *Catheter. (From Blomberg R, Olsson O: The lumbar epidural space in patients examined with epiduroscopy. Anesth Analg 68:157–160, 1989.)*

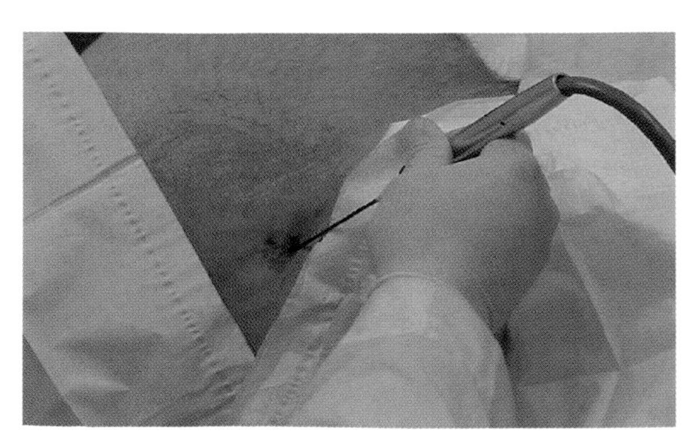

FIGURE 18–6 *Cryoablation of an anterior iliac crest bone harvest site.*

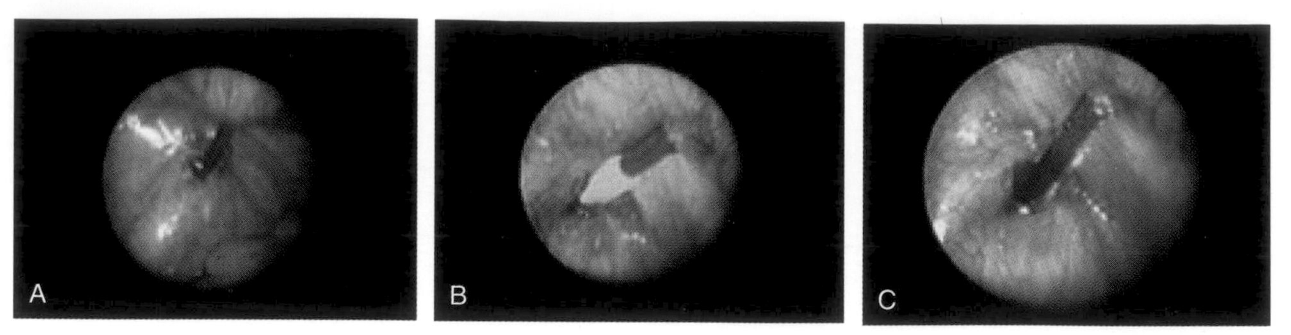

FIGURE 18–11 *A, Insertion of the Lloyd cryoprobe through the abdominal wall and fascia onto the genitofemoral nerve. B, Iceball formation for cryodenervation of the genitofemoral nerve. C, Lloyd cryoprobe immediately after defrost.*

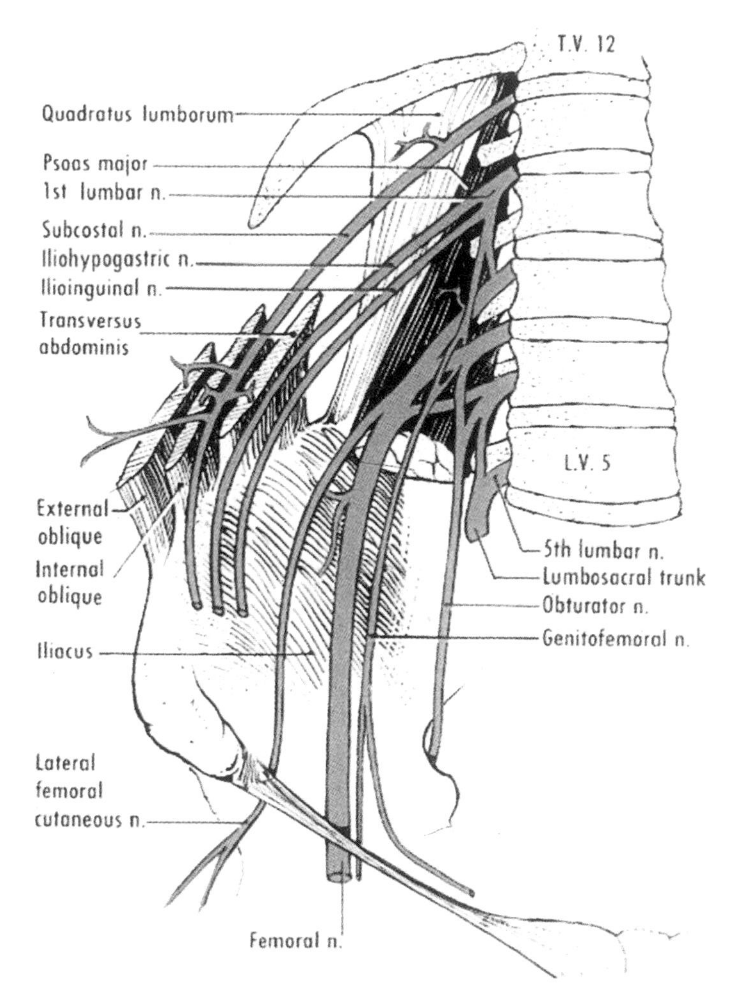

FIGURE 45–1 *Schematic drawing shows origin, course, and relations of lateral femoral cutaneous nerve. (Gardner, Gray WT, O'Rahilly R [eds]: Anatomy: A Regional Study of Human Structure, 5th ed. Philadelphia, WB Saunders, 1986.)*

PART • I

Anatomy and Physiology of Pain: Clinical Correlates

CHAPTER • 1

Toward a New Concept of Pain for the New Millennium

Ronald Melzack, PhD

Progress in science, according to historians of science such as Thomas Kuhn,[1] occurs in two ways: by the gradual accumulation of information that we call *facts* and by the rapid jumps in the integration of facts that occur when a new theory, concept, or *paradigm* is proposed. The former is normal science; the latter, a revolution. The progress occurs in a cycle that may involve generations of scientists and take centuries to complete. This historical process is depicted in Figure 1–1, with specific reference to the history of pain theories and science.

The theory of pain that we inherited in the 20th century was proposed by Descartes 300 years ago. Descartes was the first philosopher to be influenced by the scientific method that was devised in the 17th century, and he achieved a major revolution by arguing that the body works like a machine that can be studied using the experimental methods of physics. The impact of Descartes's theory, which later inspired experiments in anatomy and physiology, was enormous. The history of this era (reviewed by Melzack and Wall[2, 3]) is marked by a persistent search for pain fibers and pathways and for a pain center in the brain. The result is the well-known concept of pain as a specific projection system, which gave rise to ways of treating severe chronic pain with a multitude of neurosurgical lesions.[4, 5] Descartes's theory, then, determined the "facts" as they were known up to the middle of this century, and it even determined therapy.[6, 7]

THE GATE CONTROL THEORY OF PAIN

The gate control theory[2] has had a powerful impact on pain research and therapy.[3] When the theory was first published, in 1965, Descartes's specificity theory still dominated all thinking about pain. The specificity theory proposed that injury activates specific pain receptors and fibers, which in turn project pain impulses through a spinal pain pathway to a pain center in the brain. The psychological experience of pain, therefore, was virtually equated with physical injury. There was no room for psychological contributions to pain, such as attention, experience, and the "meaning" of the situation. Instead, pain experience was held to be proportional to peripheral injury or disease. Patients who suffered back pain without presenting signs of organic disease were labeled emotionally unstable and sent to psychiatrists. The picture, in short, was simple and, not surprisingly, erroneous. To thoughtful clinical observers such as Livingston[8] and Noordenbos,[9] the theory was clearly wrong.

Several attempts were made to find a new theory. The major opponent to specificity was labeled "pattern theory," but there were several different pattern theories, and they were generally vague and inadequate. Seen in retrospect, however, pattern theories gradually evolved to set the stage for the gate control theory (Fig. 1–2). Goldscheider proposed that central summation in the dorsal horns is one

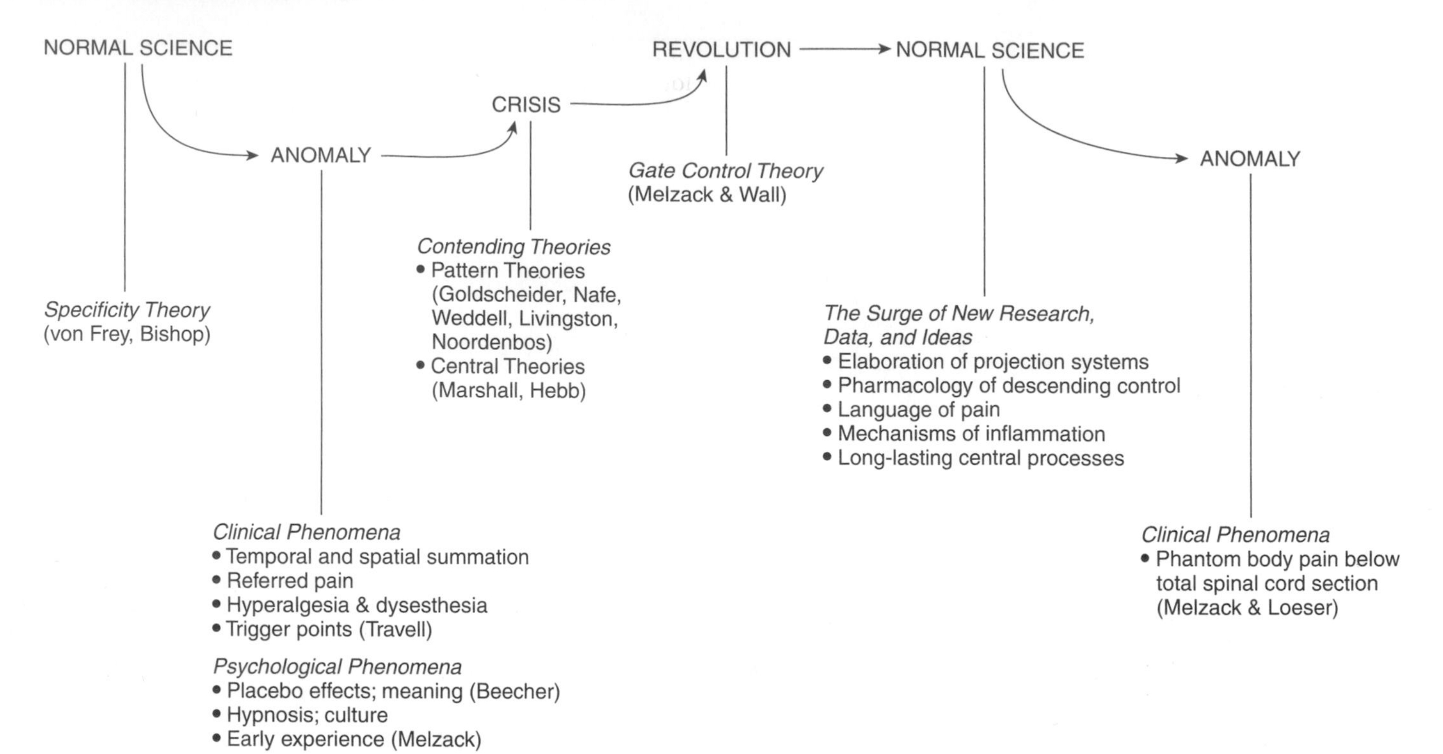

FIGURE 1–1 The pattern of scientific progress according to Kuhn.[1] Normal science *is a generally tranquil stage in which scientific data are acquired within the freamwork of a theory or paradigm that is generally accepted by all or most scientists. During this period, data are obtained that represent an* anomaly *(i.e., they do not fit the accepted paradigm). These data usually lead to the development of several new theories to explain them, producing a contentious and unsettled period* (crisis)*. Finally, a single theory emerges that becomes the new paradigm and represents a* revolution *from the old paradigm to the new one. Within this new paradigm, normal science produces new data and proceeds until a period of anomaly again arises, thus leading to a new cycle that culminates in the revolution of a new paradigm. This sequence is shown specifically for the science of pain, with the major events and scientists associated with each stage.*

of the critical determinants of pain.[3] Livingston's[8] theory postulated a reverberatory circuit in the dorsal horns to explain summation, referred pain, and pain that persisted long after healing was complete. Noordenbos's[9] theory proposed that large-diameter fibers inhibited small-diameter fibers, and he even suggested that the substantia gelatinosa in the dorsal horns plays a major role in the summation and other dynamic processes described by Livingston. None of these theories, however, posited an explicit role for the brain except as a passive receiver of messages. Nevertheless, the successive theoretical concepts moved the field in the right direction: into the spinal cord and away from the periphery as the exclusive explanation of pain (see Fig. 1–2). In the 1950s, pain was believed to be determined by nerve impulses evoked in A-delta and C fibers, direct followed by their transmission to the brain.

When Patrick Wall and I began the frequent discussions that led to a new theory of pain, we were convinced that (1) brain processes had to be integrated into the theory, including feedforward and feedback transmission, and (2) the new hypothetical spinal cord mechanism would need sufficient explanatory power to challenge spinal cord physiologists and entice them away from the concept of specificity. As a result, these two points characterize the theory.

When the gate control theory of pain was published in 1965, we were astonished by its reception. The theory generated vigorous (sometimes vicious) debate as well as a great deal of research to disprove or support it. The search for specific pain fibers and spinal cells by our opponents then became almost frantic. It was not until the mid-1970s that the gate control theory was presented in almost every major textbook in the biologic and medical sciences. At the same time, there was an explosion in research on the physiology and pharmacology of the dorsal horns and the descending control systems. The theory's emphasis on the modulation of inputs in the spinal dorsal horns and the dynamic role of the brain in pain processes had clinical as well as scientific impact. Psychological factors, which previously were dismissed as "reactions to pain," were now seen to be an integral part of pain processing, and new avenues for pain control were opened. Similarly, the cutting of nerves and pathways was gradually replaced by a host of methods to modulate the input. Physical therapists and other healthcare professionals who use a multitude of modulation techniques (including acupuncture) were brought into the picture, and transcutaneous electrical nerve stimulation (TENS) became an important modality for the treatment of chronic and acute pain.

The gate control theory's most important contribution to biologic and medical science was its emphasis on central nervous system (CNS) mechanisms. Never again, after 1965, could anyone try to explain pain exclusively in terms

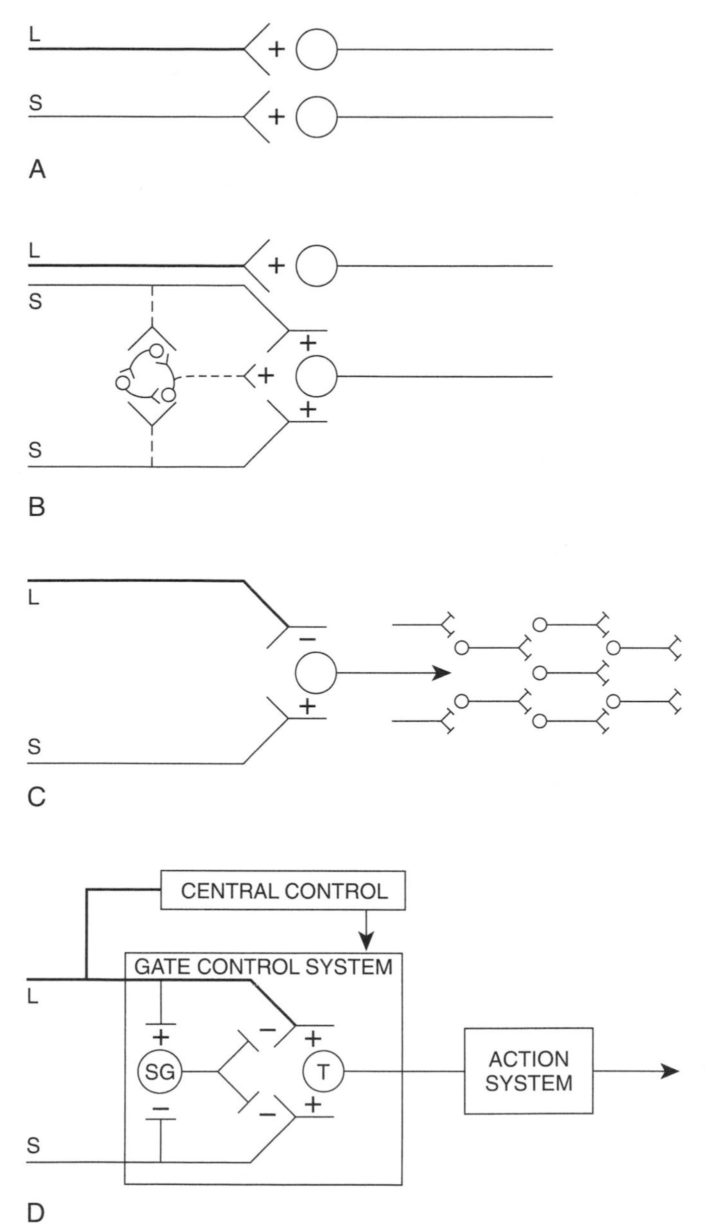

FIGURE 1–2 Schematic representation of conceptual models of pain mechanisms. A plus sign (I) indicates excitation; a minus sign ( ) indicates inhibition. A, Specificity theory. Large (L) and small (S) fibers are assumed to transmit touch and pain impulses, respectively, in separate, specific, straight-through pathways to touch and pain centers in the brain. B, Goldscheider's summation theory,[3] showing convergence of small fibers onto a dorsal horn cell. The central network projecting to the central cell represents Livingston's[8] conceptual model of reverberatory circuits underlying pathologic pain states. Touch is assumed to be carried by large fibers. C, Sensory interaction theory, in which large (L) fibers inhibit (−) and small (S) fibers excite (+) central transmission neurons. The output projects to spinal cord neurons, which are conceived by Noordenbos[9] to constitute a multisynaptic afferent system. D, Gate control theory.[2] The large (L) and small (S) fibers project to the substantia gelatinosa (SG) and first central transmission (T) cells. The central control trigger is represented by a line running from the large fiber system to central control mechanisms, which in turn project back to the gate control system. The T cells project to the entry cells of the action system.

of peripheral factors. The theory forced medical and biologic scientists to accept the brain as an active system that filters, selects, and modulates inputs. The dorsal horns, too, were not merely passive transmission stations but sites at which dynamic activities—inhibition, excitation, and modulation—occurred. This, then, was the revolution: We highlighted the CNS as an essential component in pain processes.

I believe the great challenge ahead of us is to understand brain function. Casey and I[10] made a start by trying to persuade our colleagues that specialized systems are involved in the *sensory-discriminative*, *motivational-affective*, and *evaluative* dimensions of pain. These terms seemed strange when we coined them, but they are now used so commonly and seem so "logical" that they have become part of the language. So, too, the McGill Pain Questionnaire, which taps into subjective experience—one of the functions of the brain—and is widely used to measure pain.[11, 12] We have also begun to understand the different pathways and neural mechanisms that underlie acute and chronic pain, again by invoking complex spinal and brain mechanisms, and we have gained a far better understanding of the analgesic effects of morphine.

In 1978, Loeser and I[13] described severe pains in the phantom bodies of paraplegics with verified total sections of the spinal cord and proposed a central "pattern-generating mechanism" above the level of the section. We focused more intensely than ever before on CNS mechanisms. My own efforts now are directed to exploration of new theoretical concepts to explain phantom body experiences—from pain to orgasm—in persons with total spinal sections. These experiences reveal important features of brain function because the brain is completely disconnected from the cord. In such a concept, psychophysical specificity makes no sense, and we must explore how patterns of nerve impulses generated in the brain can give rise to somesthetic experience. It comes as a shock to conclude that *you don't need a body to feel a body* or that *the brain itself can generate every quality of experience which is normally triggered by sensory input.*[14] This approach seems radical and difficult to comprehend, but I am convinced that it is the only road for us to travel on.

PHANTOM LIMBS AND PAIN CONCEPTS

It is evident that the gate control theory has taken us a long way. Yet, as historians of science have pointed out, good theories are instrumental in producing facts that eventually require a new theory that incorporates them, and this is what has happened. It is possible to make adjustments to the gate control theory, so that, for example, it includes long-lasting activity of the sort Wall[15] has described. There is a set of observations on pain in paraplegics that does not fit the theory, but this does not negate the gate control theory. All the peripheral and spinal processes obviously figure importantly in pain, and we need to know more about the mechanisms of peripheral inflammation, spinal modulation, and midbrain descending control, among others. The data on painful phantoms below the level of total spinal section[13] indicate that we also need to know more about the brain.[14]

The future of the study of pain lies in understanding the brain. Although there is still much to learn about nerves, the spinal cord, and the midbrain descending control systems, it is the brain beyond the midbrain that is almost uncharted territory and needs to be explored. The revolution created by cognitive neuroscience is teaching us new facts about brain function that simply stagger the imagination. There is no better way to enter this exciting world than to consider phantom limbs and phantom bodies: the "body-self" that is still present in experience even when input from a part of the body is gone.[15]

Phantom Limbs and the Concept of a Neuromatrix

In this exploration of new ideas, I would like to start with a case history of a patient who underwent cordectomy, total removal of a section of the spinal cord.

CASE STUDY

The patient was at work when the metal sides of a railroad car collapsed on him. He was left with total and permanent motor and sensory loss below T10–T11, and he complained of pain in the back and legs. Seven years after the accident, he underwent high thoracic cordotomy, and he was free of pain for 6 months. Two years later, he underwent thoracolumbar laminectomy and spinal cordectomy, which gave him complete pain relief for 11.5 years. At that point, he reported that the pain recurred in the lower back, radiating to both hips and down the dorsal aspect of both legs to the middle of the calves. The pain had the same properties as the pain he felt before the cordectomy: shooting pains lasting 3 to 4 seconds that, at their worst, occurred 50 to 60 times an hour. The pain was worse in humid weather.

When examined 6 months after recurrence of the pain, the patient said he had not had a single pain-free day since it returned. The pains occurred spontaneously in one or both legs without apparent triggering stimuli and without warning. The patient reported that the distribution of the pain was the same as that 12 years earlier: it began in the low back area and spread to the hips, then to the posterior thighs, and then to the calves.[13]

A New Approach

My analysis of phantom limb phenomena[9, 16] has led to four conclusions that point to a new conceptual model of the nervous system. First, because the phantom limb (or other body part) "feels" so real, it is reasonable to conclude that the body we normally feel is subserved by the same neural processes in the brain. These brain processes are normally activated and modulated by input from the body, but they can act in the absence of any input.

Second, all the qualities we normally feel from the body, including pain, are also felt in the absence of input from the body. From this we may conclude that the origins of the patterns that underlie the qualities of experience lie in neural networks in the brain. Stimuli may trigger the patterns, but they do not produce them.

Third, the body is perceived as a unity and is identified as the "self," an entity distinct from other people and the surrounding world. The experience of a unity of such diverse feelings, including the self as the point of orientation in the surrounding environment, is produced by central neural processes and cannot derive from the peripheral nervous system or spinal cord.

Fourth, the brain processes that underlie the body-self are, to an important extent that can no longer be ignored, "built in" by genetic specification, though this built-in substrate must, of course, be modified by experience. These conclusions provide the basis of the new conceptual model.

Outline of the Theory

I first present an outline of the theory and then deal with each of the components.

The anatomic substrate of the body-self, I propose, is a large, widespread network of neurons consisting of loops between the thalamus and cortex and between the cortex and limbic system. I have labeled the entire network, whose spatial distribution and synaptic links are initially determined genetically and are later sculpted by sensory inputs, a *neuromatrix*. The loops diverge to permit parallel processing in different components of the neuromatrix and converge repeatedly to permit interactions between the output products of processing. The repeated cyclic processing and synthesis of nerve impulses through the neuromatrix imparts a characteristic pattern, the *neurosignature*. The neurosignature of the neuromatrix is imparted on all nerve impulse patterns that flow through it and is produced by the patterns of synaptic connections in the entire neuromatrix. All inputs from the body undergo cyclic processing and synthesis, so that characteristic patterns are impressed on them in the neuromatrix. Portions of the neuromatrix are specialized to process information related to major sensory events (such as injury, temperature change, and stimulation of erogenous tissue) and may be labeled *neuromodules*, which impress subsignatures on the larger neurosignature.

The neurosignature, which is a continuous outflow from the body-self neuromatrix, is projected to areas in the brain—the *sentient neural hub* (*SNH*)—in which the stream of nerve impulses (the neurosignature modulated by ongoing inputs) is converted into a continually changing stream of awareness. Furthermore, the neurosignature patterns may also activate a neuromatrix to produce movement. That is, the signature patterns bifurcate so that a pattern proceeds to the SNH (where it is converted into the experience of movement), and a similar pattern proceeds through a neuromatrix that eventually activates spinal cord neurons to produce muscle patterns for complex actions.

The four components of the new conceptual nervous system, then, are (1) the body-self neuromatrix, (2) cyclic processing and synthesis in which the neurosignature is produced, (3) the SNH, which converts (transduces) the flow of neurosignatures into the flow of awareness, and (4) activation of an action neuromatrix to provide the pattern of movements to bring about the desired goal.

THE BODY-SELF NEUROMATRIX

The body is felt as a unity, with different qualities at different times, and I believe that the brain mechanism that underlies the experience also constitutes a unified system that acts as a whole and produces a neurosignature pattern of a whole body. The conceptualization of this unified brain mechanism lies at the heart of the new theory, and "neuromatrix" is the term that best characterizes it.

Matrix has several definitions in *Webster's Dictionary*,[17] and some of them imply precisely the properties of the neuromatrix as I conceive it. *Matrix* is defined as "something within which something else originates, takes form, or develops."[17] This is exactly what I wish to imply: The neuromatrix (not the stimulus, peripheral nerves, or "brain center") is the origin of the neurosignature; the neurosignature originates and takes form in the neuromatrix. Though the neurosignature may be triggered or modulated by input, the input is only a "trigger" and does not produce the neurosignature itself. *Matrix* is also defined as a mold or die that leaves an imprint on something else.[17] In this sense, the neuromatrix "casts" its distinctive signature on all inputs (nerve impulse patterns) that flow through it. Finally, *matrix* is defined as "an array of circuit elements . . . for performing a specific function as interconnected."[17] The array of neurons in a neuromatrix, I propose, is genetically programmed to perform the specific function of producing the signature pattern. The final, integrated neurosignature pattern for the body-self ultimately produces awareness and action.

For these reasons, "neuromatrix" seems the appropriate designation. The neuromatrix, distributed throughout many areas of the brain, comprises a widespread network of neurons that generates patterns, processes information that flows through it, and ultimately produces the pattern that is felt as a whole body. The stream of neurosignature output, with constantly varying patterns riding on the main signature pattern, produces the feelings of the whole body with constantly changing qualities.

The main psychological reason for postulating the neuromatrix is that it is incomprehensible to me how individual bits of information from skin, joints, or muscles can all come together to produce the experience of a coherent, articulated body. At any instant in time, millions of nerve impulses arrive at the brain from all the body's sensory systems, including the proprioceptive and vestibular systems. How can all this be integrated in a constantly changing unity of experience?

I cannot imagine how all these bits are added up to produce a whole. I can, however, visualize a genetically built-in neuromatrix for the whole body that produces a characteristic neurosignature for the body, which carries with it patterns for the myriad qualities we feel. The neuromatrix, as I conceive it, produces a continuous message that represents the whole body in which details are differentiated within the whole as inputs come into it. We start from the top, with the experience of a unity of the body, and look for differentiation of detail within the whole. The neuromatrix, then, is a template of the whole that provides the characteristic neural pattern for the whole body (the body's neurosignature) as well as subsets of signature patterns (from neuromodules) that relate to events at (or in) different parts of the body.

These views are in sharp contrast to the classic specificity theory, in which the qualities of experience are presumed to be inherent in peripheral nerve fibers. Pain is not injury: the quality of pain experiences must not be confused with the physical event of breaking skin or bone. Warmth and cold are not "out there"; temperature changes occur "out there," but the qualities of experience must be generated by structures in the brain. There are no external equivalents to stinging, smarting, tickling, itch; the qualities are produced by built-in neuromodules whose neurosignatures innately produce the qualities.

We do not learn to feel qualities of experience. Our brains are built to produce them. The inadequacy of the traditional peripheralist view becomes especially evident when we consider paraplegics with high-level complete spinal breaks. In spite of the absence of input from the body, paraplegics experience virtually every quality of sensation and affect. It is known that the absence of input produces hyperactivity and abnormal firing patterns in spinal cells above the level of the break,[18] but how, from this jumble of activity, do we get the meaningful experience of movement, the coordination of limbs with other limbs, cramping pain in specific (nonexistent) muscle groups, and so on? This must occur in the brain, where neurosignatures are produced by neuromatrixes that are triggered by the output of hyperactive cells.

When all sensory systems are intact, inputs modulate the continuous neuromatrix output to produce the wide variety of experiences we feel. We may feel position, warmth, and several kinds of pain and pressure all at once. It is a single unitary feeling, just as an orchestra produces a single unitary sound at any moment even though the sound comprises violins, cellos, horns, and other instruments. Similarly, at a particular moment in time, we feel complex qualities from all of the body. In addition, our experience of the body includes visual images, affect, "knowledge" of the self (versus not-self), as well as the meaning of body parts in terms of social norms and values. I cannot conceive of all of these bits and pieces coming together to produce a unitary body-self, but I can visualize a neuromatrix that impresses a characteristic signature on all the inputs that converge on it and thereby produces the never-ending stream of feeling from the body.

The experience of the body-self involves multiple dimensions—sensory, affective, evaluative, and postural, among many others. The sensory dimensions are subserved, in part at least, by portions of the neuromatrix that lie in the sensory projection areas of the brain; the affective dimensions, I assume, are subserved by areas in the brain stem and limbic system. Each major psychological dimension (or quality) of experience, I propose, is subserved by a particular portion of the neuromatrix, a *neuromodule*, which contributes a distinctive portion of the total neurosignature. To use a musical analogy once again, each portion of the neuromodule is like the string, percussion, woodwind, or brass section of a symphony orchestra, which constitutes a "module" of the whole. Each makes its unique contribution yet is an integral part of a single symphony that varies continually from beginning to end.

ACTION PATTERNS: THE ACTION-NEUROMATRIX

The output of the body neuromatrix, I have proposed, is directed at two systems: (1) a neuromatrix that produces awareness of the output and (2) a neuromatrix involved in overt action patterns. Just as there is a steady stream of awareness (even during the dream episodes of sleep), there is also a steady output of behavior (including movements during sleep).

Behavior occurs only after the input has been at least partially synthesized and recognized. For example, when we respond to the experience of pain or itch, it is evident that the experience has been synthesized by the body-self neuromatrix (or relevant neuromodules) sufficiently for the neuromatrix to have imparted the neurosignature patterns that underlie the quality of experience, affect, and meaning. Apart from a few reflexes (such as withdrawal of a limb, eye blink), behavior occurs only after inputs have been analyzed and synthesized sufficiently to produce meaningful experience. When we reach for an apple, the visual input has clearly been synthesized by a neuromatrix so that it has three-dimensional shape, color, and meaning as an edible, desirable object, all qualities that are produced by the brain and are not *in* the object "out there." When we respond to pain (by withdrawing or even by telephoning for an ambulance), we respond to an experience that has sensory qualities, affect, and meaning as a dangerous (or potentially dangerous) event to the body.

I propose that, after inputs from the body undergo transformation in the body-neuromatrix, the appropriate action patterns are activated concurrently (or nearly so) with the neuromatrix for experience. Thus, in the action-neuromatrix, cyclic processing and synthesis produces activation of several possible patterns and their successive elimination until one particular pattern emerges as the most appropriate for the circumstances at the moment. In this way, input and output are synthesized simultaneously, in parallel, not in series. This permits a smooth, continuous stream of action patterns.

The command, which originates in the brain, to perform a pattern such as running activates the neuromodule, which then produces firing in sequences of neurons that send precise messages through ventral horn neuron pools to appropriate sets of muscles. At the same time, the output patterns from the body-neuromatrix that engage the neuromodules for particular actions are also projected to the sentient neural hub and produce experience. In this way, the brain commands may produce the experience of movement of phantom limbs, even though there are no limbs to move and no proprioceptive feedback. Indeed, reports by paraplegics of terrible fatigue due to persistent bicycling movements (like the painful fatigue in a tightly clenched phantom fist in arm amputees) indicate that feelings of effort and fatigue are produced by the signature of a neuromodule rather than by particular input patterns from muscles and joints.

Mechanisms of Phantom Limb and Myofascial Pain

PHANTOM LIMB PAIN

The new theory of brain function, proposed on the basis of phantom limb phenomena, provides an explanation for phantom limb pain. Amputees suffer burning, cramping, and pain of other qualities. An excellent series of studies found that 72% of amputees had phantom limb pain a week after amputation and 60% had pain 6 months later.[19,20] Even 7 years after amputation, 60% still continued to suffer phantom limb pain, which means that only about 10% to 12% of amputees obtain pain relief. The pain is remarkably intractable: although more than 40 forms of treatment have been tried, none has proved to be particularly efficacious.[21]

Why is there so much pain in phantom limbs? I believe that the active body neuromatrix, in the absence of modulating inputs from the limbs or body, produces a signature pattern that is transduced in the SNH into a hot or burning sensation. The cramping pain, however, may be due to messages from the action-neuromodule to move muscles to produce movement. In the absence of the limbs, the messages to move the muscles become more frequent and "stronger" in the attempt to move the limb. The end result of the output message may be felt as cramping muscle pain. Shooting pains may have a similar origin, in which action-neuromodules attempt to move the body and send out abnormal patterns that are felt as shooting pain. The origins of these pains, then, lie in the brain.

BACK PAIN AND MYOFASCIAL PAIN

The fact that the most common kinds of pain—low back and myofascial pain—remain mysteries is testimony to the extent of our ignorance. In the case of low back pain, the majority (60% to 78%) of patients who suffer it have no apparent physical signs.[22] A variety of forms of therapy are tried, including disc surgery, trigger point injections, physical therapy, and behavior modification techniques. Yet a substantial number of people continue to suffer pain in spite of all these efforts. The search for the causes of low back pain is usually focused on the periphery: protruding discs, arthritis, pinched sensory roots, stress on ligaments and joints, spasm in muscles. Given the relatively high frequency of failures in attempts to rectify possible peripheral causes, it is reasonable to begin considering central mechanisms.

Because the action-neuromatrix maintains specific tensions on all muscles at all times, it is possible that sudden minor accidents (such as a fall) produce stresses and strains on muscles in a localized part of the body, which then send abnormal messages to the body neuromatrix. To maintain posture and balance, the action-neuromatrix may then change the tension on more distant muscles and ultimately produce a vicious circle of abnormal feedback and output for action.

A brief abnormal message, therefore, may produce a prolonged state of abnormal central outflow. The traditional trigger point and physical therapies could produce changes in inputs, which sometimes help, but the major cause may be the abnormal messages from the brain that maintain abnormal tensions on a large part of the body musculature. In the attempt to correct the inappropriate feedback, excessive tension may be put on other, distant, muscles to maintain balance and readiness for action. In this way, minor momentary injury of a shoulder may, for example, lead to pain in the upper back and the other shoulder, and eventually in the lower back and legs. In this case, the therapy that is needed may be far more complex, involving "reeducation" of the musculature of a large part of the body in the attempt to adjust the tension on muscles to normal, appropriate levels.

Myofascial syndromes such as fibromyalgia also remain a mystery and are difficult to understand. It is well-known that fibromyalgia (which has many other names) is associated with a characteristic distribution of trigger points and sleep disorder and is usually found in tense, hard-working, younger people. Here again, the initiating cause may be peripheral (muscle tension), but the sustaining cause that maintains abnormal tensions is now central. The underlying mechanism is usually sought in long repeated activities in the spinal cord, but the cause may, in fact, be in the brain, and an abnormal output thus maintains an abnormal pattern of tension on musculature throughout a large portion of the body. Therapy may require reeducation of the muscles of a large part of the body. Obviously, there are many inputs to the action-neuromatrix that may sustain the abnormal activity, such as abnormal muscle feedback, anxiety, depression, and fatigue. All of these inputs provide further avenues for health professionals to attempt to bring about a normal action neuromatrix output.

Referred Pain

Back pain and myofascial pain are often excellent examples of referred pain. They may be evoked by stimulation of tender spots at distant somatic sites.[23] Phantom limb pain may also be elicited by stimulation of distant sites,[24] or it may arise spontaneously as a result of emotional distress or even in the absence of any evident cause, but it is clearly due to brain output.

Referred pain is a complex phenomenon that must be examined at many levels. It is usually due to a combination of peripheral and central causes. Most commonly, the mechanisms are obvious and can be understood on the basis of the anatomy of the spinal cord. Sometimes, however, the mechanisms involve the brain and are complex. Even when referred pain involves trigger points that can be associated with muscles in spasm, it is likely that a spinal or brain mechanism is involved.

REFERRED PAIN DUE TO SPINAL CONNECTIONS

When the skin is injured, the pain is usually accurately localized. In contrast, visceral pain is rarely felt in the diseased viscus or in the skin above it. Nevertheless, the referred pain due to visceral disease generally follows well-known patterns. Pain due to appendicitis, for example, is usually felt in the upper abdomen in the midline above the umbilicus. Angina pectoris is generally felt as pain in the upper chest that shoots down the left arm. Inflammation of the diaphragm produces pain in the shoulder.

In all of these cases, the referred pain can be explained in terms of the convergence of visceral and somatic fibers onto dorsal horn cells in the spinal cord and the migration of nerves during embryonic development. For example, in the case of pain in the shoulder produced by an inflamed diaphragm, the explanation is that the muscle tissue of the diaphragm and the phrenic nerve that innervates it have their embryonic origin in the fifth cervical segment. Even though they migrate a considerable distance from the tissue that becomes the shoulder, the phrenic nerve activates the same spinal cells that are innervated by the fifth cervical nerve, a band of skin that includes part of the shoulder and upper arm.

The physiologic mechanisms in these cases are known to involve spinal cells at the first central synapse. Dorsal horn cells in lamina V that belong to the "wide dynamic range" (WDR) category are innervated by small-diameter fibers from the viscera and by large-diameter fibers (with low threshold) from the skin. These WDR cells provide the mechanism for referred pain in which a lesion in a deep structure seems to originate in a cutaneous area that is often tender. The tenderness, however, is due to central summation, not to peripheral injury or inflammation.

UNUSUAL CASES OF MISREFERRAL OF PAIN

At this point, referred pain becomes more complex. Sometimes, referred pain fails to occur, as in the case of the "silent" heart attack. This phenomenon suggests inhibitory neural or neurotransmitter mechanisms. Occasionally, strange referred pains occur, such as toothache that is eventually tracked down to cardiac disease.

These unusual referred pains are so well-known that they are probably due to an unusual "misinnervation" by nerve fibers that, for example, failed to stop in the shoulder and continued up into the head and jaw. Some of these anomalous cases have been studied carefully.

A few people, for reasons not known but presumably because of aberrant connections in the nervous system, find that when they scratch a body area (such as the knee) they feel a curious itchy or tickling sensation in a distant body area, such as the upper shoulder. Observations such as these underscore the complexity of central neural connections and take us far from simplistic concepts of the nervous system as little more than an old-fashioned telephone switchboard that has one plug-in connection for each telephone. As in our more complicated telecommunications networks, errors in connection occur in the human nervous system, sometimes with trivial consequences and sometimes with painful, crippling, disastrous results.

REFERRED PAIN INVOLVING TRIGGER POINTS

I have already discussed the classic case of referred pain in the upper chest and left shoulder and arm in patients who suffer anginal attacks. The story is more complex, however. Within or near (or, occasionally, at a considerable distance from) the area of referred pain, it is often possible to find small trigger points that are exquisitely sensitive and initiate severe pain when pressed with a finger or punctured by a needle.

Examination of cardiac patients by Kennard and Haugen[25] revealed that most had a common pattern of trigger points in the shoulder and chest. Pressure on the trigger points often produces intense pain that may last hours. Astonishingly, similar examination of a group of subjects who did not have heart disease revealed an almost identical distribution of tender areas.

Trigger points may involve only myofascial structures or may become associated with pathologic viscera. It is reasonable to assume that trigger points produce continuous input into the CNS. Diseased viscera, then, may evoke an input that summates with the input from the trigger points to produce pain referred to the larger skin areas surrounding the trigger points. Conversely, stimulation of the trigger points may evoke volleys of impulses that summate with low-level inputs from the diseased visceral structure, producing pain that is felt in both areas. These phenomena of referred pain, then, point to summation mechanisms that can be understood in terms of the gate control and the slower, more prolonged mechanisms.

Referred pains may also be associated with lesions of the central nervous system. Nathan[26] studied patients who had undergone unilateral or bilateral cordotomy, mostly for the relief of cancer pain, and found that pinpricks applied to analgesic parts of the body such as the leg evoked pain that was felt at distant sites on the same or the opposite side of the body.

The physiologic mechanisms of these referred pains involving trigger points undoubtedly involve spinal mechanisms. An injury may produce long-lasting activity in spinal cord cells that produce a persistently "open gate," so that inputs from many sources are summated. Coderre and I[27] have shown that a brief heat injury of a paw on one side produces a lowered threshold on the opposite side hours or days later. This condition persists even when the nerve from the injured paw is cut, thus indicating that the persistent change is in the CNS. Studies using the autotomy test show, in fact, that these central changes persist for weeks (the duration of observation), and probably much longer.

REFERRED PAIN INVOLVING THE BRAIN

Phantom limb pain is the clearest possible example of referred pain of central origin. The entire arm may have been amputated or totally denervated by a brachial plexus avulsion, yet the phantom limb (which may reside in the physical arm after avulsion) feels every quality of sensation, including agonizing pain.

The nature of these pains, which often include "memories" of injuries or other events that occurred years earlier, imply that the brain must be actively involved in these referred pains. Katz and I[28] have studied several cases and reviewed this fascinating literature. In these cases, the pain is clearly generated by the brain and is referred to the phantom or denervated limb.

Physiologic studies throw light on these mechanisms. Coderre and I[27, 29] and Katz and associates[30] have found evidence for long-lasting, persistent activity in the CNS. Coderre and colleagues[31] have reviewed the extensive literature on this problem. The early pain after an injury is critically important in initiating events in the brain that

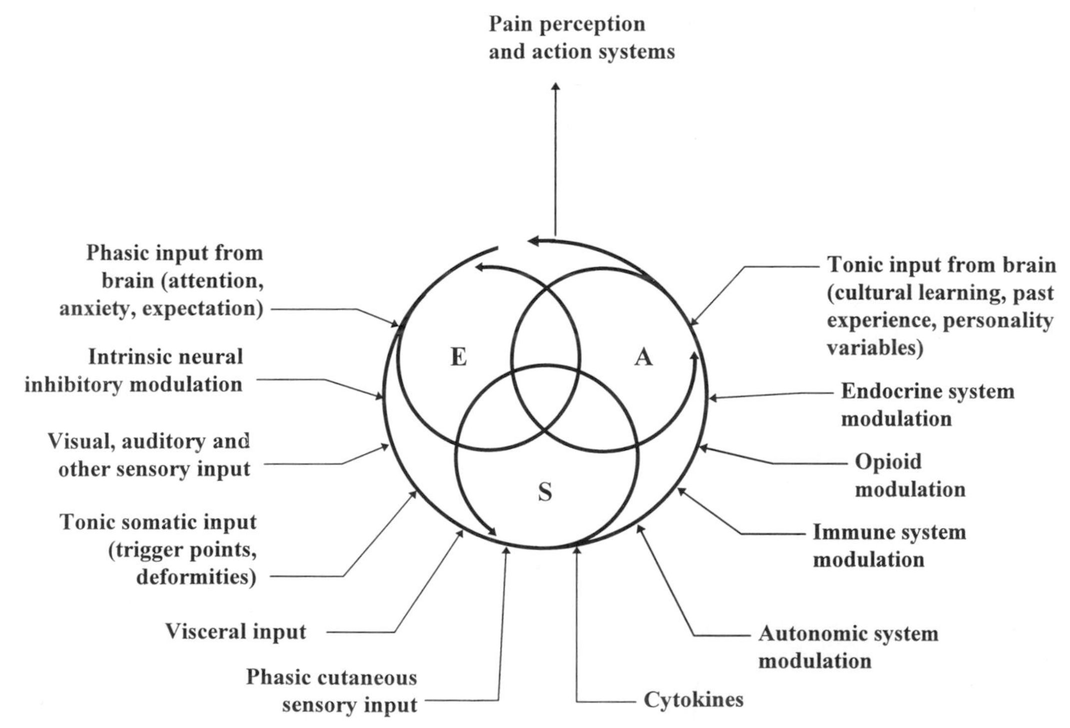

FIGURE 1–3 The body-self neuromatrix, which comprises a widely distributed neural network that includes somatosensory, limbic, and thalamocortical components, is schematically depicted as a circle containing smaller parallel networks that contribute to the sensory-discriminative (S), affective-motivational (A), and evaluative-cognitive (E) dimensions of pain experience. The synaptic architecture of the neuromatrix is determined by genetic and sensory influences. The "neurosignature" output of the neuromatrix—patterns of nerve impulses of varying temporal and spatial dimensions—which is produced by neural programs genetically built into the neuromatrix, determines the particular qualities and other properties of the pain experience and behavior. Multiple inputs that act on the neuromatrix programs and contribute to the output signature include (1) Sensory inputs from somatic receptors (phasic cutaneous, visceral, and tonic somatic inputs); (2) visual and other sensory inputs that influence the congnitive interpretation of the situation; (3) phasic and tonic congnitive and emotional inputs from other areas of the brain; (4) intrinsic neural inhibitory modulation inherent in all brain function; and (5) the activity of the body's stress-regulation systems, including cytokines and the endocrine, autonomic, immune, and opioid systems.

persist even after the peripheral nerve or spinal cord is blocked. These are referred pains that can be attributed only to central activitiy. Peripheral activity has been blocked in the spinal cord and is prevented from reaching the brain, yet pain persists.

PAIN AND STRESS

We are so accustomed to considering pain as a purely perceptual phenomenon that we have ignored the obvious fact that injury also disrupts the body's homeostatic systems, thus producing stress and initiating complex programs to restore homeostasis. When the role of the stress system in pain processes is taken into account, the scope of the puzzle of pain is greatly expanded and new pieces of the puzzle provide valuable clues in our quest to understand chronic pain.

Given the multiplicity of interacting neural and hormonal factors that contribute to homeostasis, it is not surprising that programs to restore homeostasis may go awry. The consequence is a variety of stress-related disorders, which include several chronic pain syndromes.[32–34] Recently I examined the hypothesis that stress may produce the conditions that give rise to some forms of chronic pain.[35, 36]

The neuromatrix theory of pain proposes that the neurosignature for pain experience is determined by the synaptic architecture of the neuromatrix, which is produced by genetic and sensory influences. The neurosignature pattern is also modulated by sensory inputs and by congnitive events such as psychological stress. It may also occur because stressors, physical as well as psychological, act on stress-regulation systems, which may produce lesions of muscle, bone, and nerve tissue, thereby contributing to the neurosignature patterns that give rise to chronic pain.[32–36] In short, as a result of homeostasis regulation patterns that have failed, the neuromatrix produces the destructive conditions that many give rise to many of the chronic pains that so far have resisted treatments developed primarily to manage pains that are triggered by sensory inputs. The stress-regulation system, with its complex, delicately balanced interactions, is an integral part of the multiple contributions that give rise to chronic pain.

The neuromatrix theory guides us away from the cartesian concept of pain as a sensation produced by injury, inflammation, or other tissue lesions and toward the concept of pain as a multidimensional experience produced by multiple influences. These influences range from the existing synaptic architecture of the neuromatrix, which is determined by genetic and sensory factors, to influences from within the body and from other areas in the brain. Genetic influences on synaptic architecture may determine or predispose toward the development of chronic pain syndromes.[35, 36] Figure 1–3 summarizes the factors that contribute to the output pattern from the neuromatrix that produce the sensory, affective, and cognitive dimensions of pain experience and behavior. We have travelled a long way from the psychophysical concept that sought a simple one-to-one relationship between injury and pain. We now have a theoretical framework in which a template for the body-self is modulated by the powerful stress system and by the cognitive functions of the brain in addition to the traditional sensory inputs.

REFERENCES

1. Kuhn TS: The Structure of Scientific Revolutions, ed 2. Chicago, University of Chicago Press, 1970.
2. Melzack R, Wall PD: Pain mechanisms: A new theory. Science 150:971–979, 1965.
3. Melzack R, Wall PD: The Challenge of Pain, ed 2. London, Penguin Books, 1988.
4. Drake CG, McKenzie KG: Mesencephalic tractotomy for pain. Neurosurgery 10:457–462, 1953.
5. Spiegel EA, Wycis HT: Present status of stereoencephalotomies for pain relief. Confinia Neurol 27:7–17, 1966.
6. Hebb DO: Science and the world of imagination. Can Psychologist 16:4–11, 1975.
7. Leahey TH: A History of Psychology, ed 2. Englewood Cliffs, NJ, Prentice-Hall, 1987.
8. Livingston WK: Pain Mechanisms. New York, Macmillan, 1943.
9. Noordenbos W: Pain. Amsterdam, Elsevier, 1959.
10. Melzack R, Casey KL: Sensory, motivational and central contol determinants of pain: A new conceptual model. *In* Kenshalo D (ed): The Skin Senses. Springfield, Ill, Charles C Thomas, 1968, pp 423–443.
11. Melzack R, Torgerson WR: The language of pain. Anesthesiology 34:50–59, 1971.
12. Melzack R: The McGill Pain Questionnaire: Major properties and scoring methods. Pain 1:277–299, 1975.
13. Melzack R, Loeser JD: Phantom body pain in paraplegics: Evidence for a central "pattern generating mechanism" for pain. Pain 4:195–210, 1978.
14. Melzack R: Phantom limbs, the self and the brain. The DO Hebb Memorial Lecture. Can Psychologist 30:1–14, 1989.
15. Wall PD: Introduction. *In* Wall PD, Melzack R (eds): Textbook of Pain, ed 2. Edinburgh, Churchill Livingstone, 1989, pp 1–18.
16. Melzack R: Phantom limbs and the concept of a neuromatrix. Trends Neurosci 13:88–92, 1990.
17. Webster's Seventh New Collegiate Dictionary. Springfield, Mass, G and C Merriam, 1967, p 522.
18. Tasker RR, Dostrovsky JO: Deafferentation and central pain. *In* Wall PD, Melzack R (eds): Textbook of Pain, ed 2. Edinburgh, Churchill Livingstone, 1989, pp 154–180.
19. Krebs B, Jensen TS, Kroner K, et al: Phantom limb phenomena in amputees 7 years after limb amputation. Pain Suppl 2:S85, 1984.
20. Jensen TS, Krebs B, Nielsen J, Rasmussen P: Immediate and long-term phantom limb pain in amputees: incidence, clinical characteristics and relationship to pre-amputation limb pain. Pain 21:267–278, 1985.
21. Sherman RA, Sherman CJ, Gall NG: A survey of current phantom limb pain treatment in the United States. Pain 8:85–90, 1980.
22. Loeser JD: Low back pain. *In* Bonica JJ (ed): Pain. New York, Raven Press, 1977, pp 155–162.
23. Travell JG, Simons DG: Myofascial Pain and Dysfunction. Baltimore, Williams & Wilkins, 1983.
24. Cronholm B: Phantom limbs in amputees. Acta Psychiatr Neurol Scand Suppl 72:1–310, 1951.
25. Kennard MA, Haugen FP: The relation of subcutaneous focal sensitivity to referred pain of cardiac origin. Anesthesiology 16:297–311, 1955.
26. Nathan PW: Reference of sensation at the spinal level. J Neurol Neurosurg Psychiatry 19:88–100, 1956.
27. Coderre TJ, Melzack R: Increased pain sensitivity following heat injury involves a central mechanism. Behav Brain Res 15:259–262, 1985.
28. Katz J, Melzack R: Pain "memories" in phantom limbs: Review and clinical observations. Pain 43:319–336, 1990.
29. Coderre TJ, Melzack R: Procedures which increase acute pain sensitivity also increase autotomy. Exp Neurol 92:713–722, 1986.
30. Katz J, Vaccarino AL, Coderre TJ, Melzack R: Injury prior to neurectomy alters the pattern of autotomy in rats: Behavioral evidence of central neural plasticity. Anesthesiology 75:876–883, 1991.
31. Coderre TJ, Katz J, Vaccarino AL, Melzack R: Contribution of central

neuroplasticity to pathological pain: Review of clinical and experimental evidence. Pain 52:259–285, 1993.

32. Chrousos GP: Regulation and dysregulation of the hypothalamic-pituitary-adrenal axis. Endocrinol Metab Clin North Am 21:833–858, 1992.
33. Chrousos GP, Gold PW: The concepts of stress and stress system disorders. JAMA 267:1244–1252, 1992.
34. Sapolsky RM: Neuroendocrinology of the stress-response. *In* Becker JB, Breedlove SM, Crews D (eds): Behavioral Endocrinology. Cambridge, Mass, MIT Press, 1992.
35. Melzack R: Pain and stress: Clues toward understanding chronic pain. *In* Sabourin M, Craik F, Robert M (eds): Advances in Psychological Sciences, vol. 2. Hove: Psychology Press Ltd, 1998, pp 63–85.
36. Melzack R: Pain and stress: A new perspective. *In* Gatchel RJ, Turk DC (eds): Psychosocial Factors in Pain. New York, Guilford, 1999, pp 89–106.

CHAPTER • 2

Anatomy of the Pain-Processing System

Tony L. Yaksh, PhD

ANATOMIC SYSTEMS ASSOCIATED WITH PAIN PROCESSING

Extreme mechanical distortion, thermal stimuli (>42° C), or changes in the chemical milieu (plasma products, pH, potassium at the peripheral sensory terminal will evoke the verbal report of pain in humans and efforts to escape in animals and will elicit activity in the adrenal-pituitary axis. In this chapter I discuss the circuitry that serves in the transduction and encoding of this information.[1-4] This overview emphasizes that the pain-encoding system consists of two parts. First, the stimuli already mentioned evoke activity in specific groups of small myelinated or unmyelinated primary afferents that make their synaptic contact with several distinct populations of dorsal horn neurons. Via long spinal tracts and through a variety of intersegmental systems, the information gains access to supraspinal centers that lie in the brain stem and in the thalamus. This rostrally projecting system represents the substrate by which unconditioned, high-intensity somatic and visceral stimuli give rise to escape behavior and the verbal report of pain. This circuitry constitutes the *afferent limb* of the pain pathway. Second, the encoding of a pain message depends not only on the physical characteristics of the otherwise effective stimulus but also on the properties of intrinsic systems that modulate transmission through the afferent linkage of the system.

Primary Afferents[5]

Fiber Classes

Sensory axons are classified according to their diameter, myelination, and conduction velocity (Table 2–1). Recording from fibers identified according to their conduction velocity reveals that A-beta (group II) fibers are activated at low thresholds (i.e., mechanoreceptors). Fibers that conduct at A-delta velocity (group II fibers) may belong to populations that are low or high threshold and mechanical or thermal. Low-threshold afferents may begin firing at temperatures that are not noxious (30° C) and increase their firing rate monotonically, although in this range we perceive the stimulus as warm but not noxious. Other populations of A-delta fibers may begin to fire at temperatures that are mildly noxious and increase their firing rates up to very high temperatures (52° C to 55° C). Slow-conducting afferents constitute the largest population of afferent axons. The large majority of these afferents are activated by high-threshold thermal, mechanical, and chemical stimuli and are called *C-polymodal nociceptors* (Fig. 2–1).

An important characteristic is that many of these C-polymodal afferents are activated by specific agents released into the chemical milieu. Such products can evoke direct activation of the fibers and serve to facilitate their activity. This probably represents the principal mechanism of activating afferents after the acute injury. The nature of the products is discussed later.

Afferents with High Thresholds and Pain Behavior

Electrophysiologic and correlated behavioral evidence indicate that information that can generate a pain event enters the central nervous system by the activation of small-diameter, myelinated (group III-A or A-delta) or unmyelinated (group IV or C) afferents. Thus, single-unit recording in nerve fascicles in humans reveals a close correlation between the dull pain induced by a focal high-intensity thermal stimulus (second pain) and activity in fibers conducting at velocities of less than 1 m/sec. Similarly, local anesthetics in low concentrations transiently block conduction in small, but not large, afferents, thus blocking the sensation evoked by high-threshold stimuli and leaving light touch intact. The afferent axons, particularly those derived from unmyelinated fibers, show extensive branching as they proceed distally, and the majority of the peripheral terminals of small afferents show little evidence of specialization, terminating as "free" nerve endings. Ample evidence exists to indicate that these free nerve endings, commonly designated *polymodal nociceptors*, are characteristically activated only by high-intensity physical stimuli, and this property accounts for the peripheral speci-

TABLE 2–1 **Classification of Primary Afferents by Physical Characteristics, Conduction Velocity, and Effective Stimuli**

Fiber Class*	Velocity Group†	Effective Stimuli
A-beta	Group II (>40–50 m/sec)	Low-threshold specialized nerve endings (pacinian corpuscles)
A-delta	Group III (>10 and <40 m/sec)	Low-threshold mechanical or thermal high-threshold mechanical or thermal specialized nerve endings
C	Group IV (<2 m/sec)	High-threshold thermal, mechanical, or chemical free nerve endings

* The Erlanger-Gasser A-beta/A-delta/C classification scheme is based on anatomic characteristics.
† The Lloyd-Hunt group II/III/IV classification scheme is based on conduction velocity in muscle afferents.

ficity associating A-delta/C-fiber activity with pain. This transduction specificity is best exemplified in tooth pulp and cornea, where only free nerve endings are found and local stimulation is painful.

Conditions that lead to the ability of light touch or low-intensity thermal stimuli to evoke activity in small-diameter axons result in anomalous activity that, because of the fibers that are activated, is reported as painful. Several practical examples may be cited: (1) lowering the threshold of the C-fiber terminal (peripheral hypersensitivity that develops during the release of inflammatory mediators; see later), (2) dorsal root ganglion, where local pressure can produce a continuous barrage such as associated with disc extrusion, which provides a probable source for certain focally referred pains, and (3) the neuroma that develops at the regenerating end of a cut nerve and shows local mechanical and chemical sensitivity.

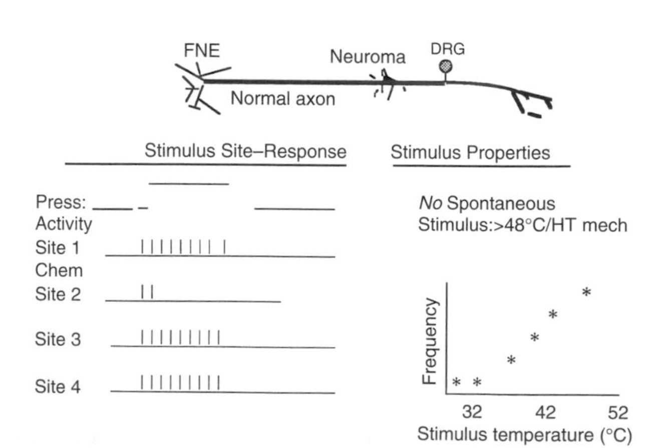

FIGURE 2–1 Transduction properties of the c-polymodal nociceptor. Top, *Schema of C fiber with peripheral free nerve ending (*FNE*), a region of normal axon and a local injury (*neuroma*), and the dorsal root ganglion (*DRG*). In this schema, a pressure stimulus was applied to the axon at sites 1 through 4.* Lower left, *the characteristic responses to the pressure stimuli are displayed. Importantly, the normal axon does not transduce the continued mechanical distortion, whereas such transduction does occur at sites 1, 3, and 4.* Lower right, *C fibers typically show little if any spontaneous activity but do show a monotonic increase in response to increasing stimulus intensities, the triggering threshold usually corresponding to temperatures that would psychophysically correspond to a pain report. (See Devor et al, 1992,[24] and Burchiel and Ochoa, 1992,[22] for* further discussion.)

Spinal Dorsal Horn[6, 7]

Anatomy of the Dorsal Horn

The spinal cord is divided into several broad anatomic regions, which are further divided on the basis of descriptive anatomy into several lamina (Rexed; Table 2–2). In the nerve, large and small afferents are anatomically intermixed. As the root approaches the spinal cord, there is a tendency for the large myelinated afferents to move medially and to displace the small unmyelinated afferents laterally. Thus, although this pattern is not absolute, large and small afferent axons enter the dorsal horn via the medial and lateral aspects of the dorsal root entry zone (DREZ), respectively. An appreciable number of unmyelinated afferent fibers that arise from dorsal root ganglion cells, however, also exist within the ventral roots, and these likely account for the pain reports evoked by ventral root stimulation in classic clinical studies.

Upon entering the spinal cord, the central processes of the afferents collateralize in two ways. First, the afferents send fibers rostrad and caudad up to several segments in the tract of Lissauer (small C fiber afferents) or into the dorsal columns (large afferents) and into the segment of entry. Second, upon penetration of the fibers into the parenchyma, the terminal fields also ramify rostrally and caudally for several segments (Fig. 2–2).

Terminals from the small myelinated fibers are located in the marginal zone or lamina I of Rexed, the ventral portion of lamina II (II inner), and throughout lamina III. Fine-caliber, unmyelinated fibers generally terminate throughout lamina II and in lamina X around the central canal (Fig. 2–3).

DORSAL HORN NEURONS

Though exceedingly complex, the second-order nocisponsive elements in the dorsal horn may be considered in four principal classes on the basis of their approximate anatomic location.

Marginal Zone (Lamina I). The large neurons of the marginal zone are oriented transversely across the cap of the dorsal gray matter. Some project to the thalamus via contralateral ascending pathways, and others project intrasegmentally and intersegmentally along the dorsal and dorsolateral white matter. Populations of these neurons respond to intense cutaneous and muscle stimulation.

TABLE 2–2 **Organization of Principal Aspects of Dorsal Horn Organization**

Anatomic Region	Rexed Laminae	Afferent Terminals	Nociceptive Cells
Marginal layer	I	A-delta/C	Marginal
Substantia gelatinosa	II	A-beta/A-delta/C	Substantia gelatinosa
	IV/V/VI	A-beta/A-delta	Wide dynamic range
Nucleus proprius	X	A-delta/C	Substantia gelatinosa–type
Central canal	VII/VIII/IX	A-beta	
Motor horn			

Substantia Gelatinosa (Lamina II). A significant proportion of the substantia gelatinosa neurons receive input from A-delta and C fibers and are frequently excited by activation of thermal receptive or mechanical nociceptive afferents. The properties of substantia gelatinosa neurons are ill-understood, but, unlike many spinal neurons, these cells exhibit complex response patterns with prolonged periods of excitation and inhibition after afferent activation.

Nucleus Proprius (Laminae IV and V). Cells in the nucleus proprius may be broadly classed as those that respond almost uniquely to innocuous (A-beta) input, or *low-threshold neurons*, and those that respond to A-beta, A-delta, and C input, or *wide dynamic range* (WDR) convergence neurons. The former class responds to brush or touch but shows no elevation in activity with prolonged pinch (Fig. 2–4). WDR neurons display several important properties:

- Light innocuous touch evokes activity that increases as the intensity of pressure or pinch is increased.
- Low-frequency (>0.33 Hz) repetitive stimulation of C fibers, but not A fibers, produces a gradual increase in the frequency discharge until the neuron is in a state of virtually continuous discharge (wind-up).
- Organ convergence: Depending on the spinal level, a neuron in the nucleus proprius may be activated by (1) stimulation of sympathetic afferents and by coronary artery occlusion, (2) stimulation of the splanchnic nerve, (3) distention of hollow viscera (bladder, small intestine, and gallbladder), (4) injection of bradykinin into the mesenteric artery, and (5) close intraarterial administration of bradykinin or the injection of hypertonic saline into muscle/tendon or group III afferent stimulation from the gastrocnemius. The same WDR neuron is always excited by cutaneous or deep (muscle and joint) input applied within the dermatome that coincides with the segmental location of the cell. Thus, T1 and T5 root stimulation activates WDR neurons that are also excited by coronary artery occlusion. These results indicate that the phenomenon of referred visceral pain has its substrate in the viscerosomatic and musculosomatic convergence onto dorsal horn neurons.

Central Canal (Lamina X). Branches of small primary afferent fibers enter the region. In this area, the presence

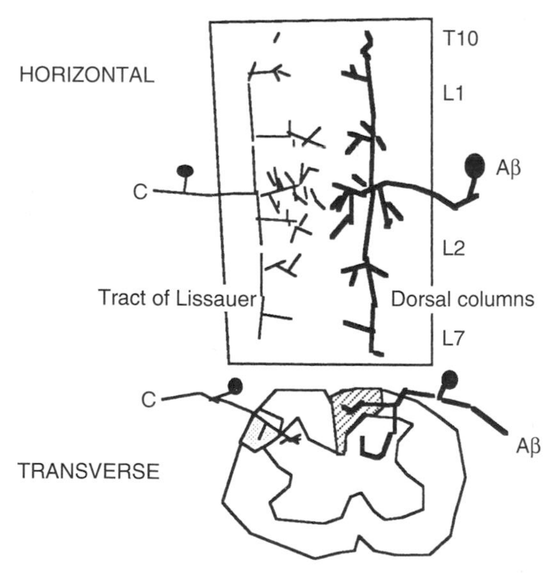

FIGURE 2–2 Schematic displaying the ramification of C fibers (left) into the dorsal horn and collateralization into the tract of Lissauer (stippled area) and of A-beta (Aβ) fibers (right) into the dorsal columns (striped area) and into the dorsal horn. Note that the densest terminations are within the segment of entry and that collateralizations into the dorsal horns at the more distal spinal segments are less dense. This density of collateralization corresponds to the potency of the excitatory drive into these distal segments. (See Wall and Shortland, 1991,[30] and Shortland and Wall, 1992,[28] for further discussion.)

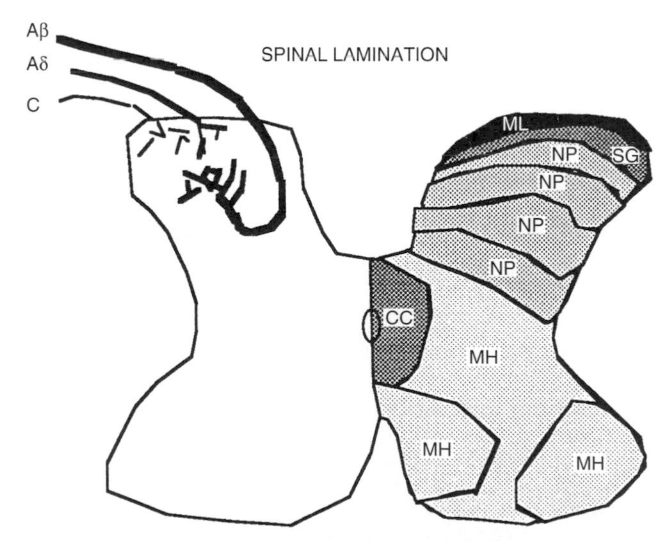

FIGURE 2–3 Schematic showing the Rexed lamination (right) and the approximate organization of the approach of the afferents to the spinal cord (left) as they enter at the dorsal root entry zone and then penetrate into the dorsal horn to terminate in the laminae I and II (Aγ/C) or penetrate deeper to loop upward and terminate as high as lamina III (Aβ). ML, marginal layer; SG, substantia gelatinosa; NP, nucleus proprius; MH, motor horn; CC, central canal.

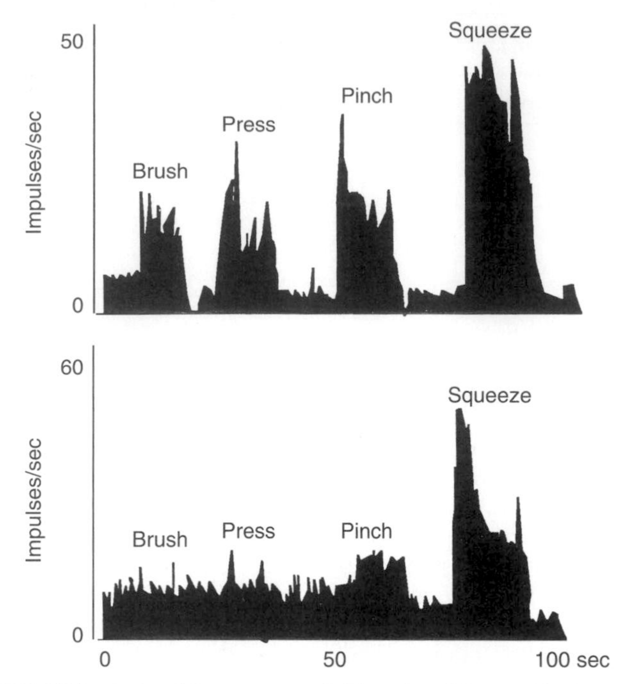

FIGURE 2–4 Firing patterns of (A) a dorsal horn wide dynamic range (WDR) neuron and (B) a high-threshold spinothalamic neuron. Graphs present the neuronal responses to graded intensities of mechanical stimulation applied to the receptive fields. (Data from Chung JM, Surmeier DJ, Lee KH, et al: Classification of primate spinothalamic and somatosensory thalamic neurons based on cluster analysis. J Neurophysiol 56:308–327, 1986.)

of cells has been demonstrated that respond principally to high-threshold temperature stimuli and noxious pinch with small receptive fields.

Ascending Spinal Tracts[7, 8]

Activity evoked in the spinal cord by high-threshold stimuli reaches supraspinal sites by several long and intersegmental tract systems that travel within the ventrolateral quadrant (Fig. 2–5).

Ventral Funicular Systems

Within the ventrolateral quadrant of the spinal cord, several systems have been identified, on the basis of their supraspinal projections, that may be relevant to the long tracts through which information characteristically associated with the pain report travels. Classic studies have shown that pain that is a "crossed pathway" in that unilateral section of the ventrolateral quadrant yields a contralateral thermal or mechanical analgesia in dermatomes below the spinal level of the section.

SPINORETICULAR FIBERS

Spinoreticular axons originating in laminae V through VIII terminate ipsilaterally and contralaterally to their spinal site of origin. In the medulla, the fibers aggregate laterally, and collaterals of these fibers terminate in the more medially situated brain stem reticular nuclei. Reticulothalamic afferents excited by these inputs then project to the thalamus.

SPINOMESENCEPHALIC FIBERS

Spinomesencephalic tracts originate primarily in lamina I; smaller components come from laminae VI, VII, VIII, and X. They project into the mesencephalic reticular formation and the lateral periaqueductal gray.

SPINOTHALAMIC FIBERS

The cells of origin of the spinothalamic tract, the most extensively studied of the ventrolateral tract systems, are not limited to the dorsal gray matter but are found throughout laminae I through VII and X of the spinal gray matter. Axons originating in the marginal layer and the neck of the nucleus proprius ascend predominantly in the contralateral ventral quadrant. Clinical experience suggests that the crossing may occur as much as several segments farther rostrad. Thus, after cordotomy, the analgesic level may be several dermatomes caudal to the section. Although crossed fibers predominate, uncrossed fibers also account for an appreciable component of the spinothalamic population. Spinothalamic axons differentiate into lateral and medial components in the posterior portion of the thalamus: the medial component passes through the internal medullary lamina to terminate in the nucleus parafascicularis thalami and intralaminar and paralaminar nuclei. The majority of fibers pass laterally through the external medullary lamina to terminate in small clusters scattered throughout the nucleus ventralis posterolateralis thalami, the medial aspect of the posterior nucleus complex, and the intralaminar nuclei.

A significant portion of the neurons projecting laterally in the thalamus (ventral posterior lateral complex) also project to the medial (central lateral nucleus or dorsal medial nucleus) portion. An additional population project solely to the medial nuclei. The importance of the ventrolateral tracts to pain is shown by the fact that ventrolateral tractotomies raise the threshold for visceral and somatic pain reports on the side contralateral to the lesion. The sensory level of the cordotomy indicates that the ascending tracts may travel rostrad several segments before crossing. Similarly, stimulation of the ventrolateral tracts in awake subjects undergoing percutaneous cordotomy results in reports of contralateral warmth and pain. Midline myelotomies that destroy fibers crossing the midline at the levels of the cut (as well as the cells in lamina X) produce bilateral pain deficits. These observations suggest that the relevant pathways for nociception are predominantly crossed. Although it is clear that spinal transmission of nociceptive information occurs in the ventrolateral funiculus, the relevance of other systems is suggested by (1) anomalous recovery of pain after 3 to 12 months, (2) persistence of contralateral pain sensations after a unilateral lesion, and (3) "breakthrough" of pain produced by afferent stimulation. Other systems may travel in the dorsal quadrant or within the central gray matter.

Dorsal Funicular Systems

In other primates and humans, lesions of the dorsolateral quadrant have been reported to produce hyperalgesia. Nociceptive cells in lamina X also project in the ventral portion of the dorsal columns. This constitutes the so-called postsynaptic dorsal column system.

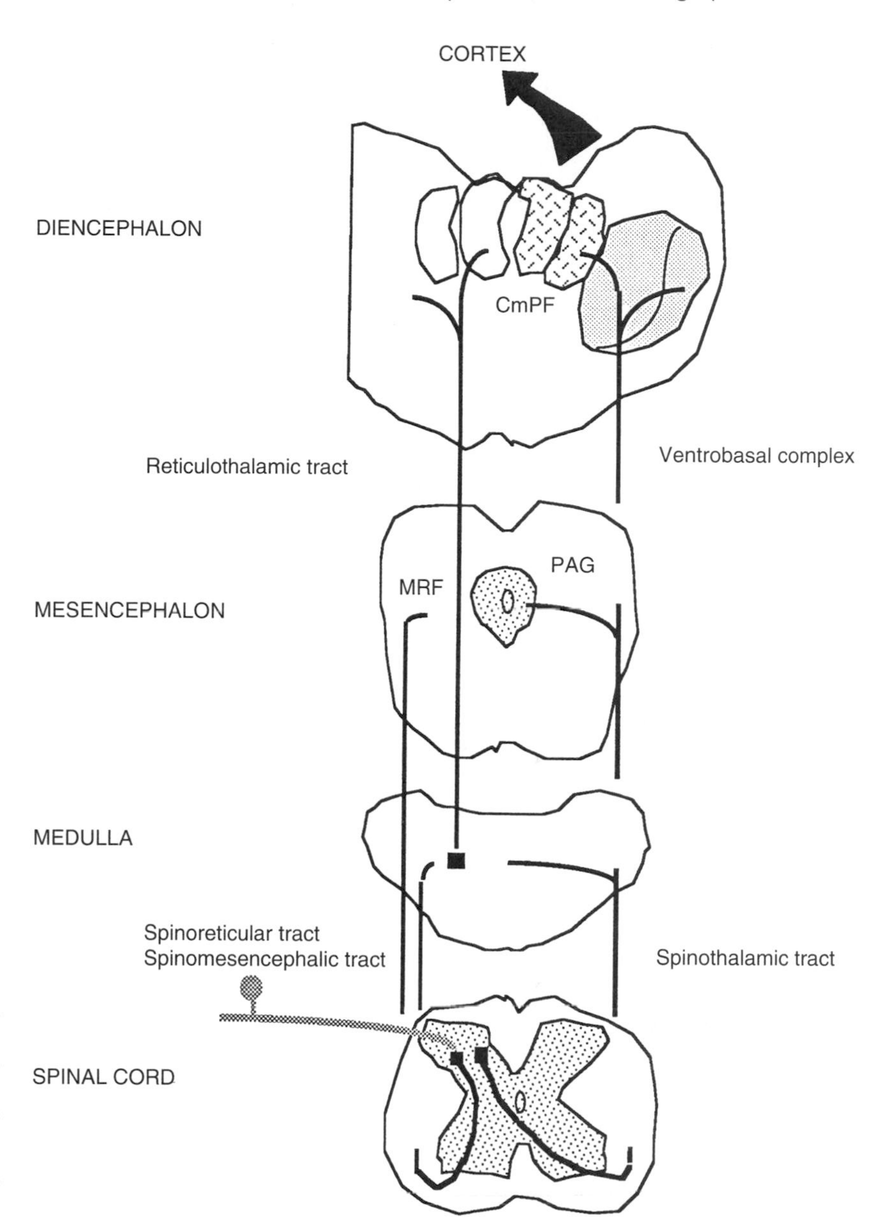

FIGURE 2–5 Schematic organization of the ascending projection systems through which nociceptive transmission is carried. Note the crossed and uncrossed fibers, multisynaptic connections for the uncrossed fibers, collaterals into the medial medullary and mesencephalic core from all ascending afferents as they progress rostrally, and potential dual projection of spinothalamic tract fibers into the medial and lateral thalamus. Cm/PF, *centromedian-parafascicular region;* MRF, *medullary reticular formation;* PAG, *periaqueductal gray;* Tr, *tract.*

Intersegmental Systems

Early studies showed that alternating hemisections poorly modify the behavioral or the autonomic responses to strong stimuli. This finding suggests that systems that project for short distances ipsilaterally may contribute to the rostrad transmission of nociceptive information. Selective destruction of the dorsal gray matter (e.g., in the vicinity of the DREZ) has proved to be clinically effective of pain management, suggesting the relevance of nonfunicular pathways traveling in the spinal gray matter. Such lesions can produce significant and prolonged relief of pain associated with nerve avulsions. Several segmental pathways relevant to the rostrad transmission of nociceptive information are the lateral tract of Lissauer, the dorsolateral propriospinal system, and the dorsal intracornual tract.

Supraspinal Systems[9–13]

Certain supraspinal regions appear to participate in the processing of relevant pain information. This relationship is based on their anatomic association with spinal tracts thought to be relevant to pain transmission and by the response to cells in those regions to peripheral stimuli that can evoke algesic behavior. As noted, on the basis of the ascending long tract projections, there are three major sites of termination: the medulla, the mesencephalon, and the diencephalon.

Medullary Reticular Formation

Because of its spinofugal input and the reticulothalamic projections from the medullary reticular neurons to the intralaminar and ventrobasal nuclei of the thalamus, the medullary reticular formation may present as a relay station for rostrad transmission of nociceptive information. Thus, medullary reticular cell bodies are activated antidromically by stimulation in the thalamus, and, conversely, stimulation of the medullary reticular formation has been reported to activate thalamic neurons. Neurons of the nucleus gigantocellularis are most effectively activated by electrical stimulation of nerves sufficient to evoke afferent volleys in A-delta and C fibers. Volleys in larger-diameter A fibers were ineffective or less effective. Electrical stimulation or lesions in the medullary reticular formation can evoke and attenuate pain behavior in animal models.

Mesencephalic Reticular Formation and Central Gray

Units in the mesencephalic central gray and the adjacent reticular formation are differentially responsive to innocuous and noxious cutaneous and electrical stimuli. Stimulation of the mesencephalic central gray and adjacent mesencephalic reticular formation can evoke signs of intense discomfort in animals, whereas in humans, autonomic responses are elicited along with reports of dysphoria.

Diencephalon

A number of nuclear groups of the thalamus receive primarily spinal projections thought to be associated with the transmission of somatic information evoked by noxious stimuli: the posterior nuclear complex, the ventrobasal complex, and the medial intralaminar nuclear complex.

POSTERIOR NUCLEAR COMPLEX

The posterior nuclear complex is a region of ill-defined cell groups extending rostrad in the medial geniculate toward the caudal pole of the ventromedial group. Populations of neurons in the perioralis region of the thalamus respond to noxious stimuli. A number of the neurons resemble the wide dynamic range neurons in the spinal cord. Lesions of monkey posterior nuclear complex reduce the responsiveness of animals to mechanical stimuli, but the literature is controversial about the analgesic effects of such lesions in humans, which seem to be only transient.

VENTROBASAL COMPLEX

The ventrobasal complex (nucleus ventralis posterior and nucleus ventralis lateralis) is situated in the ventrolateral quadrant of the thalamus. Neurons in this region project in a somatotopic manner to SI and SII of the somatosensory cortex. The majority of neurons in the ventrobasal complex are responsive to innocuous tactile or thermal stimuli or to joint movement. The number of neurons that respond to noxious stimuli is much smaller. Along the ventroposterolateral axis, large populations of neurons that respond to noxious input have been identified. Specific characterization of the projections of lamina I nociceptive neurons has revealed a surprisingly selective projection into the ventrobasal thalamus. Lesions in the ventrobasal complex in a variety of species alter somatosensory discrimination. In animals and humans, such lesions produce transient analgesia. Stimulation of the ventrobasal complex in humans commonly produces nonnoxious paresthesias and tingling.

MEDIAL AND INTRALAMINAR NUCLEI

The intralaminar nuclear complex forms a shell around the lateral aspect of the nucleus medialis dorsalis and is composed of several nuclear groups. These nuclei receive input principally from the spinothalamic tract, whereas input from the nucleus reticularis gigantocellularis terminates in the centromedian-parafascicular region. The intralaminar thalamic complex projects diffusely to wide areas of the cerebral cortex, including the frontal, parietal, and limbic regions. Lesions have been reported to raise the nociceptive threshold and relieve pain in humans suffering from neoplastic disease. Conversely, electrical stimulation of these nuclei has commonly elicited burning pain experienced contralaterally.

Cortex

The somatosensory areas (SI and SII) receive input indirectly from the three major spinal systems through which ascending sensory and noxious information may travel. Investigations have highlighted the importance of the SII area in the reception and perception of pain information. Posterior SII receives input largely from the posterior thalamic complex. These neurons are polysensory, and a number respond to high-intensity mechanical stimuli. When the region to which the posterior thalamic nuclei projects is destroyed bilaterally, the nociceptive threshold increases. Retrograde tract tracing studies in cats have also revealed strong projections from the ventrobasal complex to area 3a of the postcruciate cortex, where small populations of nociceptive neurons are observed.

Studies using positron emission tomography found that discrete regions in the anterior cingulate gyrus of the cortex were activated by noxious thermal stimuli, but not by nonnoxious ones. In contrast to previous thinking regarding the general role played by higher centers in perception, this association of a specific cortical region with nociceptive input raises the possibility of significant selectivity.

Limbic System

Whereas the preceding comments document the pathways relevant to rostrad movement of pain information (i.e., the sensory-discriminative aspects of the stimulus), it is clear that the pain response has an overriding affective-motivational component that is every bit as important to behavior as the initiating stimulus. In the space available, it is not possible to deal with this component, except to note that a variety of lesion procedures in humans and animals have been shown to psychophysically dissociate the reported stimulus intensity from its affective component. Such disconnection syndromes are produced by prefrontal lobectomies, cingulotomies, and temporal lobe–amygdala lesions.

The preceding recitation of the pathways through which afferent information evoked by high-threshold information travels reflects what is traditionally known as the *pain pathway*. In fact, this schematic, though correct, vastly oversimplifies the true organization. At every synapse, the transmission through the dorsal horn and brain stem is subject to significant modulation. We believe that, in some instances, the modulation may serve to diminish the pain message (i.e., endogenous analgesic systems). As I will discuss later, however, there are several circumstances under which repetitive afferent drive results in the involvement of an active facilitation of the message. In other cases, we will note that the nonaversive nature of large afferent stimulation (A-beta) is not noxious because of the continued presence

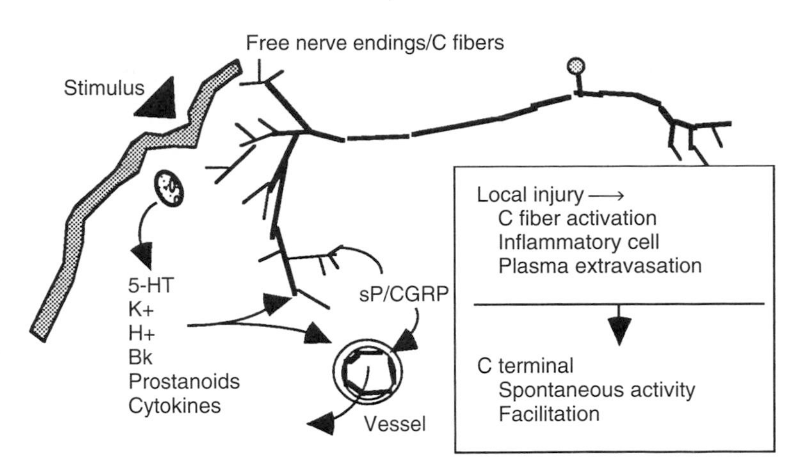

FIGURE 2–6 Schematic of complex events that occur in the vicinity of the primary afferent terminal. Local stimulus leads to the activation of the small afferent and the local activation of inflammatory cells. Afferents display antidromic release of afferent peptides (sP/CGRP). Hormones, such as prostaglandins (prostanoids) and cytokines, released from the local cells and products of plasma extravasation, such as bradykinin (Bk), hydrogen (H^+) and potassium (K^+) ions, and 5-hydroxytryptamine (5-HT), lead to the additional stimulation and sensitization of the free nerve ending.

of small inhibitory interneurons that have no effect upon activity in C fibers.

PHARMACOLOGY OF AFFERENT TRANSMITTER SYSTEMS IN NOCICEPTION

The pharmacology of the systems that process information are exceedingly complex. Significant insights have been developed into the nature of the transmitters and receptors that are at play within the peripheral afferents, spinal cord, and brain stem.

Peripheral Afferent Terminal Pharmacology[14–18]

Changes in the milieu of the peripheral terminal occur secondary to tissue damage and the accompanying extravasation of plasma owing to increased permeability of the capillary wall. These events are responsible for the "triple response": a red flush around the site of the stimulus (local arterial dilation), local edema (capillary permeability), and regional reduction in the intensity of the stimulus required to elicit a pain response (i.e., hyperalgesia). Mild damage to cutaneous receptive fields has been shown to produce significant increases in the excitability of polymodal nociceptors (C fibers) and high-threshold mechanoreceptors. These effects result from the release of algogenic agents from damaged tissue and from the peripheral terminals of sensory afferents activated by local C fiber axon reflexes. Though complex, it has become increasingly appreciated that these intermediaries may have two distinct effects (Fig. 2–6):

- Direct excitation of C fibers leads to activation of C fiber terminals and pain.
- Facilitation of C fiber activation, which results in a leftword shift and increasing slope of the frequency response curve of the C fiber axon, leads to an increase in the reported magnitude of the pain response evoked by a given stimulus (hyperalgesia).

The role of these inflammatory products in the generation of postinjury pain cannot be overstated. The majority of C fibers, referred to as *silent nociceptors*, have little or no spontaneous activity and thresholds so high as to be activated only by extremely intense physical stimuli. In the presence of the injury products, however, these terminals can be activated by relatively mild stimuli (Fig. 2–7). Several families of products are discussed next.

Histamines

Histamine (granules of mast cells, basophils, and platelets) and serotonin (mast cells and platelets) are released by a variety of stimuli, including mechanical trauma, heat, radiation, certain by-products of tissue damage, thrombin, collagen, and epinephrine, and members of the arachidonic acid cascade, leukotrienes, and prostanoids. They can stimulate free nerve endings and evoke vasodilatation.

Kinins

A variety of kinins, notably bradykinin, are released by physical trauma. The peptide is synthesized by a cascade

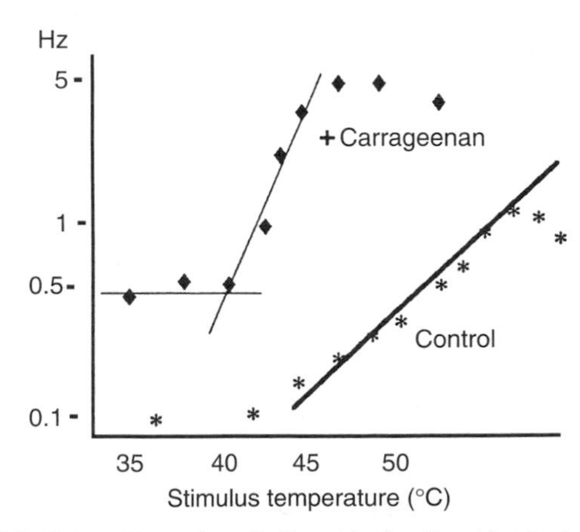

FIGURE 2–7 Firing of small afferent in the skin at increasing temperatures (asterisk curve). Following the injection of carrageenan into the skin, the afferent shows increasing spontaneous activity, a leftward shift, and an increase in the slope in the stimulus-response curve (diamonds), indicating a facilitated response to the thermal stimulus. (Data from Reeh PN: Sensory receptors in mammalian skin in an in vitro preparation. Neurosci Lett 66:141–146, 1986. With kind permission from Elsevier Science Ltd, The Boulevard, Longford Lane, Kidlington OX5 1GB, UK.)

that is triggered upon activation of factor XII by agents such as kallikrein and trypsin. Bradykinin acts by specific bradykinin receptors (B1 and B2) to activate free nerve endings.

Lipidic Acids

Lipidic acids are synthesized by lipoxygenase or cyclooxygenase (prostanoids) upon the release of cell membrane–derived arachidonic acid secondary to the activation of phospholipase A_2. A number of prostanoids, including prostaglandin E_2 (PGE_2), can directly activate C fibers. Others, such as PGI_2 and thromboxane A_2 (TXA_2), and several leukotrienes can markedly facilitate the excitability of C fibers. These effects are also mediated by specific membrane receptors. Steroids have a variety of membrane actions, one of which is to inhibit the activation of phospholipase A_2 (which frees arachidonic acid, the essential substrate for cyclooxygenase and lipoxygenase). Nonsteroidal antiinflammatory agents such as acetylsalicylic acid and indomethacin inhibit cyclooxygenase, and this inhibition is thought to account in part for their antiinflammatory and antihyperalgesic actions.

Cytokines

Cytokines such as the interleukins are formed as part of the inflammatory reaction involving macrophages and have been shown to exert powerful sensitizing effects on C fibers.

Peptides

Primary afferent peptides, such as calcitonin gene–related peptide (CGRP) and substance P (sP), are found in and released from the peripheral terminals of C fibers (see later). The role of these peripheral terminals in pain transmission is not known for certain; however, sP and CGRP are released by antidromic nerve stimulation and produce local cutaneous vasodilatation, plasma extravasation, and sensitization in the region of skin innervated by the stimulated sensory nerve. Although the classic axon reflex occurs in skin, this is not a unique situation. Thus, sP and CGRP are released by antidromic stimulation in tooth pulp and the synovial joint of the knee and increase local blood flow and capillary permeability. These agents may play an important trophic role. Thus, sP and vasoactive intestinal polypeptide (VIP) have both been shown to stimulate osteoblastic activity. In brain, the sP in plexuses surrounding cerebral vessels has been shown to originate in the trigeminal ganglion, and its anomalous release by antidromic activity has been postulated to cause the vascular response that leads to migraine.

Neurotransmitters Released from the Primary Afferent[17, 19–21]

Considerable effort has been directed at establishing the identity of the excitatory neurotransmitters in the primary afferent. Some of these are listed in Table 2–3. Antagonists of the neurotransmitter released from polymodal C fibers would provide a direct method for intervening in transmission of the pain message.

Characteristics of Primary Afferent Transmitters

Currently, excitatory amino acids such as glutamate and a number of peptides, including sP, VIP, somatostatin, a VIP homologue (phosphohexoisomerase [PHI]), CGRP, bombesin, and related peptides have been observed to possess the following characteristics:

- Peptides have been shown to exist within subpopulations of small type B dorsal root ganglion cells.
- Peptides are in the dorsal horn of the spinal cord (where the majority of primary afferent terminals are found), and these levels in the dorsal horn are reduced by rhizotomy or ganglionectomy or by treatment with the small-afferent neurotoxin capsaicin.
- Many peptides are co-contained (e.g., sP and CGRP) in the same C fiber terminal and are contained with excitatory amino acids (e.g., sP and glutamate).
- Peptides are released by activation of C fibers.
- Release of peptides is reduced by the spinal action of agents known to be analgesic, such as opiates and $alpha_2$ agonists (see later).

TABLE 2–3 ***Putative Neurotransmitters in Small Primary Afferents***

Transmitter Hyperesthesia	Small Dorsal Root Ganglion	Capsaicin Depletion	Release	Neuronal Excitation	Algesic Behavior*	
Peptides						
Substance P	+	+	Yes	Yes	+	++
Calcitonin gene–related peptide	+	+	Yes	Yes	+	+
Somatostatin	+	+	Yes	Yes/no	+	0
Bombesin	+	+	Yes	Yes	+	+
Galanin	+	+	Yes	?	?	?
Vasoactive intestinal peptide	+	+	Yes	?	0	–
Cholecystokinin	+/?	+	Yes	?	0	0
Excitatory amino acids						
Glutamate	+	0	Yes	+++	+++	+++
Aspartate	?	?	Yes	+++	+++	+++

* Algesic behavior observed after spinal administration; hyperesthesia observed after spinal administration.

From Yaksh TL, Malmberg AB: Central pharmacology of nociceptive transmission. *In* Melzack R, Wall P (eds): Textbook of Pain, ed 3. Edinburgh, Churchill Livingstone, 1994, pp 165–200.

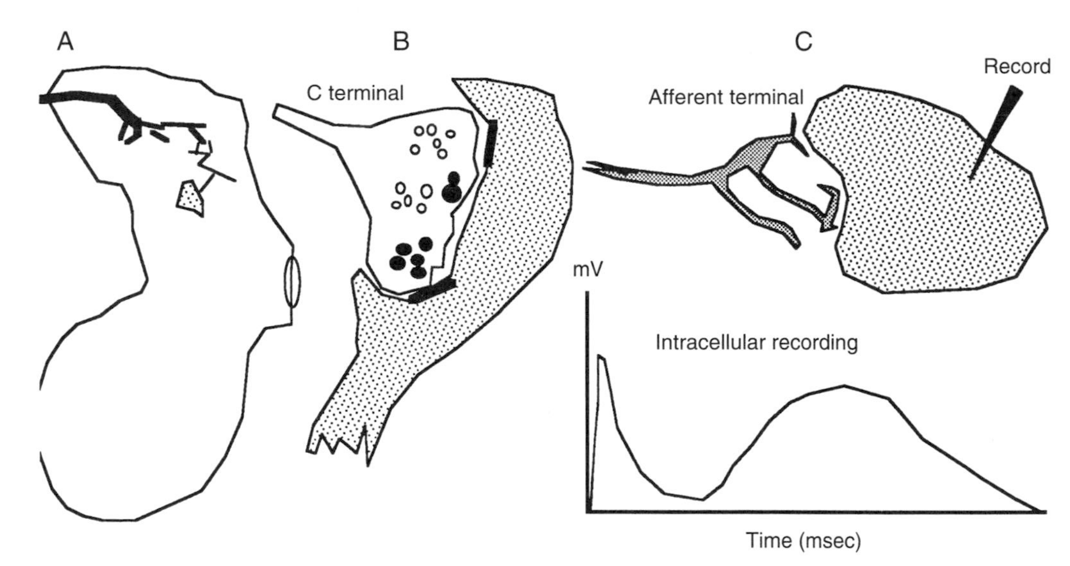

FIGURE 2–8 Schematic displays the general characteristics of the primary afferent transmitters released from small, capsaicin-sensitive, primary afferents: C primary afferents. A, *Small afferents terminate in laminae I and II of the dorsal horn and make synaptic contact with second-order neurons.* B, *Peptides and excitatory amino acids are co-contained in small primary afferent ganglion cells (type B) and in terminals in dense core and clear core vesicles, respectively, in the dorsal horn.* C, *Upon release, the excitatory amino acids are able to produce rapid, early depolarization, whereas the peptides tend to evoke long and prolonged depolarization of the second-order membrane. (See Urban and Randic, 1984,[29] Gerber and Randic, 1989,[26] and Dray, 1992,[25] for further discussion.)*

- Iontophoretic application onto the dorsal horn of the several amino acids and peptides found in primary afferents has been shown to produce excitatory effects. Amino acids produce a very rapid, short-lived depolarization. The peptides produce a delayed and long-lasting discharge.
- Local spinal administration of several agents, such as sP and glutamate, do produce pain behavior, suggesting their possible role as transmitters in the pain process.

Receptor antagonists for some of these agents (sP, VIP, glutamate) currently exist, but few have significant affinity or specificity. Substance P antagonists have been shown to have some analgesic activity after spinal administration. Given the complexity of the coding, it is likely that nociceptive information is processed by a variety of transmitters (Fig. 2–8).

Neurotransmitters Released from Ascending Projection Systems

Dorsal horn neurons projecting to brain stem sites have been shown to contain a variety of peptides (including cholecystokinin, dynorphin, somatostatin, bombesin, VIP, and sP). Glutamate has also been identified in trigeminothalamic projections, suggesting the probable role of that excitatory amino acid. Fibers containing substance P that arise from brain stem sites have been shown to project to the parafascicular and central medial nuclei of the thalamus. Given the importance of these extraspinal terminals, the relative absence of precise information currently available on the transmitters in spinofugal pathways projecting to specific supraspinal regions is surprising. In unanesthetized animals, microinjection of glutamate in the vicinity of the terminals of ascending pathways, notably within the mesencephalic central gray, evokes spontaneous pain behavior with vocalization and vigorous efforts to escape, emphasizing the presence of at least an *N*-methyl-D-aspartate (NMDA) site mediating the behavioral effects produced by NMDA in this region. Other systems will no doubt be identified as these supraspinal systems are studied in detail.

REFERENCES

1. LaMotte RH, Campbell JN: Comparison of responses of warm and nociceptive C-fiber afferents in monkey with human judgments of thermal pain. J Neurophysiol 41:509–528, 1978.
2. Torebjork HE, Schady W, Ochoa J: Sensory correlates of somatic afferent fibre activation. Hum Neurobiol 3:15–20, 1984.
3. Meyer RA, Davis KD, Cohen RH, et al: Mechanically insensitive afferents (MIAs) in cutaneous nerves of monkey. Brain Res 561:252–261, 1991.
4. Koltzenburg M, Handwerker HO: Differential ability of human cutaneous nociceptors to signal mechanical pain and to produce vasodilatation. J Neurosci 14:1756–1765, 1994.
5. Raja SN, Meyer RA, Campbell JN: Peripheral mechanisms of somatic pain. Anesthesiology 68:571–590, 1988.
6. Light AR: The organization of nociceptive neurons in the spinal grey matter. *In* Light AL (ed): The Initial Processing of Pain and Its Descending Control: Spinal and Trigeminal System. Basel, Karger, 1992, pp 109–168.
7. Willis WD, Coggeshall RE: Sensory Mechanisms of the Spinal Cord. New York, Plenum, 1991, pp 79–132.
8. Vierck CJ, Greenspan JD, Ritz LA, Yeomans DC: The spinal pathways contributing to the ascending conduction and descending modulation of pain sensations and reactions. *In* Yaksh TL (ed): Spinal Afferent Processing. New York, Plenum, 1986, pp 275–329.
9. Bushnell MC, Duncan GH: Sensory and affective aspects of pain perception: Is medial thalamus restricted to emotional issues? Exp Brain Res 78:415–418, 1989.
10. Craig AD: Supraspinal pathways and mechanisms relevant to central pain. *In* Casey KL (ed): Pain and Central Nervous Systems Disease: The Central Pain Syndromes. New York, Raven, 1991, pp 157–170.

11. Albe-Fessard D, Berkley KJ, Kruger L, et al: Diencephalic mechanisms of pain sensation. Brain Res 356:217–296, 1985.
12. Talbot JD, Marrett S, Evans AC, et al: Multiple representations of pain in human cerebral cortex. Science 251:1355–1358, 1991.
13. Vogt BA, Finch DM, Olson CR: Functional heterogeneity in cingulate cortex: The anterior executive and posterior evaluative regions. Cereb Cortex 2:435–443, 1992.
14. Handwerker HO, Reeh PW: Pain and inflammation. Pain Res Clin Manage 4:59–70, 1991.
15. Schmidt RF, Schaible HG, Messlinger K, et al: Silent and active nociceptors: Structure, functions and clinical implications. Prog Pain Res Manage 2:213–250, 1994.
16. Levine JD, Fields HL, Basbaum AI: Peptides and the primary afferent nociceptor. J Neurosci 13:2273–2286, 1993.
17. Garry MG, Miller KE, Seybold VS: Lumbar dorsal root ganglia of the cat: A quantitative study of peptide immunoreactivity and cell size. J Comp Neurol 284:36–47, 1989.
18. Smith WL: Prostanoid biosynthesis and mechanisms of action. Am J Physiol 263:F181–191, 1992.
19. Hokfelt T: Neuropeptides in perspective. Neuron 7:867–879, 1991.
20. Ju G, Hokfelt T, Brodin E, et al: Primary sensory neurons of the rat showing calcitonin gene–related peptide immunoreactivity and their relation to substance P-, somatostatin-, galanin-, vasoactive intestinal polypeptide– and cholecystokinin-immunoreactive ganglion cells. Cell Tissue Res 247:417–431, 1987.
21. Yaksh TL, Malmberg AB: Central pharmacology of nociceptive transmission. *In* Melzack R, Wall P (eds): Textbook of Pain, ed 3. Edinburgh, Churchill Livingstone, 1994, pp 165–200.
22. Burchiel KJ, Ochoa JL: Pathophysiology of injured axons. Neurosurg Clin North Am 2:105–116, 1992.
23. Chung JM, Surmeier DJ, Lee KH, et al: Classification of primate spinothalamic and somatosensory thalamic neurons based on cluster analysis. J Neurophysiol 56:308–327, 1986.
24. Devor M, Wall PD, Catalan N: Systemic lidocaine silences ectopic neuroma and DRG discharge without blocking nerve conduction. Pain 48:261–268, 1992.
25. Dray A: Neuropharmacological mechanisms of capsaicin and related substances. Biochem Pharmacol 44:611–615, 1992.
26. Gerber G, Randic M: Excitatory amino acid–mediated components of synaptically evoked input from dorsal roots to deep dorsal horn neurons in the rat spinal cord slice. Neurosci Lett 69:211–219, 1989.
27. Reeh PW: Sensory receptors in mammalian skin in an in vitro preparation. Neurosci Lett 66:141–146, 1986.
28. Shortland P, Wall PD: Long-range afferents in the rat spinal cord. II: Arborizations that penetrate grey matter. Philo Trans R Soc Lond Biol Sci 337:445–455, 1992.
29. Urban L, Randic M: Slow excitatory transmission in rat dorsal horn: Possible mediation by peptides. Brain Res 290:336–341, 1984.
30. Wall PD, Shortland P: Long-range afferents in the rat spinal cord. I: Numbers, distances and conduction velocities. Philo Trans R Soc Lond Biol Sci 334:85–93, 1991.

CHAPTER • 3

Pharmacology of the Pain-Processing System

Tony L. Yaksh, PhD

Activation of a variety of primary afferents results in activation of a number of circuits at the spinal cord and at supraspinal levels. These systems have multiple linkages (see Chapter 2). An important consequence of research in the past decade has been the appreciation that afferent input at each synaptic link is subject to modulation by a variety of specific inputs. The net result is that the response evoked by a given stimulus is subject to a variety of well-defined influences that can serve to attenuate or enhance the excitation produced by a given physical stimulus. Specifically, these interactive systems serve to alter the encoding of the afferent message and thereby change the perceived characteristics of the stimulus.

For sake of discussion, the processing of nociceptive information may be considered in three areas: (1) the response evoked by acute activation of a high-threshold, slowly conducting afferent, (2) the protracted activation of an afferent that results in the generation of a facilitated state (hyperalgesia or hyperesthesia), and (3) changes in function that lead to states in which low-threshold afferents may evoke algesic behavior (allodynia). The pharmacology and physiology of these dynamic states are considered.

ACUTE ACTIVATION OF AFFERENT PAIN PROCESSING[1-3]

Acute activation of small afferents results in clearly defined pain behavior in humans and animals. This event is believed to be mediated by the release of the excitatory afferent transmitters outlined previously and, consequently, the depolarization of projection neurons. The magnitude of the response is typically proportional to the intensity of the stimulus (or to the magnitude of the injury). The organization of this acutely driven system is typically modeled in terms of a linear relationship between activity in the peripheral afferent and the activity of neurons that project out of the spinal cord to the brain.

Modulatory Pharmacology

It has been shown that this small-afferent input is subject to modulation by a number of receptor systems, several of which are characterized in Table 3–1.[4] In most cases, as reviewed, agonists for such receptors applied by iontophoresis topically to the surface of the spinal cord or by systemic delivery in spinally transected animals reduce the magnitude of the response evoked by high-threshold afferent stimulation (Fig. 3–1). Considerable data emphasize that these agents, for example, those in the opioid class, serve to diminish the magnitude of the response evoked by small, high-threshold afferent input but have minimal effects on excitation produced by low-threshold afferents. Importantly, these agents (notably the mu/delta and $alpha_2$ receptors), when given by spinal injection, produce significant analgesia in humans and in animal models. The several mechanisms of this reduction in the response evoked by high-intensity stimulation are these:

- Where examined, the majority of these agents show predominance in binding in the dorsal horn of the spinal cord (DH). For several families of receptor systems, this binding appears to be located in part on primary afferents, as evidenced by the significant reduction induced by rhizotomy or by treatment with the C fiber neurotoxin capsaicin (see Table 3–1).
- Physiologically, agents whose receptors are thought to be located preterminally on C fibers have been shown to reduce the depolarization-evoked release of peptides believed to be contained in these unmyelinated fiber systems. Such correlations, for example, have been demonstrated with mu, delta, and $alpha_2$ receptors. Some agents, such as baclofen, have been shown to have presynaptic binding but fail to significantly alter the release of peptides such as substance P (sP). This finding suggests that the binding may be on terminals that do not contain the relevant transmitter. Such inhibition is mediated by the blockade of the opening of voltage-sensitive calcium channels responsible for transmitter release (Fig. 3–2).
- In addition to the afferent terminal actions of some classes of agents, virtually all of the compounds listed have been shown to have potent effects upon the excitation evoked by local application of an excitatory amino acid such as glutamate. Such postsynaptic effects have been described for mu, delta, kappa, gamma-

TABLE 3–1 **Spinal Receptors That Alter Activity Evoked by Acute High-Threshold Input[5]**

Receptor	Origin of System	C Fiber Binding*	Inhibits Spinal sP Release†	(-) C Fiber Evoked WDR Activity‡	Spinal Therapeutic Ratio§
Opioid					
Mu	Intrinsic	Yes	Yes	Yes	High
Delta	Intrinsic	Yes	Yes	Yes	High
Kappa	Intrinsic	??	No	Yes	Low
Adrenergic					
$Alpha_2$	Bulbospinal	Yes	Yes	Yes	High
Neuropeptide Y	Bulbospinal	Yes	Yes	?	High
Serotonin					
5HT1	Bulbospinal	Yes	Yes(?)	Yes	Medium
5HT3			No	No	Medium
GABA					
A	Intrinsic	Yes	No	Yes/no	Low
B	Intrinsic	Yes	No	Yes	Low
Adenosine					
A1	?	No	No	Yes	Low
Cholinergic					
Muscarinic	Intrinsic	Yes	No(??)	Yes	Medium

* Indicates presence on capsaicin–sensitive terminals.
† Inhibits release of substance P from spinal cord in vitro or in vivo.
‡ Blockade of C fiber evoked activity in wide dynamic range neurons.
§ Ability of agent, when given spinally, to produce analgesia without producing motor dysfunction in the rat.
(For sources of data, see reference 4, Yaksh and Malmberg, 1994.)

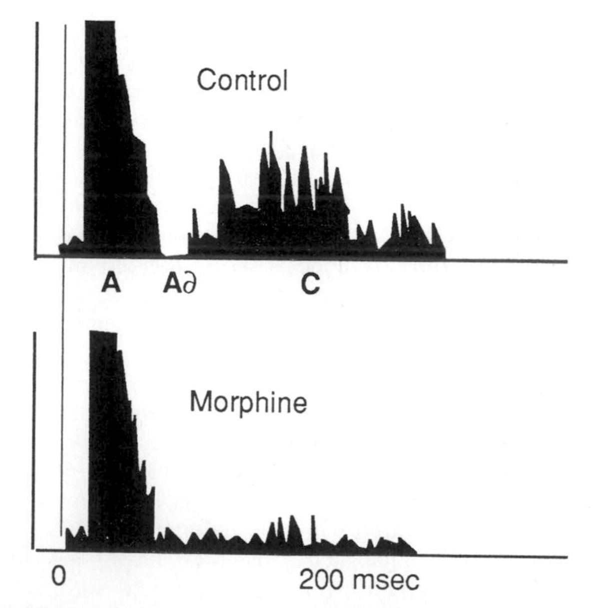

FIGURE 3–1 Poststimulus time histogram showing the effects of IV morphine on the firing of a single dorsal horn wide dynamic range (WDR) neuron after single activation of A and C fiber input in an unanesthetized decerebrate, spinal transection preparation. There is early (A-mediated) and late (Aδ/C) activation of the cell. The late phase activation is preferentially sensitive to morphine (5 mg/kg IV) as compared with the early component. These effects are readily reversed by naloxone. (Adapted from Yaksh TL: Opiate receptors for behavioral analgesia resemble those related to the depression of spinal nociceptive neurons. Science 199:1231–1233, 1978. Reprinted with permission. © 1978 American Association for the Advancement of Science.)

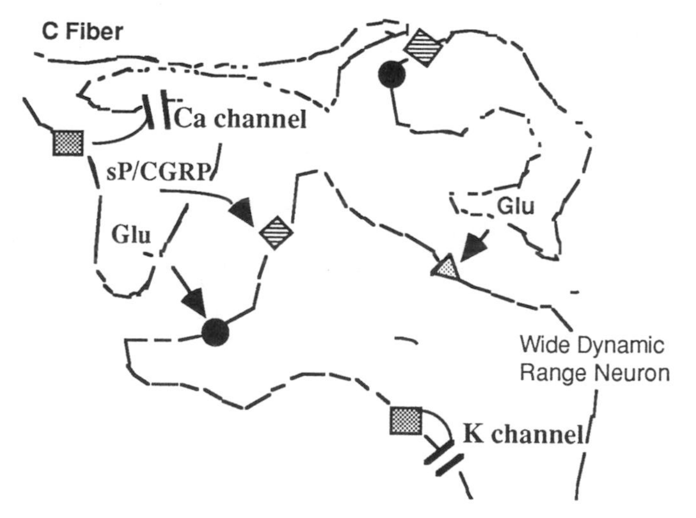

FIGURE 3–2 Schematic organization of dorsal horn shows the neurotransmitter responses discussed in the text. C fiber input releases several neuropeptides, including substance P (sP) and excitatory amino acids such as glutamate (Glu). Substance P and glutamate excite second-order neurons to induce their discharge via NK1 (striated squares) and non-NMDA (solid circles) sites. The released substances interact with interneurons, presumably in the upper lamina of the substantia gelatinosa, to stimulate release of additional agents, including glutamate, which interacts with NMDA (N-methyl-D-aspartate) receptors (stippled triangles). Mu/delta/alpha$_2$ and NPY receptors (stippled squares), acting on small primary afferents, inhibit transmitter release and hyperpolarization (K conduction, the second-order neuron). A afferents are not thought to have opioid receptors. (Adapted from Yaksh, TL, Pogrel JM, Lee YW, Chaplan SR: Reversal of nerve ligation–induced allodynia by spinal alpha$_2$-adrenoceptor agonists. J Pharmacol Exp Ther 272:207–214, 1995.)

aminobutyric acid B (GABA-B), adenosine, and several serotonin receptors.[5] The mechanism of this postsynaptic inhibition has not been defined for all agents. For receptors such as those of the mu and $alpha_2$ types, however, intracellular studies in several neuronal systems have emphasized that they may hyperpolarize the membrane by a G protein–coupled increase in potassium ion conductance (Fig. 3–3).

Origin of Modulatory Systems

The powerful regulation suggested by the effects of the intrathecally delivered transmitter agonists reflects, in many cases, upon some aspect of a role played by endogenous systems. There are two principal sources for these modulatory systems: bulbospinal pathways and intrinsic interneurons. It has long been appreciated that electrical stimulation or microinjections of opiates into the periaqueductal gray or the nucleus gigantocellularis (1) inhibit nociceptive reflexes (an effect antagonized by intrathecal administration of monoamine receptor antagonists) and (2) release serotonin or norepinephrine in the spinal cord. These observations are consistent with the presence of bulbospinal-projecting cell bodies originating in the brain stem noradrenergic (e.g., locus ceruleus) and serotoninergic (caudal raphe) nuclei. In contrast, enkephalin and GABAergic systems are believed to originate largely within local interneurons. Both monoamines and endorphins are released in spinal cord by high-intensity (but not by low-intensity) stimulation of afferent input (sciatic nerve). Importantly, spinal transections inhibit this effect, indicating that the release is mediated by a spinobulbospinal loop (Fig. 3–4). Although the principal interest thus far has focused largely on spinipetal aminergic pathways, other neurotransmitter systems have been shown to project to the spinal cord, including dopamine, sP, thyrotropin-releasing hormone, and cholecystokinin. The role of these several systems is not clear, yet together they suggest that afferent input and projections from the brain stem can regulate the processing of afferent input.

FACILITATION OF AFFERENT INPUT: INJURY-INDUCED HYPERALGESIA AND HYPERESTHESIA[6–11]

Wind-up and Central Facilitation

In animal studies, certain neurons (wide dynamic range, WDR) in the deep dorsal horn display a stimulus-dependent response to discrete (0.1-Hz) activation of afferent C fibers. Repetitive stimulation of C (but not A) fibers at a moderately faster rate (≥0.5 Hz) results in progressively facilitated discharge. This exaggerated discharge was dubbed *wind-up* by Lorne Mendell[11] in 1966 (Fig. 3–5). Intracellular recording has indicated that the facilitated state is represented by progressive, long-sustained, partial depolarization of the cell that renders the membrane increasingly susceptible to afferent input. Given the likelihood that WDR discharge frequency is part of the encoding of the intensity of a high-threshold stimulus and that many of these WDR neurons project in the ventrolateral quadrant of the spinal cord (i.e., spinobulbar projections), this augmented response is believed to be an important component of the pain message (see Fig. 3–5).

Protracted pain states, such as those that may occur with inflamed or injured tissue (leading to peripheral release of active factors), would routinely result in such an augmented afferent drive of the WDR neuron and thence to the ongoing facilitation. Such observations are consistent with the speculation that the afferent C fiber burst may initiate long-lasting events that result in changes in spinal processing, which then alter the response to subsequent input. The preceding observations regarding this dorsal horn system have been shown to have behavioral consequences.

Psychophysical studies have shown that a discrete injury to the skin of the volar surface of the arm or the direct activation of small afferents by the focal injection of a C fiber stimulant (capsaicin) results in a small area of primary hyperesthesia surrounded by a much larger area of secondary hyperesthesia. If a local anesthetic block is placed proximal to the injection site before the insult, onset of the secondary hyperesthesia is prevented. (Recall the typical

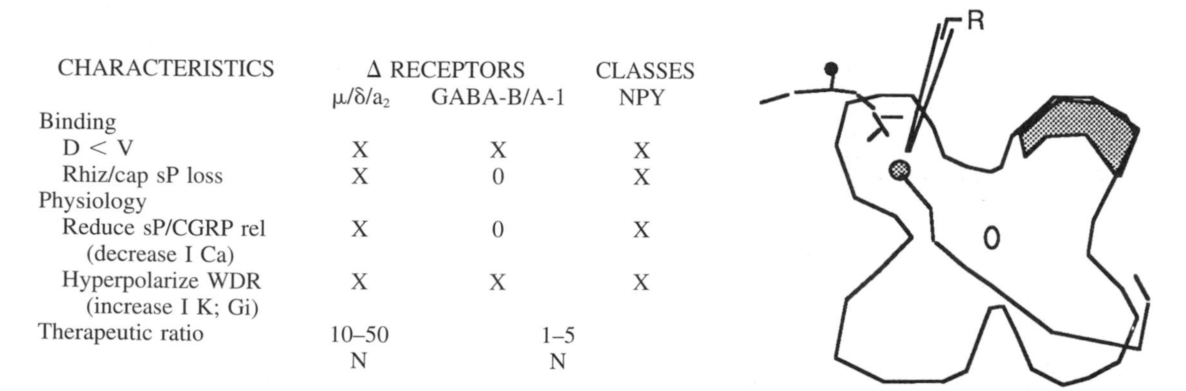

CHARACTERISTICS	Δ RECEPTORS		CLASSES
	$\mu/\delta/a_2$	GABA-B/A-1	NPY
Binding			
D < V	X	X	X
Rhiz/cap sP loss	X	0	X
Physiology			
Reduce sP/CGRP rel (decrease I Ca)	X	0	X
Hyperpolarize WDR (increase I K; Gi)	X	X	X
Therapeutic ratio	10–50 N	1–5 N	

FIGURE 3–3 *Schematic summarizing the principal characteristics of the effects of general classes of receptors (mu/delta/alpha₂, GABA B, adenosine, NPY) with respect to the following variables: D > V (binding greater in dorsal than in ventral horn); rhizotomy/capsaicin treatment reduces dorsal horn binding; release of sP/CGRP from C fibers reduced by agent through a reduction in the opening of voltage-sensitive Ca channels; hyperpolarization of the second-order membrane by an increase in K conductors. Therapeutic ratio: the spinal dose that produces analgesia divided by the dose that produces motor dysfunction.*

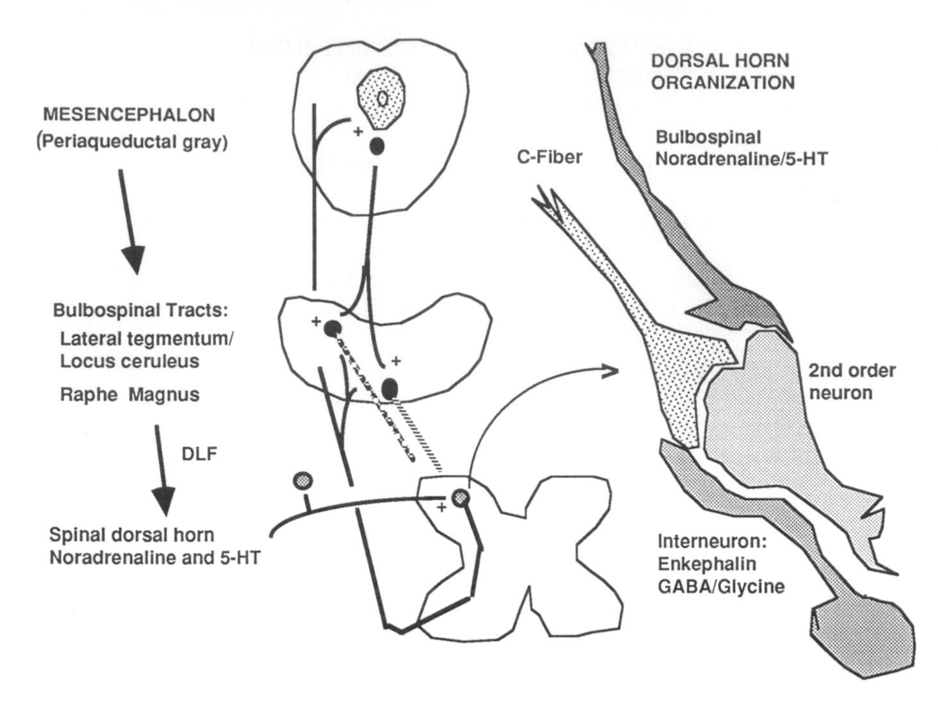

FIGURE 3–4 Left, *Schematic displays the bulbospinal projection through the dorsolateral funiculus (*DLF*) of noradrenergic and serotonergic tracts into the dorsal horn, originating from the locus ceruleus/lateral tegmentum and nucleus raphe magnus, respectively.* Right, *At the level of the dorsal horn, these bulbospinal pathways are believed to exert an action before and after synapse with the primary afferent. Also at this level, several families of local interneurons contain peptides such as enkephalin and amino acids such as GABA and glycine. These interneurons may similarly exert an action before and after synapse with the primary afferent. Both sets of systems serve to modulate the excitability of the synapse by altering the release of primary afferent neurotransmitter and the postsynaptic excitability of the second-order neuron. (See Yaksh et al, 1988.[22])*

aching of the upper arm after a local intramuscular injection.) Studies in animals have indeed shown that injection of an irritant induces an acute afferent barrage that is followed by a prolonged low level of activity. Examination of the behavior has, however, shown that the animal displays exaggerated response to the stimulus (e.g., a central facilitation; Fig. 3–6).

Single-unit studies in the dorsal horn have indeed shown that (1) the response of a WDR neuron to a fixed electrical stimulus applied to the nerve is markedly enhanced when it is administered after the local administration of a cutaneous irritant that activates C fibers and (2) the receptive field for a WDR neuron increases with a punctuate activation of C fibers in one area of the peripheral cutaneous receptive field of that cell.

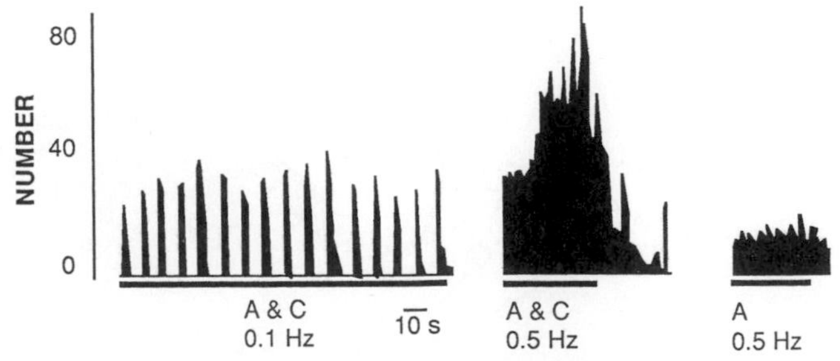

FIGURE 3–5 Right, *Single-unit recording from a wide dynamic range neuron in response to an electrical stimulus delivered at 0.1 Hz. A very reliable, stimulus-linked response is elicited at this frequency.* Left, *In contrast, when the stimulation rate is increased to 0.5 Hz, there is a progressive increase in the magnitude of the response generated by the stimulation.* Middle, *This facilitation, which results from the C fiber input (and not A fiber input), is called "wind-up." (Adapted from Dickenson AH, Sullivan, AF: Evidence for a role of the NMDA receptor in the frequency dependent potentiation of deep rat dorsal horn nociceptive neurons following C fiber stimulation. Neuropharmacology 26:1235–1238, 1987. Reprinted with kind permission from Elsevier Science Ltd, The Boulevard, Langford Lane, Kidlington OX5 1GB, UK.)*

It is important to note that WDR wind-up studies are frequently carried out in animals under 1 minimum alveolar concentration (MAC) of anesthesia. Later studies have shown that the second phase of the formalin test persists in spite of the fact that the first phase is carried out with the subject under anesthesia. The relevance of the observa-

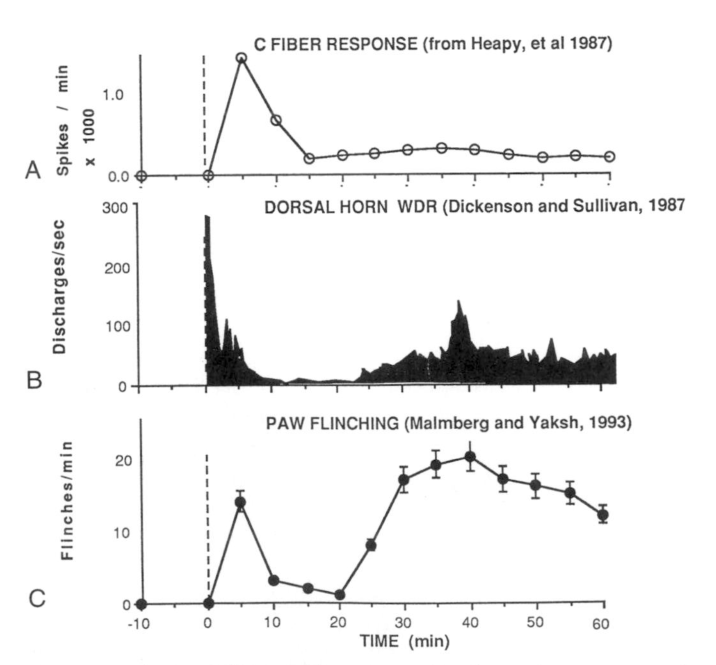

FIGURE 3–6 C fiber activity measured in the saphenous nerve of the anesthetized rat, A, *and number of flinches in the unanesthetized rat,* B *and* C, *measured before and after subcutaneous injection of formalin into the ipsilateral hind paw (*vertical dashed line*). Note the low level of input during the second phase, when behavior suggestive of pain is particularly high. (Heapy, et al, 1987[39]; Dickenson and Sullivan, 1987[37]; Malmberg and Yaksh, 1993[42]; Abram and Yaksh, 1993[34]; Wheeler-Aceto, et al, 1990.[47])*

tions to the performance of surgery on volatile "anesthetized" patients is clear. The implication of the afferent-evoked facilitation is that it is better to prevent small afferent input than to deal with its sequelae. This observation is believed to represent the basis for the consideration of the use of "preemptive analgesics" (e.g., agents and modalities that block small afferent input).

Modulatory Pharmacology

The pharmacology of this central facilitation suggests that the wind-up state reflects more than simply the repetitive activation of a simple excitatory system—it has a unique pharmacology. Aspects of the complex pharmacology in the dorsal horn are presented in Figure 3–7 and summarized here:

- The primary afferent C fibers contain and release both peptide (e.g., sP, calcitonin gene–related protein [CGRP]) and excitatory amino acid (Glu) products. Small dorsal root ganglion (DRG) cells and postsynaptic elements are diaphorase positive, which suggests that they contain nitric oxide synthase (NOS) and are thus able, upon depolarization, to synthesize and release NO.
- These peptides and excitatory amino acids, acting transsynaptically, can evoke excitation in second-order neurons. For glutamate, it is believed that the excitation is mediated by non–*N*-methyl-D-aspartate (NMDA) receptors. Antagonists for the NMDA or the sP receptor do not block C fiber–evoked excitation (i.e., the monosynaptic primary afferent excitation of WDR neurons is not mediated by the NMDA or neurokinin 1 receptor) but do prevent the development of wind-up.
- Under the appropriate circumstances, interneurons excited by the afferent barrage evoke excitation in the second-order neuron by an action mediated via an NMDA receptor. This leads to a marked increase in intracellular calcium ion and the activation of a number of kinases and phosphorylating enzymes. In this scenario, based on the effects of various enzyme inhibitors, it is believed that cyclooxygenase (COX) products (prostaglandins [PG]) and NO are formed and released. These agents move out of the cells to subsequently facilitate transmitter release from primary and nonprimary afferent terminals.
- Intervening products, such as the prostanoids, may arise from neuronal and from nonneuronal structures such as glia by the action of sP or by glutamate receptor activation.
- In certain instances, second-order neurons also receive excitatory input from large afferents. On the basis of the effects of various inhibitory amino acid antagonists, it appears that the excitatory effects of large afferents are under GABA-A/glycine modulatory control, removal of which results in an exaggerated response to low-threshold input. The behavioral correlate is called *allodynia.*
- Either interneurons containing peptides such as enkephalin or bulbospinal pathways containing monoamines (norepinephrine, serotonin) and peptides (enkephalin, neuropeptide Y) may be activated by afferent input and "reflexly" exert a modulatory effect on the release of C fiber peptides and postsynaptically to hyperpolarize projection neurons.

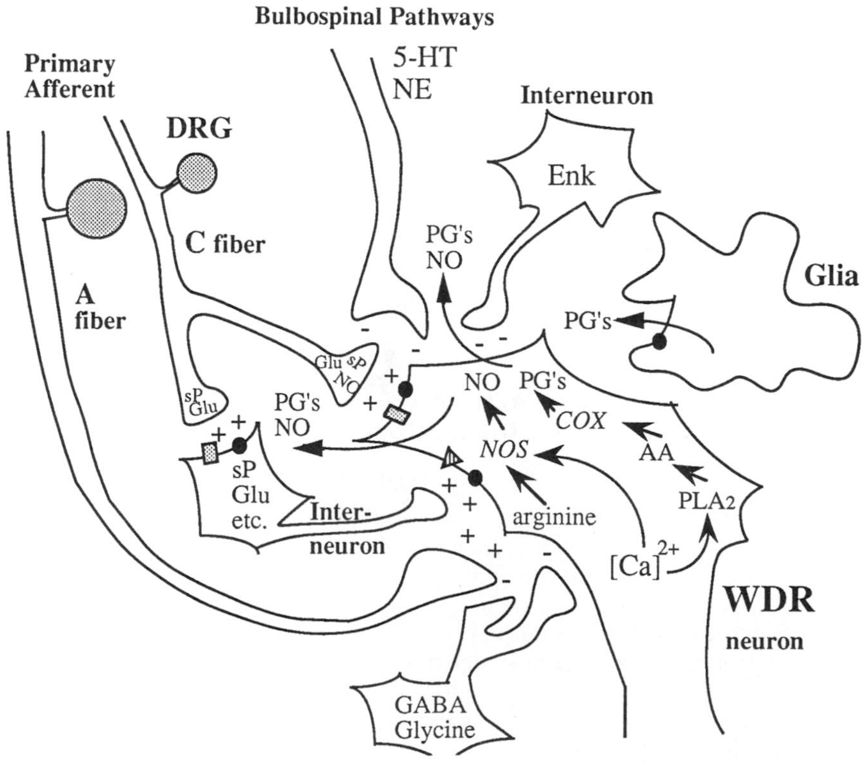

FIGURE 3–7 A schematic summary of the functional organization of elements in the dorsal horn, discussed in the text, that affect the processing of afferent input. Such an organization reflects the response to acute stimulation, development of the hyperalgesic state induced by repetitive small afferent stimulation, and development of anomalous pain states secondary to large afferent stimulation. See text for details. Solid circles *represent NK1 (sP) receptors;* striped triangles *represent NMDA receptors;* stippled rectangles *represent non-NMDA receptors. (From Yaksh TL, Malmberg AB: Central pharmacologic nociceptive transmission.* In *Wall P, Melzack R (eds): Textbook of Pain, ed 3. Edinburgh, Churchill Livingstone, 1994; see also Woolf et al, 1992,[10] and Meller and Gebhart, 1993.[44])*

The arrival of the first small afferent barrage appears to be sufficient to initiate the mechanisms that lead to an augmented response to the peripheral stimulus. Blocking the initial input or preventing the augmentation is a goal for ongoing research.

The preceding observations thus suggest that interneurons excited by C fibers may evoke the release of glutamate/aspartate from interneurons to excite, via NMDA receptors, the WDR cells, and markedly increase their sensitivity. Current thinking has emphasized that the NMDA receptor in a variety of neural systems, including the hippocampus, may play an important role in long-term potentiation (LTP). This long-lasting (minutes to hours) phenomenon is currently believed to reflect the activation of intracellular second messengers such as protein kinases, which alter membrane ion channel function to decrease membrane threshold for activation. Importantly, in animal models of protracted pain, the initial response to the injection is not attenuated by intrathecal NMDA antagonists, but the second, delayed, pain, associated with the subsequent inflammatory response, is substantially reduced when the NMDA antagonist is administered prior to the initial pain stimulus.

After activation of the NMDA sites, intracellular calcium increases, and that serves to increase activity in spinal phospholipase systems. Such activation increases intracellular arachidonic acid and the subsequent formation of prostaglandins. In addition, NMDA can induce formation of NOS, leading to the formation of NO. Both prostanoids and NO can serve subsequently to facilitate the release of primary afferent peptides and excitatory amino acids; this scenario is schematized in Figure 3–7.

ANOMALOUS PAIN MECHANISMS: ALLODYNIA[12-18]

Under normal conditions, low-threshold mechanical input, such as the input that activates A fibers, is not reported as noxious. Under certain conditions, for example after nerve injury, events clinically referred to as *causalgia* or *reflex sympathetic dystrophy* can be reported as producing extremely intense, sharp shooting pains (*allodynia*). The mechanisms of this miscoding of low-threshold afferent information are not understood, but certain phenomena should be considered. These are discussed next.

Spontaneous Generator Activity in Peripheral Terminal and Dorsal Root Ganglion Cells

After peripheral tissue injury, it has been shown in ex vivo models that there is the appearance of a spontaneous discharge in otherwise silent small axons. This spontaneous activity is blocked by lidocaine at concentrations that do not block the conducted potential. After peripheral nerve ligation or section, several events occur: (1) persistent small afferent fiber activity originating after a period from the lesioned nerve, (2) spontaneous activity from the dorsal root ganglion of the injured nerve, and (3) developing sensitivity of the terminal to a variety of products, including bradykinin, prostaglandins, and epinephrine.

Spontaneous activity originating from neuromas after intravascular lidocaine results in complete cessation of ectopic activity originating from the dorsal root ganglia and from the spontaneously active neuroma. This blockade of spontaneous activity occurs with doses smaller than those that block conduction in a normal nerve. Systemic local anesthetics thus alter the generator that leads to the facilitated state, whether that generator is the peripheral nerve terminal in the vicinity of a nerve injury or the ectopic generator of an injured nerve. These results are consistent with an increase in sodium channels in the regenerating terminal, leading to spontaneous activity originating from that terminal.

Transsynaptic Changes

In animal studies, transsynaptic changes in morphology and biochemistry in the dorsal horn have been identified after peripheral nerve lesions (Fig. 3–8). The presence of "dark-staining" neurons in the dorsal horns has been reported subsequent to chronic peripheral nerve compression. An important class of neurons in this region are the interneurons that contain GABA and glycine. Importantly, these GABA-containing terminals are frequently presynaptic to the large central afferent terminal complexes and form reciprocal synapses, and GABAergic axosomatic connections on spinothalamic cells have also been identified. Importantly, the spinal antagonism of GABA and of glycine receptors yields powerful facilitation of the response of WDR neurons to low thresholds. Thus, otherwise innocuous mechanical stimuli (e.g., light touch) yield a prominent pain behavior in the unanesthetized animal (allodynia). Im-

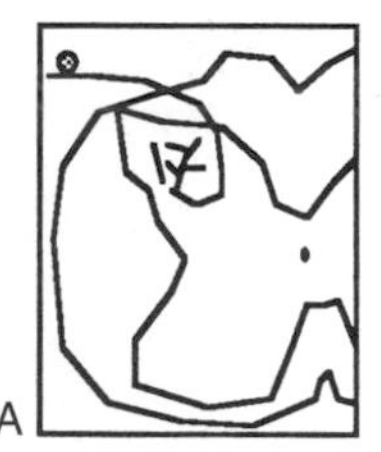

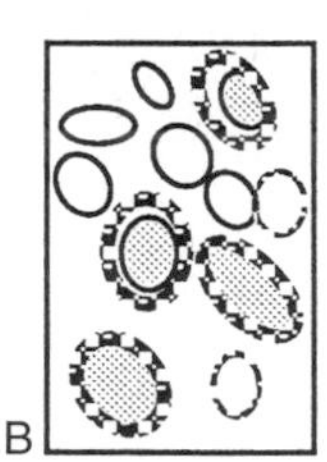

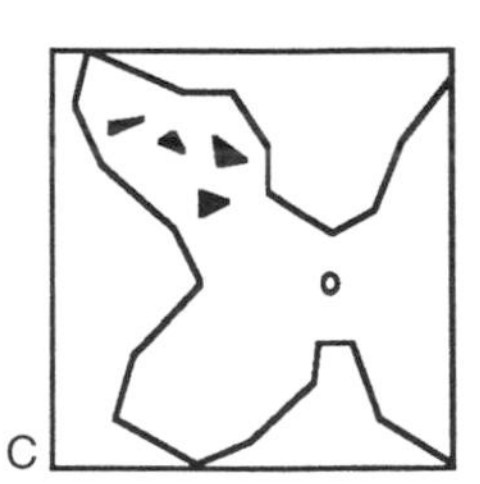

FIGURE 3–8 Schematic representations of three major events that transpire in the spinal dorsal horn after peripheral nerve injury. A, *Large primary afferents (AB fibers) sprout from lamina III into laminae I and II.* B, *Schematic of histologic section taken through the dorsal root ganglion. Type A dorsal root ganglion cells (large) display a pericellular basket composed of sympathetic sprouts. These ganglion cells also display spontaneous activity driven by preganglionic sympathetic outflow.* C, *After peripheral nerve injury, a loss of neurons and the appearance of dark-staining neurons herald cell death. This occurs in a region populated by GABA-ergic and glycinergic neurons. The loss of GABA-ergic or glycinergic tone leads to a facilitated response to low-threshold primary afferent input (i.e., allodynia). (*A *from Woolf CJ, Shortland P, Coggeshall RE: Peripheral nerve injury triggers central sprouting of myelinated afferents. Nature 355:75–78, 1992;* B *from McLachlan EM, Janig W, Devor M, Michaelis M: Peripheral nerve injury triggers noradrenergic sprouting within the dorsal root ganglia. Nature 363:543–546, 1993;* C *from Sugimoto T, Bennett GJ, Kajander KC: Transsynaptic degeneration in the superficial dorsal horn after sciatic nerve injury: Effects of a chronic constriction injury, transection, and strychnine. Pain 42:205–213, 1990; see also Yaksh, 1989.[28]* B *and* C *reprinted with permission from Nature, © 1992 and © 1993, Macmillan Magazines Limited.)*

portantly, genetic variants such as the polled Hereford calf and the spastic mouse have been shown to display particular sensitivity to even modest stimulation, and these models show a decrease of up to 90% in spinal glycine binding. The role of such interneurons in the encoding of afferent input has thus been suggested as an important mechanism involved in the allodynia and hyperesthesia evoked after spinal cord ischemia and peripheral nerve injury.

In addition to the loss of neurons, changes in dorsal horn function that occur after peripheral nerve injury include prominent increases in certain neuropeptides, such as galanin and vasoactive intestinal polypeptide (VIP), and reductions in sP and CGRP. Early immediate genes such as FOS have been shown to display significant increases over intervals of hours to days after the initiation of the lesion. The significance of the immediate early gene is that it signals changes in the cell's synthesis of products secondary to the peripheral nerve injury.

Sprouting

After peripheral nerve injury, large-diameter myelinated axons sprout from their site of termination in lamina III or deeper into the upper lamina, a region normally innervated only by small-diameter, high-threshold afferents (see Fig. 3–8). Thus, low-threshold afferents gain access to a pool of dorsal horn neurons involved in nociceptive processing that were originally accessed only by high-threshold afferent input.

Sympathetic Innervation

The role of the sympathetics in many pain states is supported by the observation that sympathectomies can attenuate the anomalous pain states leading to the diagnosis of "sympathetically dependent" pain. It has long been appreciated that, after peripheral nerve injury, there is an increase in sprouting of local sympathetic terminals at the site of injury. It has also been observed that, although the normal DRG shows little sympathetic innervation, there is a marked enhancement in the levels of sympathetic innervation within the DRG after peripheral injury. This innervation is constituted of postganglionic (catecholamine-containing) terminals and correlates with the appearance of sensitivity of DRG cells to a variety of neurohumors. The innervation forms baskets around type A cell bodies (cell bodies for large myelinated afferents). Greater sympathetic activity has been shown to increase activity originating in DRG cells.

The observations that sympathetic innervation increases in the ganglion after nerve injury and that afferent activity can be driven by sympathetic stimulation provide some link between these efferent and afferent systems and suggest that an overall increase in sympathetic activity is not necessary to evoke the activity. These observations also provide a mechanism for the action of alpha antagonists (phentolamine) and $alpha_2$ agonists (clonidine) that have been reported to be effective after topical or intrathecal delivery. Thus, $alpha_2$ receptors may act presynaptically to reduce sympathetic terminal release. Spinally, $alpha_2$ agonists are known to depress preganglionic sympathetic outflow. In either case, to the extent that pain states are driven by sympathetic input, these states would be diminished accordingly. Interestingly, this consideration provides some explanation of why opiates do not exert a potent effect on allodynia subsequent to nerve injury. Neither mu nor $alpha_2$ agonists alter large-afferent input, yet $alpha_2$ agonists may reduce allodynia. This differential action may result from the fact that opiates, unlike $alpha_2$ agents, do not alter sympathetic outflow (as indicated by the failure of spinal opiates to affect resting blood pressure).

The mechanisms associated with pain secondary to nerve injury are likely complex, but the preceding overview suggests that nerve injury may lead to an allodynic or hyperalgesic state via a number of processes, including (1) appearance of spontaneous activity in afferent input, leading to activity-dependent facilitation of dorsal horn processing, (2) sprouting of large afferents into regions originally contacted by small afferents, (3) sprouting of the sympathetic efferent into the neuroma and DRG, leading to additional evoked activity in these injured afferents, (4) loss of intrinsic modulatory systems that alter subsequent encoding of afferent evoked excitation, and (5) up-regulation of excitatory processes (e.g., dorsal horn sP receptors; Fig. 3–9). A particularly important advance in our understanding of the mechanisms of neuropathic pain states has been the development of reliable animal models in which nerve lesions can produce anomalous pain states (Fig. 3–10).

Modulatory Pharmacology

The modulatory pharmacology of experimental allodynia is clearly distinguishable from that associated with high-intensity somatic stimulation: it is relatively insensitive to opioid and $alpha_2$ agonists, and shows significant suppression in the presence of glutamate receptor antagonists of the NMDA type, adenosine receptor agonists. This distinctive pharmacology emphasizes that this pain state in hu-

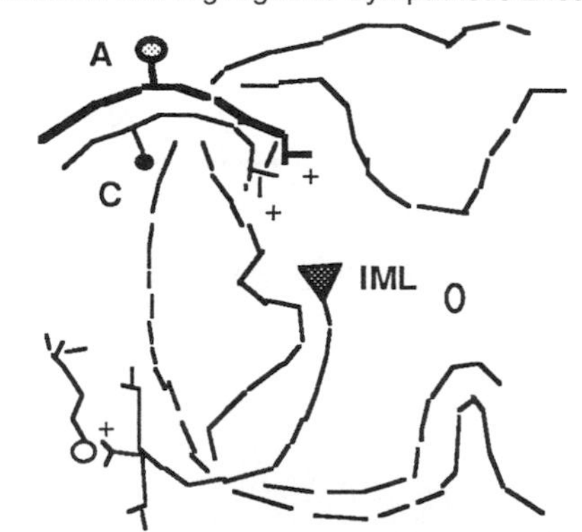

FIGURE 3–9 Schematic showing that both opiates and $alpha_2$ agonists can reduce C fiber–evoked excitation but that neither blocks A fiber excitation. The antiallodynic action of spinal $alpha_2$ agonists thus appears to depend on the fact that spinal $alpha_2$ does inhibit preganglionic sympathetic outflow whereas opiates do not. A *and* stippled circle, *A fiber;* C *and* solid circle, *C fiber;* IML *and* stippled triangle, *IML neuron. (See Yaksh et al, 1995.[50])*

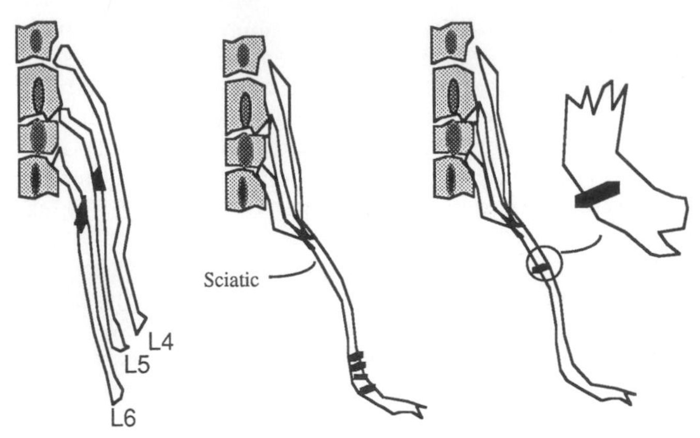

FIGURE 3–10 *Drawing summarizes the properties of the pain states induced by three models of nerve injury in the rat: A, Chung model; B, Bennett four-ligature model; C, Shir and Seltzer partial ligation. Sympathetic dependency was determined by either chemical or surgical sympathectomy. (See Kim and Chung, 1992[40]; Kim et al, 1993[41]; Chaplan et al, 1994[33]; Shir and Seltzer, 1990[45]; and Bennett and Xie, 1988[35] for details).*

mans and animals is mechanistically distinct from that activated by a primary stimulus acting through small, high-threshold afferent systems. This is emphasized by the summary of the pharmacology of analgesia as assessed by models that employ acute pain stimuli.

PRECLINICAL PAIN MODELS AND DRUG SENSITIVITY[19]

Preclinical Animal Models of Nociception

Based on the considerations discussed earlier, it is possible to establish that there are at least three principal classes of preclinical models, which employ several distinct substrates. These models are summarized in Table 3–2. It is important to recognize that these multiple models do indeed reflect on the multiplicity of the mechanisms that have been defined in the investigation of the structure of pathology and pharmacology of the pathways that lead to organized escape behavior in anesthetized and unanesthetized animals. Importantly for the study of the physiology and pharmacology of these effects, a number of preclinical animal models that reflect the function of these several underlying systems have been devised:

- *Hotplate*: The hind paw is placed on a thermally regulated surface, usually maintained at 50° to 55° C, and the interval until the animal licks that paw is measured.
- *Tail flick*: A thermal stimulus is applied to the base of the tail, and the time to reflex withdrawal of the tail is measured.
- *Paw pressure*: Pressure is applied to the hind paw, typically by using a device that permits application of stimuli of increasing intensities, and the amount of pressure required to evoke withdrawal of the paw is measured.
- *Formalin test*: A small volume of dilute irritant (formalin) is injected subcutaneously into the hind paw, and the number of flinches of the injected paw are counted. There are two phases to the response (see Fig. 3–6): acute (phase 1) and facilitated (phase 2).
- *Writhing test*: The animal is injected intraperitoneally with a dilute irritant that produces abdominal constrictures.
- *Arthritis*: An acute inflammatory stimulus is injected into a joint (ankle or knee), yielding an acute reaction in which the animal displays hypersensitivity to light pressure.
- *Spinal strychnine*: The intrathecal injection of a small dose of the glycine antagonist strychnine results in a state in which light touch evokes a powerful pain behavior.
- *Spinal ischemia*: Reversible ischemia of the spinal cord results in a time-dependent increase in sensitivity to light touch.
- *Chung's model of surgical neuropathy*: Ligation of the L5 and L6 nerves leads to a tactile allodynia, which is measured by assessing the threshold to evoke a brisk hind paw withdrawal. The thresholds are measured with "von Frey hairs" (see Fig. 3–10).
- *Bennett's model of surgical neuropathy*: The sciatic nerve is loosely compressed with four ligatures, and the ani-

TABLE 3–2 ***Nociceptive Processing and Associated Animal Models***

Neural Organization	Animal Model(s)*	Human Equivalent
Acute C fiber input (evoked activity; acute pain)	Hot Tail flick Paw pressure Phase 1 formalin test	First pain (needlestick) Second pain (incision)
Protracted C fiber input (facilitated state; facilitated response)	Phase 2 formalin test	Secondary hyperesthesia Postoperative Trauma
Acute A fiber input (tactile allodynia)	Spinal strychnine	RSD Reflex sympathetic dystrophy
Nerve injury (altered processing) (Loss of inhibitory interneurons) Sprouting (altered processing)	Spinal ischemia Chung's and Shir's models	Causalgia
Acute A-delta/C fiber input (hyperalgesia)	Bennett's and Shir's models	
"Spontaneous afferent activity"	Autotomy	Stump pain

* For description of models, see text.

mal develops a state of thermal hyperalgesia, as evidenced by a reduced latency to withdrawal (see Fig. 3–10).

- *Shir's model of surgical neuropathy*: Half of the sciatic nerve proximal to the ischial notch is tightly ligated (see Fig. 3–10).

It should be stressed that, in models of acute inflammation (e.g., the formalin, writhing, and arthritis models), the animals are sacrificed by an anesthetic overdose after data are collected, because these treatments produce significant pain from which the animals cannot escape. With the acute pain models, however, such as the hotplate and tail flick, the animals are freely able to escape the stimulus. The long-term follow-up required for the nerve injury models precludes immediate sacrifice of the animals; however, on close examination, the animals show guarding of the neuropathic paw, while otherwise, they thrive and exhibit normal behaviors and weight gain. The need to be always mindful of the welfare of the animals in these states is of great concern to the investigator.

Pharmacologic Systems That Alter the Animal's Response to Pain

Systematic studies have been carried out employing the classes of pain models just described. In Table 3–3, the effects of drugs of a variety of classes on the acute, hyperalgesic, and hyperpathic pain states are presented.[20] Several caveats are in order. First, although the mechanisms are not discussed in detail, the nature of the effect may be inferred from the previous discussions and from the consideration of the actions of drugs of certain classes in the following sections. Second, the studies reflect the *spinal* delivery of these agents, because of the extensive work carried out with this system and because the interpretation of preclinical studies with spinally delivered agents is more straightforward, in that it reduces the problem of interpreting changes in the animal's ability to provide an organized response (e.g., because of sedation).

OVERVIEW OF MECHANISMS OF ACTION OF SEVERAL COMMON ANALGESIC AGENTS

In the following section, the mechanisms by which a number of drugs exert their action to produce a change in the pain are briefly considered.

Opiates[1, 20–22]

Current data emphasize that the agents classified as opioids may interact with one or a combination of three receptors: mu, delta, and kappa. There are a number of subclasses, but currently they are less well-defined. Systemic opioids have been shown to produce a powerful and selective reduction in humans' and animals' responses to a strong and otherwise noxious stimulus. Given the widespread use of drugs of this class, the site through which these effects are mediated and the mechanisms of those actions are of interest. Direct assessment of the locus of action can be addressed initially by the focal application of the agent to the various purported sites of action, and the effects of such injections on behavior and the pharmacology of those local effects (to ensure a receptor-mediated effect) can be examined.

Sites of Action

SUPRASPINAL SITES

Microinjection mapping of the brain in animals prepared with stereotaxically placed guide cannulas has revealed that

TABLE 3–3 *Spinal Modulatory Systems: Effects of Intrathecal Injections in Rats**

Drug Classes	Experimental Pain States (Animal Models)†			
	Acute Pain (Hot Plate, Tail Flick)	*Hyperalgesia (Phase 2 Formalin, Arthritis)*	*Allodynia (Spinal Strychnine, Chung's Model)*	*Nerve Injury-Hyperalgesia (Bennett's Model)*
Agonists				
Mu/delta opioid	++	++	+/0	++
$Alpha_2$	++	++	++	++
NPY	++	++	?	?
Kappa opioid	++	++	0	±
Muscarinic	++	++	?	?
Adenosine (A1)	+M	+	++	++
Gamma-aminobutyric acid B	+M	+	++	+
Antagonists				
NMDA	+M	++P	++	++
NK1	+M	++P	0	0
Enzyme inhibitors				
Acetylcholinesterase inhibitor	+++	?	?	?
Nitric acid synthase inhibitor	+	++P	?	±
Cyclooxygenase inhibitor	0	++P	0	0

* +,; ++,; +++; +/0, positive/none; ±, 0, none; ?, unknown; M, motor; P, plateau.
† For descriptions of models, see text.
(For sources of data, see reference 20, Yaksh and Malmberg, 1994.)

opioid receptors are functionally coupled to the regulation of the animal's response to strong and otherwise noxious mechanical, thermal, and chemical stimuli that excite small primary afferents. The following discussion summarizes several of the characteristics of sites that have been identified. Table 3–4 summarizes several of the characteristics of the sites of actions as they have been identified in the rat. Of the sites so identified, the most potent is the mesencephalic periaqueductal gray (PAG). There, the local action of morphine blocks nociceptive responses in unanesthetized rats, rabbits, cats, dogs, and primates. In this region, opiates block not only spinally mediated reflexes (such as the tail flick) but also supraspinally organized responses such as the hotplate and the shock titration. This effect on a spinal reflex of a supraspinal agent emphasizes the possible activation of bulbospinal projections (discussed later). Importantly, these effects are reversed by small doses of naloxone given either systemically or into the microinjection site.

Other sites identified by microinjection techniques to modulate pain behavior in the presence of an opiate are the mesencephalic reticular formation (MRF), medial medulla, substantia nigra, nucleus accumbens/ventral forebrain, and amygdala. These sites are listed in Table 3–4 along with their distinctive properties. The pharmacology of the actions of opioids in the several sites, particularly the PAG, have been systematically examined. On the basis of the relative activity of several receptor agonists and antagonists, the effects within the PAG appear to be mediated by mu (but not delta or kappa) classes of receptors (see Table 3–4).

SPINAL CORD

Intrathecal injections of opiates have been shown to produce a powerful and dose-dependent effect on nociceptive thresholds in every species thus far examined, including humans. The characteristics of this effect and its pharmacology were discussed previously.

PERIPHERAL SITES

Classic studies by Ferreira suggested a possible action of morphine at the site of peripheral injury. It has been emphasized that the injection of morphine into the knee joint after the initiation of an inflamed site would reduce the hyperalgesic component at doses that did not redistribute. The pharmacology of this effect indicates ready naloxone reversibility and the probable role of mu and kappa receptor sites.

Mechanisms of Opiate Analgesia

Given the diversity of sites, it is unlikely that all of the mechanisms of opiates' action within the brain to alter nociceptive transmission are identical. Several mechanisms through which opiates may act to alter nociceptive transmission have been identified.

SUPRASPINAL AND SPINAL ACTIONS OF OPIATES

Bulbospinal Projections. Morphine in the brain stem inhibits spinal nociceptive reflexes. Microinjection of morphine into various brain stem sites reduces the spinal neuronal activity evoked by noxious stimuli. These effects are in accord with a variety of studies in which (1) activation of bulbospinal pathways known to contain noradrenaline or alpha 5-hydroxytryptamine (5-HT) inhibit spinal nociceptive activity, (2) pharmacologic enhancement of spinal monoamine activity (by the delivery of 5-HT agonists) leads to an inhibition of spinal activity, (3) microinjection of morphine into the brain stem increases the release or turnover of 5-HT, noradrenaline, or both at the spinal cord level, and (4) the spinal delivery of alpha$_2$ or serotoninergic antagonists reverses the effects of brain stem opiates on spinal reflexes and analgesia. These observations are in accord with the effects produced when the bulbospinal pathways are directly stimulated and emphasize that the actions of opiates in the PAG are in fact associated with increased spinofugal outflow.

Brain Stem Indirect Inhibition of Afferent Traffic. Spinomedullary and spinomesencephalic projections have been described, and they are thought to play a role in the generation of the message evoked by high-threshold stimuli. Although these projections have not been systematically examined, previous work has shown that stimulation

TABLE 3–4 ***Characteristics of Actions of Intracerebral Opiates Microinjected in the Unanesthetized Rat***

Microinjection Site	Dose Range Yielding Antinociceptive Action (g)*		Pharmacology Opioid Receptor Type
	Tail Flick/Jaw Jerk	*Hot Plate/Paw Pressure*	
Forebrain/diencephalon			
Amygdala (corticomedial)	(–)	5–15, bilateral	Mu?
Nucleus accumbens	1–5		Mu?/epsilon
Mesencephalon			
Periaqueductal gray	1–5	1–5	Mu≫delta=kappa=0
Mesencephalic reticular formation	5–5, bilateral	5–15, bilateral	Mu?
Substantia nigra	5–15, bilateral	5–15, bilateral	Mu≫delta=kappa=0
Lower brain stem			
Medial medulla	5–15	5–15	Mu=delta>0
Spinal cord	1–5	1–5	Mu=delta>kappa>0
Peripheral site (inflamed knee joint)	(–)	5–15	Mu/kappa>delta=0

* (–), inactive or prominent side effects occur at the dose.
(For references see Yaksh et al, 1988, Yaksh, 1993, and Stein, 1993.)

within the periaqueductal gray can result in inhibition of neurons in the nucleus reticulogigantocellularis. It seems probable, on the basis of the known effect of projections of these systems, that some of these cells may represent projection neurons that contribute to rostrad movement of nociceptive information.

Direct Inhibition of Brain Stem Afferent Traffic. Many of the regions in which opioids are known to exert their effects, particularly in the mesencephalon and medulla, are known to receive significant input from either direct spinobulbar projections or collaterals from spinodiencephalic projections. Cervical hemisection results in a significant reduction in the levels of 3H-dihydromorphine in the medulla and PAG/MRF ipsilateral to the cord hemisection. These observations thus provide support for the hypothesis that locally administered opiates alter nociceptive processing through presynaptic action on spinofugal terminals, thus reducing the excitation otherwise evoked by the spinofugal projections in brain stem systems relevant to the organization of the response to the noxious event.

Forebrain Mechanisms Modulating Afferent Input. Although there is ample evidence that opiates interact with the mesencephalon to alter input through a variety of direct and indirect systems, the behavioral sequelae of opioids possess a significant component that reflects on the affective component of the organism's response to the pain state. There are significant rostral projections from the dorsal raphe nucleus (5-HT) and the locus ceruleus (noradrenaline) that connect the periaqueductal gray with forebrain systems that are known to influence motivational and affective components of behavior.

PERIPHERAL ACTION OF OPIATES

Opiate "binding" sites are transported in the peripheral sensory axon, but there is no evidence that these sites are coupled to mechanisms governing the excitability of the membrane. High doses of agents such as sufentanil can block the compound action potential, but this effect is not naloxone reversible and is thought to reflect a "local anesthetic" action of the lipid-soluble agent. It is certain that the distant peripheral terminals bear opiate receptors. Opiate receptors have been shown to be on the distal terminals of C fibers, and agonist occupancy of these sites can block antidromic release of C fiber transmitters (e.g., sP/CGRP, "axon reflex"; see discussion of pharmacology of the peripheral afferent). Importantly, the models in which peripheral opiates appear to work are those that possess a significant degree of inflammation and are characterized by a hyperalgesic component. This finding raises the possibility that these peripheral actions normalize a process and lead to increased sensitivity to the local stimulus environment but do not alter normal transduction. The mechanisms of the antihyperalgesic effects of opiates applied to the inflamed regions (e.g., the knee joint) are at present unexplained. It is possible, for example, that opiates act on inflammatory cells that are present and are releasing cytokines and products that activate or sensitize the nerve terminal.

INTERACTIONS BETWEEN SUPRASPINAL AND SPINAL SYSTEMS

Opioids whose action is limited to the spinal cord and to the brain stem are able to produce a powerful alteration in nociceptive processing. There is ample evidence that the effects of opiate receptor occupancy in the brain synergize the effects produced by the concurrent occupancy of spinal receptors. A variety of studies have shown that concurrent administration of morphine spinally and supraspinally creates a prominent synergy (i.e., maximal effect with a minimum combination dose).

Nonsteroidal Antiinflammatory Drugs[23-25]

Nonsteroidal antiinflammatory drugs (NSAID) are widely prescribed agents that have been shown to have significant utility in a variety of acute (postoperative) and chronic (cancer, arthritis) pain states. Though these many agents may differ in potency, all are believed to have the same efficacy. Importantly, human and animal studies have emphasized that these agents serve, not to alter pain thresholds under normal conditions, but to reduce a hyperalgesic component of the underlying pain state. NSAID are structurally diverse but have in common the ability to function as inhibitors of the enzyme COX, the essential enzyme in the synthesis of prostaglandins. Current thinking emphasizes both peripheral and central mechanisms of action (Table 3–5).

Peripheral Actions

Prostanoids are synthesized at the site of injury and can act on the peripheral afferent terminal to facilitate afferent transduction and augment the inflammatory state. To that degree, inhibition of prostaglandin synthesis can diminish that hyperalgesic state and reduce the magnitude of inflammation. The analgesic potency of the NSAID, however, does not co-vary uniquely with the potency of these agents as inhibitors of inflammation. The best example of such a dissociation is acetaminophen, which, in contrast to aspirin, is a weak inhibitor of COX and possesses poor antiinflammatory properties; however, the clinical analgesic potencies of the two drugs do not essentially differ. Other peripheral mechanisms of action include blockade of G protein–dependent events leading to neutrophil activation.

TABLE 3–5 NSAIDs: Summary of Antihyperalgesic Actions*

Peripheral action
1. Active: Animal/human models of inflammation
2. Cyclooxygenase (COX) inhibitors stimulus (BK, K)((AAzi(COX((Prostaglandins (PG)(Lipooxygenase((leukotriene))
3. PG (stimulate/facilitate peripheral C fiber activity)
4. Reduce peripheral stimulus by reducing inflammation
Central action
1. IT COX (reduced facilitated response)
2. Repetitive C fiber input (spinal PG release)
3. IT PG (release of PA peptide (sP/glutamate))

* Analgesic efficacy does not equal antiinflammatory efficacy (e.g., acetylsalicylate versus acetaminophen, ketoprofen versus ketorolac).

Central Actions

Intracerebral or intrathecal injection of NSAID, in doses that are inactive by systemic administration, attenuates the behavioral response to certain types of noxious stimuli, indicating a central action for the agent. Central release studies have emphasized that prostaglandins are released into the extravascular extracellular space from spinal and supraspinal sites secondary to neuronal activity. Several central mechanisms may be relevant:

- Prostaglandins exert an *inhibitory* effect on noradrenergic terminals, and COX inhibitors increase turnover of monoamines. At the spinal cord level, bulbospinal pathways depress high-threshold afferent input.
- The repetitive activation of spinal neurons or the direct excitation of dorsal horn glutamate or sP receptors evokes a facilitated state of processing (see earlier) and release of prostaglandins. The direct application of several prostanoids to the spinal cord leads to a facilitated state of processing (hyperalgesia). Studies have shown that this hyperalgesic component is blocked by the spinal delivery of NSAID, thus providing an important mechanism for an alternative central action—and perhaps accounting for the characteristic antihyperalgesic effect of these agents.

NMDA Receptor Antagonists[26–28]

Ketamine is classified as a dissociative anesthetic, but there is a clinical belief that ketamine can provide a significant degree of "analgesia." The current thinking on this aspect of drug action is that it reflects on its action as an antagonist at the glutamate receptor of the NMDA subtype. The NMDA site is thought to be essential in evoking a hyperalgesic state in response to repetitive small afferent (C fiber) input. Spinal delivery of ketamine has been shown in limited studies to produce such an antihyperalgesic action in humans and animals. The toxicologic effect of spinally delivered ketamine has not been clearly defined so this route of administration remains experimental. In addition, some believe that certain states of allodynia may be mediated by a separate spinal NMDA receptor system, and the NMDA antagonists have been shown to diminish the dysesthetic component of causalgia. Considerable attention is being paid to this relationship.

Alpha$_2$-Adrenoceptor Agonists[2, 29, 30]

Systemic alpha$_2$-adrenoceptor agonists have been shown to produce significant sedation and mild analgesia. Bulbospinal noradrenergic pathways can regulate dorsal horn nociceptive processing by the release of norepinephrine and the subsequent activation of alpha$_2$-adrenergic receptors. Consequently, spinal delivery of alpha$_2$ agonists can produce powerful analgesia in humans and animal models. This spinal action of alpha$_2$ is mediated by a mechanism similar to that associated with spinal opiates, but the receptor is distinct, in the following three ways:

- Alpha$_2$ binding is presynaptic on C fibers and postsynaptic on dorsal horn neurons.
- Alpha$_2$ receptors can depress the release of C fiber transmitters.
- Alpha$_2$ agonists can hyperpolarize dorsal horn neurons through a Gi-coupled potassium channel.

Although there is some disagreement, it is generally believed that the effects of spinal alpha$_2$ adrenoceptor agonists are not naloxone reversible and do not show cross tolerance to opiates. There is a growing appreciation that clonidine may be useful in neuropathic pain states. The mechanism is not clear, but the ability of alpha$_2$ agonists to diminish sympathetic outflow, either by a direct preterminal action on the postganglionic fiber (thus directly blocking catecholamine release), or by acting spinally on preganglionic sympathetic outflow, has been suggested. This issue will be discussed further in the section on reflex sympathetic dystrophy (RSD).

Intravenous Local Anesthetics[16, 18, 31, 32]

The systemic delivery of sodium channel blockers has been shown to have analgesic efficacy in a variety of neuropathies (diabetic), nerve injury pain states (causalgia), and late-stage cancers and in lowering intraoperative anesthesia requirements. Importantly, these effects occur at plasma concentrations lower than those required to produce frank block of nerve conduction; for lidocaine, effective concentrations may be on the order of 1 to 3 g/mL. The mechanisms of this action are thought to reflect the characteristics of the pain states that are sensitive to intravenous local anesthetics. Figure 3–11 depicts the sites where local anesthetics may interfere with impulse generation.

Spontaneous Generator Activity in Peripheral Terminal Axons[33–37]

After peripheral tissue injury, it has been shown in ex vivo models that spontaneous discharge appears in otherwise silent small axons. Tanelian and MacIver[18] have shown that this spontaneous activity is blocked by lidocaine at concentrations that do not block the conducted potential.

Nerve Injury[38–46]

After peripheral nerve ligation or section, several events occur, among them (1) persistent small afferent fiber activ-

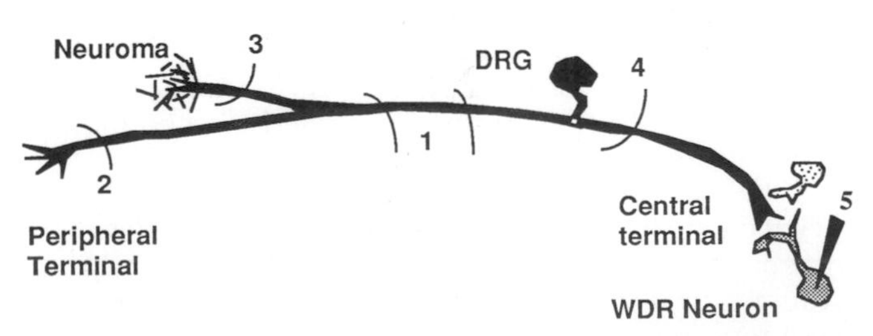

FIGURE 3–11 Four sites of potential generation of spontaneous activity (numbered 2 through 5). Table 3–2 lists the approximate plasma concentrations shown to reduce that spontaneous activity. Note that the spontaneous generators typically are blocked by lower lidocaine concentrations than those required to produce frank conduction block of an intact nerve (site 1). DRG, dorsal root ganglion; WDR, wide dynamic range.

ity originating, after a time, from the lesioned site and from the dorsal root ganglion of the injured nerve and (2) prominent morphologic changes in the spinal dorsal horn ipsilateral to the ligation. The mechanism of these changes is not known with certainty, but the possibility of persistent changes secondary to the chronic afferent barrage or to a change in factors transported from the lesioned site seems likely.[46–47]

In the wake of a peripheral nerve lesion, a state of hypersensitivity or allodynia and spontaneous pain develops. Ongoing repetitive activity like that in the injured nerve can lead not only to a constant pain state but also to dorsal horn sensitization. Moreover, the central changes that are observed after peripheral nerve injury may alter the processing of the dorsal horn. The spontaneous activity that originates from neuromas after intravascular lidocaine has been shown to result in complete cessation of ectopic activity originating from the DRG and from the spontaneously active neuroma. This blockade of spontaneous activity occurs at doses below those that block conduction in normal nerves. Systemic local anesthetics thus alter the generator that leads to the facilitated state, whether that generator is the peripheral nerve terminal in the vicinity of a nerve injury or the ectopic generator of an injured nerve. In addition, it has been shown that the generation of a central facilitated state by the spinal delivery of a glutamate agonist can be blocked by low concentrations of intravenous lidocaine. This finding offers additional likelihood of a central action.

Importantly, intravenous local anesthetics in concentrations like those described here are extremely effective in blocking the facilitated state in animal models of acute tissue injury and chronic nerve injury. Thus, after peripheral nerve blocks, in addition to the effects on conduction produced by the locally high concentrations, plasma concentrations of 1 to 3 g/mL of lidocaine may be having a central effect. Mechanistically, the state most sensitive to the local anesthetic is one in which sodium channels show a high level of activity (i.e., the blocks are frequency dependent). The hyperalgesic–hyperesthetic states described previously may result in central nervous system activity in nerve terminals, afferents, dorsal root ganglion, and small spinal interneurons that are rendered more sensitive to even low concentrations of local anesthetics.

CONCLUSION[48–50]

The brief discussions of the mechanism of nociceptive processing in Chapters 2 and 3 can only touch upon a complexly organized substrate. The common threads that connect these comments are that the complexity emphasizes that pain is not a monolithic entity and that, as in other organ systems such as the cardiovascular regulation and hypertension, multiple causes lead to the pain report. Moreover, because there are many approaches to regulating elevated blood pressure and because selecting the appropriate therapy depends on what mechanism is disordered, so too is it likely that a single approach will not be appropriate for all pain states. Our growing insight into the pharmacology and physiology of these multiple components should continue to provide new tools for the management of nociception. That has been the trend in the last decade, and it seems unlikely to end now.

REFERENCES

1. Yaksh TL: The spinal actions of opioids. *In* Herz A (ed): Handbook of Experimental Pharmacology, vol 104/II. Berlin, Springer-Verlag, 1993, pp 53–90.
2. Yaksh TL, Jage J, Takano Y: Pharmacokinetics and pharmacodynamics of medullar agents: The spinal actions of α_2-adrenergic agonists as analgesics. *In* Aitkenhead AR, Benad G, Brown BR, et al (eds): Bailliere's Clinical Anaesthesiology, vol 7, no 3. London, Bailliere Tindall, 1993, pp 597–614.
3. Price DD, McHaffie JG: Effects of heterotopic conditioning stimuli on first and second pain: A psychophysical evaluation in humans. Pain 34:245–252, 1988.
4. Yaksh TL, Malmberg AB: Central pharmacology of nociceptive transmission. *In* Wall P, Melzack R (eds): Textbook of Pain, ed 3. Edinburgh, Churchill Livingstone, 1994, pp 165–200.
5. Yaksh TL: Pharmacology of spinal adrenergic systems which modulate spinal nociceptive processing. Pharmacol Biochem Behav 22: 845–858, 1985.
6. Dickenson AH: A cure for wind-up: NMDA receptor antagonists as potential analgesics. Trends Pharmacol Sci 11:307–309, 1990.
7. Burchiel KJ, Ochoa JL: Pathophysiology of injured axons. Neurosurg Clin North Am 2:105–116, 1992.
8. Yaksh TL: The spinal pharmacology of facilitation of afferent processing evoked by high-threshold afferent input of the postinjury pain state. Curr Opin Neurol Neurosurg 6:250–256, 1993.
9. McQuay HJ, Dickenson AH: Implications of nervous system plasticity for pain management. Anaesthesia 45:101–102, 1990.
10. Woolf CJ, Chong MS: Preemptive analgesia—treating postoperative pain by preventing the establishment of central sensitization. Anesth Analg 77:362–379, 1993.
11. Torebjork HE, Lundberg LE, LaMotte RH: Central changes in processing of mechanoreceptive input in capsaicin-induced secondary hyperalgesia in humans. J Physiol 448:765–780, 1992.
12. Bennett GJ: Evidence from animal models on the pathogenesis of peripheral neuropathy and its relevance for pharmacotherapy. *In* Basbaum AI, Besson JM (eds): Toward a New Pharmacotherapy of Pain: Beyond Morphine. New York, John Wiley & Sons, 1991, pp 365–380.
13. Dubner R, Basbaum AI: Spinal dorsal horn plasticity following tissue or nerve injury. *In* Wall P, Melzack R (eds): Textbook of Pain, ed 3. Edinburgh, Churchill Livingstone, 1994, pp 225–242.
14. Todd AJ, Sullivan AC: Light microscopic study of the coexistence of GABA-like and glycine-like immunoreactivities in the spinal cord of the rat. J Comp Neurol 296:496–505, 1990.
15. Yaksh TL, Yamamoto T, Myers RR: Pharmacology of nerve compression-evoked hyperesthesia. *In* Willis WD Jr (ed): Hyperalgesia and Allodynia. New York, Raven, 1992, pp 245–258.
16. Devor M, Wall PD, Catalan N: Systemic lidocaine silences ectopic neuroma and DRG discharge without blocking nerve conduction. Pain 48:261–268, 1992.
17. Devor M, Govrin-Lippmann R, Angelides K: Na^+ channel immunolocalization in peripheral mammalian axons and changes following nerve injury and neuroma formation. J Neurosci 13:1976–1992, 1993.
18. Tanelian DL, MacIver MB: Analgesic concentrations of lidocaine suppress tonic A-delta and C fiber discharges produced by acute injury. Anesthesiology 74:934–936, 1991.
19. Yaksh TL: Preclinical models for analgesic drug study. *In* Goldberg AM, Zutphen LFM (eds): Alternative Methods in Toxicology and the Life Sciences. II: The World Congress on Alternatives and Animal Use in the Life Sciences: Education, Research, Testing. New York, Mary Ann Liebert, 1995.
20. Yaksh TL, Malmberg AB: Interaction of spinal modulatory receptor systems. *In* Fields HL, Liebeskind JC (eds): Progress in Pain Research and Management, vol 1. Seattle, IASP Press, 1994, pp 151–171.
21. Stein C: Peripheral mechanisms of opioid analgesia. Anesth Analg 76:182–191, 1993.
22. Yaksh TL, Al-Rodhan, NRF, Jensen TS: Sites of action of opiates in production of analgesia. J Neurosci 77:371–394, 1988.
23. Malmberg AB, Yaksh TL: Antinociceptive actions of spinal nonsteroidal anti-inflammatory agents on the formalin test in the rat. J Pharmacol Exp Ther 263:136–146, 1992.

24. Malmberg AB, Yaksh TL: Hyperalgesia mediated by spinal glutamate or substance P receptor blocked by spinal cyclooxygenase inhibition. Science 257:1276–1279, 1992.
25. Sawynok J, Yaksh TL: Caffeine as an analgesic adjuvant: A review of pharmacology and mechanisms of action. Pharmacol Rev 45:43–85, 1993.
26. Anis NA, Berry SC, Burton NR, Lodge D: The dissociative anaesthetics, ketamine and phencyclidine, selectively reduce excitation of central mammalian neurones by *N*-methyl-aspartate. Br J Pharmacol 79:565–575, 1983.
27. Naguib M, Sharif A, Seraj M, et al: Ketamine for caudal analgesia in children: Comparisons with caudal bupivacaine. Br J Anaesth 67:559–564, 1991.
28. Yaksh TL: Behavioral and autonomic correlates of the tactile evoked allodynia produced by spinal glycine inhibition: Effects of modulatory receptor systems and excitatory amino acid antagonists. Pain 37:111–123, 1989.
29. Pertovaara A: Antinociception induced by $alpha_2$-adrenoceptor agonists, with special emphasis on medetomidine studies. Prog Neurobiol 40:691–709, 1993.
30. Maze M, Tranquilli W: $Alpha_2$ adrenoceptor agonists: Defining the role in clinical anesthesia. Anesthesiology 74:581–605, 1991.
31. Rowbotham MC, Reisner-Keller LA, Fields HL: Both intravenous lidocaine and morphine reduce the pain of postherpetic neuralgia. Neurology 41:1024–1028, 1991.
32. Rowbotham MC, Fields HL: Topical lidocaine reduces pain in postherpetic neuralgia. Pain 38:297–301, 1989.
33. Chaplan SR, Bach FW, Pogrel JW, et al: Quantitative assessment of tactile allodynia in the rat paw. J Neurosci Methods 53:55–63, 1994.
34. Abram SE, Yaksh TL: Morphine, but not inhalation anesthesia, blocks post-injury facilitation: The role of preemptive suppression of afferent transmission. Anesthesiology 78:713–721, 1993.
35. Bennett GJ, Xie YK: A peripheral mononeuropathy in rat that produces disorders of pain sensation like those seen in man. Pain 33:87–107, 1988.
36. Dickenson AH, Sullivan AF: Evidence for a role of the NMDA receptor in the frequency dependent potentiation of deep rat dorsal horn nociceptive neurones following C fibre stimulation. Neuropharmacology 26:1235–1238, 1987.
37. Dickenson AH, Sullivan AF: Subcutaneous formalin–induced activity of dorsal horn neurones in the rat: Differential response to an intrathecal opiate administered pre or post formalin. Pain 30:349–360, 1987.
38. Garrison CJ, Dougherty PM, Kajander KC, Carlton SM: Staining of glial fibrillary acidic protein (GFAP) in lumbar spinal cord increases following a sciatic nerve constriction injury. Brain Res, 565:1–7,1991.
39. Heapy CG, Jamieson A, Russell NJW. Afferent C-fiber and A-delta activity in models of inflammation. Br J Pharmacol 90:164P, 1987.
40. Kim SH, Chung JM: An experimental model for peripheral neuropathy produced by segmental spinal nerve ligation in the rat. Pain 50:355–363, 1992.
41. Kim SH, Na HS, Sheen K, Chung JM: Effects of sympathectomy on a rat model of peripheral neuropathy. Pain 55:85–92, 1993.
42. Malmberg AB, Yaksh TL: Spinal nitric oxide synthesis inhibition blocks NMDA-induced thermal hyperalgesia and produces antinociception in the formalin test in rats. Pain 54:291–300, 1993.
43. McLachlan EM, Janig W, Devor M, Michaelis M: Peripheral nerve injury triggers noradrenergic sprouting within the dorsal root ganglia. Nature 363:543–546, 1993.
44. Meller ST, Gebhart GF: Nitric oxide (NO) and nociceptive processing in the spinal cord. Pain 52:127–136, 1993.
45. Shir Y, Seltzer Z: A fibers mediate mechanical hyperesthesia and allodynia and C fibers mediate thermal hyperalgesia in a new model of causalgia from pain disorders in rats. Neurosci Lett 115:62–67, 1990.
46. Sugimoto T, Bennett GJ, Kajander KC: Transsynaptic degeneration in the superficial dorsal horn after sciatic nerve injury: Effects of a chronic constriction injury, transection, and strychnine. Pain 42:205–213, 1990.
47. Wheeler-Aceto H, Porreca F, Cowan A: The rat paw formalin test: Comparison of noxious agents. Pain 40:229–238, 1990.
48. Woolf CJ, Shortland P, Coggeshall RE: Peripheral nerve injury triggers central sprouting of myelinated afferents. Nature 355:75–78, 1992.
49. Yaksh TL: Opiate receptors for behavioral analgesia resemble those related to the depression of spinal nociceptive neurons. Science 199: 1231–1233, 1978.
50. Yaksh TL, Pogrel JM, Lee YW, Chaplan SR: Reversal of nerve ligation–induced allodynia by spinal $alpha_2$ adrenoceptor agonists. J Pharmacol Exp Ther 272:207–214, 1995.

CHAPTER • 4

Receptors at the Spinal Cord Level: The Clinical Target

Samuel J. Hassenbusch, MD, PhD
• Meredith Dickens, MD

HISTORY AND GENERAL DISCUSSION

The pain sensation is an unpleasant yet extraordinarily complex system or chain of events with perfectly calculated receptions in the body. It is an interactive series of mechanisms that are integrated throughout all the levels of the neuroaxis from the peripheral to the dorsal horn to higher cerebral structures. Pain is the sensation that follows activation of specific nociceptors and signals the possibility of injury to sensory fibers and damage to the actual central nervous system (CNS). Pain that affects the CNS is termed *neuropathic*, which is maladaptive and harmful. Nociceptive pain, on the other hand, is a warning to the rest of the body that something is wrong, some part has been injured, or something should be investigated.[1]

Historical Perspectives

Opium was described first by the Sumerians almost 5000 years ago in writings noting its use for medicinal purposes.[2] Ancient Hebrew medicine utilized opium as an analgesic.[3] Morphine was derived first in 1803 from opium. It was named for Morpheus, the Greek god of sleep.[4] In fact, at least 25 alkaloids are derived from opium, including morphine, codeine, and papaverine.[5] Intrathecal injection of morphine was described in a Japanese report in 1901.[6] In 1906, Sherrington proposed a descending system of pain modulation.[7] In the 1960s and 1970s, however, the effects of morphine on the CNS were studied extensively.[8] The suggestion that the analgesic properties of morphine involved a descending inhibitory system originating in the brain stem and affecting dorsal horn nociceptive transmission and the description of a stereospecific opioid receptor was made only 21 years ago.[9, 10] Five years later, it was shown that opiates exert effects by selectively binding to and altering the conformation of stereospecific receptors.[11]

Specific topics in this area involve studies on (1) the first sensory nerve fibers and other pain information that is conducted into the spinal cord, (2) the anatomic representation of the spinal cord and related mechanisms, and (3) the chemicals (neurotransmitters) involved in synaptic transfer of information from the first to the second neuron in the sensory pathway to the major ascending nociceptive and corresponding descending antinociceptive pathways.

PATHWAYS OF ANTINOCICEPTIVE TRANSMISSION

To better understand the clinical significance of the receptors at the spinal cord level, a review of the receptors and transmitters involved in antinociception from brain to spinal cord levels provides a more complete picture (Fig. 4–1). This review is based heavily upon the work of Basbaum, Fields, and Gebhart.[12–14] In the periaqueductal gray (PAG), substance P neurons from ascending nociceptive systems stimulate cells that contain the opioid enkephalin. These cells, in turn, inhibit interneurons, which also are inhibited by cells containing beta-endorphin from the hypothalamus.[15] Since these interneurons inhibit the main outflow neuron of the PAG to the rostral ventral medulla (RVM),[16, 17] the action of these inhibitory interneurons allows increased transmission from outflow neurons in the PAG to the RVM. The outflow neurons appear to contain neurotensin or serotonin.

The RVM includes the nucleus raphe magnus, nucleus raphe obscurus, nucleus raphe pallidus, and nucleus magnocellularis.[18] The input from the PAG area stimulates the main output cell in the RVM, a cell that appears to contain serotonin but can also contain norepinephrine, enkephalin, and substance P as its transmitter. Norepinephrine-containing neurons in the RVM can inhibit the main outflow neuron, whereas neurons that contain a local opioid (possibly enkephalin or dynorphin) can inhibit this norepinephrine neuron.

The outflow neuron from the RVM proceeds via the dorsolateral funiculus and appears to be inhibitory via receptors on thalamic projecting neurons. These target neurons are located in the superficial dorsal horn in bilateral

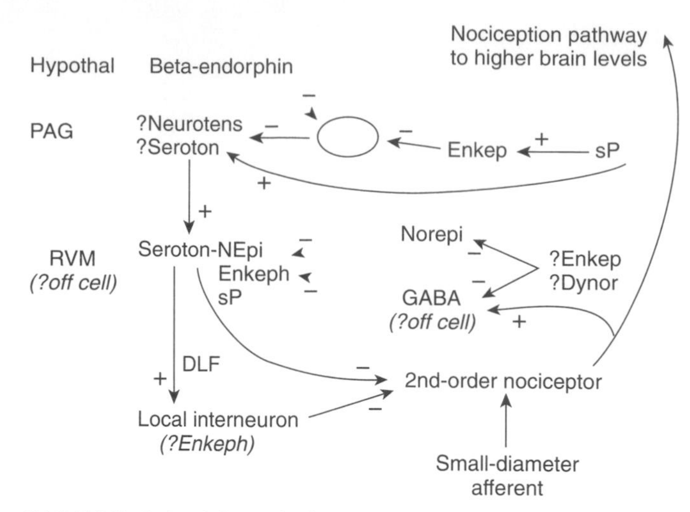

FIGURE 4–1 Schematic of various excitatory (+) and inhibitory (−) neurotransmitters involved in nociception and antinociception. Hypothal, *hypothalamus;* PAG, *periaqueductal gray;* RVM, *rostral ventral medulla;* Neurotens, *neurotensin-containing cell bodies;* Seroton, *serotonin-containing cell bodies;* Enkep, *enkephalin-containing cell bodies;* sP, *substance P–containing cell bodies;* NEpi, *norepinenephrine containing-cell bodies;* GABA, *γ-aminobutyric acid–containing cell bodies;* Dynor, *dynorphin-containing cell bodies;* DLF, *dorsal lateral funiculus;* Norepi, *norepinephrine.*

laminae I, IIo, IV, V, and near the central canal. Receptors on nociceptor neurons of the spinothalamic, spinoreticular, and spinomesencephalic tracts and interneurons in the spinal cord also appear to be targets.[19]

In the dorsal horn, small-fiber afferent nociceptors terminate in laminae I, II, and V[20, 21] and release substance P, calcitonin gene–related peptide (CGRP), and glutamate. Nociceptive, second-order neurons then project into the spinothalamic, spinoreticular, and spinomesencephalic tracts.[22] Local neurons containing opioid in the dorsal horn are inhibitory to these thalamic projecting neurons and are stimulated by input from the RVM. It is at this junction of the primary afferent fibers, second-order nociceptive neurons, and local opioid-containing neurons that theories such as the gate control theory,[23] postsynaptic inhibitory balance theory,[24, 25] and diffuse noxious inhibitory control theory[26] begin to describe the integration of the entire system of nociceptive transmission and analgesia.

After a rather slow start in understanding nociception, in the past 20 years we have markedly increased our knowledge of the various transmitters and receptors involved in nociception and antinociception. Much of this information has been based upon a variety of investigative techniques including: (1) study of neurotransmitter release caused by capsaicin, a small-diameter afferent fiber neurotoxin, or by nerve stimulation, (2) effects of analgesic agents in blocking the release of transmitters, (3) pain behavior in animals after intraspinal administration of various agents, (4) iontophoresis applied to the spinal cord, and (5) morphologic light and electron microscopic studies.

Because of this recent increase in knowledge, the nociceptive and antinociceptive receptors can be grouped into several general classes: receptors for substance P, opioid peptides (i.e., enkephalins, dynorphins, beta-endorphin), other peptides, norepinephrine, serotonin, glutamate and aspartate, gamma-aminobutyric acid (GABA), neurotensin, adenosine A1/A2, and acetylcholine. These stimuli have been applied to normal animals without hyperalgesic pain, allodynia pain, or hyperesthesia.[27] The relationship of many of these classes of receptors can also be described by pathways of antinociceptive transmission involving multiple areas of the brain and spinal cord.

Hyperalgesia is defined as extreme sensitivity to painful stimuli overall. It is pain that occurs at the site of tissue damage and can be produced by mechanical or thermal stimuli. It is also responsible for much of the peripheral sensitization of nociceptors, even though some of that appears to be caused by central mechanisms of hyperexcitability.[27]

More recently, systemic administration of cholinesterase inhibitors has been shown to enhance analgesia from opiates that have entered the spinal cord after crossing the blood-brain barrier. A major site of analgesic action of these cholinergic reactions, especially the muscarinic receptors, is in the spinal cord, deep in the neck of the dorsal horn.[28] Injection of cholinergic agonist drugs into spinal fluid causes pronounced effects on the analgesia and demonstrates muscarine receptor activation. Spinal cord release of acetylcholine can be a physiologic response after pain receptor activation in the brain stem and in the spinal cord and can result in dose-dependent analgesia.[28] Analgesia can also be produced by direct or indirect stimulation of norepinephrine and acetylcholine release through a nicotine receptor response. Descending noradrenergic neurotransmission also leads to improved analgesia via acetylcholine release by enhancing the efficacy of cholinesterase inhibitors (e.g., neostigmine) given by spinal administration.

SUBSTANCE P RECEPTORS

Substance P is an undecapeptide that was identified first in 1931 and by the mid-1950s was associated with sensory transmission.[29, 30] It is synthesized in the cell bodies of small cells (type B) of spinal ganglia and found in C-fiber primary sensory neuron cell bodies, but it is not released during stimulation of A-beta fibers. More than half of the substance P synthesized in cell bodies is transported in the peripheral direction.[31]

With the presence of substance P, it is notable that there is a marked increase in the release of various transmitters in the dorsal horn of the spinal cord. There is possible activation of the descending antinociceptive system with co-localized cholecystokinin (CCK) or serotonin. Also, substance P has been found to be nociceptive when injected into PAG.

The most likely role for substance P is to facilitate nociceptive transmission in neurons activated by noxious cutaneous stimuli. It most likely provides this facilitation by evoking slow, progressive depolarization in dorsal horn neurons,[32] thus enhancing the effectiveness of another neurotransmitter and promoting nociceptive transmission.[19] Intrathecal administration of capsaicin results in a massive discharge of primary afferent fibers that is followed by a marked decrease in substance P in the superficial layers of the dorsal horn.[33] This finding further supports the concept that substance P is a neurotransmitter in C-fiber nociceptors. Much of the evidence for the role of substance P in nociceptive transmission has been based on use of agents with high affinity for substance P receptors. Administering such an agent before intraspinal injection of substance P blocks the animal's usual responses, biting and scratching. These agents similarly block the usual animal responses to other painful stimuli.

In the spinal cord, substance P neurons make synaptic contacts with lamina I second-order neurons and local interneurons, lamina II stalked cells, and laminae III, IV, and V neurons.[19] Direct primary input of substance P to projection neurons in nociception (e.g., spinothalamic tract neurons) has not been demonstrated conclusively.[34] Substance P also has been found in the RVM. Three different subclasses of substance P receptors have been described.[35]

Substance P has actions peripherally and centrally. Mice that lack receptors for substance P (after exposure to the preprotachykinin gene) or the neurokinin-1 receptor have been bred.[27] A variety of receptors can be involved in the co-localization of substance P and other neurotransmitters in a single neuron.

Substance P and glutamate are co-localized in primary neurons, spinal neurons, and descending fibers.[27] Substance P and CGRP have been found to be co-localized in 82% to 95% of dorsal root ganglia.[36] Both transmitters have also been found in laminae I, II, and V.[37] Substance P and similar compounds like CGRP can be released into the periphery via the axon reflex. In this case, the peptide causes a degranulation of mast cells and release of histamine, vasodilatation, and plasma extravasation.[38] Other algogens are also released and other inflammatory cells activated simultaneously. Substance P is also capable of inducing production of nitric oxide and vasodilatation.[38]

OPIOID PEPTIDE RECEPTORS

Dorsal horn neuronal activity, caused by A-delta and C fiber stimulation, has been shown to be diminished by opioid peptides or endorphins as a general group. Examples of endorphins are met-enkephalin, dynorphin, and beta-endorphin. The opioids also diminish neuronal activity caused by somatic and visceral stimuli that evoke pain behavior in animals[39] and suppress the polysynaptic ventral root reflex.[40] It appears that the action of opioid peptides is always inhibitory on target neurons. Stimulation-produced analgesia has been an important technique in elucidating the effects and transmission pathways of opioids.[41]

Lamotte is credited with localizing opiate receptors in the limbic system, PAG, thalamus, and substantia gelatinosa.[42, 43] The opiate receptors in the superficial dorsal horn have been shown to have synaptic contacts with spinothalamic tract neurons.[19, 44] In 1976, three subclasses of endorphin receptors were described: mu for morphine,[45] kappa for ketocyclazocine, and sigma for SKF 10,047.[46] The delta receptors, a fourth subclass, were described by Lord,[47] and a fifth subclass, epsilon, was described based upon the selectivity of beta-endorphin.[48]

ENKEPHALINS

The enkephalin pentapeptides that contain leucine (leu-enkephalin) and methionine (met-enkephalin) were discovered in 1975.[49] The enkephalins are cleaved from proenkephalin A and bind to kappa, mu, and delta receptors.

Enkephalins are located in the dorsal horn, PAG, and nucleus raphe magnus.[50] They appear to coexist with dynorphin in dorsal horn and nucleus raphe magnus neurons.[12] In the spinal cord, enkephalins are most concentrated in laminae I, II, lateral V, VII, and X.[34, 51] Naloxone is an enkephalin antagonist, and the effects of enkephalins appear to be mediated through increased potassium conductance via the G i/o protein.

Of the enkephalin receptors in the spinal cord, 50% are kappa, 40% are mu, and 10% are delta class.[43] The binding sites for enkephalins in the dorsal horn appear to be in the central terminals of primary afferents and dorsal horn neurons.

Significant presynaptic enkephalin-binding sites have been found on small-diameter, high-threshold primary afferents for spinothalamic tract, spinoreticular tract, and spinomesencephalic tract neurons. Enkephalins cause inhibition of neuronal activity in dorsal root ganglion cultures.[52] Terminal activity in primary afferent neurons[53] is reduced after exposure to enkephalins. Enkephalins and enkephalin agonists also have been found to cause naloxone-reversible inhibition of substance P release from primary afferent neurons.[54]

Postsynaptic contacts on soma and proximal dendrites, however, appear to be more significant. This postsynaptic contact appears to form a modulating feedback loop with afferent nociceptive impulses triggering local release of enkephalin, which, in turn, inhibits the afferent nociceptive impulses.[12] Rhizotomy only partially reduces opiate binding in the dorsal horn, thus supporting the existence of postsynaptic contacts. Further support comes from study of dorsal horn neurons in which postsynaptic potentials caused by excitatory amino acids are suppressed by opiates.[55]

Neurons in lamina III of the dorsal horn that contain enkephalin may receive input from low-threshold mechanoreceptors. These same areas provide output to dorsal column postsynaptic neurons that project through the dorsal column.[51] Islet cells in lamina IIi that contain enkephalin may provide modulation upon enkephalin-containing stalked cells in lamina IIo, which provide inhibitory projections to dendrites of lamina I thalamic projecting cells.[19, 56] Neurons in lamina V also appear to provide enkephalin for lamina V neurons projecting to the thalamus.

The delta antagonist naltrindol has shown significant presynaptic binding on small-diameter, high-threshold primary afferents. The mechanism of action with these receptors appears to involve increased potassium conductance via the G i/o protein. Delta agonists also decrease substance P release from small primary afferent neurons.

DYNORPHINS

Dynorphins are cleaved proenkephalin B and bind to kappa receptors. They are found in the hypothalamus, PAG, and spinal dorsal horn.[57] Neurons containing dynorphin have been found in laminae I and V of the spinal cord, but dynorphin levels have been found to increase significantly in laminae I, II, V, and VI with peripheral inflammation.[58] Kappa agonists show a plateau effect and are most responsive to mechanical and low-intensity thermal stimulation. Intrathecal injection of kappa agonists causes analgesia.

BETA ENDORPHIN

First described by Schultz, epsilon receptors have been found to bind with beta-endorphin, which is cleaved from proopiomelanocortin.[13] The receptors appear to be located on basal hypothalamus neurons that provide axons to the limbic system, wall of the third ventricle, PAG, and the locus ceruleus.

OTHER PEPTIDE RECEPTORS

In addition to substance P and the endorphins, other neurotransmitter peptides are vasoactive intestinal peptide (VIP), somatostatin, CCK, and possibly calcitonin. Somatostatin has been found in the spinal cord in laminae IIo and very small amounts in laminae IIi, III, IV, V, and the central canal.[19, 56] Somatostatin in cells from laminae IIi and the dorsal root ganglion appears to be inhibitory to nociceptive transmission but with a longer time frame for the effects. This might provide fine tuning of nociceptive transmission.

Cholecystokinin appears to have effects and localization similar to substance P. VIP receptors have been found in lamina I, and both VIP and CCK are released from small primary afferent terminals in response to nociception. Other possible neurotransmitters include neuropeptide Y and thyrotropin-releasing hormone, which have been found in the RVM.[18]

NORADRENERGIC (ALPHA$_1$, ALPHA$_2$) RECEPTORS

Norepinephrine is a transmitter in the descending antinociceptive pathway. The concentrations of norepinephrine in the dorsal horn are not known, but there is a significant increase in the appearance of concentrations in the cerebrospinal fluid with spinal cord stimulation. Noradrenergic (e.g., norepinephrine, epinephrine) transmitters have been found in neuron axon terminals in laminae I, IIo, IV, V, VI, and X of the spinal cord dorsal horn and in axon terminals of interneurons making synapses with spinothalamic tract neurons involved in nociception.

These noradrenergic terminals make both presynaptic and postsynaptic connections with neurons involved in nociception. The presynaptic binding is especially avid on small-diameter, high-threshold (nociceptive) primary afferents. Evidence suggests that alpha$_2$-noradrenergic release is inhibitory to nociceptive transmission and critical for opiate-induced analgesia.[59–61] Application of norepinephrine to the dorsal horn produces analgesia.

Alpha$_2$-adrenergic transmitters have a depressive effect on wide dynamic range (WDR) neurons. This effect appears to involve increased potassium conductance via the G i/o protein. Agonists of alpha$_2$-adrenergic receptors (e.g., clonidine hydrochloride) decrease the release of substance P from small primary afferent neurons. Alpha$_1$ neurotransmitters can excite WDR neurons, specifically the so-called *on cells* that have a facilitatory role in transmission of nociception.[19, 62, 63] Many studies of these effects have utilized adrenergic antagonists, such as idazoxan (a selective alpha$_2$ antagonist). In the neural circuitry of antinociception within the brain and spinal cord, the locus ceruleus in the pons appears to be a key part of the noradrenergic pathway. It sends inhibitory axons containing norepinephrine to PAG and to dorsal horn neurons.[56]

SEROTONINERGIC RECEPTORS

The sensitization of nociceptors is a result of the actions of second messenger systems activated by release of the inflammatory mediators like bradykinin, prostaglandins, serotonin, and histamine. Specifically, serotonin is a transmitter in the descending system of antinociception and is contained in descending axons of neurons from the nucleus raphe magnus. Since serotonin creates activation of the pathway, it is one of the most important mechanisms in the spinal cord.

Serotonin is found in large amounts in the RVM.[18] These serotoninergic axons from the RVM make axosomatic and axodendritic connections on receptors in the spinal cord. The effects on these receptors are inhibitory in lamina I on nociceptive-specific and WDR neurons and inhibitory in lamina V. Excitatory synaptic contacts exist between the descending axons and interneurons in lamina VI that, in turn, inhibit lamina I neurons. Similar excitatory contacts are made with stalked cells in lamina II. The descending axons also can contact dorsal column postsynaptic cells in lamina IV.[19, 34, 51] With RVM activation, serotonin concentrations in the PAG remain constant, as does metabolite 5-hydroxyindoleacetic acid concentration in the RVM.

Although there is significant presynaptic binding of serotonin on small-diameter, high-threshold primary afferents, serotonin agonists do not decrease release of substance P from small primary afferent neurons. Methiothepin is a serotonin antagonist; the mechanism of action of serotonin at receptors again appears to involve increased potassium conductance via the G i/o protein.

EXCITATORY AMINO ACID RECEPTORS

Experimental evidence indicates that primary afferent neurons release excitatory amino acid neurotransmitters (most likely glutamate) at the central termina.[64] The *N*-methyl-D-aspartate (NMDA) receptor appears to be the most common target for these nociceptive neurotransmitters. Non-NMDA receptors such as the quisqualate or kainate subtype appear to be involved to a lesser degree in nociceptive transmission and descending bulbospinal sympathetic pathways.[65, 66] NMDA receptors, rather than non-NMDA receptors, appear to be the principal mediators of responses in sympathetic preganglionic neurons after stimulation of dorsal root afferent fibers.[67]

A prominent excitatory response to glutamate has been observed in motor horn cells and dorsal horn cells, which are activated by the larger myelinated A-beta fibers.[68] An excitatory response to glutamate has also been found in cuneate and gracilis nuclei neurons. These findings would appear to suggest that glutamate and aspartate are associated, not only with synapses of small-diameter primary afferents, but with larger-diameter afferents. NMDA receptor agonists have been shown to increase substance P basal outflow by 46.5% ± 10.9% without changing evoked release of the peptide.[27] It is one of the main receptors for glutamate, a substance that helps to transfer all information between neurons. The dorsal horn neurons intrinsically contain a large pool of glutamate. This is where postsynaptic activation of the dorsal horn nociceptive neurons occurs and includes a number of peptide receptors plus the receptors for the excited amino acids.

Another receptor subtype called AMPA appears to set the baseline level of nociception and to transmit its intensity and how long it is exposed to the peripheral stimulus. On the other hand, NMDA antagonists such as D, L-2-amino-5-phosphonovaleric acid and ketamine have little effect on thermal or mechanical pain at low doses that do not produce motor dysfunction. This fact suggests that the primary role of NMDA transmitters is related to their effects on small-diameter primary afferent neurons. Amino acid receptors appear to affect central or peripheral neuropathic pain transmission more than nociceptive transmission in tactile or thermal modalities.[69] Recent evidence suggests that NMDA receptors are involved in the development of tolerance to opioids infused into the spine. The NMDA receptor is most important in the synaptic events that lead to hyperalgesia.

The release of peptides such as substance P into the spinal cord could remove the magnesium block of the channel of NMDA. This action allows the glutamate to activate the NMDA receptor in varied pain states.[38] On activation of the receptor, calcium enters the neuron and can trigger involvement of other mediators from neurons in the spinal cord. This introduction of calcium can cause activation of phospholipase and lead to spinal production of prostanoids.[27] Several studies with ketamine in humans have led to theories of NMDA-controlled events that are important in chronic pain.[70]

GAMMA-AMINOBUTYRIC ACID RECEPTORS

The GABAergic network is the intrinsic circuit within the PAG. The major functions of the PAG include pain, analgesia, fear, anxiety, vocalization, and cardiovascular control. It is important to ascending pain transmission, because it is responsible for receiving afferents from all the nociceptive neurons in the spinal cord and has projections to the thalamic nuclei and other nociceptor sites. Therefore, it also projects to inhibitory neurons. In addition, the PAG works with the dorsal column and is involved in pressor responses, and the ventrolateral column mediates depressor responses.[71]

GABA is another substance that acts mainly as an inhibitor to stop the outflow neuron in descending nociception pathways. It is a major excitatory neurotransmitter in the CNS. It activates three receptors—AMPA, NMDA, and kainate (a structural analogue of glutamate)—that affect ion channels.[72] Recent work on kainate receptors in the hippocampus has indicated that repetitive stimulation of that pathway generates slow postsynaptic currents provoked by a kainate receptor–mediated excitatory action.[72] More specifically, it inhibits thin, unmyelinated primary afferents in the dorsal horn. During spinal cord stimulation, extracellular concentrations of GABA in the dorsal horn area increase but concentrations in the PAG are reduced.

In the spinal cord, neurons containing GABA make inhibitory presynaptic contacts with receptors on I_a afferents from muscle. High concentrations of GABA have also been found in areas of small-diameter primary afferents and probably cause inhibition by contacts with presynaptic receptors on the same afferents.[34] GABA has been found in stalked cells and could cause inhibition of thalamic-projecting neurons. Receptors for GABA on interneurons could cause inhibition and control of second-order nociceptors as well.[59] GABA is a substance that, when dysfunctional, can cause symptoms and reactions such as hypersensitive WDR neurons and allodynia.

There are two subclasses of GABA receptors: GABA-A and GABA-B. Muscimol is an agonist for GABA-A receptors and shows binding in spinal gray matter.[73] Benzodiazepines such as midazolam have been shown to be GABA-A agonists with some analgesic actions.[74]

Baclofen is an agonist for GABA-B receptors, which are found in the substantia gelatinosa. The concentration of these receptors is reduced by pretreatment with capsaicin, a small-afferent neurotoxin, a finding that suggests that the receptors are located on small primary afferent terminals. There appears to be significant binding of GABA-B to presynaptic receptors on small-diameter, high-threshold primary afferents, but GABA-B agonists do not reduce substance P release from similar small primary afferent neurons. Phaclofen is a GABA-B antagonist. Intrathecal administration of agonists for GABA-B (but not GABA-A) provides analgesia at doses that do not cause motor changes. The mechanism of receptor transduction appears to involve increased potassium conductance via the G i/o protein.[75]

It has been found that nociceptors can become excited with inflammation and other pathologic conditions.[76] Although adenosine triphosphate (ATP) was not detected in conjunction with glutamate, it was co-released with the inhibitory neurotransmitter GABA from a subset of GABA neurons. In one study by Jo and coworkers, 70% of the GABAergic neurons tested showed ATP being co-released.[76] At the same time, it was found that GABA and glycine are respectively, inhibitory and excitatory, to chloride channels.

These results are the first signs of co-release from the same neuron of an excitatory and an inhibitory neurotransmitter acting at ionotropic postsynaptic receptors. The neurons that most likely co-express P2X and GABA-A receptors are likely to be the postsynaptic recipients of functional fast ATP and GABA co-transmission. This co-release of chemicals may allow a reversible switch between inhibitory and excitatory roles of a given synapse without any anatomic reorganization of the neuronal circuitry. The receptor switching from inhibition to excitation occurs in the dorsal horn under certain conditions, such as mechanical analgesia or allodynic neuropathic pain (the phenomenon of normally innocuous mechanical stimulation becoming painful).[76] These situations can be explained in part on the basis of an alternation in the balance between GABAergic inhibition and P2X receptor–mediated excitation at the level of individual synapses co-releasing GABA and ATP. There are other indications of central neurons that are capable of co-releasing fast-acting excitatory and inhibitory neurotransmitters.

Different degrees of excitatory and inhibitory components of the transmission may help to describe all of the changes in the processing of sensory messages in the dorsal horn during both mechanical hyperalgesia and neuropathic pain.[76]

ADENOSINE A1/A2 RECEPTORS

Although the compound adenosine has many modulatory effects in both the central and the peripheral nervous system, current knowledge suggests that adenosine receptors of the A1 subtype are associated mainly with the modulatory effect on pain transmission at the spinal cord level. Many studies have shown that adenosine has inhibitory effects and, presumably, nociceptive reflex responses. Adenosine receptors are postulated to be located postsynaptically on interneurons in the spinal cord[77] and to act via increased potassium conductance by the G i/o protein. Methylxanthines have been found to block dorsal horn inhibition caused by high-frequency cutaneous stimulation.[78] Morphine increases release of adenosine from the spinal cord, and methylxanthines partially block morphine analgesia.[79]

At least two different receptor subclasses have been described. A1 receptors stimulate adenylate cyclase activity,[80] whereas A2 receptors inhibit adenylate cyclase activity.[81] A possible third receptor might be linked to the calcium channel.[82] L-PIA and NECA are examples of adenosine receptor agonists, whereas methylxanthines, such as theophylline, are antagonists.

OTHER RECEPTORS THAT MAY BE INVOLVED IN NOCICEPTION

In the spinal cord, neurons containing neurotensin have been found in laminae II and III. It is possible that these neurons make excitatory contacts with specific receptors on other interneurons that inhibit transmission of nociception, perhaps by controlling the release of substance P.[34] Acetylcholine has been postulated as another neurotransmitter that can be analgesic.

Spinal cord stimulation affects neurotransmitters, especially in the dorsal horn. The RVM outflow is important in these processes along with the neurochemicals that help to control the descending pain pathways on the road to pain relief. Serotonin is considered the most important neurotransmitter involved in the analgesia from spinal cord stimulation. GABA appears to exert contradictory effects on the dorsal horn and PAG. The complete role of substance P and the extent of its involvement in pain analgesia remain unclear.

REFERENCES

1. Millan M: The induction of pain: An integrative review. Prog Neurobiol 57(1):1–164, 1999.
2. Kramer SN: First pharmacopeia in man's recorded history. Am J Pharmacol 126:76–84, 1954.
3. Gordon BL: Medicine Throughout Antiquity. Philadelphia: FA Davis, 1949.
4. Fulop-Miller R: Triumph Over Pain. New York, Literary Guild of America, 1938.
5. Lewis WH, Elvin-Lewis MPF: Medical Botany: Plants Affecting Man's Health. New York, John Wiley & Sons, 1977.
6. Matsuki A: Nothing new under the sun—a Japanese pioneer in the clinical use of intrathecal morphine (editorial). Anesthesiology 58:289–290, 1983.
7. Sherrington CS: The Integrative Action of the Nervous System. New York, C Scribner & Son, 1906.
8. Way EL: Review and overview of four decades of opiate research. Adv Biochem Psychopharmacol 20:3–27, 1979.
9. Herz A, Teschemacher H: Activities and sites of antinociceptive action of morphine-like analgesics and kinetics of distribution following intravenous, intracerebral and intraventricular application. Adv Drug Res 6:79–119, 1971.
10. Goldstein A, Lowney LI, Pal PK: Stereospecific and non-specific interactions of the morphine congener levorphanol in subcellular fractions of mouse brain. Proc Natl Acad Sci USA 68:1742–1747, 1971.
11. Pert CB, Kuhar MJ, Snyder SH: Opiate receptor autoradiographic localization in rat brain. Proc Natl Acad Sci USA 73:3729–3733, 1976.
12. Basbaum AI, Fields HL: Endogenous pain control systems: Brain stem spinal pathways and endorphin circuitry. Ann Rev Neurosci 7:309, 1984.
13. Fields HL, Basbaum AI: Brain stem control of spinal pain transmission neurons. Ann Rev Physiol 40:193, 1978.
14. Gebhart GF: Opiate and opioid peptide effects on brain stem neurons: Relevance to nociception and antinociceptive mechanisms. Pain 12:93, 1982.
15. Basbaum AI: Anatomical substrates of pain and pain modulation and their relation to analgesic drug action. *In* Kuhar M, Pasternak G: Analgesics: Neurochemical, Behavioral and Clinical Perspectives. New York, Raven, 1984, pp 97–123.
16. Mantyh PW: Connections of midbrain periaqueductal gray in monkey. III. Descending efferent projections. J Neurophysiol 49:582, 1983.
17. Mantyh PW, Peschanski M: Spinal projections from the periaqueductal grey and dorsal raphe in the rat, cat, and monkey. Neuroscience 7:2769, 1982.
18. Sasek CA, Wessendorf MW, Helke CJ: Evidence for co-existence of thyrotropin-releasing hormone, substance P and serotonin in ventral medullary neurons that project to the intermediolateral cell column in the rat. Neuroscience 35:105–119, 1990.
19. Ruda MA, Bennett GJ, Dubner R: Neurochemistry and neurocircuitry in the dorsal horn. Prog Brain Res 66:219, 1986.
20. Ness TJ, Gebhart GF: Visceral pain: A review of experimental studies. Pain 41:167–234, 1990.
21. Nehuber WL, Sandoz PA, Fryscak T: The central projections of primary afferent neurons of greater splanchnic and intercostal nerves in the rat. Anat Embryol (Berl) 174:123–144, 1986.
22. Carpenter MB: Human Neuroanatomy. Baltimore, Williams & Wilkins, 1976.
23. Melzack R, Wall PD: Pain mechanisms: A new theory. Science 150:971–979, 1965.
24. Kerr FWL: Pain: A central inhibitory balance theory. Mayo Clin Proc 50:685–690, 1975.
25. Kerr FWL: Segmental circuitry and spinal cord nociceptive mechanisms. Adv Pain Res Ther 1:75–89, 1976.
26. LeBars D, Dickenson AH, Besson JM, Villaneuva L: Aspects of sensory processing through convergent neurons. *In* Yaksh TL: Spinal Afferent Processing. New York, Plenum, 1986.

27. Malgcangio M, Tomlinson DR: NMDA receptor activation modulates evoked release of substance P from rat spinal cord. Br J Pharmacol 25:1625–1626, 1998.
28. Eisenbach J: Muscarinic-mediated analgesia. Life Sci 64(6 & 7):549–554, 1999.
29. von Euler US, Gaddum JH: An unidentified depressive substance in certain tissue extracts. J Physiol 72:74, 1931.
30. Lembeck F: 5-Hydroxytryptamine in a carcinoid tumor. Nature 172:910, 1953.
31. Dockray GJ, Sharkey KA: Neurochemistry of visceral afferent neurones. *In* Cervero F, Morrison JFB, et al: Progress in Brain Research. New York, Elsevier, 1986; 67:133–148.
32. Murase K, Randic M: Actions of substance P on rat spinal dorsal horn neurons. J Physiol 346:203, 1984.
33. Jancso N, Jancso-Gabor A, Szolcsanyi J: Direct evidence for neurogenic inflammation and its prevention by denervation and by pretreatment with capsaicin. Br J Pharmacol Chemother 31:138, 1967.
34. Basbaum AI: Functional analysis of the cytochemistry of the spinal dorsal horn. *In* Fields HL, Dubner R, Cervero F (eds): Advances in Pain Research and Therapy. New York, Raven, 1985; 9:149–175.
35. Kimura S, Ogawa T, Goto K, et al: Endogenous ligands for tachykinin receptors in mammals. *In* Jordan CC, Oehme P: Substance P: Metabolism and Biological Actions. London, Taylor and Francis, 1985, pp 33–44.
36. Gibbins IL, Furness JB, Costa M: Pathway-specific patterns of the co-existence of substance P, calcitonin gene–related peptide, cholecystokinin and dynorphin in neurons of the dorsal root ganglia of the guinea pig. Cell Tissue Res 248:417–437, 1987.
37. Cuello AC: Peptides as neuromodulators in primary sensory neurons. Neuropharmacology 26:971–979, 1987.
38. Magher JW, Bennett GJ: The neurobiology of pain. Lancet 353:1610–1615, 1999.
39. Yaksh TL: Inhibition by etorphine of the discharge of dorsal horn neurons: Effects upon the neuronal response to both high- and low-threshold sensory input in the decerebrate spinal cat. Exp Neurol 60:23–40, 1978.
40. Wikler A: Sites and mechanisms of action of morphine and related drugs in the central nervous system. Pharmacol Rev 2:435–506, 1950.
41. Mayer DJ et al: Analgesia from electrical stimulation in the brain stem of the rat. Science 174:1351, 1971.
42. Lamotte C, Pert CB, Snyder SH: Opiate receptor binding primate spinal: Distribution and changes after dorsal root section. Brain Res 11:407–412, 1976.
43. Neil A, Terenius L: Receptor mechanisms for nociception. *In* Sjostrand UH, Rawal N: Regional Opioids in Anesthesiology and Pain Management. Boston, Little, Brown, 1986, pp 1–15.
44. Mayer DJ, Price DD: Central nervous system mechanisms of analgesia. Pain 2:379, 1976.
45. Martin WR, Eades CG, Thompson JA, et al: The effects of morphine- and nalorphine-like drugs in the nondependent and morphine-dependent chronic spinal dog. J Pharmacol Exp Ther 197:517, 1976.
46. Terenius L: Families of opioid peptides and classes of opioid receptors. *In* Fields HL, Dubner R, Cervero F: Advances in Pain Research and Therapy. New York, Raven, 1985; 9:463–477.
47. Lord JAH, Waterfield AA, Hughes J, Kosterlitz HW: Endogenous opioid peptides: Multiple agonists and receptors. Nature 267:495–499, 1977.
48. Schultz RE, Wuster M, Herz A: Pharmacological characterization of the epsilon-receptor. J Pharmacol Exp Ther 215:604–606, 1981.
49. Hughes J et al: Identification of two related pentapeptides from the brain with potent opiate, agonist activity. Nature 258:577, 1975.
50. Glazer EJ, Steinbusch H, Verhofstad A, Basbaum AI: Serotonin neurons in nucleus raphe dorsalis and paragigantocellularis of the cat contain enkephalin. J Physiol (Paris) 77:241, 1981.
51. Dubner R, Bennett GJ: Spinal and trigeminal mechanisms of nociception. Ann Rev Neurosci 6:381, 1983.
52. Mudge AW, Leeman SE, Fischback GD: Enkephalin inhibits release of substance P from sensory neurons in culture and decreases action potential duration. Proc Natl Acad Sci USA 76:526–530, 1979.
53. Carstens E, Tulloch I, Zieglgansberger W, Zimmerman M: Presynaptic excitability changes induced by morphine in single cutaneous afferent C- and A-fibers. Pflugers Arch 379:143–147, 1983.
54. Yaksh TL, Jessell TM, Gamse R, et al: Intrathecal morphine inhibits substance P released from mammalian spinal cord *in vivo*. Nature 286:155–156, 1980.
55. Zieglgansberger W, Bayerl H: The mechanisms of inhibition of neuronal activity by opiates in the spinal cord of the cat. Brain Res 115:111–128, 1976.
56. Dubner R: Specialization in nociceptive pathways: Sensory discrimination, sensory modulation, and neural connectivity. *In* Fields HL, Dubner R, Cervero F: Advances in Pain Research and Therapy. New York, Raven, 1985; 9:111–137.
57. Cruz L, Basbaum AI: Multiple opioid peptides and the modulation of pain: Immunohistochemical analysis of dynorphin and enkephalin in the trigeminal nucleus caudalis and spinal cord of the cat. J Comp Neurol 240(4):331, 1985.
58. Iadarola MJ, et al: Enhancement of dynorphin gene expression in spinal cord following experimental inflammation: Stimulus specificity, behavioral parameters and opioid receptor binding. Pain 35:313, 1988.
59. Dubner R, et al: Neural circuitry mediating nociception in the medullary and spinal dorsal horn. *In* Kruger L, Liebeskind JC: Advances in Pain Research and Therapy. New York, Raven, 6:151–166, 1984.
60. Hammond DL: Pharmacology of central pain-modulating networks (biogenic amines and non-opioid analgesics). *In* Fields HL, Dubner R, Cervero F: Advances in Pain Research and Therapy. New York, Raven, 9:499–511, 1985.
61. Hammond DL: Control systems for nociceptive afferent processing: The descending inhibitory pathways. *In* Yaksh TL: Spinal Afferent Processing. New York, Plenum, 1986, pp 363–390.
62. Westlund KN, Coulter JD: Descending projections of the locus coeruleus and subcoeruleus/medial parabrachial nuclei in monkey: Axonal transport studies and dopamine-beta-hydroxylase immunocytochemistry. Brain Res Rev 2:235, 1980.
63. Sagen J, Proudfit HK: Evidence for pain modulation by pre- and postsynaptic noradrenergic receptors in the medulla oblongata. Brain Res 331:285, 1985.
64. Jessell TM, Kelly DD: Pain and analgesia. *In* Kandel ER, Schwartz JH, Jessell TM: Principles of Neural Science. New York, Elsevier, 1991, pp 385–399.
65. Hong Y, Henry JL: Glutamate, NMDA and NMDA receptor antagonists: Cardiovascular effects of intrathecal administration in the rat. Brain Res 569:38–45, 1992.
66. Bazil MK, Gordon FJ: Effect of blockade of spinal NMDA receptors on sympathoexcitation and cardiovascular response produced by cerebral ischemia. Brain Res 555:149–152, 1991.
67. Shen E, Mo N, Dun NJ: APV-sensitive dorsal root afferent transmission to neonate rat sympathetic preganglionic neurons in vitro. J Neurophysiol 64:991–999, 1990.
68. Yaksh TL, Hammond DL: Peripheral and central substrates in the rostral transmission of nociceptive information. Pain 13:1, 1982.
69. Yaksh TL: Behavioral and autonomic correlates of the tactile evoked allodynia produced by spinal glycine inhibition: Effects of modulatory receptor systems and excitatory amino acid antagonists. Pain 37:111–123, 1989.
70. Dickenson A: NMDA receptor antagonists: Interactions with opioids. Acta Anaesthesiol Scand 41:112–115, 1997.
71. Behbehani M: Functional characteristics of the midbrain periaqueductal gray. Prog Neurobiol 46(6):575–605, 1995.
72. Li P, Wilding TJ, Kim SJ, Calejesan AA, et al: Kainate receptor–mediated sensory synaptic transmission. Nature 397(6715):161–164, 1999.
73. Aanonsen LM, Wilcox GL: Muscimol, γ-amino-butyric acid A receptors and excitatory amino acids in the mouse spinal cord. J Pharmacol Exp Ther 248:1034–1038, 1988.
74. Nishi S, Minota S, Karczmar AG: Primary afferent neurones: The ionic mechanism of GABA-mediated depolarization. Neuropharmacology 13:215–219, 1974.
75. Hwang AS, Wilcox GL: Baclofen, γ-aminobutyric acid B receptors and substance P in the mouse spinal cord. J Pharmacol Exp Ther 248:1026–1033, 1988.
76. Jo YH, Schlichter R: Synaptic co-release of ATP and GABA in cultured spinal neurons. Nature Neurosci 2:241–245, 1999.
77. Choco JI, Green RD, Proudfit HK: Adenosine A1 and A2 receptors of the substantia gelatinosa are located predominantly on intrinsic neurons: An autoradiography study. J Pharmacol Exp Ther 247:757–764, 1988.
78. Salter MW, Henry JL: Evidence that adenosine mediates the depression of spinal dorsal horn neurons induced by peripheral vibration in the cat. Neuroscience 22:631–650, 1987.

79. Sweeney MI, White TD, Sawynok J: Involvement of adenosine in the spinal antinociceptive effects of morphine and noradrenaline. J Pharmacol Exp Ther 243:657–665, 1987.
80. VanCalker P, Muller M, Hamprecht B: Adenosine regulates via two different types of receptors the accumulation of cAMP in cultured brain cells. J Neurochem 33:999–1005, 1979.
81. Ribeiro JA, Sebastiao AM: Adenosine receptors and calcium: Basis for proposing a third (A3) adenosine receptor. Prog Neurobiol 26:179–209, 1986.
82. Daly JW, Bruns RF, Snyder SH: Adenosine in the central nervous system: Relationship to the central action of methylxanthines. Life Sci 28:2083–2097, 1981.

CHAPTER • 5

Functional Anatomy of the Spine

Philip M. Finch, FFPM ANZCA
• James R. Taylor, MD, PhD

The erect human vertebral column is supported on the pelvis by its joints, muscles, and ligaments. Its mobile, presacral part consists of 24 vertebrae, 23 of which are united by intervertebral discs, zygapophyseal joints, and ligaments. It is straight in the frontal plane but curved in the sagittal plane. The primary, ventrally concave, spinal kyphosis of the newborn fetus changes to secondary lordotic curvatures in the cervical and lumbar regions. The cervical lordosis develops shortly after birth with extension of the head; during the second year of life, independent standing and walking with hip and pelvic extension develop the lumbar lordosis. The thoracic spine retains its primary curvature.

The spine is the central skeletal axis, and it has to adapt to a wide variety of load-bearing and movement requirements. It also acts as a protective conduit for the spinal cord and cauda equina. It is important to understand the structure, function, and innervation of the intervertebral joints and their relation to spinal nerves, to appreciate the nature of injuries to these structures and their relevance to pain syndromes.

The largest, lowest, intervertebral joints bear the greatest loads. Because the discs are the main weight-bearing shock absorbers, the lowest discs are strongest. The multiple, cylindrical sheets of collagen fibers forming the annulus fibrosus surround a nucleus pulposus with a matrix rich in proteoglycans. This gives a structure well adapted to load bearing and shock absorption.

The cervical and lumbar regions of the spine are specially adapted for wide ranges of mobility. The cervical spine shows the greatest range and variety of movements. It flexes, extends, bends, and rotates to the right and left. The lumbar spine can bend in the sagittal and coronal planes, but its capacity for twisting is limited and lumbar segments have less range of motion than cervical segments. The three joints between each pair of vertebrae make each motion segment strong with only a few degrees of intersegmental movement, but the many motion segments in each region give wide ranges of movement, especially in young persons. The wide ranges of mobility characteristic of infants and children are gradually reduced in adults. Stiffness and slow movement are characteristic of old age. With aging, the intervertebral discs lose proteoglycan and water and become thinner, less compliant, and less resilient, and the vertebrae lose bone mass and may become porotic.[1] These changes may be associated with aches, pains, and stiffness in the neck and low back. Backaches also result from industrial, motor vehicle, or sporting injuries.[2] The moving parts of the spine are most susceptible to pain-producing degenerative change or injury.

LUMBAR MOTION SEGMENT ANATOMY

The motion segment uniting two lumbar vertebrae is formed by three joints with their ligaments and muscles. This includes the intervertebral disc and two synovial facet joints. The disc is reinforced by the anterior and posterior longitudinal ligaments, and the facet joints are supported by the ligamenta flava and the interspinous and supraspinous ligaments. The discs are beautifully designed to combine the functions of a strong joint and a load-bearing shock absorber. The facet joints are like guide rails, facilitating movements in the required directions but preventing movements that would damage the disc.[2] Spinal nerves emerge from the spinal canal laterally, through paired intervertebral foramina. The C5–T1 and L2–S1 nerves are largest because they supply the limbs. They contain sensory and motor fibers in the ratio of about 3 : 1 and also sympathetic fibers.

Intervertebral Discs

Each lumbar intervertebral disc has a peripheral, multilayered annulus fibrosus of 12 to 16 circumferential lamellae enclosing a large, central nucleus pulposus (Fig. 5–1). Hyaline cartilage plates cap the vertebral end plates. The cartilage plates are integral parts of the disc structure, where the inner annulus is anchored. The adult anterior and lateral annulus has thick lamellae and is 10 to 12 mm thick. The posterior annulus has finer lamellae and it is 5 or 6 mm thick. The outer annulus fibrosus has a ligamentous function and is adapted to withstand tensile stresses. Its thick, coarse collagen lamellae unite the bony vertebral rims. The inner annulus has finer collagen lamellae, with a curved out-

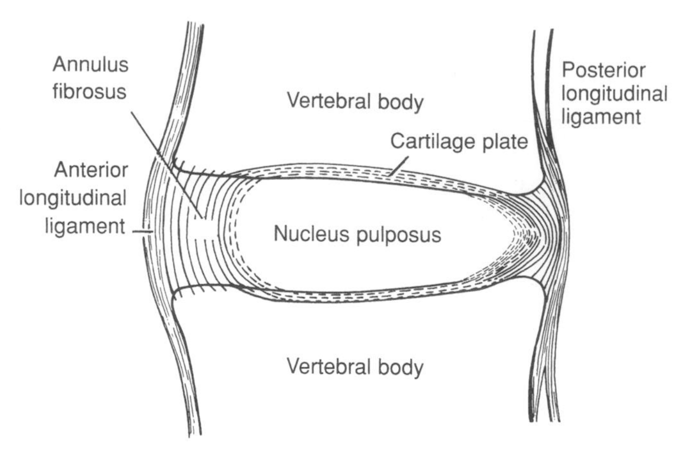

FIGURE 5–1 Diagram of an adult lumbar intervertebral disc in medial sagittal section. The outer layer of the annulus fibrosus attaches to the vertebral rim, and the inner layer is continuous with the cartilage plates.

ward convexity, enclosed in a proteoglycan-rich matrix. The lamellae of the inner annulus are continuous with the hyaline cartilage plates, and, together, these structures form a complete envelope for the nucleus pulposus. Both the nucleus and the inner annulus have high proteoglycan content, and therefore they absorb and hold water. The nucleus would absorb more water than the envelope around it allows, so that it is contained under tension within its envelope.

The inner annulus and cartilage plates, enveloping the nucleus pulposus, combine in an axial load-bearing role. When fluid is injected into a healthy disc at discography, a strong resistance to injection is felt, and injected fluid may be forced back into the syringe when the injection pressure is released.

The parallel collagen fibers of each annular lamella spiral from one vertebra to the next. The parallel fibers in alternate sheets spiral in opposite directions. This gives a strong structure that resists twisting movements. The disc is avascular in adults, except for its outermost annulus and the cartilage plate–vertebral junction.

The anterior longitudinal ligament is a broad, strong band loosely attached to the front of the discs and vertebral bodies. The posterior longitudinal ligament is a dentate structure, wide at the discs, to which it is firmly attached, and narrow opposite the vertebral bodies, from which it is separated by a space containing a venous plexus. The fibers of these ligaments bridge over several segments, forming long intersegmental ties that add to the resilience and strength of the column.

Facet Joints

Lumbar facet joints are oriented almost parallel to the long axis of the spine. Their articular surfaces are curved or biplanar, as seen in transverse sections or on computed tomography (CT) Fig. 5–2), except at the lumbosacral level, where they are often flat. The small convex facets on the downward-projecting inferior articular processes (IAP), face forward and outward, to be embraced by the wider concave facets on the upward-projecting superior articular processes (SAP). The SAP face backward and medially. The posterior joint plane approximates to the sagittal plane, and the anterior part turns toward the coronal plane. The average joint plane, as measured in CT scans (Fig. 5–3) changes from an angle of 22 degrees to the midsagittal plane at L1–L2 to an angle of 51 degrees to the sagittal plane at L5–S1.[3] The biplanar or curved orientation blocks axial rotation and prevents anterior gliding and translation of the flexed spine, movements that might damage the disc, but allows upward and downward gliding movements of the facets in flexion, extension, and lateral bending. The restraint of axial rotation is most effective when the spine is erect, because the joint surfaces are congruous; the restraint is less effective in the flexed spine, when the joint surfaces are not congruous. In the latter position, twisting and bending loads may overstretch the spiral fibers of the annulus, with the risk of an annular tear. This risk is greater for persons who work in fixed flexed postures, because under prolonged loading the discs creep so that the spine flexes beyond its "normal" end range.[4]

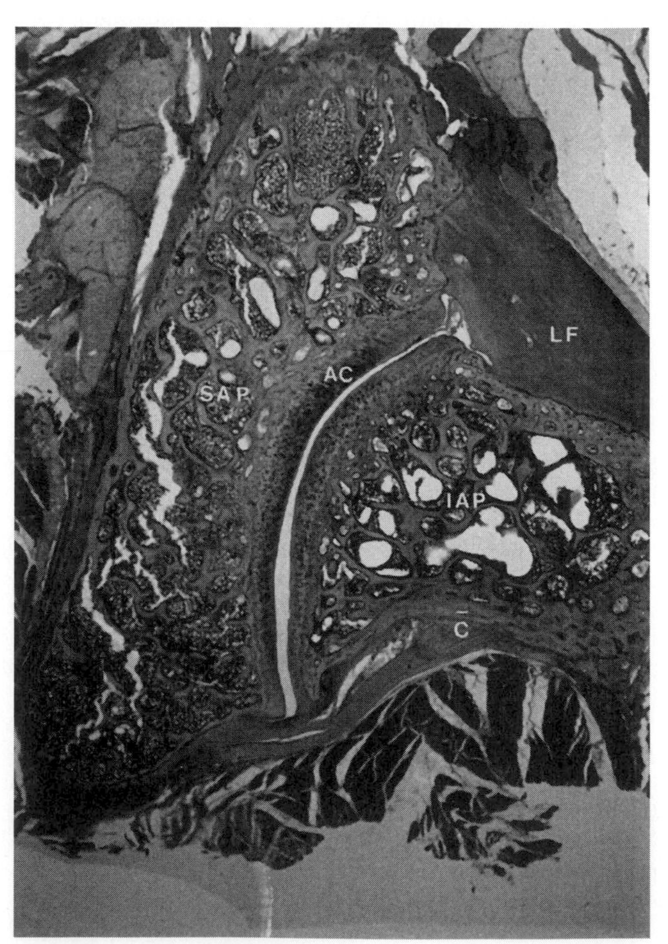

FIGURE 5–2 Transverse section of a normal young adult's L3-4 facet joint (100 μm, stained hematoxylin & light green). SAP, superior articular process of L4; AP, inferior articular process of L3; AC, articular cartilage; LF, ligamentum flavum. The posterior fibrous capsule (C) is covered by the multifidus muscle. (From Taylor J, Twomey L: Structure and function of lumbar zygapophyseal (facet) joints. In Grieve GP [ed]: Modern Manual Therapy of the Vertebral Column, 2nd ed. New York, Churchill Livingstone, 1994, pp 99–108.)

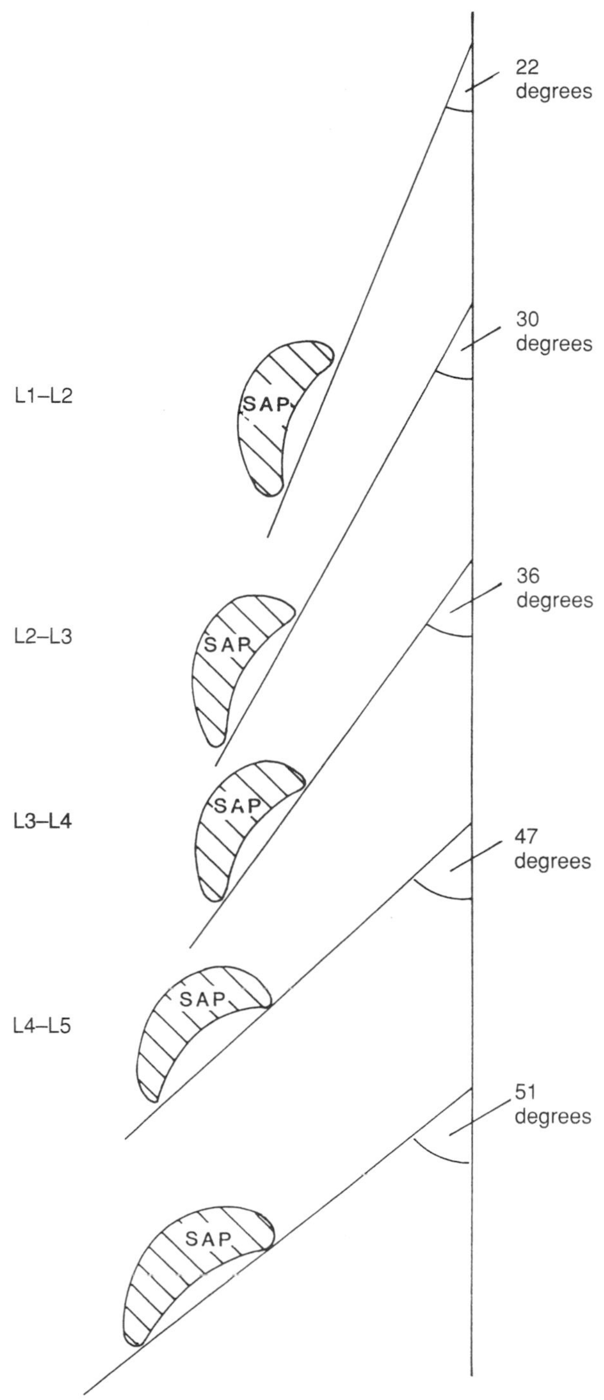

FIGURE 5–3 Diagram showing average joint planes from L1-2 to L5-S1, as measured in 260 CT scans of adults of all ages. SAP, superior articular process. (From Taylor J, Twomey L: Structure and function of lumbar zygapophyseal (facet) joints. In Grieve GP [eds]: Modern Manual Therapy of the Vertebral Column, 2nd ed. New York, Churchill Livingstone, 1994, pp 99–108.)

The posterior capsule of the facet joints is fibrous and 1 mm thick; the anterior capsule is formed by the 3-mm thick, elastic ligamentum flavum. The fibrous capsule is attached laterally to the SAP close to the joint. Medially, the capsule's long, superficial fibers pass over the posterior aspect of the IAP to be attached 7 mm or more medial to the joint line. The lumbar ligamentum flavum is partly an interlaminar ligament and partly a capsular ligament, enclosing the anterior aspect of the facet joint. Lumbar facet joints have large, fat-filled, polar recesses to allow for upward and downward gliding movements. The superior joint recess is intracapsular, between an upward extension of the ligamentum flavum and the pars interarticularis (Fig. 5–4); it contains a fat-filled vascular synovial fold. The larger fat pad of the lower recess is extracapsular; it lies in a bony hollow below the tip of the IAP, enclosed by the attachment of the multifidus muscle. Large synovial folds extend into the lower joint cavity from the inferior recess, through a hole in the capsule. This allows the fat of the extracapsular recess to enter and leave the synovial fold within the joint cavity during movement. In spondylolysis, the upper recess of one joint is in direct communication with the lower recess of the joint above through the spondylolytic defect. A facet injection into one joint spreads into

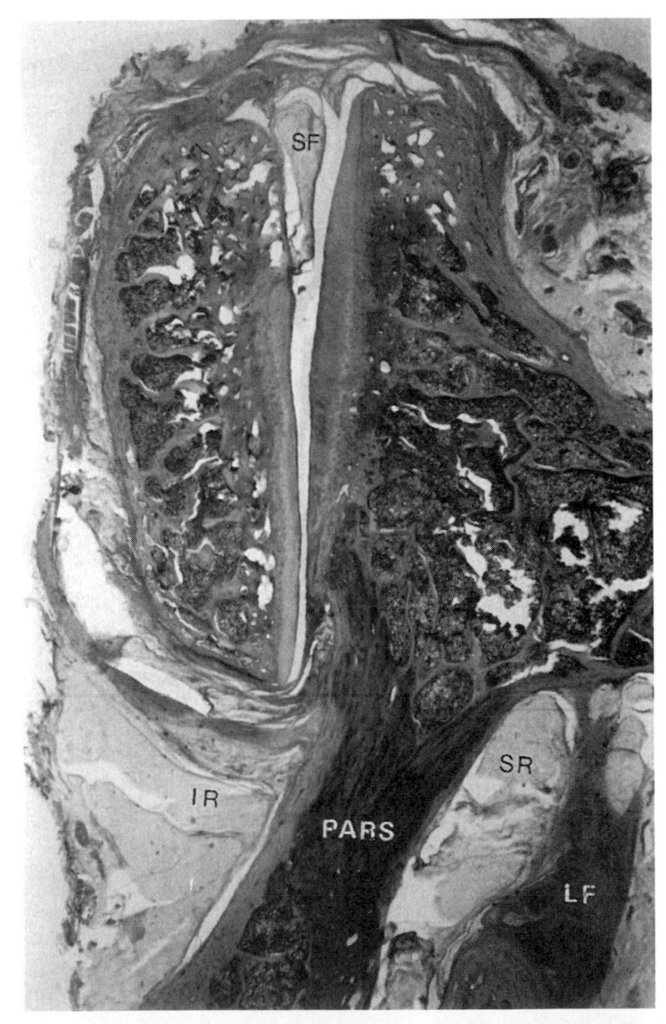

FIGURE 5–4 Sagittal section (100 μm, stained hematoxylin & light green) of the L4-5 and upper pole of L5-S1 facet joints, showing the inferior recess of L4-5 (IR), the superior recess of L5-S1 (SR), and the sclerotic pars interarticularis (PARS) intervening, in a young man. SF, synovial fold of the superior recess of L4-5; LF, capsular part of the ligamentum flavum of the L5-S1 joint. (From Taylor J, Twomey L: Structure and function of lumbar zygapophyseal (facet) joints. In Grieve GP [ed]: Modern Manual Therapy of the Vertebral Column, 2nd ed. New York, Churchill Livingstone, 1994, pp 99–108.)

an ipsilateral joint, and if the spondylolysis is bilateral, it may also spread into a contralateral joint.[5]

Spinal Nerves

The lumbar and sacral spinal nerve roots descend as the cauda equina within the subarachnoid space. The anterior and posterior nerve rootlets arise in rows from the anterior and posterior aspects of the lower spinal cord, in the thoracolumbar spinal canal. Multiple rootlets, surrounded by a small lateral extension of the meninges, come together to form single anterior and posterior roots in the inner part of each intervertebral foramen, where the posterior root swells to form the dorsal root ganglion.

The anterior and posterior roots fuse at the ganglion and pierce the dura, which forms a sleeve for the nerve as it passes out of the spinal canal through the wider, upper part of the foramen, directly under the pedicle and well above the level of the intervertebral disc and facet joint. In its intrathecal course, each nerve descends in a nerve root canal, medial to the pedicle, in the lateral recess of the spinal canal. The lumbar dorsal root ganglia (DRG) usually lie within the medial parts of the intervertebral foramina. The sacral DRG lie in the lateral recesses of the sacral spinal canal, and the sacral ventral and dorsal rami exit separately from anterior and posterior sacral foramina. The lumbar and S1 nerve roots and their dural coverings can be impinged upon in the lateral recesses of the spinal canal by a protrusion or hemiation of the disc at the level above that of their foraminal exit.

Innervation of the Motion Segment

The intervertebral discs, longitudinal ligaments, and anterior dura are innervated from the ventral rami of the spinal nerves (Fig. 5–5). Nerves penetrate the outer lamellae of the annulus fibrosus and supply its outer third with nociceptive fibers. Plexuses of nerves supply the anterior and posterior longitudinal ligaments. The nerve supply to the outer disc is derived from small branches arising directly from the origin of the ventral ramus. These pass to the posterolateral disc. Other disc branches to the lateral and anterior disc arise from the rami communicantes. These nerves tend to be distributed to the disc at the same level, or occasionally to the disc below. The sinuvertebral nerve (SVN) is a small nerve (or several small nerve filaments) arising from the anterior aspect of the origin of the ventral ramus. The SVN runs back into the spinal canal and forms a plexus or network of fine fibers, with the SVN above and below to supply the posterior longitudinal ligament, posterior outer annulus, and the anterior dura.

The facet joints and interspinous and supraspinous ligaments are supplied from the medial branches of the dorsal rami of the spinal nerves. The lateral branches of the dorsal rami supply the corresponding segments of the erector spinae muscle and the skin of the buttocks (L1 through L4). Each medial branch passes obliquely downward and backward around the SAP from the upper margin of the root of the transverse process, supplying the lower part of the facet joint capsule of the same segmental level, and then descends to supply the upper portion of the capsule of the next joint below. The medial branches also supply deep segments of the multifidus and the interspinal muscles. The fibrous capsule of each lumbar facet joint has a plentiful nerve supply; nerves, independent of vessels and staining positively for substance P, have also been observed in the fat pads within the joint's synovial folds.[6] The ligamentum flavum does not appear to have a nerve supply, except where it intermingles with the fibrous capsule at the superior and inferior joint recesses. The posterior dura has only a sparse nerve supply.

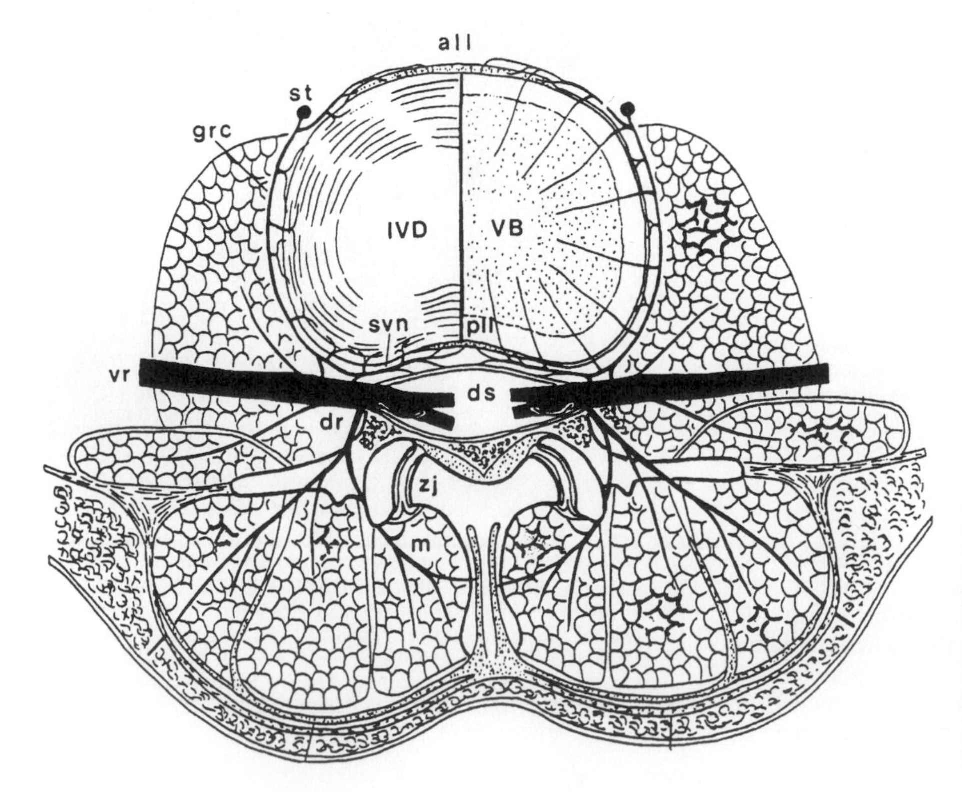

FIGURE 5–5 Innervation of the lumbar motion segment showing the vertebral body (VB) on the right and the intervertebral disc (IVD) on the left. ds, *dural sac;* zj, *zygapophyseal joint;* pll, *posterior longitudinal ligament;* all, *anterior longitudinal ligament;* vr, *ventral ramus;* dr, *dorsal ramus;* m, *medial branch;* svn, *sinuvertebral nerve;* grc, *gray ramus communications;* st, *sympathetic trunk. (From Bogduk N, Twomey LT: Nerves of the lumbar spine.* In *Clinical Anatomy of the Lumbar Spine, 2nd ed. New York, Churchill Livingstone, 1991.)*

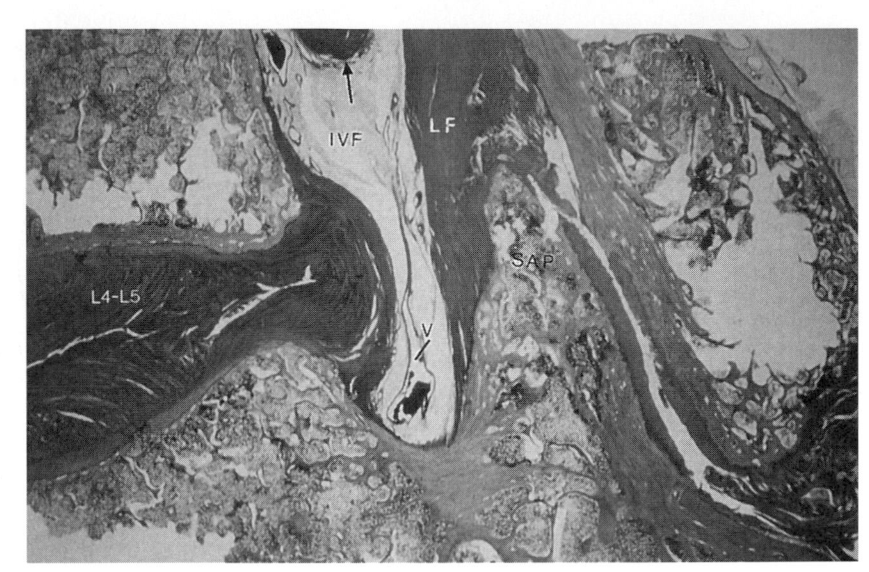

FIGURE 5–6 Sagittal section of the posterior half of an L4-5 intervertebral disc from an elderly subject shows fissuring of the disc and posterior bulging of the annulus. The intervertebral foramen (IVF) behind the disc is empty apart from a segmental vein (V). The arrow indicates the spinal nerve in the upper part of the intervertebral foramen above the disc and facets. LF, ligamentum flavum; SAP, superior articular process of the facet joint. (Also in color; see Color Plates.)

It should be noted that articular cartilages of facet joints have no innervation but the subchondral bone is innervated, so that if it is exposed by cartilage loss it may be a source of pain on load bearing.

Age Changes in Discs and Facet Joints

Intervertebral Discs

After age 50 years, discs lose some of their water and proteoglycan content and increase their collagen content,[7] especially the L4–L5 and L5–S1 discs. In a study of discs from 204 subjects, Twomey and Taylor[1] found that only about 30% of lower lumbar discs from subjects over 60 years old actually lose average thickness. There is an increase in central disc height, owing to osteoporotic bowing of the vertebral end plates, and only the peripheral parts of the discs become thinner. Histologic examination of aging discs or axial discography, however, often reveals circumferential or radial fissures in the discs of persons in middle life or older. Osti and colleagues[8] have described rim lesions in the anterior annulus of young subjects. These lesions are parallel and close to the anterior part of the vertebral end plate. They may be due to some traumatic incident, and they are occasionally observed as vacuum clefts in plain radiographs. Discs that lose proteoglycan may bulge at their posterior margins (Fig. 5–6). This is not usually a painful change unless accompanied by fissures or tears into the outer annulus, resulting from trauma. Extensively fissured discs may lose their mechanical strength, leading to instability of the motion segment. Degenerate or injured discs may be revascularized, with nerves accompanying the ingrowing blood vessels, when acute or chronic injury causes a breach in the cartilage plate or annulus and vessels and nerves grow into the breaches or fissures.[9]

Facet Joints

Facet joints of some young adults show chondromalacia in the articular cartilage of the anterior, coronally oriented part of the SAP (Fig. 5–7), probably as a reaction to repeated compressive loading of the spine in flexion.[10] In middle life, loosening of flaps of articular cartilage in the posterior parts of the lumbar facet joints may result from rotatory strains, because the capsule is often directly attached to the posterior articular cartilage margin.[3] Loose cartilage flaps may predispose to "acute locked back," if

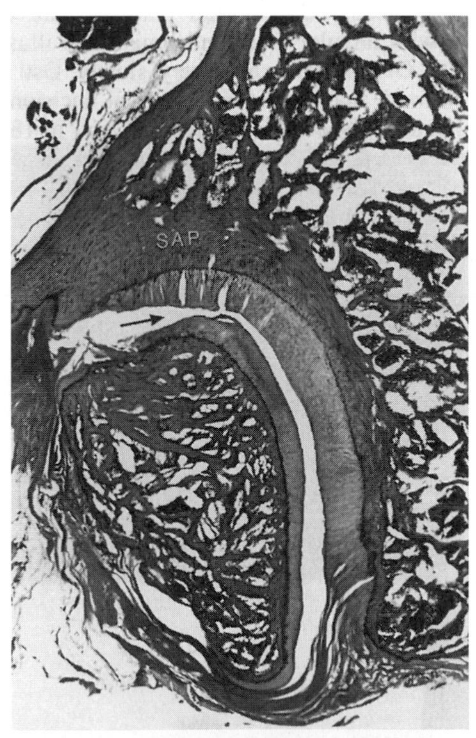

FIGURE 5–7 A 100-μm transverse section of an L3-4 facet joint from a 36-year-old man, shows chondromalacia with fibrillation of the articular cartilage of the superior articular process (SAP) in the anterior, coronally oriented part of the joint (arrow). The subchondral plate of the SAP is thickened and sclerotic. Note the continuity of the posterior capsule with the articular cartilage of the SAP. (From Taylor J, Twomey L: Structure and function of lumbar zygapophyseal (facet) joints. In Grieve GP [ed]: Modern Manual Therapy of the Vertebral Column, 2nd ed. New York, Churchill Livingstone, 1994, pp 99–108.)

they become displaced during flexion (Fig. 5–8). In unstable motion segments, there may be partial subluxation of an IAP backward from its SAP, with remodeling of the facets that are no longer held in congruous apposition. Metaplastic articular cartilage is formed around the posterior margins of the IAP and the ligamentum flavum, or a fat pad may fill an abnormal gap in the anterior joint space.[11, 12] These changes may be observed on CT. A CT scan obtained with the lumbar spine held in torsion by a wedge pillow under one hip may demonstrate loosening of the motion segment.[13]

The facets usually show hypertrophy with aging. Within the lateral recess or at the foramen of exit in older patients, grossly enlarged facets with marginal osteophytes may impinge upon, entrap, or irritate a spinal nerve in the nerve root canal (Fig. 5–9). A combination of age-related changes, such as bilateral facet hypertrophy, disc protrusion, and hypertrophy or inward buckling of the ligamentum flavum, may cause spinal stenosis, usually in the lateral recess of the spinal canal, with compression of nerve roots.

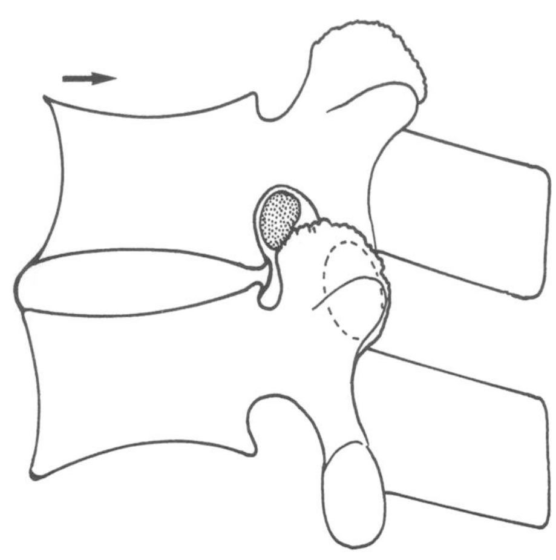

FIGURE 5–9 A diagram showing retrolisthesis (arrow) of the upper vertebra in an unstable motion segment. The combination of loss in disc height and hypertrophy of the osteophytic facets with vertebral retrolisthesis may narrow the foramen and cause entrapment or irritation of the spinal nerve. (From Taylor J, Twomey L: Structure and function of lumbar zygapophyseal (facet) joints. In Grieve GP [ed]: Modern Manual Therapy of the Vertebral Column, 2nd ed. New York, Churchill Livingstone, 1994, pp 99–108.)

Injuries to Motion Segments

We have observed, at autopsy, the lumbar motion segments of a number of victims of fatal accidents.[14] We have observed annular tears in discs, often associated with small fractures of the adjacent vertebral end plates, but injuries to the facet joints are also common. These are the most common soft tissue injuries to the capsules or ligamenta flava, but infractions of the subchondral bone plates with bleeding into the facet joints, and occult, undisplaced fractures of the facets are also seen (Figs. 5–10 to 5–12). Facet injuries would increase the likelihood of early-onset arthritis.

Major disc injuries can occur in serious accidents, but small (and potentially painful) fractures of the vertebral end plates and cartilage plates occur when the spine is forcibly flexed in flexion-compression injuries (Fig. 5–13). These may be associated with bone bruising due to multiple trabecular microfractures. A fracture of the vertebral end plate allows bleeding into the disc; the blood spreads through the soft nucleus of a disc in a younger patient or

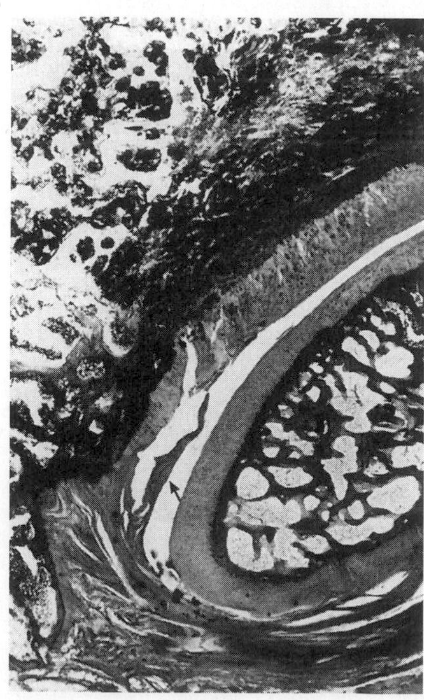

FIGURE 5–8 A transverse section of the posterior part of a lower lumbar facet joint from a 37-year-old man shows a loose fibrocartilage flap (arrow), probably a detached, torn part of the original articular cartilage. (From Twomey L, Taylor J: Physical Therapy of the Low Back, 2nd ed. New York, Churchill Livingstone, 1994, pp 1–56.)

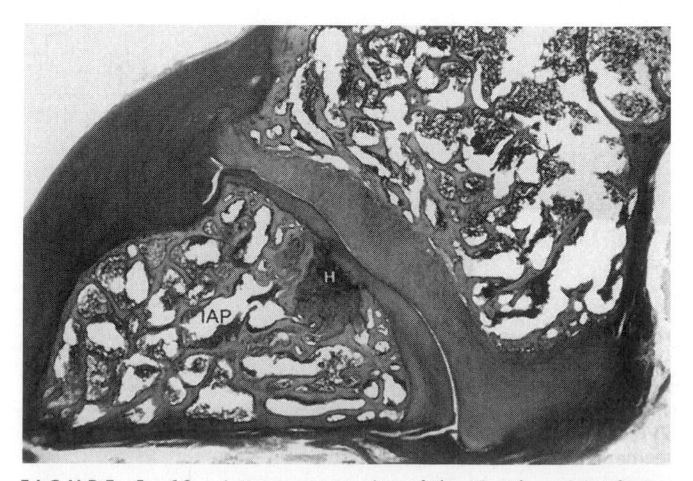

FIGURE 5–10 A transverse section of the L3-4 facet joint from a 7-year-old child who died with a subdural hematoma 3 weeks after falling from a tree. There is an infraction of the subchondral bone of the inferior articular process (IAP) with partial organization of the hematoma (H).

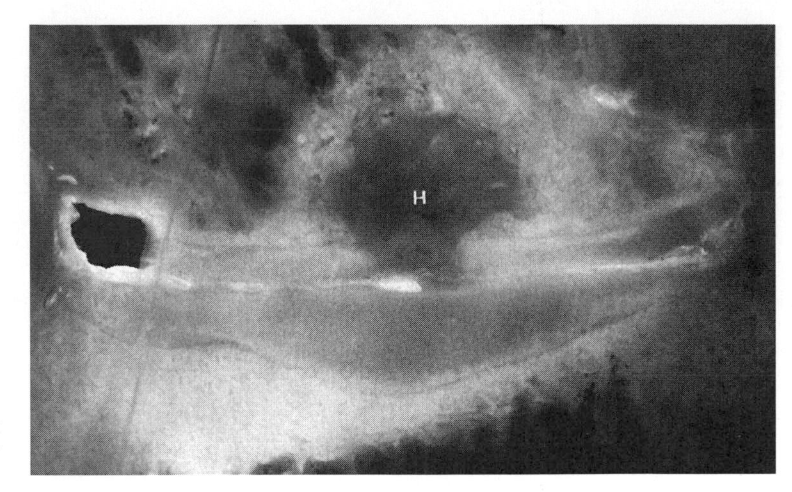

FIGURE 5–11 *A trauma-induced hemarthrosis in a lumbar facet joint of a 53-year-old woman. H, hematoma in subchondral bone. (Also in color; see Color Plates.)*

into the fissures of the disc in an older patient. This may be observed occasionally on magnetic resonance imaging (MRI) film obtained a few days or a week after the injury, at which time the blood looks like contrast in a discogram. An end plate fracture of L5 in association with annular tears and bruising is illustrated in Figure 5–14. Disc injuries heal very slowly. Osti and colleagues[8] showed that transverse surgical incisions in the anterior annulus of sheep's discs did not heal in 18 months, but the surgical fissures extended and led to premature disc degeneration. In our autopsy studies, the vast majority of disc and facet injuries described above were not visible on plain radiographs taken before sectioning.

ANATOMY OF CERVICAL MOTION SEGMENTS

The cervical region is the most mobile part of the vertebral column. It owes this quality to the nature of its motion segments, which are significantly different from lumbar segments, in both the upper and the lower cervical spine. The atlantooccipital and atlantoaxial joints are synovial joints which contribute about half of the total movement range of the head and neck. They are usually well preserved in elderly people whose lower cervical joints have become stiff.[15] While the lower cervical motion segments, from C2–C3 through C6–C7, have discs and paired facet joints like lumbar motion segments, there are important structural and functional differences between the two regions, including cervical uncinate processes with uncovertebral clefts and fissures and 45-degree angled facets, which make possible greater ranges of motion. Each lower cervical interbody joint consists of an intervertebral disc and two lateral uncovertebral clefts or "joints." The lower cervical motion segments have a flexion-extension range of 15 degrees per segment,[16] as compared with an average of 10 degrees per segment in the lumbar spine.[17] Cervical discs, though thinner than lumbar ones, have smaller horizontal dimensions and the cervical facets offer less restraint to movement than the lumbar facets, with more cervical intersegmental gliding or translation accompanying rotations in the sagittal and coronal planes and much larger ranges of axial rotation in the lower cervical segments.

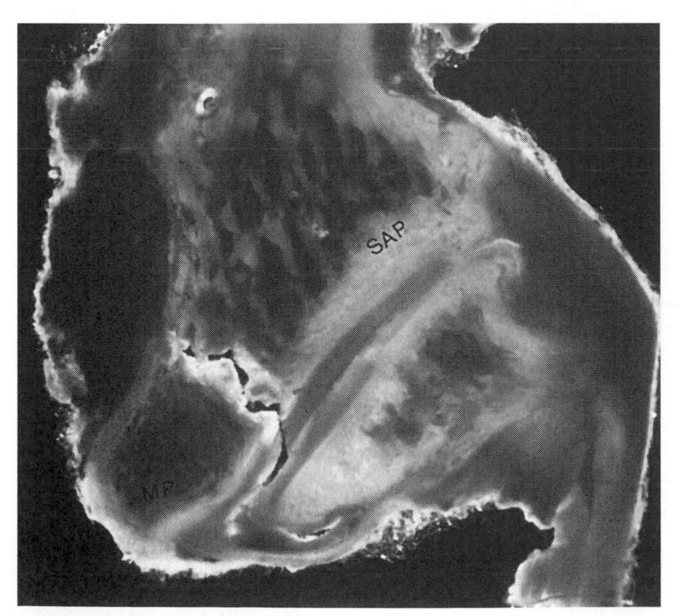

FIGURE 5–12 *A fracture of the mamillary process (MP) from the superior articular process (SAP) of L5 in a victim of a fatal traffic accident. (Also in color; see Color Plates.)*

Atlantooccipital Joint

The lateral masses of the atlas articulate with the occipital condyles. Each atlantooccipital joint is enclosed by a fibrous capsule with an inner lining of synovial membrane. The upper facets of the lateral masses of C1 are concave in the sagittal plane and they slope downward from lateral to medial. The facets are kidney shaped from front to back, and the anterior ends are higher and closer together than the posterior ends. They articulate closely with the reciprocally shaped convex occipital condyles on each side of the foramen magnum. With this configuration, axial compression would force the lateral masses apart, risking Jefferson's fracture of the anterior and posterior arches.

Injuries to the atlantooccipital (C0–C1) joint can produce high occipital pain with associated headaches. The pain is frequently worse on "nodding" motions of the head.

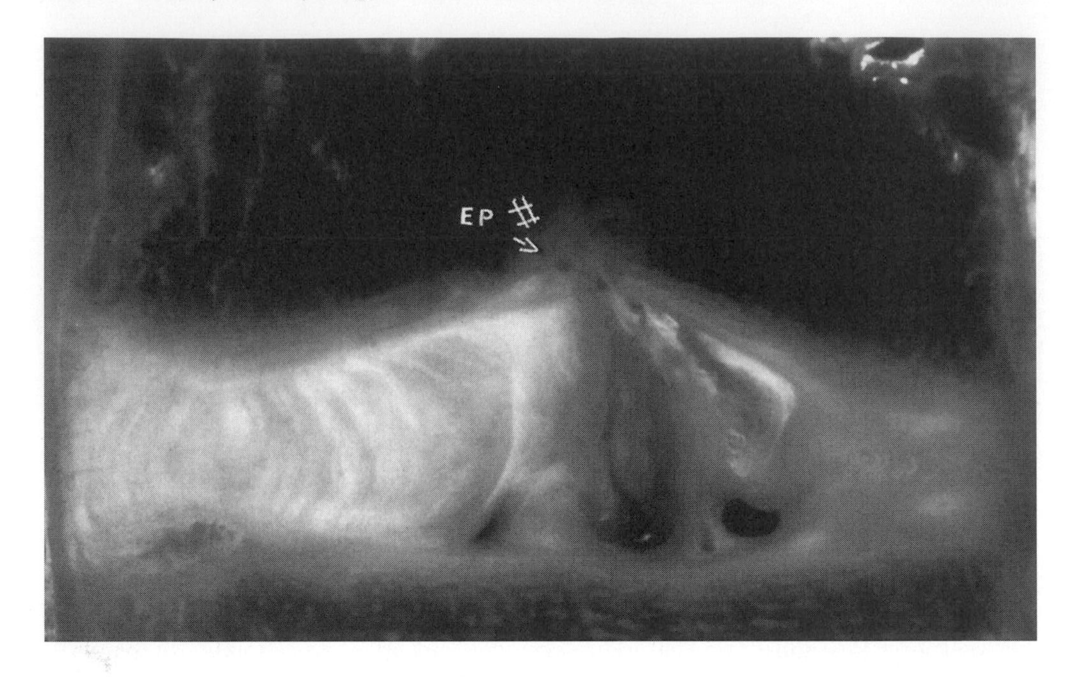

FIGURE 5–13 A fracture of the vertebral end plate of T9 (EP#) with bleeding into the disc in an 18-year-old man killed in a traffic accident. (Also in color; see Color Plates.)

Atlantoaxial Joint

This joint complex has three parts, two lateral parts between the lateral masses of the atlas and axis and a central part formed by the enclosure of the dens between the anterior arch of the atlas and the strong transverse ligament. The atlantoaxial joint (C1–C2) provides the largest component of cervical axial rotation, which is required for turning the head to direct the gaze to right or left. Stability of the joint depends on the integrity of the transverse ligament, which secures the dens. Excessive forward movement of the anterior arch of C1 from the dens in a flexion film indicates instability.

The dens is the "axis" of rotation. It articulates with the anterior arch of the atlas and the strong transverse ligament. From the apex of the dens on each side, strong alar ligaments fan up and out to the medial margins of the occipital condyles. The cruciate ligament includes the transverse ligament, a thin apical ligament from the tip of the dens to the anterior margin of the foramen magnum, and an inferior longitudinal bundle from the transverse ligament to the back of the body of C2. These are covered behind by the membrana tectoria and the anterior dura. Excessive rotation is checked by the alar ligaments, which may be injured in rotatory strains.

The lateral atlantoaxial facets are flat in the coronal plane but convex in the sagittal plane. Sagittal plane incongruity is accentuated by the greater central thickness of the articular cartilage. Almost half of the total sagittal plane flexion and extension, attributable to the occipitoatlantoaxial joint complex, occurs at C1–C2. The incongruous lateral joints of C1–C2 allow more than 20 degrees of rocking in flexion and extension.[18] The large triangular gaps between the anterior and posterior articular surfaces are filled by vascular, fat-filled synovial folds that project inward from the capsule (Fig. 5–15). The well-defined, loose fibrous capsule, 1 to 2 mm thick, is attached around the articular margins. The inferior oblique muscle of the occipital region, which has a strong fibrous lining on its anterior surface, passes transversely behind the atlantoaxial joint enclosing a space below the posterior arch of C1 which contains the C2 nerve and ganglion surrounded by a plexus of thin-walled veins. These lie medial to the vertebral artery, which is loosely attached to the lateral capsule of the joint, in its tortuous, obliquely vertical course toward the more laterally placed foramina transversaria of C1.

Muscle insertions converge on the tip of the prominent spine of C2. The facets for C2–C3, on the lower aspect of the C2 laminae, are on a more posterior plane than those of the C1–C2 joints, making the C2–C3 joints readily palpable. Injuries of the C1–C2 joint can produce chronic occipital pain and C2 pattern headaches. Diagnostic injections of the C1–C2 joint or root sleeve injections of the C2 nerve can help to confirm the diagnosis of C2 pattern pain.

Lower Cervical Mobile Segments

Uncinate Processes and Intervertebral Discs

The cervical discs do not extend the whole width of the vertebral bodies. Uncinate processes grow upward from the lateral margins of each cervical vertebra in childhood. Uncovertebral clefts, or "lateral interbody joints," are formed during early adolescence. From these lateral clefts, transverse fissures progress medially through the posterior annulus and nucleus of young adults, so that by the age of 30 years there are fine, transverse fissures across the posterior half of each cervical intervertebral disc, from one uncovertebral joint to the other. The cervical nucleus pulposus also differs from the lumbar nucleus in other respects; cervical discs have relatively little gelatinous nuclear material to begin with,[19] and the nuclear material is more firmly bound by a plentiful collagen network. Fissuring in early to middle adult life soon destroys the cervical nucleus as a discrete encapsulated entity, in marked contrast to the adult lumbar spine. A cervical nucleus is therefore less likely to herniate than a lumbar nucleus, and cervical disc herniation is usually a consequence of severe trauma.

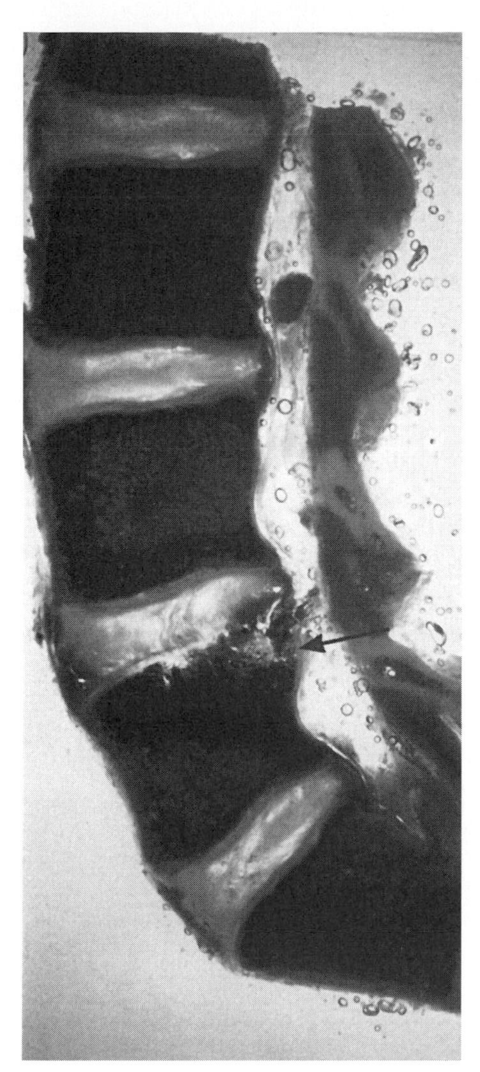

FIGURE 5–14 An unstained 2-mm sagittal section of the lumbar spine (L2 to sacrum) from a 19-year-old man who died after a traffic accident. Note the fracture of the upper posterior end plate of L5 with bleeding into the posterior annulus (arrow). There is also bleeding into the anterior annulus of L4-5 and, to a lesser degree, bleeding in the peripheral annuli of the other lumbar discs. (Also in color; see Color Plates.)

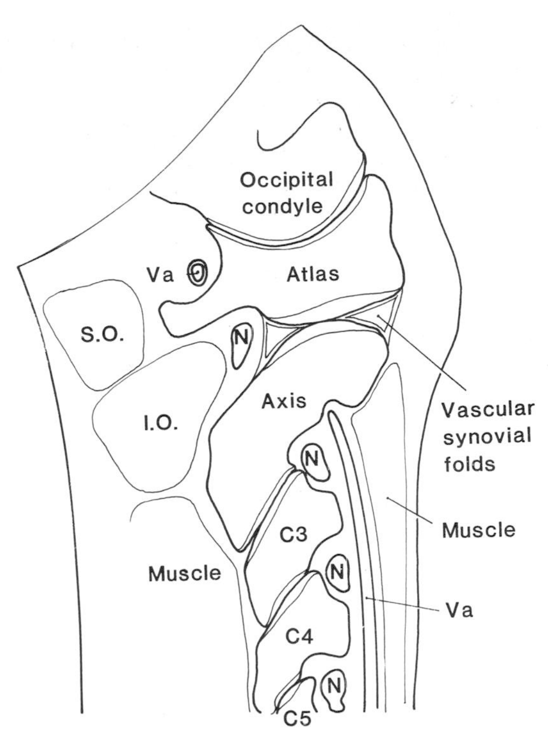

FIGURE 5–15 Tracing of a sagittal section in the plane of the facet joints: Va, vertebral artery; S.O., superior oblique muscle; I.O., inferior oblique muscle; N, dorsal root ganglion. Note the presence of vascular synovial folds which occupy the triangular gaps between the anterior and posterior parts of C1 and C2.

The cervical discs of young people—from adolescence to 25 years of age—resemble lumbar discs in most respects, except for the laterally placed uncovertebral clefts. After age 30, they have a fissure system running from one uncovertebral cleft to the other across the posterior half of the disc (Fig. 5–16), midway between the adjacent vertebral end plates so that the anterior annulus and the longitudinal ligaments are the only intact parts of middle-aged and elderly cervical discs.[10, 20] These changes would appear to be the price paid for the required range of cervical mobility. They occur so early that they may be regarded as "normal" rather than degenerative changes, but they predispose cervical discs to early degeneration. With age, the fissures become more obvious, and the posterior disc appears in sections as a bipartite structure (see Fig. 5–16), so that the cervical spine is heavily dependent, for stability in flexion, on the integrity of the facet joints, posterior muscles, and ligaments. The posterior muscles show much greater bulk than the small straplike anterior muscles of the cervical spine, making it more vulnerable to extension injury. In extension, the anterior annulus and the anterior longitudinal ligament, with the straplike longus colli and longus capitis muscles, bear the distraction strain.

Cervical Facet Joints

By their structure and orientation, the articular facets determine the directions of intervertebral movements. Their

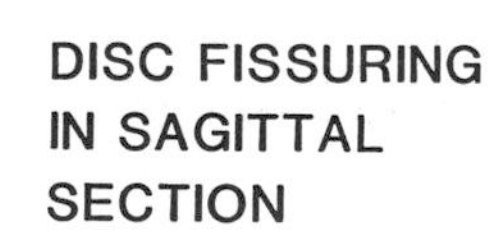

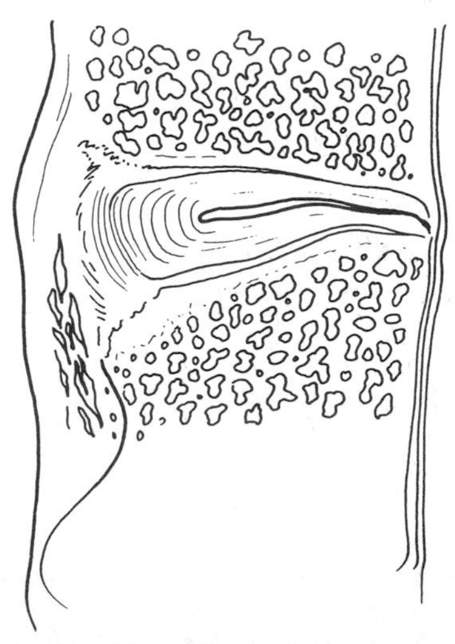

FIGURE 5–16 Diagram of midline sagittal section of a typical cervical disc in an elderly person. Note the transverse fissure through the posterior half of the disc. Only the anterior annulus and the longitudinal ligaments are intact.

articular surfaces are oriented at 45 degrees to the long axis of the spine, with a range of 30 to 60 degrees.[16] The cranial facets are directed upward and backward, and the caudal facets, downward and forward. This arrangement facilitates sagittal plane movements and requires that axial rotation and lateral bending are always coupled, whereas translation or horizontal gliding accompanies all other movements. The ligamentum flavum does not extend right across the anterior aspect of the cervical facet joints as it does in the lumbar spine. Also, the fibrous capsule is incomplete, thick, and lax laterally but virtually absent anteromedially and posteriorly. Anteromedially, each joint is isolated from the fat of the intervertebral foramen only by a plug of fat-filled synovium; the posteromedial capsule is a thin synovial fold associated with the small vascular fat pad of the inferior joint recess. This recess is enclosed by the oblique downward insertion of the multifidus muscle on the articular pillar below (see Fig. 5–23). A vascular synovial fold projects from the joint recess into the triangular space at the inferior joint margins. The lax joint capsule permits great mobility.[16, 21] In full flexion, there may only be 5 mm of facet contact remaining. Normal flexion radiographs show a "stepped" interbody arrangement because of the physiologic forward slide of each vertebra on the one below.

Spinal Cord and Cervical Spinal Nerves

The triangular cervical spinal canal is capacious, as can be seen in transverse section. It ranges from 13 to 22 mm in midsagittal diameter between C3 and C7 (mean 17 mm). The spinal cord normally occupies only 60% of this anteroposterior space.[16] In the extended position it narrows and in hyperextension, particularly with degenerative changes in the lower cervical region, disc-osteophytic bars and ligamentum flavum buckling may imperil the cord. The lateral recesses of the spinal canal are wider in the cervical spine than in the lumbar spine, so that nerve roots are less at risk in cervical lateral recesses than in lumbar ones. From C2 down, cervical nerve roots are at greater risk from osteophytes in the intervertebral canals.

On the posterior arch of C1, the small first cervical nerve passes out between the vertebral artery and the arch on each side under cover of the posterior atlantooccipital membrane. The dorsal ramus of C1 supplies the suboccipital muscles; the proprioceptive innervation of these small muscles makes them important in cervicocapital postural control. One of these small muscles is partly inserted into the posterior cervical dura to maintain its smooth outline during cervical extension.[22]

The roots of the second cervical nerve leave the spinal canal close to the medial capsule of C1–C2. They join as the spinal nerve passes transversely behind the joint, where the large dorsal root ganglion dwarfs the small anterior root. The large dorsal ramus forms the greater occipital nerve, which hooks under the inferior oblique muscle of the head to ascend through semispinalis capitis muscle into the posterior scalp.

The cervical spinal nerves pass through the lower parts of the intervertebral foramina, on the gutter-shaped transverse processes just below the levels of the facet joints and uncovertebral joints. To reach the intervertebral foramina, the cervical nerves pass obliquely forward and laterally from the spinal cord, so that in either extension or side-bending they are likely to be stretched. In the intervertebral foramina, they pass behind the vertebral arteries in grooves on the anterior surfaces of the articular pillars. The dorsal root ganglia of C5 through T1 are very large. They lie on the medial parts of the transverse process gutters, with the small anterior roots anteroinferior to them. The anatomic relationships of the cervical nerve roots in the intervertebral canal are different from those of the lumbar roots. Lumbar roots are well above the level of both the disc and the superior articular facets (see Fig. 5–6), except in advanced degenerative disease, but cervical roots pass through the canal at about the same horizontal level as the disc and facet joint line (Fig. 5–17A). They are therefore liable to be squeezed either in pincer fashion between the facet and uncovertebral osteophytes or compressed downward by the encroaching osteophytes into the lower part of the intervertebral canal (Fig. 5–17B).

Laterally directed osteophytes from the uncus also encroach on the course of the vertebral arteries, so that these normally straight vessels become tortuous with turbulent flow. These tortuous vessels are often thin-walled and affected by atheroma, making forceful cervical manipulation in elderly subjects potentially hazardous.

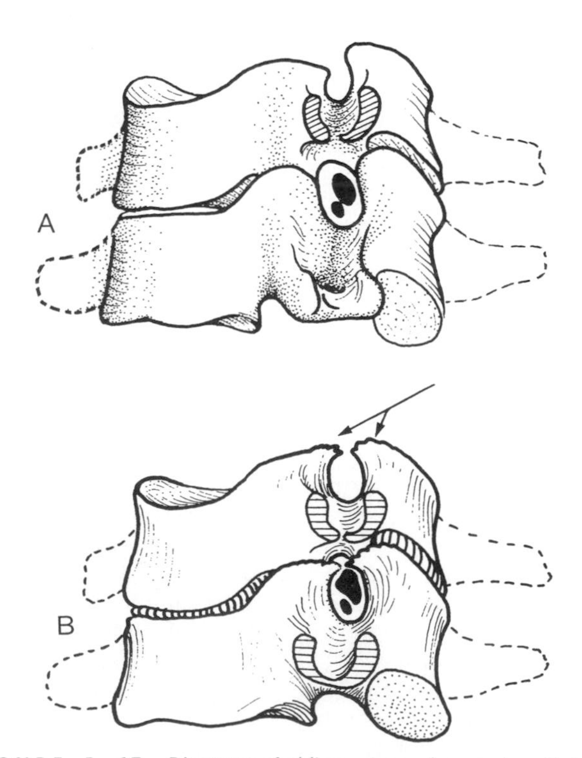

FIGURE 5–17 *Diagrams of oblique views of cervical motion segments.* A, *A young spine with a normal intervertebral foramen. Note the position of the larger dorsal root and the smaller ventral root in the medial part of the foramen.* B, *The influence of uncovertebral and facet osteophytes* (arrows) *reduces the space for the nerve roots and encloses them in the lower part of the medial foramen. (From Taylor JR, Twomey L: Functional and applied anatomy of the cervical spine.* In *Grant R [ed]: Physical Therapy of the Cervical and Thoracic Spine. New York, Churchill Livingstone, 1994.)*

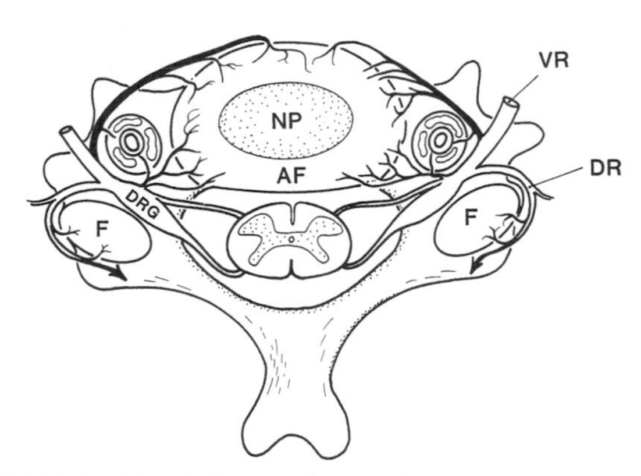

FIGURE 5–18 A diagram showing the innervation of the cervical disc and facet joints (F). The medial branch of the dorsal ramus (DR) supplies the facet joint shown and the next caudal joint. The outer annulus fibrosus (AF) is innervated, but the nucleus pulposus (NP) contains no nerves. VR, ventral ramus; DRG, dorsal root ganglion.

Innervation of the Cervical Motion Segment

The Intervertebral Disc

The longitudinal ligaments and the annulus of cervical intervertebral discs are innervated from the ventral rami, sinuvertebral nerves, and vertebral nerves (around the vertebral arteries). According to Bogduk,[23] only the outer annulus is innervated; however, Mendel and coworkers[24] claim to have demonstrated nerves through the whole thickness of the annulus (Fig. 5–18). Nerves are not found in the cartilage plates of adults or in the nucleus pulposus at any age.

The Facet Joints

The medial branch of each dorsal ramus contributes to the innervation of two facet joints.[25, 26] The medial branches of the C4 through C8 dorsal rami curve dorsally around the waists of the articular pillars. C3 (lesser occipital nerve) passes backward at a higher level in relation to C2–C3. There are often two parallel medial branches on each articular pillar. They supply articular branches to the zygapophyseal joint capsules above and below and innervate the corresponding segments of multifidus and semispinalis. The fibrous capsule and joint recesses are innervated, but the ligamentum flavum does not appear to have any nociceptive nerves.[24–27] The synovial folds projecting into the joints are probably innervated. Innervation has been demonstrated in these structures in the lumbar spine.[6]

Pain may arise from injury to any innervated part of the motion segment. It may also arise from injury to the nerves or dorsal root ganglia.[28, 29] For example, the dorsal rami of C2 and C3, which form the greater occipital nerve and the third occipital nerve, can be affected by injury. They supply skin of the medial upper neck and the occipital scalp as far as the vertex. They also supply rostral segments of postvertebral muscles and the posterior capsules of the lateral atlantoaxial joints, the C2–C3 and C3–C4 facet joints.

Degenerative Pathology of Cervical Discs

Lower cervical discs often thin with aging. When this happens the uncinate processes, compressed against the vertebral body above, are directed laterally, forming uncovertebral osteophytes which encroach on the intervertebral foramina. Facet osteophytes may also encroach on the intervertebral foramina, and together they "imprison" the cervical nerve roots in the lower part of the foramen (Figs. 5–17B, 5–19). These osteophytes, plus posterior bars

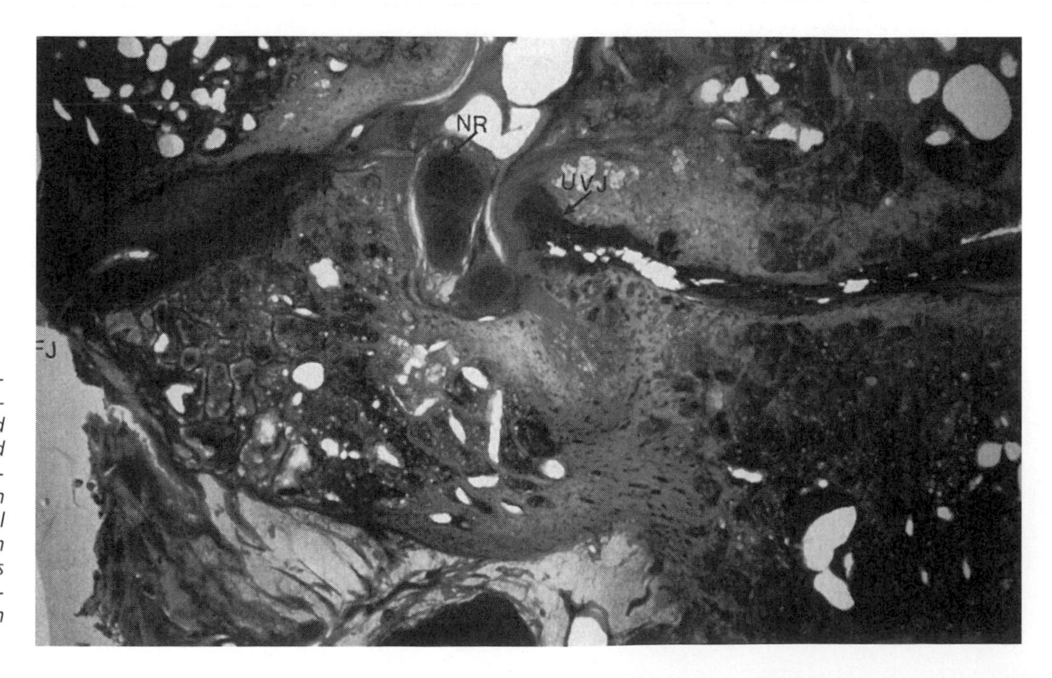

FIGURE 5–19 A 100-μm coronal section of a C6-7 motion segment, stained by hematoxylin and light green, from a 78-year-old woman, shows narrowing of the intervertebral foramen by disc resorption with laterally bulging uncovertebral osteophytes. There is an increase in the fibrous (green-stained) elements of the nerve roots (NR). UVJ, uncovertebral joint; FJ, facet joint. (Also in color; see Color Plates.)

formed by disc bulges with marginal osteophytic ridges, may impinge on the cervical nerve roots, the vertebral arteries, or the spinal cord. The extensive fissuring changes in the aging cervical disc may form a bipartite disc with a gliding joint in its posterior half. In lower cervical discs, especially C5–C6 and C6–C7, disc thinning or resorption often occurs in middle life (Fig. 5–19). This may progress in old age to spontaneous interbody fusion. Foraminal disc prolapse is rare, but disc degeneration in middle age and old age results in posterior bulging of the whole width of the disc into the spinal canal, forming a transverse "bar" or ridge. This bar extends from the uncovertebral osteophytes on one side to the contralateral uncovertebral osteophytes. These bars, especially at C5–C6 and C6–C7, may indent the spinal cord.

Cervical Injuries

Autopsy studies of 266 cervical spines, including 162 spines from two series of patients who died of nonpenetrating injuries (usually as a result of brain damage or bleeding from chest injuries), reveal that the vast majority of injuries are to the nonosseous tissues of the intervertebral discs and facets.[15, 28–32] As a rule, death was due to head or chest injuries, most often from motor vehicle accidents; almost all of the spines, even when well-aligned or normal on post-mortem radiographs, showed injuries. Often these were minor, multilevel injuries, especially when the injury was due to cervical extension or compression-extension from head impact.

Soft tissue injuries are common in the upper cervical spine.[15, 29] The soft tissues of the C1–C2 lateral joints are frequently injured with bruising of the triangular synovial folds and hematoma formation behind the joints around the C2 DRG from tearing of the vascular synovial fold or damage to the thin-walled veins which surround the nerve (Fig. 5–20). Injuries to the C2 DRG itself are sometimes observed (Fig. 5–21).

Disc injuries varied from small transverse, linear, annular tears parallel to the vertebral rim (rim lesions) to almost complete disc avulsions at the disc-vertebral junction or traumatic disc herniations into the spinal canal (Figs. 5–22, 5–23A). The majority of disc injuries were not accompanied by tears of the longitudinal ligaments, and when tears to these ligaments occurred, they were usually incomplete. Some lateral disc injuries were accompanied by small fractures of an uncinate process.

Zygapophyseal facet injuries varied from bruises to the intraarticular synovial folds with hemarthrosis (Fig. 5–23B), to articular cartilage injuries, sometimes with small fractures of the subchondral bone plate. We also observed fractures to the tips of facets, which were forced against adjacent bone in hyperextension or compression extension injuries (Fig. 5–24).

An injury observed commonly was hemorrhage into a DRG (see Fig. 5–21). The DRG is very vascular with many thin-walled veins. This injury was observed in about a third of cervical spines from those who survived from 2 hours to 2 weeks after the injury, since that afforded time for hemorrhage into the injured ganglion, drawing attention to the injury. It was rarely observed in spines after sudden roadside deaths in motor vehicle accidents. This injury was not associated as a rule with the most severe types of trauma, and the spines were generally well-aligned with relatively mild osteoligamentous injuries. In a substantial minority of the injured DRG, histologic examination showed axonal disruption in addition to hemorrhage.[32]

Vertebral artery injuries are relatively rare, even with subluxations (Fig. 5–25). The vertebral arteries are resistant to injury, except where they pierce the dura within the foramen magnum. We have observed injuries to the vertebral artery in only 5% of cases, excluding those very severe injuries with complete dislocation.[29] The arterial injuries involved dissection of the intima with ante-mortem thrombus formation.

A comparison of the appearances on post-mortem radiographs with the appearances of the sagittally sectioned

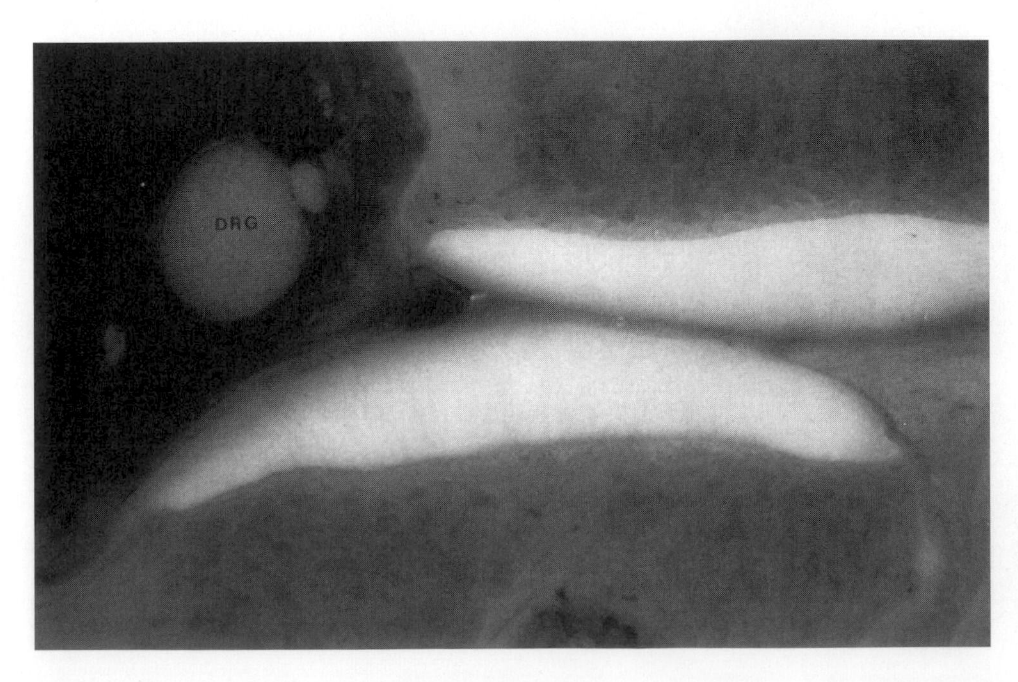

FIGURE 5–20 A 2-mm, unstained sagittal section of an injured lateral atlantoaxial joint from a 13-year-old boy shows a large hematoma behind the joint (left) and in the posterior synovial fold of the joint. The dorsal root ganglion (DRG) is surrounded by the hematoma. (Also in color; see Color Plates.)

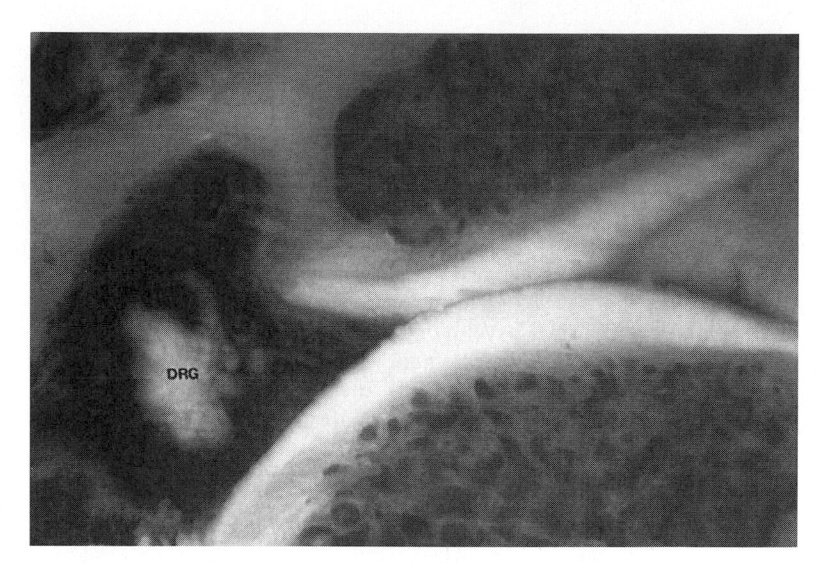

FIGURE 5–21 *A 2-mm unstained sagittal section of an atlantoaxial joint shows punctate bruising behind the joint and a bruise within the C2 dorsal root ganglion (*DRG*).*

spines shows that there is no way of suspecting the nonosseous injuries, unless gross damage to the longitudinal ligaments produces dislocation or gross widening of the disc space. The majority of the injured spines were well aligned, and the disc injuries were found only on sectioning. In addition, few of the facet fractures and none of the hemarthroses and articular cartilage injuries were visible on plain films.

In the context of pain, in survivors of similar neck injuries, it should be noted that the part of the annulus most commonly torn is well innervated, that the facet joint capsules and synovia are also innervated, and that nerve injuries can give rise to chronic intractable pain syndromes. Facet injuries have been shown to cause chronic pain after whiplash,[33] and the facet injuries we observed with articular cartilage damage would be slow to heal and likely to predispose to accelerated arthritic changes.

Thoracic Injuries

A recent unpublished study of 45 spines where cervical and upper thoracic (T1–T6) injuries could be compared showed similar incidences of facet injuries in the upper thoracic spine and the cervical spine. By contrast, in the anterior elements, vertebral end plate fracture and bone bruising were more common in the thoracic spine, whereas disc injuries predominated in the cervical spine. This raises the question whether interscapular pain is referred from the neck or arises locally. Investigations of pathology, to be correlated with the effect of local anaesthetic blocks, should enable the clinician to distinguish the true pain source.

Selective Diagnostic Injections of the Spinal Axis

Many patients are referred to our chronic pain facility without a clear diagnosis of spinal pain. In fact, previous literature would suggest that in as much as 90% of low back pain, its source and pathologic mechanism are not known[34–36] or that a suspected mechanism is not the established cause of pain.[37] One could conclude that 90% of low back pain is nonspecific, and even that it is undiagnosable.

There is also a considerable body of literature on the poor correlation between pathology and symptoms and signs of spinal pain.[34, 38–40] This has led to dissatisfaction, on the part of our patients, with their doctors,[41, 42] a perception that is compounded by much previous failed treatment. Moreover, according to Waddell,[38] advances in technology do not result in more accurate diagnoses. Spinal pain continues to defy useful classification, and it remains a symptom. The Quebec Task Force, in an attempt at classification into 11 categories, does not include such common entities as these:

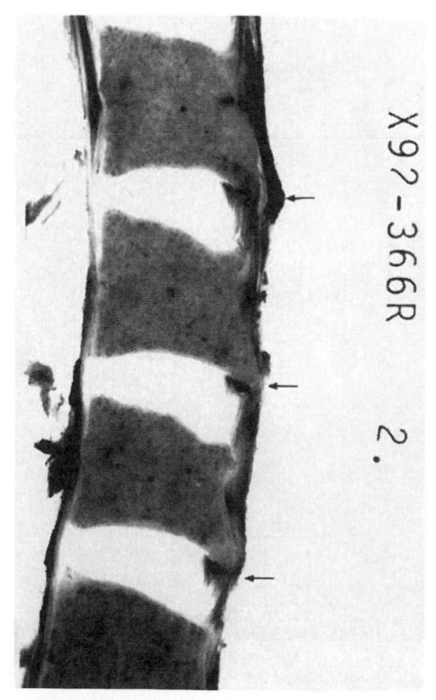

FIGURE 5–22 *A 2-mm unstained sagittal section (C3-6) of spine from the victim of a fatal motor vehicle accident shows an anterior annular tear (rim lesion) in each disc (*arrows*) with bleeding between the lamellae of the anterior annuli fibrosi.*

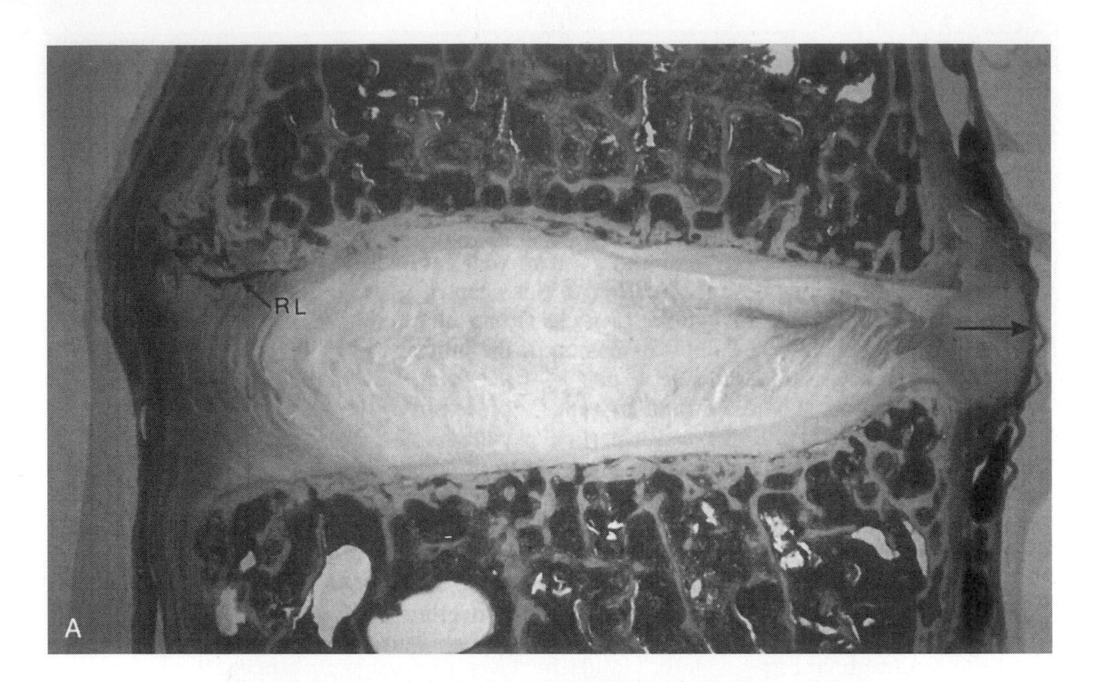

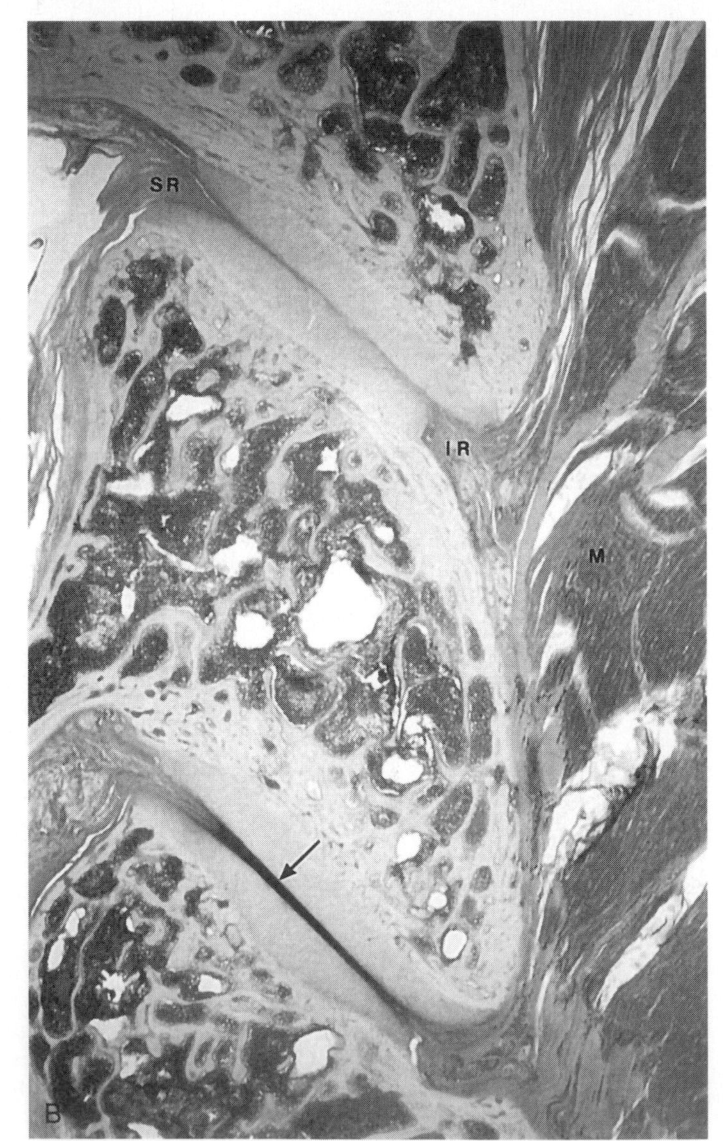

FIGURE 5–23 A, *This 100-μm section of the C6-7 disc from a 32-year-old man killed in a traffic accident shows an anterior rim lesion (*RL *and* arrow*) and a posterior traumatic disc herniation (*large arrow*) contained by a stretched but intact posterior longitudinal ligament.* B, *A 100-μm sagittal section of two facet joints from the same accident victim shows a normal joint above, with vascular synovial folds projecting into the superior recess (*SR*) and inferior recess (*IR*), which is enclosed by the multifidus muscle (*M*). The lower joint shows a traumatic hemarthrosis. (Also in color; see Color Plates.)*

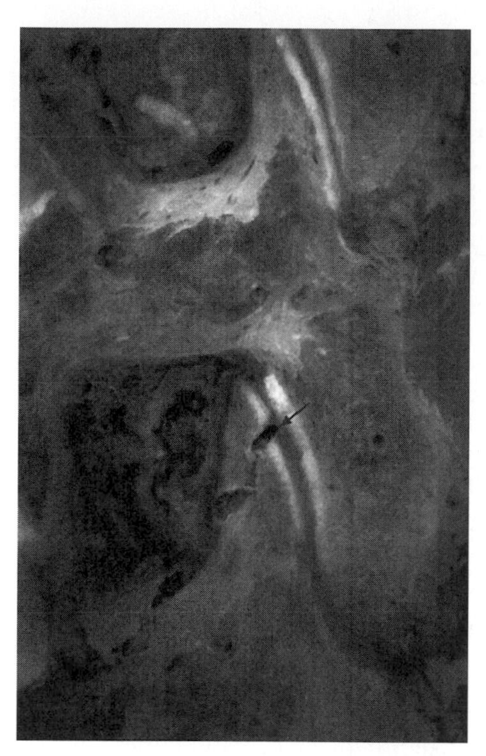

FIGURE 5–24 A 2-mm unstained sagittal section of two lower cervical facet joints from a 16-year-old youth killed by a blow behind the vertex of the skull from a baseball bat. The axial compression injury has fractured the tip of the upper facet of T1 (arrow) *and the pedicle. (Also in color; see Color Plates.)*

- Discogenic pain from internal disruption
- Zygapophyseal (facet) joint pain
- Lumbar instability pain
- Sacroiliac joint pain

Nevertheless patients with these complaints crowd our offices and daily challenge our diagnostic skills. With many of them, a segmental diagnosis can be reached using a rational approach and validated investigational tools. Rather than being defeatist, we should espouse the Hippocratic ideal of basing treatment on observation, reasoning, and experience.[43] In fact, an accurate diagnosis is a prerequisite for all good scientific management. The medical model of pain causation should apply just as much in the spine in the search for a pathologic mechanism.

Some observers of spinal pain suggest that psychosocial issues or central pain may be the reasons for the chronicity of the pain syndrome. Despite the trend away from attributing chronic pain to local nociception in a damaged spinal structure, recent research has provided evidence that a nociceptive pain source can regularly be identified in chronic spinal pain syndromes and that successful treatment of pain can cause abnormal psychological profiles to revert to normal.[44, 45] I would argue against the current trend of decrying anatomically based diagnoses and suggest that we move toward more accurate clinical assessment, including the use of selective nerve blocks in combination with advanced imaging.

The inclusion of large numbers of subjects with mild and transient pain episodes, together with the more persistent and severe pain syndromes in prevalence studies of back pain, may account for the relative rarity of accurate diagnoses. The subjects with mild short-term back pain who are not investigated are described as having *nonspecific back pain*, but it is the patients with the more severe back pain that often persists longer than 6 months who visit our pain facilities and need that accurate diagnosis. The road to such a logical diagnosis can be long and rocky. It can be restricted first by the reluctance of the patient and the physician to perform multiple, often invasive investigations, second by the skills required of the investigating physician, and last by the financial constraints present in every society. Failure to arrive at an accurate diagnosis may, however, prove even more costly to both the patient and the community over the longer term.

The current understanding of central pain owes much to the work of Melzack and Wall.[46] However, if the gate control theory is used to argue that peripheral nociception is no longer important and the further pursuit of an accurate diagnosis of a pain source is a waste of time, that approach could prevent application of treatment that could resolve the patient's pain and its behavioral sequelae.[45]

It has become common among clinicians who see patients with chronic spinal pain with depressive or other behavioral features to attribute the chronic nature of the pain to psychosocial factors and to neglect persistent physical signs of nociception. A large proportion of patients with any form of chronic pain develop secondary depressive features, which often become more intrusive and disruptive of the patient's life than the original problem. The work of Bogduk, Schwarzer and their colleagues[44] and of Jull and coworkers[47] has shown that, with chronic whiplash pain or chronic low back pain, a pain source can still be

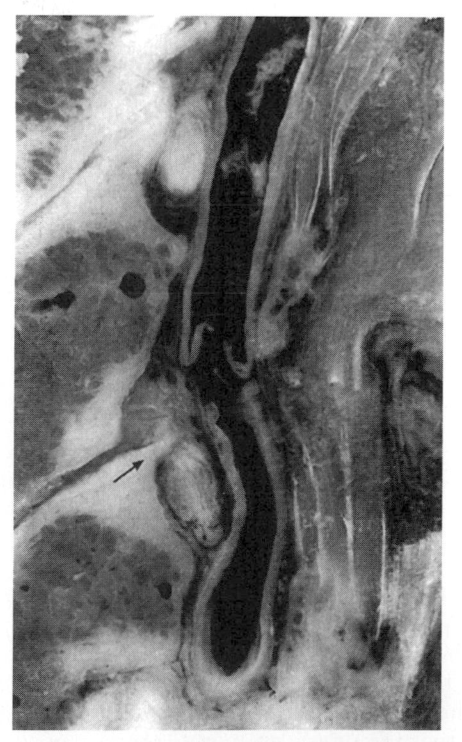

FIGURE 5–25 An osteophyte (arrow), *the result of traumatic subluxation, has injured the vertebral artery of an elderly man. Note the upward displacement of two intimal flaps, dissected by the trauma, with ante-mortem thrombus in the artery.*

identified and treated successfully and that the secondary behavioral features spontaneously disappear.[45]

For many reasons, a precise anatomic diagnosis is an immense boon to both the patient and the physician (and even their attorneys). One can, therefore, argue for further refinement of imaging techniques and use of double- or triple-block paradigms to work logically toward a diagnosis. It is this diagnosis that serves as the basis of the patient's future management and rehabilitation.

Reaching this segmental diagnosis involves piecing together a number of clues from the history, the physical examination, and various earlier investigations. To this sequence can be added the utility of precision local anesthetic nerve blocks. Abnormal radiologic findings, on the other hand, can be a trap for the unwary. Currently, the only way to test whether a morphologic abnormality is causing the pain is to place local anesthetic around or into the structure or onto its sensory nerve supply, a process that must be conducted in a logical and sequential fashion. Alternatively, a structure that has no visible abnormality, by even the most sophisticated imaging, may yet, unquestionably, be the source of pain. For example, some spinal injuries incurred in fatal traffic accidents and demonstrated by post-mortem sagittal section are not visible on radiologic examination.[30]

The spine is especially well suited for investigation by diagnostic nerve blocks. The origin of the pain in a particular spinal segment and the anatomic structure involved can often be determined by precision blocks with local anesthetic agents.[48] Usually, the preceding history and examination have provided some indication as to the structure involved, which allows the physician to make a working diagnosis. This diagnosis can then be confirmed or ruled out by of the results of precise local anesthetic blocks. Much more information can be gained if the same clinician is involved in all steps to diagnosis, from clinical examination to postblockade assessment. Surely, it is just as valid to strive for anatomic precision in the spine as it is in other organ systems? The commonly advanced argument that most spinal pain syndromes cannot be accurately diagnosed is no longer tenable, with the advent of better anatomic knowledge and the development of precision local anesthetic blocks.

Clinical History

It cannot be overemphasized how important the history is to reaching a diagnosis in the patient with chronic pain. The examiner cannot gain more than a preliminary understanding in less than 1 hour, and if the history-taking is hurried, the historian may fail to appreciate the pain problem.

How the patient presents the history provides other clues. Even though the patient might be accompanied by many relatives and proffer a folder of reports whose thickness can be measured in inches, the pain problem must be approached in the same sequential manner. In fact, being mindful that the physician might someday need to defend the chosen approach to diagnosis in court does wonders for logical thinking and record keeping. Sometimes the history is given in a simple, unembellished fashion, with a time course for events and accompanying symptoms, such as recent weight loss, that sets alarm bells ringing. When patients are asked to fill in questionnaires—and, in particular, pain diagrams—even the quickest glance gives a measure of the patient's psychological distress and the somatic nature of the complaint (Fig. 5–26). The family and work histories are just as important. The family unit may have disintegrated after endless rounds of pain, depression, and argument, which also confound the diagnostic process.

Often, chronic pain is the end result of the effects of injury or of degeneration on the workings of the spinal motion segment. The long-term history, with episodic exacerbations of low back pain, might suggest the progressive effects of degenerative changes on spinal mechanics. The patient may, over many years and in successive jobs, have experienced increasing spinal difficulties that culminated in an injury at work. This sequence of events might suggest a progressively incompetent spinal motion segment that eventually fails and develops pain. With posttraumatic pain, the mechanism of injury can assist in reaching a working diagnosis. If a lifting and rotating motion is accompanied by a sharp tearing sensation in the low back, an intervertebral disc may be disrupted. The referred symptoms can appear later. Rear-end motor vehicle collisions are particularly prone to producing certain injuries. The sudden collapse of the seatback might lead to injuries of the lumbar facet joints.[49] An unexpected "rear-ender" may well cause the cervical spine lesions described earlier in this chapter.

The current symptoms, of course, provide strong clues, but they are not conclusive. Pain on extension of the lumbar spine does not necessarily indicate a painful facet joint.[50] Very close attention should be paid to reports of sensory changes in the limbs. Paresthesias in particular patterns of segmental innervation can reveal the relevant spinal level. Global sensory changes are not necessarily an expression of a "functional disorder," but they may well have a physiologic explanation in a disturbance of autonomic function. The pattern of pain in the head and neck may implicate a particular spinal segment, but, owing to overlapping innervation by the sinuvertebral nerve, several spinal segments may be supplied by the same sensory nerve. Convergence

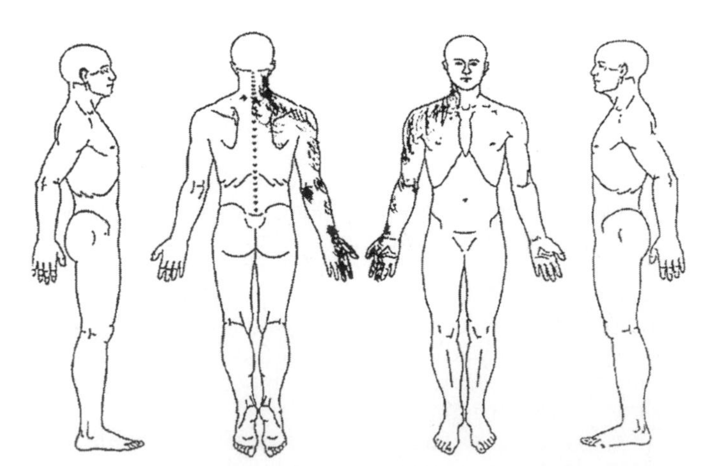

FIGURE 5–26 Markings on this somatic pain diagram were supplied by the patient to represent pain. The diagram suggests involvement of the C6 nerve root. (Also in color; see Color Plates.)

phenomena in the trigeminal nucleus may explain the mix of facial pain, headache, and cervical symptoms.[51] Also, the longer trunk muscles have multisegmental innervation (C5–T1). These muscles may generate patterns of referred pain similar to those of the underlying spinal joints. Similar patterns of pain referral from different cervical structures produce tenderness around the superior margin of the trapezius (Fig. 5–27).[52–54]

A history of injury or similar complaints can call attention to a particular spinal structure. For example, after spinal instrumentation the emergence of typical neuropathic burning limb pain with sensory changes could suggest a compromised nerve root. Similarly, the recurrence of referred pain that was previously treated by decompression of a particular nerve root foramen might trigger a critical examination of the same spinal segment.

Previous imaging results must be meticulously reviewed. Often, they are presented at the first interview, in a shopping bag containing a jumbled mess of radiographs, CT and MRI images, and scintigraphic scans. The relevant typed reports are often missing, having been removed by other physicians or otherwise lost in the mists of time. Despite the effort involved, these imaging results must be rearranged in chronologic order, with their reports. With a facsimile machine or online medical imaging, old reports and even images can be regenerated and transmitted in time for the first examination. This precious history often yields information previous observers overlooked. One should look carefully at the extension radiographs taken after a rear-end motor vehicle collision. They are frequently reported as demonstrating no evidence of injury but occasionally, lucent (vacuum) clefts can be seen adjacent to the disc–end plate margin. These clefts are seen only with the cervical spine in extension and probably represent gas in a region of the disc that has torn away from the vertebral end plate.[55] Most likely, they are the same lesion as the rim lesion seen on the post-mortem sagittal sections. These small lucent clefts with smooth outlines adjacent to the end plate should be distinguished from the vacuum phenomenon associated with disc degeneration, which has ragged borders, often extends into the degenerated disc, and is not confined to the region adjacent to the end plate (Fig. 5–28).

Physical Examination

The physical examination must be no less detailed. It commences when the questionnaire and pain diagram are handed out in the waiting room.

As the patient rises and walks across the waiting room, the examiner can observe gait and general demeanor. If the pace is slow, there may be a physical explanation, such as a demyelinating disorder; alternatively, the patient might be demonstrating an extreme form of pain behavior. Such indirect examination provides a wealth of information for the student of gait and stance. Dorsolumbar shifts and tilts can be picked up as the patient undresses. Lumbar scoliosis, visible on general physical examination, can subsequently be examined under image intensifier. The commencement of tilt at a particular spinal level reinforces the diagnosis of injury to that segment.

Spinal tenderness is often said to be totally subjective and of little help in achieving the working diagnosis. The attorney who confidently makes this assertion has not had the opportunity to gently palpate tender facet joints or sensitized nerve roots and to detect the subtle rise in protective muscle tone. Jull and associates[47] have shown that a skilled manipulative therapist can identify a symptomatic motion segment as effectively as can pain provocation and elimination techniques. Many physicians are unaware that the lumbar spine can be palpated per abdomen to detect a sensitized anterior annulus. Similar anterolateral tenderness detected in the cervical spine provides further segmental clues. Widespread areas of secondary hyperalgesia, however, can confound interpretation of spinal tenderness.[56] This referred hyperalgesia may well have its origin in disordered central neural mechanisms, but it is expressed in widespread muscle tenderness.

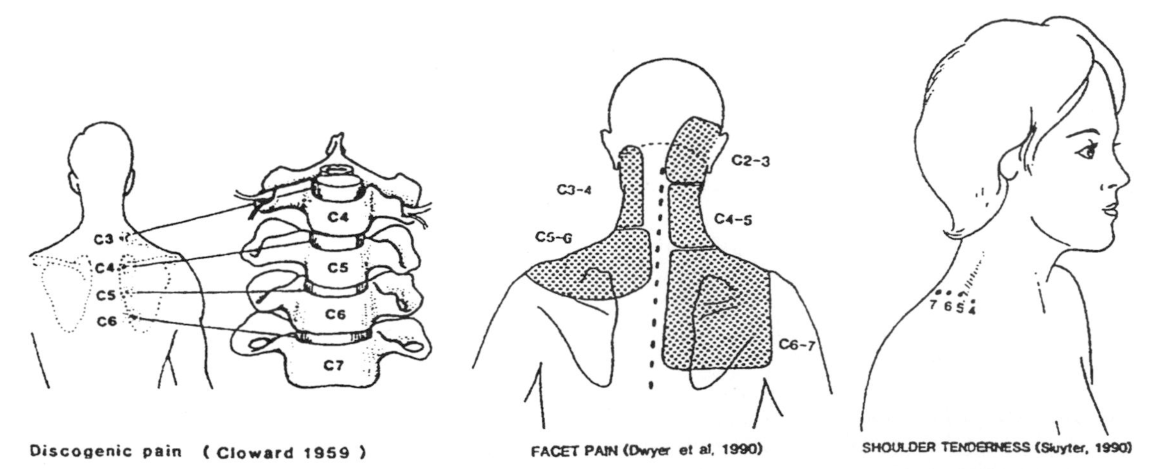

FIGURE 5–27 Similar patterns of pain referral from different cervical structures giving tenderness around the superior margin of the trapezius. (Modified and redrawn from Cloward RB: Ann Surg 150:1052, 1959(52); Dwyer A, et al: Spine 15:453, 1990(53); Sluyter ME: Procedure Technique Series 19, Radionics, 1989(54).)

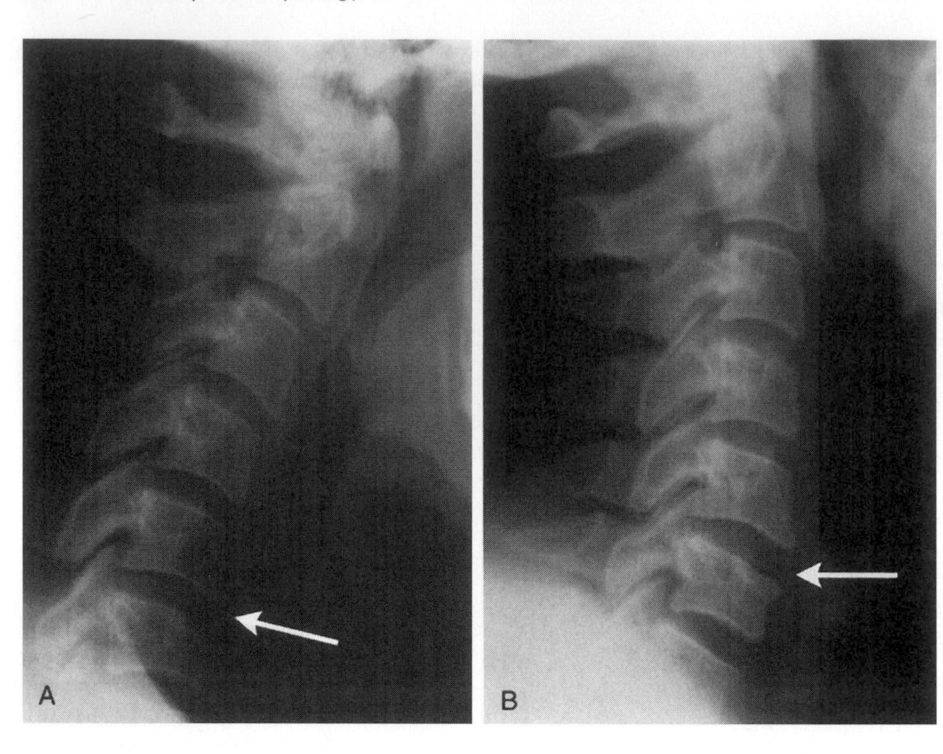

FIGURE 5–28 A, *Flexion radiograph of the cervical spine. Note that the C5-6 disc appears to be normal* (arrow). B, *Extension radiograph of the same patient's cervical spine. Note that a small lucency can be seen adjacent to the superior end plate of C6* (arrow). *This lucency represents a cleft of the C5-6 disc.*

Dural tension tests, such as the sciatic stretch test, have been described in the lower limbs.[56] Less well-known are the upper limb tests of dural irritation. Carefully performed, the brachial plexus tension test described by Elvey[57] can also provide segmental information. The patient may describe the onset of paresthesia in the upper limb at some point in this test. If the evoked paresthesia is confined to an area of particular segmental innervation, it is reasonable to direct attention to the segmental nerve supply, including the nerve root. Nerve roots can be irritated by a number of pathologic processes, including direct trauma and indirect mechanisms such as disc herniation.

Finally, the neurologic examination should include detailed reflex, motor, and sensory testing. The basis of many chronic pain syndromes is disordered neural function. The sensory testing should include more than a hasty "once-over with a blunt pin." Neuropathic pain states often feature disordered thermal sensation[58] and mechanical hyperalgesia. Perhaps it is stating the obvious to point out that the findings of such rigorous neuromuscular examinations must be recorded in detail.

Technique of Diagnostic Injection

For the purposes of nerve blocks, each spinal segment can be divided into its component disc, central neural elements, and posterior structures, such as the facet joints. The disc can be studied by using pain provocation or local anesthetic blocks. Morphologic information can be gained by placing radiopaque contrast material into the nucleus. The disc can be anesthetized by placing local anesthetic into the annulus. The individual nerve roots and facet joints can be studied in similar fashion. Ideally, the patient should be blind to the segment that is being examined, and several segments should be studied on separate occasions. Local anesthetic agents with different durations of action can be used sequentially on a given structure, to avoid the pitfall of false-positive results.[59] Blocks can produce false-negative results if the local anesthetic is inadvertently injected into a small blood vessel. This misadventure has been observed during medial branch blockade using technetium Tc-99m lidocaine, despite the use of an image intensifier and careful injection of the contrast medium (PM Finch, G Bower: Unpublished data, 1994). Multiple blocks of the same structure can greatly increase cost, so a more pragmatic approach could, perhaps, be considered.

Nerve blocks must be conducted with great accuracy and gentleness. If nerve roots are transfixed by spinal needles, the resulting neuritis can cause prolonged, and unnecessary, morbidity. The image intensifier is the basic tool for achieving this accuracy. The clinician who, by necessity, has a clear understanding of the spinal anatomy can adjust the C arm of the fluoroscope. It takes time to master the use of this machine, but, once such mastery is achieved, it is a simple task to make adjustments (whereas many words are required to explain a complex projection to a radiographer). The C arm can also be used in a general fashion to explore the spine. Subtle changes in structure become visible that are not readily apparent with static images. The C arm is adjusted around the patient so that the needle can pass down the x-ray beam and onto the structure that is about to be blocked. If the patient is moved to suit the x-ray beam, the position becomes unstable and can change for the worse during the procedure.

Directional steering of needles is greatly facilitated by deliberately placing a curve in the terminal half inch of the spinal needle. The convexity of the curve is on the same side as the cutting edge of the bevel. Directional changes on needle insertion can easily be achieved, not by repeated painful withdrawal and reinsertion but by frequent 180-degree rotations of the hub of the needle. A 25-gauge

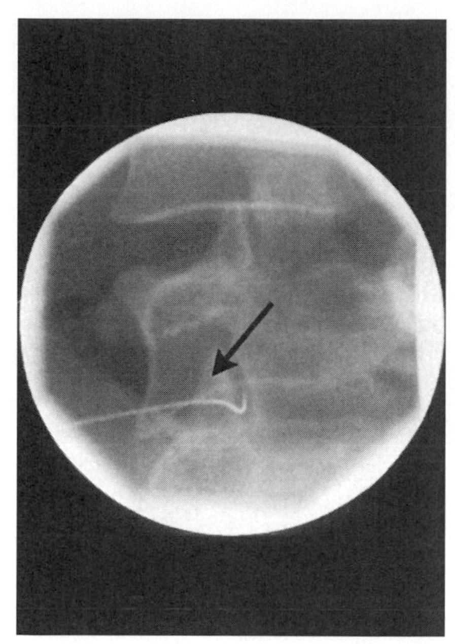

FIGURE 5–29 *A curved-needle approach to a lumbar facet joint* (arrow).

spinal needle can thus be accurately steered into narrow and relatively inaccessible parts of the spine. For example, access to the lumbosacral disc is often difficult, especially with the high pelvic brim of males or with extreme degenerative narrowing. Impaling the L5 nerve root becomes all too easy in this situation, but it can be avoided if a curvilinear path to the disc is taken and the needle tip is made to hug the outer aspect of the superior articular facet. Needles can literally be steered around corners, beneath bone graft, and past spinal fixation devices. Even greater directional changes can be achieved by using an introducing needle. A 23-gauge, 5-in discogram needle can easily be passed through a 19-gauge needle. This achieves directional control and reduces the risk of infection, because the spinal

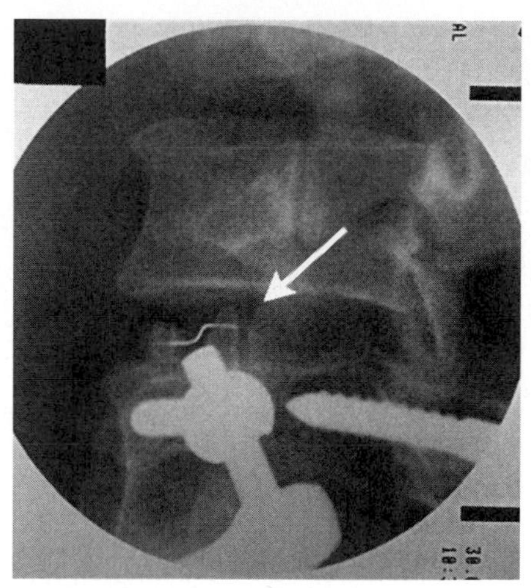

FIGURE 5–31 *A curved-needle approach to an intervertebral disc. This approach is used to avoid spinal instrumentation* (arrow).

needle does not contact the skin surface directly (Figs. 5–29 to 5–32).

The volume of local anesthetic agent injected into the spine partly dictates the extent of spread. To obtain precision, the spread must not be greater than the intended zone of influence. A fluid volume of 1.0 mL, injected slowly, does not usually spread outside any particular part of the spinal segment. The cervical disc is, perhaps, an exception, and, there, fluid volume should be restricted to 0.5 mL.[60] The approximate extent of spread can be gauged from the previously injected radiopaque contrast agent, but in some situations spread can be extensive.[61, 62] If steroid has been added to this injectate, the concentration of local anesthetic is reduced and may be inadequate to anesthetize the structure. Higher concentrations of local anesthetics must be chosen to avoid this possible cause of a false-negative result. The addition of steroid has, in any case, become somewhat traditional, but it may not much influence the outcome of spinal nerve blocks.[63, 64] Last, the extent of contrast spread

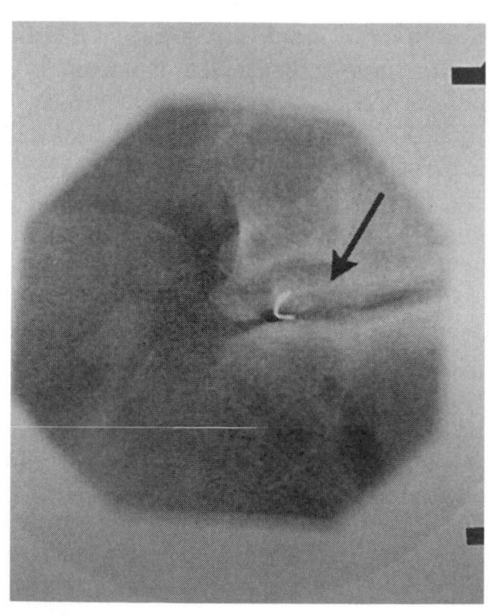

FIGURE 5–30 *A curved-needle approach to a narrowed degenerate L5-S1 disc* (arrow).

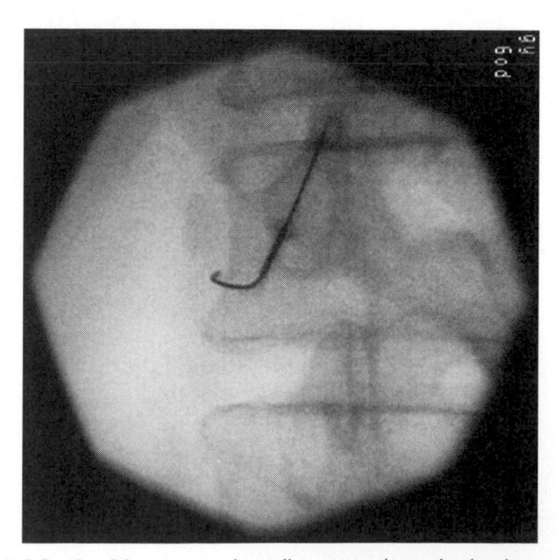

FIGURE 5–32 *A curved-needle approach to the lumbar sympathetic chain allows accurate steering around the body of a lumbar vertebra.*

must be recorded on film or computer disc for future reference and for medicolegal purposes.

Intervertebral Disc

Injection of local anesthetic agent into the cervical disc has been proposed as a sequel to the more classical pain-provoking injection of radiopaque contrast material. Roth[65] claims that this technique—cervical analgesic discography—can identify symptomatic spinal segments that might respond to surgical fusion.[60] Given the normal aging process in the cervical motion segment, it becomes apparent that transverse fissures form in the vicinity of the uncovertebral joints and, by the third or fourth decade of life, extend across to include the central regions of the disc. Therefore, a local anesthetic agent injected into a normal adult disc may find its way out of the confines of the disc. The investigator must be aware of the possibility of spread of local anesthetic substances to structures outside the segment being examined. Morphologic information can certainly be obtained by injecting radiopaque contrast material, and abnormalities, such as tears or herniations, are readily detected. Also, the pain provoked by injecting these materials may implicate a particular spinal segment. The spread of contrast material into the epidural space is of particular significance. If, subsequently, local anesthetic is injected into the same disc, it is likely to spread to other structures (Fig. 5–33).

A further difficulty in combining provocation and radiopaque contrast studies with analgesic discography is that only so much fluid can be injected into an intact cervical disc. If the disc accepts more than 0.5 mL of fluid at low injection pressure, it is possible that the injectate has spread outside the confines of the disc. At least 0.5 mL of local anesthetic agent must be injected to effectively block neural elements in the annulus. A combination of contrast agent and local anesthetic agent dilutes both, reducing their effectiveness. The resulting poor picture, the result of low contrast density and poor quality of block secondary to diluted local anesthetic, would have to be interpreted with caution. It is probably inadvisable to "overpressure" a cervical disc while striving to inject more than 0.5 mL of fluid. To inject contrast and local anesthetic agent on separate occasions might increase the risks of infection, and if local anesthetic alone were injected, spread of agent outside the disc could go undetected. It is for these reasons that results of injection of local anesthetic into cervical discs may not be as informative as provocation and contrast studies.

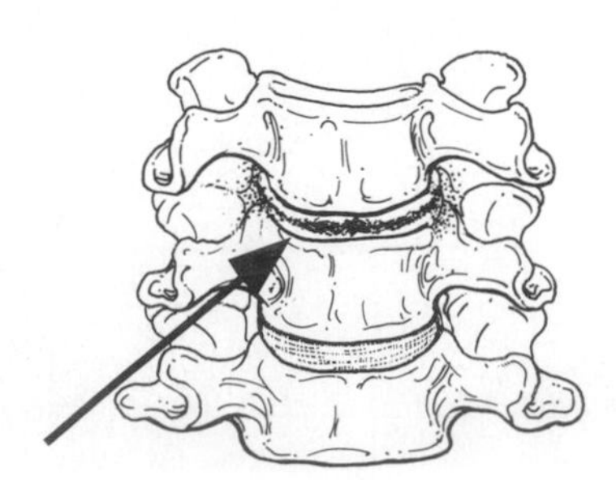

FIGURE 5–33 *An artist's drawing of the spread of contrast material within a normal cervical disc space* (arrow).

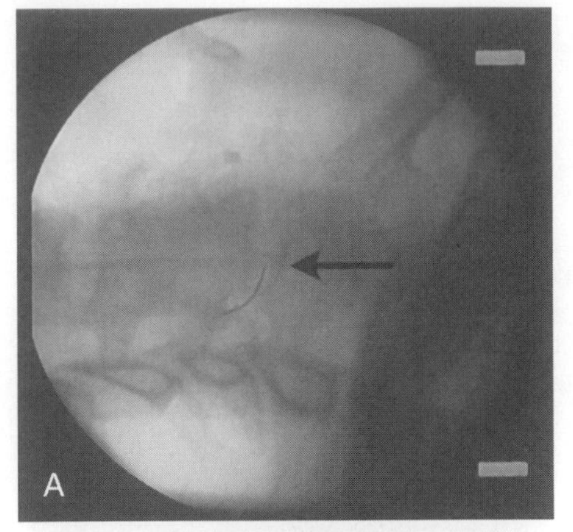

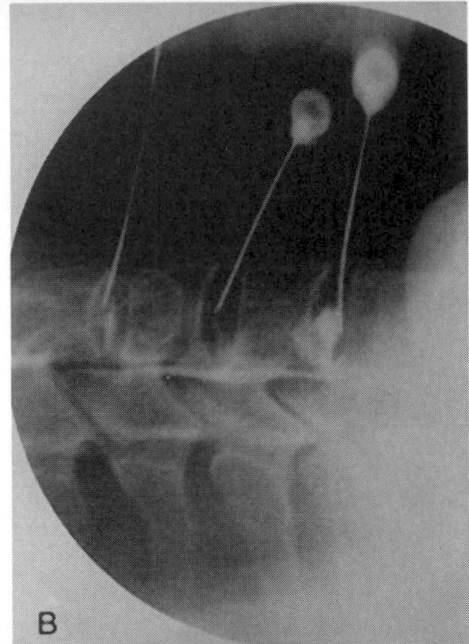

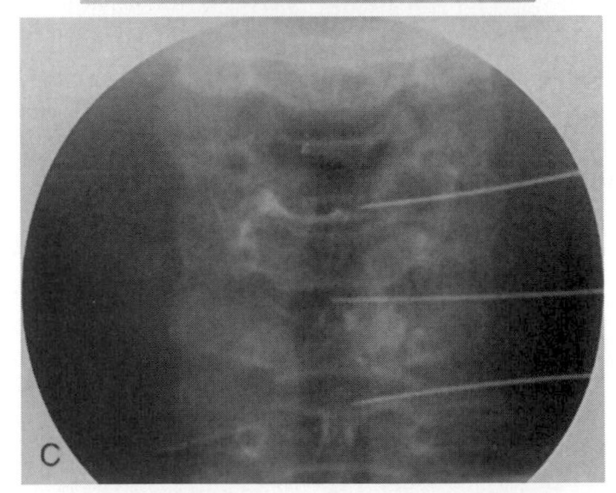

FIGURE 5–34 A, *A curved-needle approach to a cervical disc injection* (arrow), *oblique view.* B, *The spread of contrast material within a cervical disc, lateral view. Note that contrast material spreads into the epidural space from the central disc.* C, *The spread of contrast material within a cervical disc, anteroposterior view.*

Disc and facet joint pain can coexist in a particular cervical motion segment.[66] Clues from the history and physical examination findings might lead the clinician first to investigate the disc, rather than the facet joint. Radicular symptoms and signs, coupled with positive brachial tension test findings and anterolateral segmental tenderness, might point to the disc as the source of pain. Alternatively, certain patterns of posterior cervical and cranial pain with tenderness over particular facet joints could, perhaps, direct attention to the facet joints.[53] Previous abnormalities seen on CT, MRI, and other imaging investigations might also implicate a particular structure.

Cervical Discography

The approach to the cervical disc has been described by many authors. Aprill[67] has extensively reviewed this technique. It can be approached using an oblique fluoroscopy projection, from the right side to prevent the discogram needle's puncturing the esophagus and with the patient lying supine. Small amounts of propofol, injected intravenously and in sub–general anesthetic doses, can provide short-term, solid sedation. The patient emerges rapidly and can give a lucid assessment of any pain provocation. Unsedated patients often report both pain and fear during the procedure, and the use of short-acting intravenous sedative agents greatly reduces this discomfort. Because patients may be asked to return for further invasive investigations, previous experiences must not discourage them. Suitable precautions, including cardiovascular monitoring and pulse oximetry, should be undertaken. The fluoroscopy beam can be aligned so that the intervertebral foramina are displayed to their best advantage and the disc space margins lie parallel to the beam. A 25-gauge needle with a curve placed in the terminal half inch is inserted just posterolateral to the sternocleidomastoid muscle. The needle is directed to the anterolateral border of the disc, just anterior to the uncovertebral joint, and is inserted into the nuclear center. The operator can then proceed either to provocative discography using radiopaque contrast medium or to analgesic discography using a local anesthetic such as lidocaine 2%, but *not* a mixture of the two. Several segmental levels can be examined by provocative discography at one session, but analgesic discography may address only one level at a time. The quality and extent of the pain provoked must be recorded and interpreted with care. Only evoked pain responses that exactly mimic the usual pain pattern should be used to identify painful spinal segments. The observation and recording of analgesic responses is enhanced by providing charts for the patient to complete. This practice affords comparisons of results with subsequent examinations (Figs. 5–34, 5–35).

Lumbar Discography

The annulus is innervated, whereas neural structures have not been demonstrated in a normal nucleus pulposus. The pain of provocation discography is perhaps due to mechanical or chemical stimulation of nociceptors situated in the concentric layers of the annulus, where early degenerative or traumatic changes can occur. Local anesthetic agent, deposited between the lamellae and allowed to track circumferentially, might block these small sensory fibers. Annular blocks have been used to confirm that discs that appear abnormal on MRI can be painful (Fig. 5–36).[68]

The approach to the lumbar disc is posterolateral. The needle tip is passed down the fluoroscopy beam, close to the lateral border of the superior articular facet. The terminal half inch of the needle is curved, and directional changes are made by rotating the needle hub 180 degrees. Once contact is made with the superior articular facet, the needle tip is advanced in contact with the periosteum, thus avoiding contact with the nerve root. Propofol sedation can be used during needle insertion without affecting subsequent pain provocation. Based on discography findings, various stages of disc degeneration and injury have been described (Fig. 5–37).[69]

Nerve Root Sleeve

Just as discogenic pain can be studied by careful blocking of the intervertebral disc, so, too, can the central neural

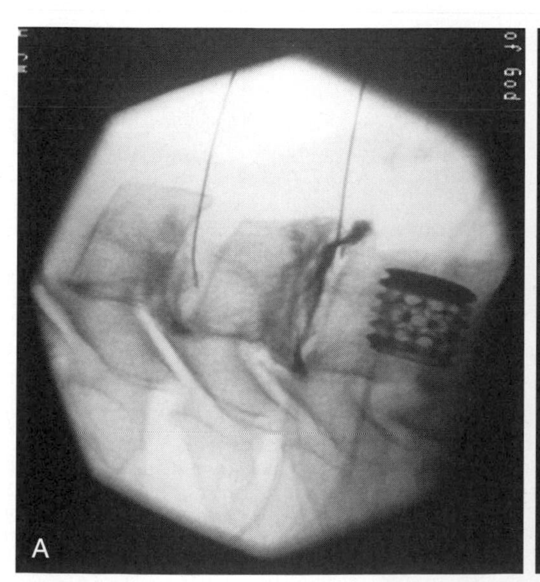

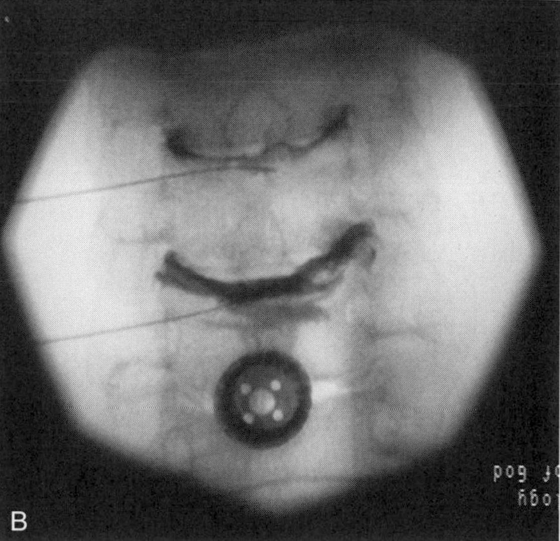

FIGURE 5–35 *A, Lateral C4-5 and C5-6 discograms. C4-5 disc shows normal age changes with uncovertebral fissure. C5-6 discs disrupted, and typical pain was provoked by injection of contrast material. C6-7 disc with a cage fixation device in situ. B, Anteroposterior discograms of the same structures.*

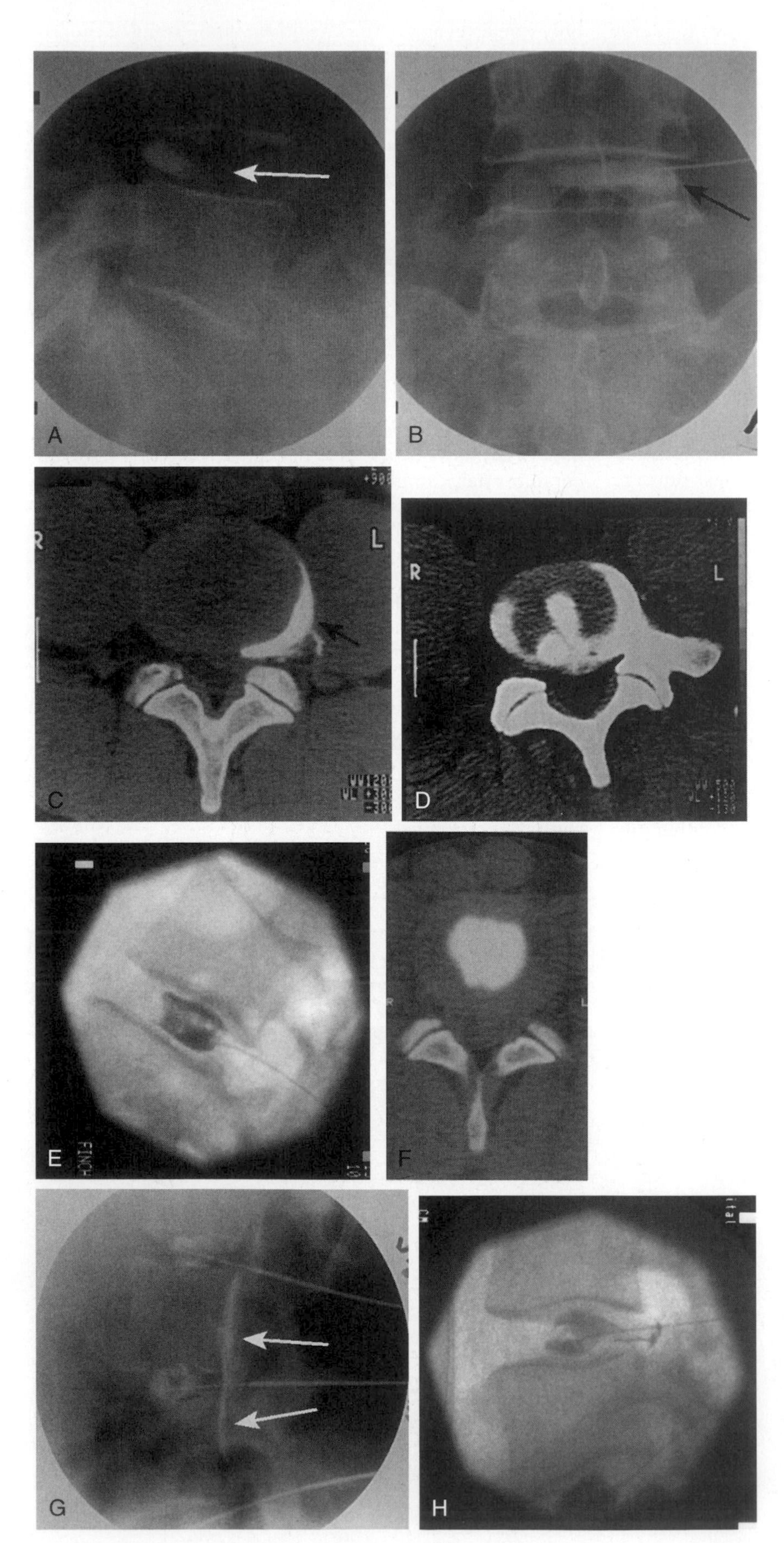

FIGURE 5–36 *A, Lateral radiograph taken after injection of contrast material into the annulus fibrosus of a lumbar disc. The contrast agent has spread smoothly around the annulus* (arrow) *without communicating with the nucleus. This is a normal annulogram.* B, *Anteroposterior view demonstrates the spread of contrast material around the right side of the annulus* (arrow). C, *CT confirms the spread of contrast material around the outer part of the annulus* (arrow). D, *CT after annular injection of contrast demonstrates the spread of contrast material to a posterior fissure that communicates with the nucleus.* E, *Lateral L4-5 discogram demonstrates normal cotton-ball spread of contrast.* F, *CT of a normal nuclear discogram.* G, *A lateral view demonstrates an L4-5 disc with a posterior tear that allows contrast material to escape into the epidural space* (arrows). H, *Abnormal discogram of an L4-5 disc demonstrates a posterior annular fissure.*

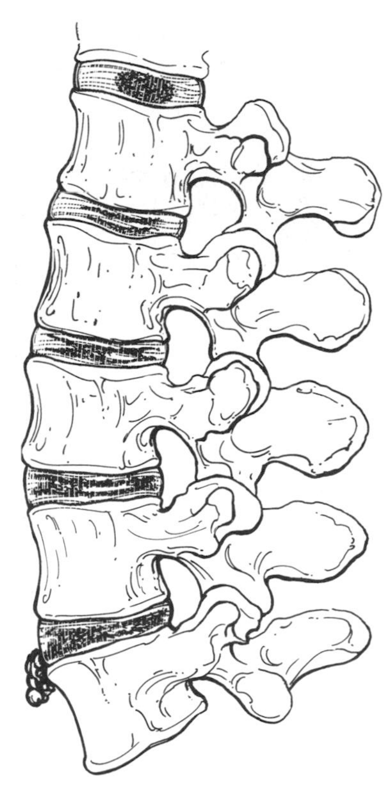

FIGURE 5–37 Drawing of the five stages of contrast spread within a lumbar disc space. The top disc has the appearance of a normal discogram. Progressive degeneration and injury are shown in lower interspaces, the extent of injury and degeneration being greatest in the lowest disc space.

elements be investigated logically and sequentially. The nerve root sleeve is particularly accessible to precise local anesthetic blocks. Segmental information gained from such nerve root blocks can be helpful in sorting out confusing patterns of referred pain to the limbs. The principles are similar, whether nerve roots are blocked in the cervical, dorsal, or lumbosacral spine. There are some regional differences in the approach to each area of the spine, however, partly as a result of the proximity of structures such as the lung or vertebral artery. The pathway for insertion of spinal needles must be planned to avoid damaging nerves. Spinal nerve roots are particularly delicate structures and do not tolerate being impaled. Also, local anesthetic or radiopaque contrast medium must be injected around spinal nerve roots slowly, to avoid the effects of a forceful injection into a confined space. Fluid volumes must be restricted to 1 mL for injection of the nerve root sleeve. Larger volumes would spread to adjacent nerve roots via the epidural space and result in loss of segmental specificity.

Cervical Nerve Root Sleeve

The cervical sleeve is approached from an oblique angle, rather like the approach to the cervical disc. It can be appreciated that large vascular structures, such as the carotid and vertebral arteries, lie close to the path taken by the spinal needle on its way to the spinal nerve root foramen. Also, at lower segmental levels, a misdirected spinal needle could enter the dome of the pleura. With the patient supine, the nerve root foramina are displayed on the image intensifier as open circles. This view is more easily achieved if the examiner remembers that the spinal nerve roots leave the cervical spine in an anterolateral and inferior direction. With the fluoroscopy beam adjusted so that the disc margins are parallel to the beam, the target point on the foramen is marked with a felt-tipped pen passed through a small hole in the end of a metal ruler (Fig. 5–38).

The skin entry point corresponds to the 12:00 o'clock position on the foramen, but the spinal needle is directed to reach the foramen at the 6:00 o'clock position. The carotid artery can be avoided by determining its position by palpation, and the vertebral artery by maintaining the needle in a posterior position once it has been positioned at the mouth of the foramen. Steering of the needle is much facilitated by placing a gentle curve in the terminal half inch of the needle. If it enters the foramen at the 6:00 o'clock position, it also avoids spearing the nerve root that exits the foramen caudally at the 3:00 to 4:00 o'clock position. With 180-degree rotations of the needle hub, the needle tip can be directed along the floor of the nerve root canal until it reaches the midpoint of the facet column, as viewed in an anteroposterior fluoroscopy projection. It is occasionally possible to inject contrast material into the facet joint from this position in the nerve root canal—if the tip of the needle has entered the anterior recess of the joint. This error can be avoided by rotating the needle tip toward the nerve root before injecting contrast agent (Fig. 5–39).

Contrast agent (Omnipaque 240) must be introduced slowly and gently, because the nerve root can be injured by an overzealous or forceful injection. Correctly placed contrast agent produces a double outline of the nerve root sleeve. There should be minimal spread into the epidural space, and the subsequent spread of contrast agent can be studied for evidence of impingement or obstruction. Local anesthetic agent is then injected in a dose not greater than 1 mL (lidocaine 2%, bupivacaine 0.5%, or ropivacaine 1%). Appropriate washout of the contrast material should be noted after the local anesthetic injection. The patient

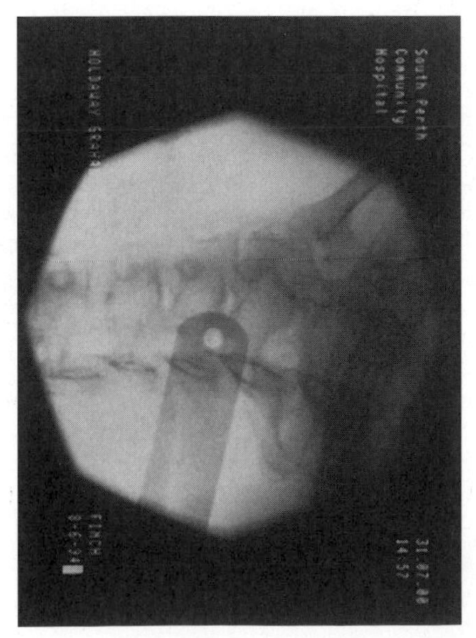

FIGURE 5–38 The skin entry point for an approach to a cervical foramen is marked through a hole in a metal ruler.

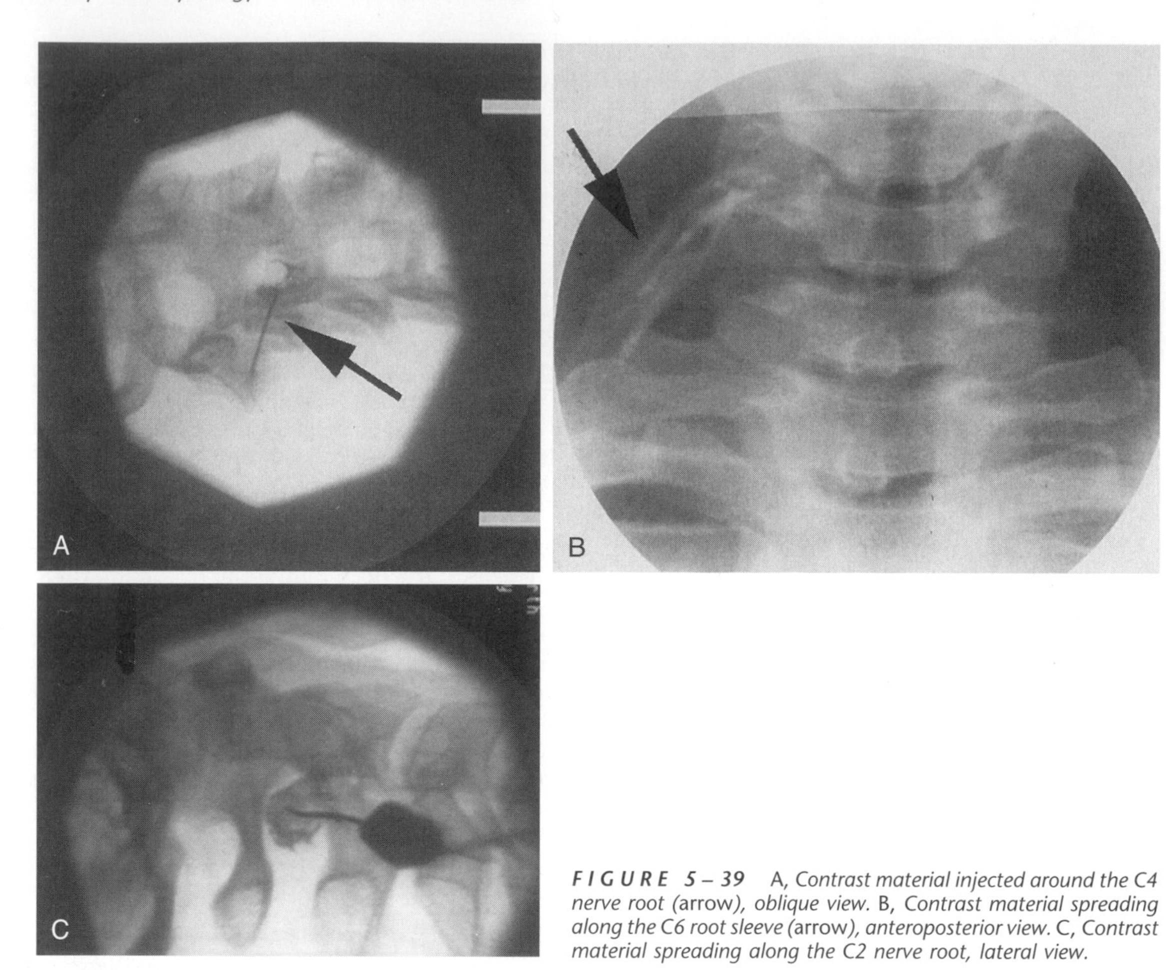

FIGURE 5-39 A, *Contrast material injected around the C4 nerve root* (arrow), *oblique view.* B, *Contrast material spreading along the C6 root sleeve* (arrow), *anteroposterior view.* C, *Contrast material spreading along the C2 nerve root, lateral view.*

should not experience paresthesia during manipulation of the spinal needle; this effect can signify penetration of the nerve root. Injection should be easy; if resistance is encountered, the needle should be repositioned. The operator must remember that the vertebral artery lies in close proximity. Finally, the patient should be observed in a recovery area that is fully equipped for cardiovascular and respiratory resuscitation, where sensory and pain pattern changes can also be observed and recorded.

Prognostic blocks of the C2 nerve are performed differently. The ovoid foraminal canals start at the C3 level. The C2 nerve exits from the arch of C2. Even though the anatomy is different, root sleeve blocks can still be performed at this level. A direct lateral approach is used, and the cannula is inserted perpendicular to the junction of the posterior two thirds with the anterior third of the C2 arch. The cannula is advanced until it is halfway across the C1–C2 joint line (on anteroposterior view). The patient's mouth must be open to provide a good anterior view of the C1–C2 joint. A paresthesia is sometimes obtained. Contrast material is injected to show the outline of the C2 root sleeve before injecting the local anesthetic.

Thoracic Nerve Root Sleeve

The thoracic nerve roots are approached in a different fashion, emphasis being placed on avoiding the parietal pleura. The first and second thoracic nerve roots are the least accessible and are approached at a point close to the lateral border of the nerve root foramen and just caudal to the transverse process, the depth of the transverse process being used as a guide. The fluoroscopy beam is anteroposterior. The spinal needle is "walked off" the transverse process inferiorly and placed just anterior to this structure before the usual contrast and local anesthetic agents are injected. More caudal thoracic nerve roots are also ap-

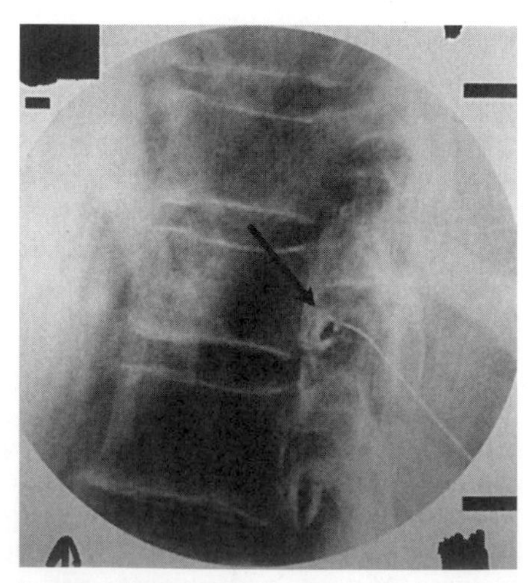

FIGURE 5-40 *A lateral view of contrast material spreading around a thoracic nerve root sleeve* (arrow). *Note curved needle tip.*

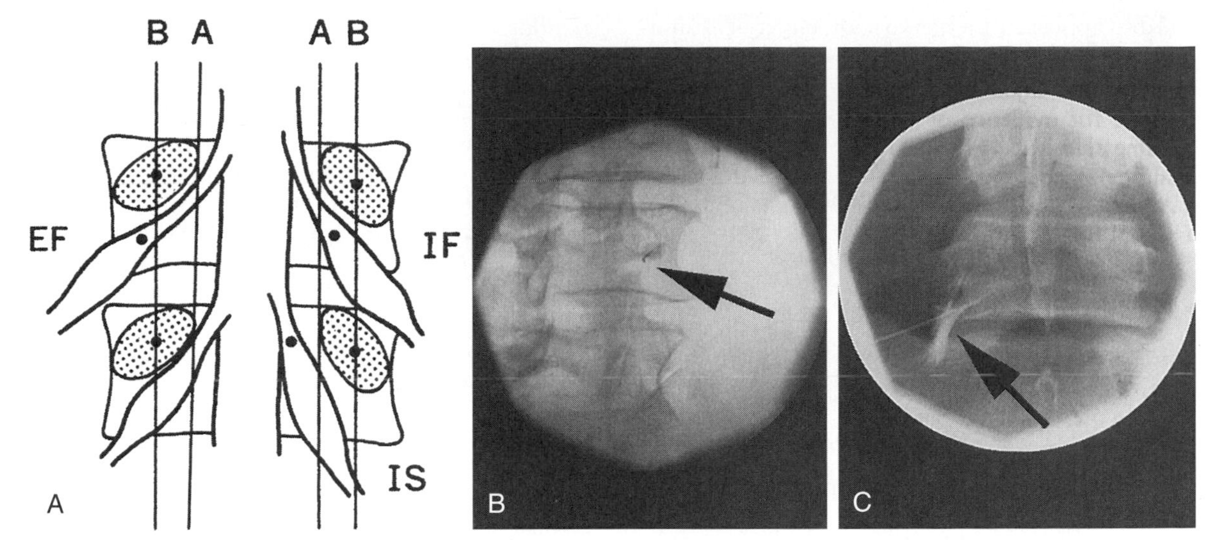

FIGURE 5–41 A, *Variation of dorsal root ganglia. If the proximal end of the dorsal root ganglion lies proximal to line* A, *it is the intraspinal (IS) type; between lines* A *and* B, *intraforaminal (*IF*); and distal to line* B, *extraforaminal (*EF*).* B, *Needle is placed at the 6:00 o'clock position just inferior to the pedicle* (arrow). C, *Spread of contrast material along the L5 nerve root sleeve* (arrow). *(A, From Kikuchi S, Sato K, Konno S, Hasue M: Anatomic and radiographic study of dorsal root ganglia. Spine 19:6–11, 1994.)*

proached with anteroposterior fluoroscopy projection and with the beam parallel to the vertebral body end plates. A spinal needle with a shallow curve placed in its tip is introduced no farther than 1 inch lateral to the vertebral body and is directed medially to strike the lateral edge of the superior articular facet. It can then be walked anteriorly until it just enters the nerve root foramen as seen on a lateral fluoroscopic projection. A satisfactory position is achieved if, on an anteroposterior fluoroscopy projection, the needle tip is seen to lie just inferior to the pedicle and halfway across this structure in a lateral-to-medial direction. Positions farther medial could penetrate the dural sheath. The needle tip should be directed so as to remain in the dorsum of the nerve root canal. Contrast and anesthetic studies can then commence (Fig. 5–40)

Lumbar Nerve Root Sleeve

There have been numerous publications on the anatomy and approach to the lumbar nerve root sleeve.[70–72] Kikuchi and associates[73] have described the anatomic variants of the dorsal root ganglia, and Derby and colleagues[74] have reviewed the techniques of blocking the lumbar nerve root sleeve.

In general, the principles of approach to these neural structures are little different from those described for the cervical region, although there are some regional differences in the fluoroscopy projection and final position of the needle tip. To avoid impaling the nerve root, the needle tip is directed to lie just inferior to the midpoint of the pedicle. This can be achieved by first aligning the fluoroscopy beam to pass squarely through the disc space. For the lumbosacral disc, a considerable degree of craniad angulation may be required. The C arm of the fluoroscope is then rotated to an oblique position so that the edges of the facet joint become clearly defined. A spinal needle with a curve in the terminal portion is then passed down the fluoroscopy beam to strike the inferior margin of the pedicle without contacting the nerve root. Derby and colleagues[74] describe this as "the 6:00 o'clock position," the oblique view of the pedicle representing the clock face. Contrast and local anesthetic agents are then injected gently and in controlled volume. If an electrically insulated

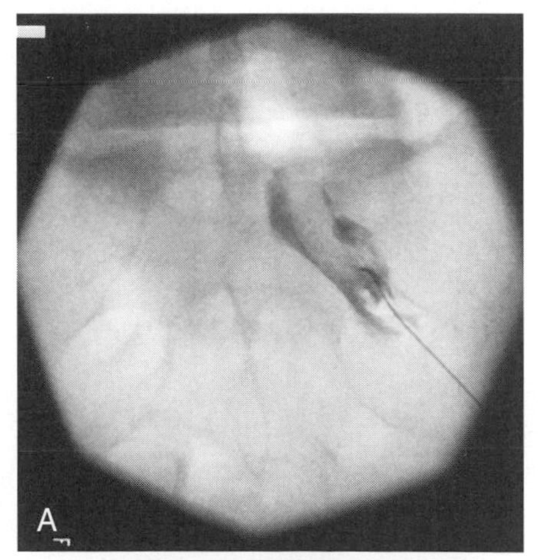

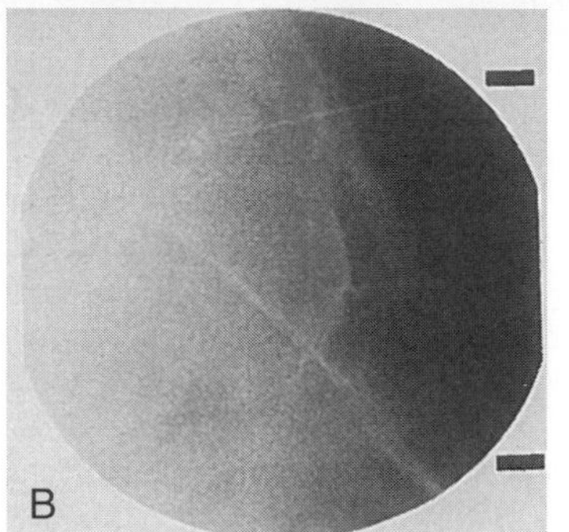

FIGURE 5–42 A, *Spread of contrast material* (arrows) *following a sacral nerve root sleeve injection, posteroanterior view.* B, *Lateral view of contrast material spreading along the S1 and S2 nerve root sleeves.*

needle is used to approach the nerve root, electrical stimulation can also be used to study patterns of referral to the lower limbs(Fig. 5–41).

Sacral nerve roots can easily be accessed by passing a spinal needle through the appropriate posterior sacral foramen. This route of access is visualized by adjusting the fluoroscopy beam to align the round posterior foramen with the curvilinear marking of the anterior foramen. The needle is passed through the epidural space onto the peripheral nerve at a point just anterior to the anterior sacral plate. Injection of contrast agent is best performed under direct fluoroscopic guidance, because veins are easily entered in the vicinity of the sacral nerve roots. Inadvertent intravascular injection of local anesthetic agent would, of course, produce a "false-negative block" and even some mild central nervous system effects (Fig. 5–42).

Facet Joints

Cervical Facet Joint

The cervical facet joint can be a source of pain.[75] Certain patterns of cervical or cranial pain and localized posterior cervical tenderness can implicate this structure. Injuries to the facet joint are seen in both the cervical and lumbar regions after motor vehicle accidents.[30, 49] Osteoarthritis of these joints is common in elderly persons. It is reasonable to investigate these structures with local anesthetic blocks as the possible source of segmental pain.

In both the cervical and lumbar regions, a small-volume arthrogram can be performed to study the morphology of the joint and its capsule. Local anesthetic agent can then be injected while the patient is observed for analgesic responses. Blocking the sensory nerve supply can provide an alternative to direct injection into the facet joint. There are several arguments for blocking the medial branches of the dorsal rami that supply these joints. We have observed spread of contrast agent from the anterosuperior joint recess of a cervical facet joint into the nerve root foramen. One could assume that, if local anesthetic agent were to follow suit, it would cause a partial block of the dorsal root ganglion or its nerve root in the nerve root canal. Although an infrequent occurrence, this would invalidate the conclusions drawn from any analgesic responses. Structural and segmental specificity would be lost. Local anesthetic agent injected slowly and in limited volume around the medial branch of a dorsal ramus, however, does not appear to spread to other segments (PM Finch, G Bower: Unpublished data, 1994). Injecting a normal joint might also pose theoretical risks, such as joint injury, chemical irritation,

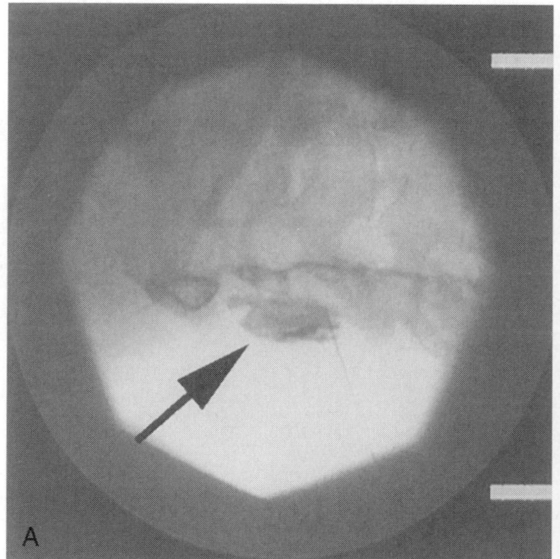

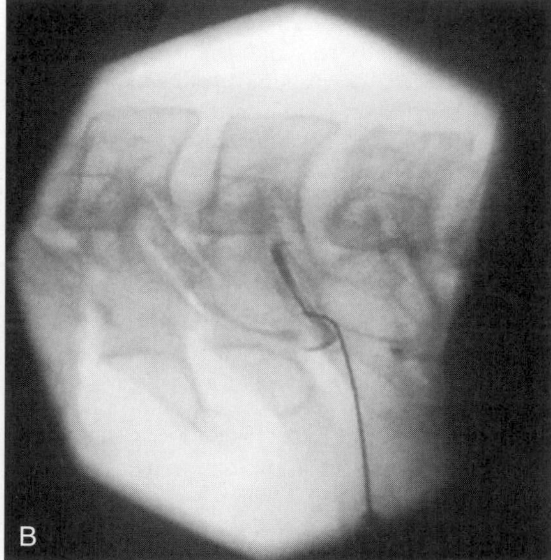

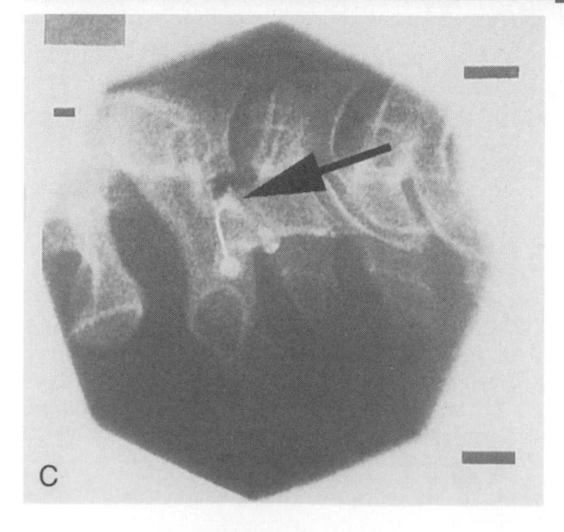

FIGURE 5–43 *A, The spread of contrast material after injection onto the medial branch of the dorsal ramus of C3-4 (arrow). B, Cervical facet arthrogram. Note the curved-needle approach to the joint and the spread of contrast material within it. C, A C2-3 cervical facet joint arthrogram with contrast material spreading to the inferior recess (arrow).*

and bacterial infection. Last, the medial branch is particularly accessible, and the introduction of a 25-gauge spinal needle onto this structure is virtually painless. If the joint is injected directly, a clearer end point is obtained, with the sensation of joint entry and the characteristic appearance of the cervical facet arthrogram (Fig. 5–43).

The technique of injecting either the joint or its medial branch is relatively simple. The cervical spine is viewed in a strictly lateral fluoroscopic projection, and the needle is introduced either into the joint, for an intraarticular injection, or onto a target point at the center of the articular pillar, at a level above and below the joint under investigation, for a medial branch block.[59] After injection of contrast agent, the patient should be closely observed for evidence of intravascular spread, and injection volume should be restricted to 0.5 mL, in the case of the medial branch, and even less for intraarticular blocks. An intact cervical facet joint does not admit much more than a total fluid volume of 0.5 mL.

Lumbar Facet Joint

There is no consensus about the utility of lumbar facet blocks.[76,77] They can be performed as part of the investigation of segmental pain but with due consideration to placebo and false-positive responses.[59] Medial branch blocks in this region may not have the advantage of restricting local anesthetic spread. Injection into the joint can provide morphologic information, including the integrity of the joint capsule or spread of contrast agent into other structures such as a fractured pars interarticularis. The lumbar facet joint is a curved structure, and the use of a needle with a curve near its tip facilitates entry into the joint. The C arm of the fluoroscope is rotated around the prone patient rather than moving the patient to suit the projection. This maneuver produces stability in the patient's position and displays the joint to best advantage. With an oblique projection, similar to the approach to the nerve root sleeve or the disc, a spinal needle is passed directly down the fluoroscopy beam and into the mouth of the joint. Steering of the needle tip is simply effected by frequent 180-degree rotations of the needle hub. As with the cervical facet joint, the operator can often detect the characteristic sensation of joint entry. Contrast agent is then observed to spread throughout the joint and into the superior or inferior joint recesses. If the joint capsule is incompetent, the spread of solution will be extensive, perhaps limiting the interpretation of any analgesic response. As with all spinal local anesthetic injections, the fluid volume injected into a lumbar facet joint must be restricted—in this case, to a total of 1 mL. Excessive injection force can even rupture the joint capsule (Fig. 5–44).

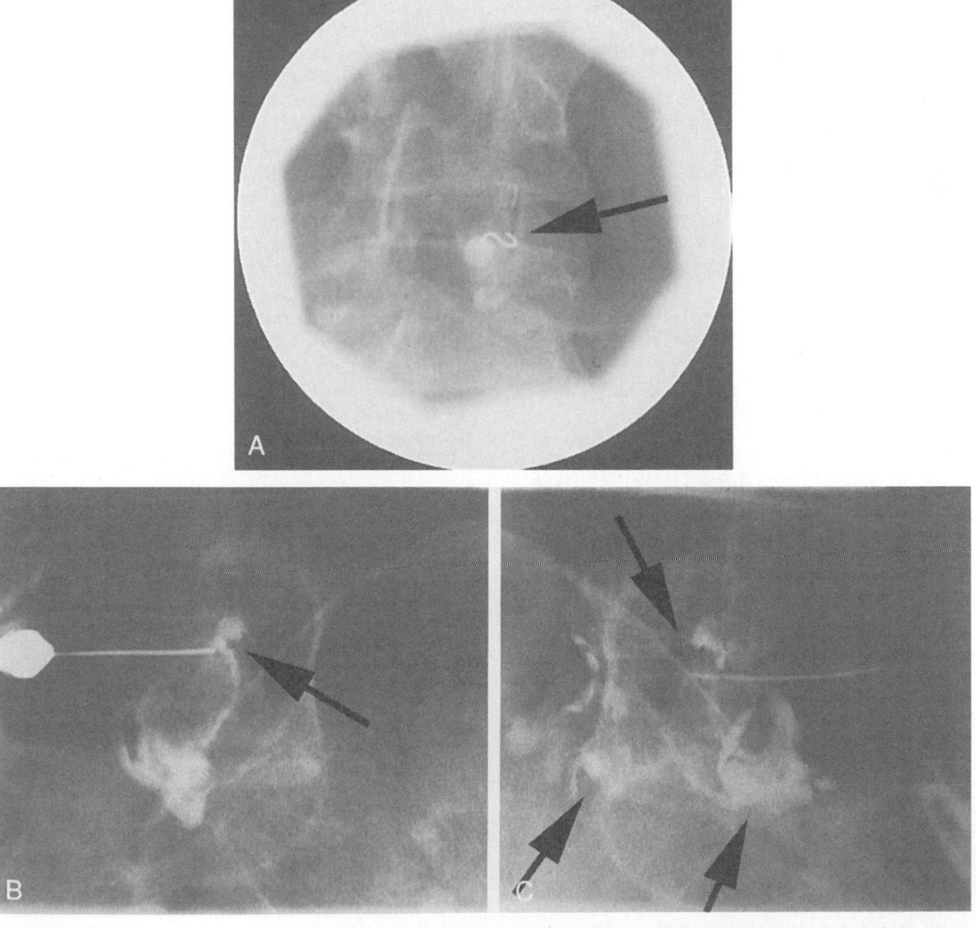

FIGURE 5–44 *A, The spread of contrast material after injection into the L4-5 facet joint (arrow). B, Normal spread of contrast material into the inferior recess of an L5-S1 facet joint. C, Spread of contrast material into the inferior recess of the contralateral L5-S1 lumbar facet joint with extracapsular spread of the contrast material on the left side of the joint (arrows).*

CONCLUSION

Although the components of the spinal motion segment have been considered separately in this discourse, the investigator should take a holistic approach to solving the problem of spinal pain. A realistic algorithm of procedures, with reasonable financial cost, must be planned with the consent and understanding of the patient. In an ideal world, multiple blocks of any given structure could be performed, utilizing different local anesthetic solutions to control for false-positive responses. The same principles could be applied to different structures in the same spinal segment, and even to adjacent segments for comparison. Such an ideal approach, although theoretically possible, can incur tremendous expense and increased risk of morbidity. A balanced and realistic approach needs to be used for day-to-day management of difficult chronic pain problems, the optimal balance being an accurate diagnosis of the underlying pathologic anatomy coupled with practical therapeutic intervention to alleviate the debilitating symptoms.

REFERENCES

1. Twomey L, Taylor JR: Age related changes in the lumbar spine and spinal rehabilitation. CRC Crit Rev Arch Phys Med Rehabil 2:153–169, 1991.
2. Twomey L, Taylor J: Physical Therapy of the Low Back, 2nd ed. New York, Churchill Livingstone, 1994, pp 1–56.
3. Taylor JR, Twomey LT: Structure and function of lumbar zygapophyseal joints. J Orthop Med 14:71–78, 1992.
4. Twomey L, Taylor J: Flexion creep deformation and hysteresis in the lumbar vertebral column. Spine 7:116–122, 1982.
5. McCormick CC, Taylor JR, Twomey LT: Facet joint arthrography in lumbar spondylolysis: Anatomic basis for spread of contrast. Radiology 171:193–196, 1989.
6. Giles LGF, Taylor JR: Human zygapophyseal joint capsule and synovial fold innervation. Br J Rheumatol 26:93–98, 1987.
7. Scott JE, Bosworth T, Cribb A, et al: The chemical morphology of age related changes in human intervertebral disc glycosaminoglycans from the cervical, thoracic and lumbar nucleus pulposus and annulus fibrosus. J Anat 184:73–82, 1994.
8. Osti OL, Frazer R, Vernon-Roberts B: Annulus tears and intervertebral disc degeneration: An experimental study using an animal model. Spine 15:762–767, 1990.
9. Freemont A, Peacock T, Goupillie P, et al: Nerve ingrowth into diseased intervertebral discs in chronic back pain. Lancet 350:178–181, 1997.
10. Taylor JR, Twomey LT: Age changes in lumbar zygapophyseal joints: Observations on structure and function. Spine 11:739–745, 1986.
11. Taylor JR, McCormick CC: Lumbar facet joint fat pads: Their normal anatomy and their appearance when enlarged. Neuroradiology 33:38–43, 1990.
12. Taylor MM, Taylor JR, McCormick CC: Features associated with subluxation in lumbar facet joints: Anatomy and radiology. *In* Bruce NW (ed): Proceedings of the Society of Human Biology, vol. 5. Perth, Center for Human Biology, University of West Australia, 1992, pp 359–373.
13. Kirkaldy-Willis WH: Managing Low Back Pain. New York, Churchill Livingstone, 1983.
14. Taylor JR, Twomey LT, Corker M: Bone and soft tissue injuries in post mortem lumbar spines. Paraplegia 28:119–129, 1989.
15. Schonstrom N, Twomey L, Taylor J: Lateral atlanto-axial joint injuries. J Trauma 35:886–892, 1993.
16. Penning L: Functional Pathology of the Cervical Spine. Baltimore, Williams & Wilkins, 1968.
17. Taylor JR, Twomey L: Sagittal and horizontal plane movements of the human lumbar vertebral column in cadavers and in the living. Rheumatology and Rehabilitation 19:223–232, 1980.
18. Panjab M, Dvorak J, Duranceau J, et al: Three dimensional movement of the upper cervical spine. Spine 13:727–730, 1988.
19. Taylor JR: Growth and development of the human intervertebral disc. PhD thesis, University of Edinburgh, 1973.
20. Tondury G: Anatomie fonctionelle des petites articulations du rachis. Ann Med Physique 15:173–191, 1972.
21. Lysell E: Motion in the cervical spine. Acta Orthop Scand Suppl 123:1–61, 1969.
22. Taylor JR, Taylor MM, Twomey LT. Muscle insertion to posterior cervical dura (Letter to editor). Spine 21(19):2300, 1996.
23. Bogduk N: The innervation of the cervical intervertebral disc. Spine 13:610–617, 1988.
24. Mendel T, Wink CS, Zimny ML: Neural elements in cervical intervertebral discs. Spine 17:132–135, 1992.
25. Bogduk N: The rationale for patterns of neck and back pain. Patient Manage 13:17–28, 1984.
26. Bogduk N, Marsland A: The cervical zygapophyseal joints as a source of neck pain. Spine 13:610–617, 1988.
27. Bogduk N, Twomey LT: Nerves of the lumbar spine. *In* Bogduk N, Twomey LT: Clinical Anatomy of the Lumbar Spine, 2nd ed. New York, Churchill Livingstone, 1991, pp 107–120.
28. Taylor JR, Finch PM: Acute injury of the neck: Anatomical and pathological basis of pain. Ann Acad Med Sing 22:187–192, 1993.
29. Taylor JR, Finch PM: Neck sprain. Aust Fam Physician 2:1623–1629, 1993.
30. Taylor JR, Twomey LT: Acute injuries to cervical joints: An autopsy study of neck sprain. Spine 18:1115–1122, 1993.
31. Taylor JR, Taylor MM: Cervical spinal injuries: An autopsy study of 109 blunt injuries. J Musculoskel Pain 4:61–79, 1996.
32. Taylor JR, Twomey LT, Kakulas BA: Dorsal root ganglion injuries in 109 blunt trauma fatalities. Injury 29:335–339, 1998.
33. Barnsley L, Lord S, Bogduk N: Whiplash injury. Pain 58:283–307, 1994.
34. Spitzer WO, Leblanc FE, Dupuis M: Scientific approach to the assessment and management of activity related spinal disorders. Report of the Quebec Task Force on Spinal Disorders. Spine 12 (Suppl. 7):1, 1987.
35. Delitto A, Cibulka MT, Erhard RE, et al: Evidence for use of an extension mobilization category in acute low back syndrome: A prescriptive validation pilot study. Phys Ther 73:216, 1993.
36. Hart LG, Deyo RA, Cherkin DC: Physician office visits for low back pain: Frequency, clinical evaluation and treatment patterns from a US national survey. Spine 20:11, 1995.
37. Boden S, Davis DO, Dina TS, et al: Abnormal magnetic resonance scans of the lumbar spine in asymptomatic subjects. J Bone Joint Surg 72A:403, 1990.
38. Waddell G: Low back pain: A twentieth century health care enigma. Spine 21:2820, 1996.
39. Jarvik JG, Haynor DR, Koepsell TD, et al: Interreader reliability of a new classification of lumbar disc disease. Acad Radiol 3:537, 1996.
40. Ito M, Incorvaia KM, Yu SF, et al: Predictive signs of discogenic lumbar pain on magnetic resonance imaging with discography correlation. Spine 23:1252, 1998.
41. Deyo RA, Phillips WR: Low back pain: A primary care challenge. Spine 21:2826, 1996.
42. Deyo RA, Diehl AK: Patient satisfaction with medical care for low back pain. Spine 11:28, 1986.
43. Marketos SG, Skiadas P: Hippocrates: The father of spine surgery, Spine 24:1381, 1999.
44. Schwarzer AC, Aprill CN, Derby R, et al: The relative contributions of the disc and zygapophyseal joint in chronic low back pain. Spine 19:801, 1994.
45. Wallis BJ, Lord SM, Barnsley L, et al: Pain and psychological symptoms of Australian patients with whiplash. Spine 21:804, 1996.
46. Melzack R, Wall PD: Pain mechanisms: A new theory. Science 150:971, 1965.
47. Jull G, Bogduk N, Marsland A: The accuracy of manual diagnosis for cervical zygapophyseal joint pain syndromes. Med J Austr 148(5):233–236, 1988.
48. Lord S, Barnsley L, et al: Percutaneous radio-frequency neurotomy for chronic cervical zygapophyseal-joint pain. N Engl J Med 335(23):1721, 1996.
49. Twomey LT, Taylor JR, Taylor MM: Unsuspected damage to lumbar zygapophyseal joints after motor-vehicle accidents. Med J Aust 151:210–217, 1989.
50. Revel ME, Listrat VM, Chevalier XJ, et al: Facet joint injection for low back pain: Identifying predictors of a good response. Arch Phys Med Rehabil 73:824–828, 1992.

51. Bogduk N: Cervical causes of headache and dizziness. *In* Grieve GP (ed): Modern Manual Therapy of the Vertebral Column. Edinburgh, Churchill Livingstone, 1986, pp 289–302.
52. Cloward RB: Cervical discography: A contribution to the etiology and mechanism of neck, shoulder and arm pain. Ann Surg 150:1052–1064, 1959.
53. Dwyer A, Aprill C, Bogduk N: Cervical zygapophyseal joint pain patterns: A study in normal volunteers. Spine 15:453–457, 1990.
54. Sluyter ME: Radiofrequency Lesions in the Treatment of Cervical Pain Syndromes. Procedure Technique Series, 19. Pain Syndromes. Burlington, Mass. Radionics, 1989.
55. Reymond RD, Wheeler PS, Perovic M, Block D: The lucent cleft, a new radiographic sign of cervical disc injury or disease. Clin Radiol 23:188–192, 1972.
56. Kellgren JH: A preliminary account of referred pains arising from muscle. Br Med J 1:325–327, 1938.
57. Elvey RL: The investigation of arm pain. *In* Grieve GP (ed): Modern Manual Therapy of the Vertebral Column. Edinburgh, Churchill Livingstone, 1986, pp 530–535.
58. Ochoa JL: The human sensory unit and pain: New concepts, syndromes, and tests. Muscle Nerve 16:1009–1016, 1993.
59. Barnsley L, Lord S, Wallis B, et al: False-positive rates of cervical zygapophyseal joint blocks. Clin J Pain 9:124–130, 1993.
60. Whitecloud TS, Seago RA: Cervical discogenic syndrome: Results of operative intervention in patients with positive discography. Spine 12:313–316, 1987.
61. Goucke CR, Lovegrove FTA, Finch PM: Lumbar sympathectomy: Spread of radiopharmaceuticals following a single-needle technique. Br J Anaesth 59:944–945, 1987.
62. Salmon JB, Finch PM, Lovegrove F, et al: Mapping the spread of epidural phenol in cancer pain patients by radionuclide admixture and epidural scintigraphy. Clin J Pain 8:18–22, 1992.
63. Carette S, Marcoux S, Truchon R, et al: A controlled trial of corticosteroid injections into facet joints for chronic low back pain. N Engl J Med 325:1002–1007, 1991.
64. Simmons JW, McMillin JN, Emery SF, et al: Intradiscal steroids: A prospective double-blind clinical trial. Spine 17(Suppl):172–175, 1992.
65. Roth DA: Cervical analgesic discograpy: A new test for definitive diagnosis of the painful syndrome: JAMA 235:1713–1714, 1976.
66. Bogduk N, Aprill C: On the nature of neck pain, discography and cervical zygapophyseal joint blocks. Pain 54:213–217, 1993.
67. Aprill C: Diagnostic disc injection. *In* Frymoyer JW (ed): The Adult Spine: Principles and Practice. New York, Raven, 1991, pp 403–440.
68. Finch PM, Khangure MS: Analgesic discography and magnetic resonance imaging (MRI). Presented at VI World Congress on Pain, Adelaide, Australia, April 5–6, 1990, IASP.
69. Adams MA, Dolan P, Hutton WC: The stages of disc degeneration as revealed by discograms. J Bone Joint Surg 68B:36–41, 1986.
70. Hasue M, Kikuchi S, Sakuyama Y, et al: Anatomic study of the interrelation between lumbosacral nerve roots and their surrounding tissue. Spine 8:50–58, 1983.
71. Kurobane Y, Takahashi T, Tajima T, et al: Extraforaminal disc herniation. Spine 11:260–268, 1984.
72. Kikuchi S, Hasue M, Nishiyama K: Anatomic and clinical studies of radicular symptoms. Spine 9:23–30, 1984.
73. Kikuchi S, Sato K, Konno S, et al: Anatomic and radiographic study of dorsal root ganglia. Spine 19:6–11, 1994.
74. Derby R, Bogduk N, Kine G: Precision percutaneous blocking procedures for localizing spinal pain. Part 2: The lumbar neuroaxial compartment. Pain Digest 3:175–188, 1993.
75. Aprill C, Bogduk N: The prevalence of cervical zygapophyseal joint pain. Spine 17:744–747, 1991.
76. Jackson R, Jacobs R, Montesano P: Facet joint injection in low-back pain: A prospective statistical study. Spine 13:966–971, 1988.
77. Helbig T, Lee C: The lumbar facet syndrome. Spine 13:61–64, 1988.

CHAPTER • 6

Pharmacologic Management and Its Limitations

Richard B. Patt, MD

RISK-BENEFIT RATIO

All medical interventions are associated with risks and benefits, which, when considered together, comprise that intervention's risk-benefit ratio. All interventions have alternatives (including no intervention), and each alternative possesses its own risk-benefit ratio. Clinical decision making involves comparing and contrasting the risk-benefit ratios of alternative interventions (relative risk-benefit ratio).

The risk-benefit ratio is derived from several variables and is usually inexact. It is in part intrinsic to a given therapy and in part dependent on the clinical situation for which treatment is under consideration. How the risk-benefit ratio is determined or interpreted is influenced by numerous factors, some of which are difficult to quantitate (e.g., provider bias, patient preference) or have subjective value (e.g., cost, suffering). As a result, the perceived risk-benefit ratio may differ profoundly based on interrelated factors pertinent to the patient (e.g., age, overall health, functional status, ethnocultural and religious background), physician (e.g., attitude, beliefs, training, financial incentives), and the system (e.g., regulatory forces, facilities, economic factors). The risk-benefit ratio is not fixed; it varies as these factors and their relationships change over time. This scenario is further complicated when applied to the treatment of pain, since, as a result of the subjective nature of pain and the newness of pain management as a specialty, few data on the outcomes of even accepted interventions are available. In the past, this has allowed wide latitude in decision making. Closer scrutiny of health care costs is likely to place greater constraints on decision making.

CONSIDERATIONS IN CHOOSING DRUGS: CANCER PAIN AND CHRONIC NONMALIGNANT PAIN

Cultural and social forces have profound influences on therapeutic decision making for pain management. A curious, but contextually understandable, dichotomy exists with respect to the treatment with opioid analgesics of pain of malignant and of nonmalignant origin.

Cancer Pain

Until recently, opioids were used only for the most desperate of medical conditions, a practice based more on cultural bias than on medical fact. Recent initiatives emphasizing the concept of comprehensive cancer care demand that attention be paid to symptom control throughout the course of a cancer illness. Contemporary approaches to managing pain in cancer patients emphasize earlier and more liberal use of opioids, citing low potential for addiction and an overall favorable risk-benefit ratio. A review of the literature suggests that these principles are grounded firmly in science.

Chronic Pain

Opioids were long considered taboo as treatment for chronic nonmalignant pain, an attitude grounded mostly in belief in the inevitability of addiction and typically a reflection not only of medical concerns but of moral ones, too. In light of data generated by the experience with opioids for cancer pain, the prohibition of opioid therapy for noncancer pain has been called into question. A spectrum of opinions currently surround the issues of the advisability and proper methods for prescribing opioids for such patients. Although both proponents and detractors cite data that support opposing views, most agree that opioid therapy is more beneficial than it is harmful in a certain portion of patients with chronic nonmalignant pain. While there is reasonable scientific support for this general contention, support for guidelines that determine the risk-benefit ratio prospectively in individual cases remains empirical.

INVASIVE PROCEDURES: SHAKY GROUND

The role of invasive and regional pain-relieving modalities is even more ill-defined than that of drugs, for the treatment of both cancer pain and other pain. The situation is analogous to that of opioids. Although there is fairly widespread agreement that procedures used to control nonmalignant pain sometimes have favorable risk-benefit ratios, no uniformly accepted, validated method has been devised for prospectively determining *in what settings which procedures* are valuable.

Cancer Pain

The U.S. Agency for Health Care Policy Research recently undertook to develop treatment guidelines for cancer pain, employing a method that utilized rigorous validation criteria. A robust review of the literature revealed considerably less compelling and less valid evidence for the value of procedures than of pharmacologic management. Unfortunately, the validity of this exercise is questionable, because its methods are so dependent on the quality of published reports, it more accurately reflects the shortcomings of the available literature than the true risk-benefit ratio. The ill-defined role of invasive procedures relates to many factors, including design problems, the historic lack of a mandate for outcome measures, and the relatively recent marriage of academic medicine and pain medicine. Notwithstanding these difficulties, the Agency's expert panel ultimately endorsed a vital role for invasive procedures. Owing to the nature of the process and the quality of data reviewed, however, recommendations for employing various procedures are somewhat vague and cite relatively narrow indications.

Chronic Pain

Debate over the role of invasive procedures for chronic nonmalignant pain is, if possible, even more contentious. Evidence has been cited supporting diametrically opposed views, and the quality of such evidence has legitimately been questioned. Factors that influence this debate are as noted above, but they also include bias (even rivalry) among specialists, financial stake, and "opiod phobia." Although there is reasonable agreement that procedures are sometimes useful, agreement on when and for whom has yet to be reached, as, likewise, has which procedures provide meaningful and durable pain relief sufficient to justify the risks and costs. There is *agreement*, however, that the outcomes for procedures are most salutary when they are "properly" integrated into a multidisciplinary matrix, although the *evidence* for even this conventional wisdom is questionable.

ADVANTAGES OF PHARMACOTHERAPY FOR CANCER PAIN

Oral opioid therapy is considered the treatment of choice for uncomplicated cancer pain, for a variety of reasons. These include the induction of analgesia that is reversible, titratable, suitable for a variety of types of pain (including multiple topographically distinct pains and generalized pain), and lack of invasiveness. The need for specialized training is modest, and efficacy is maintained when treatment is modified to apply to patients of various cultures, ages, and degrees of medical fitness.

LIMITATIONS OF PHARMACOTHERAPY FOR CANCER PAIN

It is well-recognized that, for 70% of cancer patients or more, pain relief can be achieved with uncomplicated oral or transdermal administration of opioids, especially when combined with nonsteroidal antiinflammatory drugs (NSAIDs) and adjuvant analgesics (e.g., antidepressants, anticonvulsants). As many as 30% of all patients with cancer pain, however, experience insufficient relief or dose-limiting side effects when treated with drugs alone and require alternate interventions to achieve comfort. The premise that opioids should be administered in doses sufficient to either control cancer pain or produce unacceptable side effects is widely accepted. Although the end points of opioid therapy (i.e., comfort and unacceptable side effects) are difficult to quantify, this view recognizes unacceptable side effects as one possible consequence of drug therapy. Such side effects constitute the most important limitations of drug therapy for cancer pain.

Several investigators have attempted to identify specific clinical findings that, when identified prospectively, signal that pain relief will be difficult to achieve by pharmacologic means alone. The best-validated schema, the Edmonton Staging System, suggests that a history of alcohol or drug abuse or recent tolerance, neuropathic pain, psychological distress, and movement-related pain carries a relatively poorer prognosis for controlling pain pharmacologically, whereas drug dose and the presence of delirium are not predictive. Other investigations suggest that movement-related pain is the only consistent predictor of poor outcome for pharmacotherapy. This is an extremely important focus for further study, especially with methods that target specific clinical pain syndromes. This author's experience suggests that syndromes such as tumor-mediated brachial and lumbosacral plexopathy, abdominopelvic pain, and pain due to the skin ulceration that accompanies fungating tumors are among other daunting syndromes in which pain often persists despite aggressive drug therapy. Although no single feature reliably predicts failure of pharmacotherapy, any of these findings should alert the clinician that additional resources may be needed to manage the pain effectively.

LIMITATIONS OF PHARMACOTHERAPY FOR PAIN NOT RELATED TO CANCER

The historical view that the use of opioids was *prima facie* undesirable for the management of chronic pain allowed ready determination of the risk-benefit ratio, no matter how unscientific. The contemporary view that opioid therapy is sometimes justified calls for a general reappraisal of the risk-benefit ratio and careful and individualized decision making.

The baseline limitations of drug therapy for nonmalignant pain include the same potential side effects that restrict use in cancer patients. Additional limitations in this population depend on the degree to which a given patient is perceived as being at risk for addiction and the degree to which the practitioner perceives opioid therapy as potentially effective and appropriate.

SPECIFIC LIMITATIONS

Dose-Limiting Side Effects

One set of limitations relates to the various collateral (nonanalgesic) effects of the analgesics. The most prominent side effects of the opioids are constipation, nausea, vomiting, cognitive failure (ranging from drowsiness to hallucinations), dysphoria, myoclonus, and pruritus, although, occasionally, other side effects, such as respiratory depression, supervene. Similarly, treatment with the NSAIDs and other adjuvants is limited by undesirable pharmacologic effects such as gastropathy, bleeding, renal insufficiency, masking of fever, and sedation (for NSAIDs) and constipation, dry mouth, dysrhythmias, cognitive failure, ataxia, hepatic insufficiency, and bone marrow depression (for the others).

Drug side effects, especially for the opioids, can often be managed effectively. An algorithm for managing opioid side effects in cancer patients is presented in Table 6–1. Side effects from other analgesics may be more problematic and are, in many cases, less readily reversible. Thus, an important distinction between the opioids and other analgesics is that there are few absolute contraindications to the former whereas the latter often must be avoided altogether, lest complications occur (e.g., aggravation of an ulcer, hypersensitivity, or bone marrow depression). Paradoxically, for long-term use, the opioids are both the most stigmatized of all analgesics and, on a physiologic basis, arguably the safest.

TABLE 6–1 *Strategies for Limiting the Side Effects of Opioids*

Prophylaxis	Especially for constipation; sometimes for nausea
Patient education	Informed of the potential for side effects, patients are less likely to assume they are allergic and more likely to cooperate with efforts at palliation
Patience	Nausea and sedation are usually transitory and remit with time
	Slower titration may reduce troublesome side effects
Symptomatic management	Treat with antiemetics, laxatives, psychostimulants, etc
Trials of alternative (related) analgesics	Efficacy: side effect profile of opioids is often idiosyncratic
	Trials of alternative opioids are indicated because of incomplete cross-tolerance.
Trials of adjuvant analgesics	Side effects may be due to reliance on opioids for a pain syndrome that is relatively nonresponsive to opioids.
	Successful therapy with adjuvants may allow for a reduction in opioid dose with fewer side effects
Alternate treatment modalities	Judicious application of antitumor therapy, procedures, psychotherapy, etc, may permit dose reductions with fewer attendant side effects

SPECIFIC SCENARIOS

Aside from the general category of dose-limiting side effects, a number of clinical scenarios impose specific limitations or increased risks from pharmacotherapy. Only a few such scenarios are cited here.

Neuropathic Pain

Somatic pain and visceral nociceptive pain typically respond "linearly" to escalating doses of opioid analgesics. In contrast, the dose-response relationship for neuropathic pain is often blunted, in which case higher doses become necessary and, in turn, side effects are more likely to become a problem. Once considered an "opioid-nonresponsive" set of disorders, neuropathic pain syndromes exhibit a range of responses, from which the concept of relative responsivity to opioids derives. Increasingly, neuropathic pain syndromes are successfully treated by using maintenance therapy with low dose opioids for the induction of partial analgesia and, then, conducting sequential trials of adjuvant analgesics in an effort to produce more complete analgesia.

Movement-Related (Breakthrough or Incident) Pain

Chronic pain is most often continuous, unrelenting, low-grade, basal pain punctuated by episodic exacerbations that can be unpredictable but that most often are related to activity. These superimposed flares are generally referred to as *breakthrough pain.* Typically, the basal component of pain is treated with a long-acting opioid administered "by the clock," such as an oral controlled-release formulation of morphine or oxycodone administered every 12 hours, a transdermal preparation of fentanyl applied every 72 hours, or less commonly, methadone. Breakthrough pain is then treated with symptom-contingent administration of a second, short-acting oral opioid as needed (immediate-release morphine sulfate, hydromorphone, oxycodone, oral transmucosal fentanyl citrate). The dose of long-acting medication is then titrated according to the frequency and urgency of the requirement for as-needed treatment of breakthrough pain.

Breakthrough pain that exhibits a relatively consistent temporal relationship to specific activities has come to be referred to as *incident pain.* Breakthrough pain that occurs at predictable intervals just before the next dose of an analgesic drug is scheduled is called *end-of-dose failure.* Finally, breakthrough pain that appears to be idiosyncratic and unrelated to either activity or scheduled doses of analgesics is typically referred to either as *spontaneous* or *idiopathic breakthrough pain*, or simply as *breakthrough pain*.

Pain that is exacerbated with movement is among the most difficult of syndromes to control with analgesics. The pharmacokinetics of currently available drugs, even those administered intravenously, are not complementary to the often unpredictable, rapid, and wide fluctuations in the severity of movement-related pain.

When incident pain is relatively predictable, rescue doses are provided prophylactically, about 30 minutes in advance of the pain-provoking activity. When unanticipated breakthrough pain occurs, the rescue dose should be taken as soon as possible, regardless of the timing of the basal dose. If these strategies are unsuccessful, consideration should be given to a trial of an alternative short-acting opioid or to a different route of administration. Breakthrough pain that is predictable, infrequent, of mild or moderate intensity, or slow to develop can often be managed effectively with oral analgesics such as IR morphine, hydromorphone, or oxycodone. Breakthrough pain that is severe or that occurs unpredictably, frequently, or precipitously may not be adequately relieved with currently available oral agents. Although intravenous IV and subcutaneous SC opioids are pharmacokinetically well-suited for labile or severe breakthrough pain, these attributes are offset by their invasiveness.

Oral transmucosal fentanyl citrate (OTFC), a new formulation of an established opioid analgesic, was recently approved specifically for the treatment of breakthrough pain that arises in patients who are already using opioids around the clock. A sweetened fentanyl-impregnated lozenge mounted on a stick, it is a noninvasive means of delivering a potent lipophilic opioid through the oral mucosa, which promotes rapid absorption into the circulation and analgesia of relatively fast onset and short duration of action. Extensive controlled research conducted on OTFC as a specific remedy for breakthrough pain, has confirmed its safety and demonstrated efficacy superior to that of routine oral agents for cancer patients also receiving therapy with TD and CR oral opioids for basal pain. Onset of meaningful analgesia typically occurs within 5 minutes of beginning consumption of a unit, peaks about 30 minutes later, and usually lasts about 4 hours. The duration of analgesia is slightly prolonged, because, inevitably, about half of each fentanyl dose is swallowed and subjected to hepatic first-pass effect. The availability of fentanyl in a lozenge form allows for easy self-administration and permits patients to titrate the dose to an effective level of analgesia without the need for injections. Given, however, the similarity in its kinetics with those of intravenous analgesics, it is probably an undesirable choice for patients prone to addiction.

Even with this addition to our armamentarium, prominent incident pain remains a treatment challenge, because opioid requirements vary dramatically over short intervals. Doses of opioids required to treat pain during periods of rest typically are inadequate when activity increases, and, conversely, doses required to ease movement-related pain may produce sedation and other side effects when the provocative activity ceases.

Narrow Therapeutic Window: Cachexia and Advanced Age

While a large proportion of patients with cancer are not candidates for curative therapy, palliative and supportive care may extend life. Drug-based pain control is often more difficult to achieve in patients with advanced cancer, because concomitant asthenia and cachexia increase the likelihood of side effects from opioids titrated to therapeutic effect (*narrow therapeutic window*). The sedative effects of opioids can often be countered by judicious use of psychostimulants such as methylphenidate, usually administered at starting doses of 10 mg on awakening and 10 mg with the noontime meal, which can be titrated to effect. While, theoretically, dysrhythmias and anorexia are concerns, they are rarely problematic, although this approach should be avoided in the presence of an anxiety disorder or brain metastases.

Limited epidemiologic data suggest that chronic pain is about twice as common for geriatric persons living in residential settings than in their younger counterparts (incidence 25%–50%). Although underrecognition and undertreatment of pain in nursing homes is so rampant that statistics are often misleading, targeted surveys reveal incidences of 45% to 80%.

Degenerative arthritis and other musculoskeletal disorders are the most prominent causes of pain in the elderly, although herpes zoster, decubitus ulcers, peripheral vascular disease, temporal arteritis, and polymyalgia rheumatica are disproportionately common in persons of advanced age. Since the incidence of almost every cancer increases with age, cancer pain is a particularly common problem in the geriatric population and, for them, it is an especially important problem because many of the factors that cause cancer pain to be undertreated in the general population are amplified in aging patients.

While age-associated changes in organ function of some degree are inevitable (including changes in the central nervous system), with few exceptions, they ordinarily exert little influence on pain threshold or pain tolerance, although pharmacodynamics or pharmocokinetics may be somewhat altered. Although loss of neural tissue and proliferation of glial cells occur with advancing age, there is no evidence of impairment in pain signal–processing unless dementia or delirium is clinically evident. Clinical lore suggesting that elderly patients do not experience pain as keenly as their younger counterparts is unfounded—and often is no more than a rationalization for unwillingness to spend the extra time often required to assess an elderly person.

The hospice experience has demonstrated that, when appropriate time and effort are applied, pain can usually be managed effectively, even in the frail elderly. However, drug titration should be performed with considerable caution, and, when possible, polypharmacy should be avoided.

Suffering

Pain has multiple determinants, and often persists as a result of unidentified psychosocial causes. Analgesics *per se*, are unlikely to reduce complaints of pain that are rooted in more global suffering. Psychotropic drugs combined with psychotherapy may, however, be effective in this setting.

Abdominopelvic Pain

Factors specific to patients with abdominopelvic pain that reduce the likelihood of attaining adequate pain control with systemic analgesics alone are listed in Table 6–2. NSAIDs, even of the COX-2 selective type, may be poorly tolerated or contraindicated owing to gastropathy and to general factors such as renal insufficiency, coagulopathy, bone marrow suppression, and masking of fever. The oral route may be unreliable in the presence of gastrointestinal dysfunction (e.g., dysphagia, malabsorption, intestinal obstruction, nausea and vomiting, xerostomia, and coma). Reduced gastrointestinal motility is a common upshot of tumor encroachment or sequela of surgery or radiation therapy. Even with a strict bowel protocol, opioids may exacerbate ileus or partial obstruction in patients with reduced motility. In such cases, the use of opioids, except in low doses, is undesirable. Although visceral pain is relatively opioid responsive, patients often present with pain of mixed causes. Typically pain due to nerve injury (neuropathic pain) is less sensitive to opioids, and, thus, occult microscopic deposits of perineural tumor invasion may contribute to reduced opioid responsivity.

TABLE 6–2 **Potential Limitations of the Pharmacologic Management of Abdominopelvic Pain**

Treatment Modality	Limitations
NSAIDs	Gastropathy Renal dysfunction Bone marrow depletion Concerns about masking fever
Oral analgesics	Xerostomia Dysphagia Malabsorption Obstruction Nausea Vomiting Coma
Transdermal analgesics	Dose requirements for opioids may exceed limitations of dose form
Parenteral analgesics	Inadequate household or community support to manage infusions
Opioids	Ileus Partial obstruction Intractable constipation Reduced responsivity due to neuropathic component of pain Dose-limiting side effects due to asthenia and cachexia

CONCLUSION

Notwithstanding the opioids-for-chronic-pain controversy, data support the primary role of pharmacotherapy for managing most pain syndromes. A variable proportion of patients do not, however, derive adequate comfort from systemic drug therapy alone or are not candidates for liberal use of opioids. Even for cancer pain, when addiction is less of a concern and liberal prescribing is widely endorsed, physiologic and psychological features sometimes hinder achieving an adequate pharmacologic remedy.

The most formidable limitations of drug treatment relate to their potential to produce pharmacologic side effects or complications. Careful monitoring and the use of strategies for preventing and managing drug side effects are often all that is required to maintain efficacy. Specific patient-related factors (e.g., neuropathic pain, movement-related pain, psychological distress, cachexia, alterations in gastrointestinal function) are associated with greater likelihood of limitations. The degree to which selected drugs' potential to induce habituation is an impediment to long-term use remains a topic of considerable and heated debate.

RECOMMENDED READING

American Pain Society: Principles of Analgesic Use in the Treatment of Acute Pain and Chronic Cancer Pain, ed 4. Skokie, Ill., American Pain Society, 1999.

Ashby MA, Fleming BG, Brooksbank M, et al: Description of a mechanistic approach to pain management in advanced cancer. Preliminary report. Pain 51:153–161, 1992.

Bruera E, Macmillan K, Hanson J, MacDonald RN: The Edmonton staging system for cancer pain: Preliminary report. Pain 37:203–209, 1989.

Bruera E, Schoeller T, Wenk R, et al: A prospective multicenter assessment of the Edmonton staging system for cancer pain. J Pain Symptom Manage 10:348–355, 1995.

Bruera E, Chadwick S, Brenneis C: Methylphenidate associated with narcotics for the treatment of cancer pain. Ca Treat Rep 71:120, 1987.

Christie JM, Simmonds M, Patt R, et al: Dose titration, multicenter study of oral transmucosal fentanyl citrate for the treatment of breakthrough pain in cancer patients using transdermal fentanyl for persistent pain. J Clin Oncol 16:3238–3245, 1998.

Ellison NM: Opioid analgesics: Toxicities and their treatments. *In* Patt RB (ed): Cancer Pain. Philadelphia, JB Lippincott, pp 185–194, 1995.

Ferrell BA: Pain management among elderly persons. *In* Payne R, Patt RB, Hill CS (eds): Assessment and Treatment of Cancer Pain. Seattle, IASP Press, 1998, pp 53–66.

Galer BS: Opioids and chronic nonmalignant pain. Am Pain Soc J 2:207, 1993.

Getto CJ, Sorkness CA, Howell T: Antidepressants and chronic nonmalignant pain: A review. J Pain Symptom Manage 2:9–18, 1987.

Hanks GW: Opioid-responsive and opioid-non-responsive pain in cancer. Br Med Bull. 47:718–731, 1991.

Hanks GW, Justins DM. Cancer pain: Management. Lancet 339:1031–1036, 1992.

Hogan QH, Abram SE: Epidural steroids and the outcomes movement. Pain Digest 1:269–270, 1992.

Jacox A, Carr DB, Payne R, et al (eds): Management of cancer pain: Clinical practice guideline No 9. AHCPR Publication No. 94-0592 Rockville, Md., 1994.

Jain S, Patt RB: Complications of invasive procedures. *In* Patt RB: Cancer Pain. Philadelphia, JB Lippincott, pp 443–460, 1995.

Mercadante S: Predictive factors and opioid responsiveness in cancer pain. Eur J Cancer 34:627–631, 1998.
Mercadante S, Armata M, Salvaggio L: Pain characteristics of advanced lung cancer patients referred to a palliative care service. Pain 59:141–145, 1994.
Mercadante S, Maddaloni S, Roccella S, Salvaggio L: Predictive factors in advanced cancer pain treated only by analgesics. Pain 50:151–155, 1992.
Patt RB: General principles of pharmacotherapy. *In* Patt RB: Cancer Pain. Philadelphia, JB Lippincott, pp 101–104, 1995.
Patt RB, Jain S: Therapeutic decision making for invasive procedures. *In* Patt RB: Cancer Pain. Philadelphia, JB Lippincott, pp 275–284, 1995.
Portenoy RK: Chronic opioid therapy in nonmalignant pain. J Pain Symptom Manage 5 (Suppl):S46–S62, 1990.
Portenoy RK: Chronic opioid therapy for persistent noncancer pain: Can we get past the bias? Am Pain Soc J 1:1–5, 1991.
Portenoy RK: Management of common opioid side effects during long-term therapy of cancer pain. Ann Acad Med 23:160–170, 1994.
Portenoy RK, Coyle N: Controversies in the long-term management of analgesic therapy in patients with advanced cancer. J Pain Symptom Manage 5:307–319, 1990.
Portenoy RK, Foley KM: Chronic use of opioid analgesics in non-malignant pain: Report of 38 cases. Pain 25:171–186, 1986.
Schofferman J: Long-term use of opioid analgesics for the treatment of chronic pain of nonmalignant origin. J Pain Symptom Manage 8:279–288, 1993.

CHAPTER • 7

Interventional Pain Management: Programming for Success

Steven D. Waldman, MD, JD
• Katherine A. Waldman, OTR, MBA
• Steven M. Siwek, MD

Since the publication of the first edition of *Interventional Pain Management* in 1996, the use of interventional pain management techniques has grown exponentially. With this growth has come a better understanding of what can and cannot be expected from a given interventional pain management technique. This fact has led to improved patient selection, which has, in turn, led to improved patient outcomes.

While these changes were occurring on the clinical front, the specialty of pain management saw a shift from the professional-based paradigm to the managed care–based paradigm. In today's medical care structure, it has become increasingly difficult to get reimbursement for many interventional pain management (IPM) techniques. Owing to the limitations of choice and access imposed by this new paradigm, many patients are denied the benefits that IPM might offer. In this chapter we address the new challenges facing IPM specialists and attempt to provide practical answers to often difficult questions.

PATIENT SELECTION CONSIDERATIONS

As the specialty of IPM has matured, the indications for IPM techniques have become better-defined and clinical practice more standardized among pain centers. Variations in the techniques offered at a given pain center are usually the result of the training and personal preferences of the pain clinicians caring for the patients. It should be noted that the clinician does not have a crystal ball and must bring to bear his or her cumulative expertise in the decision-making process when considering an IPM procedure. In doing so, the pain management specialist must balance several considerations when deciding whether a particular IPM technique is appropriate for a given patient: These factors include:

1. Weighing the compassionate desire to relieve the patient's pain against the likelihood that an IPM technique will, in fact, produce the desired result.
2. Assessing the risk-benefit ratio of each IPM technique contemplated, because many techniques have significant risk profiles as compared with less invasive modalities.
3. Evaluating the cost-benefit ratio for each IPM technique being contemplated.
4. Determining whether the contemplated procedure is, in fact, covered by the patient's insurance or managed care contract.
5. Providing whatever documentation or supporting literature needed to obtain appropriate precertification and authorization from the patient's insurance or managed care company.
6. Being sure that the procedure is scheduled at a facility that is covered by the patient's insurance or managed care contract.

The outcome will be less than optimal, for patient and clinician alike, if the latter fails to take all these factors into account.

VARIABLES AFFECTING OUTCOME

Patient Variables

Much has been written about the patient variables that ultimately determine the success or failure of each clinical undertaking. Because of the nature of many patients who are candidates for IPM techniques, these variables become even more important.

Motivation

Motivation is the first and foremost patient variable affecting the outcome of IPM techniques. The desire to be pain free increases the likelihood that this outcome will, in fact, occur. Conversely, patients who have secondary gain issues, such as worker's compensation, litigation, or relief of societal responsibilities, have been shown statistically to fare less well in terms of ultimate pain relief.

Chemical Dependency

The second most important patient variable affecting the outcome of IPM techniques is the presence of medication overuse and chemical dependency. Traditionally, patients who are chemically dependent on opioids, benzodiazepines, or barbiturates have been notoriously difficult to manage. They are frequently willing to undergo IPM techniques to demonstrate their desire to get better. When the technique fails to provide pain relief, such patients often resort to drug-seeking behavior. Self-medication with alcohol or controlled substances further reduces the statistical probability that the patient will obtain pain relief from an IPM technique. It is our strong belief that long-term use of opioids to manage pain not related to cancer is another negative determinative factor insofar as ultimate patient outcome is concerned and that it should be avoided at all costs. We base this statement on extensive clinical experience and our very disappointing results with patients given long-term opioid therapy for such pain.

Compliance History

Poor patient compliance with previously prescribed treatment regimens is a warning sign that the patient may not be a good candidate for many IPM techniques. In particular, spinal cord stimulation and totally implantable narcotic delivery systems require a significant level of patient compliance, especially during the early phases of treatment. Patients who have demonstrated poor compliance to previously prescribed treatment regimens may be better served with less invasive pain management techniques.

Education Level

There is a statistical correlation between the educational level of the patient and the ultimate outcome, in terms of pain relief. This relationship may be due, in part, to the work environments of less educated persons. When compensation for a disabled worker very nearly matches earnings there is little incentive to return to work. Again, secondary gain may work against a positive patient outcome and should be considered.

Coexistent Disease

When considering the use of IPM techniques, pain management specialists must identify coexistent diseases that may contribute to a poor result. For example, severe osteoporosis with progressive vertebral compression fractures may temper enthusiasm for spinal cord stimulation for peripheral vascular insufficiency. Preexisting chronic benign pain with a history of medication overuse or chemical dependency may complicate and confound management of cancer-related pain. The immunocompromised state of the patient with acquired immunodeficiency syndrome may lead the pain management specialist to avoid implantable technologies.

ASPECTS OF THE PATHOLOGIC PROCESS BEING TREATED

Chronicity

There is no question that the longer intractable pain has persisted, the less likely is a successful outcome, regardless of which IPM technique is chosen. The pain management specialist may, however, be able to treat acute exacerbations of what was a previously stable, chronic pain syndrome. For example, epidural steroids may be useful in the palliation of an acute exacerbation of pain in a patient with chronic low back pain who has slipped and fallen on ice and has reinjured his or her back. Careful use of diagnostic nerve blocks before neurodestructive procedures will not only determine whether a given procedure will in fact relieve the pain but also will give the pain management specialist time to get to know the patient. Again, it has been our experience that patients on long-term opioid therapy for nonmalignant pain fare worse after IPM, and careful assessment of such patients is indicated before an invasive therapy is attempted.

The Disease Process

When an IPM technique is under consideration, the clinician must carefully evaluate the patient to ensure that the diagnosis is correct. Some disease processes that are stable, such as failed back syndrome, may lend themselves to long-term IPM, such as spinal cord stimulation, epiduroscopy, and lysis of adhesions. Some pain syndromes are dynamic in nature and require a more hands-on approach—for example, rapidly progressive multiple myeloma involving the spine. For such patients, rapid palliation of acute pain emergencies with systemic opioids and local anesthetic nerve blocks may be more appropriate.

Sympathetic Component

Many painful conditions have both a somatic and a sympathetic component. In such cases, IPM techniques aimed only at the somatic or the sympathetic component of the pain are bound to fail. As Winnie has pointed out, unrecognized sympathetically maintained pain accounts for the largest proportion of cases of chronic benign pain for which no diagnosis has been ascertained. Failure to address this sympathetic component leads to a less than optimal outcome. Coexisting diseases such as osteoporosis, collagen vascular disease, and peripheral vascular insufficiency may also have to be treated ultimately to control the patient's pain.

PROCEDURAL FACTORS THAT AFFECT OUTCOME

Operator Skill

A frequently overlooked variable in the outcome of IPM techniques is the skill of the operator. Inadequate use of local anesthetics, repeated attempts at needle placement, and trauma to neural and vascular structures all increase periprocedural pain, which, in turn, can exacerbate any sympathetically maintained pain and contribute to a higher rate of complications, including infection.

Frequency

Frequency of nerve blocks is often a debated topic. Insurance carriers and health maintenance organizations (HMO) try to use it to deny or delay needed treatment. As with any medical treatment, diagnosis and patient progress determine the proper treatment plan. Many pain management centers follow a rigid regimen when utilizing IPM techniques. These regimens are often based on convenience of the pain management center's schedule rather than on any community standard of practice or scientific rationale. It is important that such centers have the flexibility to meet the needs of an individualized treatment plan. For example, in a pain syndrome that has a component of sympathetically maintained pain, individualizing the treatment plan by increasing the frequency of nerve blocks to daily or every other day will markedly improve the outcome.

Number of Nerve Blocks

Any pain management treatment plan should have as its basis a firm foundation in the contemporary clinical literature and, most importantly, the medical needs of the patient. Too often, managed care plans, Medicare, and other third-party payors base their utilization limitations on outdated or misinterpreted literature. In many instances, the articles used to justify claims denials are taken out of context or do not apply to the clinical situation at hand. Each patient deserves an individualized treatment plan that takes into account the diagnosis, the acuity and severity of illness, and what other treatment options are available. "Cookbook" approaches or arbitary limitations on treatment are to be avoided. Clear documentation of medical necessity is mandatory to fight such abuses by managed care plans, Medicare, and third party payors.

Staff

Many pain centers use an interdisciplinary team approach to staffing, which can include one or all of the following personnel: occupational therapist, physical therapist, psychologist, dietitian, and physiatrist. It is important that each team member understand what skills and techniques the practitioners of the other disciplines bring to the team. In addition, when interacting with the pain patient, each team member must project a positive and supportive attitude about the therapeutic techniques of the other team members. A negative attitude about a particular modality undermines the team's goals, often resulting in a poor outcome. Team meetings, patient staffings, and education in-services help to improve communication and awareness among the team members, resulting in high-quality patient care.

OTHER VARIABLES THAT AFFECT OUTCOME

The pain experience is unique to each patient, and many patients have additional emotional and physical problems that exacerbate the pain syndrome and make successful treatment of the chief complaint difficult. During the initial evaluation (follow-up visits), coexistent disease and emotional problems that contribute to the pain syndrome must be sought. The intake questionnaire and first visit must be structured so that the examiner can screen for physical ailments, family problems, personal stressors, pain management coping skills, and so on.

Treatment of coexistent disease that contributes to the patient's pain is essential for more complete pain control. For example, orthotic devices can splint vertebral compression fractures. Patients suffering from tension headaches often benefit from biofeedback, whereas patients who are concerned about being able to return to their previous occupation might benefit from vocational rehabilitation.

Hidden Agendas

No matter how well the pain management specialist knows the patients, occasionally a completely unrecognized, hidden patient agenda emerges. Issues include undisclosed malpractice litigation against other treating physicians, personal injury litigation, and the desire to obtain controlled substances for illicit use. Because of the importance of such hidden agendas, it is desirable for pain management physicians to limit the use of IPM techniques early in the course of the therapeutic relationship until any hidden agenda issues are clearly identified.

PROGRAMMING FOR SUCCESS

The following strategies should enable pain management specialists to maximize the success rate of IPM:

- Be available.
- Treat acute pain aggressively.
- Detoxify chemically dependent patients.
- Avoid narcotics for chronic pain of nonmalignant origin.
- Use adjunct treatments early.
- Project a positive attitude (physicians and staff).
- Avoid a negative attitude (do not "hang crepe").
- Do not hurt the patient.

Be Available

Pain management physicians who choose to offer IPM techniques must ensure coverage, 24 hours a day, 7 days a week, to allow immediate evaluation when problems occur. Other factors, including prompt return of phone calls and addressing patient concerns, can optimize patient satisfaction and avoid overlooking potentially serious side effects or complications related to IPM.

Treat Acute Pain Aggressively

It is the consensus among most pain specialists that the aggressive treatment of acute pain reduces the chances of development of chronic pain syndromes. For patients with a previously stable chronic pain history, the appearance of acute pain should be viewed as a harbinger of a change in the disease process or of the development of a new pain pathology. Patients should be hospitalized for pain emergencies to allow aggressive but safe pharmacologic and procedural treatment.

Detoxify Chemically Dependent Patients

It is mandatory that patients who are chemically dependent on opioids, benzodiazepines, or barbiturates and who have exhibited escalating dosage needs or drug-seeking behavior be detoxified before IPM is considered. As mentioned earlier, failure to manage chemical dependency could make the IPM technique the focus of the patient's quest for additional controlled substances. Too often, such patients report that their pain is much worse after the IPM procedure and use this excuse to press for prescription of additional controlled substances.

Avoid Narcotics for Chronic, Benign Pain

Although some pain specialists have reported success with the use of narcotics in the treatment of chronic pain, the authors' experience with this approach has been dismal. Pain management specialists should ensure that all other treatment modalities that have an acceptable risk-benefit ratio have been considered before they consider narcotic analgesics—and, even then, they must approach this treatment very cautiously.

Use Adjunct Treatments Early

The early use of adjunct drugs and of physical and behavioral modalities helps to optimize relief of the patient's pain. Treatment of sleep disturbances and underlying depression with antidepressant compounds should be the cornerstone of the treatment of chronic pain. The pain management specialist should take care to avoid polypharmacy.

Maintain a Positive Physician and Staff Attitude

It is important to ensure that all staff and treating physicians exhibit a positive attitude about the anticipated IPM procedure. If some members of the pain management team project a negative attitude about a given treatment, levels of patient satisfaction and success may decrease and the stage may be set for malpractice liability should the outcome be less than optimal.

Avoid a Negative Attitude

Although a realistic appraisal of the chances for success of a given IPM technique is appropriate, there is no reason to be unnecessarily pessimistic ("hang crepe") about the potential for pain relief. Projecting a low expectation of success increases the patient's anxiety and can contribute to the patient's feeling of hopelessness and depression.

Do Not Hurt the Patient

Care must be taken with all IPM techniques to be sensitive to how much pain the procedure itself causes. Failure to use local anesthesia, multiple attempts at needle placement, and rough technique markedly increase the incidence of periprocedural pain and complications. The use of smaller, sharper needles has become the standard of care for many pain management procedures.

CONCLUSION

In the motion picture *Dirty Harry*, Clint Eastwood's character admonishes, "A man has got to know his limitations." It is important for pain management specialists to recognize that there are limitations to our ability to provide pain relief for every patient. Even when the most sophisticated IPM techniques are utilized, the most effective therapeutic modality in the care of the patient with pain is an informed, caring, and compassionate physician.

SUGGESTED READINGS

Waldman SD: Providing pain management services: Basic considerations. Am J Pain Manage 4:86–88, 1994.

Waldman SD: Providing pain management services: Specific considerations. Am J Pain Manage 4:132–135, 1994.

Waldman SD: Setting up a pain treatment facility. *In* Warfield C (ed): Principles and Practice of Pain Management. New York, McGraw Hill, 1999.

Waldman SD: Pain management in the 21st century: An anesthesiologist's look into the crystal ball. Am J Pain Manage 1:4–5, 1991.

Waldman SD: Spinal administration of depot steroids—fact or fancy? Pain Digest 1:296–299, 1992.

Waldman SD: Motivating the pain center employee. Am J Pain Manage 3:114–117, 1993.

Waldman SD: Any willing provider laws—paradox or panacea Part I. Am J Pain Manage 6:54–61, 1996.

Waldman SD: Any willing provider laws—paradox or panacea Part II. Am J Pain Manage 6:93–96, 1996.

Waldman SD: Negotiation and the specialty of pain management—a need for reappraisal. Am J Pain Manage 6:127–131, 1996.

Waldman SD, Donohoe CD, Waldman KA: The pharmacologic management of neuropathic pain. Prog Anesthesiol 12:55–68, 1998.

Waldman SD: The current status of lumbar facet block in contemporary practice. Pain Digest 8:41–43, 1998.

Winnie AP: Differential neural blockade in pain syndrome of questionable etiology. Med Clin North Am 52:123, 1968.

PART • II

Evaluation of the Patient in Pain

CHAPTER • 8

Targeted History and Physical Examination

Charles D. Donohoe, MD

The cornerstone of accurate pain diagnosis is the medical history. In this age of technology, a disproportionate amount of time and energy is often given to testing at the expense of time spent with the patient collecting a coherent history. Indeed, it is shortcuts taken in obtaining old records, contacting prior treating physicians, calling family members of a confused hospitalized patient, and just sitting and listening to what the patient believes to be important that frequently lead to misdiagnosis of the problem and embarrassment for the pain specialist.

The bond of trust that is so integral to the relationship between patient and pain specialist is often determined by the care and thoroughness with which the initial historical material is obtained. It is my experience that, when physicians are rushed for time, the intake interview becomes abbreviated and this sets the stage for future medical errors and interpersonal dissatisfaction.

The chapters that follow this discussion highlight the utility of neurophysiologic, neuroradiologic, and selective neural blockade procedures in the evaluation of pain. Some diagnostic procedures are uncomfortable and risky. Some are extremely sensitive but lack specificity. Almost all are expensive. Most, not all, of what a pain specialist needs to know the patient can relate. By far the most cost-effective endeavor in the evaluation of the patient in pain is to be thorough in the initial targeted history taking and physical examination. If this initial consultation ends without a clear direction as to the underlying pathology or without insight into the predicament of the patient in pain, the likelihood that technology will "save the day" is very remote.

THE TARGETED PAIN HISTORY

Obtaining a history is a skill. Practice and repetition improve our skills, reduce the tendency to omit important material, and ultimately enable us to focus our questions to conserve time without sacrificing accuracy. As a starting point, the search should be directed to answer two questions,[1] "Where is the disease causing the pain—in the brain, spinal cord, plexus, muscle, tendon, or bone?" and "What is the nature of the disease?" It is the trademark of an experienced clinician to formulate an efficient line of questioning that deals with both of these issues simultaneously. I will highlight the critical elements in that process. The goal is to keep the process brief, simple, and workable.

The secret of becoming skilled at taking a history is being a good listener. The physician should put the patient at ease. The patient should never be given the impression that the physician is rushed or overworked and that only limited time is available to get the story across. The physician must remember that the patient in pain is usually anxious, if not overtly frightened, and may be inadequate in presenting the situation and having his or her plight properly perceived. Experience teaches us that the physician cannot force the pace of the interview without losing vital information and valuable mutual trust and insight. The following discussion describes the elements of the targeted history that not only define pain in a context useful for proper identification, localization, and source but also enable the physician to determine priorities about the urgency of care.

The Pain Litany

The *pain litany*—a formulaic exploration of the patient's pain history—enables the physician to identify the signature of the specific pain syndrome from its usual presenting characteristics.[2, 3]

The pain litany takes the following form*:

1. Mode of onset.
2. Location.
3. Chronicity.
4. Tempo (duration and frequency).
5. Character and severity.
6. Associated factors:
   a. Premonitory symptoms and aura.
   b. Precipitating.
   c. Environmental factors (occupation).
   d. Family history.
   e. Age at onset.
   f. Pregnancy and menstruation.
   g. Gender.
   h. Past medical and surgical history.
   i. Socioeconomic considerations.
   j. Psychiatric history.
   k. Medications, drug and alcohol use.

The targeted history also allows physicians to distinguish sick patients from well ones. If it is determined that in all probability the patient is well (i.e., has no life-threatening illness), the workup and treatment plan may proceed at a more conservative pace. From the outset, the interviewer proceeds in an orderly fashion but remains vigilant for signals of an urgent situation. Pain of uncertain origin should always be regarded as a potential emergency.

Mode of Onset and Location

The mode of onset of the pain sets the direction of the initial history and carries much weight in distinguishing sick from well. For example, the sudden, explosive presentation of a subarachnoid hemorrhage secondary to a ruptured intracranial aneurysm, manifested by severe headache, neck pain, and sense of impending doom, contrasts sharply with the chronic diffuse headache and vague neck tightness of tension-type cephalalgia.

The location of pain provides additional diagnostic information. The pain in trigeminal neuralgia, for instance, is usually limited to one or more branches of cranial nerve V and does not spread beyond the distribution of the nerve.[4] The V_2 and V_3 divisions of this nerve are much more frequently involved than V_1. The pain is rarely bilateral except in certain cases of multiple sclerosis.[5]

* (From Diamond S, Dalessio DJ [eds]: The Practicing Physician's Approach to Headache, ed 4. Baltimore, Williams & Wilkins, 1986.)

Another example of the importance of pain location is the burning, prickling dysesthesias of meralgia paresthetica. The unilateral involvement of the lateral femoral cutaneous nerve produces painful dysesthesias in the anterior thigh, more commonly in men, who notice the disturbance when they put a hand in a trouser pocket.

The physician must find out how and where the pain started. The patient should be asked to identify the site of maximum pain.

Chronicity

The duration of awareness of a painful illness targets the initial history and heavily influences the sick from well distinction. For this reason, it often serves as a starting point. "How long have you had this pain?" is an essential question. The patient should be asked to try to date the pain in relation to other medical events, such as trauma, surgery, and other illnesses.

In general, back pain that has been present for 30 years and is not associated with any progression is strong evidence of a self-limited pain syndrome; thus, the "well" determination. Conversely, a patient with severe low back pain of sudden onset or that suddenly changes in character must be assigned to the category of "sick until proved otherwise." This type of accentuated pain presentation has often been called the *first or worst syndrome.* It applies to both spinal pain and headache. Patients in this category deserve serious concern, and their pain should be viewed with medical urgency. Equating the concept of chronicity with benign disease has its pitfalls; the physician must beware of failing to:

- Identify ominous changes in a long-standing, stable pain syndrome (e.g., when a patient with chronic low back pain suddenly becomes incontinent).
- Attribute the onset of symptoms to a benign cause without adequate evaluation (e.g., dismissing a sudden increase in low back pain in the postoperative patient as muscle spasm without considering discitis and bacterial epidural abscess).
- Recognize new symptoms superimposed on chronic complaints (e.g., attributing an increase in headache with cough to chronic cervical spondylitis disease rather than considering that because the patient has a known breast malignancy, silent metastasis may be causing increased intracranial pressure).

Indeed, the characteristics of thoroughness, experience, insight into the patient's personality, and a constant resistance to being lulled into false security prevent such diagnostic disasters. As Mark Twain observed, "Good decisions come from experience and experience comes from making bad decisions."[6]

Tempo (Duration and Frequency)

The tempo of a disorder may provide one of the best clues to the diagnosis of the pain. In facial pain, trigeminal neuralgia (tic douloureux) is described as brief electric shocks or stabbing pain. Onset and termination of attacks are abrupt, and affected patients are usually pain free between episodes. Attacks last only a few seconds. It is not unusual for a series of attacks to occur in rapid succession over several hours. In contrast, the pain of temporal (giant cell) arteritis is usually described as a dull, persistent, gnawing pain that is exacerbated by chewing.[3]

In migraine, the pain is frequently throbbing and may last hours to days. Cluster headaches, by contrast, are named for their periodicity: they occur once or more often each day, last about 30 minutes, and often appear shortly after the onset of sleep. They may occur in clusters for weeks to months with headache-free intervals between. In short, the concept of pain tempo is another feature of the targeted history that is helpful in differentiating pain syndromes.

Character and Severity

Although there is considerable overlap between character and severity of pain, some generalization can be made when taking a targeted history. Vascular headaches tend to be throbbing and pulsatile and the pain intensity is often described as severe.[3] Cluster headaches may have a deeper, boring, burning, wrenching quality. This pain is reputed to be among the worst known to humans.

Trigeminal neuralgia is typically described as paroxysmal, jabbing, or shocklike, in contrast to non-neuralgic pain such as temporomandibular joint (TMJ) dysfunction, which is often described as a unilateral, dull, aching pain in the periauricular region. This TMJ pain is exacerbated by bruxism, eating, and yawning but may be patternless. The characteristic pain of postherpetic neuralgia usually includes both burning and aching superimposed on paroxysms of shocks and jabs. It usually occurs in association with dysesthesias, resulting in an unpleasant sensation even with the slightest touch over the skin (allodynia).

Many of the more common pain syndromes have a distinctive character and level of severity that is helpful in properly identifying them. Clinical insight into these characteristics comes with time and through listening to many patients describe their pain. Certain patients with cluster headaches or trigeminal neuralgia have a frantic, almost desperate demeanor that is proportionate to the severity of their pain. The patient with acute lumbar disc herniation often writhes before the physician, essentially unable to sit in a chair.

Associated Factors

Multiple associated factors round out the targeted pain history. The subtle differences between painful conditions allow us to utilize these factors to complete the various parts of the puzzle. For example, intermittent throbbing pain behind the eye would be consistent with cluster headache. If the patient is a young woman, however, the diagnosis of cluster headache is improbable because of its known male preponderance.[3] Accordingly, the combination of associated factors such as age and sex aid in the diagnosis. A dull, persistent pain over one temple in a young African American male probably is not giant cell or temporal arteritis, a disease predominant in white women older than 50 years.

Table 8–1 describes various pain syndromes according to patient age, sex, family history, precipitating factors, and occupational issues. As Osler said, "Medicine is a science of uncertainty and an art of probability."[2] Matching our knowledge about the natural history and characteristics of the various diseases that cause pain with information derived from the patient's history is our most powerful diagnostic tool. It is through this process that the physician develops confidence in the diagnosis that often exceeds that based on information from ancillary tests. An autoworker who uses an impact wrench 10 hours a day, complains of numbness in the first three digits of his right hand, and wakes up four times a night "shaking his hand

TABLE 8–1 ***Demographics of Some Common Pain Syndromes****

Pain Syndrome	Sex Preponderance (Ratio)	Family History	Age of Onset (yr)	Associated Features; Comments
Migraine				
Childhood (<10 yr)	M (1.5 : 1)	Positive	3	Abdominal pain, episodic vertigo, mood changes
Adult (>10 yr)	F (3 : 1)	Positive	15–20	Decrease by third month of pregnancy, increase with menstruation and oral contraceptives
Cluster headache	M (8 : 1)	Not positive	25–40	Common at night, precipitated by alcohol and nitrates
Multiple sclerosis	F (2 : 1)	Positive	20–40	Trigeminal neuralgia, tonic spasms, dysesthesia, extremity pain
Temporal arteritis	F (3 : 1)	Not positive	>60	Increased erythrocyte sedimentation rate (ESR), anemia, low-grade fever, jaw claudication
Trigeminal neuralgia	F (2 : 1)	Not positive	>55	V_2 (45%) >V_3, (35%) >V_1 (20%); triggered by jaw movement, heat, and cold
Ankylosing spondylitis	M (5 : 1)	Positive	20–30	Pain forces patient out of bed at night, is not relieved by lying flat
Rheumatoid arthritis	F (3 : 1)	Positive	35–50	Higher rate in nulliparous females not exposed to oral contraceptives
Thromboangiitis obliterans	M (8 : 1)	Not positive	20–40	Smoking
Carpal tunnel syndrome	F (2 : 1)	Not positive	30–60	Certain occupations, pregnancy, diabetes, hypothyroidism

* Data from references 1, 3, 4, 9, and 10.

out" has carpal tunnel syndrome, regardless of the results of nerve conduction studies and electromyography.

General Aspects of the Targeted Pain History

An old clinical maxim states, "Healing begins with the history!"[2] The clinician should be able to put the patient at ease and should then ask open-ended questions that will give the patient an opportunity to describe the pain in his or her own words. "Now, tell me about your pain" is an excellent prompt. This approach allows the patient to describe what he or she believes is most important. It is therapeutic in itself. Physicians are often leary of the open-ended question, because they are afraid that the patient will ramble. Although this can occur, a far more common problem is that the physician narrows the line of questioning after jumping to a premature conclusion.

When the pain is chronic, other doctors may already have been consulted. They probably have ordered diagnostic tests and tried therapies; indeed, it is always wise to obtain previous records or, preferably, to contact the other physicians directly. If a diagnosis seems obvious but previous doctors missed it, the physician should be cautious. When nothing has worked before, there is usually a good reason for the failures. Under these circumstances, assuming that the other physicians were competent is prudent and wise. In my experience, physicians are frequent violators of the maxim, "Do unto others as you would have them do unto you." Frank or subtle criticism of a colleague's efforts is pointless, upsets the patient, and may even initiate litigation.

One other impulse that should be resisted is the tendency to ascribe pain to psychogenic causes. Learning to believe patients who have pain averts many awkward and potentially costly errors. Once the physician projects the belief that a patient's pain is based mainly on psychogenic mechanisms, it is an extremely difficult position to recant. At all costs, the pain specialist should remain nonjudgmental, should believe in the patient's pain, and should gain the patient's confidence. The only proven "cure" for having dismissed patients' pain as psychogenic is to learn that serious organic disease was uncovered by others who saw the patient later. The pain specialist should be humble, careful, and calm.

Medication History

The importance of a thorough drug history cannot be overstated, particularly in the setting of chronic benign pain. It is not unusual, in my experience, for a patient to relate a very involved history of pain and multiple operations, diagnostic studies, and consultations. At the end of the interview, not uncommonly as the patient is preparing to leave, he or she will casually mention needing to have a prescription renewed, adding that it is "just a pain pill." It is at this very point that an otherwise pleasant consultation can become confrontational.

I believe that there is rather widespread confusion among physicians about the differences between narcotics and opioids. Many also fail to recognize that the relative analgesic, euphoric, and anxiolytic properties of a given compound are not equivalent. For example, the analgesic strength of propoxyphene (Darvon) may be equivalent to one or two aspirins, but the magnitude of its anxiolytic effects on a given patient can be considerable. It is not only opioids that pose a problem. Carisoprodol (Soma, Rela) is a noncontrolled skeletal muscle relaxant that is also available through veterinary supply catalogs.[7] Its active metabolite is meprobamate (Equanil, Miltown), an anxiolytic-sedative agent popular in the late 1950s. Patients using carisoprodol may be at risk (frequently unrecognized) for meprobamate dependency.

Ergots, aspirin, acetaminophen, nonsteroidal antiinflammatory drugs (NSAID), minor tranquilizers, and barbiturate-containing compounds (Fiorinal, Esgic, and Phrenilin) taken in varying doses can contribute to "rebound"-type headache. In this setting, the daily use of abortive drugs enhances and increases the frequency of daily headaches. The scope of this problem is difficult to assess, but in certain headache clinics taking such drugs is the single most important finding in patients with chronic refractory daily headaches.[8] Although every pharmacologic agent has some inherent risk, two practical considerations may be crucial in the targeted pain history. The first involves many individuals, particularly elderly persons who are taking anticoagulants (warfarin, heparin) or antiplatelet agents (aspirin, ticlopidine [Ticlid]) for any of a variety of reasons. Many disasters can occur in this setting. Inadvertent overdosing of an elderly, confused patient can cause intracerebral bleeding (headache) or back and radicular pain (secondary to retroperitoneal hemorrhage). Second, the physician evaluating headache symptoms should keep in mind that estrogens, progesterones, and nitrates can play major roles as provocative agents and that simply removing them can provide almost immediate improvement.

I believe that both the scope and the number of problems related to chemical dependency have been underrecognized in many clinical settings. I see some patients who are willing to subject themselves to expensive diagnostic studies, multiple nerve blocks, and even surgery to ensure an uninterrupted supply of specific medications. The specialist in pain management is uniquely positioned to recognize these problems and to offer suggestions in a compassionate, nonjudgmental fashion that may ultimately extricate patients from both their chemical dependency and their convoluted relationship with the medical system. Until such issues are fully resolved, effective inroads will not be made into the management of chronic benign pain.

Others have described a more satisfactory experience giving opioids for chronic benign pain.[9, 13] I sense that this positive experience may promote more liberal prescribing policies for a variety of primary care physicians. In my opinion, such a situation only accentuates the importance of obtaining a thorough drug history and assessing the true impact of drug use on the individual patient's pain problems. Table 8–2 lists the "red flag" agents that, when used by a patient in pain, should alert the physician to consider possible drug abuse or exacerbation of pain by medication. Information on dosage and duration of use is important. Pain specialists should make it policy to insist that patients bring all their medications at the time of the consultation.

TABLE 8–2 ***"Red Flag" Drugs in the Targeted Pain History****

Drug Class	Drug
Controlled Abused Substances†	
Schedule II narcotics	Morphine (Roxanol, MS Contin)
	Codeine
	Fentanyl (Sublimaze)
	Sufentanil (Sufenta)
	Hydromorphone (Dilaudid)
	Meperidine (Demerol)
	Methadone (Dolophine)
	Oxycodone (Percodan, Tylox)
	Opium
	Cocaine
Nonnarcotic agents	Dextroamphetamine (Dexedrine)
	Methamphetamine (Desoxyn)
	Methylphenidate (Ritalin)
	Phenmetrazine (Preludin)
	Amobarbital (Amytal)
	Pentobarbital (Nembutal)
	Secobarbital (Seconal)
	Glutethimide (Doriden)
	Secorbarbital-amobarbital (Tuinal)
Schedule III narcotics	Codeine (Tylenol w/codeine, Fiorinal w/codeine)
	Dihydrocodeine (Synalgos-DC)
	Hydrocodone (Tussionex, Hycodan, Vicodin, Lortab, Lorcet)
	Butalbital (Fiorinal, Esgic, Phrenilin, Medigesic)
Schedule IV narcotics	Propoxyphene (Darvon, Darvocet, Wygesic)
	Pentazocine (Talwin)
	Alprazolam (Xanax)
	Chlordiazepoxide (Librium)
	Clonazepam (Klonopin)
	Clorazepate (Tranxene)
	Diazepam (Valium)
	Flurazepam (Dalmane)
	Lorazepam (Ativan)
	Midazolam (Versed)
	Oxazepam (Serax)
	Quazepam (Doral)
	Temazepam (Restoril)
	Triazolam (Halcion)
Nonnarcotic agents	Phenobarbital
	Mephobarbital (Mebaral)
	Chloral hydrate
	Ethchlorvynol (Placidyl)
	Meprobamate (Equanil, Equagesic)
Schedule V narcotics	Buprenorphine (Buprenex)
	Diphenoxylate (Lomotil)
Noncontrolled Abused Substances	Carisoprodol (Soma, Rela)
	Ergotamine (Cafergot, Wigraine, Ergostat)
	Chlordiazepoxide (Librax)
	Butorphanol (Stadol)
	Nalbuphine (Nubain)
	Butalbital with acetaminophen (Fioricet)
Nonabused Drugs Important in a Targeted Pain History	Oral contraceptives
	Anticoagulants (heparin, warfarin)
	Antiplatelet agents (aspirin, ticlopidine)
	Antianginals (nitrates)

* From Brust JC: Neurological Aspects of Substance Abuse. Boston, Butterworth-Heinemann, 1993, and Missouri Taskforce on the Misuse, Abuse and Diversion of Prescription Drugs, 1994.

† *Narcotic* is a nonspecific term still used by state boards to describe a drug that induces sleep or dependence: It is not interchangeable with *opioid.* This table lists many (but not all) drugs that may be abused by patients with pain.

General Aspects of the Patient Interview

The following general but significant points enhance the patient interview process:

- The surroundings are professional, comfortable and private.
- The patient is appropriately gowned, is chaperoned if appropriate, and is sitting upright and at eye level with the interviewer, if possible.
- Old records, scans, radiographs, and consultations have been obtained and reviewed before the consultation.

- The physician listens to and does not interrupt the patient or allow outside interruptions.
- The physician remains nonjudgmental; her own moral, religious, and political beliefs are irrelevant to this process.
- The physician is honest and open with the patient; keeping information from the patient at the family's request is usually a bad decision.
- Both the patient and the physician can trust in the confidentiality of both the consultation and the medical records.

It is important to remember that the specialty of pain management is practiced by physicians from a number of disciplines. In particular, physicians trained in operating room anesthesia may not be as sensitive to some certain issues. In my own experience, as a neurologist for whom interviewing patients is a major component of practice, these basic rules of common etiquette are frequently ignored. First, the office should be both professional and comfortable. For reasons of economy, pain clinics are frequently placed in noisy and crowded additions to either the operating room suite or the emergency room. This atmosphere may not be conducive to dealing with patients with acute and chronic pain, who are often extremely apprehensive and easily frustrated.

It is important that patients have a private place where they undress and are examined. Although this may appear to be a small point, a chaotic examining site can inspire a patient's resentment, even if the medical care is of high quality. One other point that needs reinforcing is that physician and patient should always be properly chaperoned. It is not unusual, because of the hectic schedules of both physicians and ancillary personnel, for a patient and physician to be left alone in situations in which this arrangement is at best uncomfortable and at worst compromising and dangerous. Strict adherence to standardized protocol for chaperoning is really the best way of averting serious problems in this area. The keys to obtaining a complete and effective targeted pain history are as follows. The examiner should:

1. Build rapport with the patient by introducing self properly, taking an initial social history, and simultaneously assessing the patient's mood, anxiety level, and capability of giving a history on his or her own.
2. *Most importantly:* Establish the chief complaint at the outset of the history. Why is the patient here? Open-ended questions allow the patient to tell his or her own story.
3. Utilize the framework of the pain litany (discussed earlier) to further investigate the pain. Where is the pain? What is its nature?
4. Do not jump to conclusions. This is the most common cause of error, in that the interview too soon becomes too narrowly focused and important associations either are not pursued or are ignored. The examiner should ask about other doctors whom the patient has seen and their treatments.
5. Determine the impact of the pain on the patient's life—psychological fears, family issues (marriage), compensation, work record.
6. Explore past medical and family history. Using a timeline approach to establish continuity, the current pain should be placed in context with other major medical events: previous surgery, hospitalizations, cancer, medical and paramedical relationships.
7. Obtain a thorough drug history (see Table 8–2). Duration, frequency, amount, and source of medication should be asked about. The importance of this information cannot be overemphasized.

The examination should begin with the physician's introducing himself or herself to the patient and putting the patient at ease. A routine social history, such as occupation, place of employment, marital status, and number of children, should be obtained. During this interchange, the physician should be assessing the verbal and nonverbal cues that ultimately determine the caliber of the historical information. This social introduction affords the physician insight into what type of person the patient is. Over time and with the refinements of experience, this portion of the interview assumes diagnostic importance equal to that of the data-gathering portion of the consultation.

It would seem obvious that the patient's chief complaint would be the logical starting point of any history. Unfortunately, it is my experience that a great deal of time can be spent taking a history without ever addressing the chief complaint. Coming to grips with the patient's primary reason for seeking medical attention is really the crucial piece of data. Is it the pain? Is it questions about disability or worker's compensation? Is it a morbid fear of cancer? Is it that the physician who prescribed the patient's pain medications has retired and the patient is concerned about prescription renewal? Until the physician has a strong sense of the principal reason for the consultation, the history is often both misguided and aimless. Sitting in front of the patient, the physician should always ask himself or herself, "Why has this patient come to see me?" Sometimes, the patient's motives are not what they first appear to be.

Summary of the Targeted History

I cannot overstate the value of the targeted history. It affords the physician the greatest chance of understanding the nature of the pain and, more important, its effects on the patient. Diagnostic tests, laboratory reports, and other consultants' opinions often introduce error when interpreted from a perspective detached from the patient. The physician should remember that, no matter how many physicians have seen the patient earlier, historical facts critical to the diagnosis may have been overlooked or not properly sought.

Taking the targeted history is a social interaction. Courtesy, professionalism, and kindness consistently result in patient satisfaction. Issues related to compensation, returning to work, and concurrent drug use should be dealt with openly and directly, without imposing the physician's personal, political, or religious value judgments.

THE TARGETED PHYSICAL EXAMINATION

If after obtaining the targeted historical information, the pain specialist is lost, the chance that the situation may be suddenly illuminated by the physical examination findings is extremely remote. As a basic point, I emphasize that the physical examination should follow the history and, indeed, be specifically directed by clues obtained during the patient interview. For example, it makes little sense to concentrate on a detailed examination of the sensory function and individual muscle testing in the lower extremities for a patient who has diplopia, facial pain, and a family history of multiple sclerosis. The physical examination is an extension of the history, providing objective support but performed efficiently and systematically so that important findings associated with, or unrelated to, the basic disease are not overlooked.

The examination should not consume a great deal of time. Basic aspects, such as taking blood pressure, performing a screening mental status examination, and checking visual acuity, strength, and deep tendon reflexes, however, pay multiple dividends. On occasion, certain important diseases, such as unrecognized hypertension, diabetic retinopathy, and skin cancer, can be uncovered.

The very physical aspect of examining the patient imparts a reassuring sense of personal caring to the entire consultation. The benefits of this experience are considerable. Pain patients want to be examined, expect to be examined, and ultimately derive benefit from the process. As Goethe said, "We see only what we know."[11] The facility with which we examine patients is ultimately a function of our knowledge, experience, and willingness to learn.

General Aspects

The patient's temperature, pulse, and blood pressure should always be recorded, as should height and weight. The patient should be undressed and properly gowned. It is a constant source of amazement to me how frequently patients are evaluated for painful conditions, even those involving the neck and low back, while remaining fully clothed during the entire examination. The pain specialist should examine the entire body for skin lesions such as hemangiomas, areas of hyperpigmentation, and café au lait spots (neurofibromatosis); document scars from previous operations; and inquire into other scars not mentioned in the initial history. Needle marks, skin ulcerations, and tattoos (which sometimes betray drug culture orientation) may be surprising findings. The spine should be examined for kyphosis, lordosis, scoliosis, and focal areas of tenderness. Dimpling of the skin or excessive hair growth may suggest spina bifida or meningocele. The motility of the spine should also be evaluated in flexion, extension, and lateral rotation. During this period of the examination, an overall assessment of multiple joints can be done for deformities, arthritic change, trauma, and prior surgery. In short, there is much to be learned just by having the patient stand before the physician and asking the patient about abnormalities that become noticeable. No matter how inconvenient or uncomfortable it is, the physician should try never to omit this portion of the examination. Particularly in chronic pain patients, this procedure may yield revelations.

Assessment of Mental Status

Most major intellectual and psychiatric problems become apparent during the history taking. The frequency with which serious intellectual deficits are missed is, however, surprising. For example, subtle aspects of memory, comprehension, and language may not be caught unless they are specifically sought. In my experience, aphasia (a general term for all disturbances of language not the result of faulty articulation) is frequently mistaken for an organic mental syndrome or dementia. Recognition of this point not only is critical in diagnostic evaluation but also has important implications for obtaining informed consent for testing, nerve blocks, and surgical procedures.

Table 8–3 summarizes my approach to rapid assessment of the patient's mental status. Each practitioner should develop a personal set of standard questions to gain a sense of the normal versus the abnormal. Attention to these details in assessing mental status helps to avoid the embarrassment of overlooking a receptive aphasia, Alzheimer's disease, or Korsakoff's syndrome. In many of these situations, patients exhibit an unusual capacity to disguise underlying deficits by reverting to evasions or generalities or by filling in gaps with stereotypical responses that they have used before to escape detection.

One final point relates to the patient's emotional state. The examiner must remain vigilant about the patient's mood and displays of emotion. An unusually silly, euphoric, or grandiose presentation may be seen in manic states. Likewise, a discouraged, hopeless, or self-deprecating presentation may signal serious depression. As highlighted in the discussion on the targeted history, the physician must remain alert for clinical manifestations of drug use, such as slurred speech, motor hyperactivity, sweating, flushing,

TABLE 8–3 **The "Quick and Dirty" Mental Status Examination**

Orientation	Ask the following questions: What is your full name? What is today's date? What is the year? Who is the president? Who is the vice president?
Calculations	Ask the following questions: How many nickels are in a dollar? How many dollars do 60 nickles make?
Memory	Ask the following questions: What was your mother's maiden name? Who was President before Bill Clinton? Give the patient three items to remember (examples, a red ball, a blue telephone, and address 66 Hill Street). After several minutes of conversation, ask the patient to repeat the list.
Speech	Have the patient repeat two simple sentences, such as: Today is a lovely day. The weather this weekend is expected to be excellent. Have the patient name several objects in the room. Ask the patient to rhyme simple words, such as ball, pat, and can.
Comprehension	Ask the patient to: Put the right hand on the left hand. Point to the ceiling with the left index finger.

This simple screening mental status examination uncovers many (but not all) cognitive deficits. It can be performed in less than 3 minutes and is useful in evaluating basic aspects of memory, language, and general intellectual capacity.

and distractibility. In short, the physician should get to know the patient but, in the end, should vigorously resist any early impulse to suggest that stress or anxiety alone is the principal cause of the patient's pain.

Cranial Nerves

To return to the theme of keeping the targeted physical examination simple so that important points are not missed: The evaluation of cranial nerve (CN) function often overwhelms practitioners not trained in clinical neurology. It remains an important area, particularly in the evaluation of headache and facial pain. Rapid recognition of CN dysfunction may have profound significance for localizing a cerebral lesion or identifying increased intracranial pressure, or, in combination with the history, may be a strong indicator of a specific disease (e.g., explosive headache plus CN III palsy implies a ruptured aneurysm until that is ruled out).

Table 8–4 highlights an efficient approach to the clinical evaluation of the cranial nerves. Certainly, when headache and facial pain are the basic issues, particular attention should be given to this portion of the examination. The key, once again, is developing a routine that, with practice, becomes thorough. It is far beyond the scope of this chapter to describe all the nuances of cranial nerve function.[16] Anyone evaluating patients for headache or facial pain should be able at least to recognize papilledema and abnormalities of ocular motor nerve function, be familiar with the sensory division of the trigeminal nerve, and be able to recognize isolated cranial nerve palsies. More complex problems, such as diplopia, cavernous sinus disease, and complex brain stem lesions, are best left to specialists in neuroophthalmology and neurology.

In general, the pain specialist, even one whose basic training has been in anesthesia or psychiatry, can, with the proper effort, become familiar with the basics of common disorders. Ultimately, the physician who does make the effort to learn this material and incorporate it into clinical pain management practice will not have to deal constantly with feeling uneasy about a weakness in clinical aptitude. Such a physician will also avoid losing precious time in developing experience with these key physical findings associated with a variety of headache and facial pain problems.

Motor Examination

Motor examination should begin with inspection of muscle volume and contour, paying particular attention to atrophy and hypertrophy. The patient should be properly gowned so that these observations can be made without invading the patient's privacy. During this examination, fasiculations, contractures, alterations in posture, and adventitious movements may be identified. Strength is measured both proximally and distally in the upper and lower extremities and is

TABLE 8–4 ***Clinical Evaluations of Cranial Nerve Function***

Cranial Nerve(s)		
Number	*Name*	**Evaluation Procedure(s)**
I	Olfactory	Test ability to identify familiar aromatic odors, one naris at a time with eyes closed (not routinely tested).
II	Optic	Test vision with Snellen chart or Rosenbaum near-vision chart. Perform ophthalmoscopic examination of fundi. Be able to recognize papilledema. Test fields of vision using confrontation and double simultaneous stimulation.
III, IV, VI	Oculomotor, trochlear, abducens	Inspect eyelids for drooping (ptosis). Inspect pupil size for equality (direct and consensual response). Check for nystagmus. Assess basic fields of gaze. Note asymmetric extraocular movements.
V	Trigeminal	Palpate jaw muscles for tone and strength while patient clenches teeth. Test superficial pain and touch sensation in each branch: V_1, V_2, V_3.
VII	Facial	Test corneal reflex. Inspect symmetry of facial features. Have patient smile, frown, puff cheeks, wrinkle forehead. Watch for spasmodic, jerking movements of face.
VIII	Acoustic	Test sense of hearing with watch or tuning fork. Compare bone and air conduction of sound.
IX	Glossopharyngeal	Test gag reflex and ability to swallow.
X	Vagus	Inspect palate and uvula for symmetry with gag reflex. Observe for swallowing difficulty. Have patient take small sip of water. Watch for nasal or hoarse quality of speech.
IX	Spinal accessory	Test trapezius strength (have patient shrug shoulders against resistance). Test sternocleidomastoid muscle strength (have patient turn head to each side against resistance).
XII	Hypoglossal	Inspect tongue in mouth and while protruded for symmetry, fasciculations, and atrophy. Test tongue strength with index fingers when tongue is pressed against cheek.

graded according to the scale shown in Table 8–5. Detailed individual muscle testing is not carried out unless a specific nerve root or plexopathy is under investigation.

Tone is best tested by passive manipulation, note being made of the resistance of muscle when voluntary control is absent. Changes in tone are more readily detected in muscles of the arms and legs than in muscles of the trunk. Relaxation is critical to proper evaluation. Hypertonicity is usually seen with lesions rostral to the anterior horn cells. Hypotonicity is associated with diseases affecting the neuroaxis below this level. Study of the motor system should be integrated with evaluation of the sensory examination and deep tendon reflexes, to provide cumulative information critical to identifying "the site of lesion"—brain, brain stem, spinal cord, root, plexus, nerve, or muscle.

Sensory Examination

The sensory examination should be kept simple and should be targeted by clues obtained through the history. Certainly, time spent in defining sensory loss in the lower extremities would be justified in a patient complaining of pain, weakness, and numbness in the foot but not in one who has double vision and facial pain. Note in Figure 8–1 the difference between the skin areas innervated by dermatomes—specific segments of the cord, roots, or dorsal root ganglia—and the corresponding peripheral nerve cutaneous sensory distribution. Knowledge of these specific differences and of changes in motor function and reflexes clinically define a nerve root from a peripheral nerve abnormality. Tables 8–6 and 8–7 highlight comparisons between specific spinal root and peripheral nerve lesions of the upper and lower extremities. With time, experience, and persistence, the pain specialist can become confident in the evaluation of peripheral nerve root lesions. So many of the common pain syndromes (cervical radiculopathies, lumbar radiculopathies, carpal tunnel syndrome, femoral neuropathy, peroneal neuropathy) may be rapidly and accurately diagnosed without expensive and uncomfortable neurodiagnostic testing. Being persistent and resisting the fear that the task is too overwhelming results in the ability to efficiently evaluate patients in pain.

For pain syndromes of the upper extremity, the examiner should be able to differentiate sensory involvement of the radial, median, and ulnar nerves from that of specific roots (C5–T1). For pain syndromes of the lower extremities, the examiner should be able to differentiate the peroneal and tibial nerve sensory distribution from that of the L4, L5, and S1 roots. Such distinctions elucidate most of the common problems. Over time, the examiner can become more knowledgeable and may develop a stronger foundation than many neurologists, neurosurgeons, and orthopedists have.

TABLE 8–5 ***Grading of Muscle Strength***

Clinical Finding	Grade	Percent of Normal Response
No evidence of contractility	0	0
Slight contractility, no movement	1	10
Full range of motion, gravity eliminated	2	25
Full range of motion with gravity	3	50
Full range of motion against gravity, some resistance	4	75
Full range of motion against gravity, full resistance	5	100

From Chipps EM, Clanin NJ, Campbell VG: Neurologic Disorder. St. Louis, Mosby–Year Book, 1992.

Deep Tendon Reflexes

Deep tendon reflexes are actually muscle stretch reflexes mediated through neuromuscular spindles. They are the one facet of the clinical examination that is objective (Table 8–8). Responses to mental status testing and motor examination, performance on sensory testing, and even gait can be consciously altered by the patient for any of a variety of reasons. Guillain-Barré syndrome (acute inflammatory polyneuropathy), however, a condition that in its initial stages may be misdiagnosed as anxiety related, characteristically shows absence of all the deep tendon reflexes, which is an important early clue to the organic nature of the disorder.

A deep tendon reflex examination can be conducted using the numerals 1 through 8 (Fig. 8–2). I have not found testing of the superficial reflexes, such as the abdominal or cremasteric reflexes, to be of particular value in clinical assessment. The only superficial reflex I utilize is the plantar reflex (a superficial reflex innervated by the tibial nerve, L4–S2). The response to stroking the plantar surface of the foot is usually flexion of both the foot and the toes. In diseases of the cortical spinal system, there is dorsiflexion of the toes, especially the great toe, with separation or fanning of the others; this, Babinski's sign of upper motor neuron involvement (brain, brain stem, and spinal cord), is often paired with increased deep tendon reflexes and clonus (i.e., sustained muscular contractions following a stretch stimulus noted frequently in the ankle).

Unilateral absence of a deep tendon reflex implies disease at the peripheral nerve or root level. Diffuse reduction or absence of deep tendon reflexes suggests a more generalized process affecting the peripheral nerve, seen frequently in peripheral neuropathies secondary to diabetes, alcohol abuse, or inflammation. The objective data obtained quite rapidly from testing deep tendon reflexes are correlated with motor and sensory findings to determine whether a problem lies in a specific peripheral nerve, specific nerve root, diffuse peripheral nerve, or spinal cord. It should take less than 30 seconds to complete this part of the examination.

Examination of Gait

Walking is an intricate process influenced by mechanical factors such as muscles, bones, tendons, and joints and, more importantly, dependent upon nervous system inte-

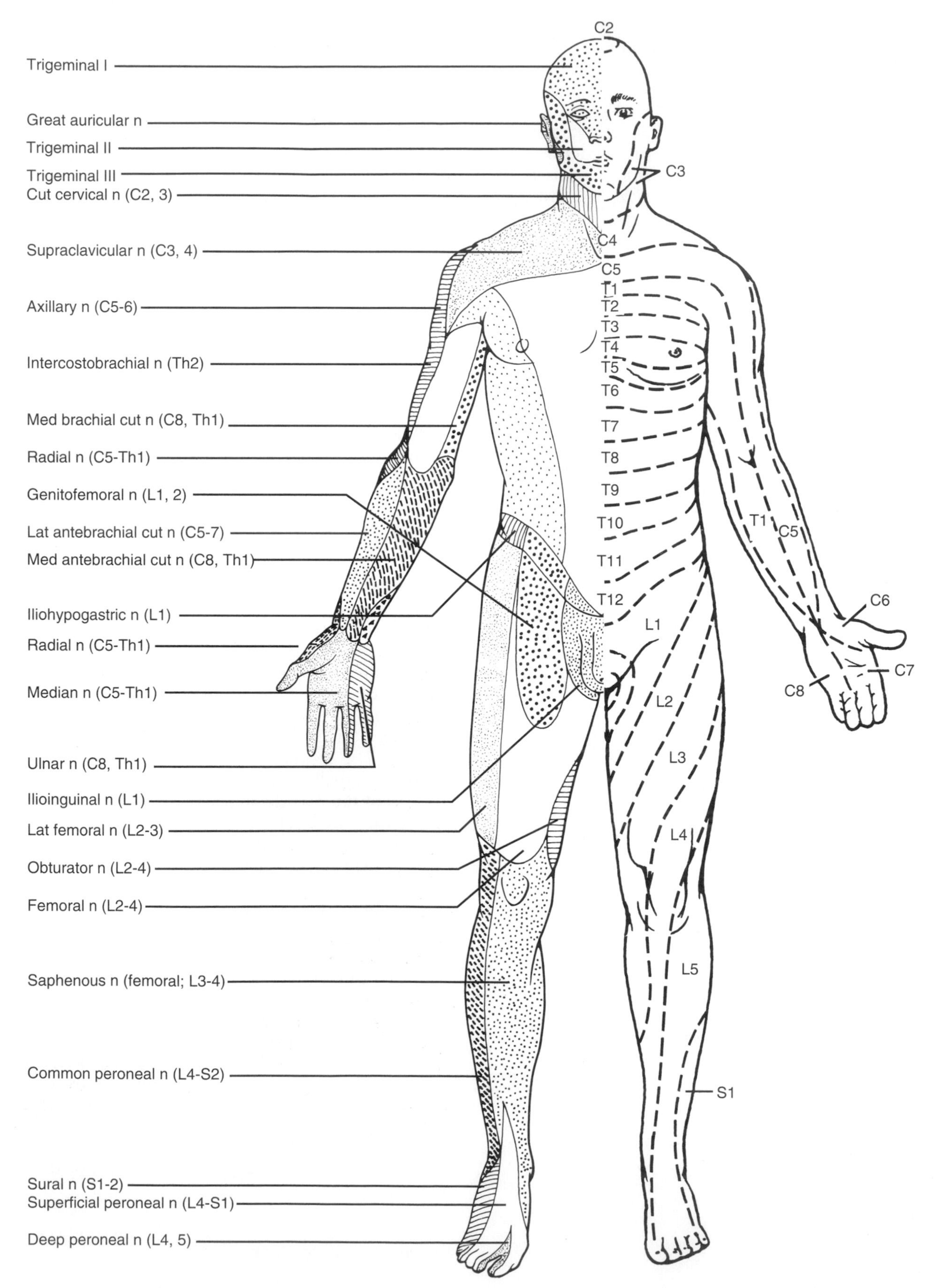

FIGURE 8–1 *Comparison of spinal segmental (dermatomal) and peripheral nerve cutaneous sensory supply. (Adapted from Haerer AF [ed]: DeJong's The Neurologic Examination, ed 5. Philadelphia: JB Lippincott, 1992.)*

TABLE 8–6 *Clinical Manifestations of Root Versus Nerve Lesions in the Arm*

Roots	**C5**	**C6**	**C7**	**C8**	**T1**
Sensory supply	Lateral border upper arm	Lateral forearm, including finger I	Over triceps, midforearm and finger III	Medial forearm to finger V	Axilla to elbow
Reflex affected	Biceps reflex	None	Triceps reflex	None	None
Motor loss	Deltoid Infraspinatus Rhomboids Supraspinatus	Biceps Brachialis Brachioradialis	Latissimus dorsi Pectoralis major Triceps Wrist extensors Wrist flexors	Finger extensors Finger flexors Flexor carpi ulnaris	Intrinsic hand muscles (in some thenar muscles through C8)
Nerves	**Axillary (C5, C6)**	**(C5, C6)**	**Radial (C5–C8)**	**Median (C6–C8, T1)**	**Ulnar (C8, T1)**
Sensory supply	Over deltoid	Lateral forearm to wrist	Lateral dorsal forearm and back of thumb and finger II	Lateral palm and lateral fingers, I, II, III and half of IV	Medial palm and finger V and medial half of finger IV
Reflex affected	None	Biceps reflex	Triceps reflex	None	None
Motor loss	Deltoid	Biceps Brachialis	Brachioradialis Finger extensors Forearm supinator Triceps Wrist extensors	Abductor pollicis brevis Long flexors of fingers I, II, III Pronators of forearm Wrist flexors	Intrinsic hand muscles Flexor carpi ulnaris Flexors of fingers IV, V

From Patten J: Neurological Differential Diagnosis. New York, Springer-Verlag, 1977.

TABLE 8–7 *Clinical Manifestations of Root Versus Nerve Lesions in the Leg*

Roots	**L2**	**L3**	**L4**	**L5**	**S1**
Sensory supply	Across upper thigh	Across lower thigh	Across knee to medial malleolus	Side of leg to dorsum and sole of foot	Behind lateral malleolus to lateral foot
Reflex affected	None	None	Patellar reflex	None	Achilles reflex
Motor loss	Hip flexion	Knee extension	Inversion of foot	Dorsiflexion of toes and foot	Plantar flexion and eversion of foot

Nerves	**Obturator (L2–L4)**	**Nerve Femoral (L2–L4)**	**Peroneal Division of Sciatic Nerve (L4, L5, S1–S3)**	**Tibial Division of Sciatic Nerve (L4, L5, S1–S3)**
Sensory supply	Medial thigh	Anterior thigh to medial malleolus	Anterior leg to dorsum of foot	Posterior leg to sole and lateral aspect of foot
Reflex affected	None	Patellar reflex	None	Achilles reflex
Motor loss	Adduction of thigh	Extension of knee	Dorsiflexion, inversion, and eversion of foot	Plantar flexion and inversion of foot

From Patten J: Neurological Differential Diagnosis. New York, Springer-Verlag, 1977.

TABLE 8–8 *Deep Tendon Reflex Scale*

Grade	**Deep Tendon Reflex Response**
0+	No response
1+	Sluggish
2+	Active or normal
3+	More brisk than expected, slightly hyperactive
4+	Abnormally hyperactive, with intermittent clonus

From Seidel HM, et al: Mosby's Guide to Physical Examination, 3rd ed. St. Louis, Mosby–Year Book, Inc., 1995.

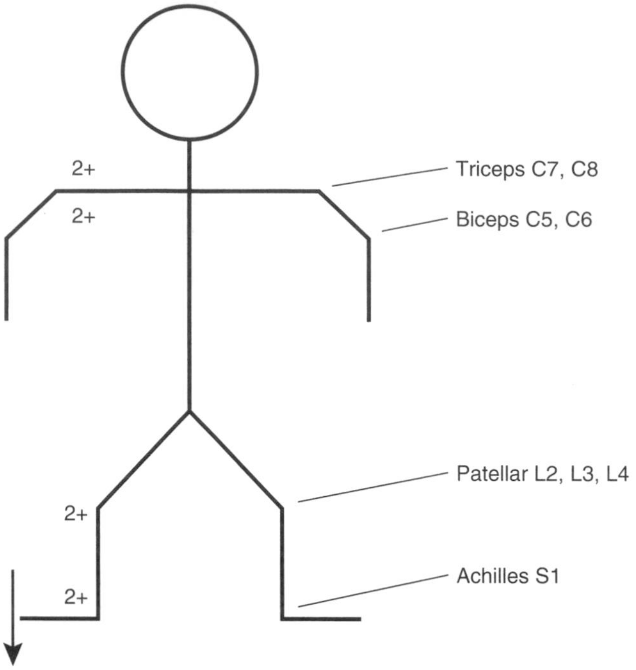

2+
Triceps C7, C8
2+
Biceps C5, C6
Patellar L2, L3, L4
2+
Achilles S1
2+

FIGURE 8–2 *A deep tendon reflex examination.*

gration. Just watching the patient walk during the examination is an extremely valuable exercise. I suggest that the patient be asked to walk with the eyes open and closed and to stand with the eyes open and closed (Romberg's sign). Gaits associated with parkinsonism, normal pressure hydrocephalus, muscular dystrophy, stroke, peripheral nerve injury, cerebellar disorder, Huntington's chorea, and hysteria (astasia-abasia) are but a few characteristic patterns of disturbed locomotion. In short, a strong measure of neuroorthopedic well-being is implied by the patient who walks well with the eyes open and closed.

CONCLUSION

The basic point of this chapter is simple. A targeted, well-organized pain history is the foundation of proper diagnosis. Advances in diagnostic technology, no matter how sophisticated, cannot replace listening to the patient's story of the illness. It is through this process that we most effectively gain insight, not only into the nature of the illness but, more important, into the personality of the patient who is in pain. The professionalism and sensitivity with which we obtain this information does much to establish our relationship with the patient and the ultimate success of our therapies. If there is anywhere room for shortcuts, it is not in this portion of the evaluation.

The targeted physical examination should be viewed as an extension of the insights derived from the history. It should be performed in a professional, thorough, but not laborious fashion. As the calling of pain management becomes more popular, physicians of various disciplines should avoid faddish technologic advances and opportunism made possible by inequities in reimbursement and should commit themselves to the very basics: obtaining historical data and eliciting physical findings. In my opinion, energy expended to this end will reduce costs, enhance patient satisfaction, and foster lasting credibility in the evolving field of pain management.

REFERENCES

1. Rowland LP (ed): Merritt's Textbook of Neurology, ed 7. Philadelphia, Lea & Febiger, 1984.
2. Judge RD, Zuidema GD, Fitzgerald FT (eds): Clinical Diagnosis: A Physiologic Approach, ed 5. Boston, Little, Brown, 1989.
3. Diamond S, Dalessio DJ (eds): The Practicing Physician's Approach to Headache, ed 4. Baltimore, Williams & Wilkins, 1986.
4. Fromm GH: Trigeminal neuralgia and related disorders. Neurol Clin 7:305–320, 1989.
5. Patten J: Neurological Differential Diagnosis. New York, Springer-Verlag, 1977.
6. Quote attributed to Mark Twain: [1835–1910].
7. Littrell RA, Haye LR, Stillner V: Carisoprodol (Soma): A new and cautious perspective on an old agent. South Med J 86:753–756, 1993.
8. Saper JR: Chronic headache syndromes. Neurol Clin 7:387–412, 1989.
9. Warfield CA (ed): Manual of Pain Management. Philadelphia, JB Lippincott, 1991.
10. Moulin DE: Pain in multiple sclerosis. Neurol Clin 7:321–332, 1989.
11. Goethe JW: Trilogy of Passion, 1824.
12. Missouri Task Force on the Misuse, Abuse and Diversion of Prescription Drugs. A Guide to Prescribing, Administering and Dispensing Controlled Substances in Missouri. Jefferson City, Mo, Missouri Task Force on the Misuse, Abuse, and Diversion of Prescription Drugs, 1994.
13. Trachtenberg AI: Opiates for pain: Patients' tolerance and society's intolerance (Letter to the editor). JAMA 271:427, 1994.
14. Brust JCM: Neurological Aspects of Substance Abuse. Boston, Butterworth-Heinemann, 1993.
15. Chipps EM, Clanin NJ, Campbell VG: Neurologic Disorders. St. Louis, CV Mosby, 1992.
16. Haerer AF (ed): DeJong's The Neurologic Examination, ed 5. Philadelphia, JB Lippincott, 1992.

CHAPTER • 9

Rational Use of Laboratory Tests in the Evaluation of Pain

Charles D. Donohoe, MD

The targeted history and physical examination remain the most effective and economical modalities for evaluating pain. We believe that routine laboratory tests are often ignored in favor of expensive radiologic and neurophysiologic studies that mesmerize clinicians. Findings such as pyuria, profound anemia, and elevation of acute phase proteins are often crucial in both identifying the cause of pain and assessing the general medical status of the patient. Although clinical laboratory medicine is a massive and rapidly evolving discipline that truly defies condensation, it is our hope that this chapter provides a practical beginning. Expertise in treating pain implies broad knowledge of medicine in general.

PITFALLS OF CLINICAL PRACTICE

There are several areas in clinical practice where mistakes are commonly made. The first involves failure to contact family members of a confused patient who is obviously unable to give a coherent history. The second is failure to obtain old records. Third, and equally tragic, is the mistaken supposition that because the patient has seen multiple physicians in the past basic laboratory work has been ordered. The ability to avoid these mistakes demands a discipline that emphasizes the critical details of the history and prior diagnostic workup. This effort is extremely effective in containing costs, conserving physicians' time, and ultimately arriving at an accurate diagnosis. In difficult patients who have seen several physicians, quality control of earlier historical data and diagnostic workup is often ignored and each additional consult simply compounds the sloppy imprecision of the preceding evaluations. It pays the clinician to take time, at the beginning, to get it right. Frequently the best use of technology is a telephone call to a concerned family member or a former treating physician.

THE BASICS

Table 9–1 lists a basic battery of laboratory tests commonly utilized to evaluate pain. We will use it as a focal point, realizing that the selection of specific tests depends on multiple factors, including age, gender, duration and location of pain, coexisting medical problems, and results of other laboratory studies. One preliminary tenet of pain practice management is that, once a physician orders lab tests, he is responsible not only for seeing that the tests are performed but for personally reviewing the results. Failure to do both can have serious medicolegal implications.

ACUTE PHASE PROTEINS

The erythrocyte sedimentation rate (ESR) and the C-reactive protein (CRP) value are the most commonly used indicators of acute phase response. This response includes numerous protein changes, including increases in the complement system, fibrinogen, serum amyloid, and acute phase phenomena including fever, thrombocytosis, leukocytosis, and anemia. A reduction in serum albumin is characteristic of the acute phase response. These complex changes are induced by inflammation-associated cytokines, particularly interleukin-6, and are seen in response to infection, trauma, surgery, burns, cancer, inflammatory conditions, and psychological stress.[1]

The ESR, the rate at which erythrocytes fall through plasma, is actually an indirect measure of plasma acute phase protein concentration and depends mainly on the plasma concentration of fibrinogen. Unfortunately, it can be influenced by other factors, including the size, shape, and number of erythrocytes, and by other plasma protein constituents such as immunoglobulins. CRP is a glycoprotein produced during acute inflammation and derives its name from its ability to react and precipitate *Pneumococcus* C polysaccharide. It has fewer associated technical problems and is resistant to the interference of anemia or plasma protein concentrations that can alter the ESR. CRP is easy to perform, and its overall utilization has recently increased.

The ESR increases steadily with age, whereas the CRP value does not. The ESR changes relatively slowly (over several days) in response to the onset of inflammation,

TABLE 9–1 **The Basic Pain Laboratory Battery**

1. Complete blood count
2. Acute phase proteins, erythrocyte sedimentation rate (ESR), C-reactive protein (CRP)
3. Blood chemistry: Glucose, sodium, potassium, chloride, carbon dioxide, calcium, phosphorus, urea nitrogen, creatinine, uric acid, total protein, albumin, globulin, bilirubin
4. Enzymes: Alkaline phosphatase, creatine kinase, lactate dehydrogenase, aspartate aminotransferase, alanine aminotransferase
5. Thyroid (TSH)
6. Vitamin B_{12}

whereas the CRP responds rapidly (several hours). CRP has certain advantages over the ESR, and both can be used in concert.

Like the CRP, ESR determination is utilized to detect inflammatory disease, follow its course, and at times in a more general fashion to suggest the presence of occult organic disease in patients who have symptoms but no definitive physical or laboratory findings. The ESR is not a specific test. The Westergren ESR method is generally more resistant than the Wintrobe method to the effects of anemia. ESR values greater than 100 mm/hr generally imply infectious disease, neoplasia, inflammatory conditions, or chronic renal disease. Realizing that the ESR is affected by age, a rough index for determining the upper limits of normal can be derived by the formula:

$$\frac{\text{Age in years} + 5}{2}$$

For an 85-year-old person, this would place the upper range of normal of a Westergren ESR at roughly 45 mm/hr. In painful conditions affecting the elderly such as temporal arteritis, use of both the ESR and CRP is encouraged.

THE COMPLETE BLOOD COUNT

The complete blood count (CBC) is a good starting point for laboratory testing in that it provides a cost-effective glimpse into a person's general health. The major emphasis in hematology is placed on cellular elements, including red blood cells (RBC), white blood cells (WBC), and platelets. Several tests form the backbone of laboratory diagnosis and can be very useful in the evaluation of both acute and chronic pain. Hemoglobin is the oxygen-carrying compound contained in red cells, and, in association with red blood cell count and hematocrit, signals anemia.

Anemia is defined as hemoglobin values less than 13g/dL for men and less than 11g/dL for women. Conditions that result in pseudoanemia include overhydration, obtaining blood specimens from an intravenous line, hypoalbuminemia, and pregnancy. Heavy smoking, dehydration, and states of extreme leukocytosis may produce elevated hemoglobin and hematocrit levels.[2] The red cell indices—mean corpuscular volume (MCV), mean corpuscular hemoglobin (MCH), mean corpuscular hemoglobin concentration (MCHC), and red blood cell distribution width (RDW)—aid in the diagnosis of a variety of conditions, including anemia, hemoglobinopathies, and spherocytosis.

The peripheral blood smear examines the size, color, and other morphologic characteristics of red and white cells important in the evaluation of hematologic disease. Reticulocyte count, serum ferritin level, serum iron, and total iron-binding capacity (TIBC) enhance the evaluation of anemia. The reticulocyte can be viewed as an intermediate between a nucleated RBC in the bone marrow and a mature, nonnucleated RBC. The reticulocyte count is an index of bone marrow activity. Hemolytic anemia, acute bleeding, and the treatment of deficiency states related to vitamin B_{12}, folate, and iron result in reticulocytosis. Anemia associated with bone marrow failure is reflected in a low reticulocyte count.[3]

Because it is the major storage compound of iron, serum ferritin is a very sensitive measure for iron deficiency. Serum TIBC is an approximation of the serum transferrin level and is elevated in iron deficiency anemia slightly before a decrease in serum iron becomes evident. Transferrin saturation (the percentage of transferrin bound to iron) declines with classic iron deficiency anemia. On the other hand, in hemochromatosis, a common genetic disorder of iron overload, persistent elevations of ferritin and transferrin saturation are effective screening tools in early recognition of this disorder.[4] The reduction in serum haptoglobin, a plasma glycoprotein that binds to oxyhemoglobin and delivers it to the reticuloendothelial system, is a useful test for evaluating intravascular hemolysis.

At birth, 80% of hemoglobin is fetal-type hemoglobin (HbF), which is replaced by the adult type (HbA) by age 6 months. An abnormal type of hemoglobin common in the Western Hemisphere is sickle hemoglobin (HbS). The heterozygous state, sickle trait (SA), is present in about 8% of African Americans. These persons are not anemic and are otherwise healthy. They rarely experience hematuria but may develop splenic infarcts during exposure to hypoxic conditions (e.g., nonpressurized airplanes). Homozygous sickle cell disease (SS) produces moderate to severe anemia. Crises secondary to small vessel occlusion with infarction often present with abdominal pain or bone pain. The disease does not present until after age 6 months with the disappearance of HbF, which has high affinity for oxygen.

Screening tests (sickle cell prep) rely on the tendency of hemoglobin S to become insoluble when oxygen tension is low, ultimately crystallizing and distorting the red cell into a sickle shape. A common screening method (Sickle Dex) avoids coverslip methods that utilize chemical (dithionite) deoxygenation and precipitation of hemoglobin S. This test is not useful before 6 months of age and does not distinguish between sickle cell disease and the trait. Definitive diagnosis requires hemoglobin electrophoresis. All African Americans with unexplained anemia, hematuria, arthralgias, or abdominal pain should be screened for sickle cell disease.[5]

White Blood Cells

WBC are the body's first line of defense against infection. Lymphocytes and plasma cells produce antibodies, whereas neutrophils and monocytes respond by phagocytosis. Alterations in the WBC provide a clue to a variety of diseases, both benign and malignant. Most individuals have WBC counts between 5000 and 10,000 per cubic millimeter. The mean WBC count in African Americans may be at least 500 per cubic millimeter less than those in Europeans, with some individuals demonstrating counts as much as 3000 per cubic millimeter lower. There are also diurnal variations in neutrophils and eosinophils. Neutrophil levels peak at about 4:00 PM at values almost 30% above those at 7:00 AM. Eosinophils more consistently parallel cortisol levels, being highest early in the morning and 40% lower later in the afternoon.

The classic picture of acute bacterial infection includes leukocytosis with an associated increased percentages of neutrophils and bands (immature forms); however the leukocytosis and increased number of bands (shift to the left) may be absent in as many as 30% of acute bacterial infections. Overwhelming infection, particularly in debilitated elderly persons, may fail to show any leukocytosis. Heavy cigarette smoking has been associated with total WBC counts that average 1000 per cubic millimeter higher than those for nonsmokers. Other causes of neutrophilic leukocytosis include metabolic abnormalities such as uremia, diabetic acidosis, acute gouty attacks, seizures, and pregnancy. Adrenal corticosteroids, even in low doses, can produce considerable increases in segmented neutrophils and total WBC count. Medications such as lithium carbonate (for bipolar disorder), epinephrine (for asthma) and the toxic effects of lead can result in leukocytosis.

Eosinophilia is most often associated with acute allergic reactions such as asthma, hay fever, and drug allergy. It is also seen in parasitic diseases, skin disorders such as pemphigus and psoriasis, and miscellaneous conditions such as connective tissue disorders, particularly polyarteritis nodosa, Churg-Strauss vasculitis, and sarcoidosis. Eosinophilia may also be a nonspecific indicator of occult malignancy.

Viral infection is most often manifested by lymphocytosis with an elevated (or relatively elevated) lymphocyte count in a person with a normal or decreased total WBC count. The usual lymphocytosis identified in viral infection is a relative one: granulocytes are reduced while the total lymphocyte number remains constant. Infectious mononucleosis is associated with absolute lymphocytosis and atypical lymphocytes. The leukemoid reaction is defined as a nonleukemic elevation in the WBC count above 50,000 per cubic millimeter. It is an exaggerated form of the nonneoplastic granulocyte reaction associated with severe bacterial infections, burns, tissue necrosis, hemolytic anemia, and juvenile rheumatoid arthritis.

Neutropenia is defined as a WBC count less than 4000 per cubic millimeter. Drug-induced agranulocytosis is a major clinical issue in pain management, particularly its association with commonly utilized medications, including phenytoin (Dilantin), carbamazepine (Carbatrol, Tegretol), nonsteroidal antiinflammatory drugs (NSAID), and many other medications used in pain management. Neutropenia should prompt an immediate review of all medications. Other conditions associated with neutropenia include aplastic anemia, aleukemic leukemia, hypersplenism, viral infections, and cyclic and chronic idiopathic neutropenia. Severe neutropenia (<1500 WBC per cubic millimeter) should be regarded as an acute emergency: careful follow-up and hematology consultation are mandatory.

In the area of hematopoietic malignancy, cells of lymphocyte origin predominate. For purposes of simplification, most lymphocytes arise from precursors in bone marrow. Of peripheral blood lymphocytes, about 75% are T cells (those lymphocytes that mature in the thymus) and 15% are B cells (those that have matured in the bone marrow, and later in the spleen or lymph nodes). All T lymphocytes develop an antigenic marker for the T cell family called CD2. The CD (cluster designation classification) applies a single CD number to all antibodies that appear to react with the same or very similar WBC antigens. Of the T cells, about 75% are of the CD4 helper-inducer type and about 25% are of the CD8 cytotoxic-suppressor type.

B cells are characterized by having a surface immunoglobulin antibody rather than the CD3 antigen receptor characteristic of mature T cells. B cells are parents of plasma cells, which can secrete specific antibodies to antigens initially recognized by the parent B lymphocyte. Initially, these antibodies are immunoglobulin M (IgM); later, the immunoglobulin changes type to IgG (or less commonly to IgA or IgE). Finally, there is a group of lymphocyte-like cells known as natural killer cells (NKC) that possess neither a T lymphocyte marker antigen A nor B lymphocyte surface immunoglobulin. NKC account for the remaining 10% of peripheral blood lymphocytes.[6]

Platelets and Blood Coagulation

An important aspect of any pain history is the identification of medications that influence coagulation. Heparin, aspirin, NSAID, warfarin (Coumadin), ticlopidine (Ticlid), and clopidogrel (Plavix) fall into this category. Any history of easy bleeding or bruising should prompt further evaluation.

Normal human platelet count generally ranges from 150,000 to 400,000 platelets per cubic millimeter. Platelet counts below 50,000 per cubic millimeter indicate severe thrombocytopenia. Platelet counts greater than 900,000 per cubic millimeter indicate thrombocytosis and a resultant hypercoagulable state. The most common causes of thrombocytopenia are immune-mediated, drug-induced, and post–blood transfusions. Many cases have no demonstrable cause. Other factors include hypersplenism, bone marrow deficiency, microangiopathic hemolytic anemia, infection, thyrotoxicosis, uremia, and preeclampsia. Drug-induced thrombocytopenia is common. Intravenous administration of heparin causes thrombocytopenia with platelet counts below 100,000 per cubic millimeter in as many as 15% of patients.[7] This effect has even been seen with heparin flushes. Other medications commonly implicated include cimetidine (Tagamet), quinine, quinidine, and furosemide (Lasix).

Thrombocytosis with platelet counts greater than 1 million are associated with myeloproliferative disorders, idiopathic thrombocythemia, and severe hemolytic anemia. Other common causes are occult malignancy, post-splenectomy, and acute and chronic infection or inflammatory disease. Both arterial and venous thrombosis can occur.

Coagulation Parameters

The prothrombin time (PT) indicates mainly defects in the extrinsic coagulation system. It is used as a liver function test and as a general screening tool for coagulation disorders. When PT is used to monitor anticoagulation therapy with warfarin, the international normalized ratio (INR) is preferred because of its ability to standardize varied thromboplastin reagents.[8] The INR is a monitoring value for warfarin after the patient has been stabilized, but it is not applied as a general marker of coagulation or liver function. Awareness of the patient's taking warfarin and of his coagulation status is critical. We have seen several patients with pain secondary to retroperitoneal hemorrhage who had marked elevations of PT and INR that went unrecognized for months.

GLUCOSE

Diabetes is a common disorder, affecting 6 million Americans. Approximately 1 million are classified as type 1 diabetics, their disease ascribed to an autoimmune process that ultimately leads to beta cell destruction. Insulin resistance, obesity, and a strong genetic predisposition characterize the more prevalent form, type 2 diabetes. The myriad painful complications to diabetes include neuropathy, foot ulceration, and Charcot's joints.

The American Diabetes Association criteria for the diagnosis of diabetes mellitus are the following (Table 9–2): (1) The classic symptoms of diabetes, including polydipsia, polyuria, and weight loss, plus a casual glucose concentration ≥200 mg/dL. (*Casual* is defined as a measurement taken at any time of day, without regard for the time since the last meal.) (2) A fasting plasma glucose value ≥126 mg/dL (fast being defined as no calorie intake for at least 8 hours). (3) An oral glucose tolerance test value, 2 hours postload, of ≥200 mg/dL. Note that, when the diagnosis is based purely on blood glucose measurements—either the fasting blood glucose or the oral glucose tolerance test—in the absence of clinical symptoms, abnormalities must be found on two different days rather than on a single occasion only.[9]

TABLE 9–2 American Diabetes Association Criteria for the Diagnosis of Diabetes Mellitus

1. Symptoms of diabetes (polydipsia, polyuria, and weight loss) plus a casual glucose ≥200 mg/dL. *Casual* is defined as any time of the day without regard to time since last meal.
2. Fasting glucose ≥126 mg/dL. *Fasting* is defined as no caloric intake for at least 8 hours.
3. Two-hour postload glucose ≥200 mg/dL on an oral glucose tolerance test. Oral glucose tolerance test is not recommended as a first-line test because the fasting glucose is easier to perform, more acceptable to patients, and less expensive.
4. In the absence of unequivocal hyperglycemia with acute metabolic decompensation, these criteria should be confirmed by repeat testing on a different day. For example, an abnormal casual glucose >200 mg/dL without symptoms should be confirmed on a different day with a fasting glucose determination.

Hemoglobin A1C determination is a valuable tool for monitoring blood sugar, but it is not recommended for the diagnosis of diabetes. In adults, hemoglobin A constitutes about 98% of normal hemoglobin. About 7% of hemoglobin A consists of molecules that have been partially modified by the attachment of glucose. Hemoglobin A1C is the major component of this glycosylated hemoglobin. It is an effective index for monitoring diabetes therapy and patient compliance, and it generally reflects the average blood glucose level during the preceding 2 to 3 months.[10]

Clinicians must be aware that medications such as glucocorticoids, nicotinic acid, and phenytoin (Dilantin) can impair insulin activity and elevate blood glucose. Another consideration is misdiagnosis of hypoglycemia. This overused label has been sensationalized in the popular press arbitrarily defined and applied in situations where there are vague protean symptoms but no objective abnormality of glucose metabolism. Those rather rare diseases in which hypoglycemia is actually a valid issue include insulinoma, nonpancreatic tumors such as fibrosarcoma and hepatoma, hepatic disease (including chronic alcoholism), and insulin overdose.[11]

ELECTROLYTES

The most frequent electrolyte abnormality involves sodium, the most important cation of the body. Hyponatremia is the most common abnormality. Symptoms related to hyponatremia, such as nausea, malaise, lethargy, psychosis, and seizures, generally do not occur until the plasma sodium value falls below 120 mEq/L. Diuretics are often implicated. Carbamazepine (Tegretol, Carbatrol) a medication commonly used in pain management, can be associated with persistent hyponatremia. The other major categories of hyponatremia include conditions of general sodium and water depletion (including gastrointestinal loss due to vomiting, diarrhea, or tube drainage), losses through skin associated with burns or sweating, endocrine loss associated with Addison's disease, and sudden withdrawal of long-term steroid therapy. Dilutional hyponatremia is associated with congestive heart failure, hyperhydrosis, nephrotic syndrome, cirrhosis, hypoalbuminemia, and acute renal failure.[12]

The syndrome of inappropriate antidiuretic hormone secretion (SIADH) is characterized by hyponatremia with reduced plasma osmolality in the face of an elevated urinary sodium value but normal extracellular volume and renal, thyroid, and adrenal function. Factitious (but actually dilutional) hyponatremia can be seen when there is marked hypertriglyceridemia, marked hyperproteinemia, or severe hyperglycemia.

Hypernatremia is much less common than hyponatremia and is usually associated with severe systemic disease in a person whose impaired mental status or physical disability prevents access to water. Other associated conditions include high-protein tube feedings, severe protracted vomiting and diarrhea, and excessive water output due to diabetes insipidus (DI) or osmotic diuresis. Sodium overload can be due to administration of hypertonic sodium solutions or to endogenous causes such as primary hyperaldosteronism (Cushing's syndrome).

DI is due to deficiency of antidiuretic hormone (ADH) or to renal resistance to ADH. Central DI results from hypothalamic or pituitary damage secondary to trauma, neoplasm, or intracranial surgery.[13] Nephrogenic DI can be seen with chronic renal failure, hyperglycemia, or medications such as lithium, chlorpromazine, and demeclocycline. To put hypernatremia in perspective, a serum sodium value above 160 mEq/L that persists longer than 48 hours carries a 60% risk of death.

Abnormalities in serum potassium concentration are very common. Its laboratory determination can be spuriously increased by a hemolyzed specimen. It is also altered by acid-base abnormalities, increased extracellular osmolality, and insulin deficiency. A fall in plasma pH of 0.1 likely corresponds to an increased plasma potassium value of 0.5 mEq/L. A rise in pH causes a similar decrease in serum potassium concentration. Hypokalemia may be associated with inadequate potassium intake seen in alcoholism, malabsorption syndrome, and severe illness. Losses can be due to diarrhea, diuretic use, vomiting, trauma, cirrhosis, and to both primary (Conn's syndrome) and secondary aldosteronism (cirrhosis), renal artery stenosis, and malignant hypertension.

Hyperkalemia is associated with renal failure, dehydration, thrombocythemia, tumor lysis syndrome, and multiple medications, including beta-adrenergic blockers such as propranolol, potassium-sparing diuretics (spironolactone triamterene), several NSAID, and cyclosporine. Overlapping clinical symptoms, including weakness, nausea, anorexia, and organic mental changes, are associated with low-sodium, low-potassium, and high-potassium states.[14]

Chloride, the most abundant extracellular anion, is affected by the same conditions that affect sodium. If the serum sodium level is low, chloride concentration is also low, with the exception of the hyperchloremic alkalosis of prolonged vomiting. When carbon dioxide is included in a serum electrolyte panel, bicarbonate accounts for most of what is actually measured. It is the opinion of many authors that neither chloride nor carbon dioxide is cost-effective as a routine assay. Most patients with abnormal serum bicarbonate values have a metabolic disturbance that would be better evaluated by blood gas determinations.

CONNECTIVE TISSUE DISEASES AND VASCULITIS

The connective tissues diseases and vasculitides are immune-mediated diseases frequently marked by pain. These disorders are often difficult to diagnose in their early stages and a basic understanding of laboratory serologic studies is essential. The connective tissue diseases (Table 9–3) are multisystem disorders that share the central feature of inflammation—whether of joints, muscles, or skin. Vasculitis is a multiorgan or organ-specific disease whose central feature is blood vessel inflammation.

TABLE 9–3 ***Common Connective Tissue Diseases and Vasculitides***

Connective tissue diseases
Systemic lupus erythematosus
Mixed connective tissue disease
Primary Sjögren's syndrome
Rheumatoid arthritis
Progressive systemic sclerosis (scleroderma)
Polymyositis and dermatomyositis
Vasculitides
Polyarteritis nodosa
Churg-Strauss angiitis
Wegener's granulomatosis
Temporal arteritis
Behçet's disease
Primary central nervous system vasculitis

Almost all patients with systemic lupus erythematosus (SLE) develop autoantibodies.[15] The immunofluorescence test for antinuclear antibodies (ANA) is the most sensitive laboratory test for detecting it. It has replaced the LE (lupus erythematosus) cell test and is positive in most patients with SLE. A negative ANA result is strong evidence against SLE. A wide variety of factors that react to either nuclear or cytoplasmic constituents have been demonstrated. Table 9–4 lists a variety of antibodies and their associated diseases. Table 9–5 lists the laboratory test abnormalities of SLE, a prototype of autoimmune disease.

The ANA is generally reported in terms of a titer and the pattern of nuclear fluorescence. Nuclear fluorescence patterns can be homogeneous (solid), peripheral (rim), speckled, nucleolar, anticentromere, or nonreactive (normal). For example, an ANA directed against nucleolar RNA suggests progressive systemic sclerosis (scleroderma), particularly when the titer is high.

ANA titers above 1 : 80 are considered positive, but, because the test is positive in many conditions, correlation with the history and with other clinical findings is mandatory. A positive ANA result alone is not sufficient to diagnose SLE. SLE can also be associated with a biologic false positive test for syphilis. Elevations of ANA titers can be seen in multiple conditions besides SLE, including infections (hepatitis, mononucleosis, malaria, subacute bacterial endocarditis), other connective tissue disorders (scleroderma, Sjögren's syndrome, rheumatoid arthritis), and thyroid disease.[16]

The ANA can be weakly positive in almost 20% of healthy adults, but a titer of 1 : 320 or higher has specificity of 97% for SLE and other connective tissue diseases. Patients can produce a positive ANA result because they are taking a variety of drugs, including hydralazine, isoniazid (INH), and chlorpromazine (Thorazine).

Additional testing for the specific autoantibody responsible for the positive ANA can help to identify a particular autoimmune disease. For example, antibodies to the DNA-histone complex suggest drug-induced lupus, whereas antibodies to double-stranded DNA (dsDNA) and to Smith (sm) antigen help to confirm SLE. Wegener's granulomatosis is associated with a positive antineutrophilic cytoplasmic antibody (ANCA) test.[17] Antibodies directed against nuclear antigens to Ro/SS-A are found frequently in Sjögren's syndrome.

Serum complement is an important component of the immune system that comprises 10% of serum globulins. Total complement (CH50) and complement fractions C3 and C4 are often reduced in SLE patients who have lupus nephritis.

TABLE 9–4 Serologic Tests for Collagen Vascular Disorders

Rheumatoid factor: 80% sensitive in rheumatoid arthritis
Antinuclear antibodies: titer ≥1 : 320 have 95% specificity for systemic lupus erythematosus
Antineutrophil cytoplasmic antibody: 90% positive in Wegener's granulomatosis
Anti-Ro: Antibodies to nuclear antigens extracted from human B lymphocytes present in 70% of patients with Sjögren's syndrome
Antinuclear (nuclear RNA): 60%–90% positive in scleroderma
Anti-SM: Highly specific for systemic lupus erythematosus
Anti-centromere: Suggest CREST syndrome (calcinosis cutis, Raynaud's phenomenon, esophageal dysmotility, sclerodactyly, telangiectasias)

Rheumatoid arthritis, a common condition in pain clinic patients, is associated with the production of immunoglobulins, including IgG, IgM, and IgA, known as *rheumatoid factors* (RF). From the laboratory standpoint, the most important of the RF is an IgM macroglobulin that combines with altered IgG antigen accompanied by complement. The average sensitivity of RF (70% to 95%) in rheumatoid arthritis is well-established.

Positive RF can be found in SLE, scleroderma, dermatomyositis, and a variety of diseases associated with increased gamma globulin production—collagen vascular disorders, sarcoidosis, viral hepatitis, cirrhosis, and subacute bacterial endocarditis. As many as 20% of persons older than 70 have a positive RF titer.

A striking example of the diagnostic crossover in autoimmune vasculitis is polyarteritis nodosa. This disease is manifested as a painful peripheral neuropathy in as many as 70% of patients. Arthritic complaints involving multiple joints have been reported in as many as 50%. These patients often exhibit various autoantibodies. The ANA test is positive in some 25% of cases, and RF in about 15%. Although sorting out the intricacies of these diseases is certainly the province of rheumatologists, pain specialists are uniquely positioned to entertain the possibility of connective tissue diseases and to initiate appropriate laboratory investigation.

THYROID

Thyroid dysfunction is a clinical problem often overlooked owing to its diverse manifestations. Elderly affected persons have a high incidence of gastrointestinal symptoms and atrial fibrillation, and even an apathetic, listless appearance that may be confused with dementia. After drug-induced encephalopathy, hypothyroidism ranks as the second most treatable metabolic cause of dementia.[18] The American College of Pathologists recommends thyroid evaluation for all women over the age of 50 who seek medical attention, all adults with newly diagnosed dyslipidemia, and all patients entering a geriatric unit, on admission and at least every 5 years thereafter.

The American Thyroid Association recommends the combination of thyroid-stimulating hormone (TSH) and free thyroxine (T_4) tests as the most efficient blood tests for the diagnosis and management of thyroid disease. The preferred method of testing for thyroid disease is a cascade starting with the TSH assay. If the TSH is normal, no further tests are performed. If TSH is abnormal, free T_4 is automatically determined. TSH usually becomes abnormal sooner than free T_4. Decreased TSH values suggest hyperthyroidism, exogenous thyroid hormone replacement, or glucocorticoid effects. Increased TSH levels usually suggest primary hypothyroidism—and only rarely a TSH-secreting pituitary adenoma or a state of thyroid resistance.

Testing of free T_4 should be ordered only when the TSH value is abnormal. In a large series of patients, no thyroid disease was detected in any patient who had normal TSH and low free T_4 levels. Accordingly, in persons with normal TSH and high free T_4 levels, almost all were monitored for thyroid replacement, thyroid suppression, or amiodarone therapy. None of the elevated T_4 levels led to a new diagnosis. Eliminating unnecessary testing can realize substantial savings.[19]

PROSTATIC SPECIFIC ANTIGEN (PSA)

Cancer of the prostate is the second most common malignancy in men and the third most common cause of cancer death in men after age 55. Unfortunately, carcinoma of the prostate may remain asymptomatic even until advanced stages. Pain is a common presenting symptom of advanced prostate cancer—dysuria and hip and back pain. Prostatic-specific antigen (PSA, a glycoprotein enzyme) testing can often detect prostate cancer 3 to 5 years before clinical symptoms would appear.[20]

The American Cancer Society and the American Urologic Association recommend annual screening for all men over 50 years of age with PSA and a digital rectal examination. The PSA value is very specific for prostate disease, but not necessarily for prostate cancer. Many conditions other than prostate cancer can increase the PSA level, such as benign prostatic hypertrophy, acute bacterial prostatitis, cystoscopy, and even use of exercise bicycles.

PSA is more sensitive than biochemical measurement of acid phosphatase, which was previously the accepted test. Annual PSA screening in combination with digital rectal examination has enhanced the detection of early localized cancer. Digital rectal exam and transrectal ultrasound generally do not have a significant effect on PSA measurements. Some 70% of men identified by PSA to have prostate cancer have organ-confined disease. In contrast, in the pre-PSA era, only one third of men diagnosed by digital

TABLE 9–5 Laboratory Findings in Systemic Lupus Erythematosus

Hemolytic anemia
Leukopenia (<4000 leukocytes/mm^3)
Thrombocytopenia (<100,000 platelets/mm^3)
Antinuclear antibody positive
Lupus erythematosus cells
Antibodies to double-stranded DNA
Antibodies to SM antigen
False-positive test for syphilis

rectal exam had organ-confined disease. PSA is one of the best tumor markers currently available.[21]

HUMAN IMMUNODEFICIENCY VIRUS 1

Pain is common in HIV disease, an RNA retroviral disorder that attacks T lymphocyte helper (CD4) cells. Common painful conditions associated with HIV include abdominal pain, painful neuropathies, oral cavity pain, headache, reactive arthritis, and neuropathic pain associated with herpes zoster. For multiple reasons, not the least of which is squeamishness in dealing with this disease directly, we find physicians reluctant to suggest laboratory testing for HIV. This observation is supported by the fact that many persons who are HIV positive are unaware of the disease. AIDS is a state of advanced infection marked by serologic evidence of HIV antigen plus opportunistic infections or neoplasms associated with immunodeficiency.

Enzyme immunoassay testing for HIV has been available since 1985. Specimens that are reactive in this initial screening test are subjective to confirmatory Western blot analysis, an immunochromatographic technique that separates the virus into its major components by electrophoresis and exposes it to the patient's serum. Seroconversion generally occurs 6 to 10 weeks after infective exposure and persists for life. Antibody detection methods and a urine test have been developed whose sensitivity is comparable to that of serum testing.

A quantitative polymerase chain reaction (PCR) assay for HIV has been available since 1996. This test, commonly referred to as *the viral load*, is used for disease monitoring. An ultrasensitive version of this analysis can detect as few as 50 copies of viral RNA in 1 mL of plasma. The patient whose HIV viral load is greater than 100,000 copies per milliliter within 6 months of serum conversion is 10 times more likely to progress to AIDS within the first 5 years than one with fewer than 10,000 copies per milliliter. Maintaining low HIV viral loads (<10,000 copies per milliliter) is currently the recommended goal of therapy.[22]

Monitoring lymphocytes is one way to assess immune system deficiency. Lymphocytes are divided into three main groups: B cells, T cells (including CD4 and CD8 cells), and NKC. B cells function via antibody-mediated immunity. T cells are involved in cell-mediated immunity. HIV-1 selectively infects and reduces the number of CD4 (helper-inducer) T lymphocytes. CD8 (suppressive-cytotoxic) T cell numbers remain normal or are increased.

Normal CD4 cell counts range between 600 and 1500 cells per cubic millimeter. Reduction in the CD4 cell count is a good indicator of when to start preventive therapy for numerous opportunistic HIV-associated infections. Generally, levels above 500 CD4 cells per cubic millimeter are not associated with significant problems. Levels between 200 and 500 signal increased risk for herpes zoster, candidiasis, sinus and pulmonary infections, and tuberculosis. When cell counts fall to 50 to 200 per cubic millimeter, the risk of *Mycobacterium avium* complex or cytomegalovirus infection and of Kaposi's sarcoma increases dramatically. Levels below 50 CD4 cells per cubic millimeter indicate profound cellular immunodeficiency.

As CD4 counts decline, the possibility of opportunistic infections increases. A ubiquitous organism that can affect the central nervous system is *Toxoplasma*. Toxoplasmosis serology (IgG) is available and is usually performed when a person is found to be HIV positive. Initial positive toxoplasmosis serology would identify a potential candidate for preventive medication. Serologic tests for hepatitis should also be performed, particularly if there are abnormalities in the routine chemistry screen such as an elevated serum transaminase level.

In summary, HIV-related disease is extremely complex. In my clinical experience, both patients and physicians consistently exhibit a tendency to ignore HIV as a possibility. Enzyme immunoassay testing for HIV antibody has been the initial screening test, followed by Western blot for confirmation. The best predictor of disease progression is not likely to be a single test but rather a combination of studies, including those for both viral load and CD4 cell count.

SPIROCHETAL DISEASES

Two spirochetal diseases that have distinguished themselves as "great imitators" because of their various manifestations include syphilis and Lyme disease. Syphilis is a sexually transmitted disease caused by *Treponema pallidum*, and Lyme disease is the most common vector-borne infection in the United States, the vector being the spirochete *Borrelia burgdorferi*, which infects *Ixodes dammini* ticks.

Serologic tests currently are the mainstay of syphilis diagnosis and management. Nontreponemal tests, including the Venereal Disease Research Laboratory (VDRL) and rapid plasma reagin (RPR), are used most often. In early primary syphilis, when antibody levels may be too low to detect, the sensitivity of nontreponemal tests ranges from 62% to 76%. As antibody levels rise in the secondary stage of syphilis, the sensitivity of nontreponemal tests approaches 100%; however, in late-stage syphilis, about a fourth of treated patients have negative VDRL results. Therefore, the combination of VDRL and RPR alone cannot be relied upon for conclusive diagnosis during the very early or very late stages of syphilis.[23]

There are many false-positive nontreponemal test results. These include collagen vascular disorders, advanced malignancy, pregnancy, hepatitis, tuberculosis, Lyme disease, intravenous drug use, and multiple transfusions, among others. Because of the high frequency of false-positive results in nontreponemal serodiagnostic testing, all positive results on asymptomatic patients should be confirmed with a more specific treponemal test such as the microhemagglutination assay for *T. pallidum* and the fluorescent treponemal antibody absorption (FTA-ABS) tests. The FTA-ABS has sensitivity of 84% in primary syphilis and almost 100% for the other stages and specificity of 96%.

Titers of treponemal tests do not correlate with disease activity, whereas nontreponemal tests (VDRL and RPR) are quite useful for monitoring response to treatment. Treponemal tests should not be used for initial screening, because they are expensive and patients with previously treated infection usually remain reactive for life. Following antibiotic treatment for syphilis, VDRL and RPR should be checked once each at 6 and 12 months. Successful treatment should produce a fourfold decline in titer, although only about 60% of patients eventually become completely negative.

The other great imitator is Lyme disease, which presents with multiple painful complaints, including headache, joint pain, cranial neuritis, unilateral or bilateral Bell's palsy, or a particularly painful syndrome of radiculitis with shooting electric pains and focal extremity weakness (Bannwarth's syndrome). Recent public awareness of Lyme disease has frequently prompted serologic testing of persons who have no clinical signs or symptoms of the disease. The pathogen, *B. burgdorferi*, is a spirochete named after Willy Burgdorfer, Ph.D., a public health researcher who identified it in 1982. A diagnosis of Lyme disease should be based primarily on the patient's symptoms and the probability of exposure to the Lyme organism. Laboratory evaluation is appropriate for patients who have the characteristic arthritic, neurologic, or cardiac symptoms. It is not warranted for patients who have nonspecific symptoms such as those frequently classified under the vague rubrics of *chronic fatigue syndrome* or *fibromyalgia*.

A true-positive result consists of a positive enzyme-linked immunosorbent assay (ELISA) or immunofluorescence assay (IFA) confirmed by a Western blot. It is essential to remember that positive results do not prove the diagnosis of Lyme disease and have little predictive value in the absence of clinical symptoms.[24]

False-positive Lyme results due to cross-reactive antibodies are associated with autoimmune disease or with infections secondary to other spirochetes such as *T. pallidum* and *Leptospira* species, and to bacteria such as *Helicobacter pylori*. Finally, because assays for antibody to *B. burgdorferi* should be used only for supporting a clinical diagnosis of Lyme disease, they are unsuitable as screening tools in evaluating asymptomatic persons or patients with nebulous complaints not characteristic of Lyme disease. There is evidence to suggest that many persons who do not actually have Lyme disease are receiving treatment for it solely because of serology results.

NEUROPATHY

A frequent issue in the evaluation of pain, particularly when the cause is not obvious, involves peripheral neuropathy. Pain, sensory loss, weakness, and dysesthesias are common clinical complaints. Even after exhaustive evaluation, the cause of as many as 50% of peripheral neuropathies remains unknown. The more common causes are diabetes, alcoholism, toxins, nutritional deficits, drugs, and renal and other metabolic disorders. Less familiar disorders include the immune-mediated hereditary neuropathies. It is important to remain aware of the immune-mediated syndromes, not only to enhance diagnostic accuracy but because these patients often respond to immunomodulatory treatments with dramatic improvements in neurologic function and quality of life.[25]

It is far beyond the scope of this chapter to discuss this rapidly evolving topic in detail. We attempt to introduce the pain specialist to this aspect of neuropathy evaluation, particularly where specific laboratory tests can be critical to diagnostic accuracy. Vitamin B_{12} deficiency is characterized by macrocytic anemia, peripheral neuropathy, and ataxia, and it may be associated with cognitive deficits. B_{12} levels above 300 ng/L are normal. Levels between 200 and 300 ng/L are borderline. Measurement of methylmalonic acid, a substrate that requires cobalamin for its metabolism, is elevated (>0.4 mmol/L) in states of true vitamin B_{12} deficiency.

Levels of vitamin B_{12} below 200 ng/L are abnormal. Serum gastrin is elevated in gastric atrophy, which is usually associated with pernicious anemia. A normal serum gastrin level effectively rules out pernicious anemia, whereas intrinsic factor–blocking antibodies are detectable in only 50% of pernicious anemia patients. The expensive and time-consuming Shilling's test should be reserved for those patients with a low level of vitamin B_{12} who test negative for intrinsic factor–blocking antibodies and have an elevated serum gastrin level.

An immune-mediated neuropathy, acute or chronic, can be associated with pain and may even present as a life-threatening emergency. The prototype of acute inflammatory demyelinating neuropathy, Guillain-Barré syndrome, may appear after any of a number of infections, surgery, vaccinations, or immune system perturbations. Chronic inflammatory demyelinating polyneuropathy may be associated with illicit drug use, vaccination, infections, autoimmune disorders, or monoclonal gammopathy. A demyelinating neuropathy associated with anti–myelin-associated glycoprotein (anti-MAG) presents as distal weakness and sensory loss, particularly in the legs. Measurement of IgM anti-MAG antibodies in the serum by the Western blot method detects this clinical disorder.[26]

Small myelinated and unmyelinated axons subserve pain and temperature. Diabetes and alcoholism, the most common causes of peripheral neuropathy in the United States, often present as a painful small-fiber neuropathy. Leprosy (Hansen's disease) is the principal cause of a treatable neuropathy worldwide. Others are amyloidosis, AIDS, and ischemic lesions such as polyarteritis nodosa, SLE, and Sjögren's syndrome. These small-fiber neuropathies often present with burning, electric shock–like or lancinating pain and uncomfortable dysesthesias. The patient may also complain of intense pain with only a minimal stimulus (allodynia), such as sheets rubbing over the feet.

Persons with a characteristic syndrome that is often dismissed as anxiety complain that "my whole body is numb and I feel tingling, painful numbness all over." In middle-aged patients, particularly those who are heavy cigarette smokers, paraneoplastic neuropathy should be considered. One indicator is serum antineuronal nuclear antibodies type I (ANNA:anti-HU). This malignant inflammatory sensory neuropathy is most often associated with small cell lung cancer, though it may associated with Hodgkin's lymphoma, epidermoid cancer, or colon or breast carcinoma. As in all areas of pain diagnosis, the clinician must resist any impulse to hastily ascribe pain to psychogenic mechanisms: Once the psychogenic arrow has been fired, it is almost impossible to retrieve it gracefully.

Nonmalignant inflammatory sensory neuropathy is a disorder that commonly affects women. It can present as distal painful dysesthesias or ataxia. Serologic markers such as ANA, rheumatoid factor, or antineutrophil cytoplasmic antibodies (ANCA) may suggest specific connective tissue disorders, such as, respectively, SLE, rheumatoid arthritis, and Wegener's granulomatosis. Certain patients with nonmalignant inflammatory neuropathy and Sjögren's syndrome test positive to extractable nuclear antigens such as ro (SS-A) and la (SS-P). Hereditary conditions, drugs, and toxins are also part of this differential diagnosis.[27]

Immune-mediated neuropathies are always worth remembering, because they can respond to immunomodulating treatments. These diagnoses are often overlooked or missed; sometimes patients suffer symptoms for years without a specific diagnosis. Frequently, pain specialists see these persons, and, not uncommonly, the patients' initial work-up was fragmented and far from thorough.

A search for serum factors associated with the immune-mediated neuropathies includes testing for monoclonal antibodies (proteins with definite antigenic targets) and for monoclonal and polyclonal antibodies that bind to specific neural components. Measurement of anti-MAG, antisulfatide, and anti-HU antibodies should be considered, as should serum and urine tests for monoclonal antibodies using immunofixation methods. Other elements of the work-up are testing serum for cryoglobulins and markers for connective tissue disorders. Table 9–6 includes a variety of specific laboratory tests that can be helpful in the evaluation of painful neuropathies. Once again, the pain specialist is in a unique position to develop expertise and knowledge, not only about the treatment of pain but in the evaluation and diagnosis of conditions that frequently escape proper identification, even by experienced subspecialists.[28]

SERUM PROTEINS

Laboratory tests involving the various components of serum proteins can be valuable adjuncts to the evaluation of

TABLE 9–6 ***Clinical and Laboratory Features of Common Neuropathies***

Neuropathic Conditions	Clinical Features	Useful Laboratory Tests (Findings)*
Diabetic neuropathy	Distal symmetric polyneuropathy Mononeuritis multiplex Diabetic amyotrophy	Fasting blood glucose HgAIC Glucose tolerance test
Alcohol neuropathy	Burning feet, ataxia Distal areflexia	Gamma-glutamyltransferase (↑) Aspartate transaminase (↑) Mean corpuscular volume (RBC macrocytosis) (↑)
Neuropathy due to renal disease	60% of dialysis patients have dysesthesias, pain, and cramps in legs	Blood urea nitrogen (↑) Creatinine (↑)
Infectious neuropathy		
Leprosy	10 million cases worldwide	Skin biopsy (+)
Lyme disease	Radiculoneuritis Bell's palsy	Lyme test with Western blot confirmation (+)
Human immunodeficiency (HIV-1)	Guillain-Barré like (acute) Mononeuritis (late) Distal painful sensory neuropathy (late)	HIV test with Western blot confirmation (+)
Neuropathy associated with malignancy		
Lung cancer	Painful sensory neuropathy	Anti-HU antibodies (+)
Myeloma	Osteosclerotic myeloma	Immunoglobulins G, A, monoclonal gammopathy
Amyloidosis	Distal painful sensory neuropathy associated with plasma cell dyscrasia	Urine Bence Jones protein monoclonal gammopathy
IgM monoclonal gammopathy	Waldenström's macroglobulinemia, chronic lymphocytic leukemia	Immunoglobulin M antibody to MAG, GMI, sulfatide
Vasculitic neuropathy		
Wegener's granulomatosis		P-ANCA (+)
Systemic lupus erythematosus		Antinuclear antibodies (+)
Hepatitis B, C		Serology cryoglobulins (+)
Sarcoid		Angiotensin-converting enzyme (↑)
Sjögren's		Anti-SSA-LA Anti-SSB-Ro antibodies
Toxic neuropathy		
Arsenic	Painful stocking and glove polyneuropathy	Urine levels >25 mg/day unless seafood was eaten recently
Lead	Abdominal pain, fatigue, wrist drop, diffuse weakness	Anemia Urine coproporphyrin (↑) Urine lead level >0.2 mg/L Blood lead levels can be misleading
Vitamin B_{12} deficiency	Burning hands and feet Cognitive impairment Posterior column loss Ataxias	Low serum B_{12} Homocysteine (↑) Methylmalonic acid (↑)

* (+), Positive; ↑, elevated.

pain. Abnormalities of the various components of serum proteins may be helpful in investigating connective tissue disorders and several malignancies. A lack of familiarity with this area of diagnosis creates a common reticence on the part of the pain specialist in ordering these studies.

Serum protein is composed of albumin and globulin. The word *globulin* is actually an old term that refers to the nonalbumin portion of serum protein, a substance that has been found to contain a varied group of proteins, such as glycoproteins, lipoproteins, and immunoglobulins. The total quantity of albumin is about three times that of globulin, and albumin acts to maintain serum oncotic pressure. Globulins tend to have more varied functions, including antibodies, clotting proteins, complement, acute phase proteins, and transport systems for various substances. Serum protein electrophoresis is utilized to screen for serum protein abnormalities. Various bands are identified that correspond to albumin, $alpha_1$ and $alpha_2$ globulins, beta globulins, and gamma globulins (Fig. 9–1).

Acute phase proteins are seen in response to acute inflammation, trauma, necrosis, infarction, burns, and psychological stress. Increases are noted in fibrinogen, $alpha_1$-antitrypsin, haptoglobin, and complement. Albumin and transferrin are often decreased in an acute stress pattern. These changes in serum proteins during acute inflammatory responses are accompanied by polymorphonuclear leukocytosis, increased ESR, and an increase in CRP, that responds very rapidly after the onset of acute inflammation.

Significant changes in albumin are usually reductions rather than elevations. These can be associated with pregnancy, malnutrition, liver disease, cachexia or wasting states such as those of tuberculosis, AIDS, or advanced cancer. Serum albumin may also be lost directly from the vascular compartment secondary to hemorrhage, burns, exudates, or protein-losing enteropathy.

Gamma globulin is composed predominantly of antibodies of the IgG, IgA, IgM, IgD, and IgE types. Marked reduction of the gamma fraction is seen in hypogammaglobulinemia and agammaglobulinemia. Secondary varieties of gamma globulin reduction may be found in patients with nephrotic syndrome, overwhelming infection, chronic lymphocytic leukemia, lymphoma, or myeloma and those on long-term corticosteroid treatment. Rheumatic and collagen vascular diseases usually demonstrate elevations in gamma globulin. Multiple myeloma and Waldenström's macroglobulinemia demonstrate a homogeneous spike or peak in a localized region of the gamma area.

Immunoglobulins are a heterogeneous group of molecules. IgG constitutes about 75% of serum immunoglobulins and the majority of antibodies. IgM represents the earliest antibodies formed and accounts for about 7% of the total immunoglobulin. The IgM class includes cold agglutinins, ABO blood groups, and rheumatoid factor. IgA constitutes about 15% of immunoglobulins. IgA deficiency, the most common primary immunodeficiency, is associated with upper respiratory tract and gastrointestinal infections. Phenytoin (Dilantin) is reported to decrease IgA levels in about 50% of patients who receive long-term therapy. IgE is elevated in certain allergic—and especially atopic—disorders.

Multiple myeloma is a malignancy of plasma cells derived from B-type lymphocytes. The disease is most common in middle-aged males and frequently presents as bone pain. Anemia is present in almost 75% of patients, and RBC rouleaux formation (cells stacked like coins) can be identified in peripheral blood smears. Elevated ESR is common, and significant hypercalcemia occurs in about a third of patients. A monoclonal gammopathy spike (M protein) is seen in about 80% of myeloma patients. Of all patients who have monoclonal protein, about two thirds have myeloma. Roughly 70% have monoclonal protein characterized as IgG; most of the others, IgA.[29]

A normal immunoglobulin molecule is composed of two heavy chains and two light chains (kappa and lambda) connected by a disulfide bridge. IgM is a pentameric configuration of five complete immunoglobulin units. In addition to normal-weight serum monoclonal protein, many myeloma patients excrete a low–molecular weight protein known as *Bence Jones protein*, which is composed only of immunoglobulin light chains. Unlike normal-weight monoclonal proteins, it can pass into the urine and, generally, is not demonstrable in the serum. Other conditions associated with Bence Jones protein include Waldenström's macroglobulinemia, a lymphoproliferative disorder

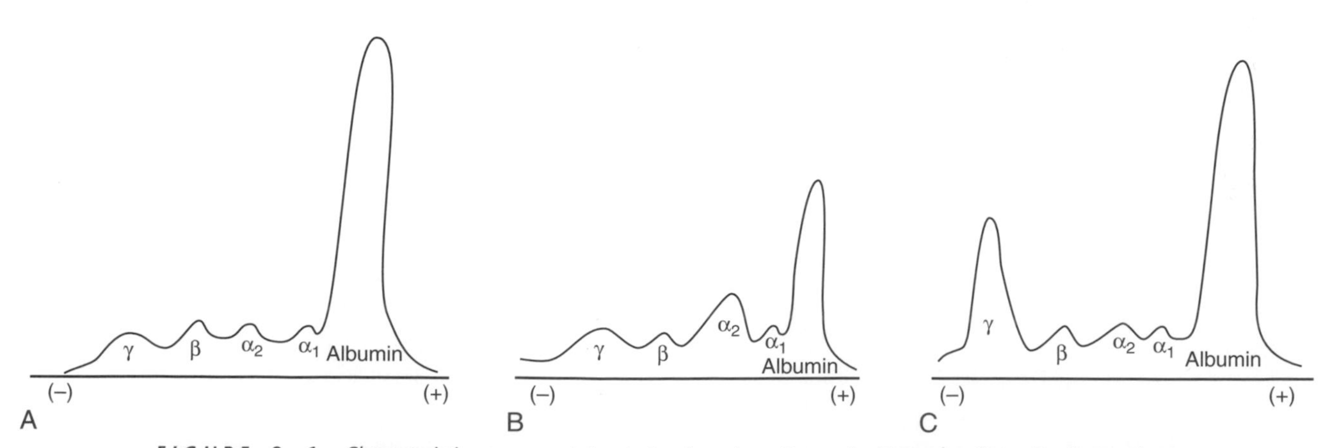

FIGURE 9–1 Characteristic serum protein electrophoresis patterns. A, Normal pattern. B, Acute phase response pattern. Note decreased albumin peak and increased $alpha_2$ globulin level, which is associated with burns, rheumatoid disease, and acute stress. C, Monoclonal gammopathy spike. Note M protein spike in gamma area. Pattern is associated with myeloma, Waldenstrom's macroglobulinemia, and idiopathic monoclonal gammopathy.

associated with monoclonal IgM production, lymphadenopathy, hepatosplenomegaly, and hyperglobulinemia. Bence Jones proteinuria is seen in monoclonal gammopathies associated with malignancies, and significant quantities (>60 mg/L) are identified. In monoclonal gammopathies of nonneoplastic origins such as rheumatic or collagen vascular disease, cirrhosis, and chronic infection, Bence Jones protein excretion is generally less than 60 mg/L.[30]

Cryoglobulins are immunoglobulins that precipitate reversibly in serum or at least partially gel at cold temperatures. The most common associated symptoms are purpura, Raynaud's phenomenon, and arthralgias. Cryoglobulins usually do not appear as discrete bands on serum protein electrophoresis. The conditions most often associated with cryoglobulins are rheumatoid and collagen vascular disease, leukemia, lymphomas, myeloma, and Waldenström's macroglobulinemia. They are also associated with a variety of infections and hepatic disease.

RENAL FUNCTION TESTS

Routine urinalysis is an indispensable part of basic clinical laboratory evaluation. Dysuria is extremely common in women; 30% experience at least one episode of cystitis during their lifetime. The differential diagnosis of painful urination includes cystitis, pyelonephritis, urethritis, vaginitis, and genital herpes. The most sensitive laboratory indicator for urinary tract infection is pyuria. The basic urinalysis should include specific gravity, albumin, hemoglobin, and microscopic evaluation for casts, crystals, and red and white cells.[31]

If no vaginal contamination occurs during urine collection, vaginitis generally does not produce pyuria. The presence of WBC casts suggests pyelonephritis. A positive leukocyte esterase test is about 90% sensitive in detecting pyuria secondary to infection. Many bacteria produce an enzyme called reductase that converts urinary nitrates to nitrites. The nitrite test enhances the sensitivity of the leukocyte esterase test in defining urinary tract infection. A positive nitrite test is 90% specific for urinary tract infections. Its sensitivity is low but can be improved by obtaining a first voided morning urine sample.

Urinary tract infection is defined as 100,000 colony-forming units per milliliter on urine culture. The microscopic examination of the urine *must* proceed promptly, generally within 1 hour after voiding. Various studies report that as many as 50% of specimens that contained abnormal numbers of white cells were considered normal after standing at room temperature only several hours.[32]

Urea is a waste product of protein metabolism that is synthesized in the liver and that contains nitrogen (BUN). Creatinine is a metabolic product of creatine phosphate in muscle. Serum levels of BUN and creatinine change only with severe renal disease. Creatinine clearance rate (the amount of creatinine that can be completely eliminated into the urine in a given time) is a much more sensitive measure of mild to moderate glomerular damage. In addition to being sensitive to function, creatinine clearance is one of the more sensitive tests available to warn of impending renal failure.

Elevations of serum BUN and creatinine generally reflect severe glomerular damage, renal tubular damage, or both. An elevated BUN level (azotemia) is not specific for renal disease. Prerenal azotemia may result from decreased renal circulation secondary to shock, hemorrhage, or dehydration. It can also be caused by increased protein catabolism like that associated with overwhelming infections or toxemia. Renal azotemia usually accompanies bilateral chronic pyelonephritis, glomerular nephritis, acute tubular necrosis, and other forms of severe glomerular damage. Postrenal or obstructive azotemia can result from any external compression of the ureter, urethra, or bladder, or, in elderly men, from prostatic hypertrophy, benign or malignant. The studies that test predominantly renal tubular function include specific gravity, osmolality, and urinary excretion of electrolytes.

OSMOLALITY

Although the very term *osmolality* evokes an imposing and esoteric image, it has practical clinical value. Serum osmolality is an indicator of total body water and generally ranges between 280 and 300 mOsm/kg of water. The principal determinants of serum osmolality are sodium, chloride, glucose, and urea. A simplified formula with excellent clinical utility is this:

$$\text{Serum osmolality} = 2\times \text{sodium} + \text{glucose}/20 + \text{BUN}/3.$$

Urine osmolality depends on an individual's state of hydration. Under normal conditions, urine osmolality ranges from 400 to 800 mOsm/kg. Profound dehydration is associated with levels above 1100 mOsm/kg, and fluid overload demonstrates values below 100 mOsm/kg. Simultaneous measurement of urine and serum osmolality is useful in diagnosing SIADH, a condition that can be induced by a variety of causes, including central nervous system tumors, infections, trauma, undifferentiated small cell lung cancer, pneumonia, and various medications, among them opiates, barbiturates, and carbamazepine (Tegretol, Carbatrol).

A typical patient with SIADH has a serum osmolality below 270 mOsm/kg and a urine osmolality that is higher than the serum value. In contrast, a patient with DI has a serum osmolality greater than 320 mOsm/kg and urine osmolality less than 100 mOsm/kg.

The osmolal gap can be used to screen for low–molecular weight toxins. The gap is determined by subtracting the calculated osmolality (from the formula cited earlier) from the actual serum osmolality. The calculated and measured values usually fall within 10 units of each other. If the measured value exceeds the calculated value by more than 10 units, other osmotically active substances that can present in an emergency room setting should be considered. These include ethanol, methanol, ethylene glycol, propylene glycol, acetone, paraldehyde, and other toxins.

CALCIUM, PHOSPHORUS, AND MAGNESIUM

Symptoms related to hypercalcemia are varied but include vomiting, constipation, polydipsia, polyuria, and encephalopathy. Hypercalcemia is often detected on routine laboratory panels in an otherwise healthy person. Primary hyperparathyroidism accounts for about 60% of outpatient abnormalities. In hospitalized patients, malignancy-associated hypercalcemia accounts for the majority. Tumors most often associated with hypercalcemia are breast, renal, and lung cancers and myeloma. Regulation of serum calcium occurs through a negative feedback loop mediated by the secretion of parathyroid hormone (PTH). A decrease in serum calcium increases secretion of PTH, whereas an increase in serum calcium reduces it. PTH also has a direct action on bone, increasing bone resorption and the release of bone calcium and phosphorus.

Other causes of hypercalcemia include dyazide diuretics, lithium therapy, sarcoidosis, hyperthyroidism, and vitamin D intoxication. The effects of PTH, vitamin D, and phosphate produce a reciprocal relationship between the serum calcium and phosphate levels, elevation of one ultimately leading to reduction of the other. Vitamin D deficiency results in low levels of both calcium and phosphorus but an elevated level of PTH.

Hypophosphatemia is seen in association with hypercalcemia as a manifestation of hyperparathyroidism. Severe hypophosphatemia can cause muscle weakness, bone pain, tremor, seizures, hypercalciuria, and decreased platelet function. Hyperventilation and respiratory alkalosis are major causes of hypophosphatemia in patients with pain, anxiety, sepsis, alcoholism, hepatic disease, heat stroke, or salicylate toxicity. Respiratory alkalosis causes plasma phosphate to shift into the cells. Life-threatening hypophosphatemia can occur if malnourished patients are administered carbohydrates rapidly.

Primary hyperparathyroidism reduces phosphate secondary to increased urinary excretion. Vitamin D deficiency causes hypocalcemia, secondary hyperparathyroidism, and increased urinary phosphate excretion in the face of decreased intestinal phosphate absorption.

Hypocalcemia and hyperphosphatemia are often seen in tandem. Renal failure accounts for more than 90% of hyperphosphatemia. Plasma phosphate levels rise when the glomerular filtration rate falls below 25% of normal. Rhabdomyolysis, hemolysis, and tumor lysis syndrome may produce severe hyperphosphatemia by releasing large amounts of intracellular phosphate. Hypoparathyroidism, acromegaly, and thyrotoxicosis reduce urinary phosphate excretion. Enemas with a high phosphate content can cause hyperphosphatemia, hypocalcemia, and, ultimately, tetany. The ill-advised practice of prolonged storage of blood samples can cause an artificial elevation in phosphate levels.

Routine serum calcium measures address total serum calcium, about 50% of which is bound calcium and about 50% ionized or free (dialyzable). Most of the bound calcium is complexed with albumin. The most common cause of "bound hypocalcemia" is a decrease in serum albumin. Although laboratory evidence of hypocalcemia is fairly common in hospitalized patients, true decreases of ionized calcium are less prevalent. Symptoms include neuromuscular irritability, mental status changes, and seizures. Causes of true hypocalcemia include primary hypoparathyroidism, pseudohypoparathyroidism secondary to diminished responsiveness of the kidney or skeleton to PTH, vitamin D deficiency, malabsorption, renal failure, chronic alcoholism, rhabdomyolysis, alkalosis, and certain drugs (large amounts of magnesium sulfate, anticonvulsant medication, or cimetidine).

After sodium, potassium, and calcium, magnesium is the fourth most common cation. It is often overlooked in patients with neuromuscular abnormalities. These symptoms include tremor, muscle cramping, seizures, confusion, anxiety, and hallucinations. Magnesium deficiency has been reported in as many as 10% of hospitalized patients. It is often associated with alcoholism, malabsorption, malnutrition, diarrhea, dialysis, diuretic use, and congestive heart failure. The most common cause of elevated serum magnesium is renal failure or a hemolyzed specimen.

URIC ACID

Hyperuricemia is defined by a serum uric acid concentration greater than 7 mg/dL. Gout, principally a disease of middle-aged men, results from the deposition of monosodium urate crystals, typically in a joint in a lower extremity, often the first metatarsophalangeal joint (a lesion called podagra). At a physiologic pH, more than 90% of uric acid exists as monosodium urate, but at levels above 8 mg/dL, monosodium urate is likely to precipitate into tissues.

Although patients with gout generally have elevated serum uric acid levels, 10% may have levels that fall within normal range. Conversely, many patients with hyperuricemia never experience an attack of gouty arthritis, and by far the most frequent cause of hyperuricemia, particularly in hospitalized patients, is renal disease with azotemia.

Serum uric acid levels may become elevated in any disorder that results in proliferation of cells or excessive turnover of nucleoproteins. Hemolytic processes, lymphoproliferative and myeloproliferative diseases, polycythemia vera, and rhabdomyolysis may result in high uric acid levels. Obesity, alcohol abuse, and purine-rich foods such as bacon, salmon, scallops, and turkey can also result in an overproduction of urate.

About 97% of all uric acid the human body produces daily is excreted through the kidneys. In about 90% of patients with gout, the primary defect is underexcretion of uric acid. This occurs with renal insufficiency, hypertension, diabetes, and various drugs, including cyclosporine, nicotinic acid, and salicylates.

In summary, although patients with gout generally have elevated serum uric acid levels, as an isolated finding that is not diagnostic for gout, nor does a normal level conclusively rule it out. A most accurate and readily available test for gout is demonstration of uric acid crystals in the synovial fluid of an acutely inflamed joint.

LIVER FUNCTION TESTS

Considerable confusion can be encountered in the interpretation of the many aspects of common liver function tests (LFT). Many of the routine tests assess liver *injury* rather than liver function. Of the LFT, only serum albumin, bilirubin, and prothrombin time provide useful information on how efficiently the liver is actually working. Certain of these findings may reflect problems arising outside the liver, such as an elevated bilirubin value, seen with hemolysis, or elevations in alkaline phosphatase associated with skeletal disorders. Normal LFT do not ensure a normal liver: patients with cirrhosis or bleeding esophageal varices can have normal LFT.[33]

The most commonly used markers of hepatic injury are the enzymes aspartate aminotransferase (AST) (formerly SGOT) and alanine aminotransferase (ALT) (formerly SGPT). AST and ALT values are higher in healthy obese patients and in males. ALT levels generally decline with weight loss. Slight elevations of the AST or ALT, within 150% of the upper range of normal, may not, in fact, indicate liver disease but rather a skewed (non–bell-shaped) distribution curve, with a higher representation on the far end of the scale (seen in blacks and Hispanics).

The highest ALT levels, often more than 10,000 units/L, are found in patients with acute toxic injury such as acetaminophen overdose or acute ischemic insult to the liver. With typical viral hepatitis or toxic injury, the serum ALT rises higher than the AST value, whereas an AST-ALT ratio greater than 2:1 is more common with alcoholic hepatitis or cirrhosis. Causes of elevated ALT or AST values in asymptomatic patients include autoimmune hepatitis, hepatitis B, hepatitis C, drugs, toxins, alcohol, fatty liver, congestive heart failure, and hemochromatosis.

Lactate dehydrogenase (LDH) is a less specific marker than AST or ALT but is disproportionately elevated after ischemic hepatic injury. AST elevations greater than 500 units/L and ALT values greater than 300 units/L are unlikely to be caused by alcohol intake alone and in a heavy drinker should prompt consideration of acetaminophen toxicity. AST and ALT are found in skeletal muscle and may be elevated to several times the normal value in conditions such as severe muscular exertion, polymyositis, and hypothyroidism.

Stoppage of bile flow (cholestasis) results from blockage of the bile ducts or from a disease that impairs bile function. Alkaline phosphatase (ALP) and gamma-glutamyltransferase (GGT) levels typically rise to several times normal after bile duct obstruction or intrahepatic cholestasis. Diagnosis can be confounded during the first few hours after acute bile duct obstruction secondary to a gallstone, when AST and ALT levels rise 500 units/L or more but ALP and GGT can take several days to rise.

Serum ALP originates from both the liver and bone. Bony metastasis, Paget's disease, recent fracture, placental production during the third trimester of pregnancy can all cause ALP elevations. ALP, like GGT, can be elevated in patients taking phenytoin (Dilantin), and this does not constitute an absolute indication for discontinuing the medication. ALP levels can be persistently elevated in asymptomatic women with primary biliary cirrhosis, a chronic inflammatory disease of small bile ducts associated with the presence of serum antimitochondrial antibodies.

The elevation of GGT alone with no other liver function abnormalities often results from enzyme induction caused by either alcohol or aromatic medications such as phenytoin or phenobarbital. The GGT level is often elevated in asymptomatic persons who take more than three alcohol-containing drinks per day. A mildly elevated GGT level in a person taking anticonvulsant medication does not indicate either liver disease or an absolute need to discontinue the medication.

Bilirubin, an indicator of liver function, is formed from the enzymatic breakdown of the hemoglobin molecule. The unconjugated bilirubin is carried to the liver, where it is rapidly transported into bile. The serum conjugated bilirubin level does not become elevated until the liver has lost half of its excretory capacity. A patient could thus have a total left or right hepatic obstruction without a rise in bilirubin.[34]

Unconjugated hyperbilirubinemia is associated with increased bilirubin production as in hemolytic anemia, resorption of a large hematoma or defective hepatic unconjugated bilirubin clearance secondary to severe liver disease, drug-induced inhibition, congestive failure, portacaval shunting, or Gilbert's syndrome. Gilbert's syndrome occurs in many healthy persons whose serum unconjugated bilirubin is mildly elevated (2 to 3 mg/dL). That is the only liver function abnormality: both the conjugated bilirubin value and the CBC remain normal. Gilbert's syndrome has been linked to an enzymatic defect in the conjugation of bilirubin.

Visible staining of tissue with bile is called *jaundice*. The three major causes are extrahepatic and intrahepatic biliary tract obstruction and hemolysis. With hemolysis, unconjugated bilirubin increases whereas the conjugated fraction remains normal or is only slightly elevated. In the case of extrahepatic biliary obstruction, usually in the common bile duct secondary to either a stone or carcinoma, initially there is an increase in conjugated bilirubin but no change in the unconjugated level. After several days, however, conjugated bilirubin in the blood breaks down to unconjugated bilirubin, eventually arriving at a ratio of 1:1.

Intrahepatic biliary obstruction is usually caused by liver cell injury from any of a variety of causes, including alcohol abuse, drugs, hepatitis, cirrhosis, passive congestion, or primary or metastatic tumors. Both conjugated and unconjugated fractions may increase, in varying proportions, in this type of obstruction. Hemolysis can be identified by measuring markers such as haptoglobin and reticulocyte count. A final word on jaundice relates to age. In persons younger than 30 years, viral infections account for 80% of cases. After age 60, cancer accounts for about 50% and gallstones for about 25%.

Another marker of hepatic synthetic capacity is serum albumin, which changes rather slowly in response to alterations in synthesis owing to its protracted plasma half-life of 3 weeks. Elevation of serum albumin usually implies dehydration. Patients with low serum albumin levels and no other LFT abnormalities are likely to have other, extrahepatic, causes, such as proteinuria, trauma, sepsis, active rheumatic disease, cancer, and severe malnutrition. During pregnancy, albumin levels progressively decrease until parturition and do not return to normal until about 3 months post partum.[35]

The PT is quite useful for following hepatic function during acute liver failure. The liver synthesizes clotting factors II, V, VII, IX, and X. Because factor VII has a short half-life (only 6 hours), it is sensitive to rapid changes in hepatic synthetic function. It is important to realize that PT does not become abnormal until more than 80% of hepatic function is lost. Vitamin K deficiency due to chronic cholestasis or fat malabsorption can prolong the PT. A therapeutic trial of vitamin K injections (5 mg/day subcutaneously for 3 days) is a reasonable option to exclude vitamin K deficiency.[36]

The measurement of blood ammonia provides a rather inexact marker for hepatic encephalopathy. Concentrations of ammonia correlate poorly with the degree of confusion. Although ammonia contributes to the encephalopathy, concentrations are often much higher in the brain than in the blood. Levels are best measured in arterial blood, because venous concentrations can be elevated as a result of muscle metabolism of amino acids. Blood ammonia determinations are most useful in evaluating encephalopathy of unknown origin rather than monitoring therapy in a person with known, hepatic encephalopathic disease.[37]

The pancreas is another vital organ that, when diseased, may cause pain. Acute pancreatitis presents with severe epigastric pain, vomiting, and abdominal distention. Two useful tests are serum amylase and lipase. Alpha-amylase is derived from both the pancreas and the salivary glands. Its sensitivity in acute pancreatitis is about 90%. Other causes of amylase elevation include biliary tract disease, peritonitis, pregnancy, peptic ulcers, diabetic ketoacidosis, and salivary gland disorders. False-normal results may be seen with lipemic serum.

The serum lipase is slightly less sensitive, but probably more specific in acute pancreatitis. The extrapancreatic disorder that most consistently elevates serum lipase is renal failure. Chronic pancreatitis is not generally a painful condition, but it reflects the end stage of acute pancreatitis, hemochromatosis, or cystic fibrosis. Diabetes, steatorrhea, and pancreatic calcification on radiographs are its signature features.

CREATINE KINASE

Creatine kinase (CK) is found in cardiac muscle, skeletal muscle, and brain. Total CK can be separated into three major isoenzymes: CK-BB, found predominantly in brain and lung; CK-MM, found in skeletal muscle; and CK-MB, found predominantly in heart muscle. Total CK elevation is seen in a number of conditions associated with acute muscle injury or severe muscular exertion. Total CK is also elevated after muscle trauma, myositis, muscular dystrophy, long distance running, or delirium tremens or seizures. Elevated levels can often be noted after intramuscular injections.

In evaluating chest pain, and particularly myocardial ischemia and infarction, total CK elevation is too often false-positive, owing principally to skeletal muscle injury. Troponin I is a regulatory protein that is specific for myocardial injury. It becomes elevated in about 4 to 6 hours, peaks at about 10 hours, and returns to reference range in about 4 days. Its major selling point is that it is highly specific for cardiac injury.

The CK-MB level begins to rise 3 to 4 hours after acute myocardial infarction, reaches a peak in 12 to 24 hours, and returns to normal in about 36 to 48 hours. The most rapid elevation after cardiac injury is that of serum myoglobin. Unfortunately, myoglobin is found in both cardiac and skeletal muscle. Elevations are noted as early as 90 minutes after cardiac injury. An analysis of myoglobin in conjunction with troponin I can be performed at intervals after the onset of myocardial infarction symptoms. Myoglobin may be viewed as a very early but not particularly specific marker for cardiac injury, whereas troponin is an extremely specific but not as rapidly responsive marker.

THERAPEUTIC DRUG MONITORING AND TESTING FOR DRUGS OF ABUSE

Particularly when the clinical information seems perplexing and contradictory, it is wise to consider the effects of prescription medications, toxic substances, and drugs of abuse. The practice of pain management inherently attracts patients prone to chemical dependency. They sometimes possess rather sophisticated pharmacologic information and present with detailed histories ultimately aimed at obtaining a specific controlled substance. It has been our experience that the treating physician often has a visceral warning about the integrity of these patients but is hampered by an overwhelming sense of social squeamishness or frank denial that ultimately misleads him to avoid drug screening and rightfully pursue a valid clinical impression.

As a practicing neurologist, I am amazed to see how many emergency room physicians faced with patients exhibiting erratic or agitated behavior fail to include toxicology screening in their evaluation. The effects of specific prescription medications or drug interactions in patients taking multiple medications should always be a primary concern.[38]

Therapeutic drug monitoring can be helpful in establishing compliance and therapeutic adequacy and avoiding toxic doses. Medications such as phenobarbital, valproic acid (Depakote), carbamazepine (Tegretol, Carbatrol), primidone (Mysoline), phenytoin (Dilantin), lithium carbonate, and the tricyclic antidepressants have readily available assays. Particularly in elderly persons, who sometimes exhibit dramatic changes in protein binding, toxicity may occur at levels normally considered therapeutic. With phenytoin, a medication that is about 90% bound to protein and that exhibits nonlinear kinetics, it is not unusual to see toxicity with a variety of symptoms, including ataxia, personality change, nystagmus, dysarthria, tremor, nausea, vomiting, and somnolence. Discovery of a toxic phenytoin level in an elderly patient with confusion and ataxia of several months' duration may not only suggest a rapid therapeutic course of action but also save several thousand dollars in unnecessary neurodiagnostic imaging studies.

Selective therapeutic drug monitoring can be very useful with phenytoin, primidone, phenobarbital, valproic acid, and carbamazepine. Valproic acid may be used for migraine prophylaxis. Carbamazepine and Dilantin are useful for trigeminal neuralgia and for neuropathic pain in general. Many of these compounds have narrow therapeutic windows, and, again particularly in the elderly, toxicity may go unnoticed and may be attributed to other causes such as cerebrovascular disease or dementia. It is not unusual to find patients with elevated medication levels who receive an incorrect diagnosis of stroke and whose drug levels consequently are allowed to remain in a protracted state of toxicity.

Lithium carbonate, used for both bipolar disorder and cluster headache management, has a distinctly narrow therapeutic window. Adverse effects include nausea, vomiting, tremor, and hypothyroidism. Lithium is excreted by the kidneys, whereas the anticonvulsant medications mentioned earlier are metabolized in the liver and interact with other drugs that are also metabolized there. Acetaminophen is a commonly used analgesic. Hepatic injury can occur with ingestion of 10 g, and 25 g has been known to be fatal. A serum level greater than 200 μg/mL is considered toxic. A pattern of acute hepatocellular injury similar to that of acute hepatitis is noted, with distinct elevations of AST and ALT.[39]

Testing for drugs of abuse is more difficult. In addition to problems with specificity and sensitivity, persistence of a drug or its metabolites in the urine varies much among individual agents and among abusers. For example, the urine can be positive for cannabinoids several days after a single casual use of marijuana. After cessation in long-term heavy users, the urine may remain positive as long as a month. All initially positive test results obtained by screening procedures should be confirmed by gas chromatography and mass spectrometry.

The different sensitivity levels of different tests must be kept in mind, as must the effect of urine concentration or dilution. It is critical to remember that detection of cannabinoids in the urine indicates that the patient has used marijuana in the past but provides no clear-cut evidence that that is related to current mental impairment or a behavioral problem. Of equal importance is the concept of chain of custody, which demands strict accountability for a specimen from its collection to its ultimate analysis. A patient could be tragically stigmatized if erroneous results were obtained in a process that was flawed.[40]

Cocaine is another popular drug of abuse. Its major metabolite, benzoylecgonine, remains detectable considerably longer than cocaine and in heavy users may be detectable for several weeks. Amphetamines, usually methamphetamine, are detectable in the urine within 3 hours after a single dose. A positive result for amphetamines in the urine usually implies use within the last 24 to 48 hours.

Opioid abuse is particularly problematic in the "pain population." Morphine and codeine are made from the seeds of the opium poppy, whereas heroin is synthesized directly from morphine. Ingestion of moderate amounts of culinary poppyseeds can result in detectable concentrations of morphine in the urine that may last as long as 3 days. A speedball (a combination of cocaine and heroin) remains popular for prolonging cocaine's effects while blunting postcocaine depression. The immediate access to opioids afforded medical personnel makes this subgroup particularly susceptible to abuse. As an overview, the most common classes of drugs found when screening trauma patients, in order of frequency, are ethanol, amphetamines, opiates, and cocaine.[41]

TOXICOLOGY

Mercury, arsenic, bismuth, and antimony are best screened by urine sampling. Hair and nails are preferred for documenting long-term exposure to arsenic or mercury. Occupational lead exposure and lead poisoning remain serious public health problems in the United States. Most exposure is in industry—in battery manufacturing, the chemical industry, smelting, soldering, and welding. Symptoms include abdominal pain, myalgias, paresthesias, general fatigue, and, ultimately, encephalopathy and death.

Arriving at the diagnosis requires a constant high index of suspicion. At present, the blood level of lead is the single best indicator of recent absorption of a large dose of lead. The blood lead level rises rapidly within hours of an acute exposure and remains elevated for several weeks. Consecutive measurements averaging 50 μg/dL or higher indicate the necessity to remove an employee from that toxic environment. A blood lead level *and* a zinc protoporphyrin level provide sufficient information to quantitate the severity and approximate chronology of the lead exposure.

Zinc protoporphyrin reflects the toxic effects of lead on an erythrocyte enzyme system. Levels usually begin to rise when the blood lead level exceeds 40 μg/100 mL. Once elevated, zinc protoporphyrin tends to remain above background levels for several months (the 120-day life span of RBC). The combination of an elevated blood lead level plus an elevated zinc protoporphyrin value suggests that exposure must have lasted longer than several days.[42]

Every year more than 100,000 Americans' deaths are associated with the use of alcohol. Intoxication is so common that physicians frequently forget that it can be fatal. Levels above 400 mg/dL are suggested lethal, but levels less than 400 mg/dL have been fatal, and levels of 800 mg/dL have been documented in alert patients. Most states define legal intoxication as a blood alcohol level of 100 mg/dL, although driving skills have been shown to become impaired at levels as low as 50 mg/dL. Alcohol is often ingested with other medications and, in combination, intoxicating levels or otherwise lethal doses may be strikingly lower. A combination of ethanol with chloral hydrate (a Mickey Finn) has a particularly devastating reputation.

Various tests have been used to screen for chronic alcoholism, including elevated GGT and AST levels, mean corpuscular volume elevation, hyperuricemia and hypomagnesemia, hyponatremia, and hypophosphatemia.[43] These indices correlate to some degree but cannot be taken as specific indicators of alcohol abuse. As in all cases with toxicology, the results should not be accepted without question. Laboratory errors do occur, and any tendency to be judgmental or punitive is strongly discouraged.

SUMMARY

The proper use of laboratory testing can be very valuable in evaluating pain. In this chapter I have highlighted only the essentials. It is presented as a starting point from which readers can expand their knowledge. In my clinical experience, lab testing is often overlooked, with embarrassing—and sometimes tragic—consequences.

These tests, along with findings of the history and physical examination form the foundation of clinical diagnosis. The pain specialist should embrace a primary care role in accurate diagnosis by ensuring thoroughness through methodical attention to detail. This approach is much preferred to the all too common mode where patients' symptoms are abruptly linked to expensive procedures without deference to diagnostic precision.

REFERENCES

1. Gabay C, Kushner I: Acute phase proteins and other responses to inflammation. N Engl J Med 340:448–454, 1999.
2. Brown RG: Anemia. *In* Taylor RB (ed): Family Medicine: Principles and Practice, ed 4. New York, Springer-Verlag, 1994, pp 997–1005.
3. Little DR: Diagnosis and management of anemia. Prim Care Rep 3:175–184, 1997.
4. Little DR: Hemochromatosis: Diagnosis and management. Am Fam Physician 53:2623–2628, 1996.
5. Ranney HM: The spectrum of sickle cell disease. Hosp Pract 27(1):133, 1992.
6. Ravel R: Clinical laboratory medicine: Clinical application of laboratory data. ed 6. St. Louis, Mosby–Year Book, 1995, pp 9–11.
7. Schmitt BP, et al: Heparin-associated thrombocytopenia. Am J Med Sci 305:208, 1993.
8. Nichols WL, et al: Standardization of the prothrombin time for monitoring orally administered anticoagulant therapy with use of the international normalized ratio system. Mayo Clin Proc 68:897, 1993.
9. The Expert Committee on the Diagnosis and Classification of Diabetes Mellitus: Report of the Expert Committee on the Diagnosis and Classification of Diabetes Mellitus. Diabetes Care 21(Suppl) 1:S5–S16, 1998.
10. Weykamp CW, et al: Influence of hemoglobin variants and derivatives on glycohemoglobin determinations. Clin Chem 39:1717, 1993.
11. Service FJ: Hypoglycemia. Endocrinol Metab Clin North Am 17:601, 1988.
12. Avus JC, et al: Pathogenesis and prevention of hyponatremic encephalopathy. Endocrinol Metab Clin North Am 22:425, 1993.
13. Halevy J, et al: Severe hypophosphatemia in hospitalized patients. Arch Intern Med 148:153, 1988.
14. Vanek VW, et al: Serum potassium concentrations in trauma patients. South Med J 87:41, 1994.
15. Systemic lupus erythematosus (SLE). *In* Ferry JA, Harris NL (eds): Atlas of Lymphoid Hyperplasia and Lymphoma. Philadelphia, WB Saunders, 1997.
16. Tan EM, Feltkamp TEW, Smolen JS, et al: Range of antinuclear antibodies in "healthy" individuals. Arthritis Rheum 1997;40:1601–1611.
17. Hoffman GS, Kerr GS, Leavitt RY, et al: Wegener granulomatosis: An analysis of 158 patients. Ann Intern Med 116:488–498, 1992.
18. Isley WL: Thyroid dysfunction in the severely ill and elderly. Postgrad Med 94:111, 1993.
19. Helfand M, et al: Screening for thyroid dysfunction: Which test is best? JAMA 270:2297, 1993.
20. Littrup PJ, et al: Prostate cancer screening: Current trends and future implications. CA 42:198, 1992.
21. Babaian RJ, et al: The relationship of prostate-specific antigen to digital rectal examination and transrectal ultrasonography. Cancer 69:1195, 1992.
22. Saag MS, Holodniy M, Kuritzkes DR, et al: HIV viral load markers in clinical practice. Nat Med 2:625–629, 1996.
23. Larsen SA, Kraus SJ, Whittington WL: Diagnostic tests. *In* Larsen SA, Hunter EF, Kraus SJ (eds): A Manual of Tests for Syphilis. Washington, DC, American Public Health Association, 1990.
24. Centers for Disease Control and Prevention: Recommendations for test performance and interpretation from the second national conference on serologic diagnosis of Lyme disease. MMWR 44:590–591, 1995.
25. Dyck PJ, Oviatt KF, Lambert EH: Intensive evaluation of referred unclassified neuropathies yields improved diagnosis. Ann Neurol 10:222–226, 1981.
26. Thomas PK, Ochoa J: Symptomatology and differential diagnosis of peripheral neuropathy. *In* Dyck PJ, Thomas PK (eds): Peripheral Neuropathy, ed 3. Philadelphia, WB Saunders, 1993, pp 749–774.
27. Kornberg AJ, Pestronk A: Immune-mediated neuropathies. Curr Opin Neurol Neurosurg 6:681, 1993.
28. Koski CL: Humoral mechanisms in immune neuropathies. Neurol Clin 10:629, 1992.
29. Boccadoro M, Pileri A: Diagnosis, prognosis, and standard treatment of multiple myeloma. Hematol Oncol Clin North Am 11:111–131, 1997.
30. Kyle RA: The monoclonal gammopathies. Clin Chem 40(11 pt 2): 2154–2161, 1994.
31. Pappas PG: Laboratory in the diagnosis and management of urinary tract infections. Med Clin North Am 75:313–325, 1991.
32. Stamm WE, Hooton TM: Management of urinary tract infections in adults. N Engl J Med 329:1328–1334, 1993.
33. Kamath PS: Clinical approach to the patient with abnormal liver function test results. Mayo Clin Proc 71:1089–1094, 1996.
34. Westwood A: The analysis of bilirubin in serum. Ann Clin Biochem 28:119–130, 1991.
35. Rothschild MA, Oratz M, Schreiber SS: Serum albumin. Hepatology 8:385–401, 1988.
36. Kaplan MM: Laboratory tests. *In* Schiff L, Schiff ER (eds): Diseases of the Liver, ed 7. Philadelphia, JB Lippincott, 1993, pp 108–144.
37. Johnston DE: Special considerations in interpreting liver function tests. Am Fam Physician 59:2223–2230, 1999.
38. McCarron MM: The use of toxicology tests in emergency room diagnosis. J Analyt Toxicol 7:131–135, 1983.
39. Kaplowitz N, Tak Yee AW, Simon FR, et al: Drug-induced hepatotoxicity. Ann Intern Med 104:826–839, 1986.
40. Schwartz JG, Zollars PR, Okorodudu AO, et al: Accuracy of common drug screen tests. Am J Emerg Med 9:166, 1991.
41. Weisman RS, Howland MA, Flomenbaum NE: The toxicology laboratory. *In* Goldfrank LR, Flomenbaum NE, Lewin NA, et al (eds): Toxicologic Emergencies, ed 4. Norwalk, Conn, Appleton & Lange, 1990, p 39.
42. Staudinger KC, Roth VS: Occupational lead poisening. Am Fam Physician 57:719–726, 1998.
43. Whitehead TP, Clarke CA, Whitfield AG: Biochemical and hematological markers of alcohol intake. Lancet 1(8071):978–981, 1978.

CHAPTER • 10

Radiologic Testing in the Evaluation of the Patient in Pain

Solomon Batnitzky, MD • Valerie R. Eckard, MD •
Bernard M. Abrams, MD • Donald A. Eckard, MD

Radiologic testing in the evaluation of the pain patient involves close collaboration and good communication between the clinician and the radiologist. The role of the radiologist is twofold:

1. Selecting the most appropriate examination.
2. Interpreting the radiographs of a particular study.

Basic considerations are an understanding of the different types of pain, the various imaging techniques, and regional diagnosis. This chapter assumes that radiologic evaluation involves pain patients whose diagnosis and management belongs in the domain of the pain specialist and not that of the primary care physician, so the discussion is directed toward entities commonly seen by pain physicians. There is considerable "turf" overlap, however, because one or more entities may be treated by different specialists.

Pain is an unpleasant sensory and emotional experience that is subjective and highly individual. It may take the following forms[1]:

- Acute (nociceptive)—somatic and visceral
- Postoperative
- Neuropathic
- Terminal
- Chronic or behavioral
- Psychogenic

Imaging of the human body can provide evidence of a pathologic process that gives strong clues to or confirmation of a pain syndrome. In some cases, however, the pain syndrome may not be amenable to anatomic delineation or the imaging technique may give irrelevant and misleading information. From past to present, clinicians have stressed caution, and as Cyriax[2] so eloquently stated, "Irrelevant radiologic appearance must be resolutely ignored," a sentiment echoed in the current literature[3–5] on potentially irrelevant data about bulging lumbar discs on magnetic resonance imaging (MRI).

The physician who cares for a patient complaining of pain must be cognizant of the fact that pain can arise from various body structures or from nonstructural or psychiatric disease. The body structures that may produce nociceptive responses are these:

- Skin
- Subcutaneous tissues
- Muscles
- Joints
- Tendinous and ligamentous attachments
- Bones, including skull, long bones, and vertebral bodies
- Central nervous system structures
- Peripheral nerves, including the sympathetic nervous system
- Viscera

In determining whether a given imaging procedure might be helpful, the first considerations are the physical examination and the clinical impression of the examining physician. Various imaging techniques lend themselves to identifying pain that originates at certain tissue sites, and, without a putative diagnosis, it is difficult if not impossible to choose the appropriate technique. A second consideration in the selection of an imaging procedure is the pattern of pain referral. Imaging of the body area to which pain is referred from a distant nerve root, nerve, or viscus can provide scant information and findings may be misleading. In addition, modern imaging techniques, including computed tomography (CT) and MRI, can reveal normal variants, congenital anomalies, and degenerative or aging processes that are present in symptomatic and asymptomatic individuals alike.[3–5] Two relevant questions remain: (1) What is the tissue site of pain production? (2) Are the radiologic findings relevant? The type of tissue damage should guide the selection of imaging techniques. Various types of processes can cause pain:

- Traumatic
- Neoplastic
- Vascular, including malformations and insufficiency
- Infectious
- Congenital, including malalignments of bony and vertebral structures

- Visceral, including ulcerations, distensions, dysfunctions, and torsions
- Impingement on normal structures by other, normal or abnormal structures (e.g., carpal tunnel syndrome, spondylolisthesis)
- Nonneoplastic bone disease, including metabolic and inherited processes
- Poorly understood neural or sympathetic mechanisms (e.g., trigeminal neuralgia, reflex sympathetic dystrophy)
- Heterotopic bone formation

IMAGING MODALITIES

Many imaging techniques are available to evaluate the pain patient: plain films, conventional tomography, CT, MRI, radionuclide scintigraphy, ultrasonography, special contrast examinations (e.g., barium enema, intravenous pyelography), arthrography, myelography, arteriography, and venography. These modalities, either alone or in combination, permit remarkable accuracy in both anatomic and pathologic diagnosis. What follows is a general discussion of the principles and limitations of current imaging modalities and their clinical applications, with particular emphasis on clinical situations in which pain is a major feature of the patient's complaints. Many pain states are encountered in clinical practice. Many are seen and treated by different specialists and are not encountered or treated in a pain clinic. The emphasis of this chapter is on the pain states that are most likely to be seen and treated in a pain clinic, although obviously there is some overlap. It is clearly impossible, owing to the limitations of a book chapter, to give anything but the briefest survey of treatment technologies. Detailed discussions can be found in standard texts.[6–15]

It is important to stress again that the choice of the proper radiologic technique for any given case depends on many variables, the most important of which are (1) the type of disease suspected to be causing the pain and the patient's other signs and symptoms, and (2) the suspected location of the disease process. Furthermore, reaching a correct diagnosis does not end the process of radiologic investigation, because the course of treatment and management depends on identifying distinguishing features and characteristics of the lesion (e.g., soft tissue or bone involvement by a particular process).

Plain Films

Plain film radiography of the human body dates back to the discovery of x-rays by Wilhelm Conrad Roentgen in 1895. It has been one of the cornerstones of radiologic investigation and remains fundamental to its practice today. Despite the technical advances in new imaging modalities such as CT and MRI, plain film radiography remains the initial imaging procedure for evaluating chest disorders, skeletal disorders, including bony, ligamentous, and joint pain, and the "acute abdomen," and in searching for opaque calculi in the kidneys, ureter, urinary bladder, and gallbladder. Plain film radiography is the least expensive, most readily available, and quickest way of visualizing these areas.

With computed tomography, metallic foreign bodies and dental fillings (in the case of the skull) cause beam hardening artifacts which often limit CT quality. This problem can be solved with plain films in which these artifacts do not occur (Fig. 10–1).

Chest Pain

Chest pain is a symptom of numerous life-threatening conditions, such as ischemic heart disease, acute myocardial

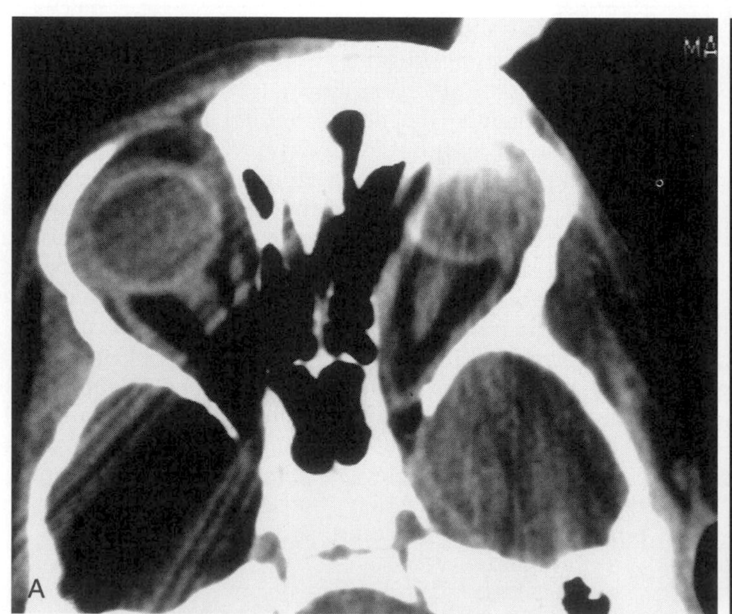

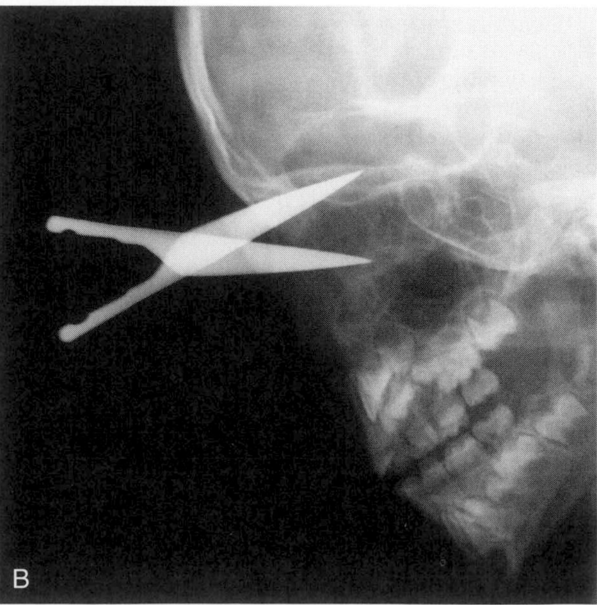

FIGURE 10–1 "Next time listen to mother." A 3-year-old boy jumped off a countertop holding a pair of scissors in his hand. He hit his elbow on the countertop, which resulted in the scissors penetrating his left orbital area. A, *Axial CT scan demonstrates metallic scissors entering the left orbit medial to the left globe, which is distorted by the scissors. The quality of the CT image is compromised and distorted by the streak artifacts caused by the metallic scissors.* B, *Lateral skull radiograph demonstrates both blades of the scissors entering the orbit.*

infarction, pulmonary embolism, and dissection of the aorta (Table 10–1).[16] Chest pain can also be a symptom of conditions with inconsequential sequelae. In many instances, plain chest film findings are nonspecific and not very helpful in the evaluation of chest pain. With lesions such as traumatic rupture of the aorta and aortic dissection, plain chest films demonstrate widening of the mediastinum, hemothorax, shift of the trachea, and widening and irregularity of the descending aorta (see section on Arteriography later).

The major value of obtaining a chest film to investigate chest pain is to exclude causes such as pneumothorax, pneumomediastinum, pneumonia, pericarditis, and fractured rib. Plain films, although they may not be diagnostic, are helpful and important in detecting and demonstrating the extent of complications of the disease process.

Musculoskeletal Disorders

Most fractures are adequately demonstrated with plain films (Figs. 10–2, 10–3). Soft tissue changes such as joint effusion and tendinous calcifications are also well demonstrated by plain films. Infections (Fig. 10–4) and inflammatory diseases of bone, changes due to arthritis, and primary and secondary tumors involving the bone can also be evaluated well on plain film radiography.

In evaluating certain areas of the body (e.g., skull), plain film radiography has been replaced by techniques such as CT and MRI that directly visualize the anatomy of the region.[17] The importance and use of plain skull films have declined markedly secondary to the widespread use of CT and MRI.[17] Today, plain skull films are reserved for secondary evaluation to answer specific questions raised by the CT or MRI findings.

TABLE 10–1 ***Disease Processes That Can Produce Chest Pain****

Organ (System)	Disease Processes
Heart	Ischemic heart disease Valvular disease Pericarditis
Aorta	Dissecting aneurysm Traumatic rupture
Pleura	Pneumothorax Pleuritis
Lungs	Pneumonia Pulmonary embolism Pulmonary infarction
Esophagus	Rupture Esophagitis Esophageal tumor Esophageal spasm
Chest wall	Rib fracture Tumor
Abdomen	Peptic ulcer Pancreatitis Cholecystitis

* Modified from Higgins CB, Lipton MJ: Chest pain. *In* Eisenberg RL: Diagnostic Imaging: An Algorithmic Approach, Philadelphia, JB Lippincott, 1988, p 30.

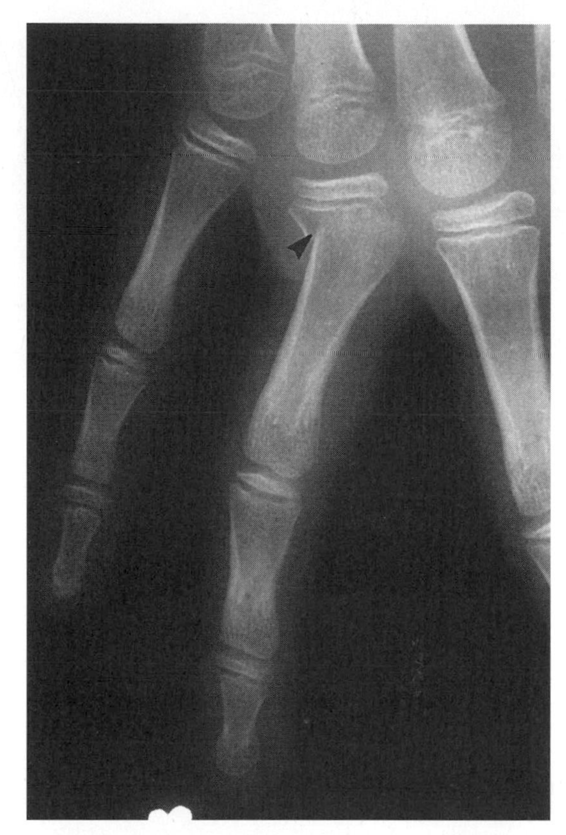

FIGURE 10–2 Fracture of the proximal phalanx of the fourth finger (arrowhead) without epiphyseal injury. The distal fracture fragment is displaced laterally.

Conventional Tomography

Conventional tomography, either linear or complex motion, is a useful adjunct to plain film radiography when better detail is needed for diagnosis. Conventional tomog-

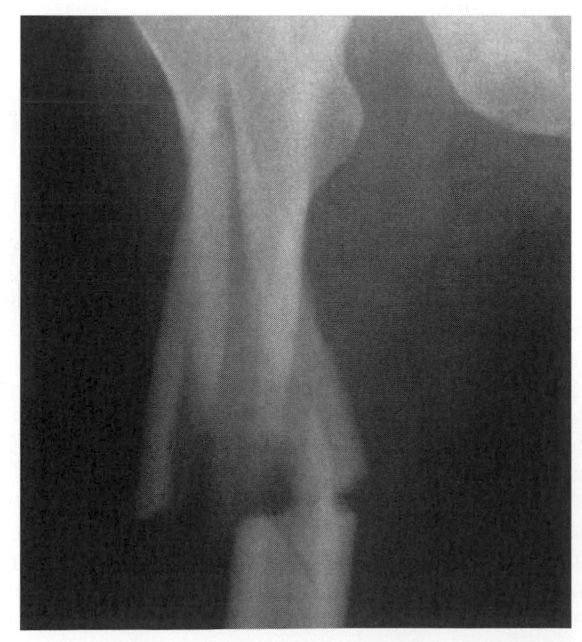

FIGURE 10–3 Comminuted fracture of the proximal third of the shaft of the right femur.

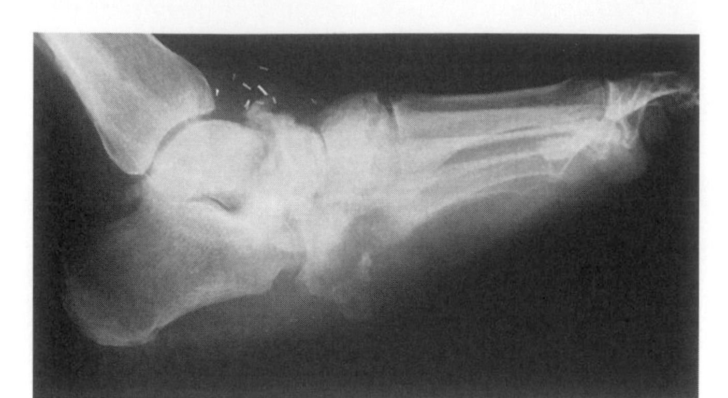

FIGURE 10–4 Osteomyelitis involving the tarsal bones of the right foot in a 54-year-old diabetic woman. Areas of irregular bone destruction and bone formation are noted in the cuboid and navicular. Surgical clips from previous surgery are visible in the ventral soft tissues of the proximal foot.

raphy can be helpful in analyzing lesions involving the joints in which the anatomy is complex, such as comminuted tibial plateau fractures. It can also be used for the detection of subtle fractures and the evaluation of osseous fusion of fractures, osteotomies, and arthrodeses. It is also very helpful for characterizing solitary bone lesions, which can suggest the correct pathologic diagnosis.

Computed Tomography

The introduction of CT for clinical use in the early 1970s revolutionized the practice of neuroradiology and profoundly affected the practices of neurology and neurosurgery. The application of CT to the evaluation of the rest of the body soon afterward proved no less revolutionary. CT is a computer-based imaging technology that permits direct visualization of anatomic structures. It provides exquisite cross-sectional images of both normal anatomy and pathologic lesions.

In the chest and abdomen CT is helpful in seeking these processes:

- Trauma
- Abscess and other manifestations of infection
- Primary neoplasm (benign and malignant)
- Metastases
- Lymphadenopathy
- Aortic aneurysm

A differential absorption of 5% or more is generally required to distinguish different soft tissues on plain radiographs.[17] CT, on the other hand, is able to differentiate among many different soft tissues for which the differential absorption may be as little as 0.5%.[17] Because of this remarkable ability to detect and display minute differences in tissue densities, CT opened up new vistas of radiologic diagnosis.

Advantages of CT over magnetic resonance imaging are rapid scan acquisition, superior bone detail, demonstration of calcium, and the demonstration of acute hemorrhage.[17] Acute intracranial hemorrhage is more reliably and easily evaluated with CT than with MRI.[13, 17] Acute subarachnoid hemorrhage due to a ruptured aneurysm or arteriovenous malformation is best imaged with CT (Fig. 10–5).[13, 18] The reported detectability on CT of subarachnoid hemorrhage due to ruptured cerebral aneurysm in the acute phase ranges from 60% to 100%.[18] In evaluating for acute intracranial hemorrhage (epidural, subdural, subarachnoid, intraparenchymal) CT scans must be obtained without the intravenous iodinated contrast material. Contrast enhancement of a lesion and fresh intracranial blood can be confused.

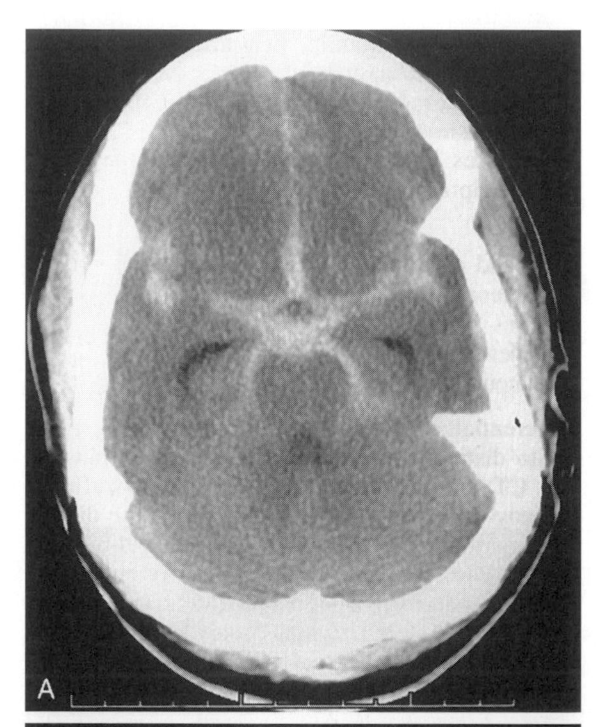

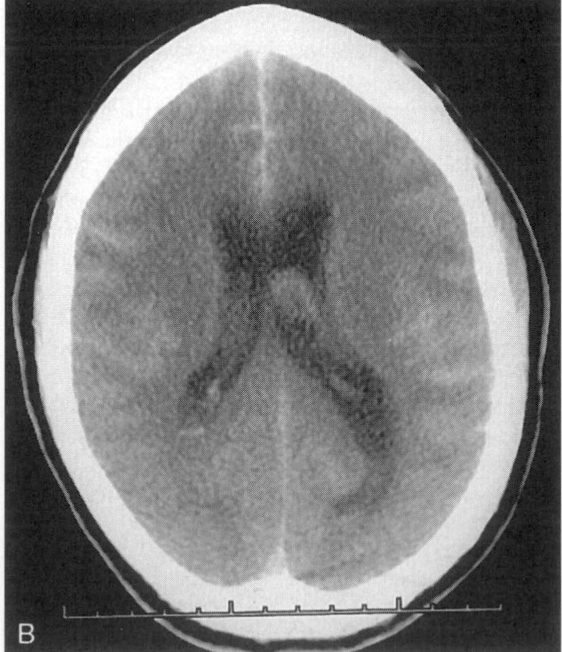

FIGURE 10–5 Subarachnoid hemorrhage secondary to rupture of intracranial aneurysm. Noncontrast axial CT demonstrates extensive subarachnoid blood in the basal cisterns, A, *and in the sulci over both cerebral convexities,* B.

Approximately 75% of all spontaneous nontraumatic subarachnoid hemorrhages are due to ruptured intracranial aneurysms. An additional 5% to 10% of nontraumatic subarachnoid hemorrhages are due to ruptured arteriovenous malformations. In approximately 15% to 20% of patients presenting with nontraumatic subarachnoid hemorrhage, no cause will be found despite a thorough diagnostic workup. Some 50% to 75% of patients who present with nontraumatic subarachnoid hemorrhage for which no cause can be found demonstrate a perimesencephalic pattern of subarachnoid hemorrhage on the initial head examination. In this condition, the subarachnoid hemorrhage is located and confined to the prepontine cistern and/or perimesencephalic cistern. No supratentorial subarachnoid blood is seen in this condition, which has been termed *perimesencephalic nonaneurysmal subarachnoid hemorrhage.* This condition is well-described in the neurosurgical literature[18a] as a benign form of subarachnoid hemorrhage that is not associated with subsequent rebleeding or cerebral infarction. The long-term prognosis is excellent and is significantly better than that for patients with subarachnoid hemorrhage associated with identifiable intracranial aneurysm (Fig. 10–6). The source of the subarachnoid bleeding is believed to be rupture of small pontine and/or perimesencephalic veins or capillaries.

Rapid scan acquisition, the demonstration of superior bone detail, and the superior and more accurate demonstration of the presence of acute hemorrhage make CT the procedure of choice in the evaluation of acute trauma (Figs. 10–7 to 10–9). MRI, on the other hand, has the ability to define subacute and chronic collections of blood much better than CT.[17] Although MRI is superior to CT for evaluating most disease processes in the central nervous system,[19] one should not underestimate the role of CT in the diagnosis of intracranial tumors (Fig. 10–10). It is still an outstanding and very accurate modality. The overall accuracy of CT, especially when performed without and then with intravenous contrast material, approaches 98% for the identification of a lesion (versus no lesion).[20] Whether CT or MRI is used as the first diagnostic study depends on the accessibility and availability of these modalities.[17]

CT, when performed without and then with intravenous iodinated contrast material, allows for greater accuracy of diagnosis and localization of various lesions by better characterizing them according to their patterns of contrast enhancement.[17] The intrathecal administration of water-soluble, nonionic myelographic contrast agents significantly increases the accuracy of CT in the evaluation of the intraspinal contents.

Magnetic Resonance Technology

MRI was the major innovation in medical imaging in the 1980s and 1990s. Like CT, MRI is a computer-based imaging modality that depicts anatomic sections in tomographic slices of varying thickness. The MRI technique is based on the effects of a large magnet and radio signals on the nuclei of hydrogen atoms present in body tissues. MRI has rapidly established itself as a noninvasive technique for evaluating the central nervous system and other parts of the body that not only rivals CT but surpasses it in many instances. Whereas CT evaluates only a single tissue pa-

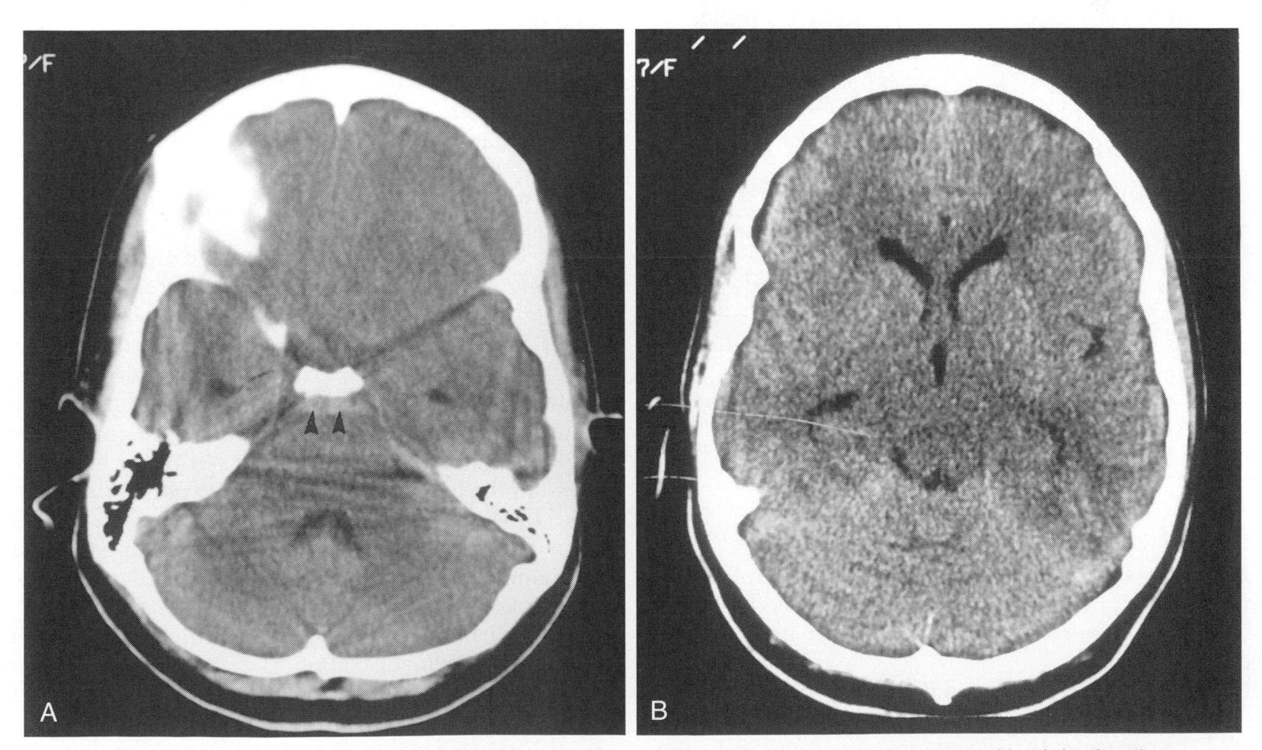

FIGURE 10–6 *Perimesencephalic nonaneurysmal subarachnoid hemorrhage. A 17-year-old girl developed severe headaches after vigorous exercise.* A, *Noncontrast axial CT scan demonstrates acute blood in the prepontine cistern* (arrowheads). B, *No supratentorial subarachnoid blood is seen. Four-vessel cerebral angiography was normal.*

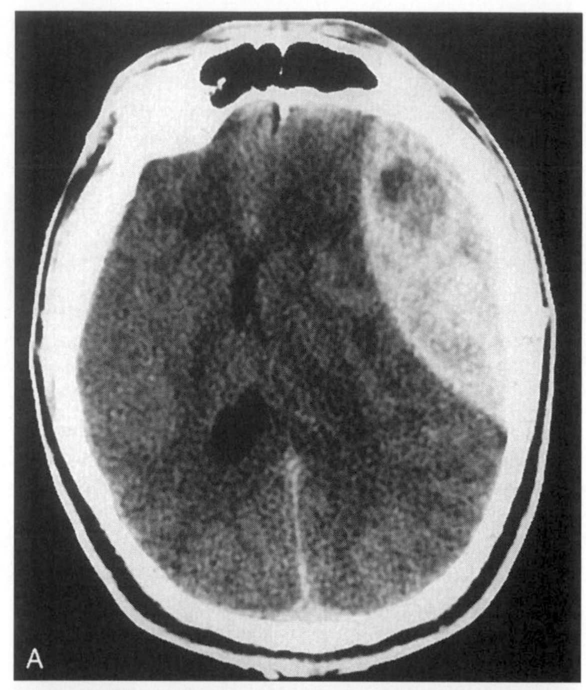

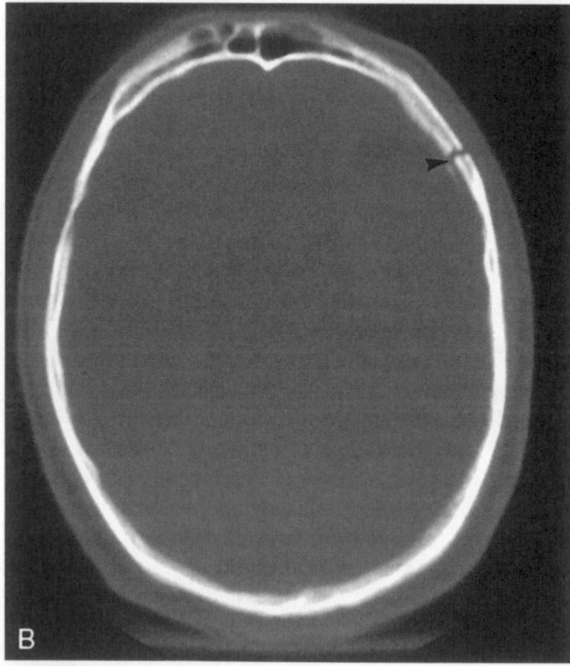

FIGURE 10–7 A, *The left-sided biconvex extradural dense mass is characteristic of an acute epidural hematoma. The ventricular system is displaced across the midline from left to right.* B, *On the bone window setting of the same CT image, an underlying skull fracture* (arrowhead) *is visible that was not appreciated on the soft tissue setting,* A.

rameter (x-ray attenuation), MRI analyzes multiple tissue characteristics. The soft tissue contrast provided by MRI is substantially better than that of any other imaging modality.

Although MR images are anatomically similar to CT scans, the MRI information is fundamentally different from x-ray CT information. In CT and in conventional radiography, the gray-scale ordering never changes. Bones always appear as the whitest tissue, followed by muscle and fat, and air always appears black. The gray-scale ordering on MRI is highly variable, however, and can be confusing. For an understanding of how an MR image is created and can be manipulated to answer clinical questions, some fundamental principles of MRI should be appreciated. It is beyond the scope of this chapter to discuss the physics of MRI; the reader is referred to the standard text for this purpose.[8–14] It should be emphasized that the description given here is very basic and simplifies the very complex physics of MRI.

As noted, the MRI technique is based on the effects that a large magnetic field and radiofrequency (RF) pulses have on the nuclei of hydrogen atoms in body tissues. Hydrogen is ideally suited for MRI because it is the most abundant atom in the body. Nuclei with odd numbers of protons, such as hydrogen, can be made to align as tiny magnetic dipoles in large magnetic fields. This alignment can be perturbed with radiopulses of certain frequencies. When this RF is terminated, the nucleus attempts to realign its axis with that of the static field by giving off the energy that it absorbed when knocked out of alignment. The released energy can be detected by an antenna. The rate of energy release is a function of the chemical environment of the nucleus. Different tissues absorb and release RF energy at different, detectable, and characteristic rates. Images are formed by encoding the spatial position of the released signal through the use of frequency and phase information.

In relaxation (i.e., the process triggered by interruption of the RF pulse), the physical changes that were caused by the pulse disappear and the tissues return to the state they were in before the application.[17] The time it takes for the voltage to decay, or for relaxation to occur, is expressed by two time constants, the T1 and T2 relaxation times.[17] These two components of relaxation proceed at different rates, depending on the nature of the tissue. Each tissue has its own peculiar T1 and T2 relaxation times. The pulse sequences can be altered to emphasize either the T1 or T2 characteristics of a tissue (i.e., to create *T1-weighted* or *T2-weighted* images).[17]

T1-weighted images produce excellent anatomic details and exquisitely demonstrate the anatomic distortion produced by mass lesions. T2-weighted images appear anatomically less aesthetic than T1-weighted images but can sharply highlight many disease processes (e.g., infarction, infection, tumors). In many instances, unless there are anatomic distortions, such pathologic processes may not be well appreciated on T1-weighted images. Magnetic resonance angiography (MRA) is based on the intensity differences between flowing blood and stationary tissue. By suppressing the background (stationary) tissue, the high signal from flowing blood can be demonstrated. In this fashion, the vascular structures can be depicted using the magnetic resonance technique. MRA is an excellent noninvasive screening modality for evaluation of the arteries and veins. It can play an important role in routine imaging by providing useful information about the vascular anatomy. In conjunction with conventional MRI studies, it can improve the overall sensitivity and specificity of such imaging. MRA is still in its developmental stage, and further technical refinements and research are needed before MRA can re-

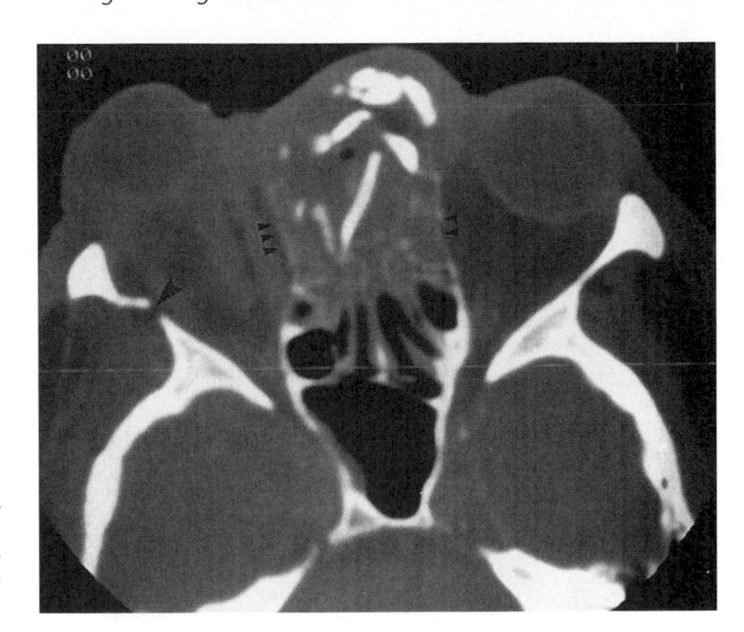

*FIGURE 10–8 Right orbital wall and complex midfacial fractures. Axial CT of the face photographed at the bone window setting exquisitely demonstrates comminuted fractures of the midface with posterior telescoping of the fracture fragments. Both medial walls of the orbits are also fractured (*small arrowheads*), as is the lateral wall of the right orbit (*large arrowhead*).*

place conventional angiography, which is still the gold standard for evaluating the vascular system.

Advantages of Magnetic Resonance Imaging

MRI has several advantages over other imaging modalities.[17] First, it has no known adverse biologic effects. Second, MRI does not use ionizing radiation; although the amount of radiation used by CT is relatively low, it is obviously preferable to avoid ionizing radiation altogether. Third, MRI produces substantially greater tissue contrast resolution than any other imaging modality. It has been reported to supply additional information not available on CT in as many as 50% of patients evaluated by both techniques. Because of the ability of MRI to detect small changes in the water content of tissues, it may identify an abnormality or define the extent of one much more readily than CT. Fourth, MRI provides significantly more information than CT about tissue characteristics, and the increased sensitivity of MRI over CT applies to metastatic disease, especially when an intravenous contrast agent is used. Fifth, beam-hardening artifacts seen with CT—for example in the posterior fossa, middle cranial fossa, and craniocervical junction—which make diagnosis difficult, if not impossible, in some patients, do not occur with MRI. Sixth, with MRI, multiple projections can be obtained with ease. Most CT images are cross-sectional, although direct coronal images of the head can be made if the patient can hyperextend the neck. Hyperextension can be difficult, cumbersome, and painful, and many patients find it impossible. The multiplanar capability of MRI allows clearer and more accurate definition of a disease process. Seventh, MRI has the ability to define subacute and chronic collections of blood much better than CT and is also superior in the

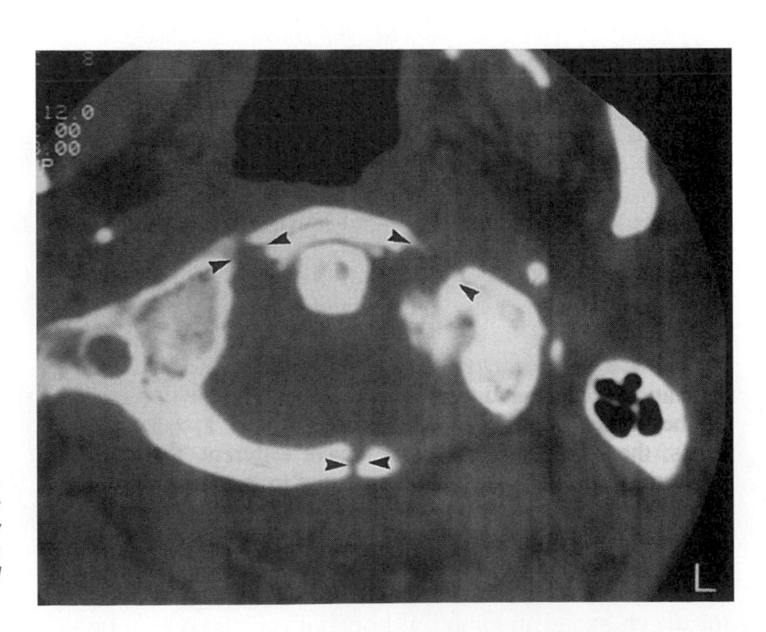

*FIGURE 10–9 Jefferson's fracture. Axial CT of the atlas demonstrates bilateral fractures of the anterior arch and a fracture of the left posterior arch of C1 (*arrowheads*). Conventional radiographs may fail to demonstrate this fracture, as they did in this patient. This fracture is optimally displayed by CT, because the entire vertebral segment can be demonstrated on a single axial slice.*

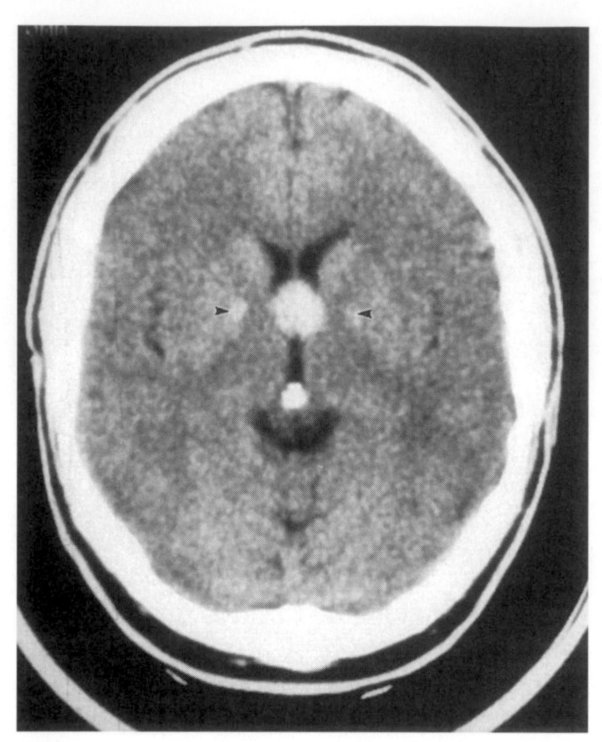

F I G U R E 10 – 10 *Colloid cyst of the third ventricle. Precontrast axial CT demonstrates a hyperdense, round midline mass in the region of the foramen of Monro. Note bilateral basal ganglia calcifications (*arrowheads*), which have no clinical significance. Postcontrast CT (not shown) did not demonstrate enhancement. Colloid cysts, benign cysts filled with mucin, are found in the roof of the third ventricle at the level of the foramen of Monro. Symptoms arise from intermittent or chronic obstruction of cerebrospinal flow from the lateral ventricles that leads to hydrocephalus. Many affected patients complain of frontal or occipital headaches. The classic positional headaches associated with colloid cysts occur in fewer than 50% of patients.*

evaluation of the contents of a cystic lesion. Eighth, patients allergic to iodinated contrast material can easily be evaluated with MRI, because the contrast agent used for this modality does not contain iodine (see later).

Indications and Contraindications

MRI is the imaging procedure of choice for the evaluation of nearly all abnormalities involving the brain (Figs. 10–11 to 10–13),[6, 9–11, 13, 14, 17, 19] spine (Figs. 10–14, 10–15),[6, 10, 13, 14, 21–23] and musculoskeletal system (Figs. 10–16 to 10–18).[7, 8] Imaging of the soft tissues of the extremities is easy with MRI. In addition to depicting muscles, fat, and blood vessels readily, it can also visualize articular cartilage. MRI is an outstanding modality for evaluating various joints, such as the shoulder, hip, and knee.[7, 8, 24] Articular cartilage of the knee is difficult to detect with CT because it lies in the plane of the section, but it can be visualized on coronal and sagittal MR images. Although inferior to CT in demonstrating bone details, MRI is the modality of choice for evaluating disorders of the bone marrow (see Fig. 10–16).[25, 26] Because a small amount of motion can decrease the spatial resolution of MR images considerably, and thus can compromise an examination, MRI is not the primary imaging modality for the chest and abdomen, although it can play an impor-

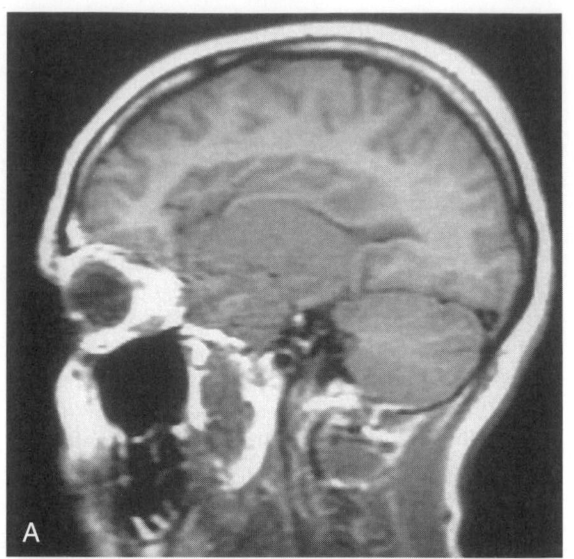

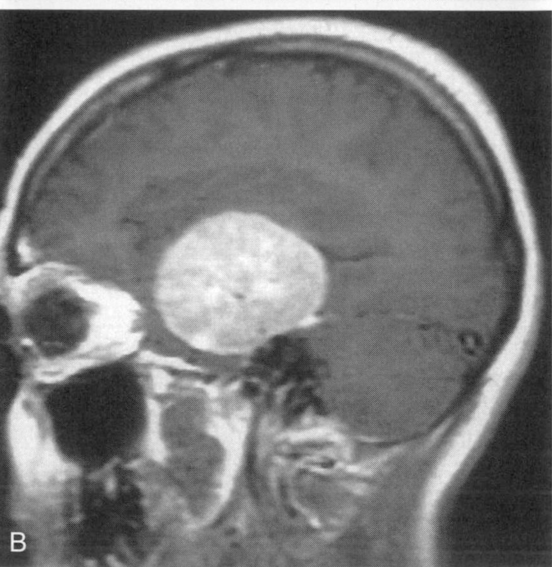

F I G U R E 10 – 11 *Sphenoid wing meningioma.* A, *T1-weighted sagittal MR image demonstrates a large, extraaxial, isointense mass.* B, *The mass enhances homogeneously after the intravenous injection of gadolinium contrast material.*

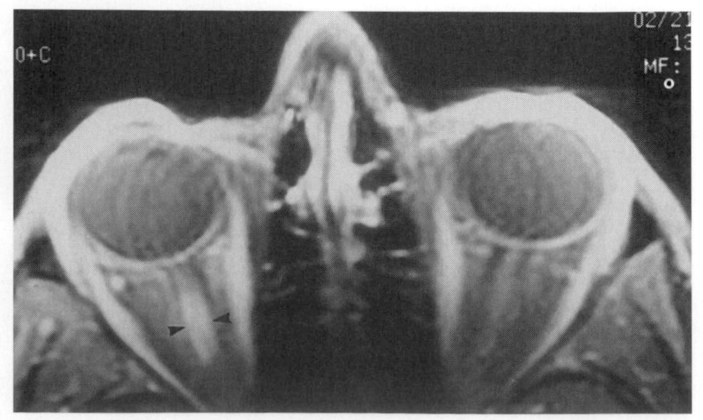

F I G U R E 10 – 12 *Optic neuritis. Fat-suppressed postgadolinium axial MR image of the orbits demonstrates a large area of enhancement in the right optic nerve (*arrowheads*). Compare with the normal left optic nerve. The patient was a 24-year-old woman who complained of right eye pain.*

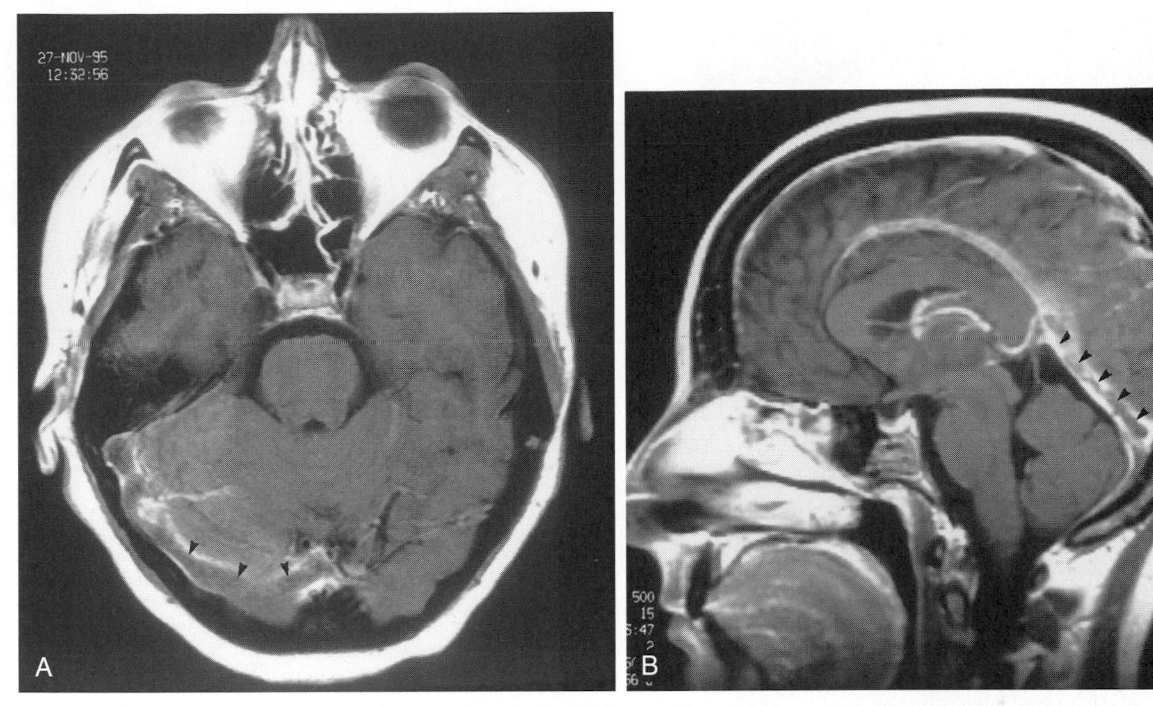

FIGURE 10–13 *Dural venous thrombosis. A 44-year-old woman presented with gradually worsening headaches over the past several weeks. Gadolinium-enhanced T1-weighted axial,* A, *and sagittal,* B, *views. The axial image shows abnormal materials of intermediate signal intensity within the right transverse sinus (*arrowheads*) surrounded by contrast enhancement, consistent with venous thrombosis. The sagittal image demonstrates thrombus within the straight sinus (*arrowheads*).*

tant role in evaluating these areas (see later). The indications for and contraindications to MRI are summarized in Table 10–2.

Contrast Agents

Gadolinium-containing contrast agents have been approved by the U.S. Food and Drug Administration for clinical use in MRI. The use of these agents has significantly improved the diagnostic armamentarium of MRI.[10, 11, 13, 14, 17, 22, 23] These contrast agents, which are administered intravenously, are paramagnetic agents that alter the magnetic environment of the tissues so that the resulting images are enhanced (see Fig. 10–11), thus providing additional information about and characterization of the lesion.[10, 17] Because these agents do not contain iodine, they may be used in patients who are allergic to iodine.[10, 17]

Limitations

Limitations of MRI include the inability to demonstrate exquisite bone detail and calcification, long imaging times, limited availability in many areas, and expense. Critically ill patients maintained with life support cannot be examined by MRI if the support equipment is ferromagnetic. Because of the physically confining space for the patient within the magnet, some patients experience claustrophobia and require sedation whereas others simply cannot tolerate the procedure.

Radionuclide Scanning

Scintigraphy detects the distribution in the body of a radioactive agent injected into a vein. Nuclear medicine is an integral part of the diagnostic armamentarium of the radiologist. The strength of radionuclide scintigraphy resides in its ability to portray the functional status of an organ or body part. The specialty of nuclear medicine has grown tremendously in the last decade through the linkage of new radioactive elements to biologic materials and via progress in the mechanics of detecting radioactivity. The radioactive-biologic element complex is localized to certain parts of the body. For example, radiolabeled sulfur colloid localizes in the liver whereas radiolabeled methylene disphosphonate localizes in bone and bypasses the liver. The radioactivity is detected from outside the body with specialized gamma cameras placed over the organs and areas of interest. Localized defects that cause either too much or too little radioactivity to be emitted from a usually homogeneous area are then detected as pathologic lesions.

Almost any organ of the body can be investigated by means of radionuclide scanning. Such imaging is used extensively in the evaluation of pathologic processes involving the brain, cerebrospinal fluid, lungs, kidneys, musculoskeletal system, hepatobiliary system, gastrointestinal tract, thyroid, spleen, and testes.

Bone Scanning

The bone scan is an excellent complement to other imaging studies of the skeletal system and in many instances can

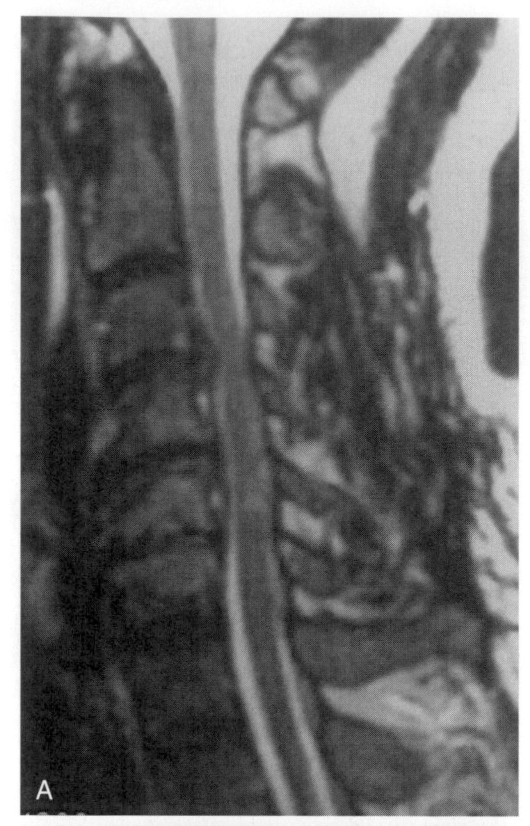

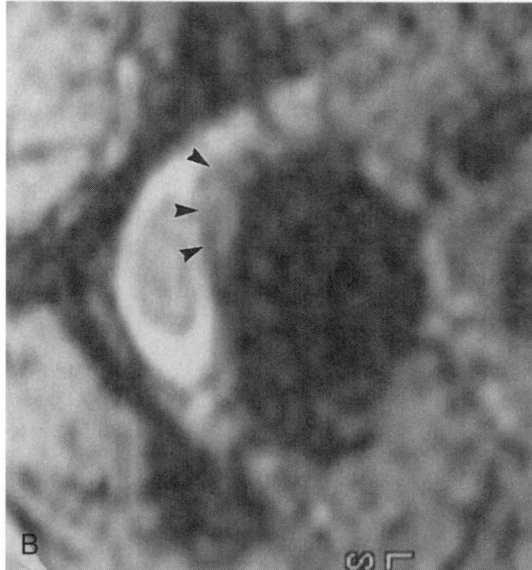

FIGURE 10–14 *Right-sided C4–C5 herniated disc.* A, *Sagittal MR image demonstrates ventral extradural mass* (arrowheads) *effacing the ventral subarachnoid space and compressing the cord at the C3–C4 level.* B, *Axial MR image demonstrates the right-sided herniated disc* (arrowheads).

be the definitive procedure.[27–30] Technetium Tc 99m is an ideal isotope for bone imaging.[27–30] Radionuclide bone imaging is an extremely sensitive but nonspecific modality for imaging the entire skeleton rapidly and inexpensively. The bone scan is a map of osteoblastic activity that occurs in response to a variety of benign and malignant conditions. Areas of increased or decreased bone turnover or remodeling can be identified by this method anywhere in the skeleton. This technique is exquisitely sensitive to very small

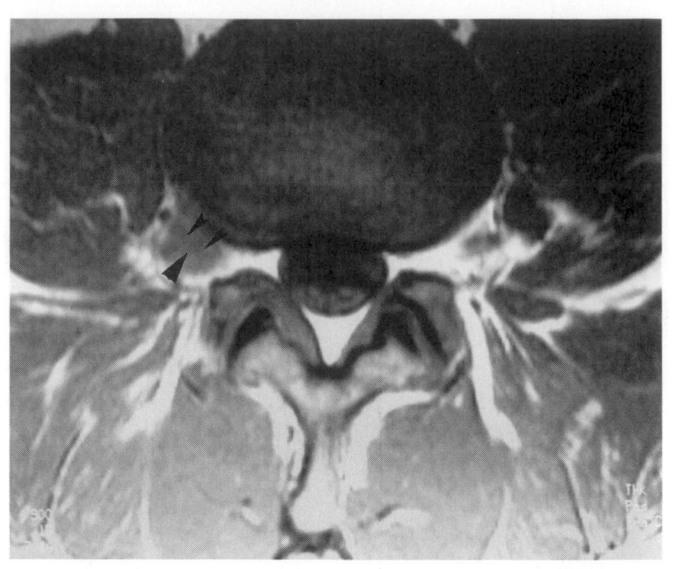

FIGURE 10–15 *A 56-year-old man presented with right lower extremity pain and tingling. T1-weighted axial MR image demonstrates a large far right lateral disc herniation* (arrowheads) *that is causing compression of the exiting nerve root.*

differences in bone turnover caused by disease processes of all kinds and allows the detection of abnormal areas long before they are visible on plain radiographs. Indications for bone scintigraphy are these:

- Evaluating bone pain when plain film findings are normal or equivocal
- Metastatic disease
- Early osteomyelitis
- Differentiating cellulitis from osteomyelitis
- Stress fractures
- Occult fractures
- Determining the "age" of compression fractures
- Primary bone tumors
- Staging of known malignancies
- Joint disease
- Early avascular necrosis
- Detecting and evaluating Paget's disease
- Evaluating bone grafts

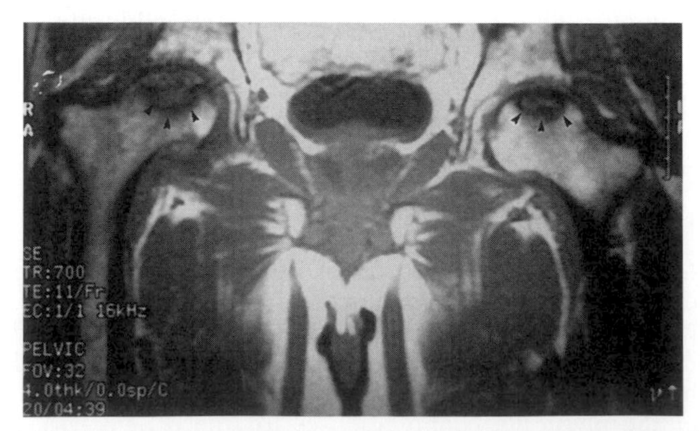

FIGURE 10–16 *Avascular necrosis of both femoral heads. Coronal T1-weighted MR image demonstrates bilateral areas of decreased signal intensity* (arrowheads) *in the femoral heads. Plain radiographs of the hip were normal in this 18-year-old male, who complained of bilateral hip pain.*

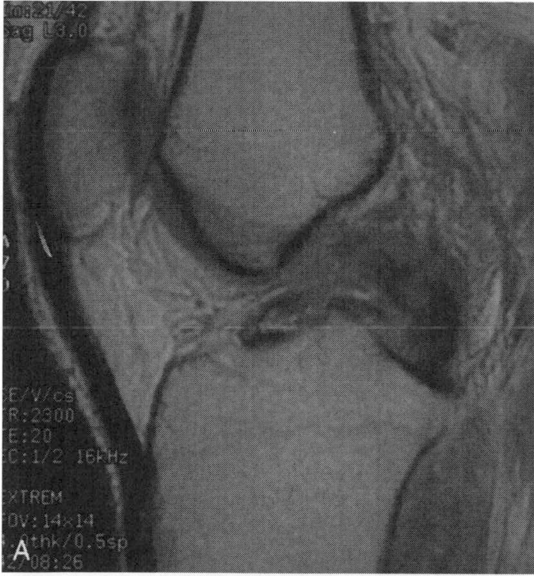

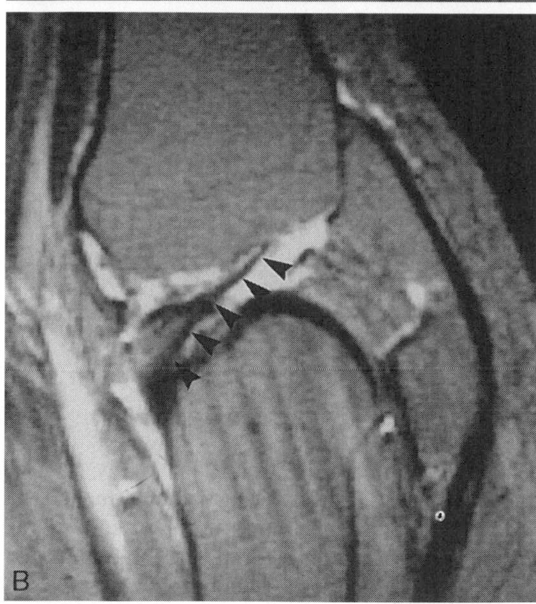

FIGURE 10–17 *Complete acute anterior cruciate ligament tear. A, Sagittal T1-weighted MR image of the knee demonstrates complete anterior cruciate ligament tear. Compare with normal anterior cruciate ligament* (arrowheads) *in* B.

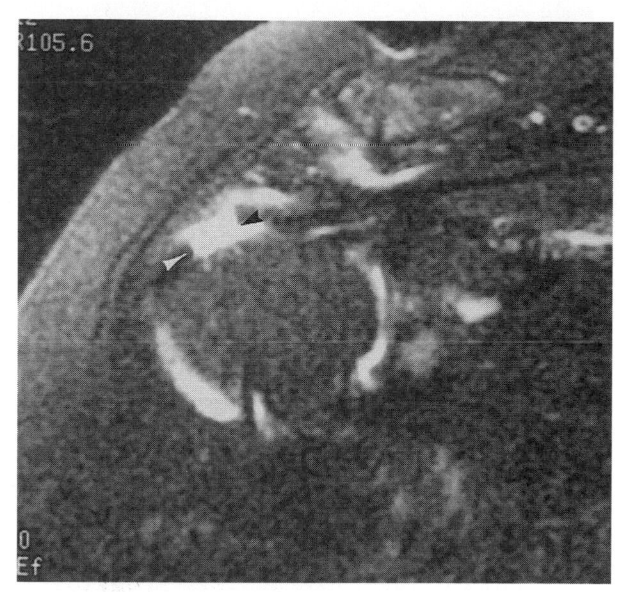

FIGURE 10–18 *Tear through supraspinatus tendon. T2-weighted coronal MR image through the right shoulder demonstrates full thickness tear through the anterior distal portion of the supraspinatus tendon. Arrowheads point to hemorrhage within the tear.*

- Evaluating painful joint prostheses
- Selecting a biopsy site

Technetium Tc 99m–labeled phosphates accumulate at metabolically active sites within the skeletal system. Deposition of the radioactive isotope occurs in areas of new bone formation of any cause. Fully calcified bone takes up relatively little radioactive tracer.

The most common use of bone scintigraphy is to detect metastatic disease (most often due to breast, prostate, lung, or renal carcinoma; Figs. 10–19, 10–20).[27–30] Lymphoma and neuroblastoma are also commonly evaluated by bone scintigraphy, and it is very helpful in follow-up during treatment of bone metastases. Bone scintigraphy is more sensitive than conventional plain radiographs for detecting lytic bone lesions.[27] Radionuclide bone scans may, however, demonstrate either no increased uptake or decreased uptake ("cold lesion") by certain aggressive tumors, such as multiple myeloma, some anaplastic carcinomas, and eosinophilic granulomas. In addition to neoplastic disease, trauma; infection; and vascular, metabolic, dysplastic, and degenerative disease of the musculoskeletal system can bc evaluated by bone scintigraphy. It is a sensitive evaluation in the initial phase of aseptic necrosis.[31]

Many fractures are easily identified and cause little or no diagnostic difficulty on conventional plain films. Some

TABLE 10–2 ***Indications for and Contraindications to MRI***

Body structures and processes for which MRI is indicated	Brain
	Spine and its contents
	Musculoskeletal system
	  Bone (neoplasm, trauma)
	  Bone marrow (osteomyelitis, neoplasm, devascularization)
	  Soft tissues (neoplasm, hematoma, abscess)
	  Muscles
	  Joints
	  Heart and great vessels
	  Focal liver masses
	  Kidney and retroperitoneum
	  Prostate
	  Gynecologic disease

Contraindications	Cardiac pacemaker Ferromagnetic cerebral aneurysm clips Metallic foreign body near the eye Cochlear implants

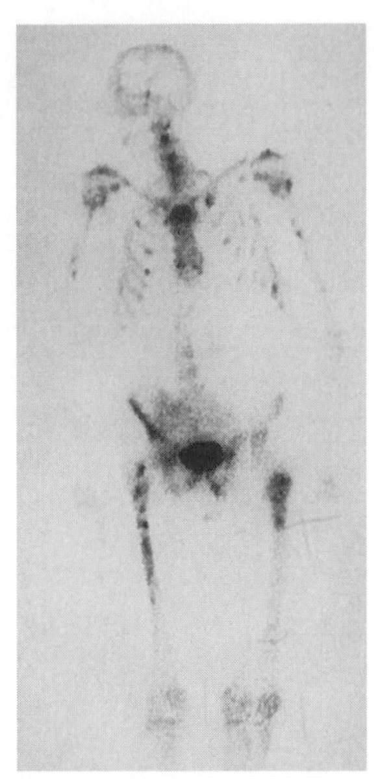

FIGURE 10–19 Diffuse skeletal metastatic disease. Whole-body bone scan of patient with prostatic cancer demonstrates markedly abnormal areas of increased uptake of the technetium Tc 99m isotope throughout the skeleton, indicative of widespread metastatic disease.

hairline fractures are very difficult to visualize on plain films (e.g., wrist, foot, face, and base of skull) but are easily seen on a bone scan.[27, 30] As many as 80% of patients with fractures have positive bone scans within 24 hours after the fracture[27] and 95% by 72 hours. The uptake of the radionuclide tracer steadily increases with time owing to greater vascularity and bone turnover at the fracture site.

The classic stress or fatigue fracture is another type of bone lesion that may not be evident on conventional plain film radiography, particularly soon after the fracture occurs, but may be obvious on the bone scan (Fig. 10–21).[27] Stress fractures may be caused by overuse of normal bone or normal use of weakened bone.

If a collapsed vertebra, whether a traumatic or nontraumatic lesion, is seen on a conventional plain radiograph, a bone scan may enable estimation of the age of the fracture (i.e., recent or old).[27] In 95% of patients younger than 65 years, a bone scan demonstrates increased bone turnover within 48 hours of such trauma, and almost all are found to have an abnormality by 72 hours. Failure of a collapsed vertebra to take up tracer indicates that the fracture is unlikely to be new.[27]

Radionuclide bone scintigraphy is more sensitive than conventional plain radiography for early detection of acute osteomyelitis or reactivation of the chronic form. The bone scan is generally positive within 24 hours. Osteomyelitis is usually evident on a radionuclide scan 7 to 10 days before changes become evident on conventional plain films (Figs. 10–22, 10–23). One difficulty in the scintigraphic diagnosis of osteomyelitis, however, is differentiating it from cellulitis. Making this distinction can be a difficult clinical problem, particularly in diabetics with nonhealing ulcers. Both conditions increase flow to the lesion, thus resulting in a higher rate of uptake of tracer by the affected bone. This problem can be resolved by modifying the routine bone scan to a three-phase or four-phase scan that involves obtaining a blood pool (early) image and, then, multiple sequential images. Osteomyelitis demonstrates increased activity of the radionuclide pharmaceutical relative to background activity over time, whereas cellulitis shows the opposite (see Fig. 10–22).

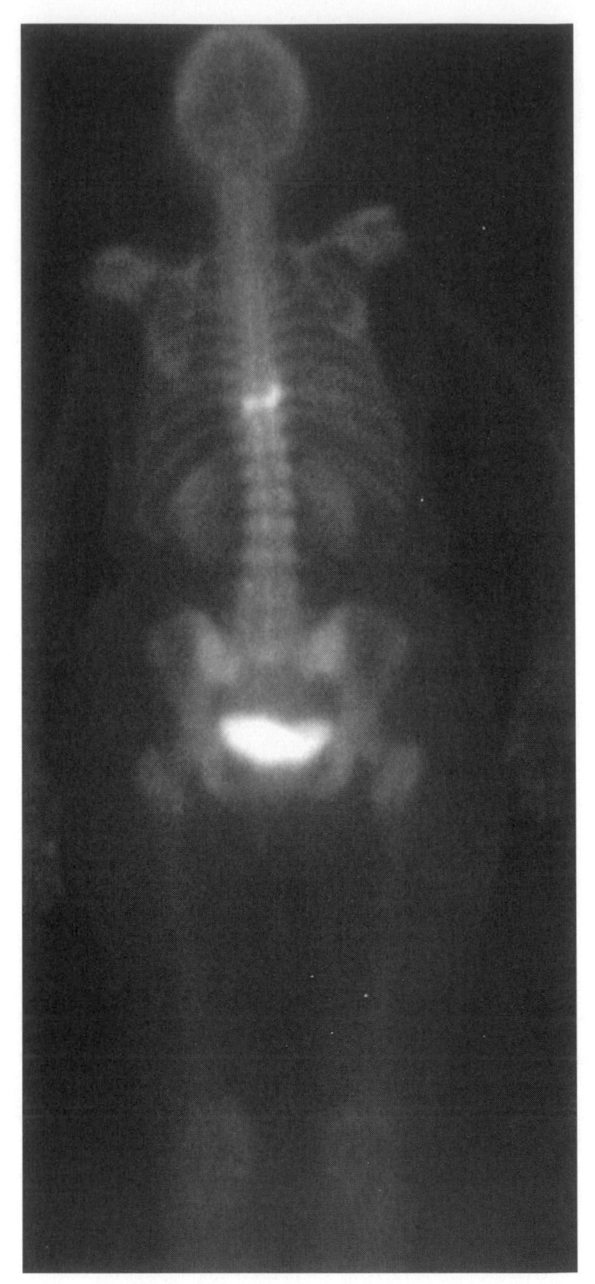

FIGURE 10–20 Solitary metastasis. A 75-year-old woman with recently diagnosed colon cancer presented with back pain of new onset. Technetium 99m MDP bone scan. Three-hour delayed planar image demonstrates markedly increased uptake in the T9 vertebral body. No additional areas of abnormal uptake are seen. The solitary lesion is nonspecific and could represent either an osteoporotic compression deformity or metastasis. It does localize the source of the patient's pain, provide direction for further imaging with CT or MRI, and exclude the presence of other metastases.

Occasionally, the scintigraphic diagnosis of osteomyelitis is difficult. This dilemma can be resolved with the use of gallium citrate Ga 67 (Fig. 10–24),[27–29] a radionuclide that is a sensitive and specific indicator of inflammatory cell

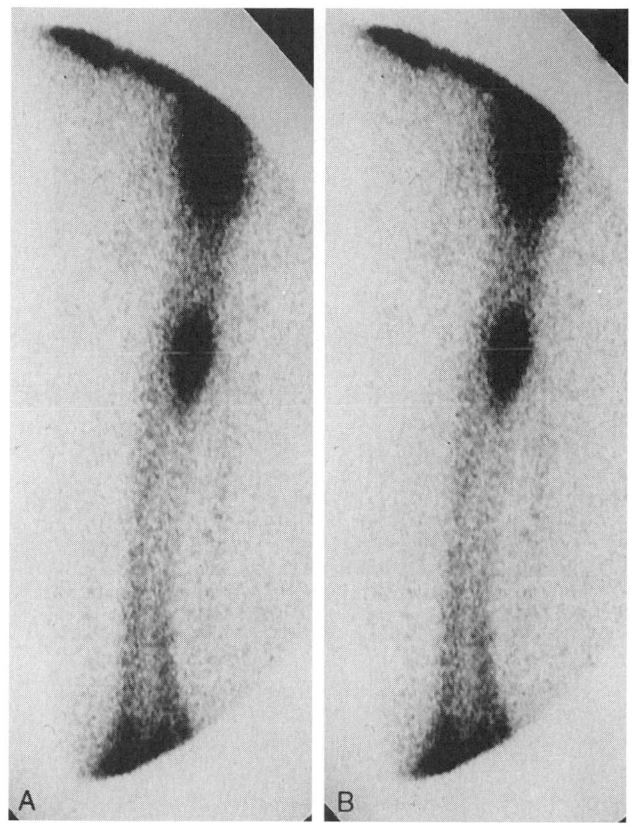

FIGURE 10–21 Stress fracture of right femur. A, B, Posterior and lateral views, respectively, of the right femur taken 3 hours after injection of technetium Tc 99m MDP show increased cortical uptake in the proximal femur. The plain film taken before the bone scan was normal.

activity, owing to its affinity for leukocytes. In some situations, particularly in infants, bone scintigraphy may fail to show an abnormality in the presence of osteomyelitis.[32] In the case of fever of unknown origin, gallium scintigraphy is probably the screening imaging procedure of choice.[27]

The detection of and differentiation between loosening and infection of a joint prosthesis may pose a diagnostic problem. In such situations, gallium citrate Ga 67 scanning can be used in conjunction with technetium 99m phosphate imaging.[33]

Indium 111–labeled white blood cells (WBC) can specifically detect infection in bone, soft tissues, and joints without localizing in uninfected granulation tissue, nonunions, degenerative arthritis, heterotopic ossification, metabolic bone disease, or inactive chronic osteomyelitis.[29] Indium 111–labeled WBC are therefore an ideal agent in the immediate postoperative period to evaluate for sepsis (Fig. 10–25). The sensitivity and specificity of the radiolabeled WBC for acute infection are superior to those of sequential technetium-gallium scanning in the diagnosis of low-grade musculoskeletal sepsis.[34]

The disadvantages of indium WBC bone scanning (which explain why it is not used routinely to evaluate osteomyelitis) are several. (1) Results of the study take at least 18 to 24 hours to develop. (2) Visualization of the thoracolumbar junction may present a problem because of overlap of activity in the liver and spleen. (3) Finally, false-positive results may occur in a patient with an accessory spleen or with areas of bowel infarction and inflammatory bowel disease, as the agent accumulates from causes other than osteomyelitis.

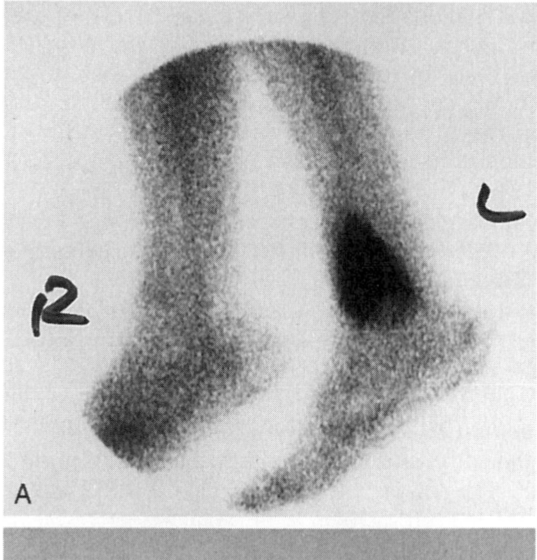

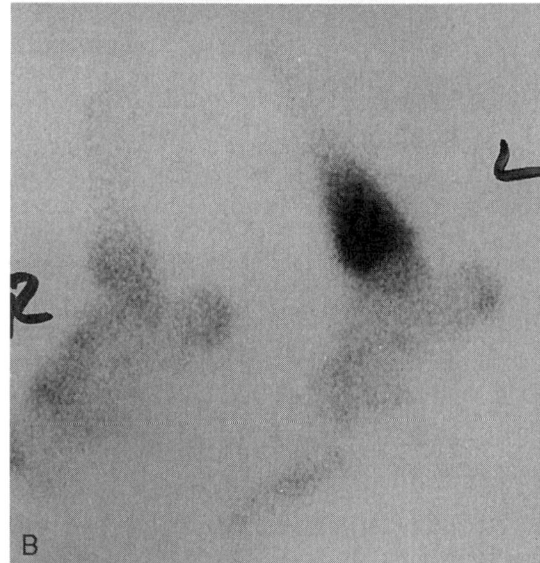

FIGURE 10–22 Osteomyelitis of distal tibia. A, Blood pool image of the left ankle after injection of technetium Tc 99m MDP in 27-year-old diabetic male. There is increased activity in the area of the distal tibia. B, Two-hour delayed image demonstrates that the activity of the technetium Tc 99m MDP does not decrease with time. Instead, it increases relative to blood background activity, reflecting osteomyelitis, not cellulitis. Initial plain films of the ankle prior to bone scintigraphy were normal.

Radionuclide Chest Scanning

A number of radionuclide examinations can be used in the evaluation of chest pain.

THALLIUM 201 MYOCARDIAL IMAGING

The thallium 201 stress test is performed during maximal or nearly maximal exercise on a treadmill or bicycle. It has limited value in the diagnosis of ischemic heart disease in patients with anginal pain. Thallium scintigraphy is positive in 90% to 100% of patients with acute myocardial infarction who are examined within 6 hours of onset.[16] Thus, a

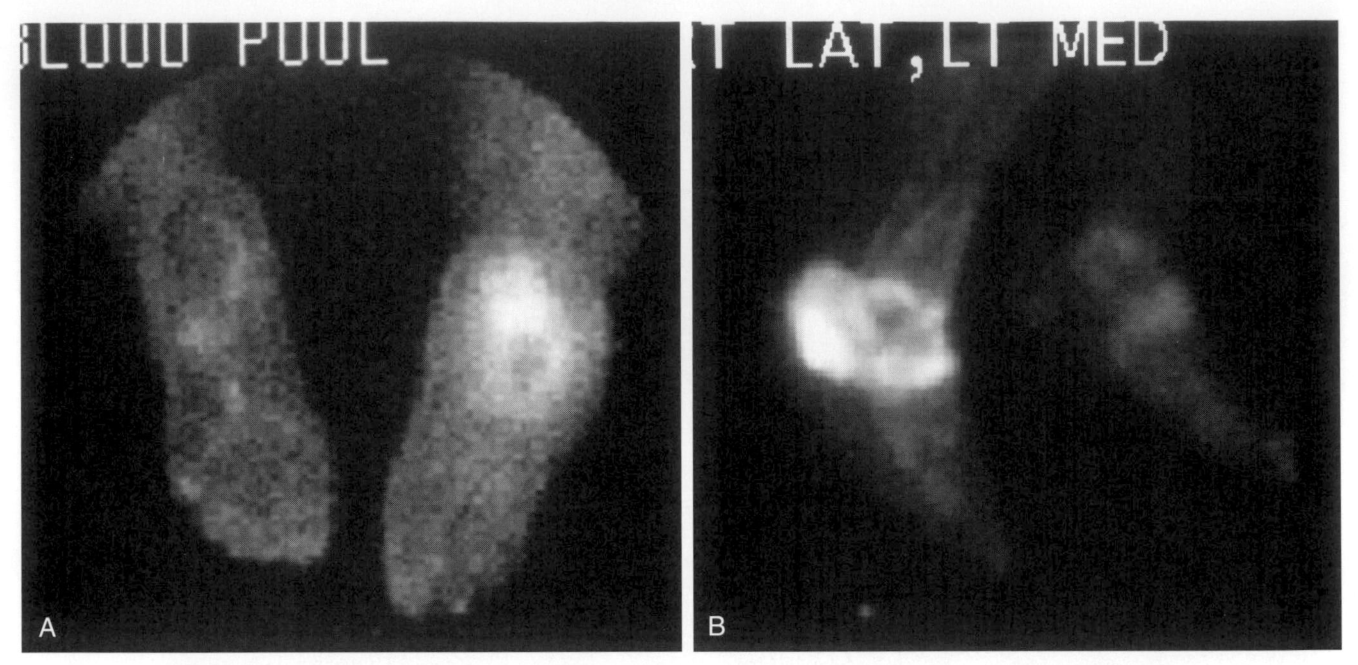

FIGURE 10–23 Osteomyelitis. A 54-year-old diabetic patient presented with right foot pain and a nonhealing ulcer. The examination was requested to exclude osteomyelitis. Three-phased bone scan with technetium 99m MDP. A, flow, blood pool and, B, delayed images demonstrate markedly increased activity throughout the right ankle consistent with osteomyelitis. The area of most intense uptake is along the inferior aspect of the calcaneus, at the site of the patient's ulcer.

normal thallium scan obtained within a few hours of the appearance of chest pain can exclude an acute myocardial infarction in most instances. Normal thallium scan findings do not rule out ischemic heart disease, however. Another disadvantage is that it does not distinguish acute myocardial infarction from an earlier infarction.

RADIONUCLIDE EXERCISE VENTRICULOGRAPHY USING RED BLOOD CELLS LABELED WITH SODIUM PERTECHNETATE TECHNETIUM TC 99M (EJECTION FRACTION)

This test is more sensitive than thallium myocardial imaging to detect ischemic heart disease.[16] The high rate of false-positive results, however, limits its usefulness.

TECHNETIUM TC 99M PYROPHOSPHATE SCINTIGRAPHY

Technetium Tc 99m pyrophosphate scans detect almost 90% of acute myocardial infarcts.[16] The radioactive tracer accumulates in areas of acute myocardial necrosis. The scan must be performed at least 12 hours after the onset of acute infarction, because the findings are usually negative during the first few hours after the onset of symptoms.

VENTILATION-PERFUSION SCANNING

In the evaluation of suspected pulmonary embolism, the radionuclide ventilation-perfusion lung scan (VQ scan) can be an effective screening test for segmental pulmonary thromboembolic disease.[35] The overall sensitivity of the VQ scan is very high, approaching 100%.[35] The perfusion scan most commonly uses technetium Tc 99m–labeled macroaggregated particles of albumin approximately 10 to 15μ in diameter. The ventilation scan is performed with xenon Xe 133 or an aerosol such as technetium Tc 99m–labeled DTPA aerosol.[35] There are four broad-based interpretations of radionuclide ventilation-perfusion examinations: (1) normal, which is considered excellent evidence for the absence of pulmonary embolism, (2) low probability of pulmonary embolism (less than 25% chance of full pulmonary embolism), (3) intermediate probability of pulmonary embolism, and (4) high probability of pulmonary embolism.[35] Pulmonary arteriography is indicated when clinical suspicion of pulmonary embolism is strong and when the ventilation-perfusion scan indicates low or intermediate probability of pulmonary embolism.[35]

Lower Extremity Pain Due to Deep Vein Thrombosis

A number of radionuclide scintigraphic studies can be used to diagnose deep vein thrombosis (DVT). Iodine 125-labeled fibrinogen scanning is the most sensitive noninvasive examination available for detection of early calf DVT.[36] Fibrinogen scanning has about 95% correlation with venographically demonstrated acute calf thrombosis, either occlusive or nonocclusive. Radionuclide venography using technetium Tc 99m–labeled macroaggregated albumin can detect approximately 80% of DVT involving the thigh, pelvis, or inferior vena cava, where the thrombus causes venous occlusion.[36] The increased background radiation from the trunk, bladder, and femoral vessels obscures DVT in the groin and pelvis. The inability to evaluate the proximal portion of the lower extremity efficiently is a major limitation of fibrinogen scintigraphy.

The combination of ultrasound (thigh and pelvis) and radionuclide studies (calf) is commonly used to evaluate for DVT.

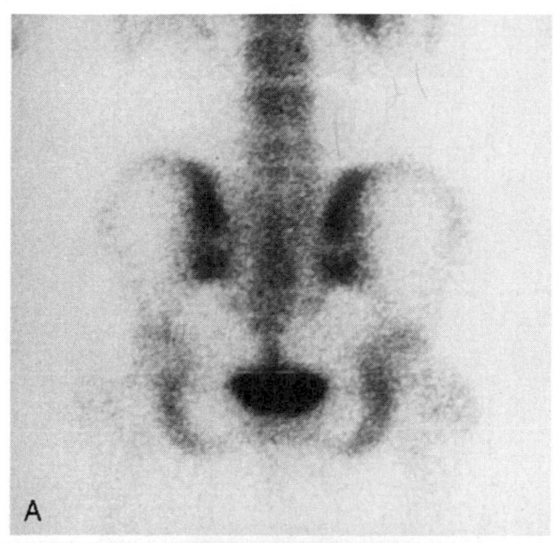

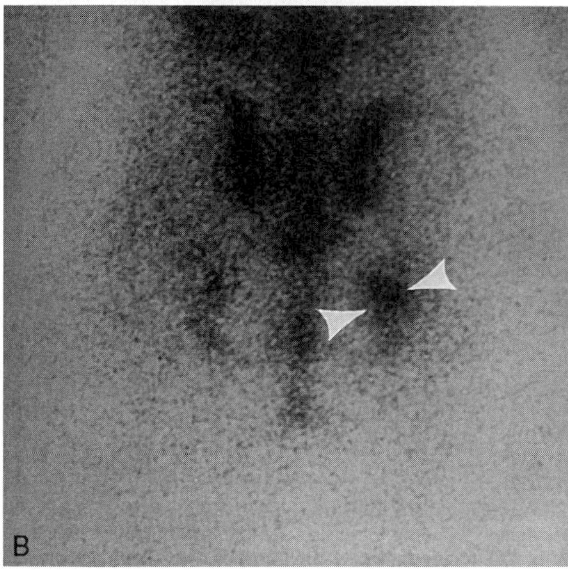

FIGURE 10–24 *Obturator abscess shown on gallium citrate Ga 67 scan.* A, *Posterior image of the pelvis after administration of technetium Tc 99m MDP is unremarkable.* B, *Posterior image of the pelvis 72 hours after intravenous administration of gallium citrate Ga 67 demonstrates an abnormal area of isotope localization (*arrowheads*) medial to the acetabulum in the region of the obturator foramen. This structure proved to be an obturator abscess.*

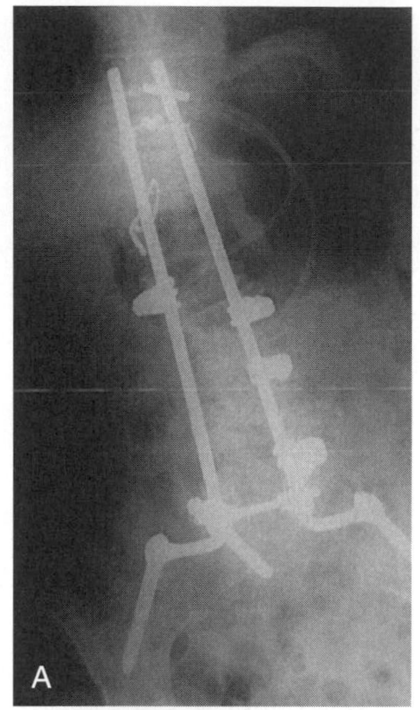

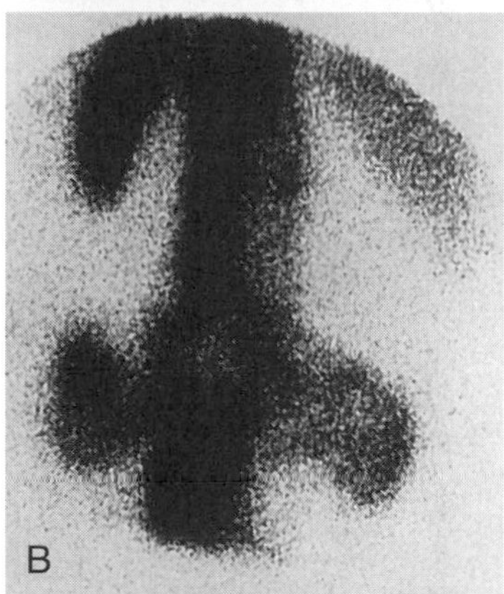

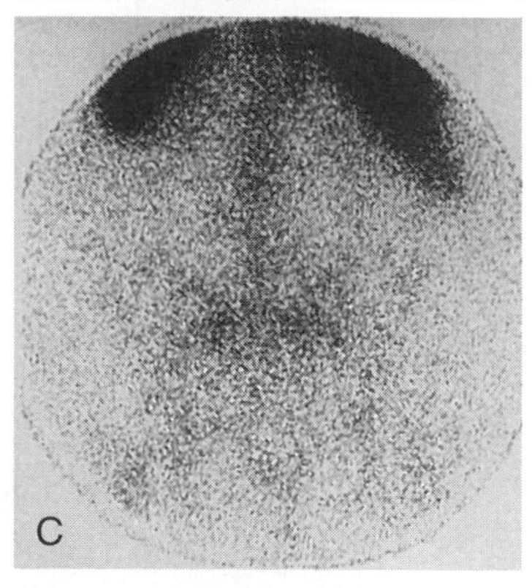

FIGURE 10–25 *Abscess status after Harrington rod placement. Value of indium 111–labeled white blood cells.* A, *Plain films of the lower thoracic lumbar spine taken 1 week after placement of Harrington rods. Clinically, infection was present at the surgical site, but plain films are unremarkable.* B, *Twenty-four-hour delayed posterior image of the back after injection of indium 111–labeled white blood cells demonstrates markedly increased activity throughout the surgical site. There is also accumulation of the tracer in the spleen and liver. Injection of indium 111–labeled white blood cells for evaluation for possible sepsis in the immediate postoperative period.* C, *Follow-up 24-hour, delayed indium 111–labeled white blood cell scan taken 3 months after treatment with antibiotics demonstrates complete resolution of the infection with no abnormal uptake of the isotope.*

Ultrasonography

Ultrasonography uses high-frequency sound waves to produce cross-sectional images of the body. The ultrasound transducer converts electrical energy to a brief pulse of high-frequency sound energy that is transmitted into the patient's tissues. The transmitted pulse encounters tissue interfaces that reflect a portion of the ultrasound beam back to the transducer, which then acts as a receiver that detects these echoes of the reflected sound energy. Most medical ultrasound transducers produce sound pulses in the frequency range of 1 to 10 mHz. The quality of all ultrasound examinations depends upon the skill and diligence of the sonographer. Ultrasound examinations generally provide the most diagnostic information when they are focused on solving a particular clinical problem.

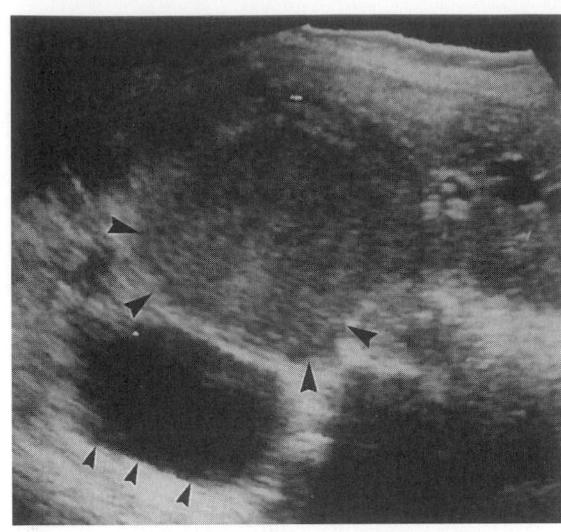

FIGURE 10–26 Multiple hepatic cysts. Axial ultrasound scan demonstrates multiple hepatic cysts. Smaller arrowheads *point to a large, echo-free cyst.* Large arrowheads *point to a larger echogenic area, a cyst filled with blood.*

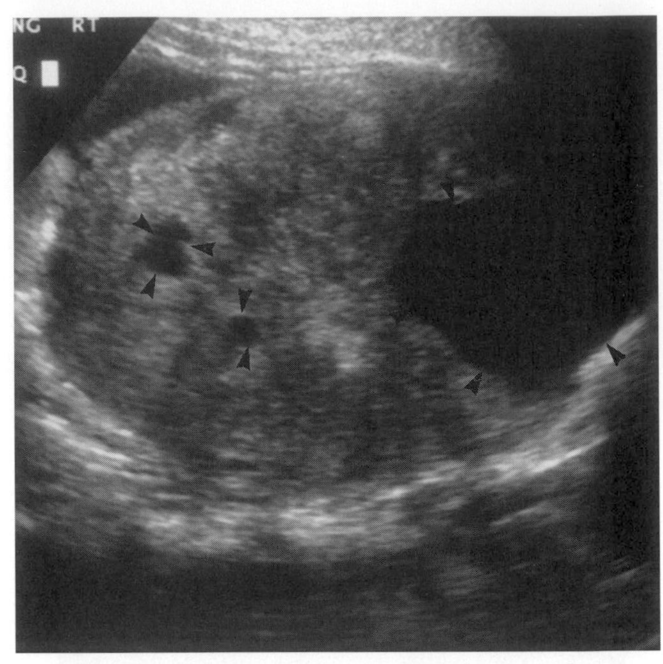

FIGURE 10–28 Acute torsion of ovarian fibroma. A 19-year-old woman with right pelvic pain of acute onset. Right parasagittal ultrasound image of pelvis demonstrates large ovarian mass with cystic components of varying sizes (arrowheads). *Other ultrasound images (not shown here) demonstrated ascites. At surgery, torsion of an ovarian fibroma was found.*

Visualization of anatomic structures by ultrasonography is severely limited by bone and by structures, such as bowel and lung, that contain gas. Ultrasound is very useful in evaluating the liver, gallbladder, kidney, ureters, urinary bladder, pancreas, pelvic organs, thyroid, breast, and soft tissue or cystic masses of the extremities. It has the unique ability to differentiate definitively between solid and cystic masses (Figs. 10–26 to 10–28). Doppler ultrasonography demonstrates not only blood flow but also its direction and velocity and thus can be very helpful in detecting vascular disorders throughout the body. It is the simplest and fastest method of evaluating the veins of the lower extremities in a noninvasive manner. The examination's accuracy depends much on the examiner's skill, experience, and attention to detail. Doppler ultrasonography is more sensitive in detecting DVT above the knee than in the calf—84% versus 25% correlation with venography, respectively.

Contrast-Enhanced Examinations

Approximately 20% to 30% of all radiologic examinations involve introduction of a contrast medium into the body for better visualization of a certain system. Contrast agents can be injected into various organs, cavities, and blood

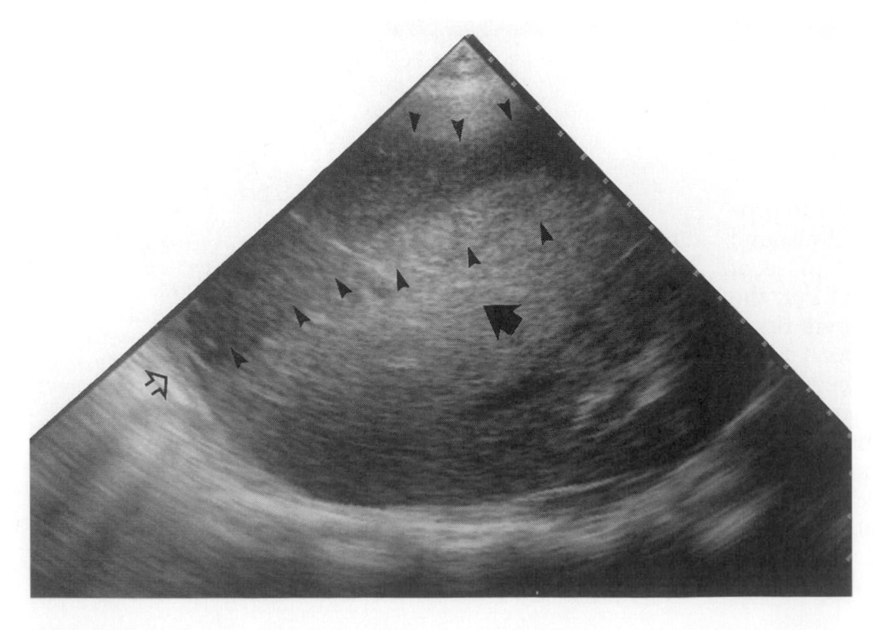

FIGURE 10–27 Subphrenic abscess. Right parasagittal ultrasound image demonstrates a heterogenous fluid-mass (arrowheads) *interposed between the diaphragm* (open arrow) *and the right lobe of the liver* (solid arrow).

vessels (both arteries and veins). Thus, it is possible to image the interior of organs and blood vessels.

Barium sulfate is used widely in radiology, in both barium meals and barium enemas, to evaluate the gastrointestinal tract (esophagus, stomach, small or large bowel). Iodinated contrast material, which is excreted by the kidneys after intravenous injection, is used to evaluate the urinary tract in intravenous pyelography. Before the advent of ultrasonography, cholecystography (for which the patient ingests contrast material) was the primary imaging modality for detecting gallstones. In most institutions, oral cholecystography has been completely replaced by ultrasonography. Intravenous iodinated contrast material is also used to enhance CT images in order to identify a soft tissue mass if the initial CT images are unremarkable or to assess the vascularity of soft tissues or a tumor.

Arthrography

Imaging after injection of contrast material into a joint space—arthrography—is a useful procedure for evaluating joints and surrounding tissues.[37] Virtually any joint can be evaluated with this technique. Arthrography can be combined with conventional tomography (arthrotomography) or with CT (CT arthrography). Shoulders, wrists, knees, ankles, and elbows are the joints most often evaluated by this technique. Arthrography is particularly effective in demonstrating rotator cuff injuries, adhesive capsulitis, abnormalities of the articular cartilage, and various ligamentous injuries.[37]

Internal derangements of the joints, such as meniscal tears, cruciate ligament tears in the knee, and rotator cuff injuries of the shoulder can now be noninvasively and painlessly demonstrated by MRI (Figs. 10–17, 10–18).[7,8,24] MRI can provide similar if not superior diagnostic accuracy. In many institutions, MRI has replaced arthrography for the evaluation of joint disease.

MRI has also rapidly replaced arthrography and CT for imaging the temporomandibular joint.[37–39] Because of its noninvasiveness and its ability to directly image internal derangements of the temporomandibular joint, MRI has become the imaging modality of choice for such an evaluation.

Myelography

For more than 50 years, myelography has been a relatively safe, accepted, and established imaging technique for the spine and its contents.[13, 14, 40–43] Performed after the introduction of a water-soluble, nonionic contrast agent into the subarachnoid space via lumbar puncture, this procedure is effective and accurate for demonstrating the subarachnoid space, spinal cord, and nerve root sheaths.[13, 14, 43] It has been, and is still being, used in some hospitals to identify surgically treatable intraspinal lesions, which may be extradural, intradural-extramedullary, or intramedullary.

The use of myelography has diminished considerably since the advent of CT and MRI, which are less costly and less invasive. Furthermore, MRI is considered superior to myelography in both sensitivity and specificity in most situations involving the spine and its contents. Today, myelography may be indicated when (1) CT or MRI fails to demonstrate an abnormality and (2) the abnormality shown by CT or MRI does not adequately explain the clinical picture. The added information provided by postmyelography CT of the spine is of great value in a large variety of situations (e.g., arachnoiditis; Figs. 10–29, 10–30).

Arteriography

In the era of CT and MRI, the emphasis of angiography has changed from diagnosis to more accurate evaluation of known processes.[17] Obviously, angiography still remains the procedure of choice for the documentation of vascular injury and disease. Preoperative angiography can provide important information by demonstrating the vascular supply to a tumor and the relationships of the major vessels with the tumor mass.[17] In many instances, the angioarchitecture of the tumor may suggest the correct pathologic diagnosis.[17] Angiography remains essential in the preliminary evaluation of potential therapeutic interventional procedures.

CORONARY ARTERIOGRAPHY

Coronary arteriography is still the gold standard for demonstrating the presence and the extent of coronary artery disease.[16] In patients with intractable angina, coronary arteriography is indicated to establish or exclude ischemic heart disease as the cause of chest pain.[16] In the diagnosis of acute myocardial infarction, coronary arteriography is of little diagnostic benefit and is not indicated.[16]

AORTOGRAPHY

Traumatic rupture of the aorta secondary to blunt chest trauma and aortic dissection are life-threatening emergen-

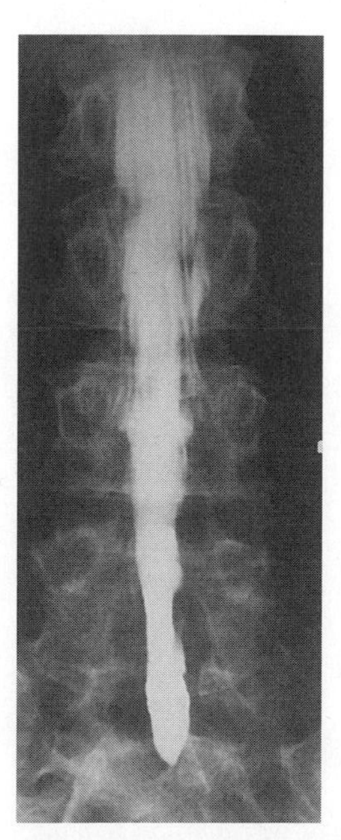

FIGURE 10–29 Arachnoiditis involving lower lumbar dural sac. Frontal projection of myelogram demonstrates marked distortion and irregularity of the lower lumbar dural sac. In addition, the contrast column exhibits the so-called empty or featureless sac, with no visualization of the individual nerve roots in the contrast column. Compare the appearance of the lower lumbar dural sac with that of the upper one, where normal nerve roots and nerves are seen within the contrast column.

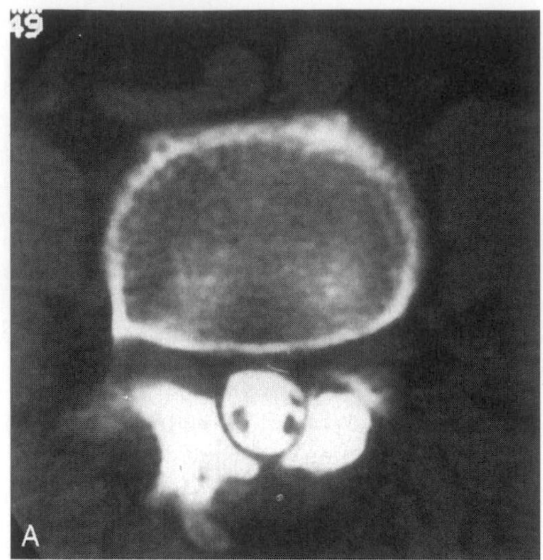

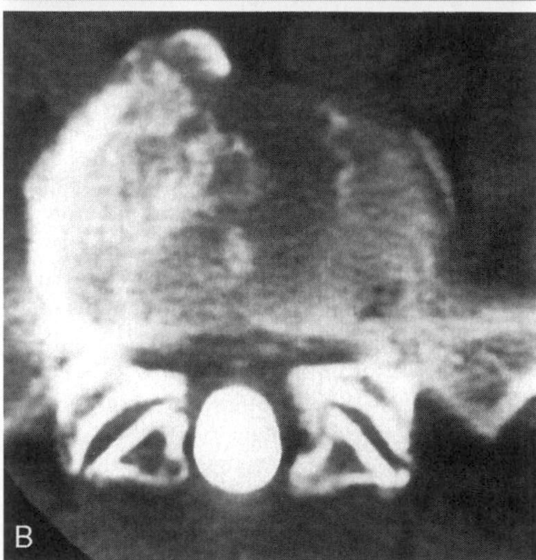

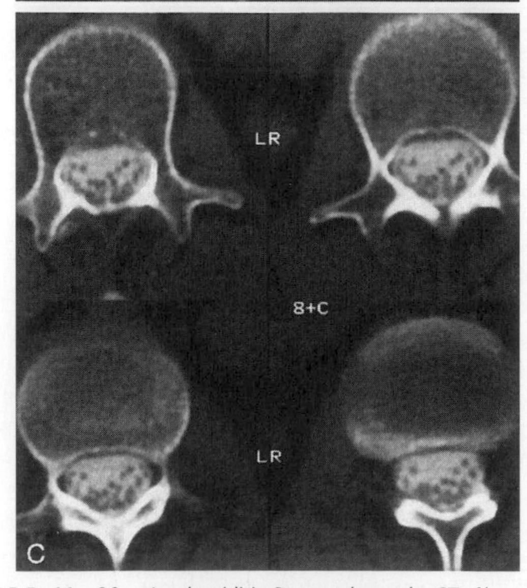

FIGURE 10–30 Arachnoiditis. Postmyelography CT of lower lumbar spine in 36-year-old man with a history of multiple back operations. Note the so-called featureless or empty sac appearance. A, The nerve roots have lost their individuality and are clumped together and appear thickened. They are seen peripherally in the dural sac. B, The nerve roots are adherent to the dura, and, in fact, no nerve roots can be seen within the contrast column. C, Normal postmyelography CT of another patient. Note how well the individual nerve roots can be seen within the contrast column. Compare this normal appearance with that in A and B.

cies[44] in which chest pain can be a dominant clinical feature. With aortic dissection, the classic finding is sharp, tearing chest pain radiating to the back and associated with loss of pulses. CT and MRI, which are reliable, rapid, and noninvasive, can provide the correct diagnosis and demonstrate the extent of the lesion in many cases[44] and are indicated when these conditions are not emergencies. In most cases, however, traumatic rupture of the aorta and aortic dissection are manifested as life-threatening emergencies for which aortography is the procedure of choice and the definitive study.[44]

PULMONARY ARTERIOGRAPHY

Pulmonary arteriography is the most definitive and specific test for pulmonary embolism.[35] It is indicated when there is strong clinical suspicion of pulmonary embolism, ventilation-perfusion scanning indicates a low or intermediate probability of pulmonary embolism, and the patient is a candidate for anticoagulant therapy. Pulmonary arteriography is also indicated for the "high-probability group" or for patients who are candidates for venous occlusion or embolectomy or would be at extremely high risk from anticoagulant therapy. Pulmonary arteriography is associated with significant mortality and morbidity.[35] The treating physician must weigh the advantages and disadvantages of making or missing the diagnosis against the potential for complications before deciding for or against a pulmonary arteriogram.

Venography

In venography, iodinated contrast material, preferably nonionic contrast, is injected into a vein in the foot, and the deep venous system of the lower extremity, pelvis, and inferior vena cava is imaged. Venography has been widely accepted as the most definitive diagnostic test for DVT and is currently the gold standard against which all other examinations are compared.

SELECTION OF RADIOLOGIC IMAGING ACCORDING TO TISSUE TYPE AND REGIONAL DIAGNOSIS

The choice of a radiologic evaluation technique is influenced by the type of tissue to be investigated (Table 10–3) and by the regional diagnosis under consideration (Table 10–4).

Regional Pain Diagnosis

Headache and Orofacial Pain

Acute, severe, and potentially catastrophic headaches (e.g., subarachnoid hemorrhage) are best imaged by CT (see Fig. 10–4).[14, 18] In most geographic areas, CT is more readily available and is the modality of choice for suspected subarachnoid hemorrhage and other intracranial hemorrhage.[17] For subacute or chronic headaches, however, MRI is the procedure of choice.[17] Orofacial pain and other related syndromes may require dental radiography, and

TABLE 10–3 ***Diagnostic Value of Imaging Procedure According to Tissue Type***

Tissue Type Requiring Evaluation	Recommended Imaging Procedure(s)
Skin	No indication for imaging: lesions can be seen and palpated
Subcutaneous tissue	Plain films and CT to demonstrate presence/absence of calcification MRI
Muscle	Plain films and CT to demonstrate presence/absence of calcification MRI
Bone	Plain films Bone scintigraphy CT MRI
Joint	Plain films MRI Arthrography
Tendon	Plain films MRI
Spine	MRI CT Myelography
Internal organs	CT MRI Ultrasonography Contrast studies (IVP, barium meal or enema)

TABLE 10–4 ***Diagnostic Value of Imaging Procedure According to Body Region***

Body Region	Recommended Imaging Procedure(s)*
Head	
Brain	**MRI** CT Angiography
Head and neck	Plain films **CT** **MRI**
Spine	Plain films **MRI** CT Myelography
Extremities	
Soft tissues (including muscle, excluding bone)	Plain films Ultrasonography CT **MRI** Venography
Bone	**Plain films** **Bone scintigraphy** **CT** **MRI**
Joint	Plain films **MRI** Arthrography
Chest	**Plain films** **CT** MRI Radionuclide studies Coronary arteriography Aortography
Abdomen	Plain films **Ultrasonography** **CT** **Contrast studies (barium meal or enema, intravenous pyelography)** MRI Radionuclide studies
Pelvis	**Ultrasonography** **MRI** CT

* Boldface indicates procedure of choice.

temporomandibular pain may require MRI or arthrography.[38, 39] Sinusitis is best investigated by CT.

Thorax and Abdomen

Thoracoabdominal pain generally is encountered by the primary care physician. Diseases such as acute angina; gastroesophageal disease; abdominal crises (including peptic ulcer disease, gallbladder disease, appendicitis, renal abnormalities, and pancreatic tumors); and prostate problems are among the many lesions for which the pain clinician is not usually consulted until they become chronic or have escaped routine detection.

Processes in the chest and abdomen for which CT is helpful are summarized in Table 10–4. As far as visceral disease is concerned, assuming that an acute lesion has been ruled out by proper clinical, diagnostic, and electrophysiologic testing (e.g., electrocardiography and echocardiography) plain radiographs are generally of limited value except to demonstrate free air from a ruptured viscus or the presence or absence of calcification. CT, ultrasound, and contrast studies (barium meal and enema) are the initial imaging procedures of choice.

MRI can play an important role in evaluating for liver,[45] kidney,[46] retroperitoneal,[46] prostate,[47] and gynecologic disease.[48, 49] Although it is not likely to become a primary imaging technique for the kidney or retroperitoneum, MRI can play an important role in detecting and staging pathologic conditions of the urinary tract.[45] It is rapidly becoming the most useful modality for evaluating the prostate and demonstrating extension of disease beyond the confines of the gland.[47] MRI imaging is also emerging as an important diagnostic tool for investigating the female pelvis and for staging endometrial and cervical cancer.[49]

Neck and Upper Extremity Pain

Neck and upper extremity pain may be neurogenic pain, soft tissue pain, referred pain from viscera, musculoskeletal pain, or sympathetic pain. In the neck, the most common causes of nerve root compression are cervical spondylosis, disc herniation (see Fig. 10–14 and later discussion on low back pain), and tumor. Routine radiography should be followed by MRI of the cervical spine. In the upper extremities, joint disease is best evaluated by MRI after plain film radiography.

Low Back and Lower Extremity Pain

Numerous entities that yield to radiologic diagnosis may be noted in the low back and lower extremities. They include referred pain from the central nervous system, lumbosacral degenerative spine disease, disease in the hip, myofascial pain, pain in the distribution of major nerves, bone disease, peripheral vascular disease, and lesions of the knees, feet, and ankles. As in the upper extremities, joint disease is best evaluated by MRI after initial plain film radiography.

LOW BACK PAIN

Disorders of the spine are probably the most common cause of disability in adults in the United States. Low back pain affects 80% of all adults at some point in their lives.[50] The diagnosis and treatment of back problems have the dubious distinction of leading the medical system in financial cost.[51]

Degenerative disorders of the spine constitute the major indication for imaging the spine in current practice. Myelography,[13, 40, 41, 43] CT,[22] and MRI[10, 13, 14, 21, 22] are all excellent modalities for the spine and its contents. MRI has had a major impact on the evaluation of the spine and its contents and is now the imaging procedure of choice for screening patients with low back pain.[10, 13, 14, 21, 22]

Overall, MRI is superior to CT and myelography in the diagnosis of herniated disc disease and spinal stenosis.[21] Considerable confusion exists among the terms *bulging disc*, *herniated disc*, *protruded disc*, and *extruded disc*. The distinction between a bulging disc and a herniated (protruded, extruded, or sequestered) disc is important.[21] Generally, a bulging disc is not associated with sciatica, whereas a herniated disc is. A bulging disc results from disc degeneration with a grossly intact but lax annulus fibrosus.[21] The disc margin extends beyond the margins of the adjacent vertebral end plates in a smooth and symmetric configuration. A protruded disc represents herniation of nucleus pulposus material through a defect in the annulus fibrosus that produces a focal extension of the disc margin.[21] The nuclear material has not broken through the entire annulus fibrosus but is still bound posteriorly by some unruptured annular fibers. With an extruded disc, there are no intact annular fibers. The nucleus pulposus material has ruptured through the annulus fibrosus and bulges into the spinal canal or intervertebral foramen. *Sequestered disc* or *free fragment* refers to disc material external to the annulus fibrosus that is no longer contiguous with the parent nucleus pulposus.[21] A free fragment can lie either anterior or posterior to the posterior longitudinal ligament.[21]

Synovial cysts usually occur in association with degenerative changes involving the facet joints. Synovial cysts often present as back pain or radicular pain. Clinical differentiation of low back pain from synovial cysts and that from a herniated disc may be difficult. Most synovial cysts develop in the lower lumbar region, most often at the L4–L5 level (Fig. 10–31). Both CT and MRI are excellent modalities to demonstrate synovial cysts.

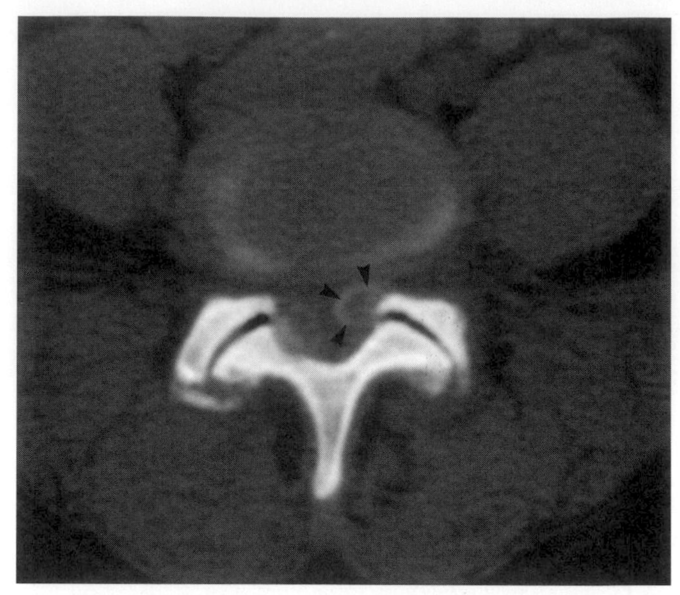

*FIGURE 10–31 Synovial cyst. A 52-year-old woman presents with chronic back pain. Non-contrast CT of the lumbar spine at the L4–L5 level demonstrates small curvilinear calcifications (*arrowheads*) within the spinal canal adjacent to the facet joint. These findings are characteristic of a calcified synovial cyst.*

CT is superior to MRI for demonstrating (1) bone and joint abnormalities in the spine and (2) foraminal bony stenosis. After spine trauma, MRI can noninvasively investigate the intervertebral discs, sites of ligamentous injury, epidural hematoma, and spinal cord injury (Fig. 10–32).[52] MRI also demonstrates vertebral alignment and the relationship of the vertebrae to the spinal cord. Thus, MRI is very helpful in evaluating the cervicothoracic junction. It is the best modality to evaluate spinal infection.[23] It is also the best primary (and often the definitive) imaging modality to demonstrate mass lesions in the intramedullary, intradural-extramedullary, or epidural compartment.[21, 22]

FAILED BACK SURGERY SYNDROME

The failed back surgery syndrome (FBSS) is a significant medical and socioeconomic problem in the United States, considering the estimated 300,000 new laminectomies performed each year. Because approximately two thirds of all patients enrolled in chronic pain centers suffer from FBSS, additional emphasis is given to this entity. By definition, FBSS is the persistence or onset of back or leg symptoms after lumbar disc surgery. The patient who has had multiple low back procedures should be assessed according to a structured and uniform scheme that differentiates initially between low back pain and leg pain.

In general, one must differentiate between mechanical and nonmechanical causes of FBSS. Mechanical lesions include recurrent herniated disc, spinal instability, and spinal stenosis, which cause symptoms by direct pressure on the neural elements and may be surgically correctable.[53] The nonmechanical entities include scar tissue (arachnoiditis or epidural fibrosis), psychosocial instability, and systemic medical diseases, which are not helped by any other type of additional spine surgery.[53]

In addition, one must differentiate among FBSS patients for whom (1) low back pain is the principal complaint, (2) leg pain is the principal complaint, and (3) the complaint is a combination of the two.[54]

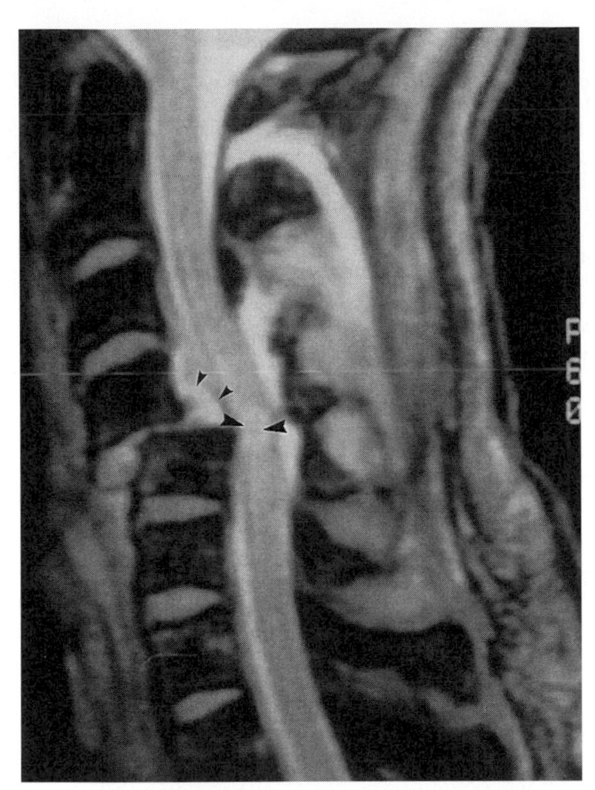

FIGURE 10–32 Traumatic dislocation of cervical spine with cord contusion. T2-weighted sagittal MR image demonstrates approximately 50% anterior subluxation of C4 on C5. The anterior and posterior longitudinal ligaments have been disrupted, and an anterior epidural hematoma is noted at the disk space (small arrowheads)*. In addition, there is an area of increased signal intensity within the spinal cord (*large arrowheads*), indicating cord contusion.*

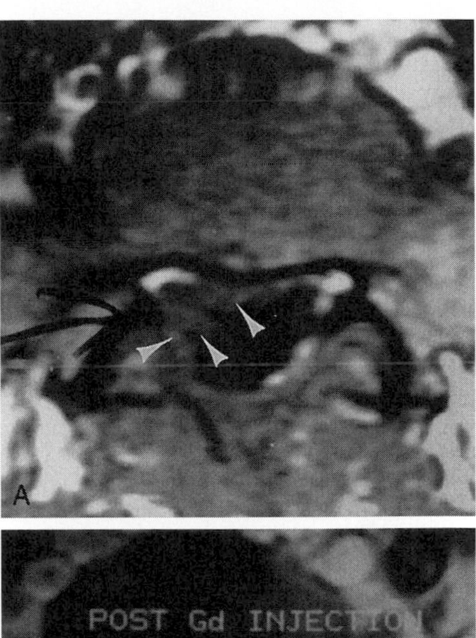

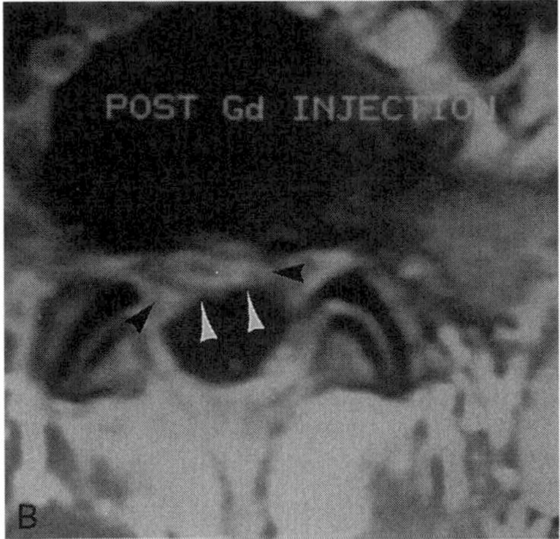

FIGURE 10–33 Epidural fibrosis. Value of postgadolinium MRI. A 27-year-old man previously had a right L4–L5 discectomy and presented with recurrent right-sided leg pain. A, *T1-weighted MR image demonstrates a right-sided ventral epidural soft tissue mass effacing and displacing the thecal sac* (arrowheads)*. On the basis of this MR appearance, recurrent L4–L5 disc or epidural fibrosis cannot be differentiated.* B, *After the administration of intravenous contrast medium containing gadolinium, T1-weighted axial MR image demonstrates enhancement of the right-sided epidural mass* (arrowheads)*, confirming that the ventral epidural mass is epidural fibrosis, and not a recurrent disc.*

Among the major causes of the FBSS are recurrent disc herniation (12%–16%), preoperatively unrecognized stenosis (lateral recess 50%, central stenosis 7%–40%), epidural fibrosis or scar (6%–8%; Fig. 10–33), and arachnoiditis (6%–16%; Figs. 10–29, 10–30.)[55–57] Less common causes include lateral or central stenosis from postoperative bone overgrowth, extrusion of a bone fusion fragment into the canal, severe nerve injury from a herniation or postoperative trauma, pseudomeningocele, postoperative spondylolisthesis, operation at the wrong level, unrecognized sequestered fragment, incomplete excision of a herniated disc, and failed fusion.[56]

MRI with the use of intravenous contrast material is the best overall imaging technique to investigate FBSS.[55, 58] Myelography may demonstrate an extradural defect at the surgical site, but it cannot differentiate between scar and herniated disc.[59, 60] CT is the best technique for foraminal stenosis and other bone abnormalities.

Although CT[61] and MRI[58] (both performed after contrast injection) can demonstrate arachnoiditis, myelography (see Fig. 10–29), especially when followed by CT myelography, is often the best and definitive diagnostic modality to demonstrate arachnoiditis and epidural fibrosis (see Fig. 10–33). It should be remembered that, as far back as 1968, Hitselberger and Witten[62] pointed out that 37% of asymptomatic patients had abnormalities on iophendylate myelography. Therefore, clinical correlation remains the watchword. In addition, on CT examination,[56, 63] it is extremely difficult to determine prospectively who will have pain postoperatively. In a study of the lumbar spine with postoperative surface coil MRI,[58] early postoperative spine changes were dramatic and affected every portion of the neural canal. Immediately after discectomy, the rent in the annulus that was the site of discectomy and curettage was easily demonstrated. The soft tissue changes seen in the first 10 days after surgery on MRI are secondary to the surgery and severely limit the usefulness of this modality during that time to investigate persistent or new symptoms. The exception to this is postoperative hemorrhage whose distinctive MRI signal characteristics make identification possible.[64]

CONCLUSION

Selection of an imaging technique according to (1) body region and (2) the putative tissue and mechanism involved in the production of pain usually results in a cost-effective, productive examination that then can be correlated with clinical findings.

REFERENCES

1. Wilson PR, Lamer TJ: Pain mechanisms: Anatomy and physiology. *In* Raj PP (ed): Practical Management of Pain, ed 2. St. Louis, Mosby–Year Book, 1992.
2. Cyriax JH: Diagnosis of soft tissue lesions. *In* Textbook of Orthopedic Medicine, ed 7, vol I. London, Bailliere Tindall, 1978.
3. Penning L, Wilmink JT, Woerden HH, et al: CT myelographic findings in degenerative disorders of the cervical spine: Clinical significance. AJNR 7:119, 1986.
4. Teresi LM, Lufkin RB, Reicher MA, et al: Asymptomatic degenerative disk disease and spondylosis of the cervical spine: MR imaging. Radiology 164:83, 1987.
5. Jensen MC, Brant-Zawadski MN, Obuchowski N, et al: Magnetic resonance imaging of the lumbar spine in people without back pain. N Engl J Med 331:69, 1994.
6. Taveras JM, Ferrucci JT: Radiology: Diagnosis, Imaging, Intervention. Philadelphia, JB Lippincott, 1989.
7. Resnick D: Bone and Joint Imaging. Philadelphia, WB Saunders, 1989.
8. Berquist TH: MRI of the Musculoskeletal System, ed 2. New York, Raven, 1990.
9. Edelman RR, Hesselink JR: Clinical Magnetic Resonance Imaging. Philadelphia, WB Saunders, 1990.
10. Atlas SW: Magnetic Resonance Imaging of the Brain and Spine. New York, Raven, 1991.
11. Stark DD, Bradley WG Jr: Magnetic Resonance Imaging, ed 2. St Louis, Mosby–Year Book, 1992.
12. Brant WE, Helms CA: Fundamentals of Diagnostic Radiology. Baltimore, Williams & Wilkins, 1994.
13. Grossman RI, Youssem DM: Neuroradiology: The Requisites. St Louis, Mosby–Year Book, 1994.
14. Osborne AG: Diagnostic Neuroradiology. St Louis, Mosby–Year Book, 1994.
15. Putman CE, Ravin CE: Textbook of Diagnostic Imaging, ed 2. Philadelphia, WB Saunders, 1994.
16. Higgins CB, Lipton MJ: Chest pain. *In* Eisenberg RL (ed): Diagnostic Imaging: An Algorithmic Approach. Philadelphia, JB Lippincott, 1988, p 30.
17. Batnitzky S, Eckard DA: The radiology of brain tumors: General considerations and neoplasms of the posterior fossa. *In* Morantz RA, Walsh JW (eds): Brain Tumors: A Comprehensive Text. New York, Marcel Dekker, 1994, p 213.
18. Sadato N, Numaguchi T, Rigamonti D, et al: Bleeding in ruptured posterior fossa aneurysms: A CT study. J Comput Assist Tomogr 15:612, 1991.
18a. Schwartz PH, Solomon RA: Perimesencephalic nonaneurysmal subarachnoid hemorrhage: Review of the literature. Neurosurgery 39:433–440, 1996.
19. Packer RJ, Batnitzky S, Cohen ME: Magnetic resonance imaging in the evaluation of intracranial tumors of childhood. Cancer 56:1767, 1985.
20. Baker HI, Houser OW, Campbell JR: National Cancer Institute Study: Evaluation of CT in the diagnosis of intracranial neoplasms. Radiology 136:91, 1980.
21. Modic MT, Masaryk TJ, Ross JS: Magnetic Resonance Imaging of the Spine. Chicago, Year Book Medical, 1989.
22. Rao KCV, Williams JP, Lee BCP, Sherman JL: MRI and CT of the Spine. Baltimore, Williams & Wilkins, 1994.
23. Eckard DA, Batnitzky S, Price HI: Infection. *In* Rao KCV, Williams JP, Lee BCP, Sherman JL (eds): MRI and CT of the Spine. Baltimore, Williams & Wilkins, 1994, p 251.
24. Dalinka MK, Kricun ME, Zlatkin MB, et al: Modern diagnostic imaging in joint disease. AJR 152:229, 1989.
25. Moore SG, Sebag GH: Primary disorders of bone marrow. *In* Cohen MD, Edwards MK (eds): Magnetic Resonance Imaging of Children. Philadelphia, BC Decker, 1990, p 765.
26. Moore SG: MR imaging of bone marrow. *In* Kressel HY, Modic MT, Murphy WA (eds): MR 1990. Oak Brook, Ill., RSNA Publications, 1990, p 219.
27. Alazraki MP, Mishkin FS: Fundamentals of Nuclear Medicine. New York, Society of Nuclear Medicine, 1984.
28. Pinsky SM: A Categorical Course in Nuclear Medicine. Oak Brook, Ill., RSNA Publications, 1985.
29. Mandell G: Radionuclide imaging. *In* Kricun ME (ed): Imaging Modalities in Spinal Disorders. Philadelphia, WB Saunders, 1988, p 503.
30. Alazraki N: Radionuclude techniques. *In* Resnick D (ed): Bone and Joint Imaging, Philadelphia, WB Saunders, 1989, p 185.
31. D'Ambrosia RD, Shoji H, Riggins RS, et al: Scintigraphy in the diagnosis of osteonecrosis. Clin Orthop 130:139, 1978.
32. Ash JM, Gilday DL: The futility of bone scanning in neonatal osteomyelitis. J Nucl Med 21:417, 1980.
33. Kirchner PT: Nuclear Medicine Review Syllabus. New York, The Society of Nuclear Medicine, 1980.
34. Merkel KD, Brown ML, Dewanjee MK, et al: Comparison of indium-labeled leukocyte imaging with sequential technetium gallium scanning in the diagnosis of low-grade musculoskeletal sepsis: A prospective study. J Bone Joint Surg 76A:465, 1985.
35. Julien P: Pulmonary embolism. *In* Eisenberg RL (ed): Diagnostic Imaging: An Algorithmic Approach. Philadelphia, JB Lippincott, 1988, p 49.
36. Holden RW, Mail JT, Becker GJ: Deep venous thrombosis. *In* Eisenberg RL (ed): Diagnostic Imaging: An Algorithmic Approach. Philadelphia, JB Lippincott, 1988, p 659.
37. Resnick D: Arthrography. *In* Bone and Joint Imaging. Philadelphia, WB Saunders, 1989, p 154.
38. Katzberg RW: Temporomandibular joint imaging. Radiology 170:297, 1989.
39. Helms CA: Temporomandibular joint. *In* MRI of the Musculoskeletal System, ed 2. New York, Raven Press, 1990, p 75.
40. Batnitzky S: Negative contrast myelographic agents. *In* Miller RE, Skucas J (eds): Radiographic Contrast Agents. Baltimore, University Park Press, 1977, p 419.
41. Batnitzky S: Positive contrast myelography: Water insoluble iodinated organic agents. *In* Miller RE, Skucas J (eds): Radiographic Contrast Agents. Baltimore, University Park Press, 1977, p 429.
42. Amundsen P: Water soluble myelographic agents. *In* Miller RE, Skucas J (eds): Radiographic Contrast Agents. Baltimore, University Park Press, 1977, p 437.
43. Batnitzky S: Intraspinal disorders. *In* Sarwar M, Azar-Kia B, Batnitzky S (eds): Basic Neuroradiology. St Louis, Warren Green, 1983, p 758.
44. Ovenfors CO, Godwin JD: Aortic aneurysms and dissections. *In* Eisenberg RL (ed): Diagnostic Imaging: An Algorithmic Approach. Philadelphia, JB Lippincott, 1988, p 72.
45. Kressel HY: MR imaging of the liver. *In* Kressel HY, Modic MT, Murphey WA (eds): MR 1990. Oak Brook, Ill., RSNA Publications, 1990, p 147.
46. Choyke PL: MR imaging of the kidneys and retroperitoneum. *In* Kressel HY, Modic MT, Murphey WA (eds): MR 1990. Oak Brook, Ill., RSNA Publications, 1990, p 165.
47. Rifkin MD: MR imaging of the prostate gland. *In* Kressel HY, Modic MT, Murphey WA (eds): MR 1990. Oak Brook, Ill., RSNA Publications, 1990, p 175.
48. McCarthy SM: MR imaging of the female pelvis: Normal anatomy and benign disease. *In* Kressel HY, Modic MT, Murphey WA (eds): MR 1990. Oak Brook, Ill., RSNA Publications, 1990, p 183.
49. Hricak H: MR imaging in gynecologic oncology. *In* Kressel HY, Modic MT, Murphey WA (eds): MR 1990. Oak Brook, Ill., RSNA Publications, 1990, p 191.
50. Nachemson A: The lumbar spine: An orthopedic challenge. Spine 1:59, 1976.
51. Burton CV: High resolution CT scanning: The present and future. Orthop Clin North Am 14:539, 1983.
52. Murphey MD, Batnitzky S, Bramble JM: Diagnostic imaging of spinal trauma. Radiol Clin North Am 27:855, 1989.
53. Boden SD, Wiesel SW, Laws ER Jr, et al: The multiply operated low back patient. *In* The Aging Spine: Essentials of Pathophysiology, Diagnosis, and Treatment. Philadelphia, WB Saunders, 1991.
54. Wilkinson HA: The role of improper surgery in the etiology of the failed back syndrome. *In* The Failed Back Syndrome: Etiology and Therapy. Philadelphia, Harper and Row, 1983.
55. Ross JS, Hueftle MG: Postoperative spine. *In* Modic MT, Masaryk TJ, Ross JS (eds): Magnetic Resonance Imaging of the Spine. Chicago, Year Book, 1989, p 120.

56. Teplick JG: Lumbar spine CT and MRI. *In* the Postoperative Lumbar Spine. Philadelphia, JB Lippincott, 1992.
57. Burton CV, Kirkaldy-Willis WH, Young-Hing K, et al: Causes of failure of surgery on lumbar spine. Clin Orthop 157:191, 1981.
58. Ross JS, Masaryk TJ, Modic MT, et al: Lumbar spine: Postoperative assessment with surface coil MR imaging. Radiology 164:851, 1987.
59. Cronqvist S: The postoperative myelogram. Acta Radiol 157:191, 1959.
60. Quencer RM, Tenner M, Rothman L: The postoperative myelogram. Radiology 123:667, 1977.
61. Teplick JG, Haskin ME: Computed tomography of the postoperative lumbar spine. AJR 141:865, 1983.
62. Hitselberger WE, Witten RM: Abnormal myelograms in symptomatic patients. J Neurosurg 28:204, 1968.
63. Jensen TT, Overgaard S, Thomsen NOB, et al: Prospective computed tomography three months after lumbar disc surgery: A prospective single-blind study. Spine 16:620, 1991.
64. Boden SD, Davis DO, Dina TS, et al: Contrast-enhanced MR imaging performed after successful lumbar disc surgery: Prospective study. Radiology 182:59, 1992.

CHAPTER • 11

Discography in Clinical Practice

Steven M. Siwek, MD •
Steven D. Waldman, MD, JD

The intervertebral disc is recognized as a source of chronic axial pain.[1] Before the advent of imaging studies such as computed tomography (CT) and magnetic resonance imaging (MRI), discography was often used as a complementary study to myelography. Studies have demonstrated the accuracy of discography in delineating both disc herniations and disc degenerations.[2–4] Discography is not, however, a procedure that seeks to compete with modern imaging modalities in a search for disc lesions. The purpose of modern discography is to determine whether the intervertebral disc is a source of clinical symptoms. While interpretation of images obtained with discography is important, in current clinical practice discography is primarily a provocative clinical test rather than a radiographic procedure.[5] The International Association for the Study of Pain (IASP) has published diagnostic criteria for discogenic pain, which includes that the stimulation of the putative symptomatic disc reproduce the patient's accustomed pain, but provides that provocation of at least two adjacent intervertebral discs clearly not produce discomfort.[6]

Discography is predominantly a diagnostic modality utilized to obtain information about the potential source of a patient's pain. The premise of discography is that a stimulus is applied that replicates the clinical noxious stimulus responsible for the patient's symptoms and that reproduction of the patient's symptoms during the injection confirms that the stimulated disc is the source of pain. The stimulus has a chemical component—the injected contrast medium, which contacts sensitized tissue—and a mechanical component—stretching of tissue as fluid is injected into the disc.

Identifying a particular disc as the source of pain is challenging because of overlapping pain patterns from a number of anatomic structures that are potential sources of pain, including intervertebral discs, myofascial structures, and facet joints. The primary objective of provocative discography is to delineate, if possible, the source of chronic spinal pain. The limitations of discography must be recognized if the information is to be used to make clinical therapeutic decisions. Notably, the presence of a sensitive disc does not rule out other intercurrent pain generators, nor does it exclude patients with pain magnification or various psychosocial factors. In this regard, Carragee and associates stressed the importance of identifying coexisting sources of pain before considering therapeutic options.

HISTORICAL CONSIDERATIONS

Lumbar discography evolved as a complementary modality for studying the lumbar intervertebral discs.[7] It was developed at a time when oil-based myelography was associated with an unacceptably high false-negative rate, notably at the lumbosacral junction. Schmorl is credited with being the first to inject a lumbar disc for radiographic visualization. Knut Lindblom, a radiologist in Stockholm, Sweden, first described diagnostic disc puncture and coined the term *discography*.[7] It was Carl Hirsch who employed the procedure to identify painful discs in patients with lumbago and sciatica. The diagnostic parameter of the procedure was the pain response; thus, the concept of provocative discography. Lindblom continued to modify the technique to utilize the injection of contrast material to visualize the radial ruptures of the discs, and the diagnostic criteria were expanded to include the radiographic appearance of the disc and the patient's response to the injection (i.e., to provocation).

Wise and Weiford were the first in the United States to visualize and study internal disc morphology.[8] Cloward and Busade continued the work and described the technique and indications for discography in their 1952 paper on the evaluation of normal and abnormal discs.[9] Ulf Fernstrom suggested mechanical and biomechanical causes for symptoms, based on cases of back and leg pain in which no nerve compression was detectable.[10]

The diagnostic merits and applications of discography have been challenged frequently, and the modality remains highly controversial. In 1968, Holt questioned the validity of discography, reporting a 36% rate of positive findings in asymptomatic subjects.[11] His study, however, had flaws that included using prisoners as all of his study subjects, using a very irritating contrast medium, and, importantly, failing to include a positive pain response as a criterion for a positive result. Positive results were based primarily on radiographic appearance. Walsh and coworkers refuted Holt's findings in a well-designed study demonstrating a zero rate of false-positive results in asymptomatic volunteers.[12] Unfortunately, Walsh's study did not address the validity or sensitivity of discography.

Caragee, in a study of selected patients without low back complaints, concluded that the rate of false positives is very low when strict criteria are applied and subjects have normal psychometrics and no chronic pain. The false-positive rate was greater among patients with abnormal psychometrics and increased annular disruption.

CERVICAL DISCOGRAPHY

Indications

Cervical discography is indicated as a diagnostic maneuver for a carefully selected subset of patients suffering from neck and cervical radicular pain. Patients who may benefit from discography include:

1. Patients with persistent neck and/or cervical radicular pain when traditional diagnostic modalities, such as MRI, CT, and electromyography (EMG), have failed to identify the cause of the pain
2. Patients in whom findings, such as bulging cervical discs identified on traditional diagnostic modalities, are equivocal (to determine whether such abnormalities are, in fact, responsible for the pain)
3. Patients who are to undergo cervical fusion (to help to identify which levels need to be fused)
4. Patients who have previously undergone fusion of the cervical spine (to help to identify whether levels above and below the fusion are causing persistent pain)
5. Patients in whom traditional imaging techniques cannot distinguish recurrent disc herniation from scar tissue.

For each of these patient populations, the pain management specialist must correlate the data obtained from the injection itself, the provocation of pain on injection, the radiographic appearance of the discogram, and, in certain ones, relief of pain after the disc is injected with local anesthetics. Failure to carefully consider all of this diagnostic information in the context of the patient's clinical presentation can lead to misinterpretation of the results of discography and can adversely affect clinical decision making.

Clinically Relevant Anatomy

From a functional anatomic viewpoint, cervical discs must be thought of as distinct from lumbar discs insofar as their being sources of pain is concerned. Radicular symptoms attributable solely to disc herniation are much less common in the cervical region than in the lumbar region. The reasons for this are two. First, for the cervical disc to impinge on the cervical nerve roots, it must herniate posteriorly and laterally. The cervical nerve roots are protected from impingement from cervical disc herniation in part by the facet joints, which interpose a bony wall between the disc and the nerve root. Second, the disc is completely enclosed posteriorly by the dense, double-layered posterior longitudinal ligament. This ligament is much more developed than its lumbar counterpart, which is thinner in its lateral aspects and composed of a single layer.

In the cervical disc the nuclear material lies farther anterior than it does in its lumbar counterpart. The anterior portion of the cervical disc space is larger than the posterior portion, which makes it difficult for the nuclear material to move posteriorly unless great forces are applied to the disc. The tough outer annulus is also thicker in the posterior portion of the cervical disc, so posterior bulging is less likely. It is this annular layer that receives sensory innervation from a variety of sources. Posteriorly, the annulus receives fibers from the sinovertebral nerves, which also provide sensory innervation to the posterior elements, including portions of the facet joints. Laterally, fibers from the exiting spinal nerve roots provide sensory innervation, and the anterior portion of the disc receives fibers from the sympathetic chain. Whether some or all of these fibers play a role in discogenic pain is a subject of controversy among pain specialists.

The cervical nerve roots leave the spinal cord and travel laterally through the intervertebral foramina. If the posterior cervical disc herniates laterally, it can impinge on the cervical root as it travels though the intervertebral foramen, producing classic radicular symptoms. If the cervical disc herniates posteromedially, it may impinge on the spinal cord itself, producing myelopathy that may cause upper and lower extremity, and bowel and bladder symptoms. Severe compression of the cervical spinal cord may result in quadriparesis or, rarely, quadriplegia.

Technique of Cervical Discography

The patient is placed supine with the neck in neutral position, as if for a stellate ganglion block. The anterior right side of the neck is usually chosen for needle entry, as the esophagus tracks to the left as it descends through the neck. The skin of the anterior neck is then prepared with antiseptic solution. If CT guidance is utilized, views are taken through the discs to be imaged and the relative positions of the carotid artery, esophagus, and trachea are noted. If fluoroscopy is utilized, a skin weal of local anesthetic is placed at the medial border of the sternocleidomastoid muscle at the level to be evaluated. A 22-gauge, 13-cm stylet needle is then advanced toward the superior margin of the vertebral body just below the disc of interest, carefully to avoid the carotid artery, jugular vein, trachea, and esophagus (Fig. 11–1).

After the needle impinges on bone, the depth at which bone contact is made is noted and the needle is withdrawn into the subcutaneous tissues and then advanced in a more superior trajectory into the anterior disc annulus. The needle is advanced in increments into the nucleus. Sequential scanning or fluoroscopy is indicated to avoid advancing the needle completely *through* the disc and into the cervical spinal cord. Water-soluble contrast medium suitable for intrathecal use is then slowly injected through the needle into the disc in a volume of 0.2 to 0.6 mL. The resistance to injection should be noted: intact discs offer firm resistance to these volumes. Simultaneously, the patient's pain response during injection is noted. The site of the pain and

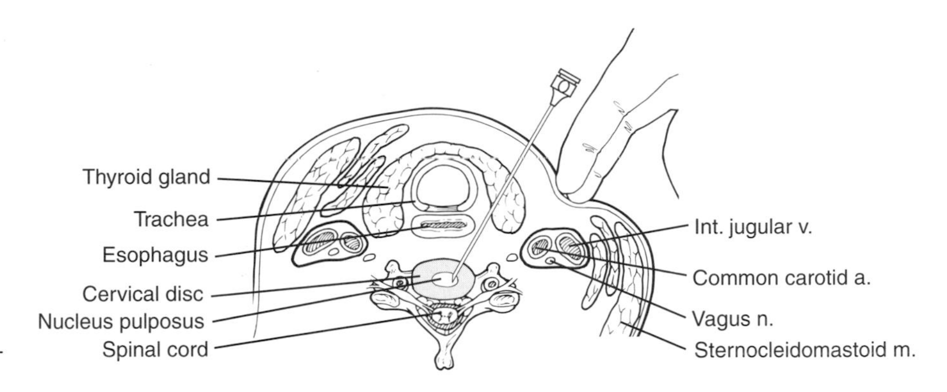

FIGURE 11–1 Technique of cervical discography.

its quality and similarity to the patient's ongoing clinical complaint are evaluated. A verbal analogue scale may be useful to help the patient quantify the degree of pain as compared with that from injection of adjacent discs.

The nucleogram of a normal cervical disc shows a lobulated mass with posterolateral clefts, which develop as part of the normal aging process of the disc. In a damaged disc, the contrast material may flow into tears in the inner annulus, producing a characteristic transverse pattern. If the tears in the annulus extend to the outer layer, a radial pattern is produced. Contrast material may also flow between the layers of annulus, producing a circumferential pattern. Complete disruption of the annulus allows the contrast medium to flow into the epidural space or into the cartilaginous end plate of the vertebra itself. While the likelihood that the disc being evaluated is the source of the patient's pain is directly proportional to the damage to the annulus, the pain management specialist must evaluate all information obtained during the discography procedure in the context of the pain symptoms. After evaluation of the nucleogram, a decision must be made to proceed with discography of adjacent discs or to inject local anesthetic into the disc currently being imaged. Analgesic discography is useful when the clinical pain pattern is reproduced or provoked during injection of contrast medium. If the pain that was provoked during the injection of contrast medium is relieved by a subsequent injection of local anesthetic into the disc, the inference can be drawn that the disc is the likely source of the patient's pain. It must be remembered that, if the annulus is disrupted, the injected local anesthetic may spread into the epidural space and anesthetize somatic and sympathetic nerves that may subserve discs at adjacent levels. Should that occur findings obtained from subsequent discography on adjacent discs may be misleading.

After injection procedures are completed, the patient is observed for 30 minutes before discharge. The patient should be warned to expect minor postprocedure discomfort, including some difficulty swallowing. Ice packs placed on the injection site for 20-minute periods help to decrease these untoward effects. The patient should be instructed to call immediately if any fever or other systemic symptoms develop that might suggest infection.

THORACIC DISCOGRAPHY

Indications

Although thoracic discography is performed less frequently than cervical or lumbar discography, it probably provides the most clinically useful information of the three. The reasons for this paradox are three: (1) less is known about the thoracic disc in health and disease; (2) thoracic disc herniation is less common than lumbar or cervical disc herniation; and (3) clinicians are less comfortable attributing pain symptoms to thoracic discogenic disease. For these reasons, thoracic discography can help the clinician to determine whether a damaged thoracic disc is, in fact, the true source of the patient's pain. This information is extremely valuable, given the difficulty and risks associated with surgery on the thoracic discs.

Thoracic discography is indicated as a diagnostic maneuver for a carefully selected subset of patients suffering from thoracic radicular—and occasionally myelopathic—pain. Patients in several situations may benefit from discography:

1. Patients with persistent thoracic radicular or myelopathic pain, when traditional diagnostic modalities such as MRI, CT, and EMG have failed to identify the cause
2. Patients in whom equivocal findings, such as bulging thoracic discs, are identified by traditional diagnostic modalities, to determine whether such abnormalities are, in fact, responsible for the pain
3. Patients who are to undergo instrumentation and fusion of the thoracic spine, when discography may help to identify which levels need to be fused
4. Patients who have previously undergone instrumentation and fusion of the thoracic spine, to help to identify whether levels above and below the fusion are responsible for persistent pain
5. Patients in whom recurrent disc herniation cannot be distinguished from scar tissue with traditional imaging techniques.

For each of these patient groups, the pain specialist must correlate the data obtained from the injection itself, the provocation of pain on injection, the appearance of the discogram, and, in certain patients, relief of pain after the disc is injected with local anesthetics. Failure to carefully consider all diagnostic information in the context of the patient's clinical presentation can lead to misinterpretation of results of discography and can adversely influence clinical decision making.

Clinically Relevant Anatomy

The gelatinous nucleus pulposus of the thoracic disc is surrounded by a dense, laminated fibroelastic network of fibers known as the annulus. The annular fibers are arranged in concentric layers that run obliquely from adjacent vertebrae. It is this annular layer that receives sensory innervation from a variety of sources. Posteriorly, the annulus receives fibers from the sinovertebral nerves, which also provide sensory innervation to the posterior elements, including portions of the facet joints. Laterally, fibers from the exiting spinal nerve roots provide sensory innervation, and the anterior portion of the disc receives fibers from the sympathetic chain. Whether some or all of these fibers play a role in discogenic pain is a subject of controversy among pain specialists. Each thoracic disc is situated between the cartilaginous end plates of the vertebrae above and below it.

The thoracic nerve roots leave the spinal cord and travel laterally through the intervertebral foramina. If the posterior thoracic disc herniates laterally, it can impinge on the thoracic root as it travels though the intervertebral foramen, producing classic radicular symptoms. If the thoracic disc herniates posteromedially, it may impinge on the spinal cord itself, producing myelopathy that may cause thoracic, lower extremity, and bowel and bladder symptoms. Severe compression of the thoracic spinal cord may result in paraparesis or, rarely, paraplegia.

Technique of Thoracic Discography

The patient is placed prone with a pillow under the lower chest to slightly flex the thoracic spine as if for a thoracic sympathetic block. CT or fluoroscopic views are taken through the discs to be imaged, and the relative positions of the pleural space, lung, ribs, nerve roots, and spinal cord are noted. The spinous process of the vertebra just above the disc to be evaluated is palpated. At a point just below and 1.5 inches lateral to the spinous process, the skin is prepared with antiseptic solution, and the skin and subcutaneous tissues are infiltrated with local anesthetic.

A 22-gauge, 13 cm styleted needle is introduced through the skin under CT or fluoroscopic guidance, the target being the middle of the disc of interest. Given the proximity of the somatic nerve roots, paresthesia may be elicited in the distribution of the corresponding thoracic paravertebral nerve (Fig. 11–2). If this occurs, the needle should be withdrawn and redirected slightly more cephalad. The needle is again readvanced in steps under CT or fluoroscopic guidance, care being taken to keep the needle trajectory medial, to avoid causing pneumothorax.

The needle is advanced in incremental steps into the central nucleus. Sequential CT scanning or fluoroscopy is indicated to avoid advancing the needle completely through the disc and into the thoracic spinal cord or to

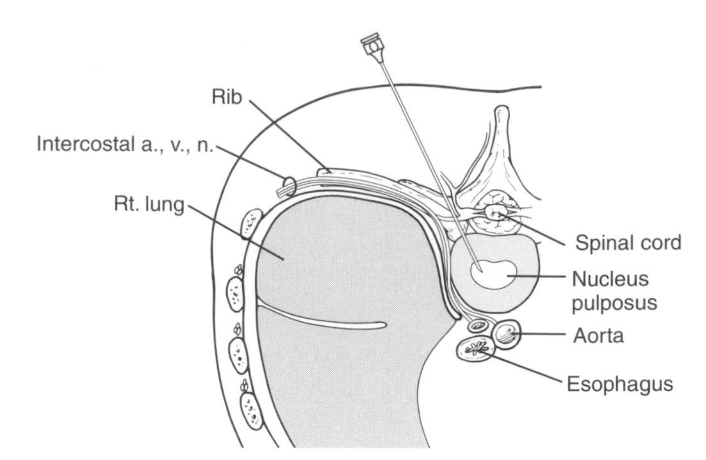

FIGURE 11–2 Technique of thoracic discography.

allow the needle to track too laterally into the pleural cavity. Water-soluble contrast medium suitable for intrathecal use is then slowly injected through the needle into the disc in a volume of 0.2 to 0.6 mL. The resistance to injection should be noted, as an intact disc offers firm resistance at these volumes. Simultaneously, the patient's pain response during injection is noted. The site of the patient's pain and its quality and similarity to the ongoing clinical symptoms are evaluated. A verbal analogue scale may be useful to help the patient to describe the degree of pain as compared with that of injection of adjacent discs.

The nucleogram of a normal thoracic disc appears as a lobulated mass with occasional posterolateral clefts, which develop as part of the normal aging process of the disc. In a damaged disc, the contrast material may flow into tears of the inner annulus, producing a characteristic transverse pattern. If the tears in the annulus extend to the outer layer, a radial pattern is produced. Contrast material may also flow between the layers of annulus, producing a circumferential pattern. Complete disruption of the annulus allows contrast material to flow into the epidural space or into the cartilaginous end plate of the vertebra itself. Although the damage to the annulus is directly proportional to the likelihood that the disc is the source of the patient's pain, the specialist must evaluate all information obtained from discography in the context of the patient's symptoms.

After evaluation of the nucleogram, a decision must be made to proceed with discography of adjacent discs or to inject local anesthetic into the disc currently being imaged. Analgesic discography is useful in patients whose clinical pain pattern is reproduced or provoked during the injection of contrast medium. If the pain that was provoked during the injection is relieved by a subsequent injection of local anesthetic into the disc, the inference can be drawn that the disc is the likely source of the patient's pain. It must be remembered that, if the annulus is disrupted, the injected local anesthetic may spread into the epidural space and anesthetize somatic and sympathetic nerves that may subserve discs at adjacent levels. If this occurs, erroneous information may be obtained if discography is then performed on adjacent discs.

After injection procedures are completed, the patient is observed for 30 minutes before discharge. The patient should be warned to expect minor postprocedure discomfort, including some soreness of the paraspinous musculature. Ice packs placed on the injection site for 20-minute periods help to decrease these untoward effects. The patient should be instructed to call immediately if any fever or other systemic symptoms occur that might suggest infection.

LUMBAR DISCOGRAPHY

Indications

Lumbar discography is indicated as a diagnostic maneuver in a carefully selected subset of patients suffering from back and lumbar radicular pain. Patients who may benefit from discography include these:

1. Patients with persistent back and/or lumbar radicular pain, when traditional diagnostic modalities such as MRI, CT, and EMG have failed to determine the cause
2. Patients in whom equivocal findings, such as bulging lumbar discs, are identified by traditional diagnostic modalities, to determine whether such abnormalities are, in fact, responsible for the pain
3. Patients who are to undergo lumbar fusion, when discography may help to identify which levels need to be fused
4. Patients who have previously undergone fusion of the lumbar spine, when discography may help to identify whether levels above and below the fusion are responsible for persistent pain
5. Patients in whom recurrent disc herniation cannot be distinguished from scar tissue with traditional imaging techniques.

For each of these patient populations, the specialist must correlate the data obtained from the injection itself, the provocation of pain on injection, the appearance of the discogram, and, in certain patients, relief of pain after the disc is injected with local anesthetics. Failure to carefully consider all of this diagnostic information in the context of the patient's clinical presentation can lead to misinterpretation of the results of discography and adversely influence clinical decision making.

Clinically Relevant Anatomy

From a functional anatomic viewpoint, lumbar discs must be thought of as distinct from cervical discs insofar as their being sources of pain is concerned. Radicular symptoms attributable solely to disc herniation are much more common in the lumbar region than in the cervical or thoracic region. The reasons for this are two. First, for the lumbar disc to impinge on the lumbar nerve roots, it must herniate posteriorly and laterally. The lumbar nerve roots are not protected from impingement from lumbar disc herniation by the bony wall of the facet joints as the cervical nerve roots are. Second, the posterior longitudinal ligament in the lumbar region is only a single layer, which is thinner and less well developed in its lateral aspects. It is in this lateral region where lumbar disc herniation with impingement on exiting nerve roots is most likely.

The nuclear material in the lumbar disc lies farther posterior than that in its cervical counterpart. The gelatinous nucleus pulposus of the lumbar disc is surrounded by a dense, laminated fibroelastic network of fibers known as the *annulus.* The annular fibers are arranged in concentric layers that run obliquely from adjacent vertebrae. It is this annular layer that receives sensory innervation from a variety of sources. Posteriorly, the annulus receives fibers from the sinovertebral nerves, which also provide sensory innervation to the posterior elements, including portions of the facet joints. Laterally, fibers from the exiting spinal nerve roots provide sensory innervation, and the anterior portion of the disc receives fibers from the sympathetic chain. Whether some or all of these fibers play a role in discogenic pain is a subject of controversy among pain specialists.

The lumbar nerve roots leave the spinal cord and travel laterally through the intervertebral foramina. If the posterior lumbar disc herniates laterally, it can impinge on the lumbar root as it travels though the intervertebral foramen, producing classic radicular symptoms. If the lumbar disc herniates posteromedially, it may impinge on the spinal cord itself, producing myelopathy that may cause lower extremity, bowel, and bladder symptoms. Severe compression of the lumbar spinal cord may result in cauda equina syndrome, paraparesis, or, rarely, paraplegia.

Technique of Lumbar Discography

The patient is placed prone with a pillow under the abdomen to slightly flex the lumbar spine, as if for lumbar sympathetic block. CT or fluoroscopic views are taken through the discs to be imaged, and the relative positions of the lung, ribs, aorta, vena cava, kidneys, nerve roots, and spinal cord are noted. The spinous process of the vertebra just above the disc of interest is palpated. At a point just below and 1.5 inches lateral to the spinous process, the skin is prepared with antiseptic solution, and the skin and subcutaneous tissues are infiltrated with local anesthetic (Fig. 11–3).

A 22-gauge, 13-cm styleted needle is introduced through the skin under CT or fluoroscopic guidance toward the target, the middle of the disc to be imaged. Given the proximity of the somatic nerve roots, paresthesia may be elicited in the distribution of the corresponding lumbar paravertebral nerve. If this occurs, the needle should be withdrawn and redirected slightly more cephalad. Then the needle is advanced in incremental steps under CT or fluoroscopic guidance, care being taken to keep the needle trajectory medial to avoid pneumothorax.

The needle is advanced in incremental steps into the central nucleus. Sequential CT scanning or fluoroscopy is indicated to avoid advancing the needle completely through the disc and into the lower limits of the spinal cord or cauda equina. The clinician must also take care lest the needle track too far laterally into the lower pleural or the retroperitoneal space. Water-soluble contrast medium suitable for intrathecal use is then slowly injected through the needle into the disc in a volume of 0.2 to 0.6 mL. Resistance to injection should be noted: an intact disc offers firm resistance at these volumes. Simultaneously, the patient's pain response is noted. The site of the pain

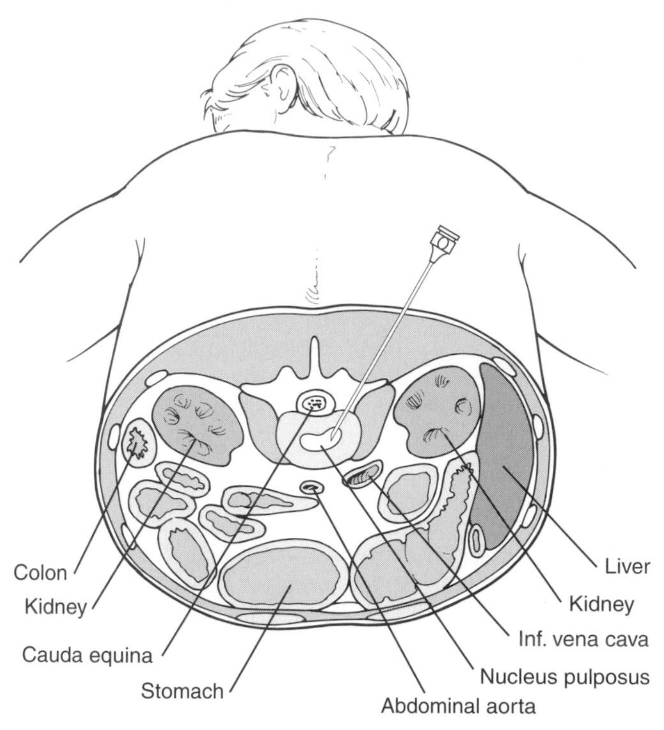

FIGURE 11–3 Technique of lumbar discography.

and its quality and similarity to the ongoing clinical symptoms are evaluated. A verbal analogue scale may be useful to help the patient to describe the degree of pain as compared with that of injection of adjacent discs.

The nucleographic appearance of a normal lumbar disc is a globular mass with occasional posterolateral clefts, which develop as part of the normal aging process of the disc. In the damaged disc, the contrast material may flow into tears in the inner annulus, producing a characteristic transverse pattern. If the tears in the annulus extend to the outer layer, a radial pattern is produced. Contrast medium may also flow between the layers of annulus, producing a circumferential pattern. Complete disruption of the annulus allows the contrast material to flow into the epidural space or into the cartilaginous end plate of the vertebra itself. Although the likelihood that the disc of interest is the source of the patient's pain is directly proportional to the damage to the annulus, the pain specialist must evaluate all information from the discography in the context of the patient's symptoms.

After evaluation of the nucleogram, a decision must be made to proceed with discography of adjacent discs or to inject local anesthetic into the disc currently being imaged. Analgesic discography is useful in patients whose clinical pain pattern is reproduced or provoked during injection of contrast medium. If the pain that was provoked during the injection is relieved by a subsequent injection of local anesthetic into the disc, the inference can be drawn that the disc is the likely source of the patient's pain. It must be remembered that, if the annulus is disrupted, the injected local anesthetic may spread into the epidural space and anesthetize somatic and sympathetic nerves that may subserve discs at adjacent levels. Should that occur, subsequent discography on adjacent discs may be misleading.

After injection procedures are completed, the patient is observed for 30 minutes before discharge. The patient should be warned to expect minor postprocedure discomfort, including some soreness in the paraspinous musculature. Ice packs placed on the injection site for 20-minute periods help to decrease these untoward effects. The patient should be instructed to call immediately if any fever or other systemic symptoms occur that might suggest infection.

Side Effects and Complications

Complications directly related to discography are generally self-limited, although, occasionally, even in the best of hands, serious complications can occur. The most common severe complication of discography is infection of the disc, commonly referred to as *discitis.* Because of the limited blood supply of the disc, such infections can be extremely hard to eradicate. Discitis usually presents as an increase in spine pain several days to a week after discography. At first, there is no change in the patient's neurologic findings as a result of disc infection.

Epidural abscess, which occasionally follows discography, generally presents within 24 to 48 hours. Clinically, the signs and symptoms of epidural abscess are high fever, spine pain, and progressive neurologic deficit. If either discitis or epidural abscess is suspected, blood and urine cultures should be taken, antibiotic treatment started, and emergent MRI of the spine obtained to allow identification and drainage of any abscess before an irreversible neurologic deficit develops.

In addition to infectious complications, pneumothorax can complicate cervical, thoracic, or lumbar discography. This complication should be rare if radiographic guidance is utilized during needle placement. A small pneumothorax after discography can often be treated conservatively, and tube thoracostomy can be avoided. Trauma to retroperitoneal structures, including the kidney, may also occur if thoracic or lumbar discography is undertaken without radiographic guidance.

Direct trauma to the nerve roots and the spinal cord can occur if the needle is allowed to traverse the entire disc or is placed too far lateral. These complications should be rare if serial CT or fluoroscopic views are taken while the needle is advanced. Such needle-induced trauma to the spinal cord and cauda equina can result in devastating neurologic deficits.

CONCLUSION

Discography is a straightforward technique that may provide useful clinical information on carefully selected patients. The information obtained from discography must always be analyzed in the context of the clinical presentation. Failure to do so can lead to a variety of clinical misadventures, including additional spine surgeries, which are doomed to failure. CT guidance affords an additional measure of safety, as compared with fluoroscopy, because it allows the pain specialist to clearly identify anatomic structures and monitor the needle position. These advantages may outweigh the additional cost as compared with fluoroscopically guided procedures.

REFERENCES

1. Coppes MH, Marani E, Thomeer RTWM, Groen GJ: Innervation of "painful" lumbar discs. Spine 22:2342–2350, 1997.
2. Brodsky AE, Binder WF: Lumbar discography—its value in diagnosis and treatment of lumbar disc lesions. Spine 4:110–120, 1979.
3. Jackson RP, Glah JJ: Foraminal and extraforaminal lumbar disc herniation: Diagnosis and treatment. Spine 12:577–585, 1987.
4. Milette PC, Raymond J, Fontaine S: Comparison of high-resolution computed tomography with discography in the evaluation of lumbar disc herniations. Spine 15:525–533, 1990.
5. O'Neil C, Derby R, Ryan DP: Precision injection techniques for diagnosis and treatment of lumbar disc disease. ISIS Sci Newslett 3:34–43, 1999.
6. Merskey H, Bogduk N (eds): Classification of Chronic Pain: Descriptions of Chronic Pain Syndromes and Definitions of Pain Terms, ed 2. Seattle, IASP Press, 1994, p 178.
7. Bernard T: Lumbar discography followed by computed tomography: Refining the diagnosis of low back pain. Spine 15:690–707, 1990.
8. Wise RE, Weiford EC: X-ray visualization of the intervertebral disc. Cleve Clin Q 18:127–130, 1951.
9. Cloward RB, Busade LL: Discography: Technique, indications and evaluation of the normal and abnormal intervertebral disc. Am J Roentgenol 68:552–564, 1952.
10. Fernstrom U: A discographical study of ruptured lumbar intervertebral disc. Acta Chir Scand (Suppl) 258:1–60, 1960.
11. Holt EP: The question of lumbar discography. J Bone Joint Surg 50A:720–726, 1968.
12. Walsh TR, Weinstein JN, Spratt KF, et al: Lumbar discography in normal subjects. J Bone Joint Surg 72A:1081–1088, 1990.

CHAPTER • 12

Spinal Endoscopy: Current Concepts

Lloyd R. Saberski, MD

HISTORICAL CONSIDERATIONS

Endoscopy plays a role in the diagnosis and treatment of many different conditions. The endoscopy platforms continue to grow into areas amenable to endoscopic visualization, particularly the epidural space, spinal cord, and contiguous structures. A review of medical literature shows that clinicians have been working with various types of endoscopes for more than 60 years, with varying degrees of success. Today, fiberoptic technology has been combined with computer-enhanced imaging to provide a new medium for viewing the central nervous system. The initial results are promising and will likely pave the way for newer, less invasive means of diagnosis and treatment of central nervous system (CNS) disease.

Direct visualization of the spinal canal and its contents was born in 1931 from the pioneering work of Michael Burman.[1] With each decade since then, myeloscopists and epiduroscopists have attempted to develop a means of fiberoptic visualization that would be easy and safe for application in medical practice. This was not achieved until the 1980s, when both flexible fiberoptic light sources and optics became available.[2] Burman removed 11 cadaver vertebral columns and examined them using rigid arthroscopic equipment with an incandescent light source.[1] As might be expected, the diameter of the trocar in which the lamp was mounted was greater than the average width of the spinal canal (approximately 3/8 inch, or 9.5 mm). Thus, the viewing lens was not completely within the spinal canal. In a few locations, the spinal canal was wide enough to accommodate the endoscope, permitting visualization of spinal canal contents, dura mater, blood vessels, and cauda equina. The endoscope's field of view was limited by its large size to only 1 inch (2.54 cm). In 1931, Burman[1] concluded that myeloscopy was limited by the available technology. With higher-quality instrumentation, a better post-mortem examination of the cauda equina could be performed in situ. He believed visualization of the contents of cadaver spinal canals would be especially important in establishing a diagnosis of tumor or inflammation. He did not anticipate that a more sophisticated device might allow for in situ, in vivo, minimally invasive therapies.

In 1936, Elias Stern[3] of Columbia University's Department of Anatomy was among the first to describe a "spinascope." A working model was built by American Cystoscopes Makers. The spinascope was designed for in vivo examination of spinal canal contents with adjunctive spinal anesthetic (Fig. 12–1). The instrument was never actually used, but Stern[3] did envision direct observation of the posterior roots for rhizotomy in patients with intractable pain and sectioning of anterior roots for incurable spastic conditions. He predicted that technologic improvements might allow the endoscopic platform to replace exploratory laminotomy.

In March of 1937, the first anesthetized subject was examined with a myeloscope by J. Lawrence Pool[4] of New York (Figs. 12–2 to 12–4). Unfortunately, hemorrhage obscured the field of vision, permitting only a fleeting glimpse of the lumbosacral nerve roots. Subsequently, seven patients were examined without complication. The cauda equina and blood flow through epidural vessels were observed. In 1942, Pool published in the journal *Surgery* a summation of 400 cases.[5, 6] In the era before computed tomography (CT) and magnetic resonance imaging (MRI), he reconstructed graphics that established or confirmed a diagnosis via the myeloscope. With images in hand, he approached operations with expectation and avoided extensive explorations. He identified neuritis, herniated nucleus pulposus, hypertrophic ligamentum flavum, primary and metastatic neoplasms, varicose vessels, and arachnoid adhesions.

Despite these successes and the relative ease of performing such examinations, no further reports of similar technique are found in the literature until 1967. This is because of widespread acceptance and simplicity of myelography and the need to sketch observations if performing spinal endoscopy. There was no automatic graphic capture; photographic equipment of the era did not provide sufficient light for image formation. Dr. Pool, a talented artist, documented his observations with beautiful hand-drawn sketches (Fig. 12–5).

In the late 1960s and early 1970s, Yoshio Ooi and colleagues,[7–11] working without knowledge of the American experience, developed an endoscope for intradural and extradural examinations. Fiberoptic light source technology was available in the 1970s. This allowed for minaturization and the transmission of more lumens of light without gen-

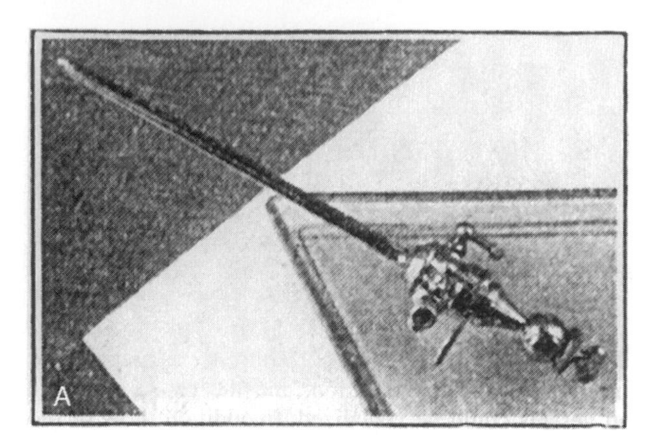

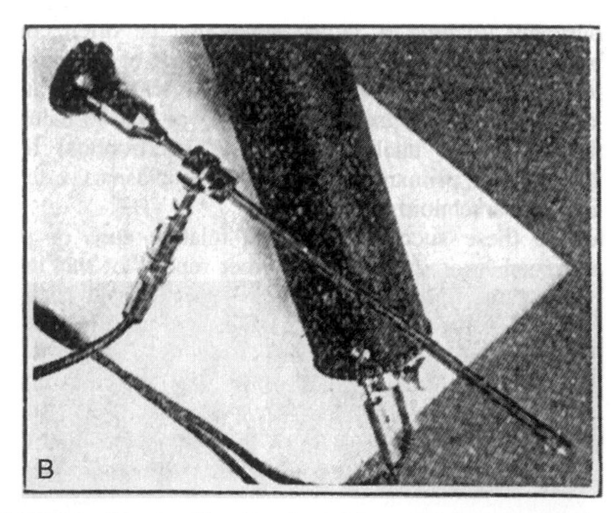

FIGURE 12–1 Elias Stern's stainless steel introducer with side flushport. A, Trocar now removed from introducer. B, The rigid optical system inserted with flush system and light source attached. (From Stern EL: The spinascope: A new instrument for visualizing the spinal canal and its contents. Med Rec 143:31–32, 1936.)

erating more heat. The fiberoptic light source technology protected tissues from heat injury, because fiberoptic fibers absorbed infrared rays and reflected visible rays. The myeloscope could now be miniaturized, since large size was not necessary to carry sufficient light. The smaller size allowed the myeloscope to be inserted between lumbar spinous processes just as a needle for percutaneous lumbar puncture is.[12] The procedure was now greatly simplified, and no serious complications were reported from the initial 86 patients. Postspinal cephalalgia was a common, albeit temporary, feature (prevalence 70%). Dr. Ooi and colleagues[13] recorded detailed descriptions of normal and abnormal anatomy as well as blurry black-and-white photographic images of ligamentum flavum, epidural adipose tissue, the surface of the dural sac, and the cauda equina.

From 1967 to 1977, Ooi and colleagues[13, 14] performed 208 myeloscopies using various types of equipment. Their progress was reported in several publications, culminating in 1981 with their publication on myeloscopy and blood flow changes of the cauda equina during Lasègue's test.[15] The intrathecal space was regularly entered with a 1.8-mm rigid scope (Fig. 12–6). The fiberoptics were used only as the light source; fiberoptic myeloscopes with fiberoptic light sources for direct visualization were still a decade away. The authors noted changes in the blood flow in vessels accompanying the cauda equina during straight leg–raising tests. During this maneuver, caudad anterior displacement of the cauda equina was observed, which led to temporary cessation of blood flow. Presumably, this is clinically associated with pain in susceptible patients. Abdominal straining, coughing, and sneezing did not alter blood flow but did cause slight up-and-down movement of the cauda equina in the lateral position. Unfortunately, with the decrease in diameter of the scope, the amount of light available for good-quality pictures was reduced. A larger myeloscope (2.5 mm) was needed to visualize the epidural space. Myeloscopy (epiduroscopy) therefore continued to have limited value in the diagnosis of spinal stenosis but was an important aid in the diagnosis of lesions associated with spinal pain syndromes such as arachnoiditis, tumors, and vascular abnormalities. Procedures such as removal of a herniated nucleus pulposus were considered, but, owing to the inflexibility of the rigid scope, insufficient light, and difficulty distinguishing normal from abnormal tissue, the surgical use of spinal endoscopic equipment remained limited. A flexible myeloscope was envisioned to have many advantages, but another decade passed before the invention of the micromyeloscope.

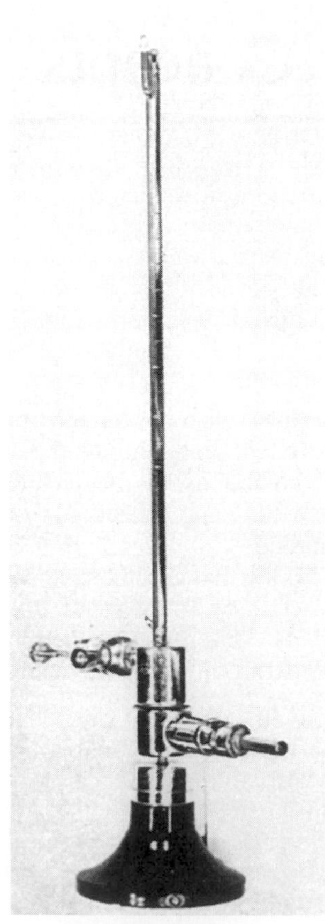

FIGURE 12–2 J. Lawrence Pool's myeloscope assembled for visualization. (From Pool JL: Myeloscopy: Intraspinal endoscopy. Surgery 11:169–182, 1942.)

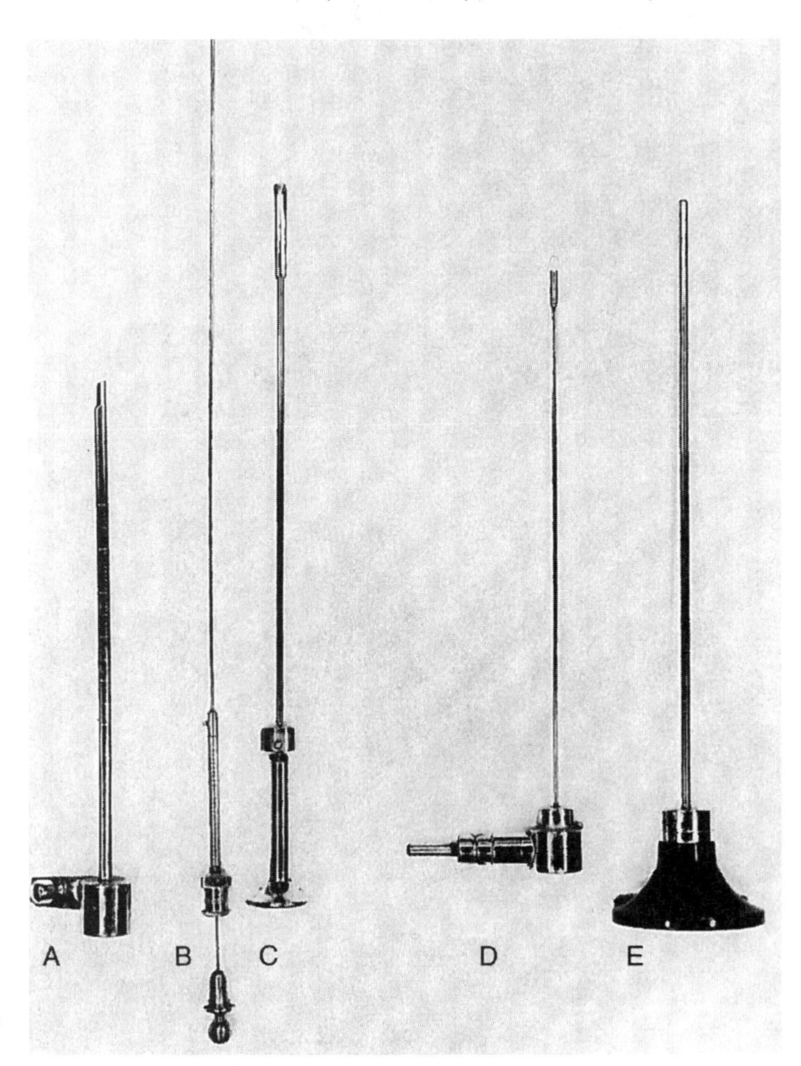

FIGURE 12–3 *J. Lawrence Pool's myeloscope disassembled.* A, *Cannula.* B, *Guide needle (stylet partially withdrawn).* C, *Obturator.* D, *Lighting system.* E, *Lens system with eyepiece. (From Pool JL: Myeloscopy: Intraspinal endoscopy. Surgery 11:169–182, 1942.)*

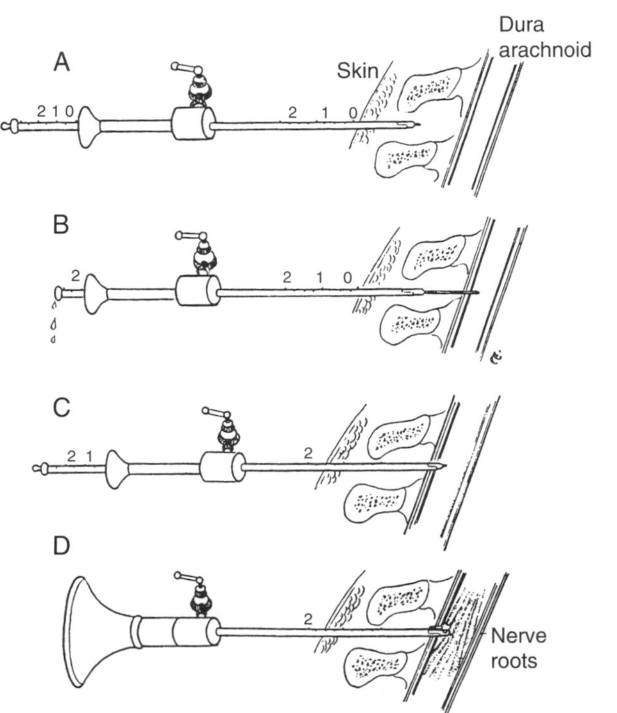

FIGURE 12–4 A, *The first step in the introduction of the Pool myeloscope: Cannula with obturator and guide needle penetrate interspinous ligament.* B, *Second step: Guide needle is advanced until cerebrospinal fluid is obtained. Millimeter scale on handle of needle then indicates distance from the obturator tip to subarachnoid space.* C, *Third step: With guide needle returned to original neutral position, the entire instrument is advanced the required distance.* D, *Final step: Obturator and guide needle are replaced by lighting and lens systems. (From Pool JL: Myeloscopy: Intraspinal endoscopy. Surgery 11:169–182, 1942.)*

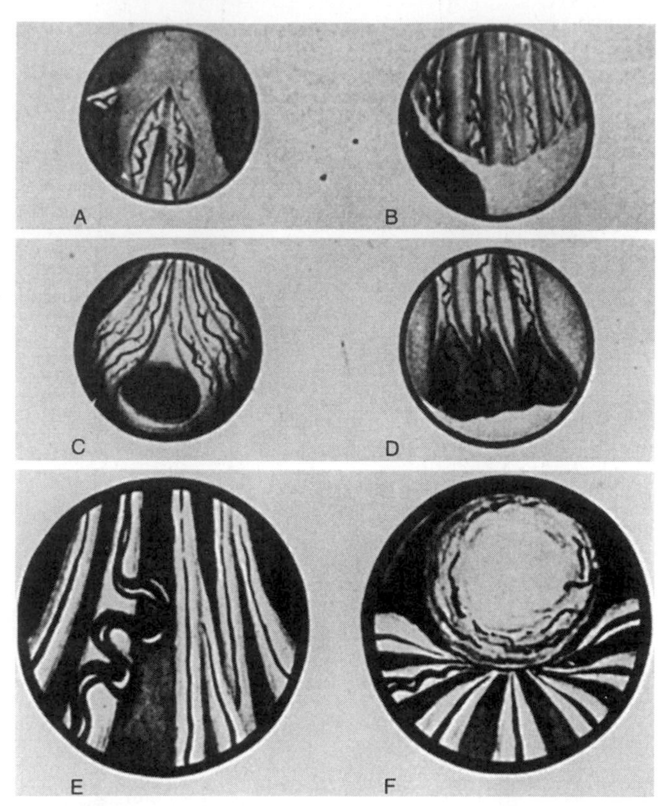

FIGURE 12–5 *A, Normal anatomy with dura mater open and cauda equina visualized. B, Neuritis with reddened, inflamed-looking nerve roots. C, Herniated nucleus pulposus. D, Ventral disc herniation (not seen) with dorsally displaced, broadened nerve roots. E, Hypertrophic ligamentum flavum caused compression of the nerve root near its foramen of exit. The lesion itself was not visualized, but the greatly dilated vessel indicated pressure on that nerve at a lower level. F, Tumor. (From Pool JL: Myeloscopy: Intraspinal endoscopy. Surgery 11:169–182, 1942.)*

Rune Blomberg[16] (1985) of Sweden was the next to describe a method of epiduroscopy and spinaloscopy. It was his interest to study anatomic variations of the epidural space, so that a better understanding of epidural anesthesia could be gained. Using a fiberoptic light source with a small, rigid endoscope, he determined that the contents of the epidural space varied widely among humans, especially in the amounts of fat and connective tissue. In 12 of 30 post-mortem examinations, the epidural contents limited visibility of the epidural space. Adhesions between dura mater and ligamentum flavum restricted opening of the epidural space despite flushing with normal saline. Dr. Blomberg was able to position the epiduroscope (which was still similar to Stern's spinascope) to visualize entry of a Tuohy needle through ligamentum flavum into the epidural space. Dural tenting was seen when an epidural catheter was threaded through the Tuohy needle into the epidural space. Once in the epidural space, the orientation of the catheter varied greatly and was ultimately determined by surrounding structures. Dr. Blomberg surmised that it was "too early to decide to what extent clinical application is possible with epiduroscopy. Under all circumstances it would be necessary to improve lighting conditions, and to shorten shutter speeds in order to make the method more easily handled."[16]

In 1989, Blomberg and Olsson[17] performed 10 epiduroscopies on patients scheduled for partial laminectomies for herniated lumbar discs. They believed that the conclusions drawn from previous autopsy work were not necessarily transferable to the clinical setting. Their concerns pertained to the absence of circulation in cadavers and to the possible impact of low or no cerebrospinal fluid (CSF) pressure on the appearance of the epidural space.[17] They determined that the epidural space was, indeed, only a potential space that remained open for brief periods when fluid or air was injected. Blomberg and Olsson[17] confirmed the presence of a dorsomedian connective tissue band that divided the epidural space into compartments. They determined that the midline approach to the epidural space was often associated with bleeding and that a paramedian approach was less likely to cause this complication.[18] Blomberg recorded his internal images with a VCR on videotape. The fiberoptic light source, combined with computer-assisted exposures, allowed for adequate video capture.

Koki Shimoji and associates[2] were the first group to publish their endoscopic experience utilizing both a fiberoptic light source and a flexible fiberoptic catheter (instead of traditional rigid metal endoscopes) for myeloscopy. Their experience using small (0.5- to 1.4-mm) flexible fiberoptic scopes was published in 1991 (Fig. 12–7).[18] The continued availability of camcorders and VCRs made it possible to have simultaneous video images and a recording of all aspects of the internal procedure. In 10 patients with chronic, intractable spinal pain syndromes, they placed flexible fiberoptic myeloscopes and epiduroscopes into either the subarachnoid space or the epidural space, or both, via a lumbar paramedian approach through a Tuohy needle. The epidural space was visualized only after the myeloscope was withdrawn from the subarachnoid space. This happened because the passage of CSF into the potential epidural space gently distended the space, permitting tissues to be less adherent and allowing the lens to achieve its focal length of 3 to 5 mm. (With the tissues adherent to the lens, the tissue bed was obliterated.) The procedures were performed without sedatives or local anesthetics, to investigate patients' discomfort. There was interest in whether chronic pain sources could be identified via a mechanical stimulus. Accurate identification of the spinal level was determined by the simultaneous use of radiography. In four of the study patients, subarachnoid fiberoptic scopes were advanced to the cisterna magna. In patients with a diagnosis of adhesive arachnoiditis, nerve roots were matted or clumped by filamentous tissue, but there was no evidence of other structural lesions. The excessive connective tissue made observation of the subarachnoid space difficult. Three of the five patients diagnosed with adhesive arachnoiditis before the procedure reported either a reduction or complete remission of their pain after the procedure. Although the myeloscopic examinations did not establish the anatomic cause of pain, the authors believed that further study was warranted. There were minimal complications, mainly transient post–dural puncture headaches and fever; the few cases of dysesthesia during the procedure were rectified by slowly withdrawing the scope from the nerve root in question.

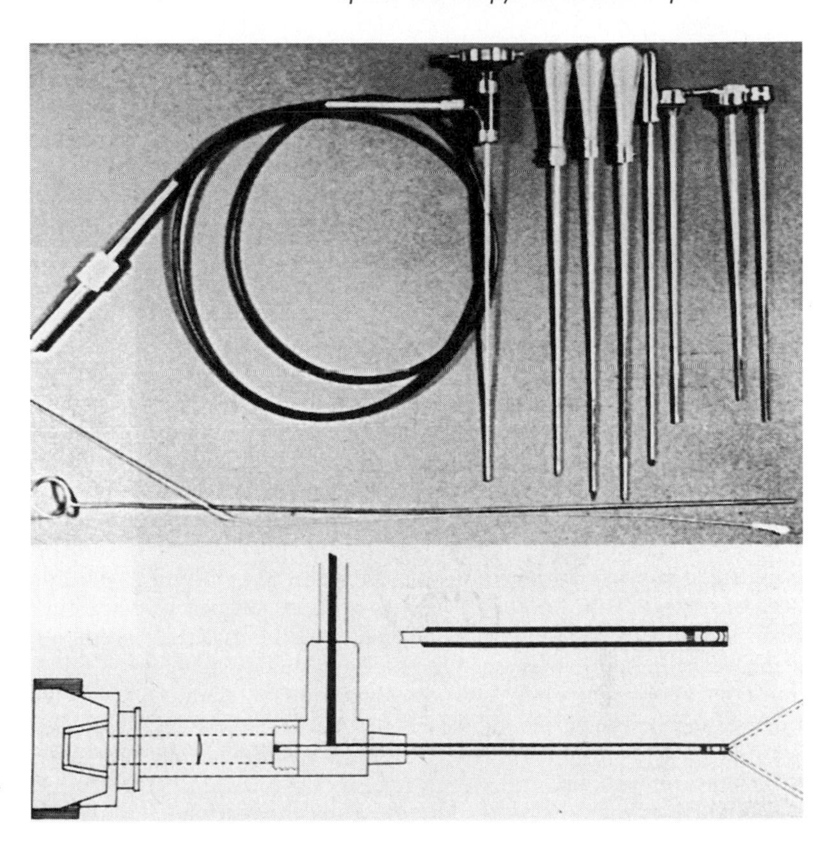

FIGURE 12–6 Yoshio Ooi's rigid myeloscope with flexible fiberoptic light source. (From Ooi Y, Satoh Y, Inoue K, et al: Myeloscopy. Int Orthop 1:107–111, 1977.)

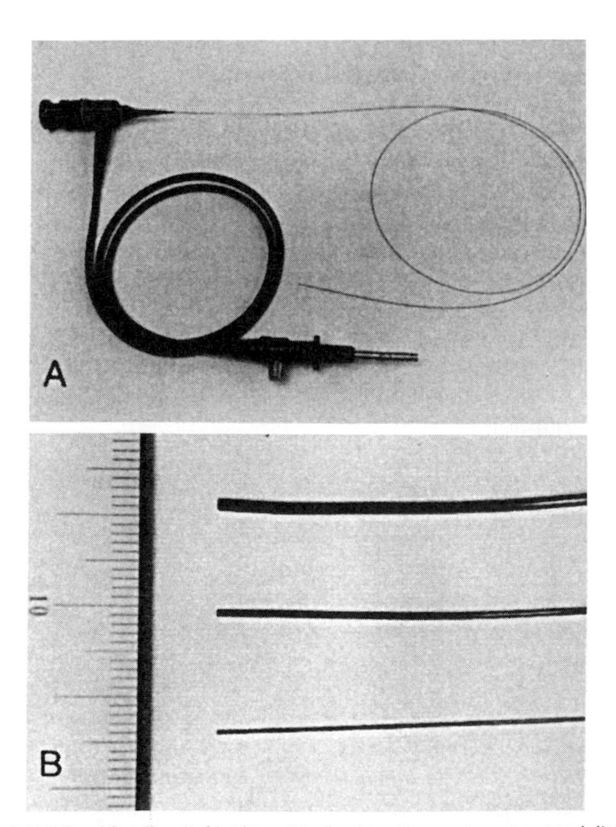

FIGURE 12–7 Koki Shimoji's flexible fiberoptic scope and light source. A, The fiberscope with its lead to a high-intensity light source. B, Tips of three types of fiberscopes with diameters of 1.4, 0.9, and 0.5 mm (from top to bottom). (From Shimoji K, Fujioka H, Onodera M, et al: Observation of spinal cord and cisternae with the newly developed small-diameter, flexible fiberscopes. Anesthesiology 75:341–344, 1991.)

In 1991, Saberski and Kitahata began evaluations of several fiberoptic endoscopes for epiduroscopy. The technology had improved, but appropriate indications for epiduroscopy were still not clearly established. Uncertainty persisted about whether epiduroscopy provided a diagnostic advantage over noninvasive imaging procedures such as CT and MRI.[19] A number of technologic problems needed to be surmounted before clinical use of such devices could be seriously considered. The fiberoptic endoscopes could visualize tissue immediately in front of the lens when the 2-mm focal length was maintained. This focal distance was difficult to achieve in a potential space like the epidural space. There were also difficulties getting the endoscopes into the epidural space without causing damage, even with fluoroscopic guidance. The original fiberoptic endoscopes did not have working channels for tissue sampling or delivery of medication. The ideal device had to be maneuverable, have a working lumen, and have a lens with a short focal length or incorporate a mechanism that prevented tissue from obstructing the lens. By using the caudal approach, Saberski and Kitahata were able to steer a fiberoptic, though with great difficulty, to specific sites and to deliver steroid medication to nerve roots via the introducer after removing the fiberoptic device.[20]

To achieve steering capability, Saberski and Kitahata curved the naked fiberoptic by wrapping it gently over a finger. Then, when the tip was inside the epidural space, they rotated the proximal end of the fiberoptic, which caused exaggerated rotation inside the epidural canal. This afforded visualization of more epidural space.

These early therapeutic successes indicated that spinal canal endoscopy was not only possible but had the advantage of delivering medications directly to structures of concern. This contrasted sharply with the widely accepted technique of epidural steroid injection, which took the path of least resistance. Saberski and Kitahata found that normal saline irrigation easily distended the epidural space and allowed the fiberoptic to assume the necessary focal length. Once the initial 15 to 20 mL of normal saline was injected, only slight positive pressure on the syringe was sufficient to keep the epidural space distended.

Saberski and Kitahata also observed that nerves identified for visualization, because of symptoms, electrodiagnostic studies, response to local anesthetic root blocks, and imaging studies often appeared with spinal canal endoscopy to have fluffy connective tissue over them. These tissues had never been appreciated before spinal canal endoscopy, because earlier techniques for entering the spine always did so at the level of interest and were associated with local bleeding. The spinal canal endoscope was floated from the caudal epidural space into position to observe lumbar epidural anatomy. Any bleeding was far removed from the area of interest. The "cottony" tissues at times seemed to float in the saline. Some of this material could be irrigated aside, revealing denser connective tissue attached to nerves and contiguous structures. On occasion, an erythematous hue was seen in the perineural tissue after the fluffier tissues were irrigated away. These changes are likely an inflammatory immune response.

Concurrent with the work done at Yale, Heavner and colleagues[21] reported in 1991 on flexible endoscopic evaluation of the epidural and subarachnoid spaces in rabbits or dogs and in human cadavers. The technique employed flexible endoscopes with outside diameters of 2.1 and 1.4 mm, respectively. In 1992, Mollmann and associates[22] published details of spinaloscopy with a rigid 4-mm endoscope on nonfixed preparations from human cadavers. At the Seventh World Congress on Pain in 1993, Heavner and coworkers[23] reported that, in anesthetized dogs, endoscopes could be passed freely from their lumbar epidural insertion sites to the cervical epidural space without producing motor or cardiovascular responses. Significant difficulties with orientation suggested that further modifications would be necessary before the vast potential of epiduroscopy could be exploited.[23] In 1994, Rosenberg and colleagues[24] demonstrated epiduroscopy in anesthetized dogs with a thin, flexible and deflectable (steerable) fiberscope. The same year, Schutze and Kurtze[25] published their experience with epiduroscopy in 12 patients who had various pain syndromes. They were able to visualize normal and abnormal anatomic structures. Pronounced adhesions and fibrosis were observed in two patients whose back surgery had failed. Three permanent epidural catheters were implanted with epiduroscopic control.[25]

Although they represented multiple breakthroughs in technology, these devices had limitations that needed to be addressed before further human clinical trials could begin in earnest. A channel for instrumentation and refinements in steering were necessary. An easy-to-steer system with multiple lumens for instrumentation, irrigation, and fiberoptics had to be developed. In response to these needs, Catheter Imaging Systems, Myelotec, Clarus, K. Storz, and EBI have manufactured or supplied various devices that were used for spinal canal endoscopy throughout the 1990s (Fig. 12–8).

By 1996, epidural spinal canal endoscopy was used frequently for delivery of epidural steroid medication. Many providers throughout the world modified the Saberski-Kitahata techniques for lysis of adhesions with blunt dissection, volumetric injection, lasers, and balloons. There was a sense that these techniques were preferable to percutaneous, blind techniques, but there were few studies to support the idea. By 1998, various versions of the technique were

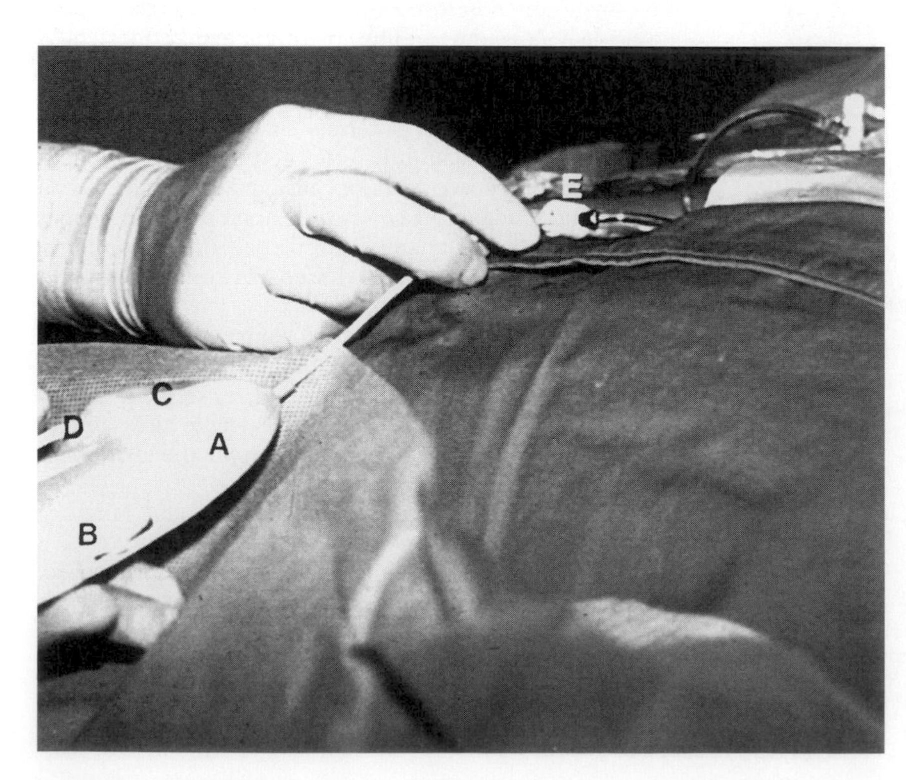

FIGURE 12–8 A, *Steerable handle with 2.7-mm catheter.* B, *Steering lever turns catheter right and left in the position pictured, and up and down when the lever is rotated 90 degrees.* C, *Auxiliary working channel.* D, *Flushport.* E, *A 3-mm introducer with flush system attached. (Not pictured is opening at base of handle for fiberoptic cable; see Fig. 12–14* F.*)*

common. Insurance carriers began to review whether literature supported continuing reimbursement for such services, despite strong advocacy by patients and physicians. Many concluded that peer reviewed literature (randomized controlled studies) was insufficient and that these technologies were experimental; they denied reimbursement for service to physicians, hospitals, and surgery centers.

Although there was considerable interest in continuing research, a number of factors impeded progress. First of all, the first company to manufacturer and distribute a commercial flexible fiberoptic endoscope system for spinal canal endoscopy (Myelotec) had limited funds for research. Although Myelotec was aware of the need to fund research, it hoped that commercial sales and widespread use of the technologies would generate enough revenue to underwrite future research. Unfortunately, simultaneous growth in the United States of managed care slowed expansion of the endoscopy field and limited funds for research. It was also extremely difficult to develop randomized controlled studies, even with funding. Most patients were not interested in randomization and opted for surgery or endoscopy, depending on personal preference and clinical circumstance. The demands of the insurance review boards for randomized controlled studies seemed particularly harsh in regard to endoscopy, since other surgical and minimally interventional procedures were performed in the United States with a dearth of outcome data. Although the platform for endoscopy was easy to use, was relatively safe, and made perfect sense as an option before consideration of a surgical procedure involving discs, inflammation, and pain, it was a paradigm shift that required reeducating physicians, surgeons, insurance companies, and the people. Before the work of McCarron, Saberski, the Saals, and others, disc-related spine disease was usually conceptualized in terms of nerve compression. That disc disease and spine pain could be partially or completely a medical inflammatory condition controlled by the immune system was not even considered. The focus was on anatomic causes of pain. Physicians looked at an MRI and expected the size of a herniated disc to reflect the degree of pain. In fact, this specificity theory (i.e., size determines pain) was debunked for more than 30 years, yet some still subscribe to it. Now we know that chemical and cell signal changes at the tissue bed level, in conjunction with changes in receptivity of the CNS, determine the degree of pain. Thus, a patient with an apparently small injury can be debilitated and in pain, and that pain is every bit real—and organic.

The 1990s concluded with several studies that took advantage of the spinal endoscopic platform. They looked at living anatomy (Igarashi of Japan[26]); the risk of dural puncture during combined anesthetic technique[27]; effects of epidural fat on epidural catheter placement[28]; changes in epidural anatomy after epidural anesthesia[29–31]; and the relative effects of age on epidural fat content and local anesthetic dose requirements.[28] Dr. Kurtze from Germany reported on the Internet observations of 139 patients' epidural space. He placed epidural catheters and electrodes with spinal endoscopic guidance.[32] Numerous case reports showcased the potential of the endoscopic platform.[19,20,33–35] A distinction was made between management of acute pain and chronic pain syndromes. It is recognized that a multitude of different pathophysiologic mechanisms constitute the spinal pain syndrome. Thus the platform was used in many different ways, for many different pathologies. Dr. Saberski indicated that immunoinflammation secondary to acute disc irritation was regularly observed.[36] This phenomenon appears to be independent of disc compression and may represent leaky disc syndrome or an autoimmune response.[36] This raises the likelihood of developing specific chemotherapies to interfere with immunochemical "events" in epidural tissue beds. It has been suggested, but not substantiated, that environmental factors (e.g., infectious disease) may influence the immune system response to disc antigen or chemical. Animal work was begun to analyze cell signals and immune response. This work, when "mature," could define many common spine afflictions as medical diseases (not surgical disorders).[36] Dr. Richardson published a review of spinal canal endoscopy in the *British Medical Journal* during the autumn of 1999.[37] The millennium wrapped up with Dr. Saberski reporting, at the World Foundation for Pain Conference in New York, that medical management of acute herniated disc by spinal canal endoscopy is less expensive and more likely to a return a patient to work than is laminectomy or discectomy.[38]

Terminology

The original term for the endoscopic evaluation of the epidural space was *epiduroscopy*. The coining of the term is credited to Rune Blomberg. In the United States, there was considerable reluctance from insurance carriers to reimburse for epiduroscopy, because they were not familiar with the term (which did not appear in insurance coding books). The term *spinal canal endoscopy* was adopted because American insurers were familiar with *endoscopy* in other body cavities. Today, spinal canal endoscopy refers to epiduroscopy, fiberoptic evaluation in the peridural position, or myeloscopy for subarachnoid visualization.

Epiduroscopy/Spinal Canal Endoscopy Consensus

On 17 September, 1998 in Iserlohn, and 3 October 1998 in Bad Durkheim, an international group of experts drew up a consensus paper entitled "Standards for Epiduroscopy."[32] The participants in the working group agreed on general principles governing the clinical application of spinal canal endoscopy (cited next). The scientific basis for these recommendations was derived from publications and clinical experience of Groll (Dortmund, Germany), Heavner (Lubbock, Tex.), Kurtze (Bad Durkheim, Germany), Leu (Zurich), Mollmann (Munster), Rawal (Oreboro, Sweden), Saberski (New Haven, Conn.), and Schutze (Iserlohn, Germany).

Spinal canal endoscopy (epiduroscopy) was defined as percutaneous, minimally invasive endoscopic investigation of the epidural space to enable color visualization of anatomic structures inside the spinal canal: dura mater, blood vessels, connective tissue, nerves, fat, and pathologic structures, including adhesion (fibrosis), inflammation, and stenotic change. General indications were established for spinal canal endoscopy and diagnosis and treatment of spinal pain syndromes:

1. Observation of pathology and anatomy
2. Direct drug application
3. Direct lysis of scarring (with medication, blunt dissection, laser, and other instruments)
4. Placement of catheter and electrode systems (epidural, subarachnoid)
5. An adjunct to minimally invasive surgery

RATIONALE FOR THE CAUDAL APPROACH

The caudal approach to the epidural space seemed to offer advantages over the paramedian approach. The straight entry into the epidural space contrasted sharply with the approximately 45-degree bend required to pass a catheter into the lumbar epidural space. Thus, there was less chance of fracturing the fiberoptic device. Straight caudal canal placement also made it easier to add channels for future surgical procedures and to steer.

The previous work of Odendaal and van Aswegen[39] supported the caudal approach on an entirely different basis—the kinetics of injected fluids. They injected a radionuclide admixture into the lumbar epidural space of patients, some of whom had had laminectomy and some of whom had not. By following the radioactive tracer, the researchers were able to demonstrate poor caudal spread of injectate in the patients who had had laminectomies. In the nonoperated control group, however, there was a uniform spread of fluid throughout lumbar and sacral nerve roots. Thus, an injection into the lumbar epidural space took the path of least resistance and would not necessarily deliver steroids to their intended target in the sacral nerve roots. For these reasons, Cyriax[40] intuitively advocated volumetric caudal injections during the 1960s to 1980s. With such epidural injections, the injectate (normal saline, local anesthetic, steroid) was more likely to spread cephalad. Some injectate did escape through the sacral foramen. Using volumes of 25 to 50 mL containing local anesthetic, normal saline, and steroid, Cyriax[40] claimed lasting results in more than 40% of his patients. These results were attributable to the better spread of steroid, improved irrigation of the epidural tissue bed, and hydrostatic pressure gradients mobilizing adherent tissues. It is presumed that the dramatic response was reported by patients with relatively acute inflammatory disc processes rather than failed-back-surgery syndromes. The effect of Dr. Cyriax's personal choice for local anesthetic, procaine, on long-term outcome is unknown, but its role cannot be discounted.

The work of Gabor Racz and associates[41] in Lubbock, Texas, suggested that lysis of epidural adhesion produced significant benefit for many patients with refractory lumbar radiculopathies. Their pioneering work indicated that scar adhesions formed in the epidural space of many who have chronic spine pain syndromes, after surgery or perhaps from inflammation, and that they were responsible for pulling and tugging nerve roots and dural sac. Their innovative technique involved placement of a catheter through the sacral hiatus into the epidural space close to the root of the adhesion in question, which was identified on an epidurogram. A total volume of 30 to 40 mL of a local anesthetic, steroid, and nonionic contrast was then injected. The results showed significant variability between study groups, likely a consequence of the heterogeneous nature of persistent lumbar radiculopathy. Nonetheless, approximately 50% of the patients had marked improvement as measured by decreased need for medication, enhanced function, and reduced visual analogue scale (VAS) scores for 1 to 6 months. Racz and associates[41, 42] concluded that overlooked epidural adhesions could cause pain, perhaps from compression and irritation of nerves. With spinal canal endoscopy, it is hoped that a three-dimensional color view of the adhesion and adjacent structures will afford the operator advantages over two-dimensional, black-and-white fluoroscopic projections (epidurograms). Thus, spinal canal endoscopy seems to have potential as a platform for management of chronic spinal canal–based diseases in addition to management of acute inflammatory canal diseases.

Work by Serpell and associates[43] showed that sustained pressure applied epidurally is transmitted intrathecally and might compromise perfusion or cause barotrauma at remote sites. They noted initial leakage of fluid into the large sacral root foramina and sheaths. After capacity was achieved (around 20 mL in ewes), there was an abrupt increase in CSF pressure with each injection. The range was variable and was reflective of each study animal and CNS compliance. The researchers concluded that instillation of saline into the epidural space eventually resulted in a significant increase in CSF pressures. CNS compliance was variable and seemed to deteriorate after instrumentation (surgery). Thus, scarring associated with surgery predisposed animals to neurologically dangerous pressures. Serpell and colleagues[43] recommend continuous monitoring of CSF pressures in humans. However, Cyriax[40] reported no major long-term complications after 50,000 volumetric caudal injections. Certainly, with these injections, even when given slowly, increases in CSF pressures were observed, but without apparent ill effect. At volumes greater than 100 mL, Cyriax did note potential for retinal hemorrhage with the single-shot caudal injection technique (i.e., injection completed in minutes). Dr. Cyriax indicated that retinal hemorrhages resolved without consequence. Other reports indicate that retinal hemorrhage can occur with routine epidural injections.[44] A few reports have now been published of retinal and macular hemorrhages and varying degrees of blindness after spinal canal endoscopy. In the cases I know of, the patients were deeply anesthetized. Thus the most sensitive monitor for elevated pressures, the patient's own complaint of pain, was "disconnected." Patients that have a noncompliant spinal canal will have resistance to injection and will complain of significant pain, both local and remote. The pain often begins in the lumbar spine and migrates cephalad. As a precaution, all injections into the spinal canal (both endoscopic and routine epidural injections) should be given gradually while the operator maintains constant dialogue with the patient. When the patient reports that pain or discomfort has moved cephalad, the managing physician must take appropriate action, as determined by the clinical circumstance: alter technique, infuse less injectate, stop the procedure, drain or decompress the epidural space, or use some other measure. The total volume that can be injected into a spinal canal with a series of injections or endoscopic procedures often increases with each subsequent injection (presumably from stretch of the more compliant spinal canal). An injection rate of 1 mL/sec is recommended. Previous work at Yale has determined that rapid injection of fluid (> 1 mL/sec) is more likely to be associated with high peak epidural pressures, at times in excess of 300 mm Hg. (Rate of injection, size of syringe, volume of injectate, compliance of the spinal canal [epidural space], and turbulence of the injection are all determinants of peak pressures.) As a rule, the peak pressures drop off abruptly to preinjection levels with disconnection of the syringe when total volume is less than 30 to 40 mL.

CLINICALLY RELEVANT ANATOMY

The spinal canal extends from the foramen magnum to the sacrum. It is bounded posteriorly by the ligamentum flavum and periosteum and anteriorly by the posterior longitudinal ligament that lies over the dorsal aspect of the vertebral bodies and discs. The size of the canal is approximately twice the size of the cord. It is largest in the cervical and lumbar regions, corresponding to enlargements in the spinal cord. At C4–C6, it measures 18 mm in anteroposterior dimension. The transverse diameter at C4–C6 is 30 mm. The thoracic canal is 17 mm in both anteroposterior and transverse measurements. The lumbar canal is 23 mm and 18 mm, respectively.[46] The canal in cross section appears triangular at the cervical and lumbar levels and more cylindrical at the thoracic level.

The spinal cord is continuous with the brain and ends with the conus medullaris at the lower border of the L1 vertebra. The dural sac containing the spinal cord and conus, however, runs down to the level of S2. The cauda equina consists of the terminal fibers of the conus that extend inside the dural sac from L1–S2. In the fetus, the spinal cord extends down to the coccyx, but, as development proceeds, it is drawn upward, owing to the greater growth of the vertebral column, so that, at birth, the spinal cord extends only to L3. Flexing the column draws the cord temporarily higher.[47] In nerves that are not freely movable, like those affected by arachnoiditis, flexion can cause lancinating pain.

The epidural space surrounds the dural sac. It is bordered posteriorly by ligamentum flavum and periosteum and anteriorly by the posterior longitudinal ligament. Laterally, the pedicles and the 48 intervertebral foramina bound it. The epidural space extends from the foramen magnum to the end of the dural sac at S2. Technically, the sacral canal is not part of the epidural space because it has no dural sac.

The size of the posterior epidural space varies greatly. It averages 2 mm at the cervical level, 3 to 5 mm at the thoracic level, and 4 to 6 mm at the lumbar level.[46] The epidural space narrows considerably at L4–S2. The epidural space anterior to the dura is uniformly narrow (1 mm) cephalad through caudad.

The epidural space is rich in content. At midline, connecting the dura to the periosteum posteriorly, there is usually a dorsal median connective tissue band, which can be complete or weblike.[48] Through the epidural space run the internal vertebral venous plexus, the spinal branches of the segmental arteries, the lymphatics, and the dura-arachnoid projections that surround the spinal nerve roots.[49] In addition, fat is abundant, and the amount seems to have no relationship to the patient's body fat percentage (Figs. 12–5, 12–9 to 12–13).[50]

The dura mater covering the spinal cord is a tough elastic tube that forms a loose sheath around the spinal cord. It is composed principally of longitudinal connective tissue fibers, and a relatively small amount of circular yellow elastic tissue fibers. The spinal dura mater extends from the foramen magnum, to which it is closely adherent by its outer surface, to the S2 vertebra, where it ends in a cul-de-sac. Below this level, the dura mater forms the filum terminale and descends to the coccyx, where it fuses with the periosteum.[49]

The paramedian approach for lumbar epidural injections has been advocated by anatomists (spinal endoscopists), because vessels concentrate at midline. It is remarkable to note the success of epidural anesthetic technique despite the plethora of fat and connective tissue. Even catheters are threaded more easily than one might predict. As demonstrated by Blomberg and colleagues,[17] the dura is fairly tough and deflects catheters, usually cephalad or caudad, depending on the direction of the bevel of the needle and the surrounding anatomic structures.

INDICATIONS

In selecting patients for spinal canal endoscopy the provider must realize there are symptoms pertaining to chief complaint and anatomic diagnosis. Both symptoms and anatomic variables need be taken into consideration in selecting the technique. Symptoms attributed to nerve irritation (from a variety of causes) may be responsive to directed irrigation and placement of antiinflammatory steroid medication. The chemical mediators responsible for the immune-mediated inflammation may come from herniated nucleus pulposus, synovium, or another source. Such irritants can be associated with radiculopathy, canal stenosis, fibrous adhesions, and cysts. Symptoms typically amenable to spinal canal endoscopy include those related to lumbar and sacral radiculopathy, neuralgias, and plexopathies from nerve root irritation without a significant compressive component. Presence of a compressive lesion with signs of progressive neurologic impairment is a contraindication to

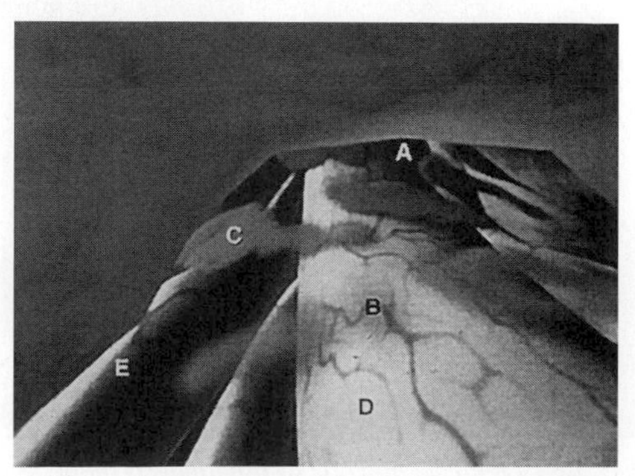

FIGURE 12–9 Artist's rendering of the contents of the lower lumbar epidural space. A, Epidural space. B, Blood vessel. C, Epidural fat. D, Dura mater. E, Nerve root. (Also in color; see Color Plates.)

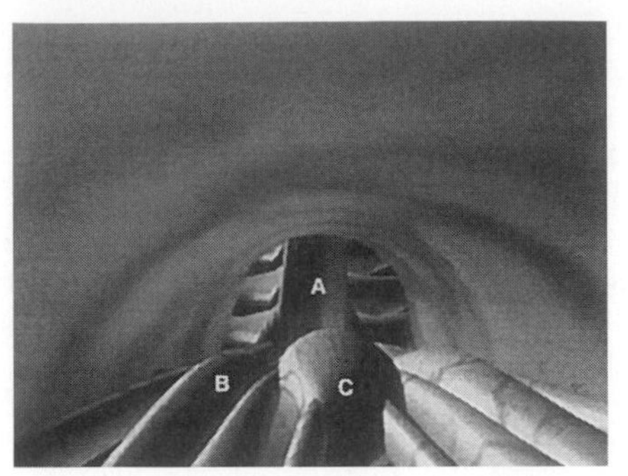

FIGURE 12–10 Artist's rendering of the contents of the epidural space at the level of the conus medullaris (L1). A, Epidural space. B, Nerve root. C, Conus medullaris. (Also in color; see Color Plates.)

placement of more fluid into the epidural space. Patient selection based on case reports suggests better results in the subgroup who have acute or subacute disc-related spinal pain syndrome but have not undergone back surgery and exhibit no associated pain behaviors.[19,20,33–35] This subgroup of patients may be more likely to be responsive to "washout" of chemical irritants and corticosteroid antiinflammatory effect. These patients may not have developed changes in CNS plasticity or secondary hyperalgesia and may thus be responsive to peripheral treatment with washouts alone. Spinal canal endoscopy is not indicated for patients suffering from biomechanical pain syndromes such as lumbar facet syndrome, sacroiliac joint dysfunction, or myofascial pain syndromes.

Widely Accepted Indications: Irritative neuralgias, new-onset radiculopathy, and radiculopathy associated with the postlaminectomy pain syndrome.

Probable Indications: Adhesion related, postlaminectomy epidural adhesion, low back pain, Tarlov's cyst.

Ideal Candidate Characteristics: Healthy, working, not involved in litigation, minimal medication, no dependent behaviors.

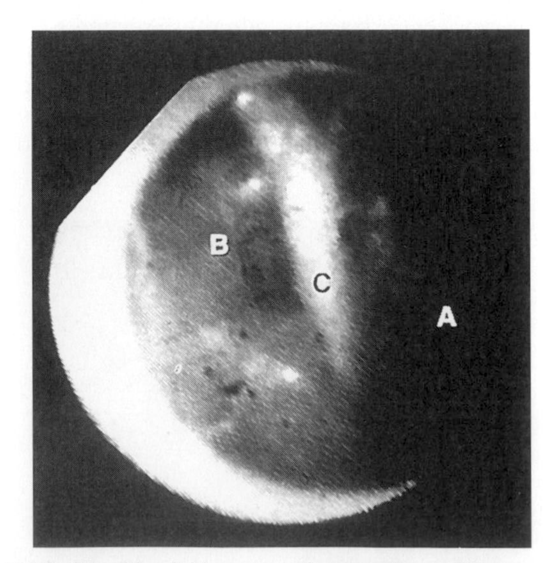

FIGURE 12–11 Epiduroscopy of a normal sacral nerve root. The fiberoptic scope, introduced from the sacral hiatus, is on the right side, looking left toward a normal nerve root. A, Epidural space. B, Dura mater. C, Sacral nerve root. (Also in color; see Color Plates.)

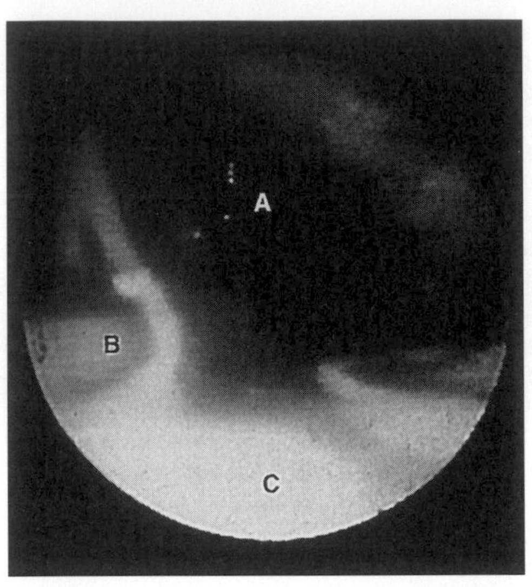

FIGURE 12–12 Photograph of the lumbar epidural space caudad to the conus. A, Epidural space. B, Nerve root. C, Dura mater. See Figure 12–13 for an artist's rendering. (Also in color; see Color Plates.)

Contraindications: No consent, cauda equina syndrome, urinary dynamic problem, sphincter dysfunction, foot drop, pilonidal cyst, osteomyelitis, and fissure, raised intracranial pressure, pseudotumor cerebri, CNS tumor, coagulopathy, no sacral hiatus, obstruction to placing a skinny needle into sacral canal, untreated addictive behavior, unstable angina, severe chronic obstructive pulmonary disease, meningocele/meningomyelocele, inability to lie prone (owing to chronic obstructive pulmonary disease, congestive heart failure, angina, back pain, etc.), inadequate facilities, allergy to necessary medications.

Relative Contraindications: Multiple different complaints of pain, active untreated psychiatric disorders[51], somatoform process, unrealistic expectations, retinal disease, partial blindness.

Facilities Required: Operating room, dedicated anesthesiologist providing monitored anesthetic care, postanesthesia care unit.

TECHNIQUE: A STEP-BY-STEP APPROACH

Before spinal canal endoscopy, all patients must undergo a thorough physical examination and give a complete history.

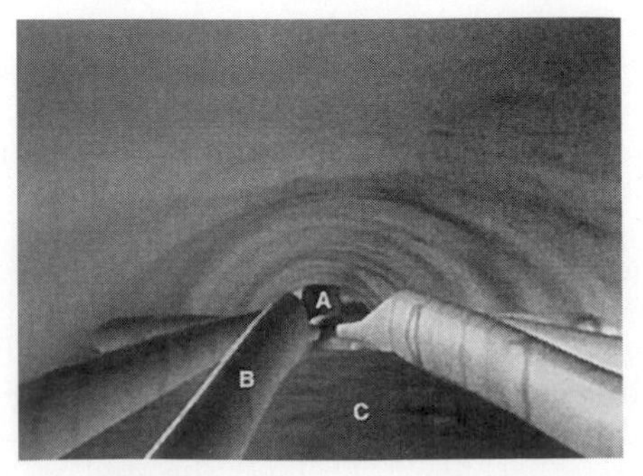

FIGURE 12–13 Artist's rendering of the lumbar epidural space caudad to the conus shown in Figure 12–12. A, Epidural space. B, Nerve root. C, Dura mater. (Also in color; see Color Plates.)

Care should be taken to document this examination carefully with special attention to a full neurologic examination. Imaging studies should be reviewed, as should special tests such as EMG and nerve conduction studies. Lumbosacral, flexion, extension, and oblique plain x-ray views should be reviewed for lesions that are not amenable to epidural procedures. MRI of the lumbar and sacral spine should be considered to assess the contents of spinal canal and seek spinal stenosis. If the decision is made to offer spinal canal endoscopy, all contraindications and relative contraindications must be addressed and documented in the medical record.

Preparation

Nonsteroidal antiinflammatory drugs, aspirin, and anticoagulants should be discontinued before spinal canal endoscopy.[52] Appropriate laboratory studies should be considered. As a rule, bleeding associated with spinal canal endoscopy is limited and occurs distally at the introducer's entrance at the sacral hiatus. The patient should use an antibacterial scrub during a shower the previous evening and should carefully cleanse the lumbar spine and sacral areas. The patient is directed to take nothing by mouth after midnight.

Equipment should be inspected, including disposables, several days in advance to ensure that all needed equipment is available. Fluoroscopy capability and a postanesthesia care unit must be available. Preprocedure discussion with the anesthesiologist should include patient positioning (prone) and the need for the patient to be awake and responsive. We recommend that voice contact be maintained with the patient throughout the procedure so as to monitor the patient's responses to manipulations. Informed consent must be obtained, and it is preferable to do this before the day of the procedure. A standard consent form can be found on the worldwide web at http://gasnet.med.yale.edu/local/pain.

Procedure

1. Preprocedure prophylactic antibiotic coverage should be considered. The patient lies prone with a pillow under the abdomen, the feet internally rotated. Such positioning provides better exposure of the sacral hiatus. The sacral hiatus is identified anatomically by palpating for the sacral cornua, which lie on either side of the midline, just above the natal crease. When the cornua are not palpable, firm midline palpation just above the natal crease should reveal the spinal canal. A midline position is confirmed with posteroanterior (PA) fluoroscopy.
2. With a 25-gauge or smaller needle, 3 to 5 mL of local anesthetic with epinephrine is placed into the floor of the sacral canal. The small needle is passed cephalad and should slide easily into the sacral canal.
3. A 17-gauge Tuohy needle is inserted into the sacral hiatus and advanced cephalad (Fig. 12–14A). The loss-of-resistance technique can be used to determine entry into the canal. A lateral fluoroscopic projection will show the needle in the canal. If it is dorsal to the canal (false passageway), it should be withdrawn and repositioned.
4. An injection of nonionic contrast medium, 5 to 15 mL, followed by PA fluoroscopy will provide an epidurogram that outlines nerve roots, scar adhesions, and other spinal canal structures (Fig. 12–14B).
5. The flexible end of the guidewire is threaded through the Tuohy needle (Fig. 12–14C). The guidewire should be threaded cephalad and its progress checked with PA fluoroscopy. Repositioning and flushing the Tuohy needle with normal saline may be necessary to facilitate passage of the guidewire toward the nerve root(s) of interest. After proper positioning of the wire is confirmed with PA and lateral fluoroscopy, the Tuohy needle is removed.
6. The dilator and sheath are carefully introduced over the wire (Fig. 12–14D). With a no. 11 scalpel, the wire's aperture is widened to allow easier passage of the introducer (Fig. 12–14E). (A similar technique is employed to place a central line.) If there is significant bleeding, firm pressure is applied with gauze. Additional local anesthetic with epinephrine can be given. Rotary movement facilitates passage of the dilator through the soft tissues. As dilator and sheath are passed cephalad, the wire should be tested frequently to see whether it moves freely. If the guidewire cannot be moved easily, there may be a kink in the wire, which PA and lateral fluoroscopy can help to check. If a kink is present, it is best to remove both dilator and sheath and slide the Tuohy needle back over the guidewire so that the wire can be removed and inspected. If the wire is kinked, a new wire should be used. (A kinked wire could misdirect passage of dilator and introducer catheter.)
7. After the dilator and sheath are inserted, the dilator is removed, leaving the introducer sheath (Fig. 12–14F).
8. The sidearm of the introducer sheath is flushed with 5 to 10 mL of preservative-free normal saline. The fiberoptic cable is then placed through one of the two lumens in the steering handle (Fig. 12–14G). Normal saline for irrigation into the spinal canal/epidural space is attached to the second steering handle lumen via tubing. The clinician should next orient himself or herself as to steering direction and focus the fiberoptic onto a sterile rule or other recognizable structure (Fig. 12–14H).
9. The steering handle containing the fiberoptic scope and preservative-free normal saline irrigation are inserted through the introducer (Fig. 12–14I). The camera and the video recorder are started. The steering handle with the fiberoptic device is advanced cephalad through the sacral canal into the epidural space. To keep the epidural space distended and achieve the proper focal length for fiberoptic visualization, gentle pressure is applied to the normal saline syringe. Complementing gentle pressure on the syringe can be the use of a 100 mL bag of preservative-free normal saline pressurized to less than systole for brief periods (1 to 2 minutes). This often frees hands for steering. Care should always be taken to ensure

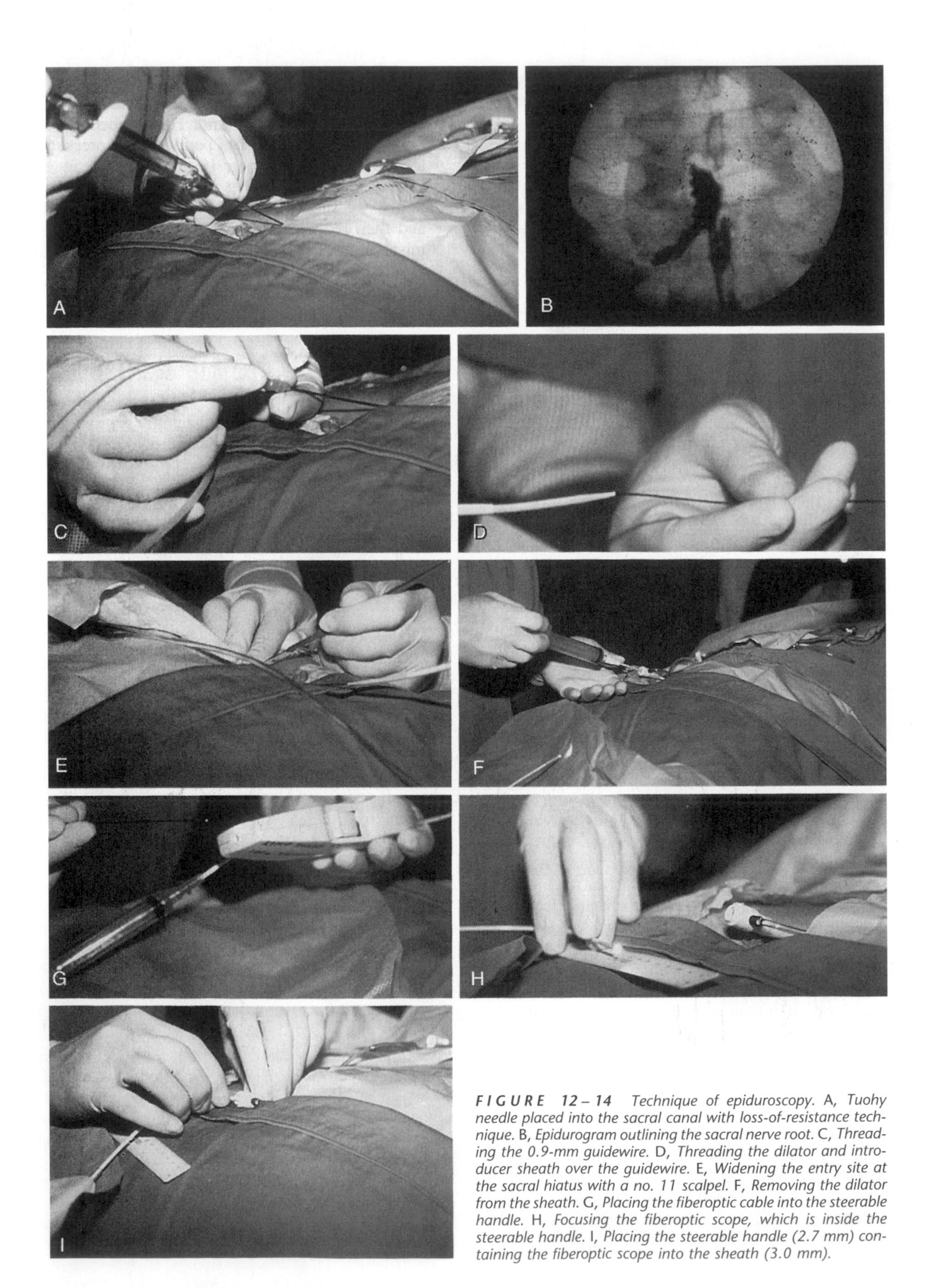

FIGURE 12–14 *Technique of epiduroscopy.* A, *Tuohy needle placed into the sacral canal with loss-of-resistance technique.* B, *Epidurogram outlining the sacral nerve root.* C, *Threading the 0.9-mm guidewire.* D, *Threading the dilator and introducer sheath over the guidewire.* E, *Widening the entry site at the sacral hiatus with a no. 11 scalpel.* F, *Removing the dilator from the sheath.* G, *Placing the fiberoptic cable into the steerable handle.* H, *Focusing the fiberoptic scope, which is inside the steerable handle.* I, *Placing the steerable handle (2.7 mm) containing the fiberoptic scope into the sheath (3.0 mm).*

against infusion of excess normal saline. For this reason, small bags of normal saline are chosen. High pressures in the epidural space may be safe for brief periods in some patients with a compliant spinal canal. (The pressures generated by a bolus from a 10-mL syringe injected at 1 mL/sec can be greater than 300 mm Hg.) Using a pressurized bag, we sustain pressure for 1 to 2 minutes, then reduce it to resting pressure to prevent compromise in perfusion. The amount of fluid injected must be accurately monitored. The amount of preservative-free normal saline used is approximately 60 mL per procedure. Most procedures last 30 to 45 minutes after the fiberoptic scope has been placed. Insertion of the introducer can at times be prolonged depending on the patient's anatomy and the skill of the operator.

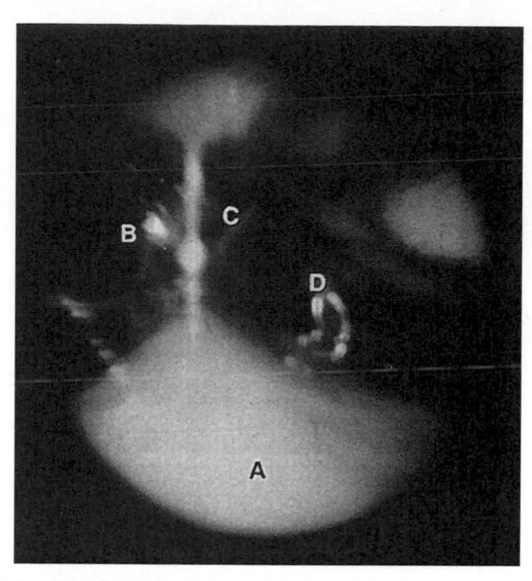

FIGURE 12–15 Tuohy needle placed into the epidural space. A, Dura mater. B, Epidural space. C, Connective tissue band. D, Ligamentum flavum. (From Blomberg R, Olsson O: The lumbar epidural space in patients examined with epiduroscopy. Anesth Analg 68:157–160, 1989.) (Also in color; see Color Plates.)

Postprocedure

After the procedure is completed, a dressing is applied and the patient is taken to the recovery area, where a postprocedure neurologic examination is performed. Any new deficits should be detailed and followed serially, and MRI and neurosurgical consultation should be considered. Patients are instructed not to bathe for 5 days, but showers are allowed after day 2. Hygiene instructions are important. In cleaning the perineum after bowel movements, wipes should be directed away from the procedural site. The patient should be discharged with a driver and should be observed by a friend or family member for the immediate postprocedure period. A 2- or 3-day supply of a short-acting opioid such as hydrocodone or oxycodone is appropriate.

EPIDURAL IMAGES

To follow the internal spinal canal (epidural) anatomy, it is critical to maintain proper orientation. Simultaneous use of fluoroscopy allows the operator to distinguish one level of epidural anatomy from the next. If the operator is confused about the location or orientation, needles can be inserted into the posterior epidural space. Blomberg's photographs of epidural catheters passing into the spinal canal (epidural space) illustrate this nicely. The needle identifies the dorsal epidural space (Figs. 12–13, 12–15, and 12–16). It is best to direct each spinal canal endoscopy to one or more specific areas instead of conducting a generalized exploration of canal, epidural space, and contents. In this way, the time a spinal canal is subjected to insufflation with normal saline—and potentially hazardous hydrostatic pressures—is minimized.

PITFALLS AND COMPLICATIONS

For spinal canal endoscopy to be performed, the epidural space must be distended with preservative-free normal saline. This makes room for the fiberoptic scope to achieve the focal length necessary to reveal intricate epidural structures that would not otherwise be visualized. A possible complication of this technique is significant epidural pressures that could affect local perfusion (L. R. Saberski, unpublished data, 1990). The epidural pressures generated can be transmitted cephalad through CSF and affect perfusion at more remote levels.[43] For these reasons, it is essential that the procedure be performed on lightly sedated, well-informed, cooperative patients, who are capable of informing the operator of pain at remote sites. If such a complaint is reported, the provider should consider adjusting the technique or terminating the procedure. An example of such a complication is spontaneous development of headache or altered vision during endoscopy.

Potential Complications

Complications of spinal canal endoscopy generally pertain to improper needle placement and/or generation of excessive epidural hydrostatic pressures.[53] Excessive pressure has the potential to affect both local and distant perfusion. Scapular or neck pain of new onset during the procedure suggests elevated pressures and may portend retinal hemorrhage. Patient complaints of pain from distention of the epidural space with a small volume of fluid usually signifies a noncompliant epidural space and may herald transmission of pressure far from the site of fluid deposition via the CSF. The operator must be very careful to keep epidural fluid volumes low and to maintain contact with the patient throughout the procedure. An alert patient can inform the operator of bodily sensations and changes as they occur. The operator uses clinical judgment during the procedure to determine whether an adjustment to or termination of the procedure is necessary.

Other potential complications are pain at and remote from the surgical site, transient dysesthesias, paresis, paralysis, blindness, other visual changes, post–dural puncture headaches, local surgical site bleeding, infection, and aller-

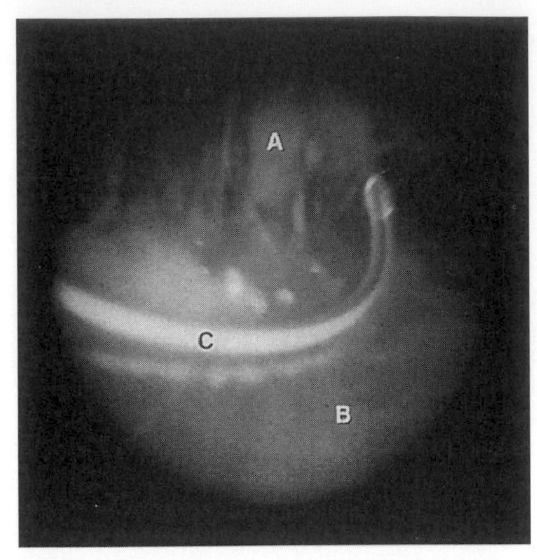

FIGURE 12–16 Catheter passing into the epidural space from Tuohy needle. A, Ligamentum flavum. B, Dura mater. C, Catheter. (From Blomberg R, Olsson O: The lumbar epidural space in patients examined with epiduroscopy. Anesth Analg 68:157–160, 1989.) (Also in color; see Color Plates.)

gic reactions. Pain at the surgical site is generally self-limited. Pain elsewhere requires evaluation and documentation in the medical record: severe headache, dysesthesia, and acute back pain. Such symptoms may be representative of epidural hematoma, cord ischemia, and elevated hydrostatic pressure. Paresis, paralysis, and pain can complicate needle trauma, epidural hematoma, elevated hydrostatic pressures, ischemia, or nerve injury (avulsion, traction, transection). Visual changes and even blindness have been reported. Their incidence is rare and they have been reported with routine epidural injections, presumably resulting from transmission of spinal canal pressures cephalad into the brain via CSF and effecting retinal perfusion or macular hemorrhage. Bleeding at the local surgical site is unlikely to cause neurologic complications, since it is just above the coccyx. Bleeding can predispose to infection, though infection is rare. Suggestions are a soapy scrub by patient before procedure, prophylactic antibiotics, sterile preparation and draping, keeping wound dry for 3 days, and wiping rectum after bowel movement away from surgical site (posterior to anterior).

OUTCOME

The initial study was designed to assess the outcome and safety of epidural steroid injection made with fiberoptic assistance (improved targeting) on patients with persistent lumbar radiculopathy that did not respond to physical therapy after two or three caudal injections. It was the premise of the initial study that an epidural injection might fail because medication was not delivered to the proper area, owing to scar, fat, or another morphologic anomaly adjacent to the nerve roots in question. Unfortunately, despite widespread acceptance of spinal canal endoscopy for delivery of targeted injections, outcome data are hard to come by, owing largely to the limited funds available for research. Clinical data have been collected from tens of thousands of procedures worldwide. Case reports and retrospectives have started to be published, and findings have been presented at various symposia. There have been no controlled studies, to date, comparing the outcomes of early spinal canal endoscopy and discectomy. In one study, pre- and postprocedural survey data from 77 patients demonstrated decreased need for medication and improved functional capacity up to 6 months after spinal endoscopy (Table 12–1).[54]

A Retrospective Pilot Study and Analysis of Spinal Canal Endoscopy and Laminectomy Outcome Data

There has been no demonstrable increase in the prevalence or severity of low back pain in the general population for the past 40 years. Despite this plateau, several studies have shown that disability from back pain has increased at a steady pace since the 1950s.[55–57] Interestingly, no study has associated chronic disability with physical factors such as height, weight, mobility, strength, or severity of injury.[58] In contrast, there are numerous studies that correlate chronic disability with psychosocial factors such as anxiety, depression, drug and alcohol abuse, low job satisfaction, poor job performance, and altered family dynamics.[59–63] Surprisingly, a factor strongly—and positively—associated with chronic disability is surgical intervention.[56, 64, 65] A well-designed study from Oregon related rising costs in workers' compensation to high rates of surgical failure.[66, 67] The most common surgical interventions were for spinal pain secondary to herniated discs, although many studies have demonstrated that only 1% of severe episodes of low back

*TABLE 12–1 Changes in Function and Complaints in Patients Before and After Spinal Canal Endoscopy**

	Baseline	2 Weeks	6 Months	Percentage Change (%)
Sad/blue	3.21	2.04	1.95	−39.3
Poor sleep	4.25	2.68	2.22	−42
Bend/stoop	2.79	3.49	3.69	32
Mile walk	2.21	3.49	3.69	60
Sit 20 min	3.03	3.43	3.62	20
Moderate activity	2.12	2.64	2.88	36
Climb stairs	3.12	3.51	3.62	16
Pain (sharp/stab)	3.62	2.22	1.92	−47
Sexual activity	2.36	3.42	3.42	44
Narcotic use†	14	6	4	−71

* Pre- and postprocedural survey data from 77 patients collected on 70 attributes. Data were graded on a 5-point scale: 1 never; 2 rarely; 3 sometimes; 4 often; 5 always. Tabulated scores are simple averages.
† Narcotic use was scored as number of patients.[55, 56]

pain are attributable to herniated discs. The associated sciatica is usually self-limited and resolves with conservative care in 80% to 85% of the cases.[68–72] Even in patients with a herniated disc who have neurologic deficit (numbness and weakness), there is equal resolve with conservatively treated patients compared with surgically managed ones.[69, 70] A large-scale English study showed that 86% of patients with herniated disc and sciatica had a good outcome with conservative, nonsurgical treatment.[72] Another study demonstrated that 83% of patients for whom urgent surgery was recommended could avoid surgical intervention and still achieve a good or excellent outcome.[71] Even more fascinating was the fact that the discs most amenable to surgery showed the greatest tendency toward regression on follow-up MRI. In other developed countries, surgery is utilized less—and only when there is evidence of cauda equina compression or multiradicular symptoms. As a result, outcomes are better. On the strength of clinical and epidemiologic studies cited earlier, we must recognize that only between 15 and 50 of every 10,000 cases of acute low back pain should require surgery; the others should be managed conservatively. Thus, low back pain qualifies as a medical disease, not necessarily a surgical problem, even in cases of herniated disc.

To date, medical management of disc-related complaints consists of oral medications and exercise programs. With the advent of spinal canal endoscopy, other options are now available for medical care of disc disease. Spinal canal endoscopy represents a platform that permits medical management of disc-related inflammation in the spinal canal. McCarron established that disc material when placed into the spinal canal of dogs caused an inflammatory response.[73] This response is initiated by various inflammatory mediators, including phospholipase A. The patient's immune system will continue to respond in the presence of inflammatory mediators.

Spinal canal endoscopy as currently practiced can irrigate, dilute, and remove inflammatory mediators, decreasing the chance of reactivity to chemical and biologic mediators. In addition, spinal canal endoscopy can direct corticosteroid medication precisely to the site of action. Such directed injection suppresses components of the inflammatory response and is the first chemotherapeutic modality to target the disc-related inflammatory response.

Materials and Methods: Pilot Study I

Data collection was performed in one geographical area of the United States. The initial sample population consisted of 35 patients aged 35 to 55 years who had radicular spinal pain as determined by history, physical examination, and MRI. The patients were divided into two groups: group 1 (n = 22) were treated via spinal endoscopy and group 2 (n = 13) with laminectomy. Group 1 patients were treated with 8 weeks of physical therapy and oral analgesic medication before spinal canal endoscopy. Group 2 patients were treated with 8 weeks of physical therapy, oral analgesic medication, and lumbar and caudal epidural steroid injections, before data collection.

While there were additional elements to the treatment regimens, this report is restricted to statistical analysis of the results. Basic descriptive statistics consisted of generating contingency tables (Tables 12–2 to 12–4). Tables 12–2 to 12–4 are arranged for ready comparison of each group's response. In the tables, preprocedure is self-explanatory; postprocedure is 8 weeks' follow-up. Demographic data were not complete from the presented data. No analysis or correlations with demographic factors were conducted. This report contains the results of statistical analysis only. Any other interpretation is at the discretion of the reader. Data were not deleted from the analysis.

Results

Data analysis compared the two groups for the significance of their responses to opiates and for return-to-work rates. Neuromedication was not tested owing to the 100% response rates in each group. Table 12–5 and Figure 12–17 illustrate the statistical testing. Chi-square analysis was performed using summary data with two nominal variables (procedure at two levels and response at two levels for each procedure). Using a significance level of 0.05, the responses are significantly independent between treatment groups. A similar approach was used to compare the return-to-work rates (Table 12–6, Fig. 12–18).

In group 1, 14 of the 22 patients were receiving opioid medication preprocedure. In Group 2, all 13 patients (63.5%) were receiving opioid medication preprocedure. After spinal canal endoscopy (group 1), seven patients

*TABLE 12–2 Contingency Table for Comparison of Opiate Use Rates**

	Group 1 Spinal Endoscopy				Group 2 Open Laminectomy			
	Preprocedure		*Postprocedure*		*Preprocedure*		*Postprocedure*	
Contingency	**Count**	**Rate (%)**	**Count**	**Rate (%)**	**Count**	**Rate (%)**	**Count**	**Rate (%)**
No	8	36.4	15	68.2	0	0	1	7.7
Yes	14	63.6	7	31.8	13	100	12	92.3
Totals	22	100	22	100	13	100	13	100

* Neuropathic medication was utilized in all 22 patients from group 1 before and after spinal canal endoscopy. In Group 2, three patients were on neuropathic medication before the procedure and 13 were on neuropathic medication after the procedure.

TABLE 12–3 ***Contingency Table: Neuropathic Medication Use/Rate Comparison****

	Group 1 Spinal Endoscopy				**Group 2 Open Laminectomy**			
	Preprocedure		*Postprocedure*		*Preprocedure*		*Postprocedure*	
Contingency	**Count**	**Rate (%)**	**Count**	**Rate (%)**	**Count**	**Rate (%)**	**Count**	**Rate (%)**
No	0	0	0	0	10	76.9	0	0
Yes	22	100	22	100	3	23.1	13	100
Totals	22	100	22	100	13	100	13	100

* Sixteen patients (72%) from group 1 returned to work and four patients (28%) from group 2 returned to work.

(31.8%) continued taking opioid medication; after laminectomy (group 2), 12 patients (92.3%) did.

Discussion

A relatively small number of postlaminectomy patients returned to work as compared with the spinal canal endoscopy group managed medically. The reasons are several:

1. The relatively atraumatic nature of spinal canal endoscopy as compared with laminectomy
2. The relatively short recovery times for spinal canal endoscopy as compared with laminectomy
3. The medical management of patients (not surgical candidates) with several modalities, including medication and spinal canal endoscopy

Although similar retrospective and preliminary data collected earlier indicated that spine disability is associated with laminectomy,[56, 64, 65, 74–81] these data suggest that avoidance of laminectomy in favor of a medical protocol built around spinal canal endoscopy is associated with a high return-to-work rate. This represents substantial savings in health care and disability expenditures. The cost savings, when extrapolated to an entire population, suggests that substantial amounts can be saved by using medical programs that emphasize medical care and spinal endoscopy. It is estimated that 1 year of disability costs the system $15,171. Disability savings alone (not even considering costs of surgery, hospitalization, and recovery) for 100 patients can exceed $1 million. Add to this the savings from *surgery not performed*, and the total savings are multimillions of dollars.

Conclusion

This pilot study suggests a remarkable difference in outcomes for medically managed patients with the benefit of spinal canal endoscopy and for a similar population of patients treated by laminectomy. A prospective study is now needed to compare the outcomes and cost savings of spinal canal endoscopy and laminectomy.

CODING FOR SPINAL CANAL ENDOSCOPY

Insurers typically cover procedures that meet certain criteria: The procedure must be medically necessary to treat the patient's condition and the device used according to labeled indications approved by the U.S. Food and Drug Administration. Individual insurance companies honor only certain procedural codes. It is important that providers communicate with individual payers to learn their respective requirements. In this changing health care environment, insurance coverage is never a guarantee of payment. Insurers vary widely in the services they cover. Even among patients insured by the same insurance company, benefits may vary according to specific plans. Some plans may be unfamiliar with spinal canal endoscopy and may require submission of additional information with the claim before making a coverage decision. For this reason, it may be prudent to file a claim manually with a complete operative report and hard copy of all supporting radiographs.

No existing CPT codes are specific to epidural diagnostic and therapeutic procedures that use the spinal endoscope. CPT codes vary from insurer to insurer. Several possible codes are listed below. Individual payers may have their own policies regarding the use of CPT codes.

TABLE 12–4 ***Contingency Table for Return-to-Work Rates***

	Spinal Endoscopy		**Open Laminectomy**	
Contingency	*Count*	*Rate (%)*	*Count*	*Rate (%)*
No	6	27.3	9	69.2
Yes	16	72.7	4	30.8
Totals	22	100	13	100

TABLE 12–5 ***Results of Chi-Square Test of Post-procedure Opiate Use Rates***

Statistic	**Value**
Degree of freedom	1
Chi-Square	12.048
P value	.0005

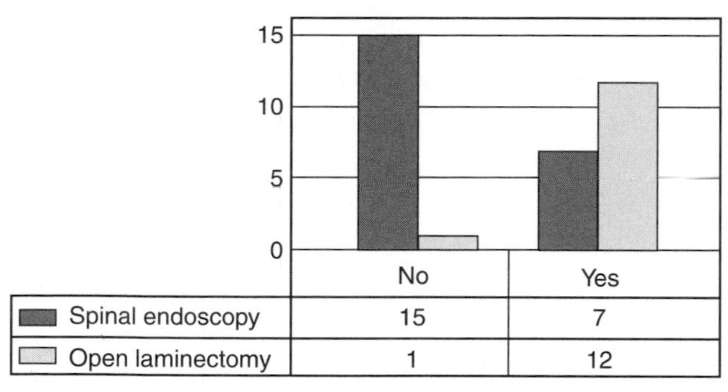

FIGURE 12–17 Postprocedure comparison of opiate use.

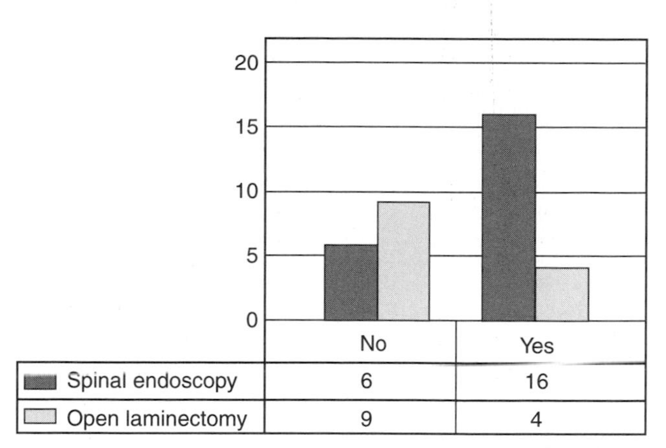

FIGURE 12–18 Postprocedure comparison of return-to-work rates.

Coding for Diagnosis (ICD-9-CM)

Diagnosis and the diagnostic codes must be supportive of the medical necessity for procedures and service rendered. The diagnostic codes below may be appropriate for epidural endoscopy.

- 353.1 Lumbosacral plexus lesions
- 353.4 Lumbosacral root lesions, not elsewhere classified
- 722.83 Postlaminectomy syndrome; lumbar region
- 724.4 Lumbosacral radiculitis
- 724.9 Other unspecified back disorder; compression of spinal nerve root, NEC
- 953.2 Injury to lumbar nerve root
- 953.3 Injury to sacral nerve root
- 953.4 Injury to lumbosacral plexus

CONCLUSIONS AND FUTURE DIRECTIONS

The technology of spinal canal endoscopy developed slowly over the twentieth century. Contributions were made by many, but only recently has the technique been refined sufficiently to be clinically useful. Further study is needed to determine whether this technique holds advantages over other currently used techniques for delivering medication into the epidural space. Real-time direct visual examination of epidural anatomy currently enables identification of epidural lesions and localization of pain generators there. This capability to examine the epidural space without operative trauma and to direct the delivery of medication is not currently available with any other technique.

The future may hold the promise of minimally invasive and effective therapy for both radicular and perhaps other forms of disabling back pain. Other exciting possibilities for this technology may include removal of extradural and intradural scar tissue, cyst drainage, biopsies, studies of cell biology and inflammatory mediators, and retrieval of foreign bodies. We feel that the possibility of modifying the inflammatory process by blocking the mediators of inflammation holds the greatest promise. Today, the technique can be used to safely and effectively deliver medication under direct vision. It opens new doors for the diagnosis and treatment of disease accessible through the epidural space.

TABLE 12–6 ***Results of Chi-Square Testing of Postprocedure Return-to-Work Rates***

Statistic	Value
Degree of freedom	1
Chi-Square	5.874
P value	.0154

REFERENCES

1. Burman MS: Myeloscopy or the direct visualization of the spinal cord. J Bone Joint Surg 13:695–696, 1931.
2. Shimoji K, Fujioka H, Onodera M, et al: Observation of spinal canal and cisternae with the newly developed small-diameter, flexible fiberscopes. Anesthesiology 75:341–344, 1991.
3. Stern EL: The spinascope: A new instrument for visualizing the spinal canal and its contents. Med Rec (NY) 143:31–32, 1936.
4. Pool JL: Direct visualization of dorsal nerve roots of the cauda equina by means of a myeloscope. Arch Neurol Psychiatry 39:1308–1312, 1938.
5. Pool JL: Myeloscopy: Intraspinal endoscopy. Surgery 11:169–182, 1942.
6. Pool JL: Myeloscopy: Diagnostic inspection of the cauda equina by means of an endoscope. Bull Neurol Inst NY 7:178–189, 1938.
7. Ooi Y, Morisaki N: Intrathecal lumbar endoscope. Clin Orthop Surg (Jpn) 4:295–297, 1969.
8. Ooi Y, Satoh Y, Morisaki N: Myeloscopy. Igakuno Ayumi (Jpn) 81:209–212, 1972.
9. Ooi Y, Satoh Y, Morisaki N: Myeloscopy. Orthop Surg (Jpn) 24:181–186, 1973.
10. Ooi Y, Satoh Y, Morisaki N: Myeloscopy: Possibility of observing lumbar intrathecal space by use of an endoscope. Endoscopy 5:91–96, 1973.
11. Ooi Y, Satoh Y, Morisaki N: Myeloscopy: A preliminary report. J Jpn Orthop Assoc 47:619–627, 1973.
12. Ooi Y, Satoh Y, Morisaki N: Myeloscopy. Int Orthop 1:107–111, 1977.
13. Ooi Y, Satoh Y, Inoue K, et al: Myeloscopy. Acta Orthop Belg 44:881, 1978.
14. Satoh Y, Hirose K, Ooi Y, Mikanagi K: Myeloscopy in the diagnosis of low back pain syndrome. Presented at The Third Congress of International Rehabilitation Medicine Association, Basel, Switzerland, July 2–9, 1978.
15. Ooi Y, Satoh Y, Inoue K, et al: Myeloscopy with special reference to blood flow changes in the cauda equina during Lasègue's test. Int Orthop 4:307–311, 1981.

16. Blomberg R: A method for spinal canal endoscopy and spinaloscopy: Presentation of preliminary results. Acta Anaesthesiol Scand 21:113–116, 1985.
17. Blomberg R, Olsson S: The lumbar epidural space in patients examined with epiduroscopy. Anesth Analg 68:157–160, 1989.
18. Blomberg R: Technical advantages of the paramedian approach for lumbar epidural puncture and catheter introduction. Anesthesiology 43:837–843, 1988.
19. Saberski LR, Kitahata LM: Direct visualization of the lumbosacral epidural space through the sacral hiatus. Anesth Analg 80:839–840, 1995.
20. Saberski LR, Kitahata LM: Review of the clinical basis and protocol for epidural endoscopy. Connecticut Med 50(2): 71–73, 1995.
21. Heavner JE, Cholkhavatia S, Kizelshteyn G: Percutaneous evaluation of the epidural and subarachnoid space with the flexible fiberscope. Reg Anesth 15S1:85, 1991.
22. Mollman M, Host D, Enk D: Spinaloskopie zur Darstellung von Problemen bei der Anwendung der kontinuierlichen Spinalanaesthesie. Anaesthesist 41:544–547, 1992.
23. Heavner J, Chokhavatia K, McDaniel K, et al: Diagnostic and therapeutic maneuvers in the epidural space via a flexible endoscope (Abstract 1534). *In* Abstracts of the Seventh World Congress on Pain, Paris, August 1993.
24. Rosenberg P, Heavner J, Chokhavatia K, et al: Epiduroscopy with a thin flexible and deflectable fiberscope. Br J Anaesth 72 (Suppl 1):74–75, 1994.
25. Schutze G, Kurtze H: Direct observation of the epidural space with a flexible catheter–secured epiduroscopic unit. Reg Anesth 19:85–89, 1994.
26. Igarashi T, Hirabayashi Y, Shimizu R, et al: Thoracic and lumbar extradural structure examined by extraduroscope. Br J Anaesth 81:121–125, 1998.
27. Holmstrom B, Rawal N, Axelson K, Nydahl PA: Risk of catheter migration during combined spinal epidural block: Percutaneous epiduroscopy study. Anesth Analg 747–753, 1995.
28. Igarashi T, Hirabayashi Y, Shimizu R, et al: The lumbar epidural structure changes with increasing age. Br J Anaesth 78:149–152, 1997.
29. Igarashi T, Hirabayashi Y, Shimizu R, et al: Inflammatory changes after extradural anaesthesia may effect the spread of local anaesthetic within the extradural space. Br J Anaesth 77:347–351, 1996.
30. Kitamura A, Sakamoto A, Shigemasa A, et al: Epiduroscopic changes in patients undergoing single and repeated epidural injections. Anesth Analg 82:88–90, 1996.
31. Wulf H, Streipling E: Postmortem findings after epidural anaesthesia. Anaesthesia 45:357–361, 1990.
32. Schmerztherapeutisches Kolloquiurn e. V., Iserlohn, Dr. med. G. Sch, tze, Hagenerstr. 121, 58642 Iserlohn., http://pain.de/pages/pub102.html
33. Saberski LR, Kitahata LM: Persistent radiculopathy diagnosed and treated with epidural endoscopy. Jpn Anesth 10: 292–295, 1996.
34. Saberski LR, Brull SJ: Spinal and epidural endoscopy: A historical review and case report. Yale J Biol Med 68: 7–17, 1995.
35. Saberski LR: Technical workshop: Epiduroscopy. J Back Musculoskel Rehabil 11:149–152, 1998.
36. Saberski LR, Fredericks R, Dunn EL, et al: Bovine model for studying nucleus pulposus–related immunoinflammation in spinal canals. (Submitted for publication 2000).
37. Richardson J: Realizing visions (Editorial). BJA 83: 1999.
38. Saberski LR: Current application of spinal canal endoscopy: Is it a diagnostic tool or a therapeutic modality? Syllabus: The World Foundation for Pain Relief and Research: Current Concepts in Acute, Chronic and Cancer Pain Management, New York, December 1999. pp 177–181.
39. Odendaal CL, van Aswegen A: Determining the spread of epidural medication in post laminectomy patients by radionuclide admixture (Abstract 1487). *In* Abstracts of the Seventh World Congress on Pain, Paris, Raven, August 1993.
40. Cyriax J: The Illustrated Manual of Orthopedic Medicine. London, Butterworth, 1983.
41. Racz GB, Holubec JT: Lysis of adhesions in the epidural space. *In* Racz GB (ed): Techniques of Neurolysis. Boston, Kluwer Academic, 1989.
42. Arthur J, Racz G, Heinrich R, et al: Epidural space: Identification of filling defects and lysis of adhesions in the treatment of chronic painful conditions (Abstract 1485). *In* Abstracts of the Seventh World Congress on Pain, Paris, Raven, August 1993.
43. Serpell MG, Coombs DW, Colburn RW, et al: Intrathecal pressure recordings due to saline instillation in the epidural space (Abstract 1535). *In* Abstracts of the Seventh World Congress on Pain, Paris, Raven, August 1993.
44. Kushner FH, Olson JC: Retinal hemorrhage as a consequence of epidural steroid injection. Arch Ophthalmol 113:309–313, 1995.
45. Saberski LR, Garfunkel D: Unpublished data, 1991.
46. Clemente CD (ed): Gray's Anatomy of the Human Body. Philadelphia, Lea & Febiger, 1985.
47. Basmajian J: Grant's Method of Anatomy, ed 8. Baltimore, Williams & Wilkins, 1993, p 41.
48. Shimoji K, Fujioka H, Onodera J, et al: Observation of spinal cord and cisternae with the newly developed small-diameter, flexible fiberscopes. Anesthesiology 75:341–344, 1991.
49. Bonica JJ: The Management of Pain. Philadelphia, Lea & Febiger, 1990, pp. 1411–1413.
50. Holmstrom B, Raawal N: Epiduroscopic study of risk of catheter migration following dural puncture by spinal and epidural needles: A Video Presentation. American Society of Anesthesiology, 1992.
51. Levin SC, Stacey BR, Cantees K: Preoperative and postoperative back pain management. *In* Welch WC, Jacobs GB, Jackson GP (eds): Operative Spine Surgery, ed 1. Norwalk, Appleton & Lange, 1999.
52. Odoom JA, Sih IL: Epidural analgesia and anticoagulant therapy. Experience with 1000 cases of continuous epidurals. Anaesthesia 38:254–259, 1983.
53. Serpell MG, Coombs DW, Colburn RW, et al: Intrathecal pressure recordings due to saline instillation in the epidural space (Abstract). 7th world congress on pain. # 1535, 8/93
54. Unpublished data, Myelotec Incorporated, Alpharetta, GA, 1998
55. Social Security Bulletin: Annual Statistical Supplement. Washington, DC, U.S. Government Printing Office, 1986.
56. Waddel GA: A new clinical model for the treatment of low-back pain. Volvo award in clinical sciences. Spine 12:632–644, 1987.
57. Workers' Compensation Board of British Columbia: Vancouver, Canada, 1986. (Unpublished data.) Myelotec, 1998.
58. Rybock JD: Industrial low back pain. *In* Bleecker ML (ed): Occupational Neurology and Clinical Neurotoxicology. Baltimore, Williams & Wilkins 1994, pp 335–343.
59. Bigos SJ, Battie MC, Sprengler NM, Guy DP: *In* Weinstein JN, Wiesel SW (eds): The Lumbar Spine. Philadelphia, WB Saunders, 1990, pp 846–859.
60. Helander E: Back pain and work disability. Social Med Times 50: 398–404, 1973.
61. Lee PWJ, Chow SP, Lieh-Mak F, et al: The psychosocial factors influencing outcomes in patients with low back pain. Spine 14:838–846, 1989.
62. Magora A: Investigation of the relation between low back pain and occupation: 5 Psychological aspects. Scand J Rehabil Med 5:186–190, 1973.
63. Waddwll G, Mani CJ, Morris EW, et al: Chronic low back pain, psychological distress and illness behavior. Spine 9:209–213, 1984.
64. Frymoyer JW, Cats-Baril WL: An overview of the incidence and costs of low back pain. Orthop Clin North Am 22:263–271, 1991.
65. Frymoyer JW, Rosen JC, Clements J, et al: Psychologic factors in low back pain disability. Clin Orthop 195:178–184, 1985.
66. Norton WL: Chemonucleolysis versus surgical discectomy: Comparison of costs and results in workers' compensation claimants. Spine 11:440–443, 1986.
67. Antonakes JA: Claim costs of back pain. Best's Review September:1981.
68. Hakelius A: Prognosis in sciatica: A clinical follow-up of surgical and non-surgical treatment. Acta Orthop Scand Suppl 129:1–76, 1970.
69. Javid MJ, Nordby EJ, Ford LT: Safety and efficacy of chymopapain in herniated nucleus with sciatica: Results of a randomized double blind study. JAMA 249:2489–2494, 1983.
70. Weher H: Lumbar disc herniation: A controlled prospective study with 10 years of observation. 1983;8:131–139, Spine.
71. Saal JA, Saal JS: Non-operative treatment of herniated intervertebral discs with radiculopathy: An outcome study. Spine 14:431–437, 1989.
72. Bush K, Cowan N, Katz DE, Gishen P: The natural history of sciatica associated with disc pathology. Spine 17:1205–1212, 1991.
73. McCarron RF: Epidural fibrosis: Experimental model and therapeutic alternatives, techniques of neurolysis. *In* Racz GB (ed): Techniques of Neurolysis. Boston, Kluwer, 1989.
74. Robertson JT: The rape of the spine. Surg Neurol 39:5–12, 1993.

75. Dicksen RA: The surgical treatment of low back pain. Corr Orthop 1:387–390, 1987.
76. Ferran A: One day back operations could save NHS millions. Observer July 22:6, 1990.
77. Kane WJ: The incidence rate of laminectomies in the USA. Proceedings of the International Society for the Study of the Lumbar Spine Meeting, New Orleans, Louisiana, May 1980.
78. National hospital discharge survey. 1986.
79. Office of Health Economics. Back Pain. London, 1985.
80. Spamgfort EV: The lumbar disc herniation: A computer aided analysis of 2504 operations. Acta Orthop Scand Suppl 142:1–95, 1972.
81. New Haven Register, November 1995.
82. Kirschner CG, Davis SJ, Duffy L, et al (eds): CPT 99. Chicago, American Medical Association, 1998.

CHAPTER • 13

Differential Neural Blockade for the Diagnosis of Pain

Alon P. Winnie, MD • Kenneth D. Candido, MD

Clinically, differential neural blockade is the selective blockade of one type of nerve fiber without blocking other types of nerve fibers. It is an extremely useful diagnostic tool that allows the clinician to observe the effect of a sympathetic block, a sensory block, and, for that matter, a block of all nerve fibers by local anesthetic agents on a patient's pain, and to compare that effect with the effect of an injection of an inactive agent (placebo). There are two clinical approaches to the production of differential neural blockade, an anatomic approach and a pharmacologic approach. The anatomic approach is based on sufficient anatomic separation of sympathetic and somatic fibers to allow injection of local anesthetic to block one type only (see later). The pharmacologic approach is based on the presumed difference in the sensitivity of the various types of nerve fibers to local anesthetics, so that the injection of local anesthetics in different concentrations selectively blocks different types of fibers.

Since pain is a totally *subjective* phenomenon, what is needed to identify the neural pathway that subserves it is some sort of *objective* diagnostic test, and differential neural blockade is just such a test. While differential neural blockade is not intended to replace a detailed history, a complete physical examination, and appropriate laboratory, radiographic, and psychological studies, in our practice it has been a rewarding diagnostic maneuver that has been effective in delineating the neural mechanisms subserving many puzzling pain problems, and it has been particularly useful in patients who have intractable pain with no apparent cause.

TECHNIQUES

As stated above, there are two basic approaches to the performance of differential neural blockade, a pharmacologic approach and an anatomic one.

THE PHARMACOLOGIC APPROACH

A differential spinal is the simplest pharmacologic approach with the most discrete end points. The first clinical application of this technique[1] was based on the seminal work of Gasser and Erlanger,[2,3] and, while these investigators were wrong about the site of conduction (they believed it took place within the axoplasm), they established forever the relationship between fiber size, conduction velocity, and fiber function. Their classification of nerve fibers based on size is still used today (Table 13–1). In a simple but elegant experiment, these researchers showed that when a nerve is stimulated and the response is recorded only a few millimeters away, the record shows a single action potential. Then they demonstrated that, as the recording electrode is moved progressively farther away from the stimulating electrode, the action potential can be shown to consist of several smaller spikes, each representing an impulse traveling at a different rate along a nerve fiber of a different size. The action potentials might be compared to runners in a race who become separated along the course as the faster contestants outstrip the slower. Thus, in a record obtained by a recording electrode 82 mm from the point of stimulation, three waves can be seen, whereas at 12 mm, the potentials are fused, and only one large wave appears (Fig. 13–1). It may be seen in Table 13–1 that the diameter of a nerve fiber is its most important physical dimension, so it is on that basis that they have been subdivided into three classes, A, B, and C fibers, A fibers being subdivided into four subclasses, alpha, beta, gamma, and delta. Furthermore, it may be seen that the fiber diameter is an important determinant of conduction velocity, the conduction velocity of A fibers (in meters per second) being approximately six times the fiber diameter (in micrometers).[4] In addition, the diameter and myelination of a nerve fiber also determine to some degree the modality or modalities subserved by that fiber[5]: A-alpha fibers subserve motor function and proprioception; A-beta fibers subserve the transmission of touch and pressure; and A-gamma fibers subserve muscle tone. The thinnest A fibers, the A-delta group, convey pain and temperature sensation and signal nociception (tissue damage). The myelinated B fibers are thin, preganglionic, autonomic fibers, and the nonmyelinated C fibers, like the myelinated A-delta fibers, subserve pain, temperature transmission, and nociception. C fibers are thinner than

TABLE 13–1 **Classification of Nerve Fibers by Fiber Size and the Relation of Fiber Size to Function and Sensitivity to Local Anesthetics***

Group/Subgroup	Diameter (μm)	Conduction Velocity (m/sec)	Modalities Subserved	Sensitivity to Local Anesthetics (%)†
A (myelinated)				
A-alpha	15–20	8–120	Large motor, proprioception	1.0
A-beta	8–15	30–70	Small motor, touch, pressure	↓ ↓
A-gamma	4–8	30–70	Muscle spindle, reflex	↓
A-delta	3–4	10–30	Temperature, sharp pain, nociception	0.5
B (unmyelinated)	3–4	10–15	Preganglionic autonomic	0.25
C (unmyelinated)	1–2	1–2	Dull pain, temperature, nociception	0.5

* Subarachnoid procaine.
† Vertical arrows indicate intermediate values, in descending order.

the myelinated fibers and have a much slower conduction velocity than even A-delta fibers.

Though the relationship between fiber size and sensitivity to local anesthetics originally proposed by Gasser and Erlanger was challenged recently, the "bathed length principle" proposed by Fink[6,7] has restored the functional relationship between fiber size and sensitivity to local anesthetics, since the larger the nerve fiber, the greater is the internodal distance. Furthermore, it has been postulated that the density of the distribution of sodium channels at the nodes of Ranvier increases with fiber size, so that the "denser channel packing at the nodes" may also result in increased minimum blocking concentration (C_m), so this may be another reason why larger fibers require a higher concentration of local anesthetic for blockade than do smaller fibers.[8]

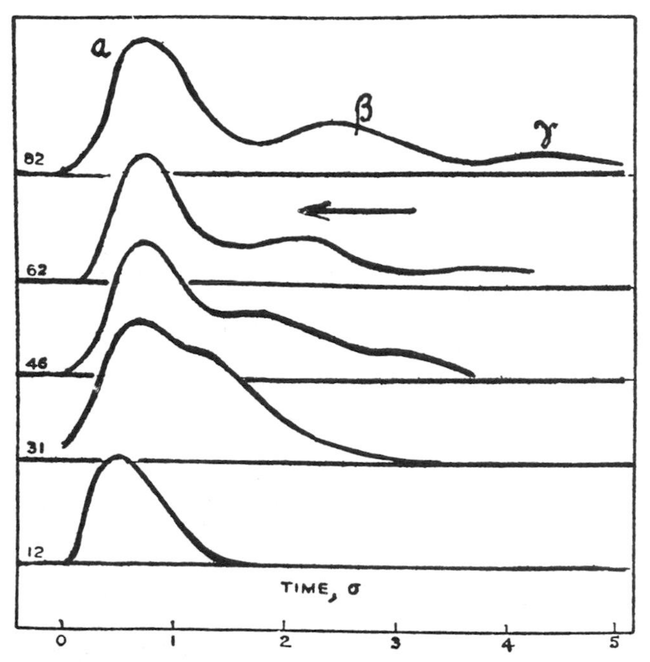

FIGURE 13–1 Cathode ray oscillograph records of the action current in a bullfrog's sciatic nerve after conduction from the point of stimulation through the distances (mm) shown at the left. The delta wave is not shown in the record. (Modified from Gasser HS, Erlanger J: Role of fiber size in establishment of nerve block by pressure or cocaine. Am J Physiol 88:587–591, 1929.)

Conventional Sequential Differential Spinal Block

The conventional sequential technique of differential subarachnoid block[9,10] is a refinement of the techniques first used by Arrowood and Sarnoff[1] and later by McCollum and Stephen.[11] The technique has certain inherent shortcomings (see later), which have caused it to be replaced in our practice by the modified technique, but, because this is the prototype of differential neural blockade, understanding the technique and the problems it presents provides insight into the usefulness and the limitations of diagnostic differential spinal blockade using the pharmacologic approach.

Procedure

After detailed informed consent is obtained from the patient, an intravenous infusion is started and prehydration with crystalloid is begun, as for any spinal anesthetic. Similarly, all of the monitors routinely utilized for spinal anesthesia are applied, including blood pressure, electrocardiography (ECG), and pulse oximetry, and baseline values are recorded. Four solutions are prepared (Table 13–2), and the patient is placed in the lateral position with the painful side down, if possible. After the usual sterile preparation and draping of the back, a 25- to 27-gauge spinal needle is introduced into the lumbar subarachnoid space at the L2–L3 or L3–L4 interspace. The patient is shown the four prepared syringes, all of which appear identical, and is told that each of the solutions will be injected sequentially at 10- to 15-min intervals. The patient is instructed to tell the physician which, if any, of the solutions relieves the pain. The solutions are referred to as *A* through *D*, so that the physicians can discuss the solutions freely in front of the patient without using the word *placebo.*

Solution A, which contains no local anesthetic, is the placebo. Solution B contains 0.25% procaine, which is the mean sympatholytic concentration of procaine in the subarachnoid space,[1] that is, the concentration that is suffi-

TABLE 13–2 **Preparation of Solutions for Conventional Sequential Differential Spinal Blockade**

Solution	Preparation of Solution	Yield	Blockade
D	To 2 mL of 10% procaine add 2 mL of normal saline	4 mL of 5% procaine	Motor
C	To 1 mL of 5% procaine add 9 mL of normal saline	10 mL of 0.5% procaine	Sensory
B	To 5 mL of 0.5% procaine add 5 mL of normal saline	10 mL of 0.25% procaine	Sympathetic
A	Draw up 10 mL of normal saline	10 mL of normal saline	Placebo

cient to block B fibers but is *usually* insufficient to block A-delta and C fibers. Solution C contains 0.5% procaine, the mean sensory blocking concentration of procaine, that is, the concentration *usually* sufficient to block, in addition to B fibers, A-delta and C fibers but is insufficient to block A-alpha, A-beta, and A-gamma fibers. Finally, solution D contains 5.0% procaine, which provides complete blockade of all fibers.

To prevent bias, it is extremely important that all of the injections be carried out in exactly the same manner, so that to the patient they are identical to and indistinguishable from one another. It is equally important that the physician make exactly the same observations after each injection (Table 13–3). Furthermore, the observations must be carried out in an identical manner after each injection so that the observations themselves do not influence the patient's response. Obviously, an inexperienced clinician who checks only the blood pressure after the sympatholytic injection, who checks only the response to pinprick after the sensory-blocking injection, and who checks only the motor function after the motor-blocking injection would clearly reveal the expectation that each sequential injection will produce progressively increasing effects. This would clearly compromise the validity of the information obtained from the procedure.

Interpretation

The conventional sequential differential spinal is interpreted as follows: If the patient's pain is relieved after solution A (the placebo), the patient's pain is classified as "psychogenic." It is well known that some 30% to 35% of all patients with true, organic pain obtain relief from an inactive agent.[12] Therefore, relief in response to the normal saline may represent a placebo reaction, but it may also indicate that an entirely psychogenic mechanism is subserving the patient's pain. Clinically, these two can usually be differentiated, because a placebo reaction is usually short-lived and self-limiting, whereas pain relief provided by a placebo to a patient suffering from true, psychogenic pain is usually long-lasting, if not permanent. If the difference between the two is not clinically evident, evaluation by a clinical psychologist or psychiatrist may be necessary.

If the patient does not obtain relief from the placebo but does obtain relief from the 0.25% procaine, the mechanism subserving the patient's pain is tentatively classified as sympathetic, provided that concurrent with the onset of pain relief signs of sympathetic blockade are observed *without* signs of sensory block. Obviously, although 0.25% procaine is the *usual* sympatholytic concentration in most patients, in some patients (who may have a reduced C_m for A-delta and C fibers) relief may be due to the production of analgesia and/or anesthesia. The finding that a sympathetic mechanism is subserving a patient's pain is extremely fortuitous for the patient, because if the pain is truly sympathetically mediated, if treated early enough, it may be completely and permanently relieved by a series of sympathetic nerve blocks.

If 0.25% procaine does not provide pain relief but the 0.5% concentration does, this usually indicates that the patient's pain is subserved by A-delta and/or C fibers and is classified as somatic pain, *provided that* the patient did exhibit signs of sympathetic blockade after the previous injection of 0.25% procaine and that the onset of pain relief is accompanied by the onset of analgesia and/or anesthesia. This is important because if a patient has an elevated C_m for B fibers, the pain relief from 0.5% procaine could be due to sympathetic block rather than to sensory block.

If pain relief is not obtained by any of the first three injections, 5% procaine is injected to block all modalities. If the 5% concentration *does* relieve the patient's pain, the mechanism is still considered somatic, the presumption being that the patient has an elevated C_m for A-delta and C fibers. If, however, the patient obtains no relief in spite of complete sympathetic, sensory, and motor blockade, the pain is classified as "central" in origin, although this is not a specific diagnosis and may indicate any one of the four possibilities in Table 13–4.

TABLE 13–3 **Observations After Each Injection**

Sequence	Observation
1	Blood pressure and pulse rate
2	Patient's subjective evaluation of the pain at rest
3	Reproduction of patient's pain by movement
4	Signs of sympathetic block (temperature change, psychogalvanic reflex)
5	Signs of sensory block (no response to pinprick)
6	Signs of motor block (inability to move toes, feet, legs)

Disadvantages

The conventional sequential differential spinal technique just described was utilized by the authors for many years and was effective in pinpointing the neural mechanisms subserving pain syndromes in a multitude of patients. It was particularly effective in establishing a diagnosis in patients with pain syndromes of questionable or unknown etiology. However, the technique has several obvious draw-

TABLE 13–4 *Diagnostic Possibilities of "Central Mechanism"*

Diagnosis	Explanation/Basis of Diagnosis
Central lesion	The patient may have a lesion in the central nervous system that is above the level of the subarachnoid sensory block. For example, we have seen two patients who had a metastatic lesion in the precentral gyrus, which was the origin of the patient's peripheral pain and was clearly above the level of the block.
Psychogenic pain	The patient may have true "psychogenic pain," which obviously is not going to respond to a block at any level. This is an even more uncommon response in patients with psychogenic pain than a positive response to placebo.
Encephalization	The patient's pain may have undergone "encephalization," that poorly understood phenomenon whereby persistent, severe, agonizing pain, originally of peripheral origin, becomes self-sustaining at a central level. This usually does not occur until severe pain has been endured for a long time, but once it has occurred, removal or blockade of the original peripheral mechanism fails to provide relief.
Malingering	The patient may be malingering. One cannot prove or disprove this with differential blocks, but if a patient is involved in litigation concerning the cause of his pain and anticipates financial benefit, it is unlikely that any therapeutic modality will relieve the pain. However, empirically, it is our belief that a previous placebo reaction from solution A followed by no relief from solution D strongly suggests that the patient whose pain ultimately appears to have a "central mechanism" is not malingering, since the placebo reaction, depending as it does on a positive motivation to obtain relief, is unlikely in a malingerer. Clearly, there is no way to document the validity of this theory, but it certainly suggests greater motivation to obtain pain relief than to obtain financial gain.

backs. First of all, it is quite time-consuming, because of the fact that the physician must wait long enough after each injection for the response to become evident. Second, occasionally a patient is encountered whose C_m for sympathetic blockade is greater than 0.25, so when relief is produced by 0.5% procaine, one *might* erroneously conclude that this is somatic pain rather than sympathetic pain. Similarly, a patient may occasionally be encountered who has a lower C_m for sensory blockade than 0.5%, and when 0.25% procaine produces relief, one *might* erroneously conclude that the mechanism is sympathetic rather than somatic. Third, each successive injection with this technique deposits more procaine in the subarachnoid space, so that after the final injection, when all modalities are blocked, it takes quite a while for full function to return. Full recovery is absolutely essential, at least in our pain center, because the vast majority of the patients are outpatients and must be fully able to ambulate before they are discharged. Finally, this technique demands that the needle remain in place throughout the entire procedure, so the patient must remain in the lateral position throughout the test. Occasionally this is a serious problem, especially when the patient's pain is associated with a particular position that he cannot assume with the needle in situ.

The "Modified Differential Spinal"

In an effort to overcome the disadvantages just described, the conventional technique has been modified in a way that both simplifies it and increases its utility.[13-16] For the modified technique, only two solutions need to be prepared, as summarized in Table 13–5, namely, normal saline (solution A) and 5% procaine (solution D).

Procedure

As in the conventional technique, after informed consent has been obtained, an infusion started, and the monitors applied, the back is prepared and draped, and a small-bore spinal needle is utilized to enter the subarachnoid space. At this point 2 mL of normal saline is injected, and observations are made as in the conventional technique (see Table 13–3). If the patient obtains no relief or only partial relief from the placebo injection, 2 mL of 5% procaine is injected, the needle is removed, and the patient is returned to the supine position. Because the injected 5% procaine is hyperbaric, the position of the table may have to be adjusted to obtain the desired level of anesthesia. Once this is accomplished, the same observations are made as after the previous injection (see Table 13–3).

Interpretation

If the patient's pain is relieved after the injection of normal saline, the interpretation is the same as if it were relieved by placebo in the conventional differential spinal—that is, the pain is considered to be of psychogenic origin. Again, when the pain relief is prolonged or permanent, the pain is probably truly psychogenic, whereas if relief is transient and self-limited, the response probably represents a placebo reaction.

When the patient does not obtain pain relief after injection of 5% procaine, the diagnosis is considered to be the same as that when the patient obtains no relief after injection of all of the solutions with the conventional technique—that is, the mechanism is considered to be "central." As in the conventional technique, this diagnosis is

TABLE 13–5 *Preparation of Solutions for Modified Differential Spinal Blockade*

Solution	Preparation and Solution	Yield
D	To 1 mL of 10% procaine add 1 mL of procaine	2 mL of 5% procaine (hyperbaric)
A	Draw up 2 mL of normal saline	2 mL of normal saline

not specific; rather, it indicates one of four possibilities (see Table 13–4).

On the other hand, when the patient does obtain complete pain relief after the injection of 5% procaine, the cause of the pain is considered to be organic. The mechanism is considered to be somatic (to be subserved by A-delta and/or C fibers) if the pain returns when the patient again perceives pinprick as sharp (recovery from analgesia); whereas it is considered sympathetic if the pain relief persists long after recovery from analgesia.

Fundamental Differences Between the Conventional Technique and the Modified Technique of Differential Spinal

The conventional sequential differential spinal sought to block specific types of nerve fibers with specific concentrations of local anesthetics. At the time when we modified the conventional technique, evidence was accumulating that the exact concentrations of local anesthetics required to block different fiber types are unpredictable, to say the least. Thus, we abandoned the practice of injecting predetermined concentrations of local anesthetics in an attempt to selectively block one fiber type at a time and utilized a technique not unlike that used to produce surgical spinal anesthesia, a technique that was much better understood. With that technique, after a placebo injection, a concentration of local anesthetic sufficient to produce surgical anesthesia is injected into the subarachnoid space to block all types of fibers, and the patient is observed as the concentration of local anesthetic in the cerebrospinal fluid decreases and the fibers recover sequentially, motor fibers first, followed by sensory fibers, and then sympathetic fibers. Thus, whereas the conventional sequential technique attempted to correlate the *onset* of pain relief with the *onset* of blockade of the various fiber types, the modified technique attempts to correlate the *return* of pain with the *recovery* of the various blocked fibers.

It readily becomes apparent that this modified technique of differential spinal block simplifies the differentiation of sympathetic from somatic mechanisms considerably. With the conventional technique, occasionally the concentration required to produce sympathetic blockade is somewhat greater or somewhat less than the usual mean of 0.25%, and the concentration of procaine required to produce a sensory block is greater or less than the usual mean of 0.5%. Significant diagnostic confusion can result. With the modified technique, when a patient recovers sensation, the only fibers that remain blocked are the sympathetic fibers; thus, pain relief that persists beyond the recovery of sensation clearly indicates a sympathetic mechanism.

Advantages Over the Conventional Technique

The major advantage of the modified differential spinal block over the conventional technique is that it takes less time. The modified technique has consistently provided diagnostic information identical to that provided by the conventional technique, but in approximately one third of the time. The conventional differential technique requires a series of injections of progressively increasing concentrations of local anesthetic into the subarachnoid space, so that when the study is complete, the patient has a high level of anesthesia that takes a long time to dissipate. The modified technique requires only a single injection of active drug, so in addition to the test's taking less time, the time for recovery is likewise reduced, a fact of great importance in a busy pain center. The modified technique also minimizes the extent and duration of discomfort for the patient, who does not have to lie so long in the lateral position with the needle in place. In addition, the modified technique allows a better evaluation of the subjective nature of a patient's pain. Because there is no need to keep the needle in the back throughout the procedure, the patient can lie supine, and positional changes or passive movement of the legs that may be necessary to reproduce the pain are much easier. The advantage of the modified approach over the traditional one in differentiating sympathetic from somatic pain has already been described.

Differential Epidural Block

More than 20 years ago, Raj[17] suggested using sequential differential epidural block instead of the conventional sequential differential spinal to avoid spinal headaches after the procedure. With his proposed technique, solution A was still to be the placebo, but solution B was 0.5% lidocaine, which was presumed to be the mean sympatholytic concentration of lidocaine in the epidural space; solution C was 1% lidocaine, the presumed mean sensory blocking concentration in the epidural space; and solution D was 2% lidocaine, a concentration sufficient to block all modalities. In short, the technique Raj proposed for differential epidural block was virtually identical to that used for the conventional differential spinal block, except that the local anesthetic doses were injected sequentially into the epidural space and the concentrations were modified as described earlier.

There were two problems with the technique proposed by Raj. First, because of the slower onset of blockade after each injection of local anesthetic into the epidural space, more time would be required between injections before the usual observations could be made. So a differential epidural block, as proposed by Raj, would take even longer than the conventional differential spinal technique, for complete recovery. An even more serious drawback of this approach, however, relates to the fact that, if local anesthetics occasionally fail to give discrete end points when injected into the subarachnoid space, the endpoints are even less discrete with injections into the epidural space. For example, 0.5% lidocaine provides sympathetic blockade when injected epidurally, but it commonly causes sensory block too. Similarly, whereas 1% lidocaine injected epidurally almost always produces sensory block, it frequently also produces paresis, if not paralysis. As a matter of fact, it was the failure of this technique to provide definitive end points that led Raj to decide not to publish it.

Nonetheless, *conceptually*, a differential epidural approach is inherently appealing, because it avoids lumbar puncture and the possibility of post–lumbar puncture headache in a predominantly outpatient population. The major problem with the technique Raj proposed, the lack of discrete end points, was due to the attempt to inject a different concentration of local anesthetic to block each type of nerve fiber, something we had attempted with our conventional differential spinal. Since our modified differential spinal eliminated the occasional confusing end points of the conventional technique, we decided to modify Raj's proposed differential epidural as we had modified our differential spinal. This technique as we perform it is as follows[14–16]:

Informed consent is obtained, an infusion is started, and the various monitors are applied. The patient is placed in the lateral (or sitting) position, and the back is prepared and draped in the usual manner. After a 20-gauge Husted needle has been placed in the epidural space by the modified loss-of-resistance technique, equal volumes of normal saline and 2% chloroprocaine (or lidocaine) are injected sequentially 15 to 20 minutes apart, and the needle is removed. The volume of each is that required to produce the desired level of anesthesia. After each injection, exactly the same observations are made as for a differential spinal (see Table 13–3).

The interpretation is virtually identical to that of a modified differential spinal. If the patient experiences pain relief after the injection of saline, the presumptive diagnosis is "psychogenic pain," a designation that indicates the possibility of either a placebo reaction or true psychogenic pain. If the patient does not experience pain relief after the injection of 2% chloroprocaine (or lidocaine) into the epidural space *in spite of complete anesthesia of the painful area*, the diagnosis is considered to be "central pain," that diagnosis again including the four possibilities described earlier (see Table 13–4). When the patient does experience pain relief after the injection of 2% chloroprocaine (or lidocaine), however, the pain is considered organic. It is presumed to be somatic (subserved by A-delta and C fibers) when the pain returns with the return of sensation, and sympathetic when the pain persists long after sensation has been recovered. This approach to differential epidural blockade has been used extensively at our institution and has provided the same valuable information obtained from the modified differential spinal technique without the usual risk of spinal headache. In addition, differential epidural is a useful alternative to differential spinal when a patient refuses spinal anesthesia or when spinal anesthesia is contraindicated, although both of these situations are rare. A catheter can be placed through a larger epidural needle if it is anticipated that supplemental injections may be necessary to achieve the proper level, but in our experience this has rarely been necessary.

Differential Brachial Plexus Block

Performed in a manner analogous to that of differential epidural block, a differential brachial plexus block can be extremely useful in evaluating upper extremity pain.[18] Two successive injections are made into the perivascular compartment using an approach appropriate to the site of the patient's pain, one injection consisting of normal saline and the other 2% chloroprocaine. Again, the same observations are made after each injection (see Table 13–3). If the patient is somewhat naive with respect to the injections carried out at a pain center, it may be sufficient for the placebo injection to consist of local infiltration over the anticipated site of injection of the active agent, as long as all of the appropriate observations are made after the injection. If this does not provide relief, the brachial plexus block is carried out with local anesthetic, inserting the needle through the anesthetized skin. If the patient obtains pain relief from the placebo injection, as with a differential spinal or epidural, the pain is considered psychogenic, whereas if the pain disappears after injection of chloroprocaine into the brachial plexus sheath, it is labeled organic. If the pain returns as soon as the sensory block is dissipated, the mechanism is somatic (i.e., it is subserved by A-delta and C fibers); if the relief persists long after recovery from the sensory block, the mechanism is presumed to be sympathetic. Finally, of course, if the pain does not disappear, even when the arm is fully anesthetized, the diagnosis is central pain, and the same four possibilities are again associated with that response (see Table 13–4).

It is significant to note that Durrani[19] has reported on 25 patients referred to our pain control center with a clinical diagnosis of "classic" reflex sympathetic dystrophy of the upper extremity, all of whom obtained no relief from a series of three stellate ganglion blocks, even though each patient developed Horner's syndrome after each block. The significance of this report is that, when these patients were subjected to differential brachial plexus block by one of the perivascular techniques, 16 of the 25 patients (who had not obtained relief from three stellate ganglion blocks) exhibited a typical sympathetic response to the brachial plexus block. Furthermore, and perhaps more importantly, 12 of the 19 patients so treated obtained complete and permanent relief from a series of therapeutic brachial plexus blocks, even though they had failed to do so after a series of stellate ganglion blocks. Thus, it would appear that perivascular brachial plexus blocks provide more complete sympathetic denervation of the upper extremity than do stellate ganglion blocks. The success of brachial plexus block and the failure of stellate ganglion blocks in this report might be explained by the fact that the local anesthetic injected at the stellate ganglion failed to reach the nerve of Kuntz, the nerve by which ascending sympathetic fibers may bypass the stellate ganglion.[20, 21] Since all of the stellate ganglion blocks at our institution are carried out using a minimum of 8 mL of local anesthetic, however, this is unlikely. A more likely explanation is that stellate ganglion block interrupts only those sympathetic fibers that travel with the peripheral nerves, whereas perivascular brachial plexus block interrupts the sympathetic fibers traveling by both neural and perivascular pathways.[22]

Summary

Controversial aspects aside, the pharmacologic approach to differential neural blockade remains a simple but useful technique, whether carried out at a subarachnoid, epidural, or plexus level, because it provides reproducible, objective, and definitive diagnostic information on the neural mechanisms subserving a patient's pain. Obviously, the results of this test must be interpreted in the light of other diagnostic tests (including psychological tests) and the results must be integrated with the information obtained from the patient's history and the findings on physical examination. Not infrequently the results of a differential spinal, a differential epidural, or a differential plexus block provide the missing piece in the complex puzzle of pain.

THE ANATOMIC APPROACH

To obviate the problems inherent in high spinal (or epidural) anesthesia, particularly in an outpatient or a patient whose pain is in the upper part of the body, it is occasionally safer and more appropriate to use an anatomic approach to differential neural blockade. In this approach, after the injection of a placebo, the sympathetic and then the sensory and/or motor fibers are blocked sequentially by injecting local anesthetic at points where one modality can be blocked without blocking the other. The procedural sequences by which differential nerve blocks are carried out in this approach for pain in the various parts of the body are presented in Table 13–6.

Procedure

For pain in the head, neck, and upper extremity, if a placebo injection fails to provide relief, a stellate ganglion block is carried out with any short-acting, dilute local anesthetic. If the sympathetic block cannot be carried out without spillover onto somatic nerves innervating the painful area, the sequential blocks should be carried out on two separate occasions, allowing the sympathetic block to wear off before proceeding with the somatic block. In any case, if the patient does not obtain relief from the stellate ganglion block, then a block of the somatic nerves to the painful area should be carried out.

For pain in the thorax, after a placebo injection, the safest procedure (and the one that causes the least discomfort to the patient) is a differential segmental epidural block, as described previously. It must be remembered, however, that, with thoracic pain, relief after an extensive sympathetic block, in addition to suggesting a possible sympathetic mechanism, may indicate visceral rather than somatic pain, because visceral pain is mediated by sympathetic fibers. If it is unwise to carry out a differential thoracic epidural block in a particular patient because of cachexia, hypovolemia, or dehydration, an alternative is the anatomic approach, using paravertebral or intercostal blocks of the appropriate dermatomes. Failure of these somatic blocks to provide relief implies (but does not prove) a visceral origin for the pain; however, if the blocks provide complete relief and if the pain returns immediately after recovery, a peripheral somatic mechanism is indicated. If the relief provided by the blocks persists long after recovery of sensation, this may indicate a sympathetic mechanism.

When a placebo injection fails to provide relief for abdominal pain, before a celiac block is considered, paravertebral or intercostal blocks of the appropriate dermatomes should be done to make certain that the pain is not somatic (body wall). Patients have a great deal of difficulty localizing "abdominal pain," and therefore, they usually cannot differentiate pain due to body wall extension of a lesion from that due to true visceral involvement. If the paravertebral or intercostal blocks produce complete anesthesia of the body wall overlying the patient's pain but fail to provide relief, celiac plexus block should be carried out to confirm that the pain is truly visceral in origin.

If a placebo injection fails to provide relief for pelvic pain, before a superior hypogastric plexus block is attempted, paravertebral or appropriate sacral blocks should be carried out to make certain that the pain is not somatic. If these blocks produce appropriate anesthesia but fail to provide relief, a superior hypogastric block is carried out to establish that the pain is visceral.

For pain in the lower extremities, the pharmacologic approach (differential spinal or epidural) is preferable, as it is both more precise and less painful than are peripheral nerve blocks. Differential peripheral blocks, however, can be utilized if the pharmacologic approach is contraindicated or undesirable or if subsequent neurolytic blocks are

TABLE 13–6 ***Anatomic Approach: Procedural Sequence for Differential Diagnostic Nerve Blocks***

Site of Pain	Technique		
Head	Placebo Block	Stellate ganglion block	Block of C_2 Block of trigeminal I, II, III (or specific nerve block)
Neck	Placebo Block	Stellate ganglion block	Cervical plexus block (or of specific nerve)
Arm	Placebo Block	Stellate ganglion block	Brachial plexus block (or specific nerve block)
Thorax*	Placebo Block	Thoracic paravertebral sympathetic block	Lumbar paravertebral somatic block
Abdomen†	Placebo Block	Celiac plexus block	Paravertebral somatic or intercostal block
Pelvis†	Placebo Block	Superior hypogastric plexus block	Paravertebral somatic or intercostal block
Leg	Placebo Block	Lumbar paravertebral sympathetic block	Lumbosacral plexus block (or specific nerve block)

* In our opinion, thoracic paravertebral sympathetic blocks carry such a high risk of pneumothorax that a pharmacologic approach should be utilized.

† Because of the simplicity of intercostal blocks, as compared with celiac plexus and superior hypogastric plexus blocks, the procedural sequence is altered for abdominal pain (i.e., somatic before sympathetic).

anticipated. After a placebo block, lumbar paravertebral sympathetic blocks are performed at the levels L2–L4, and if these fail to provide relief, lumbosacral plexus block (or any appropriate specific peripheral nerve block) is carried out.

Interpretation

Interpretation of the results achieved with differential nerve blocks for head, neck, arm, and leg pain is self-evident. Relief after a placebo injection indicates a psychogenic mechanism, but, as with the pharmacologic approaches, it could indicate either a placebo reaction or true psychogenic pain. Relief after sympathetic blocks indicates a sympathetic mechanism, usually reflex sympathetic dystrophy (complex regional pain syndrome I [CRPS I]), and relief after blockade of somatic nerves indicates an organic, somatic mechanism. Failure to obtain relief in spite of the establishment of complete anesthesia in the appropriate area would tend to indicate a central mechanism, which could be any of the four possibilities in Table 13–4. Interpretation of the results of differential blocks for thoracic and abdominal pain has already been discussed.

DISCUSSION

In spite of the clinical success of the various techniques of differential neural blockade, in many centers over the last 25 years, the validity of the results has become very controversial. There are two reasons for this: (1) The changes in our understanding of the factors that determine the process of nerve conduction and blockade are believed by some to invalidate the concept of differential neural blockade. (2) The even greater changes in our understanding of the complexities of chronic pain and the physiologic, anatomic, and psychosocial factors involved are believed to limit the diagnostic utility of neural blockade. To establish both the validity and utility of differential neural blockade in the diagnosis of pain mechanisms, it is essential to understand the bases of this controversy by answering two questions:

1. Do the Factors Recently Found to Determine Nerve Conduction and Blockade Invalidate the Concept of Differential Neural Blockade?

The pharmacologic approach to differential neural blockade is based on the assumption that local anesthetic agents can selectively produce conduction block of one type of fiber in a nerve while sparing the other types in that nerve.[23] Although the concept of differential block was introduced more than 70 years ago by Gasser and Erlanger,[24] in vitro and in vivo studies carried out over the past 25 years have indicated that the basis of Gasser and Erlanger's explanation of this commonly observed clinical phenomenon was totally erroneous, as was their explanation of the process of nerve conduction itself. From the classic studies Gasser and Erlanger carried out on the peripheral nerves of dogs they concluded that, in general, small-diameter fibers were more readily blocked by cocaine than were larger-diameter fibers. At that time, however, it was believed that the site of action of conduction was the axonal protoplasm. Thus, the higher ratio of surface to volume in small-diameter fibers was supposed to make them more "sensitive" (easier to enter and render unexcitable) than large ones. Since that theory was articulated in one form or another this "size principle" has influenced the concept of differential block, has led to clinical use of differential spinal block,[1] and has provided an explanation for the persistent differential losses of function observed during subarachnoid[25] and epidural[26] anesthesia.

It was almost 50 years before the concept of Gasser and Erlanger was challenged. Studies by Franz and Perry in vivo[27] and by Fink and Cairns in vitro[28] indicated that all mammalian axons require about the same blocking concentration of local anesthetic, regardless of their diameter, and the issue was rendered even more confusing when Gissen and coworkers[29] demonstrated that the larger the diameter of an axon, the more susceptible it was to conduction block by local anesthetics, a finding diametrically opposed to Gasser and Erlanger's traditional concept. However, as de Jong pointed out,[30] a major flaw in Gissen's study was that the experiments were carried out at room temperature. Because conduction in large fibers is more affected by cold than is conduction in small fibers, relatively little anesthetic may be needed to block large fibers in conditions cooler than body temperature. Subsequently, Palmer and coworkers,[31] using a preparation maintained at body temperature, showed that C fibers were, in fact, more susceptible to conduction block by bupivacaine than were A fibers, but they were unable to demonstrate such differential effects with lidocaine. This study introduced a new complexity: different anesthetics may affect various axon types differently. In two sequential in vitro studies, Wildsmith and colleagues[32,33] compared the differential nerve-blocking activity of a series of amide-linked local anesthetics with that of a series of ester-linked agents. These studies confirmed Gissen's finding that, in general, A fibers are the most sensitive and C fibers the least sensitive to blockade by local anesthetics but that the absolute and relative rates of development of A fiber blockade were directly related to lipid solubility and inversely related to pK_a. On the basis of the findings of these two in vitro studies, Wildsmith postulated that, in vivo, C fibers could be blocked differentially by an agent of low lipid solubility and high pK_a, because a compound with these properties (such as procaine) might produce blockade of C fibers relatively quickly, but before it could penetrate the great diffusion barriers around A fibers, it would be removed by the circulation. Ford and Raj[34] tested this hypothesis, studying several local anesthetics in a cat model in vivo and found that, regardless of the local anesthetic, A-alpha fibers were consistently less sensitive to blockade than either A-delta or C fibers, thus reaffirming the original scheme of Gasser and Erlanger.

It remained for Fink[6] to elucidate the importance of two other factors subserving differential neural blockade. First, he pointed out the importance of the nodes of Ranvier, the internodal distance, and the number of nodes bathed by a local anesthetic to differential neural blockade. It has long been known that to block conduction an adequate concentration of local anesthetic (C_m) applied to a myelinated axon must bathe at least three consecutive nodes.[35] Since the internodal distance increases as the thickness of the axon increases, the probability of three successive nodes of Ranvier being bathed quickly by an injected local anesthetic solution decreases as the internodal distance increases, that is, as the size of the fiber increases (Fig. 13–2). In other words, the chance of a local anesthetic solution blocking a given nerve fiber decreases with increasing fiber size. For example, the internodal distance of small A-delta fibers ranges from 0.3 to 0.7 mm, so a puddle of local anesthetic solution only 2 mm long will fully cover three successive nodes. In contrast, large A-alpha fibers have an internodal distance of 0.8 to 1.4 mm, so their *critical blocking length* is at least 5 mm.[27] Thus, because the internodal distance increases with thickness of the axon, the minimal blocking length ranges from 2 to 5 mm.

Next, Fink demonstrated that the differential blockade of the sympathetics observed clinically with spinal anesthesia is probably due, at least in part, to decremental block with a superimposed frequency-dependent effect.[36] Decremental block occurs when a nerve is bathed by a weak concentration of local anesthetic ($<C_m$): Both thick and thin axons have more than three nodes covered by local anesthetic (Fig. 13–3), but, because of the difference in the internodal distance, fewer nodes are bathed by local anesthetic in the thick fiber than in the thin one. Thus, when an impulse arrives at the incompletely blocked thick fiber, though there is a progressive reduction in conduction velocity and elevation of firing threshold as it traverses the incompletely blocked segment, it resumes full speed when it reaches a segment of normally conducting membrane. In other words, too few nodes were partially blocked to completely halt conduction. However, in the thin axon, a sufficient number of nodes are partially blocked so that the

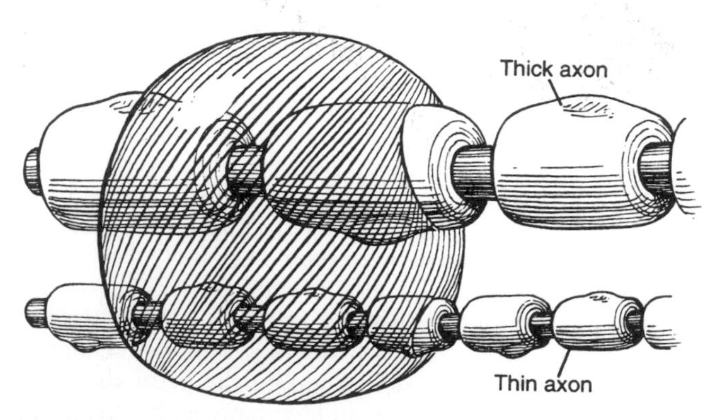

FIGURE 13–2 Differential nerve block based on different internodal intervals. Two axons, one thin and one thick, are depicted lying side by side in a puddle of local anesthetic at or above the minimum blocking concentration *(C_m). The internodal interval of the thick fiber is twice that of the thin one, so whereas the local anesthetic solution covers three successive nodes of the thin axon, it covers only one node of the thick one. Nerve impulses can skip easily over one node, and even over two, rendered inexcitable by the local anesthetic,[35] so conduction along the thick axon will continue uninterrupted. In the thin axon, however, because three nodes are covered by the local anesthetic solution, impulse conduction is halted. Thus, conduction appears to proceed normally in the thick (motor) fiber but is blocked in the thin (sensory) fiber. Such a differential block of thin versus thick nerve fibers occurs in spinal roots during spinal anesthesia (see text). (Modified from de Jong RH: Local Anesthetics. St. Louis, Mosby–Year Book, 1994, p 89.)*

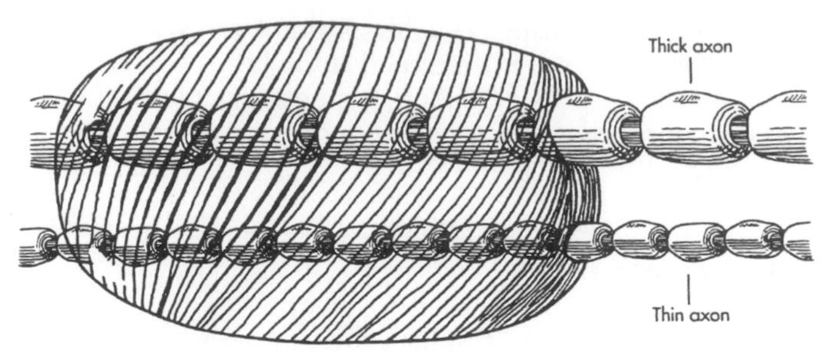

FIGURE 13–3 Differential decremental nerve block and frequency-dependent block. When both thick and thin axons have more than three nodes covered by a local anesthetic solution, if the solution is at or above C_m, all of the sodium channels are occupied and conduction is blocked in both fibers. However, if the concentration of local anesthetic is below *C_m, a significant portion (but not all) of the sodium channels are blocked, so that at each node the action potential undergoes a progressive reduction in amplitude, with resultant decremental slowing of impulse conduction. Such decremental conduction will ultimately extinguish the impulse in the nine exposed nodes of the thin fiber* (decremental block)*; but, though slowed in its passage along the five incompletely blocked nodes of the thick fiber, it will resume at full speed when normally conducting membrane is reached again. The lower the concentration of the local anesthetic, the longer must be the exposure length (the number of nodes of Ranvier exposed) to yield complete impulse blockade. Conversely, the more concentrated the local anesthetic solution, the shorter is the exposure length required for complete blockade, up to the point of C_m, when the "three-node principle" again applies. In other words, below C_m the blocking concentration of local anesthetic is inversely proportional to the length of the nerve it bathes. In addition, the greater the frequency of nerve stimulation, the shorter is the exposure length (the number of incompletely blocked nodes) required to yield complete impulse blockade. Such a* frequency-dependent block *superimposed on decremental block is operant clinically in the zone cephalic to the level of somatic block in a spinal anesthesia (see text). (Modified from de Jong RH: Local Anesthetics. St. Louis, Mosby–Year Book, 1994, p 91.)*

progressive reduction in the action current at each node ultimately causes the impulse to be blocked. Because the action current decreases in decrements, the phenomenon is referred to as *decremental conduction block*, and since the block is complete in the small axon and incomplete in the large one, this represents a differential (decremental) block.

In this example, decremental block of single impulses has been described, and single impulses allow enough time for membrane recovery. In reality, impulses occur in rapid sequential bursts that allow little time for recovery, and it has been demonstrated repeatedly that, as the rate of stimulation increases, so does the intensity of the block. Presumably, this phenomenon, called *frequency-dependent block*, is due to the fact that, at rapid rates of stimulation, the time between impulses is insufficient for the local anesthetic to unbind, so a fraction of the sodium channels are still blocked when the next impulse arrives. Obviously, frequency-dependent block superimposed on decremental block enhances conduction block by local anesthetics in concentrations considerably below C_m. Since the conditions necessary for frequency-dependent block include a weak concentration of local anesthetic ($<C_m$) and a train of repetitive stimuli,[37] clearly, both conditions are present in the zone cephalad to the level of somatic block in spinal anesthesia: The cerebrospinal fluid concentration of local anesthetic is too low to block somatic axons, but the preganglionic sympathetic fibers carry a normal tonic flow of rapid vasoconstrictor impulses. As a result, frequency-dependent

block of the sympathetic fibers is superimposed on decremental block. Another observation of clinical importance is that highly lipid-soluble local anesthetics require more repetitive stimuli to reach maximal frequency-dependent blocking than less lipid-soluble agents,[38] so differential blockade of the sympathetic fibers without blockade of somatic fibers is easier to accomplish with agents of low lipid solubility such as procaine.

Applying these two concepts, Fink pointed out that the anatomy of the spinal roots in the spinal canal of an adult varies considerably at different levels, because the spinal cord is substantially shorter than the dural sac that surrounds it. Thus, proceeding cephalocaudad, the length of the spinal roots from the point where they leave the cord to the point where they exit the dura increases from 0.5 cm for the C1 root to 15 cm for the S4 root. With spinal anesthesia, the densest concentration of local anesthetic is nearest the lumbar puncture site. Here the length of the lumbosacral nerve roots allows many nodes of Ranvier of all sizes of fibers to be exposed to the local anesthetic, so a solid block of the lumbosacral roots is rapidly achieved. Progressively farther craniad, the local anesthetic solution is increasingly diluted by spinal fluid until the cephalad salient is "watered down" to C_m. At that point, fibers with a short internodal distance may still fall within the blocking zone, whereas the distal nodes of thicker fibers with a longer internodal distance may well fall outside the blocking potency range. In other words, small autonomic and nociceptive fibers are still blocked, but the thick touch and motor fibers no longer are.[39] As fibers cephalad to the C_m zone are exposed to sub-threshold local anesthetic concentrations, decremental block and/or frequency-dependent block begins to play a role. The short-to-long internode-blocking gradient still holds, but now a longer string of nodes must be bathed before an impulse is halted (see Fig. 13–3). Because of the shorter internodal intervals of thin fibers, the segment of a thin nerve that needs to be bathed to block conduction is shorter than the segment required to block thick nerves. Thus, differential spinal block is observed at threshold-blocking concentrations.[7] The other contribution of Fink, based on the same "bathed length" concept, is seen during epidural anesthesia. The length of the nerve segments from dural sac to intervertebral foramen is both shorter and less variable than that of the intrathecal roots. In fact, the few millimeters of root exposed in the cervical and thoracic epidural space barely span the three-node length of thin nerves, let alone that of thicker nerves. Differential block with epidural analgesia thus can be quite pronounced, a property used to great advantage in providing "pure" postoperative analgesia with epidural infusions of a weak local anesthetic solution.

In an editorial accompanying Fink's article, Raymond and Strichartz[40] summarized the impact of Fink's "innovative" observations on the concept of differential block as follows:

> They link clinical observations to anatomical findings in both humans and animals and to measurements made in vitro on isolated nerves, thereby generating interesting predictions and possibilities. They lead the discussion of differential block away from a broad susceptibility to LA [local anesthetics] according to fiber size to focus on the number of nodes per unit length, which is correlated with fiber size. Clinically, this permits retention of familiar interpretations (based on the size principle) of phenomena consistently seen during epidural and spinal anesthesia; and it does not deny the single fiber data showing similar LA susceptibility across the fiber spectrum (for long exposed segments). The ideas are, in this sense, an extension of the size principle, not a renunciation of it.

From all of the above, it is clear that differential neural blockade is a reality. While the size principle (the thicker the fiber, the harder it is to block) has been replaced by the length principle (the fewer nodes bathed, the harder it is to block), as indicated by de Jong,[41]

> The clinical outcome remains functionally the same. For, the thicker the nerve fiber, the broader the internode and the fewer nodes per exposure length. Thus, blocking a thick nerve fiber requires a supra-C_m local anesthetic solution, as there are too few nodes accessible for decremental block to come into play. In other words, for a given local anesthetic concentration, there will be an interim transition phase where nociception (pain) conducted by thin fibers is blocked, but touch and motor function conducted by thick fibers remain virtually intact.

Thus, though inconsistencies and contraindications about the mechanisms of differential neural blockade persist, it is conceptually valid, and in our hands, it has proved an invaluable clinical tool for identifying the mechanism subserving a patient's pain.

2. Do the Complexities of Chronic Pain and the Physiologic, Anatomic, and Psychosocial Factors Involved Limit the Diagnostic Utility of Differential Neural Blockade?

No one could deny that over the last 25 years basic research in the field of pain has produced important insights into the pathophysiology of chronic pain, the anatomic pathways involved in the processing and conduction of pain, and the important psychosocial issues that affect a patient's perception of pain. It is not readily apparent, however, why increases in our understanding of the complexities of pain should invalidate the diagnostic information provided by differential neural blockade. As a matter of fact, better understanding of the mechanisms involved in the pain process should actually enhance our ability to interpret the information gained from diagnostic nerve blocks. Yet, in a recent review of neural blockade for diagnosis and prognosis,[42] the authors state categorically that "complex physiologic events may confound the simple interpretation of diagnostic blocks"; that "compelling evidence with regard to placebo responses leads to the conclusion that the ambiguity created by these reponses is a major impediment to the valid use of neural blockade for diagnosis"; and that "anatomic uncertainties with regard to neuroconnections and structural variability degrade the accuracy of diagnostic information obtained by neural blockade." Furthermore, the author of an editorial supporting these views states that "several factors, such as the improper use of pain measurement scales, observer errors, problems of placebo effects, and bias introduced by patient expectations, confound the interpretation of studies on the usefuless of neural blockade in the diagnosis of chronic pain," and that "because the treatment [of pain] and prognosis often depend on accurate diagnosis, the incorrect interpretation of the results of a nerve block may result in inappropriate therapy."[43] These platitudes and attitudes denigrate, not differential neural blockade, but the intelligence, knowledge, and clinical judgment of anesthesiologists who are in the practice of pain management. There are few (if any) diagnostic techniques in all of medicine that are infallibly positive or negative or, taken by themselves, invariably indicative of a specific etiology. All such tests give false-positive and false-negative results, and knowing this, the experienced clinician integrates the result of any one test with the results of others, with the information gained from a careful history, and with the findings of the physical examination. Of course, caution must be used in interpreting any tests, but, interpreted intelligently, the results of differential neural blockade not infrequently provide the missing piece of the puzzle of pain, and the reward for the patient (and the concerned physician) is pain relief.

To abandon differential nerve blocks for the diagnosis of pain until the precise mechanisms subserving pain and its relief are understood would be as foolish as to abandon general anesthesia until the precise mechanism by which general anesthetics work is understood. Even those who decry diagnostic blocks admit that "experienced and observant clinicians have found that these procedures may, on certain occasions, provide information that is helpful in guiding subsequent therapy, so we should not be in haste to dismiss the accumulated judgement of [the] practitioner," and that "the confusion and complexity that typify the diagnosis of chronic pain may justify the selective use of diagnostic blocks that make anatomic and physiologic sense, even if their validity is incompletely proved."[42] It goes without saying that the clinician who employs diagnostic nerve blocks must exercise great care in carrying out the technique, in confirming observed effects in interpreting the results, and in applying them to clinical decisions.

ROLE OF DIFFERENTIAL NEURAL BLOCKADE

Many patients seeking pain relief at a pain control center present no diagnostic problem whatsoever; however, anyone experienced in the diagnosis and management of chronic pain problems has seen many apparently clear-cut diagnoses completely and unexpectedly refuted when one of the techniques of differential neural blockade was utilized to "confirm" the diagnosis. The concern in such cases is that *if this diagnostic approach had not been utilized* because the clinician felt that with his or her "experience and expertise in pain management" such supportive evidence was unnecessary, *the true diagnosis would have been missed*, and the patient's therapy, based on the clinical diagnosis, would have been unsuccessful. Human limitations being what they are and pain being the complex process that it is, no one ever develops enough experience or expertise to make the correct diagnosis 100% of the time. Differential neural blockade provides an objective means of *confirming* a diagnosis when the cause of pain appears obvious, and, perhaps more importantly, a means of *establishing* a diagnosis when there appears to be no demonstrable cause.

TABLE 13–7 **Results of Differential Neural Blockade in 100 Patients Referred Because of "No Demonstrable Cause for Pain"[9]**

Diagnosis	Incidence (%)
"Psychogenic mechanism"	5
Sympathetic mechanism	74
Somatic mechanism	18
"Central mechanism"	3

Thirty years ago we retrospectively reviewed a series of 100 patients referred to our pain control center "because all diagnostic attempts had failed to discover a cause for the patient's pain."[9] Reviewing these difficult cases, we were impressed by the fact that differential neural blockade was effective in identifying the mechanism as sympathetic, somatic, or central in all of these patients (Table 13–7). Even more impressive and surprising was the fact that in 74% of the patients differential neural blockade indicated the mechanism to be sympathetic. A somatic mechanism was implicated in only 18% and a central (including psychogenic) mechanism in only 8%. These findings were important because in the vast majority of these patients, patients in whom a sympathetic mechanism was *unexpectedly* identified, the diagnosis was established early enough that complete and permanent relief could be provided by a series of sympathetic blocks. These data provide convincing evidence that, at least in patients suffering from pain syndromes of questionable cause, sympathetically maintained pain (sympathetically maintained pain, reflex sympathetic dystrophy, complex regional pain syndrome) is not uncommon. All of these patients were referred by specialists who could find no cause for the pain, and indeed, in most of the cases the signs and symptoms were either so bizarre or so seemingly unrelated to any precipitating factor that, had differential blocks not been carried out, we (like the referring physicians) would probably have considered the pain to be psychogenic. The importance of establishing a diagnosis in this group of patients was emphasized 50 years ago by de Takats[44] and 10 years later by Bonica,[45] both of whom pointed out that if such patients are not properly diagnosed and treated in time, they often become addicted to narcotics or become psychotic or even suicidal.

In short, in view of the difficulty of establishing a precise diagnosis in many patients suffering intractable chronic pain and in view of the efficacy of differential neural blockade, in doing so, it has been and continues to be our practice to use differential neural blockade to confirm the diagnosis in many cases, even when the mechanism appears to be obvious on clinical grounds, and even more frequently to establish a diagnosis when the mechanism is in question or is not known.

REFERENCES

1. Arrowood JG, Sarnoff SJ: Differential block. V. Use in the investigation of pain following amputations. Anesthesiology 9:614–622, 1948.

2. Gasser HS, Erlanger J: The compound nature of the action current of nerve as disclosed by the cathode ray oscilloscope. Am J Physiol 70:624, 1924.
3. Gasser HS, Erlanger J: The role played by the size of the constituent fibers of a nerve trunk in determining the form of its action potential wave. Am J Physiol 80:522–547, 1927.
4. Gasser HS, Grundfest H: Axon diameters in relation to the spike dimensions and the conduction velocity in the mammalian A fibers. Am J Physiol 127:393–414, 1939.
5. Collins WF, Hulsen FE, Randt CT: Relation of peripheral nerve fiber size and sensation in man. Arch Neurol 3:381–385, 1960.
6. Fink BR: Mechanisms of differential axial blockade in epidural and subarachnoid anesthesia. Anesthesiology 70:851–858, 1989.
7. Fink BR: Toward the mathematization of spinal anesthesia. Reg Anesth 17:263–273, 1992.
8. de Jong RH: Differential nerve block. *In* Local Anesthetics. St. Louis, Mosby–Year Book, 1994, p 84.
9. Winnie AP, Collins VJ: The pain clinic. I: Differential neural blockade in pain syndromes of questionable etiology. Med Clin North Am 52:123–129, 1968.
10. Winnie AP, Ramamurthy S, Durrani Z: Diagnostic and therapeutic nerve blocks: Recent advances in techniques. Adv Neurol 4:455–460, 1974.
11. McCollum DE, Stephen CR: Use of graduated spinal anesthesia in the differential diagnosis of pain of the back and lower extremities. South Med J 57:410–416, 1964.
12. Beecher HK: The powerful placebo. JAMA 159:1602–1606, 1955.
13. Akkineni SR, Ramamurthy S: Simplified differential spinal block. Presented at the Annual Meeting of the American Society of Anesthesiologists, New Orleans, October 15–19, 1977.
14. Winnie AP: Differential diagnosis of pain mechanisms. ASA Refresher Courses in Anesthesiology 6:171–186, 1978.
15. Ramamurthy S, Winnie AP: Diagnostic maneuvers in painful syndromes. Int Anesth Clin 21:47–59, 1983.
16. Ramamurthy S, Winnie AP: Regional anesthetic techniques for pain relief. Semin Anesth 4:237–246, 1985.
17. Raj PP: Sympathetic pain mechanisms and management. Presented at the Second Annual Meeting of the American Society of Regional Anesthesia, Hollywood, Fla, March 10–11, 1977.
18. Winnie AP: Differential neural blockade for the diagnosis of pain mechanisms. *In* Waldman SD, Winnie AP (eds): Interventional Pain Management. Philadelphia, WB Saunders, 1996, pp 129–136.
19. Durrani Z, Winnie AP: Role of brachial plexus block after negative response from stellate ganglion block for RSD. Anesthesiology 73:A837, 1990.
20. Kuntz A: Distribution of the sympathetic rami to the brachial plexus: Its relation to sympathectomy affecting the upper extremity. Arch Surg 15:871–877, 1927.
21. Kirgis HD, Kuntz A: Inconstant sympathetic neural pathways: Their relation to sympathetic denervation of the upper extremity. Arch Surg 44:95–102, 1942.
22. Kramer JG, Todd TW: The distribution of nerves to the arteries of the arm: With a discussion of the clinical value of results. Anat Rec 8:243–255, 1914.
23. Raymond SA, Gissen AJ: Mechanisms of differential nerve block. *In* Strichartz G (ed): Local Anesthetics. New York, Springer-Verlag, 1987, pp 95–164.
24. Gasser HS, Erlanger J: Role of fiber size in establishment of nerve block by pressure or cocaine. Am J Physiol 88:581–591, 1929.
25. Greene NM: Area of differential block in spinal anesthesia with hyperbaric tetracaine. Anesthesiology 19:45–50, 1958.
26. Bromage PR: An evaluation of bupivacaine in epidural analgesia in obstetrics. Can Anaesth Soc J 16:46–56, 1969.
27. Franz DN, Perry RS: Mechanisms for differential block among single myelinated and non-myelinated axons by procaine. J Physiol (Lond) 236:193–210, 1974.
28. Fink BR, Cairns AM: Differential slowing and block of conduction in individual afferent myelinated and unmyelinated axons. Anesthesiology 60:111–120, 1984.
29. Gissen AJ, Covino BG, Gregus J: Differential sensitivities of mammalian nerve fibers to local anesthetic agents. Anesthesiology 53:467–474, 1980.
30. de Jong RH: Differential nerve block by local anesthetics (Editorial). Anesthesiology 53:443–444, 1980.
31. Palmer SK, Bosnjak ZJ, Hopp FA, et al: Lidocaine and bupivacaine differential blockade of isolated canine nerves. Anesth Analg 62:754–757, 1983.
32. Wildsmith JAW, Gissen AJ, Gregus J, Covino BG: Differential nerve blocking activity of amino-ester local anaesthetics. Br J Anaesth 57:612–620, 1985.
33. Wildsmith JAW, Gissen AJ, Takman B, Covino BG: Differential nerve blockade: Esters V. Amides and the influence of pK_a. Br J Anaesth 59:379–384, 1987.
34. Ford D, Raj PP, Singh P, et al: Differential peripheral nerve block by local anesthetics in the cat. Anesthesiology 60:28–33, 1984.
35. Tasaki I: Nervous Transmission. Springfield, Charles C Thomas, 1953, p 164.
36. Fink BR, Cairns AM: Differential use-dependent (frequency-dependent) effects in single mammalian axons: Data and clinical considerations. Anesthesiology 67:477–484, 1987.
37. Scurlock JE, Meyaris E, Gregus J: The clinical character of local anesthetics: A function of frequency-dependent conduction block. Acta Anaesthesiol Scand 22:601–608, 1978.
38. Courtney KR, Kendig JJ, Cohen EN: Frequency-dependent conduction block. Anesthesiology 48:111–117, 1978.
39. Brull SJ, Green NM: Time courses of zones of differential sensory blockade during spinal anesthesia with hyperbaric tetracaine or bupivacaine. Anesth Analg 69:343–347, 1989.
40. Raymond SA, Strichartz GR: The long and short of differential block (Editorial). Anesthesiology 70:725–728, 1989.
41. de Jong RH: Differential nerve blocks. *In* Local Anesthetics. St. Louis, Mosby–Year Book, 1994, p 96.
42. Hogan QH, Abram SE: Neural blockade for diagnosis and prognosis. Anesthesiology 86:216–241, 1997.
43. Raja SN: Nerve blocks in the evaluation of chronic pain: A plea for caution in their use and interpretation (Editorial). Anesthesiology 86:4–6, 1997.
44. de Takats G: Nature of painful vasodilation in causalgic states. Arch Neurol Psychiatry 50:318–326, 1943.
45. Bonica JJ: Causalgia and other reflex sympathetic dystrophies. *In* Bonica JJ (ed): The Management of Pain. Philadelphia, Lea & Febiger, 1953, p 956.

CHAPTER • 14

Neurophysiologic Testing in the Evaluation of the Patient in Pain

Howard J. Waldman, MD, DO

ELECTROMYOGRAPHY AND NERVE CONDUCTION STUDIES

Electromyography (EMG) is an extension of the clinical examination utilized in the assessment of neuromuscular disease. EMG testing can help to determine the presence of nerve or muscle disease and its anatomic location, the type of injury, and its severity. Sequential studies can help to monitor progression or regression of neuropathic processes as well.[1, 2] The EMG test typically consists of two parts, the EMG needle-electrode examination and nerve conduction studies (NCSs). These two tests, which provide complementary information on neuropathology, are commonly described together by the term *electromyography*.

Generally, EMG testing is utilized to evaluate function of the lower motor neuron (LMN) and has limited utility in evaluation of central nervous system (CNS) disease.[1, 3] The LMN consists of the anterior horn cell, nerve axon, neuromuscular junction, and muscle. (A motor neuron, its axon, and the muscle fibers it innervates, referred to as a *motor unit*, make up the functional unit of the LMN system.) The EMG is most often indicated in evaluation of persons with symptoms of LMN disease, such as numbness, weakness, and pain. Pathology of any portion of the LMN may be associated with EMG abnormalities.[1, 3, 4]

Information obtained from EMG testing must be utilized in conjunction with data from other evaluations, such as clinical, laboratory, and radiographic examinations. EMG testing is complementary to, and not exclusive of, radiologic evaluation. EMG reflects the physiology of nerve function, whereas radiographic testing evaluates the anatomy of nerves and related structures. The ability to properly utilize EMG information depends on viewing it as part of the data about the total patient.[1–3]

Electromyographic Instrumentation and Evaluation

The EMG apparatus amplifies and displays biologic information derived from surface- and needle-recording electrodes. Electrical information recorded from muscles and nerves is amplified, is displayed on an oscilloscope, and may undergo audio amplification to be heard over a loudspeaker. Various digital analyses of EMG data are possible, and data can be recorded to produce hard-copy records. An electrical nerve stimulator is part of the EMG apparatus and is utilized to stimulate nerves for nerve conduction testing. Contemporary EMG equipment has been standardized to allow reliable and reproducible testing by different electrodiagnostic laboratories. It must be noted that normal values may differ among individual laboratories.[1, 3, 5]

For the EMG needle-electrode examination, a fine needle recording electrode is inserted into a skeletal muscle. Electrical information produced by the muscle is evaluated for abnormalities, the type and anatomic distribution of which reflect the disease process (e.g., neuropathic abnormalities in C6-innervated musculature reflect a C6 radiculopathy). Disease of any portion of the LMN may result in EMG abnormalities. In the needle-electrode examination, electrical activity associated with needle insertion is examined for abnormal spontaneous activity (e.g., fibrillations and positive sharp waves) and to evaluate motor unit potentials and their recruitment.[1, 3, 6–8]

Insertional Activity

At rest, the muscle is electrically silent. When a needle-electrode is inserted into the muscle, the needle mechanically deforms and injures muscle fibers, producing a short burst of electrical activity referred to as *insertional activity*. Normally, insertional activity is short-lived (<300 msec) and ceases after needle movement stops.[1, 2, 7, 9] Duration of insertional activity may increase with loss of innervation or primary disease of muscle fibers.[1, 7, 10] Reduction of insertional activity may occur in myopathies or more advanced denervation when muscle tissue has been replaced by fat or connective tissue and the number of functioning muscle fibers is reduced.[1, 3, 7, 10]

Abnormal Spontaneous Potentials

The muscle is electrically silent after cessation of needle movement. Any electrical activity recorded during this quiescent period may constitute abnormal spontaneous activity. Abnormal spontaneous activity of single muscle fibers may be recorded as fibrillations or positive sharp waves. *Fibrillations* and *positive sharp waves* reflect muscle membrane irritability associated with spontaneous discharge of a single muscle fiber. These two phenomena reflect essentially the same abnormality and differ only in the position of the recording needle-electrode tip in relation to the abnormal muscle fiber: fibrillations are recorded when the needle tip is near the denervated fiber, whereas positive sharp waves arise from fibers that have been injured by the tip of the needle. Generally, in denervation of recent onset, positive sharp waves precede the appearance of fibrillation potentials by several days. Fibrillations and positive sharp waves may be seen in a variety of neuropathic and myopathic processes (Fig. 14–1) and are neither specific to nor diagnostic of a single disease process.[1–3, 7, 8, 11]

Fasciculation potentials are spontaneous activity that reflects spontaneous discharge of all or a portion of a motor unit. Fasciculations may be visible to the naked eye as muscle twitching under the skin. Traditionally they have been associated with motor neuron diseases such as amyotrophic lateral sclerosis (ALS), but they can occur in a variety of neuropathic disorders, most notably chronic ones. Fasciculations may occur in normal humans in conjunction with the taking of some medications (e.g., theophylline) and in those who have metabolic disorders.[1, 3, 7, 11, 12]

Complex repetitive discharges (formerly known as *bizarre high-frequency potentials*) consist of trains of spikelike potentials that fire at high frequencies, starting and ending abruptly. They are thought to occur when ephaptic or direct electrical activation occurs between groups of adjacent muscle fibers. Complex repetitive discharges are seen in a variety of chronic neuropathic and myopathic disorders, including chronic radiculopathies, neuropathies, motor neuron diseases, and inflammatory and familial myopathies.[1, 3, 7, 13]

Myokymic discharges are associated with fine, quivering or rippling motions of muscles at rest. Electromyographically, these appear as repetitively discharging groups of fasciculations. Myokymia of facial muscles may be associated with multiple sclerosis (MS), brain stem tumors, and Guillain-Barré syndrome. Myokymia in limb muscles may occur in chronic entrapment and peripheral neuropathies, but typically it is associated with postradiation plexopathies.[1, 2, 6, 7]

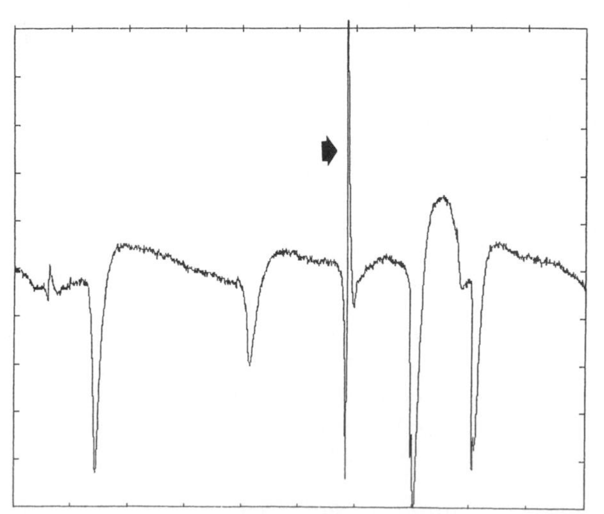

FIGURE 14–1 *EMG needle recording of positive sharp waves and a fibrillation potential (arrow) recorded from the tibialis anterior muscle of a person with L5 radiculopathy.*

Myotonia occurs in disorders with continuous muscle fiber activity associated with impaired muscle relaxation. Electromyographically, myotonia appears as waxing and waning trains of positive sharp wavelike potentials that vary in amplitude and frequency. They produce a characteristic "dive bomber" sound over the audio monitor. Myotonic discharges may follow voluntary muscle contractions or with mechanical or electrical stimulation of the muscle. Myotonia occurs in myotonic dystrophy, myotonia congenita, paramyotonia, acid maltase deficiency, and hyperthyroidism.[1–3, 11, 14]

Cramps are frequently painful contractions lasting from seconds to minutes. They appear on EMG as high-frequency motor unit discharges. Cramps may occur in normal persons, either spontaneously or in association with exercise or ischemia. Cramps also occur in a variety of disorders, including peripheral neuropathies, motor neuron disease, and sciatica.[1, 6, 11]

Motor Unit Potentials

Motor unit potentials (MUP) are seen with voluntary muscle contraction and reflect the summation of the electrical activity of the individual muscle fibers innervated by a single motor neuron (e.g., a motor unit).[1, 2, 8, 15] During weak voluntary muscle contraction, only a few motor neurons and their corresponding muscle fibers are activated to contribute to the contractile strength. To strengthen the contraction, increasing numbers of motor units must be recruited (Fig. 14–2). The manner in which MUP appear is referred to as the *recruitment pattern.*

In addition to motor unit recruitment, evaluation of individual motor unit morphology is important. Of the various measurements of MUP configuration, the most important are duration, amplitude, and phases (the number of crossings of the isoelectric baseline). Neuromuscular disease frequently alters MUP morphology. MUP of reduced duration and amplitude (myopathic MUP) are usually seen in disorders associated with loss or atrophy of muscle fiber, such as myopathies, muscular dystrophies, and neuromuscular junction disorders, and in association with early reinnervation.[1, 10, 11, 15, 16] MUP of increased duration and amplitude (neuropathic MUP) may be found with radiculopathies, neuropathies, motor neuron disease, and polymyositis. In these disorders, opportunity for reinnervation may occur so that an increased number of motor fibers are included in the motor unit. This may result from axonal sprouting of regenerating neurons that includes muscle fibers from motor units other than its own.[1, 2, 10, 16–18]

A normal motor unit has less than 5 phases (baseline crossings). A motor unit potential with more than five phases is referred to as *polyphasic* (Fig. 14–3). Although a small percentage of MUP may be polyphasic in normal humans, increased proportions of polyphasic potentials may be seen in those with any of a variety of neurogenic and myopathic disorders.[1, 7, 17, 19]

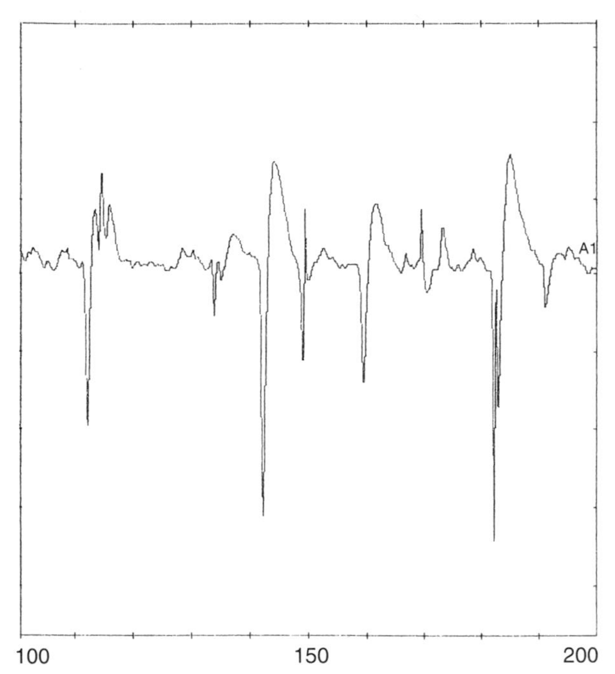

FIGURE 14–2 EMG needle recording of normal motor unit potentials from a biceps muscle during a voluntary muscle contraction of moderate strength.

The morphology of an individual motor unit may also vary during activation. MUP variation is secondary to blocking or failure of activation of fibers within a motor unit. This abnormality may occur with neuromuscular junction disorders, with reinnervation after nerve injury, and with myositis.[1, 11, 17]

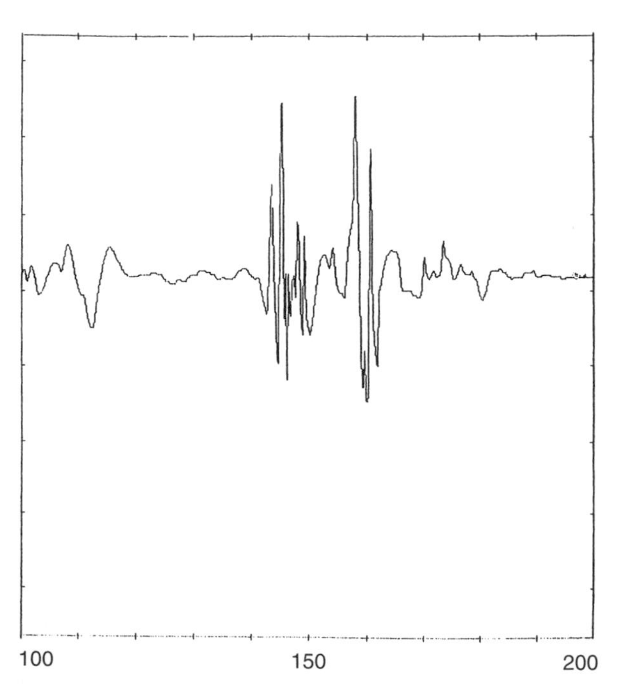

FIGURE 14–3 EMG needle recording of a polyphasic motor unit potential from the soleus muscle of a person with a chronic S1 radiculopathy.

Motor Unit Potential Recruitment

In normal muscles, the strength of a voluntary muscle contraction is directly related to the number of individual motor units that have been recruited and to their firing rate.[2, 15, 16] The increase in recruitment of motor units occurs in a graded fashion. During strong contractions, so many MUP may be seen that individual potentials are no longer distinguishable on the EMG display; this condition is referred to as a *complete* or *full interference pattern.* With weaker voluntary muscle contractions, individual MUP are distinguishable, and evaluation of numbers and firing rates is possible. With neuromuscular disease, less than complete interference patterns may be seen with full muscle contraction. In disorders associated with loss of MUP, the remaining motor units must fire more rapidly to offset the loss in total numbers of motor units. During EMG examination, this process results in a loss of MUP and the remaining MUP fire at a rate disproportionate to their numbers, a condition referred to as *reduced recruitment.* Reduced recruitment is most often associated with neuropathic disorders such as motor neuron disease and disease of the nerve root or peripheral nerve.[1, 2, 11, 13]

In contrast to reduced recruitment, *early recruitment* occurs in primary muscle disorders. Owing to loss or atrophy of muscle fibers, greater numbers of motor units must be recruited to produce a given muscle contraction. An inordinate number of MUP are observed in relationship to the strength of muscle contraction.[1, 10, 11, 14, 20]

Nerve Conduction Studies

Because nerve tissue is able to propagate an electrical stimulus along its course, testing of nerve function by electrical stimulation and recording of responses is possible. In its most basic form, nerve conduction testing consists of applying an electrical stimulus at various sites along the course of the nerve and recording responses from a distal or, less frequently, proximal point on the nerve (Fig. 14–4). NCS results may be abnormal because of local nerve compres-

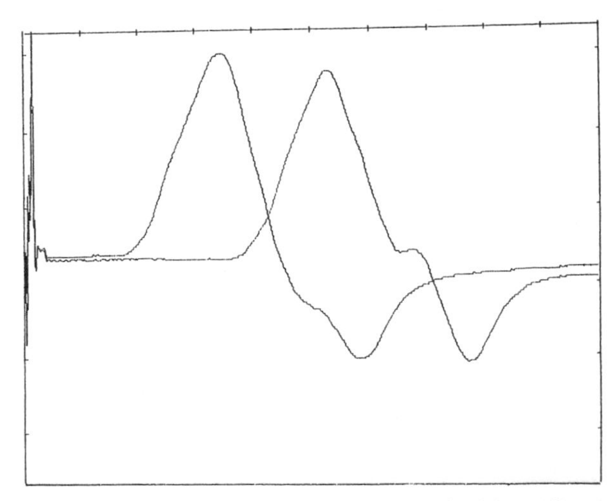

FIGURE 14–4 Normal nerve conduction study of the median nerve demonstrates responses obtained from stimulation at the wrist (left peak) and the antecubital fossa (right peak).

sion or disruption or disease affecting the myelin sheath or axonal structures of the nerve. Abnormalities of nerve conduction between two sites of stimulation allow anatomic localization of the lesion. Additionally, the types of abnormalities observed may provide information on the underlying abnormalities (e.g., "axonal" versus "demyelinating" neuropathy). NCS generally reflect conduction in the larger, faster-conducting myelinated nerve fibers. Testing of motor, sensory, and mixed nerves is possible.[1, 3, 4, 21]

The propagated electrical activity that travels along a nerve axon is referred to as a *nerve action potential.* In the case of motor nerves, the propagated nerve action potential is recorded from a distal muscle innervated by the nerve being tested, and muscle fiber activation produces a *compound muscle action potential* (CMAP). The nerve action potential recorded from a sensory nerve is referred to as a *sensory nerve action potential* (SNAP). Because there is no muscle to record from during sensory nerve conduction testing, the SNAP must be recorded from the sensory axon itself. The recorded response is of much lower amplitude than those recorded in motor nerve conduction testing.[1, 3, 22, 23] Sensory nerve conduction abnormalities only occur in lesions distal to the dorsal root ganglion, which may be helpful in differentiating pre- and postganglionic lesions.[1, 2, 17]

Sensory NCS may be recorded in the same direction as physiologic conduction (e.g., distal to proximal); it is referred to as *orthodromic conduction.* Recording SNAP from a distal site in response to proximal stimulation is referred to as *antidromic conduction.* The speed of propagation of a nerve action potential along a nerve is referred to as *conduction velocity.* Nerve conduction velocity is calculated as a function of time over distance between two stimulation sites and is expressed in meters per second (m/sec). In general, conduction velocities greater than 50 m/sec in the upper extremities and 40 m/sec in the lower extremities are normal.[1, 3] The amplitude, duration, and latency of compound motor and sensory nerve action potentials are evaluated. Normal values for these nerve action potential parameters have been established, but they can vary, depending on what techniques a given neurodiagnostic laboratory uses.[5]

In general, reduction of nerve action potential amplitude reflects axonal damage or dysfunction, although atrophy of the muscle from which the response is being recorded can also reduce amplitude. Slowing of conduction velocity or increased duration of nerve action potentials (temporal dispersion) is indicative of demyelination.[1, 2, 4, 24]

The interval between the electrical stimulus and the resultant nerve action potential, referred to as the *distal latency,* is important in the evaluation of many entrapment neuropathies. For example, prolongation of the distal latencies of the median nerve across the wrist is common in carpal tunnel syndrome[25] (CTS; Figs. 14–5, 14–6). Abnormalities of nerve conduction between two stimulation sites reflect nerve disease in that segment. For example, slowing of nerve conduction in the across-elbow segment of the ulnar nerve may reflect a tardy ulnar nerve palsy.[26] More diffuse nerve conduction abnormalities affecting multiple nerves may reveal a polyneuropathy.[27] As noted, slowing of conduction velocity and temporal dispersion are seen in demyelinating neuropathies, whereas reduction of nerve

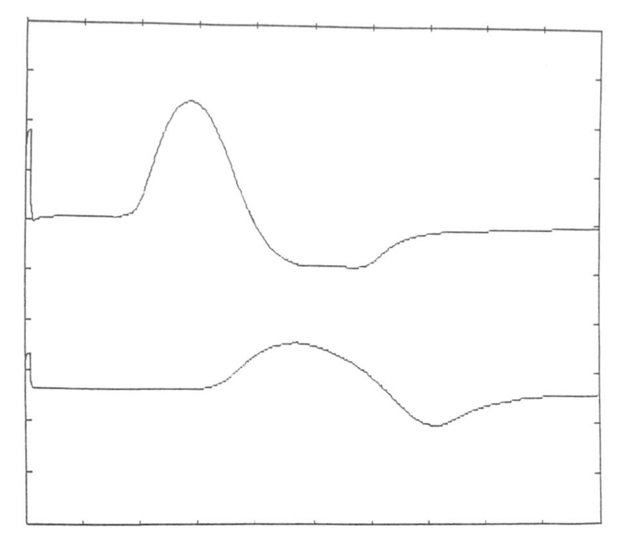

FIGURE 14–5 Upper trace, *Normal median nerve response obtained from stimulation at the wrist is evidence of normal distal motor latency.* Lower trace, *Median nerve response from stimulation at the wrist demonstrates prolonged distal motor latency and reduced amplitude in a person with carpal tunnel syndrome.*

action potential amplitudes is indicative of axonal neuropathies. A combination of these last two abnormalities is common in neuropathies of mixed type (e.g., diabetic neuropathy).[1, 4, 17] Absence of recordable nerve conduction responses may be associated with severe neuropathies or nerve disruptions. Additionally, responses may also be difficult to record in the presence of edema or excessive adipose tissue and from some nerves in elderly subjects.[1, 3]

Proximal Nerve Conduction Studies, the H Reflex, and the F Wave

Conventional NCS are able to evaluate nerve function in the more accessible peripheral segments of nerves. The more proximal segments of nerves (e.g., roots and plexus) are anatomically inaccessible and cannot readily be tested by conventional nerve conduction testing.[13, 28, 29] NCS that use deep needle stimulation of nerve roots and plexus are possible, and they provide information on nerve function in more proximal nerve segments. Unfortunately, these techniques are painful and technically difficult, can result in nerve injury, and do not provide information concerning the most proximal portions of the LMN.[13, 21, 30] The H reflex and F wave are proximal or "late response" nerve conduction techniques that allow evaluation of the entire course of the neuron.

The *H reflex* is the electrophysiologic equivalent of the deep tendon stretch reflex obtained by tapping over a tendon. This monosynaptic reflex consists of an afferent arc from the Ia muscle spindle fibers that synapse with an efferent arc consisting of alpha motor neuron fibers. In adults, the H reflex is obtainable from the gastrocnemius and soleus muscles (tibial nerve/S1 nerve root; Fig. 14–7) and the flexor carpi radialis muscle (median nerve/C6–C7 nerve roots).[1, 13, 28, 31, 32]

Unlike the H reflex, the *F wave* is recordable for many muscles throughout the body. Electrical stimulation of the peripheral portions of motor nerves results in antidromic

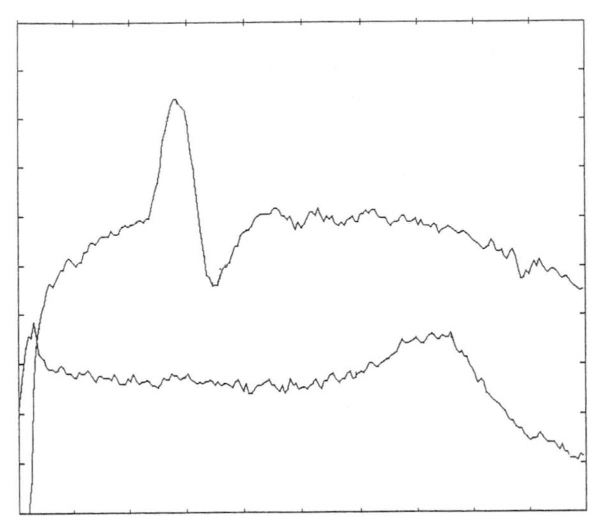

FIGURE 14–6 Upper trace, *Normal median nerve distal sensory response from stimulation at the wrist.* Lower trace, *Prolonged distal sensory response demonstrates prolonged distal sensory latency, a finding obtained from stimulation at the wrist from a person with carpal tunnel syndrome. This response also demonstrates reduced amplitude and temporal dispersion of the evoked response.*

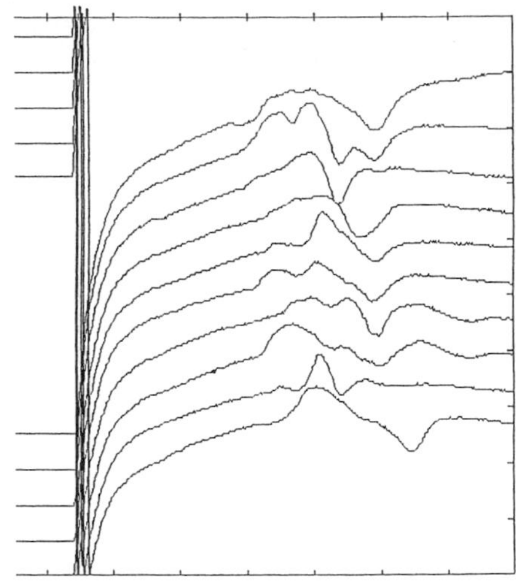

FIGURE 14–8 Normal F-wave responses obtained by stimulation of the median nerve at the wrist, recorded from the abductor pollicis brevis muscle. Note that the latency of each response varies slightly.

stimulation of anterior horn cells, which causes "backfiring" of the motor neurons. This backfiring results in an orthodromically conducted response recorded distally, reflecting conduction throughout the length of the axon (Fig. 14–8).[1, 2, 28]

The H reflex and F wave may be abnormal in disorders such as radiculopathy, plexopathy, motor neuron disease, and polyneuropathy. These late responses are particularly helpful in evaluating disorders that involve only the proximal portion of axons, such as Guillain-Barré syndrome and thoracic outlet syndrome. The H reflex has additional utility in the diagnosis of S1 and C6–C7 radiculopathies.[1, 3, 13, 28]

Neuromuscular Junction Testing

Repetitive nerve stimulation techniques are commonly helpful in the diagnosis of neuromuscular junction disorders such as myasthenia gravis and Lambert-Eaton myasthenic syndrome.[11, 17, 33, 34] In normal persons, repeated stimulation of motor nerves results in recorded CMAP of the same amplitude (Fig. 14–9). In persons who have myasthenia gravis, partial blocking of neuromuscular transmission results in decreasing amplitude of the evoked CMAP after a few repetitive nerve stimuli (*decremental response*). Lambert-Eaton myasthenic syndrome consists of proximal muscle weakness and fatigability and is frequently seen in association with oat cell carcinoma of the lung. In affected persons, rapid, repetitive stimulation results in a significant increase of CMAP amplitude after an initial low-amplitude response (*incremental response*).[33, 34] A similar response is seen with botulism poisoning.[35, 36]

Single-fiber EMG (*SFEMG*) is a technique for recording action potentials from single muscle fibers. It can be utilized

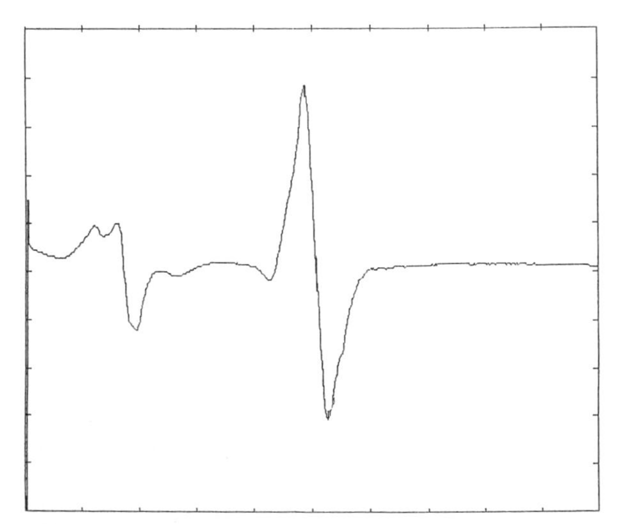

FIGURE 14–7 Normal H-reflex response from stimulation of the tibial nerve at the popliteal fossa recorded from the soleus muscle.

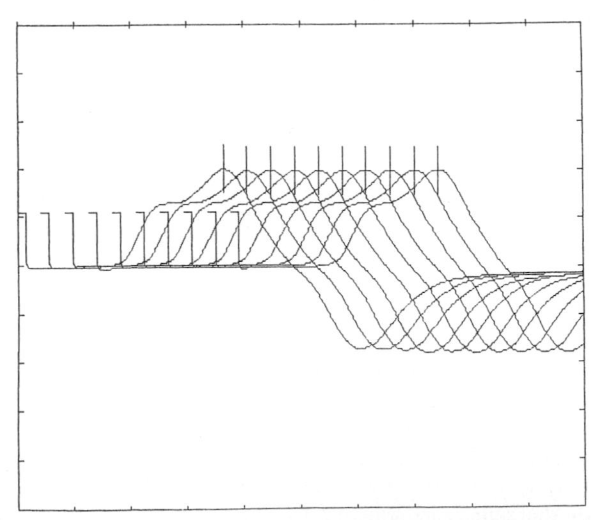

FIGURE 14–9 Normal repetitive stimulation neuromuscular junction testing recorded from the abductor digiti minimi muscle after stimulation of the ulnar nerve. Incremental or decremental changes in response amplitude are associated with diseases that affect the neuromuscular junction.

to evaluate synaptic delay at the neuromuscular junction and is therefore useful in the diagnosis of neuromuscular junction disorders.[1, 18, 33–35]

Diagnosis by Electromyography and Nerve Conduction Studies

The diagnosis of neuromuscular disorders by EMG and NCS is based on the type and distribution of abnormalities. Information on the patient's history, physical examination findings, and results of complementary testing is often also necessary to formulate an accurate diagnosis.[3, 9, 37, 38] Unfortunately, in some patients, definitive diagnosis based solely on EMG testing may not be possible, particularly in those who have subtle or incomplete lesions. In addition, adequate time must have elapsed for nerve degeneration to take place before EMG abnormalities become apparent. For example, it can take 14 to 21 days after onset of a radiculopathy before EMG abnormalities appear.[1, 21, 29] Nerve conduction abnormalities may be seen immediately across the site of total nerve disruption or within 4 to 7 days after less severe nerve injury.[1, 3, 4]

Central Nervous System Disorders

Conventional EMG and NCS have limited utility in the evaluation of CNS disorders. Unless a CNS disorder involves a portion of the lower motor neuron, nerve conduction findings will not be abnormal. In the same clinical setting, EMG needle examination generally reveals only changes in temporal firing or recruitment of motor unit potentials. In some acute CNS disorders, such as a cerebrovascular accident, fibrillation potentials and positive sharp waves in the involved muscles may be detectable approximately 2 to 4 weeks after the CNS insult and can persist for about 4 to 6 months.[17, 18] Evaluation of some aspects of CNS function is possible,[2, 39] especially cranial nerve assessment. EMG needle examination of muscles innervated by the spinal accessory, facial, trigeminal, and hypoglossal nerves is possible. NCS of the facial, spinal accessory, and sensory portions of the trigeminal nerves can also be performed.[1, 3, 40] Unfortunately, EMG and NCS have been of limited utility in patients with trigeminal neuralgia (tic douloureux).[40, 41] Specialized blink reflex testing may be abnormal in several disorders, such as Raeder's paratrigeminal syndrome, Bell's palsy, multiple sclerosis, Wallenberg's syndrome, and some polyneuropathies that affect the cranial nerves.[1, 3, 41]

Spinal Cord Disorders

Disorders of the spinal cord that involve the motor neurons or their axons may be manifested as EMG abnormalities. The central cavitation of the spinal cord that occurs with syringomyelia can be manifested as weakness and atrophy of upper extremity musculature (especially in the hands) with disassociated sensory loss in a capelike distribution over the neck, shoulders, and arms. In this disorder, EMG needle abnormalities are commonly seen in atrophic muscles and, generally, the lower extremities are spared, as they are not in ALS, which usually involves both upper and lower extremities. NCS usually are not affected, except possibly by reduction of CMAP amplitude.[1, 8, 34]

Significant EMG abnormalities may not be detected in persons with midline intervertebral disc herniation or spondylosis that does not involve the motor neurons of the spinal cord or their associated nerve roots.[8, 13, 29] More severe disease may cause symptoms of myelopathy, and the presentation may be similar to that of motor neuron disorders, with signs of denervation in involved musculature.[1, 8, 42]

Lesions involving the spinal canal below the T12 vertebral level may affect the conus medullaris or cauda equina. With midline lesions, several lumbar or sacral roots may be affected, which condition produces radicular pain, numbness, weakness, and possibly sphincter and sexual dysfunction.

Electrophysiologically, evidence of denervation of affected muscles is seen with reduced CMAP amplitudes on motor nerve conduction testing. Sensory nerve action potentials remain unaffected as the lesion is proximal to the dorsal root ganglion. Various tumors, midline disc herniations, infections, and spinal stenosis may be associated with cauda equina involvement.[1, 17, 43]

Motor Neuron Disorders

Motor neuron disorders such as ALS frequently involve upper and lower motor neurons. Affected persons may have asymmetric, progressive weakness and muscle atrophy. Muscle cramping, fasciculations, hyperreflexia, and bulbar signs may also be seen. Sensory abnormalities are absent. Typical EMG findings in motor neuron disease are diffuse changes of denervation such as fibrillations, positive sharp waves, neuropathic MUP, and reduced MUP recruitment. Mild slowing of motor nerve conduction velocity is the only significant NCS abnormality. Cervical spondylosis and syringomyelia may closely mimic motor neuron disorders and should be excluded by radiographic evaluation.[1, 8, 42–45]

Various infectious diseases, such as poliomyelitis,[1] human immunodeficiency virus infection,[46] herpes zoster,[14, 47] and Lyme disease,[48] and paraneoplastic[3, 44, 48] and idiopathic[1, 8, 44] disorders may be associated with myelitis and can involve other nervous system structures. The presence of associated EMG and NCS abnormalities depends on the extent and anatomic site of neuronal involvement.

Disorders of the Nerve Roots

Disorders of spinal nerve roots are commonly associated with EMG abnormalities. The most common ones are radiculopathies secondary to herniated intervertebral discs, spondylosis, and spinal stenosis. The prevalence of EMG abnormalities in radiculopathies with root compression and concomitant denervation of supplied musculature approaches 90%.[3, 13] EMG abnormalities may be absent with mild disease without significant root compression or with slowly progressive disease (e.g., spinal stenosis) or with midline disease (e.g., disc herniation) with myelopathic (rather than radiculopathic) involvement.[13, 29] With radicular disease, NCS results are usually normal, although in severe, chronic, or more extensive disease, reduction of MUP amplitude secondary to associated axonal degeneration may be seen.[1, 13] H-reflex abnormalities may be seen early in S1 and C6–C7 radiculopathies.[3, 28, 32] Prolongation, blocking, or chronodispersion of F-wave responses may occur in more severe or chronic radiculopathies.[1, 3, 17] EMG abnormalities of denervation should occur in the myotome supplied by the involved nerve roots.

Abnormalities initially consist of positive sharp waves followed by fibrillation potentials and polyphasic and neuropathic MUP. MUP recruitment may also be reduced.[1, 13, 29] The presence of paraspinal muscle EMG abnormalities is important in the diagnosis of radiculopathies, because it confirms involvement at the root level. EMG diagnosis of radiculopathy based on abnormalities limited to the paraspinal musculature should be viewed with suspicion, because local degenerative changes, placement of the EMG needle in neural structures, or local trauma (e.g., following epidural nerve blocks or laminectomy) may also cause EMG changes in the paraspinal region.[1, 32]

Within the first day after onset of radiculopathy there may be a reduction in the number of MUP recruited in the involved myotome and H-reflex abnormalities. EMG abnormalities may be seen in the paraspinal musculature after 7 to 8 days. At 13 to 14 days, EMG changes can appear in proximal limb musculature. It can take as along as 21 days after onset of radiculopathy for EMG abnormalities to be seen throughout an involved nerve root myotome.[29, 32] Although this temporal progression of denervation has been generally accepted, recent studies have disputed its invariability.[49]

Radiculopathies may be incomplete, involving only a portion of the affected myotome; therefore, absence of EMG abnormalities in a given muscle or muscles supplied by a compressed nerve root does not exclude a diagnosis of radiculopathy.[13, 29] Chronicity is suggested by MUP of increased amplitude and duration, polyphasic MUP, and complex repetitive discharges.[1, 29, 48] Bilateral involvement suggests midline disc herniation or more diffuse disease such as spinal stenosis. Involvement of several nerve root levels suggests the likelihood of multiple disc herniations or spinal stenosis.[29] Some neuropathies (e.g., diabetic neuropathy) may involve the peripheral nerves and nerve roots, presenting as polyradiculoneuropathy. Neoplasms, infections such as herpes zoster, and idiopathic disorders can also be associated with radiculopathy.[1, 8, 17]

Plexus Lesions

Lesions of the plexus may occur secondary to trauma, to space-occupying or compressive lesions, or radiation, and some are idiopathic. EMG evaluation of plexopathies is often challenging, especially in differentiating plexopathies from more proximal root lesions and more peripheral neuropathies. History and physical examination findings may suggest a plexopathy, which can be confirmed by EMG and associated tests such as radiographic studies.[1, 50] Brachial plexopathies are more common because anatomically the brachial plexus is more susceptible to injury. With severe injuries, profound flaccid weakness often occurs, whereas with lesser lesions, physical findings may be quite subtle.

The clinical and EMG findings associated with plexopathy depend on what portion of the plexus is affected. In general, EMG abnormalities associated with brachial and lumbosacral plexopathies include (1) denervation in muscles supplied by the involved portion of the plexus but not involving paraspinal muscles or muscles supplied above the level of the lesion; (2) slowing of conduction velocities across the site of injury, with normal or slightly slowed conduction upon stimulation distal to the site of involvement (F waves may also be prolonged); (3) reduction of SNAP amplitude (which does not occur in radiculopathies or root avulsions); and (4) possibly, CMAP amplitude reduction.[1, 9, 50] Of particular importance is the spread of a superior sulcus (Pancoast's) tumor, which may invade the lower brachial plexus or cervicothoracic nerve roots. With this tumor, pain in the chest wall and arm with paresthesias, numbness, and weakness in the distribution of involved neural structures may occur. Horner's syndrome, due to invasion of the cervicothoracic sympathetic nerves, may also be present.[1, 8, 49]

Idiopathic brachial neuritis (also referred to as *neuralgic amyotrophy* or *Parsonage-Turner syndrome*) is a disorder of the brachial plexus that may mimic acute cervical radiculopathy or another brachial plexus disorder. This disorder most often appears in males after the third decade; it may occur following viral illness, immunization, or trauma. Clinically, severe pain followed by more persistent weakness and atrophy of involved musculature occurs most frequently in the C5 and C6 nerve root distributions. EMG findings are similar to those of other brachial plexopathies.[1, 37, 50, 51]

Thoracic outlet syndrome may occur secondary to compression of nerve roots or brachial plexus trunks by anomalous structures such as cervical ribs or fibrous bands. Vascular or neurologic symptoms may occur together or independently. True neurogenic thoracic outlet syndrome is rare and affects principally females, who present with pain, paresthesias, and muscle atrophy, usually involving the distribution of the lower trunk of the brachial plexus or the C8–T1 nerve roots. EMG abnormalities may include denervation of intrinsic hand muscles, absence or reduction of ulnar SNAP, and absence or prolongation of ulnar nerve F-wave response.[1, 8, 37, 43, 50, 52]

Postirradiation plexopathy may occur months to years after treatment. The disorder may be progressive and is frequently associated with myokymia and complex repetitive discharges in addition to EMG abnormalities generally associated with plexopathies.[1, 3, 50] Recurrence of neoplasms must be excluded as the cause of plexopathy.

Neuropathies and Disorders of Peripheral Nerves

Disorders of the peripheral portion of nerves include traumatic nerve injuries, entrapment neuropathies, and a wide variety of mononeuropathies and polyneuropathies of various causes. EMG and NCS can help to identify the site of involvement and the type of nerve lesion and can assist in monitoring progression and recovery.[1, 3, 8, 17, 43] Nerve injuries may be classified by degree and type of injury.

Neurapraxia, the mildest form of nerve injury, consists of conduction loss without associated axonal structural changes. This form of conduction block often occurs with compressive or ischemic injuries of nerves, such as mild entrapment neuropathies. With neurapraxic injuries, focal demyelination occurs. As a result, nerve conduction is slowed or absent across the site of neurapraxic injury, but conduction proximal and distal to the site of injury is normal. Serial nerve conduction determinations along the course of the nerve are able to locate the site of conduction block. When the cause of nerve compression is removed, recovery generally occurs within days or weeks. The prognosis for complete recovery is usually excellent. With neurapraxic injuries, motor weakness or paralysis may occur. If sensory symptoms are present, they tend to be mild with some sparing. EMG needle examination tends to reveal only reduced MUP recruitment with little in the way of abnormal spontaneous potentials.[1, 3, 22, 43, 53]

In *axonotmesis*, a more severe form of nerve injury, there is disruption of the axon and its myelin sheath. The neural tube (endoneurium, perineurium, and epineurium) remains intact. The nerve undergoes wallerian degeneration with fragmentation of the axon distal to the site of injury. After nerve injury with axonotmesis, motor and sensory paralyses occur with associated atrophy of supplied muscles. After approximately 4 to 5 days, the distal segments of the nerve become inexcitable. In 1 to 2 weeks, positive sharp waves are seen; fibrillations in involved muscles occur in 2 to 3 weeks. The intact neural tube "guides" the regenerating axon, generally resulting in a good prognosis for recovery. The recovering axon regenerates at a rate of 1 to 3 mm/day.[1, 3, 4, 22, 43, 53]

Neurotmesis, the most severe form of nerve injury, is associated with severe disruption or actual transection of the nerve. Nerve regeneration and recovery are often incomplete and may require surgical reanastomosis or nerve graft. Neuroma formation may occur and is commonly associated with pain. Clinically and electrophysiologically, neurotmesis and axonotmesis are indistinguishable, except that, in the recovery phase of axonotmesis, electrophysiologic evidence of reinnervation is seen.[1, 3, 22, 43, 53]

In nontraumatic neuropathies, segmental demyelination is generally associated with slowing of nerve conduction velocities and temporal dispersion of evoked responses. With axonal degeneration, however, reduction of the evoked response amplitudes with mild or minimal slowing of nerve conduction velocities is typical. Unless axonal degeneration has occurred, significant EMG needle abnormalities are usually absent. Pure demyelinating or axonal neuropathies are uncommon; mixed patterns occur more frequently.[1, 3, 8, 54, 55] Polyneuropathies are most often heralded by distal dysesthesias often in a stocking or stocking-and-glove distribution. The causes of nontraumatic neuropathies are protean: toxic, inherited, infectious, metabolic, paraneoplastic, and idiopathic.[1, 8, 54–57] An individual discussion of each of these neuropathies is beyond the scope of this chapter. A disease such as diabetes that is frequently associated with the development of neuropathy often indicates the cause. Despite the ability of electrophysiologic, laboratory, and nerve biopsy studies to aid in identifying the cause of the neuropathy, no definitive cause may be determined in as many as 25% of patients.[8]

Mononeuropathies, ones involving a single nerve, also occur concomitantly with disorders commonly associated with the development of *poly*neuropathies.[1, 27, 37] Mononeuropathies may occur in the extremities or may involve the thoracic nerves. In mononeuropathy multiplex, several individual nerves may be involved concurrently; this disorder is commonly associated with collagen vascular disease, diabetes mellitus, leprosy, and vasculitis of other causes.[1, 8, 17, 19] A preexisting polyneuropathy often renders individual nerves more vulnerable to the development of mononeuropathies, especially entrapment neuropathies (vulnerable nerve syndrome).[1, 9, 37] It has been hypothesized that proximal compression of a peripheral nerve might interfere with axoplasmic flow and increase the susceptibility of more distal nerve segments to injury or compression (e.g., C6 radiculopathy increasing susceptibility to CTS).[58] This predisposition has been referred to as the *double crush hypothesis*. Recent clinical studies have failed to confirm the existence of this disorder.[43, 59, 60] In older, poorly controlled diabetics, diabetic amyotrophy may develop. This truncal neuropathy is commonly associated with pain, weakness, and atrophy of the pelvic and anterior thigh musculature.[37, 61, 62]

Entrapment neuropathies are common mononeuropathies. The most common entrapment neuropathy is CTS, which is associated with dysesthesias, pain, and numbness in the median nerve distribution. Electrophysiologically, CTS presents with prolongation of the distal motor and sensory latencies of the median nerve with normal NCS results proximal to the site of entrapment. Mild CTS is associated with neurapraxia; therefore, only in severe cases of CTS associated with axonal degeneration are EMG needle abnormalities seen.[1, 3, 25, 37] The diagnosis of early or very mild CTS may be aided by special NCS techniques, such as determination of nerve conduction from the midpalm across the carpal tunnel (transpalmar study) and differential studies.[17, 43, 63] Transpalmar studies evaluate median nerve conduction across the short transpalmar segment involving the carpal tunnel and thus are more sensitive than conventional nerve conduction techniques. Differential nerve studies record distal sensory latencies from the ring finger. The ring finger is usually supplied by both the median and the ulnar nerve, but only the median nerve passes through the carpal tunnel. In the presence of CTS, there is prolongation of the median latency as compared with the ulnar latency (which is not prolonged by entrapment in the carpal tunnel). The same technique may be performed by recording from the thumb, which is supplied by both the median and radial nerves. Transpalmar and differential studies are more sensitive than conventional latency determinations, and findings may be abnormal even in the presence of normal median nerve distal motor and sensory latencies.[3, 63–66]

Entrapment neuropathies involving more proximal segments of peripheral nerves, such as ulnar nerve entrapment at the elbow (tardy ulnar palsy), also occur frequently. With these entrapments, slowing of nerve conduction velocity across the involved segment is seen, with normal nerve conduction proximal to the site of entrapment. Nerve conduction distal to the site of entrapment may be normal, but in more severe cases, slowing of conduction and changes of axonopathy may occur with associated EMG needle abnormalities in the muscles supplied distal to the site of entrapment.[1, 3, 4, 21, 53] Entrapment neuropathies have been reported to occur in many of the peripheral nerves. Diagnosis of individual entrapment neuropathies is based on their clinical presentation and is confirmed by electrodiagnostic studies.[1, 11, 17, 43]

Neuromuscular Junction Disorders

Neuromuscular junction (NMJ) disorders are frequently associated with fatigability and muscle weakness. Often, the weakness is exacerbated by exercise and strength improves after periods of rest. The two most common NMJ disorders are myasthenia gravis and myasthenic syndrome (Eaton-Lambert myasthenic syndrome).

Myasthenia gravis is an autoimmune disorder often associated with thymoma. Patients present with progressive paresis of muscles undergoing repeated or progressive contraction. Initially, ocular musculature is involved by ptosis and diplopia. Weakness of facial and bulbar muscles is also common. Proximal muscles, particularly those of the neck, are involved more often than distal ones. Electrophysiologically, decrement of CMAP amplitude is seen on repetitive nerve stimulation testing. Single-fiber EMG reveals increased jitter and blocking.[11, 33, 62, 67]

Myasthenic syndrome of Eaton-Lambert is usually associated with small cell carcinoma of the lung or other malignancies. Unlike myasthenia gravis patients, those with myasthenic syndrome are often weak at rest but show transitory improvement in strength after brief exercise. Weakness primarily involves the proximal musculature, especially in the lower extremities. The extraocular, bulbar, and neck muscles are rarely involved. Upon repetitive nerve stimulation testing, an incremental increase in CMAP amplitude is seen after a brief period of muscle contraction. Single-fiber EMG reveals increased jitter and blocking, which improve after brief muscle contraction. Other diseases associated with NMJ dysfunction are botulism, tick paralysis, and drug-associated myasthenia (e.g., secondary to aminoglycoside).[33, 62, 67, 68]

Periodic paralysis describes a group of hereditary disorders of episodic weakness that are characterized by reversible inexcitability of muscle membranes and are generally associated with abnormalities of potassium metabolism.[1, 8, 17, 20]

Myopathies

Myopathies may be associated with inflammatory, toxic, and genetic causes. The most common inflammatory myopathies are dermatomyositis and polymyositis. These disorders often occur in association with other collagen vascular diseases and in the presence of malignancies. Clinical features include progressive, symmetric weakness and aching pain, most frequently involving proximal musculature. In dermatomyositis, a lilac-colored rash (heliotrope rash) over the eyelids and malar area is often seen. In both diseases, creatine kinase is elevated, a finding helpful in determining the diagnosis and monitoring the clinical course. EMG evaluation of involved muscles reveals fibrillations, positive sharp waves, and complex repetitive discharges in association with MUP of reduced amplitude and duration (myopathic MUP) with polyphasia.[1, 8, 20, 69]

Congenital myopathies include the various muscular dystrophies in association with several inborn errors of metabolism and with other genetic disorders that involve morphologic abnormalities of muscle fibers. Most of these myopathies are characterized by certain EMG features: myopathic MUP, polyphasic MUP, and abnormal spontaneous potentials. Myopathies may also occur in association with malignant hyperpyrexia, alcoholism, hypoparathyroidism and hyperparathyroidism, and infectious diseases such as trichinosis, and some viral infections.[1, 8, 14, 20, 70]

MAGNETIC STIMULATION

The inability of conventional NCS to practically and directly evaluate anatomically inaccessible structures (e.g., the lumbar plexus) has prompted a search for alternative methods to allow evaluation of these deep-seated structures. It had long been known that a magnetic field is able to induce electric current flow in the neural tissue and cause generation of an action potential. Not until the 1980s, however, was a feasible method developed. This technique of magnetic stimulation of neural structures allowed not only stimulation of deep-seated structures but, more importantly, transcranial stimulation of the motor portions of the brain, enabling determination of nerve conduction through central motor pathways.[71, 72] Magnetic stimulation has the added advantage of being essentially painless.

Magnetic NCS are performed much as conventional electrical NCS are, except that a magnetic coil provides a time-varying magnetic field to induce nerve conduction. Because of the difficulty in determining the exact site along a nerve where the action potential is initiated, magnetic stimulation is generally not utilized for determining nerve conduction along the more peripheral portions of a nerve.[71, 72] Magnetic stimulation has been used to aid in the diagnosis of radiculopathies and plexus lesions but has found its greatest utility in evaluating central motor nerve conduction.[39, 73–79]

Magnetic transcortical stimulation of the cortex of the brain allows measurement of CNS conduction through the central motor pathways. In direct magnetic stimulation of the cortex, the evoked action potential (motor evoked potential) is recorded from peripheral sites, such as muscles of the upper and lower extremities. Determination of motor conduction throughout the entire length of the motor pathway is therefore possible. Magnetic stimulation testing has been found useful in the diagnosis of multiple sclerosis, cervical spondylitic myelopathy, ALS, cerebrovascular disorders, cerebellar ataxia, and polyneuropathies with proximal involvement (e.g., Charcot-Marie-Tooth disease). The primary abnormality in these disorders is prolongation of central motor conduction or absence of motor evoked potentials.[71–79] Central sensory pathways are evaluated by somatosensory evoked potentials.

EVOKED POTENTIAL TESTING

Evoked potentials (EP) are electrophysiologic responses of the nervous system to externally applied sensory stimuli. EP testing can provide information on the peripheral and the central sensory nervous system pathways that is unobtainable by EMG and magnetic stimulation evaluations. EP testing provides objective and reproducible data to delineate sensory system lesions that are unsuspected or are clinically ambiguous on the basis of history and physical examination findings alone. EP testing can provide information on the anatomic location of nervous system lesions and help to monitor progression or regression.[74, 80–82]

EP responses are of very low amplitude (0.1 to 20 μV) and are obscured by random electrical "noise" such as muscle artifact, electroencephalographic activity, and interference from surrounding electrical devices. Extraction of the EP response is accomplished by computer averaging. This technique summates the EP response, which is "time-locked" to the applied sensory stimuli, and minimizes unwanted noise interference.[74, 81]

A variety of stimuli may elicit evoked potentials, but the most commonly employed are visual, auditory, and somatosensory. These three stimuli give rise to visual evoked potentials (VEPs), brain stem auditory evoked potentials (BAEPs), and somatosensory evoked potentials (SEPs), which evaluate functions of their respective sensory systems.[81, 83]

EP responses consist of a sequence of peaks and waves characterized by latency, amplitude, configuration, and interval between individual peaks (interpeak latency). In this manner, EP responses are similar to conventional NCS responses and magnetically stimulated motor EP.

There is a standardized nomenclature for the individual peaks and waves of the various EP responses.[84–87] The peaks and waves may be identified by *polarity* (positive or negative), *latency* (e.g., the positive wave occurring at 100 msec in VEP testing is designated P100), by the *anatomic site* where the response was recorded (e.g., Erb's point), or by simple numbering in sequence (e.g., waves I through V in the BAEP). Normal values for EP responses are generally established by each electrophysiology laboratory, utilizing 2.5 or 3.0 standard deviations from mean values as the upper limits of normal.[74, 81, 88]

Instrumentation

The EP equipment, like that for EMG, is a biologic amplifier. In its most basic form, EP equipment consists of recording electrodes attached to specific areas over the scalp, spine, and extremities. Input from the electrodes is routed to an amplifier, which filters, averages, displays, and records data.[81] Electrodes are placed on the scalp much as for conventional electroencephalography, following the international 10–20 system according to which electrodes are located at distances 10% or 20% of the total distance between bony landmarks of the skull.[89] The configuration of electrode placement for a specific test is referred to as a *montage*.

Specific Evoked Potential Tests

The three most commonly utilized EP tests are the VEP, BAEP, and SEP. For most patients who consult a pain specialist, SEP have the most clinical utility. A fourth test, cognitive evoked potentials, is also discussed briefly.

Visual Evoked Potentials

VEP are utilized to evaluate pathology affecting the visual pathways. They are primarily generated in the visual cortex and, therefore, may be affected by pathology anywhere along the visual pathways, from the corneas to the visual cortex.[84, 90] A reversing checkerboard pattern projected through a video monitor is most often utilized to stimulate the visual pathways (pattern-reversal VEP). Each eye is tested individually to localize abnormalities to the affected side. Generally, 100 pattern reversals (trials) are required to obtain a clearly defined response. The test is repeated to confirm reproducibility of responses. The resultant VEP consists of three peaks: The primary peak of interest occurs at approximately 100 msec, has positive polarity, and is thus referred to as the *P100 peak*. The remaining two peaks have negative polarities and latencies of approximately 75 and 145 msec, respectively.[74, 88] The upper limits of normal for the P100 response are about 117 to 120 msec, with a differential latency between eyes of no more than 6 to 7 msec.[81]

VEP testing is useful in the diagnosis of many conditions that affect the visual pathways but is most often used in the diagnosis of MS (Fig. 14–10). The demyelination of the optic nerve that occurs in MS has the same effect as demyelination in peripheral nerves (i.e., slowing of conduction velocity), resulting in increased response latency. If axonal loss also occurs, response amplitude is also reduced.[74, 91–93] These abnormalities correspond to the changes seen in demyelination and axonopathy found in conventional NCS. In MS patients, the most common abnormalities are increased P100 latency and increased interocular latencies. Reduction of P100 amplitude may also occur, although this is generally associated with compressive or ischemic lesions.[74] In patients suspected to have MS, VEP abnormality rates are approximately 63%, and they approach 85% in patients with confirmed MS.[74] VEP abnormalities may antedate typical changes of MS seen on magnetic resonance imaging.[74] MS may also produce abnormalities of BAEP and SEP; therefore, testing all three may improve the diagnostic yield over that of VEP alone.[94, 95]

Ocular disorders, tumors, inflammatory conditions, and ischemia of the optic pathways may be associated with VEP abnormalities.[96–98] VEP abnormalities have also been reported in a variety of cerebral degenerative disorders and neuropathies with CNS involvement.[74, 98] There are a few reports of VEP abnormalities in patients with migraine headaches.[99–103] VEP testing has been used for visual screen-

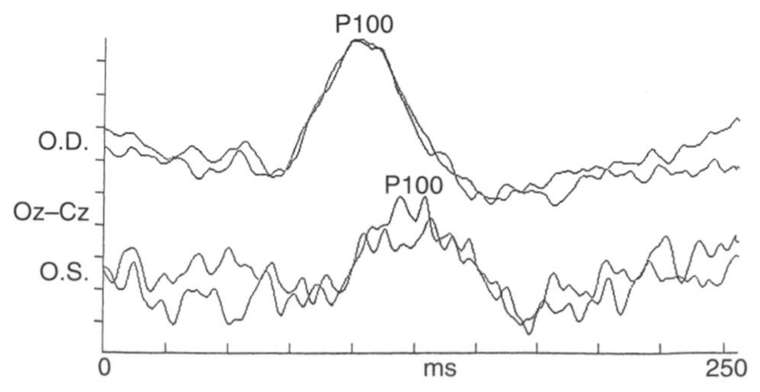

FIGURE 14–10 Upper trace, *Normal visual evoked potential response.* Lower trace, *Abnormal visual evoked potential response demonstrates prolonged latency and reduced amplitude in a person with multiple sclerosis.*

ing of infants and persons who are suspected of having visual pathway disease but are unable to respond to or comply with conventional ophthalmologic or optometric testing.[88, 100]

Brain Stem Auditory Evoked Potentials

In the manner that visual stimuli are used to evaluate visual pathways, auditory stimuli are utilized to assess the auditory pathways. The auditory pathway extends from the middle ear structures through the eighth cranial nerve and brain stem to the auditory cortex.[74, 81, 88] Auditory stimuli presented to each ear individually produce the BAEP, which consist of a series of waves that correspond closely to these auditory pathway structures. BAEP evaluation, therefore, allows relatively specific localization of auditory pathway pathology. BAEP responses are recorded from electrodes placed on the scalp, near or on each ear. The most commonly utilized auditory stimulus is brief, electrical pulses, referred to as *clicks*, which are presented to each ear through audiologic earphones. (Earphones that fit *into* the auditory canal can also be used.) These click stimuli may be varied in frequency, intensity, and rate. A well-defined BAEP response generally requires 1000 to 2000 stimuli.

The typical BAEP response consists of a sequence of seven positive waves, of which the first five are used clinically. They are numbered sequentially by Roman numerals I through V and occur within the first 10 msec after presentation of auditory stimuli. Each wave closely corresponds to structures along the auditory pathway that are believed to generate it. Wave I is thought to be generated by CN VIII; wave II by CN VIII and the cochlear nucleus; wave III by the lower pons; and waves IV and V by the upper pons and lower midbrain.[74, 80, 88, 104] Diagnosis of the anatomic site of pathology is based on which wave or waves demonstrate increased latency or are absent (Fig. 14–11). Determination of interpeak latency is important, because disorders such as peripheral hearing loss may increase the latency of the entire BAEP response but do not change the interpeak latency relationships. Severe hearing loss may render recording of the BAEP impossible owing to degradation of the response.[74, 104] BAEP response amplitudes vary considerably among normal subjects. To reduce intersubject variability, the ratio of wave I and wave V amplitudes is calculated. If the wave V amplitude is reduced in comparison to wave I, an intrinsic brain stem impairment is implied.

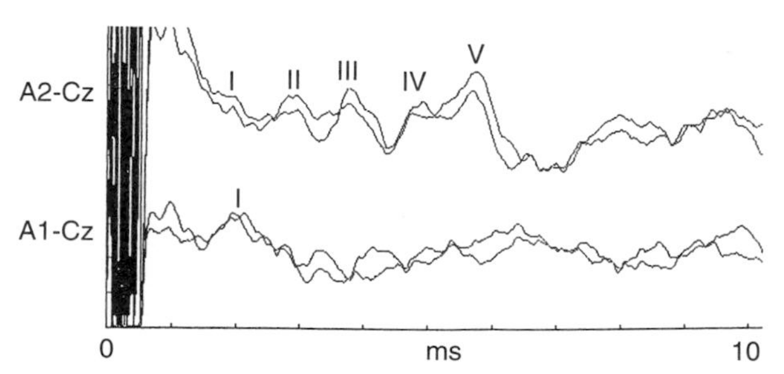

FIGURE 14–11 Upper trace, *Normal brain stem auditory evoked potential response demonstrates waves I through V.* Lower trace, *Abnormal brain stem auditory evoked potential response obtained from a patient with a left acoustic neuroma. Wave I is present, but waves II through V are absent.*

A reduction of wave I to wave V amplitude ratio suggests possible hearing impairment.[17, 82]

BAEP may aid in the diagnosis of a variety of diseases affecting the auditory pathways. The BAEP may be abnormal in 32% to 64% of persons with MS,[104, 105] although it is less sensitive than either VEP or SEP testing.[93, 106, 107] BAEP are particularly useful in the diagnosis of cerebellopontine angle tumors such as acoustic neuromas (see Fig. 14–11). BAEP testing has been found to be superior to routine audiometry and computed tomography in the diagnosis of cerebellopontine angle tumors[108, 109] and appears to be at least as sensitive as, and less expensive than, MRI for this diagnosis.[74] BAEP are also useful in (1) the evaluation of strokes and tumors involving the auditory pathways,[88, 90, 106, 110] (2) the evaluation of, and as a predictor of outcome for, comatose and head-injured persons,[111–113] and (3) the diagnosis of a variety of neurodegenerative disorders, such as Friedreich's ataxia, in which the responses are abnormal.[114] BAEP abnormalities have been reported in association with Arnold-Chiari malformations, postconcussion syndrome, vertebrobasilar transient ischemic attacks, basilar migraines, and spasmodic torticollis.[115, 116] These responses are utilized in audiometric screening of infants and of patients with mental deficiency who are unable to undergo routine audiometric testing.[104, 117]

Somatosensory Evoked Potentials

SEP assess the function of somatosensory pathways by stimulation of sensory nerves. SEP may be recorded by stimulation of mixed or pure sensory nerves in the upper and lower extremities, in dermatomal areas of the skin, and from some cranial nerves with sensory function. The somatosensory pathway consists of the peripheral nerve, dorsal columns of the spinal cord, medial lemniscus, ventroposterior lateral thalamus, and primary sensory cortex.[74, 88, 118] SEP appear to be related to the senses of joint position, touch, vibration, and stereognosis but are not related to pain and temperature sensation.[74, 84]

Typically, SEP are obtained through electrical stimulation of a peripheral nerve after recording electrodes are placed at sites along the somatosensory pathway. In upper and lower extremity SEP, stimulation is generally applied at the more distal portion of major nerves, with recording sites along the extremity, over certain spinous processes, and on the scalp over regions that correspond to the somatosensory cortex. In SEP evaluation of dermatomal sensory areas, stimulation is performed over an area of skin that is innervated by a given dermatome (e.g., lateral foot for the S1 dermatome), and recording is usually limited to the scalp.[74, 81, 119]

SEP responses consist of a group of waveforms, each corresponding to the anatomic site of the recording electrode (e.g., Erb's point; Figs. 14–12, 14–13). Abnormalities are manifested as increased latency, reduced amplitude, or absence of a given wave. The anatomic site of the lesion is determined by the point at which the abnormality is seen in a wave corresponding to recording electrode sites along the somatosensory pathway.[74, 88, 118] The SEP is analogous to conventional nerve conduction testing, in which the site of the NCS abnormality corresponds to the site of disease. Because peripheral nerve disorders may prolong response

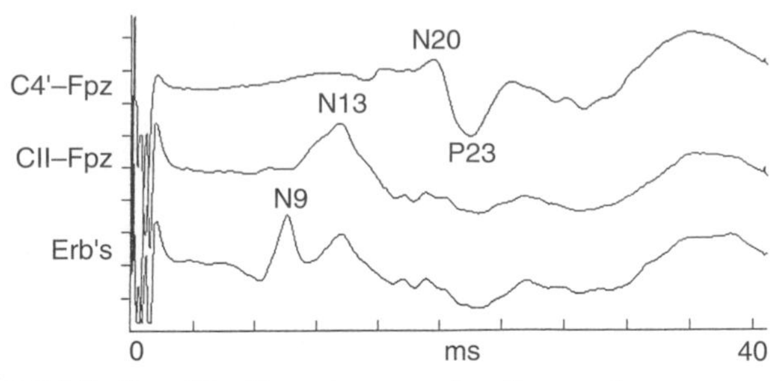

FIGURE 14–12 Normal upper extremity somatosensory evoked potential response obtained by stimulating the median nerve at the wrist demonstrates responses recorded from Erb's point (N9), the second cervical vertebra (N13), and the cortex (N20-P23).

latencies along the entire length of the somatosensory pathway, interpeak latency determinations are important.[118, 120] Additionally, conventional nerve conduction testing of the peripheral portions of the nerve can help to exclude peripheral neuropathy.

SEP are often abnormal in persons with MS. SEP testing is frequently performed in conjunction with VEP and BAEP testing to enhance diagnostic sensitivity, SEP being the most sensitive of the three modalities.[8, 74, 88] SEP abnormalities are more often seen in MS patients with sensory symptoms and are more common in the lower extremities.[121] Generally, conventional NCS are utilized in evaluation of sensory disturbances of the peripheral nerve, although SEP may be recordable from the scalp (owing to amplification effects of the cerebral cortex) when SNAP are unrecordable. This amplification effect may be particularly useful in evaluating some entrapment neuropathies, such as meralgia paresthetica, in which recording of the response from the peripheral nerve is technically difficult or impossible.[118, 122, 123] SEP are useful in the diagnosis of brachial plexus lesions and may be complementary to conventional EMG.[120, 122, 124] SEP may help to confirm axonal continuity and to determine whether lesions are preganglionic or postganglionic.[103, 104] Ulnar nerve SEP may be useful in the diagnosis of thoracic outlet syndrome and appear to be complementary to EMG testing.[125–129]

The use of SEPs in the diagnosis of radiculopathy has been controversial.[81, 122, 130–140] Many studies utilizing SEP of peripheral nerves in the diagnosis of radiculopathy have found the test to be of limited utility. This limitation was attributed to "overshadowing" of abnormalities in a single nerve root by contributions from uninvolved nerve roots that supply the same peripheral nerve. Recording of SEP from a dermatomal area supplied by a single nerve root (e.g., the webbed space between the great and first toes innervated by the L5 nerve root) represents an attempt to circumvent this problem.[131–135] Dermatomal SEP have been generally found to improve diagnostic yield; however, EMG testing remains the most sensitive electrodiagnostic test for radiculopathy.[74, 81, 122, 131, 134, 141]

Somatosensory EP are frequently abnormal in patients with myelopathy, and they may be abnormal in the presence of normal EMG evaluation.[126, 142–145] Serial SEP have been found useful in determining the extent of spinal cord trauma and may help to determine prognosis for recovery.[121, 146]

SEP recorded from the trigeminal nerve have been reported to be abnormal in persons with MS-related trigeminal neuralgia and with parasellar and cerebellopontine angle tumors affecting the trigeminal nerve. Alterations of trigeminal SEP also relate well to successful treatment of trigeminal neuralgia by retrogasserian injection of glycerol and thermocoagulation-induced lesions. Trigeminal SEP generally have not been found useful in the diagnosis of "idiopathic" trigeminal neuralgia.[147–150]

Other uses of SEP are evaluation of spinal cord syndromes such as transverse myelitis, syringomyelia, and spinal cord ischemia, and of tumors, infarctions, and hemorrhages involving the somatosensory pathways of the brain stem and cortex.[74, 88, 121] Some neurodegenerative disorders, such as Huntington's chorea, and some neuropathies involving the central somatosensory pathways may also be associated with SEP abnormalities.[74, 88]

Cognitive Evoked Potentials

Cognitive EP, or endogenous event-related potentials, are long-latency EP related to cognitive processing. Testing consists of random presentations of infrequent stimuli (*rare* stimuli) interdispersed with different, more frequently occurring stimuli (*common* stimuli). The subject is instructed to attend to the infrequent stimuli only. Normal persons produce a P300 response with a latency of approximately 300 msec and positive polarity. The P300 response latency may be abnormally prolonged or reduced in amplitude in disorders that impair cognition, such as dementias, autism, schizophrenia, and Huntington's chorea.[74, 81, 88, 151–153]

SUMMARY

EMG and EP testing are essential tools in the diagnosis of neuromuscular disorders. They provide reliable and reproducible information on function of the nervous system that would not be obtainable through other means. They provide an extension of the clinical examination and are complementary to laboratory, radiologic, and other evaluations. Development of new techniques and improvements in old ones continue to expand the clinical utility of these tests. For example, the addition of transcranial magnetic stimulation has allowed evaluation of central motor pathways that had not been possible with EMG or other EP

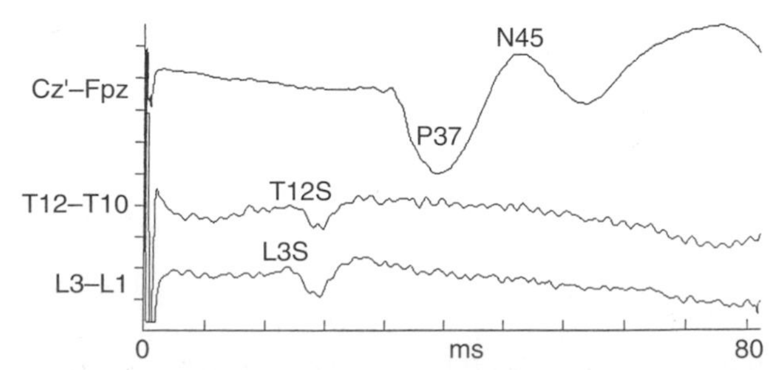

FIGURE 14–13 Normal lower extremity somatosensory evoked potential response obtained by stimulation of the tibial nerve at the ankle demonstrates responses recorded from the third lumbar vertebra (L3S), the twelfth thoracic vertebra (T12S), and the cortex (P37-N45).

testing. Further refinements in cognitive EP testing may allow greater understanding of the nature and complexity of cognitive processing. The clinical neurophysiology laboratory is an increasingly important part of the total clinical milieu. With this thought in mind, the prudent practitioner will find greater utility and put more reliance on these tests for evaluation of patients, now and in the future.

REFERENCES

1. Kimura J: Electrodiagnosis in Diseases of Nerve and Muscle: Principles and Practice. Philadelphia, FA Davis, 1983.
2. Brown WF: The Physiological and Technical Basis of Electromyography. Boston, Butterworth, 1984.
3. Oh SJ: Clinical Electromyography: Nerve Conduction Techniques, ed 2. Baltimore, Williams & Wilkins, 1993.
4. Brown WF: Negative symptoms and signs of peripheral nerve disease. *In* Brown WF, Bolton CF (eds): Clinical Electromyography, ed 2. Boston, Butterworth-Heinemann, 1993.
5. Guidelines in Electrodiagnostic Medicine. Muscle Nerve, Supplement 8, 1999.
6. Sivak M, Ochoa J, Fernandez JM: Positive manifestations of nerve fiber dysfunction: Clinical, electrophysiologic, and pathologic correlates. *In* Brown WF, Bolton CF (eds): Clinical Electromyography, ed 2. Boston, Butterworth-Heinemann, 1993.
7. Johnson EW: The EMG examination. *In* Johnson EW (ed): Practical Electromyography, ed 2. Baltimore, Williams & Wilkins, 1988.
8. Adams RD, Victor M: Principles of Neurology, ed 5. St Louis, McGraw-Hill, 1993.
9. Chu-Andrews J, Johnson RJ: Electrodiagnosis: An Anatomical and Clinical Approach. Philadelphia, JB Lippincott, 1986.
10. Ball RD: Basics of needle electromyography: An AAEE workshop. Rochester, Minn, American Association of Electromyography and Electrodiagnosis, 1985.
11. Daube JR: Clinical Neurophysiology. Philadelphia, FA Davis, 1996.
12. Litchy WJ: Needle examination in electromyography. *In* AAEE Course B: Practical EMG. American Association of Electromyography and Electrodiagnosis 10th Annual Continuing Education Course, San Antonio, Oct 15, 1987, pp 7–17.
13. Wilbourn AJ, Aminoff MJ: Radiculopathies. *In* Brown WF, Bolton CF (eds): Clinical Electromyography, ed 2. Boston, Butterworth-Heinemann, 1993.
14. Wiechers DO: Motor unit potentials in disease. *In* Johnson EW (ed): Practical Electromyography, ed 2. Baltimore, Williams & Wilkins, 1988.
15. Wiechers DO: Normal and abnormal motor unit potentials. *In* Johnson EW (ed): Practical Electromyography, ed 2. Baltimore, Williams & Wilkins, 1988.
16. Jablecki C: Physiologic basis of electromyographic activity. *In* AAEE Course C: Standard Needle Electromyography of Muscles. American Association of Electromyography and Electrodiagnosis 11th Annual Continuing Education Course, San Diego, Oct 6, 1988, pp 15–21.
17. Dumitru D: Electrodiagnostic Medicine. St. Louis, Mosby–Year Book, 1995.
18. Stalberg E, Falck B: The role of electromyography in neurology. Electroenceph Clin Neurophysiol 103:579–598, 1997.
19. Wilbourn AJ, Levin KH: Ischemic neuropathy. *In* Brown WF, Bolton CF (eds): Clinical Electromyography, ed 2. Boston, Butterworth-Heinemann, 1993.
20. Jablecki CK: Myopathies. *In* Brown WF, Bolton CF (eds): Clinical Electromyography, ed 2. Boston, Butterworth-Heinemann, 1993.
21. Weber RJ: Motor and sensory conduction and entrapment syndromes. *In* Johnson EW (ed): Practical Electromyography, ed 2. Baltimore, Williams & Wilkins, 1988.
22. Kimura J: Basic nerve conduction studies. *In* AAEE Course A: Fundamentals of EMG. American Association of Electromyography and Electrodiagnosis. 7th Annual Continuing Education Course, Kansas City, Mo, Sept 19–29, 1984. pp 7–15.
23. DeLisa JA: Basic motor and sensory nerve conduction. *In* AAEE Course A: Basic Nerve Conduction and Electromyography. American Association of Electromyography and Electrodiagnosis, 9th Annual Continuing Education Course, Boston, Sept 24, 1986, pp 19–29.
24. Albers JW: Principles of defining the location and severity of focal peripheral nerve lesions. *In* AAEE Course A: Basic Electrophysiologic Testing in Mononeuropathy. American Association of Electromyography and Electrodiagnosis 8th Annual Continuing Education Course, Las Vegas, Oct 24, 1985, pp 7–16.
25. Kimura J, Shivapour E: The Carpal Tunnel Syndrome. AAEE Case Report #2. Rochester, Minn, American Association of Electromyography and Electrodiagnosis, undated.
26. Kincaid JC: The Electrodiagnosis of Ulnar Neuropathy at the Elbow. AAEE Minimonograph #31. Rochester, Minn, American Association of Electromyography and Electrodiagnosis, 1988.
27. Donofrio PD, Albers JW: Polyneuropathy: Classification by Nerve Conduction Studies and Electromyography. AAEM Minimonograph #34. Rochester, Minn, American Association of Electrodiagnostic Medicine, 1990.
28. Kraft GH, Johnson EW: Proximal Motor Nerve Conduction and Late Responses: An AAEE Workshop. Rochester, Minn, American Association of Electromyography and Electrodiagnosis, Sept 1986.
29. Wilbourn AJ, Aminoff MJ: The Electrophysiologic Examination in Patients with Radiculopathies. AAEE Minimonograph #32. Rochester, Minn, American Association of Electromyography and Electrodiagnosis, 1988.
30. MacLean IC: Spinal nerve stimulation. *In* AAEE Course B: Nerve Conduction Studies—A Review. American Association of Electromyography and Electrodiagnosis 11th Annual Continuing Education Course, San Diego, Oct 6, 1988, pp 27–35.
31. Miller T, Pardo R, Yaworski R: Clinical utility of reflex studies in assessing cervical radiculopathy. Muscle Nerve 22:1075–1079, 1999.
32. Johnson EW: Electrodiagnosis of radiculopathy. *In* Johnson EW (ed): Practical Electromyography, ed 2. Baltimore, Williams & Wilkins, 1988.
33. Keesey JC: Electrodiagnostic approach to defects of neuromuscular transmission. AAEM Minimonograph #33. Rochester, Minn, American Association of Electrodiagnostic Medicine, 1989.
34. Jablecki CK: Myasthenia Gravis. AAEM Case Report #3. Rochester, Minn, American Association of Electrodiagnostic Medicine, 1991.
35. Rivner MH, Swift TR: Electrical testing in disorders of neuromuscular transmission. *In* Brown WF, Bolton CF (eds): Clinical Electromyography, ed 2. Boston, Butterworth-Heinemann, 1993.
36. Pickett JB: Botulism. AAEE Case Report #16. Rochester, Minn, American Association of Electromyography and Electrodiagnosis, 1988.
37. Dawson D, Hallett M, Millender LH: Entrapment Neuropathies, ed 3. Philadelphia, Lippincott-Raven, 1999.
38. Nardin R, Patel M, Gudas T, et al: Electromyography and magnetic resonance imaging in the evaluation of radiculopathy. Muscle Nerve 22:151–155, 1999.
39. Komori T, Brown WF: Central electromyography. *In* Brown WF, Bolton CF (eds): Clinical Electromyography, ed 2. Boston, Butterworth-Heinemann, 1993.
40. Kimura J, DeLisa JA, Hallett M: Cranial Nerve Testing: An AAEE Workshop. Rochester, Minn, American Association of Electromyography and Electrodiagnosis, May 1984.
41. Ongerboer de Visser BW, Cruccu G: Neurophysiologic examination of the trigeminal, facial, hypoglossal, and spinal accessory nerves in cranial neuropathies and brain stem disorders. *In* Brown WF, Bolton CF (eds): Clinical Electromyography, ed 2. Boston, Butterworth-Heinemann, 1993.
42. Eisen A, McComas AJ: Motor neuron disorders. *In* Brown WF, Bolton CF (eds): Clinical Electromyography, ed 2. Boston, Butterworth-Heinemann, 1993.
43. Stewart J: Focal peripheral neuropathies, ed 3. Philadelphia, JB Lippincott, 2000.
44. Preston DC, Kelly JJ: Atypical motor neuron disease. *In* Brown WF, Bolton CF (eds): Clinical Electromyography, ed 2. Boston, Butterworth-Heinemann, 1993.
45. Daube JR: EMG in Motor Neuron Diseases. AAEE Minimonograph #18. Rochester, Minn, American Association of Electromyography and Electrodiagnosis, 1982.
46. Lange DJ: Neuromuscular Diseases Associated with HIV-1 Infection. AAEM Minimonograph #41. Rochester, Minn, American Association of Electrodiagnostic Medicine, 1994.

47. Cioni R, Giannini F, Passero S, et al: An electromyographic evaluation of motor complications in thoracic herpes zoster. Electromyogr Clin Neurophysiol 34:125–128, 1994.
48. Johnson EW: Electrodiagnosis of radiculopathy. *In* Course B: Advanced Concepts in Evaluating Focal Neuropathies. American Association of Electromyography and Electrodiagnosis 8th Annual Continuing Education Course, Las Vegas, Oct 24, 1985, pp 19–24.
49. Pezzin L, Dillingham T, Lauder T, et al: Cervical radiculopathies: Relationships between symptom duration and spontaneous EMG activity. Muscle Nerve 22:1412–1418, 1999.
50. Eisen AA: The electrodiagnosis of plexopathies. *In* Brown WF, Bolton CF (eds): Clinical Electromyography, ed 2. Boston, Butterworth-Heinemann, 1993.
51. Subramony SH: Neuralgic Amyotrophy (Acute Brachial Neuropathy). AAEE case report #14. Rochester, Minn, American Association of Electromyography and Electrodiagnosis, 1988.
52. Felice K, Butler K, Druckemiller W: Cervical root stimulation in a case of classic neurogenic thoracic outlet syndrome. Muscle Nerve 22:1287–1292, 1999.
53. Berry H: Traumatic peripheral nerve lesions. *In* Brown WF, Bolton CF (eds): Clinical Electromyography, ed 2. Boston, Butterworth-Heinemann, 1993.
54. Bolton CF: Metabolic neuropathy. *In* Brown WF, Bolton CF (eds): Clinical Electromyography, ed 2. Boston, Butterworth-Heinemann, 1993.
55. Kraft GH: Peripheral neuropathies. *In* Johnson EW (ed): Practical Electromyography, ed 2. Baltimore, Williams & Wilkins, 1988.
56. Brown WF: Acute and chronic inflammatory demyelinating neuropathies. *In* Brown WF, Bolton CF (eds): Clinical Electromyography, ed 2. Boston, Butterworth-Heinemann, 1993.
57. Nielsen VK: Toxic neuropathies. *In* Brown WF, Bolton CF (eds): Clinical Electromyography, ed 2. Boston, Butterworth-Heinemann, 1993.
58. Golovchinsky V: Double crush syndrome in lower extremities. Electromyography Clin Neurophysiol 38:1115–1120, 1998.
59. Johnson E: Double crush syndrome: A definition in search of a cause. J Phys Med Rehab 76:439, 1997.
60. Richardson J, Forman G, Riley B: An electrophysiologic exploration of the double crush syndrome. Muscle Nerve 22:71–77, 1999.
61. Wilbourn AJ: Diabetic neuropathies. *In* Brown WF, Bolton CF (eds): Clinical Electromyography, ed 2. Boston, Butterworth-Heinemann, 1993.
62. Chokroverty S: Diabetic Amyotrophy. AAEE Case Report #13. Rochester, Minn, American Association of Electromyography and Electrodiagnosis, 1987.
63. Sander H, Quinto C, Saadeh P, et al: Sensitive median-ulnar motor comparative techniques in carpal tunnel syndrome. Muscle Nerve 22:88–98, 1999.
64. Kimura J: Median nerve. *In* Brown WF, Bolton CF (eds): Clinical Electromyography, ed 2. Boston, Butterworth-Heinemann, 1993.
65. Stevens JC: The electrodiagnosis of carpal tunnel syndrome. *In* Course A: Basic Electrophysiologic Testing in Mononeuropathy. American Association of Electromyography and Electrodiagnosis 8th Annual Continuing Education Course, Las Vegas, Oct 24, 1985, pp 17–26.
66. Liveson JA, Ma DM: Laboratory Reference for Clinical Neurophysiology. Philadelphia, FA Davis, 1992.
67. Keesey JC: Electrodiagnostic approach to defects of neuromuscular transmission. *In* Course B: Practical EMG. American Association of Electromyography and Electrodiagnosis 10th Annual Continuing Education Course, San Antonio, Oct 15, 1987, pp 23–34.
68. Hulley WC: Paraneoplastic syndromes: Their EMG features. *In* Course C: Neuromuscular Complications of Cancer. American Association of Electromyography and Electrodiagnosis 8th Annual Continuing Education Course, Las Vegas, Oct 24, 1985, pp 27–35.
69. Robinson LR: Polymyositis. AAEM case report #22. Rochester, Minn, American Association of Electrodiagnostic Medicine, 1991.
70. Gilroy J: Basic Neurology, ed 2. New York, Pergamon Press, 1990.
71. Pascual-Leone A, Meador K: Is transcranial magnetic stimulation coming of age? J Clin Neurophysiol 15:285–287, 1998.
72. Zwarts M: Magnetic stimulation of the peripheral nervous system: Local versus generalized disorders. Electromyogr Clin Neurophysiol 38:309–316, 1998.
73. Tavy D, Franssen H, Keunen R, et al: Motor and somatosensory evoked potentials in asymptomatic spondylotic cord compression. Muscle Nerve 22:628–634, 1999.
74. Chiappa KH: Evoked Potentials in Clinical Medicine, ed 2. New York, Raven, 1990.
75. Barker AT: Basic principles of magnetic stimulation of the central and peripheral nervous system. Presented at American Electroencephalographic Society and American Association of Electromyography and Electrodiagnosis Joint Symposium on Somatosensory Evoked Potentials and Magnetic Stimulation, San Diego, Oct 5, 1988, pp 25–30.
76. Chiappa KH: Transcranial motor evoked potentials. Electromyogr Clin Neurophysiol 34:15–21, 1994.
77. Eisen AA, Shtybel W: Clinical experience with transcranial magnetic stimulation. AAEM Minimonograph #35. Rochester, Minn, American Association of Electrodiagnostic Medicine, 1990.
78. Tavy DLJ, Wagner GL, Keunen RWM, et al: Transcranial magnetic stimulation in patients with cervical spondylotic myelopathy: Clinical and radiological correlations. Muscle Nerve 17:235–241, 1994.
79. Daube JR: Selected applications of magnetic stimulation. Presented at American Electroencephalographic Society and American Association of Electromyography and Electrodiagnosis Joint Symposium on Somatosensory Evoked Potentials and Magnetic Stimulation, San Diego, Oct 5, 1988, pp 31–35.
80. Nuwer MR: Evoked Potential Monitoring in the Operating Room. New York, Raven Press, 1986.
81. Waldman HJ: Evoked potentials. *In* Raj PP (ed): Practical Management of Pain, ed 2. St. Louis, Mosby–Year Book, 1992.
82. Nuwer M: Fundamentals of evoked potentials and common clinical applications today. Electroencephalog Clin Neurophysiol 106:142–148, 1998.
83. Starr A: Natural forms of somatosensory stimulation that can evoke cerebral, spinal, and peripheral nerve potentials in man. Presented at American Association of Electromyography and Electrodiagnosis International Symposium on Somatosensory Evoked Potentials, Rochester, Minn, 1984.
84. Braddom R: Somatosensory, brainstem, and visual evoked potentials. *In* Johnson EW (ed): Practical Electromyography, ed 2. Baltimore, Williams & Wilkins, 1988.
85. Celesia G: Somatosensory evoked potentials: Nomenclature. Presented at American Association of Electromyography and Electrodiagnosis International Symposium on Somatosensory Evoked Potentials, Rochester, Minn, 1984.
86. American Electroencephalography Society Clinical Evoked Potential Guidelines. J Clin Neurophysiol 1:6–62, 1984.
87. Guidelines for Somatosensory Evoked Potentials. Rochester, MN, American Association of Electromyography and Electrodiagnosis, 1984.
88. Spehlmann R: Evoked Potential Primer. Boston, Butterworth, 1988.
89. Jasper HH: The ten-twenty electrode system of the International Federation: Report of the Committee on Clinical Examination in Electroencephalography. Electroencephalogr Clin Neurophysiol 10:371–375, 1958.
90. Chiappa K, Ropper A: Evoked potentials in clinical medicine: Part I. N Engl J Med 306:1140–1150, 1982.
91. Halliday A: Visual evoked responses in the diagnosis of multiple sclerosis. Br Med J 4:661–664, 1973.
92. Halliday A: Visual evoked potentials in demyelinating disease. *In* Waxman S, Ritchie J (eds): Demyelinating Disease: Basic and Clinical Electrophysiology. New York, Raven, 1981.
93. Hume AL, Waxman SG: Evoked potentials in suspected multiple sclerosis: Diagnostic value and prediction of clinical course. J Neurol Sci 83:191–210, 1988.
94. Aminoff M: The Clinical Role of Somatosensory Evoked Potential Studies: A Critical Appraisal. AAEE Minimonograph #22. Rochester, Minn, American Association of Electromyography and Electrodiagnosis, 1984.
95. Chiappa K, Ropper A: Evoked potentials in clinical medicine: Part II. N Engl J Med 306:1205–1211, 1982.
96. Halliday A, Mushin J: The visual evoked potential in neuroophthalmology. Int Ophthalmol Clin 20:155–183, 1980.
97. Halliday A, Halliday E, Kriss A, et al: The pattern-evoked potential in compression of the anterior visual pathways. Brain 99:357–374, 1976.
98. Ikeda H, Tremain K, Sanders M: Neurophysiological investigation in optic nerve disease: Combined assessment of the visual evoked response and electroretinogram. Br J Opthalmol 62:227–239, 1978.

99. Marsters JB, Good PA, Mortimer MJ: A diagnostic test for migraine using the visual evoked potential. Headache Sept:526–530, 1988.
100. Muller-Jensen A, Zschocke S: Pattern-induced visual evoked response in patients with migraine accompagnée. Electroencephalogr Clin Neurophysiol 50:37, 1980.
101. Polich J, Maung A, Dalessio D: Pattern-shift visual evoked responses in cluster headache. Headache Sept:446–451, 1987.
102. Raudino F: Visual evoked potential in patients with migraine. Headache 28:531–532, 1988.
103. Afra J, Cecchini P, Pasqua V, et al: Visual evoked potentials during long periods of pattern-reversal stimulation in migraine. Brain 121:233–241, 1998.
104. Hood L, Berlin C: Auditory Evoked Potentials. Austin, Tx, Pro-Ed, 1986.
105. Hammond S, Yiannikas C: The relevance of contralateral recordings and patient disability to assessment of brainstem auditory evoked potential abnormalities in multiple sclerosis. Arch Neurol 44:382–387, 1987.
106. Donohoe C: Application of the brainstem auditory evoked response in clinical neurologic practice. *In* Owen J, Donohoe C (eds): Clinical Atlas of Auditory Evoked Potentials. New York, Grune & Stratton, 1988.
107. Kirshner HS, Tsai SI, Runge VM, et al: Magnetic resonance imaging and other techniques in the diagnosis of multiple sclerosis. Arch Neurol 42:859–863, 1985.
108. Deka R, Kacker S, Tandon P: Auditory brainstem evoked responses in cerebellopontine angle tumors. Arch Otolaryngol Head Neck Surg 113:11647–11650, 1987.
109. Musiek F, Josey A, Glasscock M: Auditory brain-stem response in patients with acoustic neuromas. Arch Otolaryngol Head Neck Surg 112:186–189, 1986.
110. Facco E, Behr A, Munari M, et al: Auditory and somatosensory evoked potentials in coma following spontaneous cerebral hemorrhage: Early prognosis and outcome. Electroencephalog Clin Neurophysiol 107:332–338, 1998.
111. Newton P, Greenberg R: Evoked potentials in severe head injury. J Trauma 24:61–65, 1984.
112. Stone J, Ghaly R, Hughes J: Evoked potentials in head injury and states of increased intracranial pressure. J Clin Neurophysiol 5:135–160, 1988.
113. Chiappa K, Hill R: Evaluation and prognostication in coma. Electroencephalogr Clin Neurophysiol 106:149–155, 1998.
114. Jewett D: Auditory evoked potentials: Overview of the field. *In* Barber C, Blum T (eds): Evoked Potentials III. Boston, Butterworth, 1987.
115. Drake M: Brainstem auditory-evoked potentials in spasmodic torticollis. Arch Neurol 45:174–175, 1988.
116. Yamada T, Dickins Q, Arensdorg K, et al: Basilar migraine: Polarity-dependent alteration of brainstem auditory evoked potentials. Neurology 36:1256–1260, 1986.
117. Jerger J, Oliver T, Stack B: ABR testing strategies. *In* Jacobson J (ed): The Auditory Brainstem Response. San Diego, College Hill Press, 1984.
118. Aminoff M, Eisen A: Somatosensory evoked potentials. AAEM Minimonograph 19. Muscle Nerve 21:277–290, 1998.
119. Assessment: Dermatomal somatosensory evoked potentials. Neurology 49:1127–1130, 1997.
120. Jones S: Clinical applications of somatosensory evoked potentials: Peripheral nervous system. Presented at American Association of Electromyography and Electrodiagnosis International Symposium on Somatosensory Evoked Potentials, Rochester, Minn, 1984.
121. Oken B, Chiappa K: Somatosensory evoked potentials in neurological diagnosis. *In* Bodin-Wollner I, Cracco RQ (eds): Evoked Potentials: Frontiers of Clinical Neurophysiology. New York, Alan R Liss, 1986.
122. Eisen A: SEP in the evaluation of disorders of the peripheral nervous system. *In* Cracco R, Bodis-Wollner I (eds): Evoked Potentials. New York, Alan R Liss, 1986.
123. Aminoff M: Use of somatosensory evoked potentials to evaluate the peripheral nervous system. J Clin Neurophysiol 4:135–144, 1987.
124. Yiannikas C, Shahani B, Young R. The investigation of traumatic lesions of the brachial plexus by electromyography and short latency somatosensory evoked potentials evoked by stimulation of multiple peripheral nerves. J Neurol Neurosurg Psychiatry 46:1014–1022, 1983.
125. Machleder H, Moll F, Nuwer M, et al: Somatosensory evoked potentials in the assessment of thoracic outlet compression syndrome. J Vasc Surg 6:177–184, 1987.
126. Oh SJ: Clinical Electromyography: Nerve Conduction Studies. Baltimore, University Park Press, 1984.
127. Synek V: Diagnostic importance of somatosensory evoked potentials in the diagnosis of thoracic outlet syndrome. Clin Electroencephalogr 17:112–116, 1986.
128. Yiannikas C, Walsh J: Somatosensory evoked responses in the diagnosis of thoracic outlet syndrome. J Neurol Neurosurg Psychiatry 46:234–240, 1983.
129. Cakmur R, Idiman F, Akalin E, et al: Dermatomal and mixed nerve somatosensory evoked potentials in the diagnosis of neurogenic thoracic outlet syndrome. Electroencephalogr Clin Neurophysiol 108:423–434, 1998.
130. Aminoff M, Goodin D, Parry G, et al: Electrophysiologic evaluation of lumbosacral radiculopathies: Electromyography, late responses, and somatosensory evoked potentials. Neurology 35:1514–1518, 1985.
131. Perlik S, Fisher M, Patel D, et al: On the usefulness of somatosensory evoked responses for the evaluation of lower back pain. Arch Neurol 43:907–913, 1986.
132. Aminoff M, Goodin D, Barbaro N, et al: Dermatomal somatosensory evoked potentials in unilateral lumbosacral radiculopathy. Ann Neurol 17:171–176, 1985.
133. Katifi H, Sedgwick E: Dermatomal somatosensory evoked potentials in lumbosacral disk disease: Diagnosis and results of treatment. *In* Barber C, Blum T (eds): Evoked Potentials III. Boston, Butterworth, 1987.
134. Katifi H, Sedgwick E: Evaluation of the dermatomal somatosensory evoked potential in the diagnosis of lumbosacral root compression. J Neurol Neurosurg Psychiatry 50:1204–1210, 1987.
135. Eisen A, Hoirch M, Moll A: Evaluation of radiculopathies by segmental stimulation and somatosensory evoked potentials. Can J Neurol Sci 10:178–182, 1983.
136. Machida M, Asai T, Sato K, et al: New approach for diagnosis in herniated lumbosacral disc. Spine 11:380–384, 1985.
137. Rodriguez A, Kanis L, Rodriguez AA, et al: Somatosensory evoked potentials from dermatomal stimulation as an indicator of L5 and S1 radiculopathies. Arch Phys Med Rehabil 6.366–368, 1987.
138. Scarff R, Dallmann D, Roleikis J: Dermatomal somatosensory evoked potentials in the diagnosis of lumbosacral root entrapment. Surg Forum 32:489–491, 1981.
139. Schmid U, Hess C, Ludin H: Somatosensory evoked potentials following nerve and segmental stimulation do not confirm cervical radiculopathy with sensory deficit. J Neurol Neurosurg Psychiatry 51:182–187, 1988.
140. Seyal M, Palma G, Sandhu L, et al: Spinal somatosensory evoked potentials following segmental sensory stimulation: A direct measure of dorsal root function. Electroencephalogr Clin Neurophysiol 69: 390–393, 1988.
141. Yazicioglu K, Ozgul A, Kalyon T, et al: The diagnostic value of dermatomal somatosensory evoked potentials in lumbosacral disc herniations: A critical approach. Electromyogr Clin Neurophysiol 39:175–181, 1999.
142. Stolov W, Slimp J: Dermatomal somatosensory evoked potentials in lumbar spinal stenosis. Presented at American Association of Electromyography and Electrodiagnosis/American Electroencephalographic Society Joint Symposium of Somatosensory Evoked Potentials and Magnetic Stimulation, Rochester, Minn, 1988.
143. Yiannikas C, Shahani B, Young R: Short-latency somatosensory evoked potentials from radial, median, ulnar, and perioneal nerve stimulation in the assessment of cervical spondylosis. Arch Neurol 43:1264–1271, 1986.
144. Yu U, Jones S: Somatosensory evoked potentials in cervical spondylosis. Brain 108:273–300, 1985.
145. Noordhout A, Myressiotis S, Delvaux V, et al: Motor and somatosensory evoked potentials in cervical spondylotic myelopathy. Electroencephalogr Clin Neurophysiol 108:24–31, 1998.
146. Toleikis J, Sloan T: Comparison of major nerve and dermatomal somatosensory evoked potentials in the evaluation of patients with spinal cord injury. *In* Barber C, Blum T (eds): Evoked Potentials III. Boston, Butterworth, 1987.
147. Chiappa K: Clinical applications of short latency somatosensory

evoked potentials to central nervous system disease. Presented at American Association of Electromyography and Electrodiagnosis International Symposium on Somatosensory Evoked Potentials, Rochester, Minn, 1984.

148. Buettner U, Rieble S, Altenmuller E, et al: Trigeminal somatosensory evoked potentials in patients with lesions of the mandibular branches of the trigeminal nerve. *In* Barber C, Blum T (eds): Evoked Potentials III. Boston, Butterworth, 1987.
149. Iraguy V, Wiederholt W, Romine J: Evoked potentials in trigeminal neuralgia associated with multiple sclerosis. Arch Neurol 43:444–446, 1986.
150. Leandri M, Parodi C, Favala E: Early trigeminal evoked potentials in tumors of the base of the skull and trigeminal neuralgia. Electroencephalogr Clin Neurophysiol 71:114–124, 1988.
151. McCallum WC: Some recent developments in ERP research related to cognitive function. *In* Barber C, Blum T (eds): Evoked Potentials III. Boston, Butterworth, 1987.
152. Polich J: P300 clinical utility and control of variability. J Clin Neurophysiol 15:14–33, 1998.
153. Keren O, Ben-Dror S, Stern M, et al: Event-related potentials as an index of cognitive function during recovery from severe closed head injury. J Head Trauma Rehabil 13:15–30, 1998.

CHAPTER • 15

Psychological Evaluation of the Patient in Pain

Donald W. Hinnant, PhD • C. David Tollison, PhD

It has long been recognized that the perception, intensity, and reaction to pain, as subjective phenomena, are influenced by a variety of factors other than tissue damage or organic dysfunction. Pain intensity, reactions, suffering, and overt pain behaviors are thought to be subject to a variety of influences, including personality variables, attention, sociologic and cultural variables, litigation and financial considerations, psychological state, biochemical profile, environmental contingencies, and others.[1]

The gate control theory of Melzack and Wall emphasizes the importance of including assessment of the motivational-affective, sensory-discriminative, and cognitive-evaluative processes in the comprehensive evaluation of the patient in pain. Our awareness of multiple pathways and the effects of interacting systems on nociceptive impulses at the level of spinal integration has been confirmed. We know that the transmission of pain impulses may be inhibited by peripheral large fiber impulses. Similarly, neurotransmitters, including neuropeptides and serotoninergic mechanisms, have been discovered that are capable of inhibiting the perception of painful sensation. Higher cortical processes are known to modify the meaning of an emotional reaction to nociceptive stimulation. Related research demonstrates varying correspondence between the subjective experience of pain and the physiologic functions involved in the somatosensory cortex, the limbic system, and the frontal lobes. As clinicians, we are often confronted with the conspicuous finding that no simple correlation exists between the extent of tissue damage and the level of suffering expressed by the patient. Thus, recognition of emotional variables, particularly dysfunctional ones, in the causation, maintenance, exacerbation, and disability of pain has promoted the "psychology of pain" to a level of scientific and clinical prominence equal to that of sensory-physiologic models and treatments.

Although there is little consensus and even less empirical basis for choosing an appropriate psychological instrument for pain assessment, it is accepted that evaluation of pain is facilitated by a combination of measures. Thus, the psychological evaluation of a person in pain may comprise a variety of behavioral, observational, and assessment devices. It is our opinion that combined behavioral and physical assessment improves identification of multiple factors that influence pain perception and diagnostic accuracy. It is recommended that the pain physician have available both biologic and psychological data for simultaneous weighing, evaluation, diagnosis, and treatment.

Our purpose in this chapter is to outline current assessment techniques and provide an overview of a variety of methods for assessing pain and its psychological correlates. There is considerable overlap among the many available assessment devices, and clinicians are confronted with the task of selecting pain instruments appropriate to the particular patient. Formal psychological testing is usually helpful but may not always be indicated, depending on the patient's status and the treatment setting. An overview and description of several of the most current and commonly utilized assessment instruments and psychological tests are offered later in this chapter.

PURPOSE

Psychological evaluation of the patient in pain is considered standard protocol in the majority of pain centers and clinical practices today. Guidelines for cancer pain assessment and pain control, which include psychological assessment, have been developed and published by the U. S. Agency for Health Care Policy and Research[2] and the American Pain Society.[3] A presurgical psychological evaluation of candidates for implantation of a spinal cord stimulator or morphine pump is required by Medicare. A growing number of spine surgeons routinely obtain psychological evaluations of patients before surgery. In addition, psychological evaluation is a required component of pain treatment centers accredited by the Commission on Accreditation of Rehabilitation Facilities (CARF).[4]

The primary goal of psychological evaluation of a patient in pain is to identify emotional and behavioral factors that may be complicating or perpetuating the clinical pain presentation. As evaluation is often requested when the pain patient's symptoms or subjective reports of pain are disproportionate to the physical findings. A psychological evaluation may also be helpful when a patient is "overusing" the healthcare system, "doctor shops," pursues additional diagnoses, fails to respond to appropriate treatments, or suffers an obvious psychological disturbance or exhibits unusual behavior. Other indications include ineffective coping mechanisms, tendency toward drug abuse or dependence, and motivational problems.

Unfortunately, a psychological evaluation is occasionally requested by a physician who wonders whether a patient's pain and related symptoms are *functional* or *organic*. It is important to recognize that physical and psychological symptoms are not mutually exclusive. Furthermore, it is good to avoid diagnostic labels such as hysterical, hypochondrical, and functional. Psychogenic pain is recognized to be relatively rare in the general population, and such labels may potentiate confusion and inappropriate treatment protocols. We recommend an evaluation that addresses abnormal "illness behavior" as well as emotional, cognitive, and behavioral factors that provide useful information and assist in developing effective treatment. An appropriate question that should be answered by psychological testing and evaluation is, How likely is a patient to respond favorably to intervention, whether surgical, medical, or psychological? The functional-versus-organic dichotomy is essentially meaningless.[5]

An important question is, When should referral for psychological evaluation be made? Often, psychological referral of the patient in pain is delayed until the physician believes that all traditional, and sometimes nontraditional methods for pain control have been exhausted and, therefore, that psychological factors *must* be involved and be perpetuating the patient's complaints. Even physicians who specialize in pain management do not always recognize behavioral and psychological symptoms and, consequently, fail to make appropriate referrals for evaluation and psychological treatment in conjunction with physical interventions. It is now well-recognized that delayed delivery of appropriate treatment results in exorbitant and unnecessary costs to society through additional compensation payments and medical costs. Delays in psychological referral and treatment place the acute pain patient at high risk for long-term disability and associated personal and financial costs. In addition, comorbid problems such as major depression, family stress, legal involvement, and secondary physical and psychological symptoms can lead to chronic symptoms that are sometimes refractory to any type of intervention. For example, research has demonstrated that prolonged low back pain is associated with a high risk of clinical depression. Although this association may be predicted by the experienced pain practitioner, estimates of depression in clinical back pain patient samples are surprisingly high (30% to 74%).[5]

Yet, despite its morbidity, even when diagnosed, often, major depression is not recognized as a legitimate complication of pain and treatment is not approved by insurance carriers or managed care programs. Many algorithms for evaluation of the patient in pain, including the need for timely referrals for specific consultations, have been developed and are applicable for various types of pain and patient populations.

PSYCHOLOGICAL RISK FACTORS FOR PATIENTS IN PAIN

Although it is widely accepted that psychological factors play a role in medical syndromes and painful conditions, findings from a number of studies suggest that common mental disorders are often overlooked in the diagnosis and treatment of pain syndromes. One study published in the *Journal of the American Medical Association*[6] evaluated approximately 26,000 subjects from 14 countries and concluded that psychological factors were more closely associated than medical factors with patient-reported physical disability. The most common psychosocial and psychological factors found to be related to persistent pain are job dissatisfaction,[7] hysteria, antisocial personality, workers' compensation, childhood trauma, anger, and somatization disorders.[8]

Personality Disorders

According to the *Diagnostic and Statistical Manual of Mental Disorders*, 4th edition (DSM IV, 1994),[9] a personality disorder is defined as "an enduring pattern of inner experience and behavior that deviates markedly from the expectations of the individual's culture, is pervasive and inflexible, has an onset in adolescence or early adulthood, is stable over time, and leads to distress or impairment" (p. 629). Kinney and coworkers[10] described a well-designed study in which 60% of their sample of chronic pain patients met the diagnostic criteria for personality disorder. Most prevalent of the characterologic disorders were paranoid, passive-aggressive, avoidant, and borderline disorders. Although personality disorders are marked by long-standing behavioral characteristics that predate an injury or development of a pain syndrome, such disorders are particularly influential in a patient's response to pain management and rehabilitation. A significant number of persons with dependent or obsessive-compulsive personality are particularly difficult to treat owing to their anxious/fearful coping style. They tend to engage in a cycle of avoidance and inactivity, thus increasing their pain and the likelihood of developing a chronic pain syndrome. Obviously, someone with antisocial personality will demonstrate impulsive, erratic, and aggressive behavior, and the clinician should carefully monitor for potential drug abuse. Failure to comply with treatment is common. In addition, a patient with antisocial personality often has a negative influence on other pain patients in rehabilitation settings. Characteristics for several of the more common personality types are listed in Table 15–1.

The Somatoform Disorders

It has been estimated that as many as 75% of all visits to primary care providers involve manifestations of psychosocial problems in physical complaints.[11] The primary features of the somatoform disorders are physical symptoms that suggest a medical condition that cannot be fully explained by organic findings or known physiologic mechanisms. Although the symptoms of somatoform disorders

TABLE 15–1 Common Personality Types

The Dependent, Avoidant, Fearful Patient
- History of anxiety, evidence of high emotional arousal and fear
- Evidence of clinical anxiety and nervousness, including hypervigilance, motor tension, pressured speech, and impatience
- Excessive dependence on physicians or other clinicians for continued guidance and support
- Tendencies toward obsessive-compulsive behaviors such as persistent focus on diagnostic test results, medications, or, in some case, overworking and persistent anxiety about underachievement
- Unfounded resistance to the use of medications or particular combinations of medications
- History of activity that has been powerfully reinforcing
- Tendencies toward impulsive behavior and, possibly, denial of bodily needs, proper rest, and nutrition
- These persons may be more open to acknowledging the role of psychological influences in their pain.

The Dramatic, Borderline, or Histrionic Patient
- Few or no objective organic findings to explain pain
- Often a female with a long history of problems with relationships
- Overly dramatic and excitable, labile emotions, persistent changes in emotional reactions
- Possible attention-seeking behaviors such as exaggerated statements of pain and other physical problems
- Tendencies to demonstrate helplessness
- Tendencies toward numerous phone calls to the physician, personal crises, and negative responses to treatment or interventions
- Tendency to "doctor shop"

The Antisocial/Sociopathic Patient
- Usually, little objective organic evidence for pain
- Probable history of multiple injuries or claims
- History of "doctor shopping" or demands for changing physicians
- Frequent negative comments about prior treatment or physicians, case managers, or treatments rendered
- History of substance abuse, problems with legal system
- History of family problems
- Tendency to demonstrate distrust and negative reactions toward those who have offered treatment or recommended treatment
- Exaggerated pain response to interventions
- History of violent or aggressive behavior, particularly reckless behavior with denial of responsibility for consequences
- Tendency to convince the physician that "down time," rest, or other passive activity is reinforcing
- Indirect or direct evidence of a history of malingering or manipulation of the healthcare system

are physical, there is usually some evidence of a significant psychological influence. It is important, however, to note that the production of physical symptoms and complaints is not a conscious and intentional act on the part of the patient. The DSM IV includes seven categories of somatoform disorders, four of which are commonly encountered by those who evaluate and treat patients in pain.

Patients with *somatization disorder*, which, historically, has been referred to as hysteria or 'Briquet's syndrome,' report recurrent and multiple somatic complaints for which medical attention has been repeatedly sought. Symptoms typically have no clear relationship to any physical or medical disease. This disorder appears before age 30 and extends over a period of years. Typically, there is a combination of pain, gastrointestinal symptoms, sexual dysfunction, and vague neurologic complaints. Anxiety and affective symptoms are associated features. Differential diagnosis is often difficult: Usually, it is necessary to rule out physical disorders that are charactized by vague, multiple, and confusing clinical features, such as myofascial and neurologic disorders, among others. Diagnostic criteria for somatization disorder are outlined in Table 15–2.

The possibility of *conversion disorder* should be entertained when patients present with neurologic or other medical symptoms that suggest or reveal deficits in voluntary motor or sensory function. Typically, conversion symptoms *suggest* a physical disorder, but the symptoms are considered an expression of psychological conflict or need. Conversion disorder is not diagnosed when conversion symptoms are limited to pain. The most common and traditional conversion symptoms are not, in fact, pain but, rather, signs that suggest neurologic disease such as seizures, paralysis, coordination disturbance, dyskinesia, akinesia, blindness, and paresthesias. Symptoms typically develop during times of particular psychological stress, and the effect of the conversion disorder on the patient's life is usually marked. Prolonged loss of function may produce obvious and serious complications, such as contractures or disuse atrophy. Antecedent physical disorders or serve psychological stress is considered a predisposing factor (Table 15–3).

The essential feature of *pain disorder* is preoccupation with pain in the absence of physical findings that fully

TABLE 15–2 Diagnostic Criteria: Somatization Disorder (DSM IV, 1994, pp. 446–503)

A. A history of numerous physical complaints beginning before age 30 that occur over a period of several years and result in treatment being sought or significant impairment in social, occupational, and other important areas of functioning.
B. Each of the following criteria must have been met, with individual symptoms occurring at any time during the course of disturbance:
   1. Four pain symptoms
      a. History of pain related to at least four different sites or functions (e.g., head, abdomen, back, joints, extremities, chest, rectum, during menstruation, during sexual intercourse, or during urination).
   2. Gastrointestinal symptoms: a history of at least two gastrointestinal symptoms other than pain (e.g., nausea, bloating, vomiting, diarrhea, or intolerance of several foods).
   3. One sexual symptom: a history of at least one sexually reproductive symptom other than pain.
   4. One pseudoneurologic symptom: a history of at least one symptom or deficit suggesting a neurologic condition not limited to pain (e.g., conversion symptom such as impaired coordination or balance, paralysis or localized weakness, difficulty swallowing or lump in throat, aphonia, urinary retention, hallucinations, loss of touch or pain sensation, double vision, blindness, deafness, seizures, dissociative symptoms such as amnesia, loss of consciousness other than fainting).
C. Either 1 or 2
   1. After appropriate investigation of each of the symptoms in criteria B, the symptoms cannot be fully explained by known medical conditions or the effects of a substance (e.g., a drug of abuse, a medication).
   2. When there is a related general medical condition, the physical complaints are resulting in social or occupational impairment that is in excess of what would be expected from the history, physical examination, or laboratory findings.
D. The symptoms are not intentionally produced or feigned (as in factitious disorder or malingering).

Reprinted with permission from the Diagnostic and Statistical Manual of Mental Disorders, Fourth Edition. Copyright 1994 American Psychiatric Association.

TABLE 15–3 Diagnostic Criteria: Conversion Disorder (DSM IV, 1994, pp. 453–457)

A. One or more symptoms or deficits affecting voluntary motor or sensory function that suggests a neurologic or other general medical condition.
B. Psychological factors are judged to be associated with symptoms or deficits because the initiation or exacerbation of the symptom or deficit is preceded by conflicts or other stressors.
C. The symptoms or deficits are not intentionally produced or feigned (as in factitious disorder or malingering).
D. The symptoms or deficit cannot, after appropriate investigation, be fully explained by a general medical condition, or by the direct effects of a substance or as a culturally sanctioned behavior experience.
E. The symptom or deficit causes clinically significant distress or impairment in social, occupational, or other important areas of functioning or warrants medical evaluation.
F. The symptom or deficit is not limited to pain or sexual dysfunction, does not occur exclusively during the course of a somatization disorder, and is not better accounted for by another mental disorder.

Reprinted with permission from the Diagnostic and Statistical Manual of Mental Disorders, Fourth Edition. Copyright 1994 American Psychiatric Association.

account for a cause of the pain or its intensity and ramifications. In this disorder, pain symptoms are inconsistent with the anatomic distribution of nerves or, when the pain mimics that of another disease, symptoms cannot be adequately accounted for after extensive diagnostic assessment. Psychological factors are judged to play a significant role in the onset, exacerbation, severity, and maintenance of pain. Behavioral signs include frequent visits to physicians despite medical reassurance and excessive use of analgesic that do not, however, produce adequate pain relief. Pain disorder patients often refuse to seriously consider that psychological factors might be influencing the clinical picture, adamantly asserting that there cannot be an organic cause. Symptoms of depression are common, and, in many cases, symptoms are severe enough to warrant a diagnosis of major depression. Subtypes of pain disorder include these:

1. *Pain Disorder Associated with Psychological Factors.* This subtype is used when psychological factors are judged to play a major role in onset, severity, exacerbation, or maintenance of pain. General medical conditions may not be involved or may play a secondary role in onset or maintenance of pain.
2. *Pain Disorder Associated with Both Psychological Factors and a General Medical Condition.* This subtype is considered when psychological factors and a general medical condition in combination play important roles in the onset, severity, exacerbation, or maintenance of pain.
3. *Pain Disorder Associated with a General Medical Condition.* This subtype is considered when no mental disorder is evident and pain is believed to be a function of a general medical condition. Consequently, psychological factors play a minor and insignificant role in the onset and maintenance of pain.

The category of *psychological factors affecting physical condition* applies to any physical condition to which psychological factors are contributory. This diagnostic category is used to describe disorders that, historically, have been referred to as either *psychosomatic or psychophysiologic.* This category is used only when pain from a known organic lesion is exacerbated by psychological factors. Diagnostic criteria for pain disorders are outlined in Table 15–4.

Factitious Disorders and Malingering

Factitious disorders are physical or psychological symptoms that are intentionally produced or feigned so that the "patient" can assume the "sick role." External incentives for assuming a sick role, such as economic gain and avoiding legal responsibility, are absent. Similar to factitious disorder is malingering, which is characterized by intentional presentation of false or grossly exaggerated physical or psychological symptoms that is motivated by external incentives such as work avoidance, financial compensation, evading criminal prosecution, or obtaining drugs. According to the *DSM IV* (p. 683), malingering should be strongly suspected if any combination of the following findings is noted:

1. Medicolegal context of presentation (e.g., the patient is referred by an attorney to the clinician for examination).
2. Marked discrepancy between the patient's claim, stress, or disability and the objective findings.
3. Lack of cooperation during the diagnostic evaluation and noncompliance with the prescribed treatment regimen.
4. The presence of antisocial personality disorder.

Malingering is differentiated from factitious disorder by the intentional production of symptoms and by obvious external incentives. Malingering is not considered a mental disorder.

Affective Disorders

There is substantial evidence that depression is the most common emotional disorder among patients with chronic pain. Although the majority of patients in acute pain demonstrate some degree of anxiety and fear, they may not exhibit symptoms of clinical depression. With persistent pain, psychological symptoms may become more complicated—depression, anxiety, anger, and generalized hostil-

TABLE 15–4 Diagnostic Criteria for Pain Disorder (DSM IV, 1994, pp 458–462)

A. Pain in one or more anatomic sites is the predominant focus of the clinical presentation and is of sufficient severity to warrant clinical attention.
B. Pain causes clinically significant distress or impairment in social, occupational, or other important areas of functioning.
C. Psychological factors are judged to have an important role in the onset, severity, exacerbation, or maintenance of the pain.
D. The symptom or deficit is not intentionally produced or feigned (as in factitious disorder or malingering)
E. Pain is not accounted for by a mood, anxiety, or psychotic disorder and does not meet the criteria for dyspareunia. The disorder is determined acute if the duration of pain is less than 6 months, and chronic if there is a duration of pain greater than 6 months.

Reprinted with permission from the Diagnostic and Statistical Manual of Mental Disorders, Fourth Edition. Copyright 1994 American Psychiatric Association.

ity. Although depression may occur as a reaction to intense or chronic pain and alterations of lifestyle, it is not unusual to find patients with depression that antedates the onset of pain. Depression may confound a patient's response to physical treatment and response to analgesic medications, and can actually increase analgesic requirements. Anxiety may lead to use or overuse of analgesic medications when the pain patient desires sedation and reduction of anxiety and tension. The wise clinician carefully differentiates psychological from physical symptoms and avoids using analgesic medications to treat depressive and anxiety symptoms.

In chronic pain syndromes, the patient may exhibit neurovegetative signs of depression, including insomnia or hypersomnia, appetite change, diminished libido, withdrawal, and excessive use of alcohol or other substances. A vicious cycle of pain, depression, and insomnia can develop, and patients often mistake emotional distress for pain. Fortunately, more effective medications have been developed, such as the serotonin-specific reuptake inhibitors and other antidepressant drugs that reduce symptoms of both depression and anxiety. These medications do not, however, have a direct pharmacologic impact on pain as did the older antidepressants, such as the tricyclics.

Perhaps the most popular screening instrument for depression is the Beck Depression Inventory.[12] The BDI is based on questions about common features of depression, such as sleep disturbance, fatigue, weight gain or loss, sexual dysfunction, and cognitive components of depressive illness. Other popular screening instruments useful for evaluating affective states are the Symptom Checklist 90 Revised (SCL-90-R),[13] Brief Symptom Inventory (BSI), which is based on the SCL-90-R, the Coping Strategies Questionnaire,[14] and the Pain Patient Profile (P-3).[15] Anger and hostility should also be included in the assessment of affective functioning.

TABLE 15–5 ***Multiple Dimensions of the Pain Experience***

Physiologic dimensions
Location
Onset
Duration
Cause
Syndrome
Sensory dimensions
Intensity
Quality
Pattern
Affective dimensions
Mood state
Anxiety
Depression
Well-being
Cognitive dimensions
Meaning of pain
View of pain
Coping skills and strategies
Previous treatments
Attitudes and beliefs
Factors influencing pain
Behavioral dimensions
Communications
Interpersonal interaction
Physical activity
Pain behaviors
Medications
Interventions
Sleep
Sociocultural dimensions
Ethnocultural background
Family and social life
Work and home responsibilities
Recreation and leisure
Environmental factors
Attitudes and beliefs
Social influences

PSYCHOSOCIAL AND BEHAVIORAL ASSESSMENT OF PAIN

The most important features of pain assessment are severity and location of pain, pain behavior, physical capacity, emotional symptoms, psychosocial influences of pain (on work and family), coping skills, and perceived disability. Identification of emotional factors involved in the constellation of symptoms presented by pain patients may be beneficial. If emotional symptoms go undetected or ignored, even the best medical or surgical intervention can result in treatment failure. The psychological evaluation should describe treatment variables that specifically address behaviors and personality characteristics that affect response to treatment. The multidimensional aspects of pain assessment have been described by McGuire[16] and are a helpful guide to pain assessment (Table 15–5).

Many personality features have been described in the literature that help to predict treatment complications or failure. Certain personality features and disorders are described in the section on Risk Factors.

PSYCHOLOGICAL/BEHAVIORAL INTERVIEW

In the clinical evaluation of the patient in pain, the interview is conducted first, before the physical examination. The purpose of the interview is not only to diagnose physical disease but also to learn about the patient and his response to pain. We must, of course, understand the patient's medical history and learn not to rely on subconscious impressions that may be inaccurate, difficult to validate, and impossible to interpret entirely in the context of the patient's presenting pain symptoms. It is critical to accurately distinguish the symptoms and signs of illness behavior from those of physical disease or benign pain problems.

Interview topics should include descriptions of the patient's pain and experience. The pattern, intensity, and quality of pain should be elicited. It is important to ask the patient how the pain relates to function and what factors increase or decrease pain after certain behaviors and activities. The pain history must inquire into the onset and course of the pain and the patient's current experience with pain. The treatment history and response to interventions are critical. Many patients have undergone numerous attempts to control their pain before they consult a pain specialist, and this area of inquiry can be very cumbersome. Care must be taken to elicit clear descriptions of treatments, as chronic pain patients tend to report simply that nothing has worked or been successful. Medications and side effects, drug and alcohol use, and problems with sleep and sexual functioning should be reviewed.

The psychosocial history should be comprehensive. Sometimes patterns of chronic pain are common in certain family systems. Information about the patient's family background—education, occupation, and the physical status of other family members—is helpful. In the social history, work status, including issues related to litigation, workers' compensation, and the potential for continuing to work or returning to work, are critical. Job satisfaction is important. Issues of emotional and physical abuse are helpful. Compelling findings have demonstrated the influences of childhood psychological and physical trauma on treatment outcomes, especially surgical treatment of the lumbar spine.[17].

In the psychosocial history, quality of past and current relationships with spouse, family, and friends is an important indication of how much pain is affecting the patient and his behavior, as are leisure activities. It is important to look for recent or current stressors that may have a relationship to the pain complaint or earlier failed treatment responses.

The patient's perception of pain and the patient's beliefs, expectations, and concepts about the causes of pain should be evaluated. In addition, the patient's concept of her role in treatment and mastery of the ability to manage pain independently is important information for the clinician. The patient's willingness to communicate and to assume responsibility for managing the pain is essential. If the patient is not motivated to actively participate in his care, treatment outcome is negatively affected.

Behavioral and mental status can be obtained through observations during the physical examination and observations of the patient's behavior while waiting for the appointment and walking into the examination room. During the interview, problems with memory and concentration and difficulty making decisions and solving problems should become evident. For elders or persons who seem to be impaired, a brief cognitive examination, the Mini-Mental State Examination, is reliable and widely used.[18]

MEASURES OF PAIN INTENSITY, SENSATION, AND LOCATION

Various methods for measuring pain intensity and location have traditionally focused on assessment through verbal rating scales, numerical scales, and visual analogue scales. These devices appear particularly popular in hospitals, clinics and physicians' offices. Measures of pain complaints have been used in numerous clinical studies and in countless research publications; however, it should be noted that little normative information is available in such instruments. The upshot is that a raw score on any simple unidimensional device or instrument is essentially meaningless without additional information.

There are four primary types of self-report measures for pain: visual analogue scales, pain drawings, numerical rating scales, and verbal rating scales. Verbal rating scales use adjectives to describe the quality of pain, such as *burning* and *throbbing*. The most popular of these has been the McGill Pain Questionnaire.[19] The advantage of this type of instrument is the fact that the patient may choose words to qualify the characteristics of pain that, in turn, may lead to a more accurate diagnosis based upon the patient's sensory experience. Disadvantages include the fact that the patient may not understand the adjectives or may choose words that are not accurate.

Visual analogue scales and numerical rating scales utilize a numerical scale (e.g., 0 to 10, or 1 to 100) to reflect pain intensity. Strengths of such scales are their clarity and simplicity. They are useful with children and elderly persons and are versatile for measuring pretreatment post-treatment pain. They are also adaptable to various cognitive levels and can be used in a variety of settings. Furthermore, they are brief and easy to administer. Limitations derive from the fact that there is great variability in the numerical scales utilized. For example, clinicians may for their own purposes utilize a 0 to 10 scale for pain assessment but work in hospitals and settings where scales such as 0 to 5 or 0 to 100 are popular. In addition, pain patients often give a pain rating that is unreliable or highly embellished. In our clinical practices, we find it not uncommon to encounter patients who report pain intensity of 10 or even 11 on a 0- to 10-point scale! Embellished responses obviously require further assessment with other instruments plus behavioral observations. Some such patients may embellish pain ratings in an effort to impress upon their physician that they are truly suffering or need more intensive treatment or medications. The clinician should keep in mind that research indicates that little is gained in reliability using rating scales with more than seven levels. In other words, there is little to be gained in using a 0 to 100 scale over a 0 to 10 scale. In practice, the 0 to 10 scaling method has been the most widely accepted.[20]

Problems inherent with self-report, and particularly unidimensional measures, include the fact that, while it may be assumed that a single dimension, such as pain intensity, is being measured, the individual's rating is easily influenced by emotional states and other factors that compound the pain description. As we know, pain intensity usually changes over time and is affected by motivation, medications, and psychological factors. Thus, it is wrong to assume that we can measure a multidimensional phenomenon with a linear technique or a ratio.

Pain drawings are helpful in assessing pain patterns and locations. Although scoring systems for pain drawings have been devised, experienced pain clinicians typically use pain drawings in combination with some type of sensory assessment system. Pain drawings with the use of indicators for pain patterns and sensory markings can be particularly helpful in diagnostics *and* in identifying a person's tendency to embellish symptoms or identify pain patterns not associated with clear physiologic derangements or anatomic lesions. Picture scales utilize line drawings that illustrate facial expressions of persons experiencing pain. Facial drawings are most helpful with children, older adults, and patients who have language or other communication problems.

In conclusion, efforts to improve evaluation of both acute and chronic pain often include patient self-reports along with certain sensory and descriptive instruments. Although these instruments are simple and easily administered, it is recommended that pain behavior also be observed and considered. Pain behavior during the examination and careful observation of physical maneuvers in the office or medical setting are extremely helpful. Techniques for eliciting the pain response and physical examination are described in other chapters of this text.

ASSESSMENT OF FUNCTIONAL STATUS AND TREATMENT OUTCOME

Several instruments are purported to measure the patient's own perceptions of health, pain, and psychological functioning related to pain. The Oswestry Disability Questionnaire contains 10 multiple-choice items that address nine areas of daily living and the use of medications.[21] The Oswestry is most often used to assess patients with low back pain. The Health Status Questionnaire 2 (HSQ) is designed to be used in multiple settings. This instrument measures a patient's own perceptions of his health status before, during, and after treatment. It allows for comparison of treatment results across settings and has been standardized. The HSQ is based on a normative population of patients and nonpatients. The HSQ groups eight health attributes under three major divisions, namely, Overall Evaluation of Health, Functional Status, and Well-Being. The HSQ is an effective new instrument for measuring a patient's perception of health status in a general sense, but it is not specific to pain.

McGrath and associates[21] examined the use of the MMPI in the evaluation of chronic pain patients and found that higher scores on the K scale suggested less of a psychological contribution to pain complaints. Gatchel and coworkers evaluated 324 low back pain patients in an effort to predict which ones would subsequently report chronic pain disability problems.[22] Results indicate the predictive importance of three factors: self-reported pain and disability, a personality disorder, and elevations on Scale 3 of the MMPI.

The Pain Patient Profile (P-3) is specifically "normed" on patients in pain and measures somatization, depression, and anxiety associated with pain. Test results may be compared to a national sample of patients in pain and to a national sample of patients who had no significant pain problems (community subjects). Because the P-3 is brief and simple to administer, it may be used before, during, and after treatment, for comparison purposes.[15]

ASSESSMENT OF COGNITIVE COPING MECHANISMS

Cognitive assessment is important because many patients in pain tend to distort their perception of it. Common cognitive distortions include catastrophization, overgeneralization, and misinterpretation of the cause of pain symptoms. The experienced pain clinician knows that patients in pain often anticipate the worst outcome and frequently generalize symptoms to future experiences. The Cognitive Error Questionnaire[23] helps to identify cognitive distortions and misinterpretation in chronic pain patients. After assessing cognitive distortions, it is often helpful to implement cognitive-behavioral treatment techniques such as cognitive restructuring and self-instructional training. Cognitive techniques in conjunction with behavioral techniques, such as relaxation training, imagery training, and rational interpretation of symptoms, are often effective in combination with medications and physical interventions. A common misinterpretation and/or catastrophization is equating *pain* with *tissue damage*. Educational techniques are an effective adjunct to physical treatment. Medications, nerve blocks, and even surgery may not be effective if cognitive errors are not detected and treated. Cognitive beliefs, which are often catastrophized and exaggerated, may lead the patient to mistrust the medical professional and to request additional diagnostic tests or referral to another physician. Some patients lack sophistication with regard to their pain symptoms. It is often difficult for such patients to understand medical information that has been provided without detailed (and time-consuming) education.

The Vanderbilt Multidimensional Pain Coping Inventory assesses seven distinct coping strategies.[24] This instrument evaluates both positive and negative psychological adjustment, demonstrating whether the patient is relying on internal or external resources for pain management. Passive strategies have been linked with poor treatment response and outcome. Studies of coping strategies have determined that clinically depressed subjects often show more passive and avoidance behaviors. Active coping strategies are associated with more adaptive adjustment and positive treatment outcome.

The West Haven–Yale Multidimensional Pain Inventory[25] consists of 12 scales that measure the impact of pain on a patient's life, communication of pain experience, and extent to which a patient participates in activities of daily living. Patient profiles on this instrument may be descriptive of dysfunctional, interpersonally distressed, and minimizer/adaptive coping. The instrument has successfully predicted physical improvement after pain treatment.

COMPREHENSIVE ASSESSMENT INSTRUMENTS

Minnesota Multiphasic Personality Inventory (MMPI-2)

Despite criticism and unparalleled research examination, the MMPI remains the instrument most widely used in psychological assessment. The updated MMPI-2 preserves the most valuable features of the original MMPI while providing descriptive and diagnostic information that is more helpful to clinicians.[26] The MMPI-2 provides computerized scoring and interpretation for a variety of disorders and settings, including an interpretative report for chronic pain patients. Several analytic studies have provided consistent replications with chronic pain patients. The use of cluster analysis in multivariant statistical studies has shown statistically reliable and valid interpretations of test results. Depressive symptoms have been identified in association with increased pain symptoms, and the intensity of depression has been found to be a significant negative predictor of treatment outcome. Several studies have identified negative emotions as contributory to the relationship between pain-related impairment and disability. Patients with a high score on somatization have had higher scores on pain-related disability. In a recent study, Vendrig and coworkers revealed underlying factors with the MMPI-2, which include psychological disturbance, extroversion/extroversion, passivity, and somatic complaints.[27] Results of this study support the work of Deardorff and associates with correlations to a number of factors, including the number of painful areas on the body, Waddell signs, and fear of movement.[28] The authors concluded that MMPI-2 research with chronic pain patients should include clinical correlates with a clear conceptual framework of distress and personality relevant to chronic pain and pain treatment.

Many psychologists find the original work of Fordyce[29] helpful in assessment. Fordyce presented MMPI interpretations that indicated (1) to what degree a patient with pain finds pain rewarding and (2) how great is the gain or reward (secondary gain) derived from having painful symptoms. The patient with a high score on Depression (Scale 2) is less likely to find pain reinforcing than is the patient whose profile demonstrates a very low Scale 2 score. Persons with elevations on scales measuring Hypochondriasis (Scale 1) and Hysteria (Scale 3) in conjunction with a proportionately low Scale 2 score are likely to report pain but often have a low level of emotional concern and distress about pain. This classic configuration is referred to as the *conversion V profile*, but the clinician should remember that this profile does not necessarily demonstrate that physical problems are not actively involved in causing the pain. Chronic pain patients also frequently have elevations on scales of Paranoia (Scale 6) and/or Schizophrenia (Scale 8). Elevations on these psychiatric scales have various causes, including sensory disturbance, confusion due to medications, easy distractability and difficulty maintaining concentration and attention over time, somatic distractability and subsequent distractability, unusual interpretations of pain and somatic symptoms, and other symptoms associated with pain and treatment.[30] In summary, the MMPI-2 profile of a patient in pain has significantly different meaning than that of an identical test profile of a person who presents with primary symptoms other than pain. It is our opinion and experience that to properly use the MMPI-2 with patients in pain requires specific and advanced training and experience in pain psychology.

The Battery for Health Improvement

The Battery for Health Improvement (BHI) is a self-report inventory designed to identify multiple factors that interfere with a patient's normal course of recovery from a physical injury.[31] The test has proven reliability and validity and provides a comprehensive assessment for psychological and psychosocial factors that interfere with a patient's recovery from physical injury. Measures that identify the impact of physical, environmental, and psychological factors are included in the report, and it has been used for orthopedic, occupational, and other injuries. The test is helpful with workers' compensation patients because it gathers information about a patient's readiness for vocational training or job placement. It is also helpful for evaluating emotional readiness for surgery and, so, may be used to enhance physician-psychologist communication. Specific clinical scales are symptom dependency, chronic maladjustment, family dysfunction, job satisfaction, doctor satisfaction, muscular bracing, somatic complaints, pain complaints, and perseverance. An added attribute is that the test was normed on a large community sample *and* a large sample of physical rehabilitation patients. The report compares the patient being tested to both norm samples and uses the average of physical rehabilitation patients as a benchmark for interpretation and treatment recommendations. An interesting study was performed using the BHI that identified violent ideation and dysfunctional, angry behavior in patients involved in medical treatment.[32] Obviously, hostility and aggressiveness are important to consider when we clinicians press patients to perform exercises that, for example, may temporarily increase pain or urge them to assume more responsibility for managing their painful conditions independently. A short form of the BHI is currently being developed that should improve the utility of the instrument. When a patient exhibits significant elevations on the short form, the full BHI should be administered.

Behavioral Assessment of Pain

The Behavioral Assessment of Pain (BAP) is a comprehensive self-report questionnaire test that offers excellent reliability and validity plus internal consistency.[33] The authors of the questionnaire have used a biopsychosocial framework to develop the instrument, which include data often ignored by other assessment instruments. It evaluates potential influences on the patient's pain problems, including physician influences, spousal influences, and cognitive beliefs and has traditional scales of mood and activity level. The principal drawback of the BAP is that completing the lengthy battery takes time. The instrument appears to be particularly useful for research purposes. The BAP should be used with other measures of psychological disturbance and measures of physical capacity.

Pain Patient Profile (P-3)

Developed in 1993, the P-3 is a clinically effective instrument for briefly assessing for personality and psychological characteristics that are known to affect pain perception and treatment response of patients in pain.[15] The P-3 consists of 48 items, each having three response options that collectively comprise four clinical subscales: validity, somatization, depression, and anxiety. A computerized profile is produced with an interpretation that compares the pain patient to a national sample of patients in pain. Patient responses also are compared to those of a large community sample of "nonpatients." The computerized report offers treatment recommendations based on each patient's responses and profile configuration.

The P-3 offers several advantages to pain professionals. Administration time is brief (12 to 15 min), and items are inoffensive and relevant to patients in pain. The P-3 profile compares individual test responses to those of a large group of patients in pain. This comparison allows the clinician to evaluate a patient relative to other pain patients. T scores are provided for comparison of a patient to both pain patients and the nonpatient group. The test may be used to assess the presence and severity of psychological symptoms before, during, and after treatment, thereby serving as a tool to evaluate clinical outcome and treatment effectiveness.

The P-3 has been used in clinical research with patients suffering from a variety of painful disorders. In a recent study of neurosurgery patients, data analysis based solely upon initial P-3 profiles was predictive of: (1) insurance status (workers' compensation or "other"), (2) gender, and (3) smoker/nonsmoker status. Symptoms of depression and somatization were significant predictors of medical and psychological factors that affected treatment outcome. Multiple regression and bivariate analysis for P-3 subscale scores were analyzed and demonstrated the predictive utility of the P-3 in this study. At 6-month follow-up, P-3 scale elevations had declined in response to various types of therapeutic intervention. Several trends were detected, including decreased somatization scores with psychological/behavioral intervention, medication, epidurals, and surgery. Depression scale scores also decreased with psychological intervention, epidurals, medications, and surgery. Although the P-3 measures psychological symptoms associated with pain, changes following various forms of intervention showed reductions on the clinical scales. Thus, the P-3 has added value as an objective measure of overall treatment improvement. Final results of this longitudinal study should provide additional information on the utility—predictive and overall—of the P-3 as a measure of treatment outcome.[34]

SCREENING PATIENTS FOR SURGERY AND OTHER INTERVENTIONS

Social, psychological, and job-related variables appear to be of greater significance in predicting a return to work following injury than physical factors. As studied previously, Waddell presented evidence that the correlations between impairment and pain, impairment and disability, and pain and disability were relatively weak, suggesting that disability is related more to nonphysical factors than to structural pathology.[35] The concept of "psychological readiness" may be an important determinant in the successful outcome of patients undergoing surgery. Recognized high-risk factors for presurgical patients include tobacco use, obesity, and psychopathologiatric disease. Smoking and obesity have been shown to have great influence on the outcome of spinal fusions. Doxey and coworkers[36] used an assessment protocol with back pain patients that provided an 82% prognostic success rate. The predictor variables that most significantly correlated with surgical outcome were English language proficiency, nonorganic signs/tests (Waddell), back pain (versus leg pain), Hypochondriasis scale of the MMPI, and pain drawings. Block[37] produced an excellent text for presurgical evaluation of pain patients. He presents a thorough rationale for psychological investigation of candidates for surgery for chronic pain, and he developed a classification system for assessment of risk. In addition to techniques for presurgical assessment of the patient, Block provides a clear summary of major psychological and medical factors that affect the outcome of spine surgery (Table 15–6).

TABLE 15–6 ***Risk Factors for Poor Surgical Outcome***

Risk Factor	Risk Level
Pending legal actions related to injury	High risk
Workers' compensation	High risk
Job dissatisfaction	
Moderate	Moderate risk
Extreme	High risk
Heavy job demands (frequent lifting >50 lb)	High risk
Substance abuse	
Preinjury	Moderate risk
Current	High risk
Reinforcement of disability by family members	Moderate/high risk
Marital dissatisfaction	Moderate risk
Physical or sexual abuse	
Preinjury	Moderate risk
Current	High risk
Preinjury psychological problems	
Outpatient treatment	Moderate risk
Inpatient	High risk

From Block AR: Presurgical psychological screening in chronic pain syndrome: A guide for the behavioral health practitioner. Mahwah, NJ: Lawrence Erlbaum Associates, 1996.

CONCLUSIONS

Psychological assessment of the patient in pain should include multidimensional evaluation and measures of compliance, motivational factors, and the social influences of pain on the patient. Special pain populations, such as children and elders, require certain evaluation methods, as their cognitive problems may prevent accurate communication. Specialists who assess pain in children and the elderly should be experienced with these techniques and methods. Instruments have been developed specifically to evaluate pain in children and persons with communication deficits through the Agency for Health Care Policy and Research, U.S. Department of Health and Human Services, Public Health Service, 1994.

In the future, our ability to evaluate patients in pain will be enhanced by better understanding of pain responses and evaluation of the physiologic changes that correlate with pain symptoms. At the present time, however, it is recommended that we use assessment techniques that have proven validity and reliability, and use them in combination with physical and objective behavioral measures. Evaluation of pain requires special training and experience for both psychological and medical practitioners. Fortunately, there is growing interest—and continued specialized training is available—in the ever growing specialty of pain management.

REFERENCES

1. Polatin PB, Kinney R, Gatchel RB, Mayer TG: Psychiatric Illness and Chronic Lower Back Pain: The Mind and the Spine—Which

Goes First? Paper presented at the Seventh Annual Meeting, North American Spine Society, Boston, July 1992.
2. Pain Management. Clinical Practice Guidelines. Washington, D.C., Agency for Health Care Policy and Research, Public Health Service, U.S. Department of Health and Human Services, 1992.
3. American Pain Society: Principles of Analgesic Use in the Treatment of Acute Pain and Cancer Pain, ed 3. Skokie, Ill, American Pain Society, 1992.
4. Standards Manual for Organizations Serving People with Disabilities. Tucson, Commission on Accreditation of Rehabilitation Facilities (CARF), 1986.
5. Atkinson JH, Slater MA, Patterson TL: Prevalence, onset and risk of psychiatric disorders in men with chronic low back pain: A controlled study. Pain 45:111–121, 1991.
6. Ormel J, Voncorff M, Ustun TB, Pini S, Korten A, Oldehinkel T: Mental disorders and disability across cultures. JAMA 272(22):1741–1748, 1994.
7. Bigos SJ, Spengler DM, Martin NA: Back injuries in industry: A retrospective study: Employee-related factors. Spine 11:252–256, 1986.
8. Elliott TR, Jackson WT, Layfield M, Kendall D: Personality disorders in response to outpatient treatment of chronic pain. J Clin Psychol Med Settings 3(3):219–233, 1996.
9. American Psychiatric Association: Diagnostic and Statistical Manual of Mental Disorders, ed 4. Washington, DC, American Psychiatric Association, 1994.
10. Kinney RK, Gatchel RJ, Polatin, PB, Fogarty WT, Mayer TG: Prevalence of psychopathology in acute and chronic low back pain patients. J Occup Rehab 3:95–103, 1993.
11. Shelton JL: Psychological Considerations. *In* Cole AJ, Herring SA (eds): The Low Back Pain Handbook: A Practical Guide for the Primary Care Physician. Philadelphia, Hanley and Belfus, 1997, pp 245–252.
12. Beck AT, Beck RW: Screening depressed patients in family practice: A rapid technique. Post Grad Med 52(6):81–85, 1972.
13. Derogatis LR: SCL-90-R. Towson, Md, Clinical Psychometric Research, 1997.
14. Rosenstiel AK, Keefe FJ: Use of coping strategies in chronic low back pain patients: Relationship to patient characteristics and current adjustment. Pain 17:33–44, 1983.
15. Tollison CD, Langley JC: Pain Patient Profile (P-3) Manual. Minneapolis, National Computer Systems, 1995.
16. McGuire DB: Comprehensive and multidimensional assessment and measurement of pain. J Pain Symptom Mgmt 7:312–319, 1992.
17. Schofferman J, Anderson D, Hines R, Smith G, White A: Childhood sexual trauma correlates with unsuccessful lumbar spine surgery. Spine 17(6, Suppl) S138–S144, 1992.
18. Folstein MF, Folstein SE, McHugh PR: Mini-mental state: A practical method for grading the cognitive state of outpatients for clinicians. J Psychiatr Res 12:189–198, 1975.
19. Melzack R: The McGill Pain Questionnaire: Major properties in scoring methods. Pain 1:275–299, 1975.
20. Hinnant DW: Psychological evaluation and testing. *In* Tollison CD, Satterthwaite, JR, Tollison JW (eds): Handbook of Pain Management, ed 2. Baltimore: Williams & Wilkins, 1994, pp 18–36.
21. McGrath RE, Sweeney M, O'Malley WB, Carlton TK: Identifying psychological contributions to chronic pain complaints with the MMPI-2: The role of the K scale. J Personality Assessment 70(3):448–459, 1998.
22. Gatchel RJ, Polatin PB, Kinney RK: Predicting outcomes of chronic back pain using clinical predictors of psychopathology: A prospective analysis. Health Psychol 14(5):415–420, 1995.
23. Lefebvre MF: Cognitive distortion and cognitive errors in depressed, psychiatric, and low back pain patients. J Consult Clin Psychol 49:515–517, 1984.
24. Snow-Turek, A, Norris MP, Tan G: Active and passive coping strategies in chronic pain patients. Pain 64:455–462, 1996.
25. Kerns RD, Turk DC, Rudy TE: The West Haven–Yale Multidimensional Pain Inventory (WHYMPI). Pain 23:345–356, 1985.
26. Butcher JN, Dahlstrom WG, Graham JR, Tellegen AM, Kaemer B: MMPI-2 Manual for Administration and Scoring. Minneapolis: University of Minnesota Press, 1989.
27. Vendrig AA, deMay HR, Derksen JL, Akkerveeken PF: The assessment of chronic back pain patient characteristics using factor analysis of the MMPI-2: Which dimensions are actually assessed? Pain 76(1–2):179–188, 1998.
28. Deardoff WW, Chino AF, Scott DW: Characteristics of chronic pain patients: Factor analysis of the MMPI-2. Pain 54:153–158, 1993.
29. Fordyce WE: Use of the MMPI in the assessment of chronic pain. In Butcher J, Dahlstrom G, Gynther W, Schofield W (eds): Clinical Notes on the MMPI. LaRoche, NJ: Hoffman. 1979.
30. Riley JL, Robinson ME: Validity of the MMPI-2 profiles in chronic back pain patients: Differences in path models of coping and somatization. Clin J Pain 14:324–335, 1998.
31. Bruns D, Disorbio JM, Copeland-Disorbio J: Manual for the Battery for Health Improvement. Minneapolis: NCS Assessments, 1996.
32. Bruns D, Disorbio JM: Violent ideation in medical patients in four insurance systems. Paper presention. Annual Meeting of the American Psychological Association, 1998.
33. Tearnan DH, Lewandowski MJ: The behavioral assessment of pain questionnaire: The development and validation of a comprehensive self-report instrument. Am J Pain Mgmt 2:181–191, 1992.
34. Hinnant DW, Tollison CD: The Pain Patient Profile (P-3) used as a screening instrument and outcome measures with neurosurgical patients. Unpublished manuscript, 1999.
35. Waddell G, Main C, Morris E, diPaola M, Gray I: Chronic low back, psychological distress, and illness behavior. Spine 9:209–215, 1984.
36. Doxey NC, Dzioba RB, Mitson GL: Predictors of outcome in back surgery candidates. J Clin Psychol 44:611–622, 1985.
37. Block AR: Presurgical Psychological Screening in Chronic Pain Syndromes: A Guide for the Behavioral Health Practitioner. Mahwah, NJ: Lawrence Erlbaum Associates, 1996.

PART · III

Neural Blockade and Neurolytic Blocks

CHAPTER · 16

Local Anesthetics in Clinical Practice

Rudolph H. de Jong, MD

CLINICAL PHYSIOLOGY

Nerve Block Basics

Local anesthetics are sodium channel–blocking drugs that completely halt electrical impulse conduction—proximally (pain) and distally (motor)—in excitable neural tissues such as peripheral nerves, spinal roots, and autonomic ganglia. As a result, and depending on the particular nerve's function (i.e., sensory, motor, autonomic), pain sensation, muscle contraction, autonomic effector activity, or all of these, are interrupted (blocked) in the body part innervated distal to the site of local anesthetic application. Unlike neurolytic agents (see Chapter 17), local anesthetics produce an impulse conduction block that is painless and completely reversible: the nerve block dissipates (wears off) spontaneously with time as drug is released from its bond with sodium channel receptors. Local anesthetics thus are unique in interventional pain management, for they permit precise neurotopic identification of structures targeted for destructive procedures. Temporary blockade lets the patient experience the sensation of numbness before it becomes a permanent annoyance and, critical before resort to permanent neurolysis, is a convenient and spontaneously reversible assessment tool before potentially ineffective often irreversible nerve damage is produced.

Unique, too, is that the transitory neural quiescence provided by local anesthetic block, repeated at intervals, often is sufficient to gradually wind down activity of spontaneously discharging hyperactive neurons, thereby relieving pain effectively far beyond the few hours' duration of the drug's blocking action. Examples of such therapeutic action are treatment of scar neuromas, sympathetic plexus block for reflex sympathetic dystrophy, and muscle trigger point injections. In short, local anesthetics (1) are both diagnostic and therapeutic in the invasive management of pain, (2) not infrequently obviate altogether the need for permanent neurolysis—whether chemical, thermal, or surgical, and (3) synergistically reinforce and potentiate the analgesic action of spinal opioids.

Brief History

The mouth-numbing property of cocaine—extracted from the leaves of the coca shrub, grown as a crop in the Andean foothills—has been known for centuries. In 1855, Gaedicke extracted the alkaloid erythroxylin from coca leaves. Albert Niemann later isolated cocaine from the erythroxylin extract in 1860 and reported that the bitter crystals numbed his tongue.

Sigmund Freud (best known for founding psychoanalysis) became intrigued by the new drug's vast medicinal potential and shared these insights with Karl Koller, a fellow intern at Vienna's City Hospital. Numbing of the tongue came as a "eureka" experience to Koller, who had the vision to expand that idle curiosity into surgical anesthesia of the eye, first reported in 1884. News of the discovery spread like wildfire through the medical world, and cocaine soon was tested on the upper airway for otolaryngologic surgery. Although his contribution to ophthalmology is uncontested, Koller failed to receive the coveted Assistantship to the Vienna Eye Clinic; he died a bitter man.

When, some 60 years later, Sweden's Erdtman discovered that the alkaloid gramine (much like cocaine) numbed his tongue, a fresh track leading to quality local anesthesia was carved from amino amide derivatives that culminated in Löfgren's description of lidocaine in 1948. Lidocaine (Xylocaine), a potent and stable local anesthetic, combines high tissue penetrance with acceptably low toxicity. Ten years later, Löfgren's countryman Ekenstam introduced the first of the pipecoly1 xylidides (PPX), mepivacaine (Carbocaine). To this day, Sweden remains the undisputed birthland of new local anesthetics, among them long-acting bupivacaine (Marcaine) and monomeric ropivacaine (Naropin).

Pharmacodynamics

Resting Membrane Potential

Reduced to essentials (see references 1, 2 for details), the key to local anesthetic action is locked in the thin lipoprotein *nerve membrane* that, like the skin of a hot dog, separates a nerve's internal stable axoplasm from the ever changing extraneural environment. Traversing the nerve membrane are sparsely distributed, protein-lined, voltage-responsive ion-transmitting channels that render the membrane excitable and, so, capable of generating and conducting tiny electrical currents (impulses). In general, the nerve's resting potential is generated by the cross-membrane potassium ion concentration gradient and the action potential by the sodium ion concentration gradient maintained across the nerve membrane.

The metabolically fueled *sodium-potassium pump* restores and maintains these cross-membrane ionic gradients—and, thus, nerve excitability—by continuously pumping sodium out of, and potassium into, the axoplasm. Metabolic poisons such as cyanide (and similar neurotoxic agents) cripple the pump, killing off nerve activity as the vital electrostatic gradient runs down. By the way, local anesthetics most emphatically are *not* metabolic poisons and, in fact, do not at all alter the nerve's resting potential.

Local Anesthetic Nerve Blockade

Stabilization (deactivation) of the sodium channel lies at the heart of local anesthetic conduction block. Local anesthetics suppress impulse generation and, so, halt bidirectional signal propagation by preventing generation of the so-called sodium current, the first step in initiating a nerve action potential. Impulse block is caused by closing off transmembrane sodium channels, that normally provide transient current paths, thus rendering them impermeant to the inward membrane-depolarizing surge of sodium ions. Thus, although the resting potential is maintained and the blocked nerve proper remains fully polarized, the local anesthetic has rendered the nerve completely inexcitable. Local anesthetic blockade is a nondepolarizing (stabilizing) type of block, comparable, in a sense, to neuromuscular block by curare.

Deep within the sodium channel lies a polar binding site that becomes uncovered, and thus periodically accessible to local anesthetic cation, during voltage-induced conformational changes of channel proteins. Electrostatic binding of the positively charged local anesthetic molecule to oppositely charged fatty acid tails now "locks" the movement of helical protein subunits that normally open and close ("gate") the channel to transmembrane sodium ion traffic. The channel-gating binding site can be reached by local anesthetic cation only by detouring via the internal (axoplasmic) ion channel "mouth," necessitating prior entry by lipophilic local anesthetic base into, and its passage through, the lipid nerve membrane (Fig. 16–1).

The uncharged local anesthetic molecule (the base configuration) also contributes to sodium channel receptor block: being highly lipid soluble, it functions as a carrier that traverses the lipid nerve membrane. On emergence at the membrane's internal (axoplasmic) surface, the base form dissociates into local anesthetic cation, which thereupon ascends into the sodium channel to rigidly lock up the mobile gating structures. Concurrently, the local anesthetic base also diffuses laterally through the membrane in a sidewise direction, creeping up on the sodium channel binding site via the membrane-channel interface (Fig. 16–2). This alternate lateral approach route to the sodium channel–gating receptor site does *not* invoke prior ion pore entry, functions independently of voltage-mediated channel state, and becomes the dominant blocking mechanism for poorly dissociable topical local anesthetics such as benzocaine.

Minimum Blocking Concentration

As we know well from clinical practice, bupivacaine is severalfold more potent than lidocaine, which, in turn, is severalfold more potent than procaine. To provide a measure of relative potency, the *minimum blocking concentration* (C_m) of local anesthetic is defined as the drug concentration that is just sufficient to halt impulse traffic (i.e., the lowest concentration that blocks the nerve and relieves pain). In practice, measurement of C_m in myelinated axons is complicated by the observation that an electrical impulse can skip over one and two—perhaps even three—solidly blocked

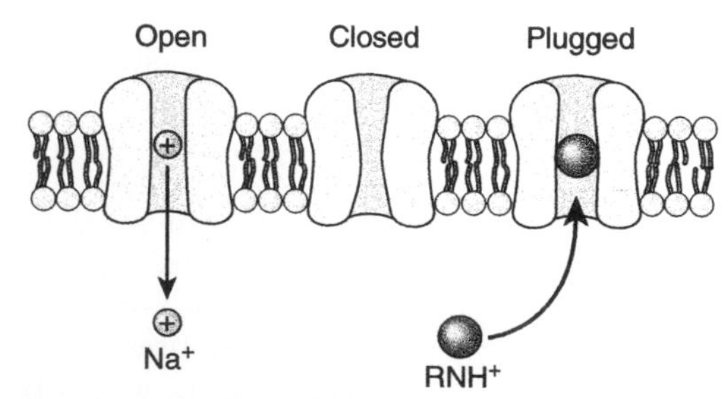

FIGURE 16–1 Channel entry. On the left is an open transmembrane channel, permeable inward to sodium ion. The center channel is in the resting, closed, configuration. Though impermeant to sodium ion as shown, the closed channel remains voltage responsive. The channel on the right, though in open configuration, has been rendered impermeant to sodium ion because local anesthetic cation is bound to the gating receptor site. Note that local anesthetic enters the channel from the axoplasmic (internal) side; the channel's proximally sited filter precludes direct entry via the exterior mouth. Local anesthetic renders the membrane impermeant to sodium ion and thus inexcitable by local action currents; that is, the nerve is blocked. *(From de Jong RH: Local Anesthetics, St. Louis, CV Mosby, 1994.)*

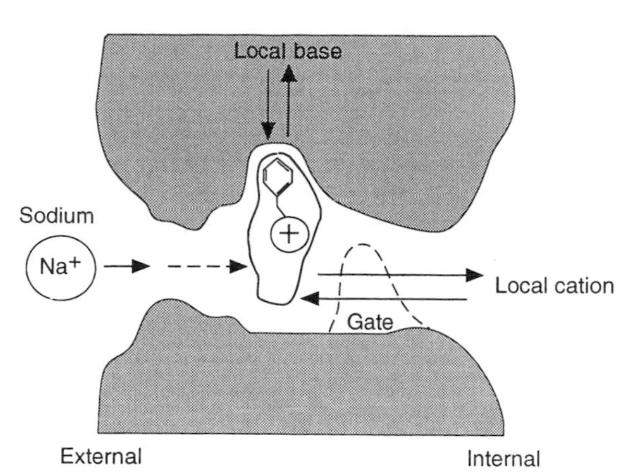

FIGURE 16–2 Interaction at membrane-binding site. Protonated hydrophilic local anesthetic species ("local cation") reaches the sodium channel binding site indirectly via the pore's internal mouth; the uncharged local anesthetic species ("local base") approaches the channel binding site directly via the lipophilic lateral intramembrane route. Hydrophilic pore access is optimal when channel proteins are in the open state. Hydrophobic undissociated local anesthetic bases (e.g., benzocaine) also bind to the gating receptor, reaching it via the membrane-channel interface; such intramembrane blockade is independent of channel state and ambient pH. Captured local anesthetic narrows the transmembrane channel pore, freezes channel protein realignment, and repels like-charged sodium ions. Though the dominant mechanism may vary with spatial channel configuration, the net result is sodium ion impermeability and membrane inexcitability. (Modified from Gintant GA, Hoffman BF: The role of local anesthetic effects in the actions of antiarrhythmic drugs. Handb Exp Pharmacol 81:213–251, 1987.)

successive nodes of Ranvier. At the C_m of local anesthetic, then, propagation of a single impulse is halted by bathing three successive nodes of a myelinated axon or a comparable length (perhaps 5 to 6 mm) of a nonmyelinated nerve fiber. For the sake of both uniformity and convenience, the C_m is commonly measured in a 10-mm length of mixed peripheral nerve for a specified exposure time.

Counter to common clinical teaching, the experimental C_m has proved to be independent of fiber diameter at steady-state conditions and at slow rates of nerve stimulation, at least in the laboratory. As one might surmise, the C_m represents a dynamic equilibrium between channel-bound and channel-released drug. At C_m, the net transmembrane sodium current is reduced below the nerve's firing threshold, and thus cannot marshal sufficient energy to generate an action potential. Clinically, a multitude of real-life variables, such as nerve exposure length, rate of impulse traffic, speed of drug diffusion, and concentration and volume of local anesthetic solution, largely obscure ideal laboratory conditions.

Critical Blocking Length

Nerve impulses can skip over one and two (perhaps even three) consecutive blocked nodes. Anatomically, the thicker a nerve fiber, the longer is the distance between one node and the next. Thus, the internodal interval is considerably greater in large-diameter motor fibers than in small, thin, pain-conducting fibers. Each nerve fiber thus has a *critical blocking length* (CBL), which is proportional to its diameter, spanning three successive nodes that must all be coated by local anesthetic to ensure solid impulse blockade.

Frequency-Dependent Nerve Block

Local anesthetic ions preferentially bind to sodium channel receptors in the open state, whereas they are released faster than they are bound when sodium channels are in the resting state. Thus, the receptor accessibility status of the channel state (open, inactivated, closed, or resting), of itself, affects the quality (depth) of nerve block. This membrane voltage-dependent variability in quality of block is called *state-dependent block*.

When the frequency of stimulation is increased, membrane ion channels are open, and thus accessible to local anesthetic, a greater proportion of the time. Opportunities for sodium channel drug binding are enhanced (and those for drug release reduced) accordingly, and frequency-dependent (also known as *use-dependent* or *phasic*) block ensues. Said plainly, the faster the nerve is made to fire, the more profound will be the block. Fibers that carry rapidly flowing impulse packet traffic—that is, nociceptive and sympathetic nerves—thus require a less concentrated local anesthetic solution to interrupt neural traffic than do motor nerves. *State dependence* and *frequency dependence* are useful concepts, too, in clarifying the curious difference in cardiotoxicity between local anesthetics such as lidocaine and bupivacaine, as we shall see later.

Differential Nerve Block

As mentioned, the critical blocking length of a large-diameter fiber is several times that of a thin-diameter nerve fiber. Thus, a large A-alpha motor fiber may remain functional at a time that pain-related barrages in thin A-delta and C fibers have been blocked by local anesthetic. During such differential nerve block the patient feels no pain yet still can perceive touch and pressure and can contract striated muscles at will (Fig. 16–3). It is that unique character-

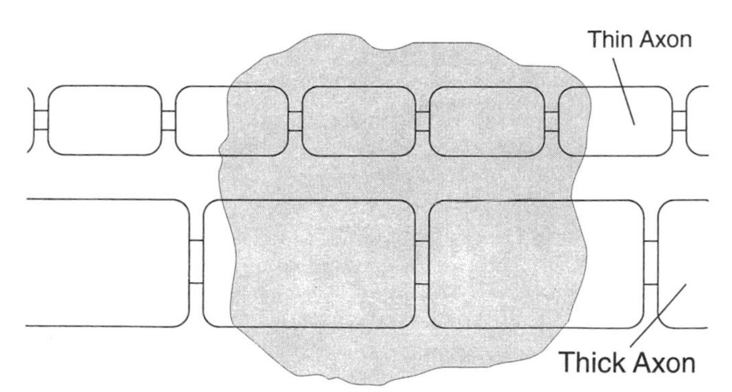

FIGURE 16–3 Nodal interval longitudinal (length-dependent) blockade. Two side-by-side axons—one thin, one thick—are bathed in a puddle of local anesthetic at the minimum blocking concentration (C_m); the internode *(internodal interval) of the thick fiber is twice that of the thin one. The local anesthetic solution covers three successive nodes of the thin axon (*top*) but only one node of the thick axon (*bottom*). Impulses can easily skip over one and even two inexcitable nodes; thus, conduction along the thick axon continues uninterrupted. In the thin axon, its three nodes covered by local anesthetic, impulse conduction is halted. A sufficient volume should be injected to coat with local anesthetic at least three successive nodes (about 1 cm) of even the thickest axon. Longitudinal block is the main operand in threshold differential block of thin (as against thick) nerve bundles (spinal roots, for instance). (From Franz DN, Perry RS: Mechanisms for differential block among single myelinated and non-myelinated axons by procaine. J Physiol 236:193–210, 1974.)*

istic of differential nerve block that allows us to offer nerve blocks to ambulatory patients in chronic pain: the pain has vanished, yet the patient can walk out of the office.

The critical blocking length of spinal B fibers (preganglionic autonomic axons) approximates that of the smallest sensory (cold) fibers. Thus, the sympathetic (and sacral parasympathetic) block that inevitably accompanies spinal or epidural analgesia extends several segments higher, and persists longer, than nociceptive block. The extent of the sympathetic component can be approximated by dermatomal mapping for cold sensation, as with an alcohol sponge. Similar considerations of low C_m and short CBL apply to the fine postganglionic autonomic fibers like those in the paravertebral sympathetic chains and the pelvic parasympathetic nerves.

Because an electrical impulse can readily skip over two successive inexcitable (i.e., blocked) nodes, at least 5 mm (and preferably 8 mm or more) of nerve length must be bathed in local anesthetic solution to ensure solid blockade of even the thickest nerve fibers. As the internodal distance increases with the thickness of the axon, nonuniform longitudinal diffusion further contributes to erratic local anesthetic distribution, and thus to differential block of small and large myelinated fibers. Uneven radial penetration toward, and erratic axial spread through, the core of a major nerve trunk are additional contributors to incomplete anesthesia or differential block. Because pain-relieving nerve blocks are given with the weakest possible local anesthetic solution (to minimize locomotor impairment), larger volumes of more dilute local anesthetic are necessary to ensure deep, wide, and solid penetration of thick nerve trunks, thus to lessen the chance of an incomplete block yet retain the considerable advantages of differential nerve block.

Physicochemical Parameters

Local anesthetics are organic amines, with an intermediary ester or amide linkage separating the lipophilic ringed head from the hydrophilic hydrocarbon tail. The weakly basic local anesthetic amine is lipid soluble, but water insoluble and unstable. Crystalline salts (commonly the hydrochloride) of the local anesthetic base, conversely, are water soluble and stable, but lipid insoluble.

Drug Dissociation

Dissolved in water, the local anesthetic salt crystals ionize to yield anesthetic cation (and chloride or another acid anion). The anesthetic cation (positively charged quaternary amine), in turn, is in dissociation equilibrium with the anesthetic base (uncharged tertiary amine). The proportions of local anesthetic cation and base are governed by the drug's fixed dissociation constant (pK_a) and the variable ambient hydrogen ion concentration (pH). The more acid the solution is (i.e., the lower the pH), the greater the proportion of anesthetic cation in the numerator and the less that of anesthetic base in the denominator:

$$\log\left(\frac{[cation]}{[base]}\right) = pK_a - pH$$

where [*cation*] and [*base*] denote "concentration of" local anesthetic cation and base, respectively.

The lipid-soluble uncharged local anesthetic base species diffuses from the extraneural injection site through dense nerve sheath toward component nerve fibers, eventually to penetrate individual neural membranes. Arriving in the (internal) axoplasm, the anesthetic base then dissociates to local anesthetic cation that, in turn, moves upward in the sodium channel to bond to receptor sites, so locking the gating system that barricades sodium ion influx. The cation-base ratio, determined from the preceding equation, allows only a narrow window for nerve conduction block: Too little base, and too few local anesthetic molecules, will reach the neural target; too little cation, and too few sodium channels, will be closed to sodium ion traffic. Dissociation constants of common local anesthetics are shown in Table 16–1.

The clinical significance of the dissociation constant and the dissociation equation is illustrated by the well-known difficulty of anesthetizing infected tissues. Lactic acidosis (low pH) accompanying tissue infection, though it raises the active channel-blocking cation numerator in the equation, at the same time lowers the concentration of diffusable lipid-soluble local anesthetic base carrier, often rendering anesthesia partial or incomplete.

Pharmacokinetics

The plasma concentration–time profile provides a snapshot of the seesawing balance between local anesthetic absorption from the injection site, interim uptake in (and storage by) tissue reservoirs, drug biotransformation, and ultimate excretion of metabolites. Pharmacokinetic equations are derived from sequential plasma drug concentrations, so they permit construction of drug disposition models. The terminology is a bit arcane. Some plain-English explanations helpful to clinicians follow.

TABLE 16–1 ***Dissociation Constants (Rounded)***

Local Anesthetic	pK_a
Benzocaine	3.5
Mepivacaine	7.7
Lidocaine	7.8
Etidocaine	7.9
Prilocaine	7.9
Ropivacaine	8.1
Bupivacaine	8.1
MEGX (des-ethyl lidocaine)	8.1
Tetracaine	8.4
PPX (pipecolyl xylidide)	8.6
Cocaine	8.6
Dibucaine	8.8
Procaine	8.9
Chloroprocaine	9.1
Hexylcaine	9.3
Procainamide	9.3
Piperocaine	9.8

(From de Jong RH: Local Anesthetics, ed 2. St. Louis, CV Mosby, 1994.)

The total apparent drug storage capacity of human organ reservoirs is called the *volume of drug distribution. Clearance* expresses the rate at which local anesthetic is removed from this huge reservoir. *Half-time* is a convenient composite measure of how quickly (or slowly) the local anesthetic plasma concentration is halved. After some four or five half-times have elapsed, the drug is, for all practical purposes, cleared completely from storage sites.

ABSORPTION

Absorption delivers local anesthetic into the bloodstream, which then distributes it all through the body. While the local anesthetic is bloodborne, a considerable portion is bound to plasma albumin and globulin fractions (mainly A_1AG), limiting the quantity of unbound (free) drug available for outward diffusion into perfused tissues. Human organs have both greater affinity and larger storage capacity for local anesthetic than does the plasma compartment; the extravascular compartment thus provides a high-capacity reservoir that smooths the blood level. During continuous local anesthetic infusion, the tissue buffers eventually become saturated (after about 2 days in the case of bupivacaine) and the drug's blood level increases sharply, and, with it, the risk of drug toxicity.

The rate of local anesthetic absorption into the bloodstream depends on the vascularity of the injection site: The more vascular the tissue is, the faster will be absorption, the higher the blood level rises, and the sooner it peaks. For any given site, drug absorption reflects the net balance between total drug dose injected and tissue perfusion; thus, absorption is essentially independent of concentration. Local vasoconstriction, as with epinephrine, slows absorption, so more local anesthetic is retained longer at the target site, producing both more profound and more prolonged nerve impulse blockade.

DISPOSITION

In general, local anesthetic disposition in humans is approximated by a two-compartment model composed of two phases. Initially there is rapid dilution of absorbed drug into blood and subsequent spread to well-perfused organs (e.g., brain). That rapid dilution phase is followed by a phase of slower, steady distribution into the capacious buffer of less-perfused organs (e.g., muscle). Thus, two half-times are defined: one (alpha) for the rapid initial dilution phase and a second (beta) describing the slow but steady distribution phase. The second phase (beta) parameters have immediate clinical application, as they represent essentially steady-state conditions. Rapid lowering of blood level (i.e., short drug half-time) shortens the duration of a toxic reaction.

Amino amide local anesthetics depend on hepatic blood flow for clearance. Incompletely protein-bound amino amides such as lidocaine and mepivacaine have a substantial free plasma fraction; their disposition is almost entirely hepatic flow–dependent. Strongly plasma protein–bound amino amides such as bupivacaine and ropivacaine have little free (unbound) drug to contribute to hepatic clearance; their elimination is rate-dependent on the free fraction concentration. Urinary and biliary (fecal) elimination is minor for intact local anesthetic; metabolites and conjugates, conversely, are largely excreted renally.

Tissue Diffusion

To reach the neural target site, local anesthetic must diffuse through tissue barriers. In peripheral nerve, the main diffusion barrier is the perineurium[2]; comparably, in transmeningeal diffusion, the arachnoid mater is the principal barrier.[3] An interesting clinical application of drug migration is intravenous regional anesthesia, resulting from reverse diffusion of local anesthetic across the blood-nerve barrier so that the blocking agent reaches nerve trunks as well as terminal nerve branches.[4] During gestation, local anesthetic diffuses transplacentally to reach the fetal circulation; the usual first-trimester precautions apply.

Ultralong Neural Blockade—The Holy Grail

The limited duration of action of local anesthetic neural blockade—measured in hours rather than in days or weeks—is at once its finest attribute, for it allows patients to recover quickly and fully, and its greatest shortcoming, as when treating chronic persistent pain. Although certain benign pain syndromes (e.g., muscle trigger points, scar neuromas) respond favorably to repeated injections of local anesthetic, that is rarely the case with cancer pain, for which nonspecific tissue-destructive neurolytic procedures (see Chapter 17) may produce longer-lasting results.

In the attempt of providing the best of both worlds—prolonged yet nondestructive and painless neural blockade—the search for neurospecific ultralong-acting local anesthetics continues. One promising pharmaceutical approach is modification of the delivery vehicle from aqueous solution to high-payload lipid or crystal encapsulation, to ensure steady and prolonged drug release.[5] Concurrently, chemists continue to modify existing blocking agents that bind more firmly to channel receptors and are less readily leached from the injection site.[6] Taking an altogether different tack are efforts at taming highly lethal natural neurotoxins, such as the infamous puffer fish toxin (tetrodotoxin), to provide semipermanent impulse blockade.[7] The attractive option of providing long-lasting yet reversible pain relief without resort to chemical, surgical, or thermal nerve destruction remains as yet a promise unfulfilled.

Tachyphylaxis

Tachyphylaxis—decreasing response to a drug given repeatedly—to local anesthetics turns out to be more of a mechanical than a physicochemical phenomenon, for it is seen not infrequently with intermittent "top-up" catheter injections but not with continuous infusion. Quite to the contrary, rather than reducing apparent potency (as would be expected with physicochemical tachyphylaxis), continuous drug infusion proves to enhance local anesthetic potency, eventually raising the nerve to supra-C_m steady-state, and so actually decreasing the net local anesthetic requirement as drug uptake approaches losses to drug disposition.[8] Gradually reducing the concentration of infused local anesthetic to the near-C_m range can maintain solid analgesia, with little or no motor block, for days on end without risking spillover from saturated tissue buffers; witness the popular "walking epidural" infusion used for labor analgesia.

Molecular Configuration

Local anesthetics form a class of drugs remarkably homogeneous both in biologic properties and in molecular structure. Other than chemical variations on a common structural theme, three distinguishing features individualize various local anesthetics: (1) *linkage* (ester or amide), which separates the aromatic lipophilic head from the hydrophilic tail; (2) *binding* to lipids and plasma proteins, which controls spread, penetration, duration of action, and toxicity; (3) *dissociation constant* (pK_a; see Table 16–1), which governs the proportions of diffusable lipid-penetrating mobile local anesthetic base and neurally active, but nonmobile, cation for any given pH (see preceding equation).

Most injectable local anesthetics in common use are weakly basic tertiary amines. Exceptions are the secondary amines prilocaine (a partner, with lidocaine, in EMLA cream) and articaine (see later). (Conceptually, a tertiary amine is derived from ammonia [NH_3] each one of its three hydrogen atoms being replaced by an organic substitute.) The fundamental properties of local anesthetic amines (Fig. 16–4) derive from three building blocks: lipophilic aromatic head, hydrophilic aminoalkyl tail, and an intermediate ester or amide carboxy linkage that chains the tail to the head.

The bulky hydrophilic aromatic head is (with rare exception) derived either from benzoic acid (ester family) or from aniline (aminoacyl family). The hydrophilic hydrocarbon tail, which contains dissociable amino nitrogen, is less readily categorized, as it comprises various amino derivatives of ethyl alcohol, acetic acid, or ringed piperidine. Local anesthetics lacking the hydrophilic tail and linkage are hydrophobic and, thus, virtually insoluble in water (e.g., it takes 2500 parts water to dissolve 1 part benzocaine). Although unsuitable for injection, these local anesthetics are instead well-suited for topical application to mucosal surfaces.

Ester and Amide Linkages

The length of the four- or five-atom intermediate linkage has proven to be critical in providing proper planar orientation for the local anesthetic's unique affinity for sodium channel receptors. Some compounds, antihistaminic and anticholinergic drugs, for example, have a similar head-linkage-tail configuration but, because of different linkage orientation, exhibit only weak local anesthetic effects at best. Even the probability of an allergic reaction to local anesthetic turns out to be linkage-dependent.

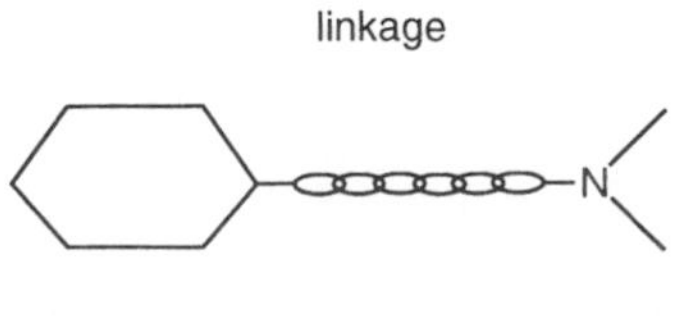

FIGURE 16–4 Fundamental structure. Local anesthetic molecule with lipophilic aromatic (head) and hydrophilic amino (tail) fractions joined together by a five-carbon amino-ester or amino amide connecting "linkage." (From de Jong RH: Local Anesthetics. St. Louis, CV Mosby, 1994.)

A cardinal structural attribute of the linkage is determination of the course of biotransformation, an importance underscored by noting that local anesthetics are classified as either *ester-linked* or *amide-linked* compounds. Ester-linked local anesthetics, characterized by procaine, are readily hydrolyzed by appropriate plasma esterases, whereas amide-linked local anesthetics, characterized by lidocaine, generally require preliminary enzymatic dismantling to ready them for eventual hydrolysis in the liver. Consequently, a somewhat greater proportion of amino amides is excreted partially intact, or nearly so.

Structural Characteristics

Of the literally hundreds of local anesthetics synthesized, few have survived beyond the pharmaceutical laboratory, and even fewer beyond clinical trial. Some initially promising drugs proved to be either very systemically toxic or irritating to tissues; others were too insoluble in water or too unstable once in solution. Finding the proper balance of high potency, low toxicity, just-so dissociation constant, and reasonable balance between solubility in water and diffusibility in lipids remains a largely unpredictable and costly trial-and-error process.

Lengthening the para-amino chain of the aromatic ring makes the compound more resistant to hydrolysis, offering longer duration of action albeit at the price of greater toxicity (e.g., tetracaine). Substitution elsewhere along the aromatic ring alters the three-dimensional configuration of the molecule and imparts new traits. The methyl groups occupying the two ortho positions of the xylidine ring convey great stability to the molecule (e.g., lidocaine, bupivacaine). Their molecular bulk also shields access to the amide linkage, rendering these drugs resistant to first-order immediate enzymatic hydrolysis.

Stereoisomerism

CHIRALITY

When each of the four valences of a carbon atom is linked to a different atom or group, the carbon atom is said to be *asymmetric* or *chiral.* The molecule can be configured around the chiral carbon in either of two three-dimensional mirror images (see ropivacaine, later), each having different physicochemical (and often biologic) properties, including opposite rotation of the axis of polarization of a light beam in a counterclockwise direction (left) or clockwise (right). The two stereoisomers are designated as *S* (*sinister*, or left) and *R* (*rectus*, or right) enantiomers and the axis of light rotation shown as (−) for counterclockwise and (+) for clockwise beam deflection.

Various local anesthetics (e.g., bupivacaine, prilocaine, cocaine) contain a chiral carbon, and thus have *S* and *R* configurations. Lidocaine, conversely, is symmetrically configured and is nonchiral. During routine manufacture of a chiral local anesthetic, equal proportions of each enantiomer are formed; that mixture is said to be *racemic* because the oppositely rotated light axes cancel out. Interestingly, cocaine, the botanically derived original local anesthetic, is a purely levorotatory *monomer* (beta cocaine).

MONOMERIC LOCAL ANESTHETICS

The stereospecificity of local anesthetics was not seriously explored until bupivacaine cardiotoxicity became a public health concern in the 1970s. For instance, *R*(+) bupivacaine has a much longer dwell time (i.e., binds more firmly and is released more slowly) in cardiac sodium channels than the *S*(−) form, accounting for the former's nearly fourfold greater cardiotoxicity.[9] Of additional clinical significance is the more potent depressant effect of *R*(+) bupivacaine, not only directly on the heart but also indirectly on brain stem cardiorespiratory neurons, as compared with its *S*(−) enantiomer.[10] Notable, though of as yet uncertain clinical implication, is the striking stereoselectivity for *R*(+) bupivacaine of an obscure ("flicker") potassium channel (*R/S* affinity ratio 73).[11]

As the two bupivacaine enantiomers are approximately equipotent local anesthetics, the *S*(−) monomer is the preferable choice as it is considerably less cardiotoxic than its *R*(+) mate.[12] Commercial exploration of enantiospecificity took two directions. The more obvious one, synthesis of monomeric L-bupivacaine, was introduced in Europe, whereas a levorotatory monomeric sister of bupivacaine and mepivacaine became the dominant product in the United States (ropivacaine, see later).

Metabolism (generic)

As noted, the intramolecular linkage chain determines certain cardinal pharmaceutical properties, such as course, direction, and rapidity of the first stage(s) of metabolism. Ester-linked local anesthetics (e.g., procaine, tetracaine) are readily hydrolyzed in plasma to the parent aromatic acid and aminoalcohol. In contrast, amide-linked tertiary amines (e.g., lidocaine) resist direct plasma hydrolysis and require one or more preliminary degradation steps before eventual hepatic hydrolysis. In fact, the amide bond is so resistant to nonenzymatic hydrolysis that amino amide local anesthetics can be autoclaved without significant loss of potency; procaine, conversely, tolerates autoclaving only briefly, and poorly at that, before becoming biologically inert. Tetracaine, probably because it is hydrolyzed much more slowly than procaine, can be autoclaved repeatedly with little loss of potency.

Amino amides with a nonlinear cyclic amino tail (e.g., bupivacaine) are even more hydrolysis resistant than the linear-chained ones (e.g., lidocaine) and stoutly defy any attempt at further cleavage. Thus, they are eliminated as incomplete intermediaries with the amide linkage still intact.[2] The cardiotherapeutic use of systemic lidocaine and the long-term epidural infusion of bupivacaine in the control of pain provided a field day for biochemical mapping of their fate in man, well beyond the scope of studies in volunteer subjects. As a result, pronounced differences between biotransformation in humans and laboratory animals have become apparent and will be discussed under individual headings.

CLINICAL PHARMACOLOGY

Classification by Linkage

As noted (see Molecular Configuration), the physicochemical characteristics of the four- or five-atom long linking bridge that chains a local anesthetic's aromatic head to its amino tail are so fundamental as to determine key clinical characteristics such as potency, biotransformation, duration of action, and even drug allergy. In fact, the distinction is so sharp and so predictable that local anesthetics, a unique sodium channel–blocking family of drugs, are subdivided into two major classes: ester-linked and amide-linked or more precisely, *amino ester* and *amino amide* local anesthetics.

The amino amide local anesthetics, in turn, are further subdivided into two classes, once again according to linkage structure. An amino amide linkage can be forged either by fusing an aromatic amine with an alkylamino acid or, the other way around, by joining an aromatic acid to an alkylamino alcohol. The former yields an aminoacyl amide as typified by lidocaine and mepivacaine; the latter, an aminoalkyl amide as represented by dibucaine and procainamide. As only aminoacyl local anesthetics are used in pain management, the reader is referred elsewhere for consideration of aminoalkyl amides.[2]

The dominant aminoacyl class is further subdivided, based on whether the hydrophilic amino tail is a straight carbon chain (like that of lidocaine) or whether the amino nitrogen is captured within a ringed structure (as in mepivacaine). The PPX-ringed local anesthetics (e.g., mepivacaine and bupivacaine) differ from the aminoalkyl xylidide class (e.g., lidocaine and prilocaine) by being even more strongly resistant to hydrolytic cleavage of the amide linkage. The massive piperidine ring, like a large umbrella, evidently shields the linkage from ready enzymatic access.

Amino Ester Local Anesthetics (Procaine Series)

The members of this major class of local anesthetics (Fig. 16–5) have in common ester linkage to benzoic acid or its derivatives. As cocaine, the original botanically derived local anesthetic, turned out to be a complex dual organic acid amino ester, subsequent synthetic local anesthetics (e.g., procaine) mimicked that successful amino ester mold. Not until some 60 years later would a whole new class of local anesthetics—the amide-linked amino amide group—come to the fore.

Ester-linked local anesthetics are cleaved by hydrolysis at the ester linkage, but the rates of the hydrolysis reaction vary considerably among amino esters. Tetracaine, for example, in human plasma, is hydrolyzed some four or five times more slowly than procaine, and other amino esters are affected more by hepatic than by plasma enzymes. As a rule, esters of para-aminobenzoic acid (PABA) or its derivatives (e.g., procaine or tetracaine) are more readily hydrolyzed by plasma than by liver enzymes, as against local anesthetic esters of other aromatic acids (e.g., piperocaine or articaine), which are hydrolyzed more readily in the liver than in plasma. Cocaine, being both a benzoic acid and a methyl ester, straddles the divide; it requires both plasma and liver esterases for complete disposition.[2]

Procaine

Procaine (Novocaine), godfather of the synthetic para-amino benzoic acid ester family, long was synonymous

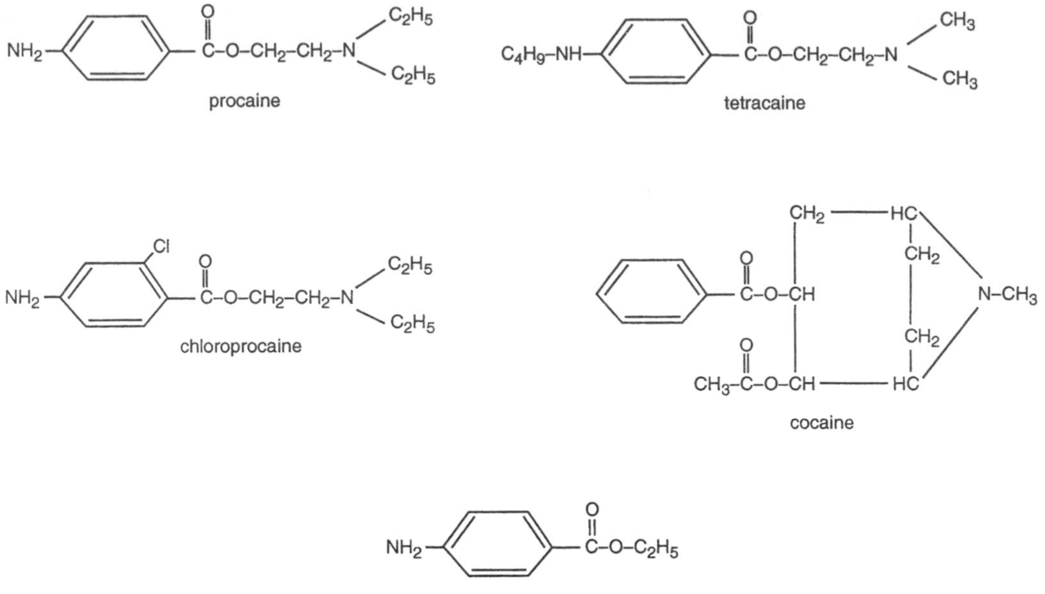

procaine

tetracaine

chloroprocaine

cocaine

benzocaine

FIGURE 16–5 Representative ester-linked local anesthetics. (From de Jong RH: Local Anesthetics. St. Louis, CV Mosby, 1994.)

with local anesthesia. Though its relatively low toxicity permitted extensive regional block procedures, it has long since been replaced by more potent, longer-acting, and more readily diffusible ester- and amide-linked local anesthetics.

Procaine is hydrolyzed by plasma enzymes to form PABA and diethylaminoethanol (DEAE). "Procainesterase" later was identified as serum pseudocholinesterase (which also hydrolyzes succinylcholine): certain patients with low plasma pseudocholinesterase levels potentially could suffer protracted amino ester toxicity. When this enzyme deficiency is suspected, a nonhydrolyzable local anesthetic such as lidocaine might be the better choice.

Chloroprocaine

Rather trivial alterations to the procaine molecule can produce substantial changes in biologic activity. To illustrate, chloroprocaine (2-chlorprocaine or Nesacaine; see Fig. 16–5) is hydrolyzed some four times faster than procaine in human plasma and thus on unintended intravenous injection is less toxic than procaine. Yet nagging issues have surfaced in the past about potential myelo- and neurotoxicity that, for a while, caused chloroprocaine to yield ground.

The 1970s formulation Nesacaine incorporated an acid antioxidant to ensure stable shelf life; the sodium metabisulfite later was implicated in causing neural damage.[13] Nesacaine was reformulated subsequently by substituting ethylene diamine tetraacetic acid (EDTA) stabilizer for bisulfite (Nesacaine MPF). That switch shortly was hounded by reports of severe lumbar muscle spasm after uneventful epidural analgesia, possibly because of the calcium-chelating action of EDTA.[13] Even so, solid blocking potency, fast onset, and rapid disposition by the fetus commend chloroprocaine for analgesic nerve blocks in pregnant patients.

Tetracaine

Substituting a butylamino radical for the para-amino group on procaine's aromatic ring (and shortening the alkylamino tail) yields tetracaine (Pontocaine, Amethocaine). This simple modification (see Fig. 16–5) spawns a profoundly different local anesthetic that is some ten times more potent, and hydrolyzed some three to four times more slowly, than procaine. Pity that it is also just about ten times more toxic than procaine. The therapeutic advantages of tetracaine—long duration of action and intense neural blockade—are mitigated somewhat by tediously slow tissue diffusion and delayed onset. At century's end, however, tetracaine reemerged as the gold standard for subarachnoid analgesia because of its enviable track record of safety, reasonable speed of onset, predictable duration of blocking action, and negligible incidence of transient postspinal radicular pain in ambulatory patients. Synergism of tetracaine with intrathecal opioids (in contrast to bupivacaine's) remains to be explored.

Tetracaine is hydrolyzed slowly but completely by cleavage at the ester linkage. Neither of its hydrolysis products—para-butylaminobenzoic acid and dimethylamino ethanol—are thought to be toxic; the fragments and their conjugates are eliminated in the urine. Though tetracaine hydrolysis is some four times slower than that of procaine, it still is fast as compared with that of amino amide local anesthetics.

Benzocaine

The ethyl ester of PABA differs from injectable water-soluble amino esters in that it lacks the cardinal connecting linkage and attached hydrophilic amino tail. Even so, benzocaine retains a rudimentary linkage sufficient to impart elemental anesthesiophoric characteristics (see Fig.

16–5). Being a very weak nonionizable base (pK_a 3.5), it exists almost entirely as the uncharged (neutral) free base species at physiologic pH. Accordingly, benzocaine is barely soluble in water (1 part in 2500) and, in fact, causes tissue irritation on injection. Benzocaine is used extensively as a topical anesthetic in products like burn nostrums, mucosal sprays, hemorrhoid salves, and throat lozenges. Benzocaine's most likely metabolic pathway is simple hydrolysis to PABA and ethanol. Rare methemoglobinemia, of undetermined cause, has been described after use as a laryngotracheal topical spray.[2]

Amino Amide Local Anesthetics (Lidocaine and Mepivacaine Series)

The amide-linked local anesthetics (Fig. 16–6) are much more resistant to hydrolysis at the linkage join than their ester-linked cousins, longer duration of action being the most immediate benefit. In most instances, a tertiary amino amide must be converted first to a simpler (secondary amine) form before the linkage can be cleaved at all. The common first step is dealkylation of the amino nitrogen, which transforms a tertiary amine to a secondary one: for example, lidocaine to monoethylglycinexylidide (MEGX). Indeed, a secondary amine such as prilocaine is more readily hydrolyzed by amidases than are tertiary amines.

Because the predominant configuration of an amino amide local anesthetic remains virtually intact during opening metabolic skirmishes, one might well wonder about the biologic activity and toxicity of complex intermediary products. Metabolism of lidocaine and bupivacaine are singled out because these local anesthetics, or close congeners, are commonly given for pain relief, either by mouth or as a continuous infusion. Efficient drug disposition is desirable, because if it is not cleared promptly, parent drug or metabolites or both can accumulate to cause unexpected, and perhaps unwanted, toxic side effects.

Aminoalkyl Xylidide Local Anesthetics (Lidocaine Family)

Lidocaine

In the half century since its discovery lidocaine (Xylocaine), named *lignocaine* in the *British Pharmacopeia*, has supplanted procaine as the standard local anesthetic. Though its activity-toxicity ratio is not much different from that of procaine, lidocaine diffuses farther and faster, yields a more solid and longer-lasting block, and raises nary a concern about allergy.

Widespread use and diversity of applications (e.g., antiarrhythmic, tumescent liposuction, anticonvulsant) of lidocaine led to detailed study. More is known about its fate in

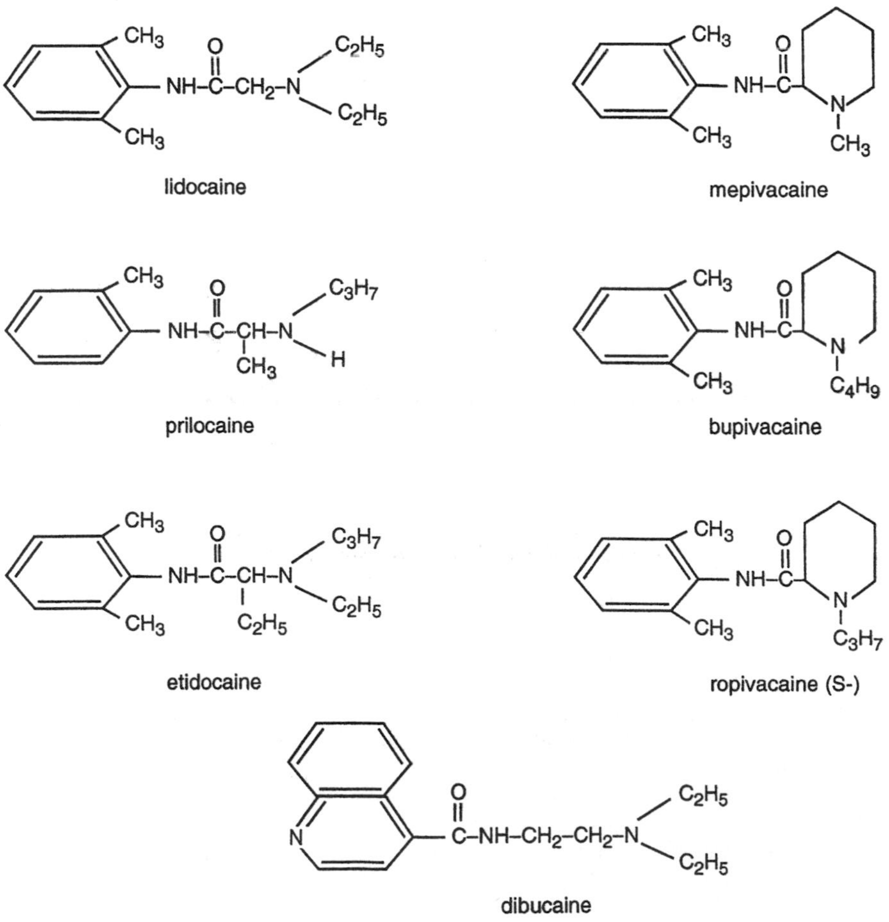

lidocaine

mepivacaine

prilocaine

bupivacaine

etidocaine

ropivacaine (S-)

dibucaine

FIGURE 16–6 Representative amide-linked local anesthetics. (From de Jong RH: Local Anesthetics. St. Louis, CV Mosby, 1994.)

humans than that of any other local anesthetic. Lidocaine's duration of action is several hours, a desirable attribute for rapid recovery (as in ambulatory pain management) but less desirable when prolonged pain relief is needed. One workaround for short duration is to slow drug absorption with a vasoconstrictor such as epinephrine; another is repeated injection or continuous infusion through an implanted catheter. Opening new vistas in invasive pain management is the demonstration of profound synergistic antinociception when subclinical amounts of local anesthetic are added to spinal opioid.[14]

VASOCONSTRICTOR

Adding a vasoconstrictor to lidocaine solution reduces blood flow in the target region, thus slowing drug absorption. Retaining the drug longer on target prolongs duration of lidocaine block by as much as 50%, and, because there is less dilution with tissue fluid, nerve block is more intense. Thus, one can obtain the same "depth" of block with a lower lidocaine concentration and thereby reduce the total drug dose. Similarly, systemic toxicity is reduced because less lidocaine is absorbed per unit of time, so that drug release is slowed. The net result is a lower peak blood level (as compared with the same dose of plain lidocaine) that occurs later.

Though numerous vasoconstrictors and adrenergic agents have been tested (e.g., neosynephrine, octapressin, clonidine), epinephrine has remained the first-line choice. Empirically, the optimal concentration of epinephrine is 5 μg/mL (also expressed as 1 : 200,000). More epinephrine (i.e., 10 μg/mL) provides little, if any, longer duration of action, and raises the ante for epinephrine side effects.[2] Quite the opposite, *less* epinephrine (1 μg/mL or 1 : 1,000,000) has made possible the subcutaneous infiltration of gargantuan (35 mg/kg and up) doses of lidocaine for so-called tumescent liposuction.[15]

PAIN MANAGEMENT

Management of central pain states has emerged as a challenging corollary to lidocaine-induced systemic analgesia. Experimentally, lidocaine profoundly suppresses injury-induced spinal nociception and secondary sensitization ("windup") of wide dynamic range (WDR) neurons in the spinal cord's dorsal horn.[16] This has been corroborated clinically in a highly effective lidocaine infusion protocol for treating chronic refractory neuropathic pain.[17]

Lidocaine itself, when taken orally, has poor bioavailability because of extensive hepatic first-pass extraction. But more metabolism-resistant lidocaine derivatives (e.g., mexiletine) are used increasingly as ancillary drugs in managing diabetic neuropathy, for instance. Oral dose regimens of 10 mg/kg per day have relieved a variety of other neuropathic pain syndromes as well: postamputation stump pain, chemotherapy neurotoxicity, postirradiation plexopathies, and even the agony of thalamic pain.[18, 19] Tinnitus, an early sign of cerebrotoxicity, has been observed as a side effect of mexiletine.

METABOLISM

Lidocaine is transformed in the human liver by microsomal mixed-function oxidases and amidases, largely the cytochrome P_{450} 3A4 isoenzyme cluster.[20] Lidocaine metabolism is (hepatic blood) flow-limited, with better than 70% extraction. Nearly 80% of a single dose of lidocaine eventually can be accounted for as hydroxylated and conjugated products in human urine. With its favorable hepatic extraction ratio, only advanced liver disease might hamper lidocaine metabolism enough to cause the blood level to rise. Even so, concern has been expressed by advocates of ultra-high lidocaine dosing that hepatic enzyme competition with drugs such as selective serotonin inhibitors (e.g., sertraline) could cause unexpectedly high, potentially toxic, lidocaine blood levels.[21] That concern appears to be speculative at best, as the premise was inferred from studies in vitro rather than evidence based on solid clinical grounds.[22]

In humans, biotransformation of lidocaine begins with oxidative de-ethylation of the amino nitrogen to monoethylglycinexylidide (MEGX). MEGX, a secondary amine, is then further dismantled by shearing the remaining ethyl radical off the amino nitrogen to form glycinexylidide (GX), a primary amine. MEGX is excreted more than adequately by the kidneys; surprisingly, seeing its simpler chemical structure, the renal capacity for GX elimination is rather marginal. In fact, the GX plasma level continues to increase perceptibly during continuous lidocaine infusion because its rate of elimination approaches renal transport saturation. Even a modest reduction in renal function could lead to accumulation, raising the (remote) specter of delayed GX cardio- or cerebrotoxicity in the renally impaired.[2]

Prilocaine

Prilocaine (Citanest), named *propitocaine* by the *British Pharmacopeia*, is a lidocaine homologue local anesthetic (see Fig. 16–6). When first introduced, it received considerable acclaim, for prilocaine is approximately as potent as lidocaine yet, being a secondary amine, is more readily hydrolyzed to ensure lower systemic toxicity. Yet biotransformation eventually was its undoing, as prilocaine's aminophenol metabolites oxidize hemoglobin to methemoglobin. While methemoglobinemia of minor degree has occasionally followed the use of lidocaine or benzocaine, prilocaine reduces the blood's oxygen-carrying capacity in a dose-dependent manner—at times enough to cause visible cyanosis. Despite undeniable advantages, prilocaine was doomed for interventional nerve block procedures by its metabolites.

EMLA CREAM

That said, prilocaine has made a stunning comeback because of an altogether different physicochemical attribute: miscibility. When mixed in equal proportions, lidocaine and prilocaine base form an oily substance with a melting point lower than either of its parents. This *e*utectic *m*ixture of *l*ocal *a*nesthetics (EMLA) is picked up by the transdermal transport system to anesthetize terminal sensory nerve fibers underneath the skin. EMLA cream's main drawback is slow transdermal migration; dermal analgesia sufficient for venipuncture requires an hour's application under an occlusive skin dressing.

Because of its profound blocking action on subdermal nerve endings, topical application to spontaneously discharging nociceptors seems a logical therapeutic extension.

In informal clinical trials, EMLA cream has produced encouraging results in the treatment of postherpetic allodynia, superficial scar neuromas, and atypical facial pain; encouraging in that regard is the observation that EMLA cream effectively penetrates any skin, regardless of thickness or pigmentation.[23] Nevertheless, the uncertainties surrounding prolonged low-level aminophenol metabolite exposure remain to be resolved before long-term application, as for burn treatment, can be recommended.

Articaine

Articaine (Carticaine, Ultracaine) was introduced in the 1970s as a low-toxicity replacement for lidocaine. It has found favor as a regional anesthetic in dentistry, but dependence on adding epinephrine (without it, articaine block can be altogether unpredictable) nullified evanescent advantages in nerve block therapy. Overall, articaine (with epinephrine) has little to distinguish it from lidocaine or mepivacaine, whose proven track records give them the advantage.[24] Articaine is an amide-linked local anesthetic unique in two ways. First, like prilocaine, it is a secondary amine; second, unlike the six-membered xylidine aromatic ring of other aminoacyls, it has a five-membered thiophene ring that contains sulfur. Also different is articaine's metabolism: oxidation of the lipophilic thiophene ring is given priority over the more usual dealkylation of the hydrophilic secondary amino nitrogen tail.

Etidocaine

Etidocaine, yet another offshoot of lidocaine (see Fig. 16–6) initially seemed promising because of long duration of action (comparable to bupivacaine), short latency of onset (comparable to lidocaine), and profound motor nerve blockade. But, like bupivacaine, etidocaine soon was found cursed with refractory cardiotoxicity. Worse yet, etidocaine selectively blocked motor fibers more intensely than sensory fibers, giving rise to the anomalous situation of a motor-impaired patient suffering incomplete analgesia. That latter shortcoming, alone, doomed etidocaine for outpatient nerve blocks.[2]

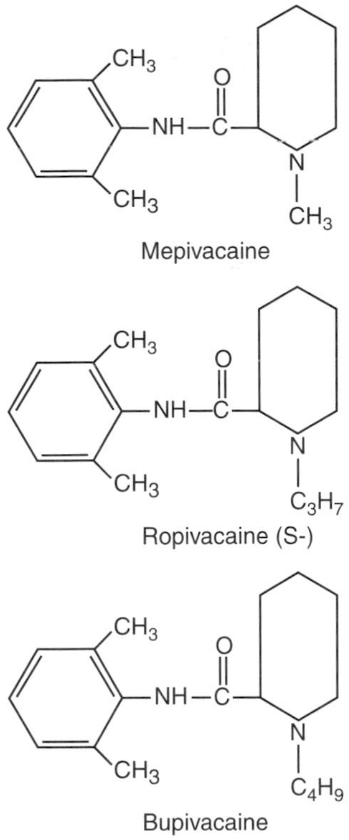

FIGURE 16–7 *Pipecolyl xylidides. The members of the mepivacaine family are alike in fundamental structure, differing solely in the length of the alkyl tail trailing from the piperidine nitrogen. The drug's generic name reflects its alkyl appendage; that is, mepivacaine (methyl) and bupivacaince (butyl). Ropivacaine (*center*) originally was named propivacaine (propyl); potential confusion with propitocaine eventually dictated renaming. While mepivacaine and bupivacaine are racemic (RS) mixtures, ropivacaine and* L*-bupivacaine both are pure S-monomers.*

Pipecolyl Xylidide Local Anesthetics (Mepivacaine Family)

The PPX series, like the aminoalkyl xylidide series a decade earlier, traces its birth roots to Sweden. Though structurally different in tail assembly, the common amide linkage component bestows comparable local anesthetic qualities to mepivacaine and lidocaine, the respective family patriarchs. Differences arise from the more complex and bulky nitrogen-containing piperidine ring, as compared with the structurally simpler straight-chained amino alkyl portion of the lidocaine family. First, PPX metabolism is more circuitous and less complete because of extensive steric shielding of the amide linkage by the ringed structure at either end (Fig. 16–7). Second, the carbon atom joining the piperidine ring to the amide linkage is chiral. Hence pipecolyl xylidides exist in two mirror-image three-dimensional structural configurations: *R* (rectus) and *S* (sinister). Experimentally, the *S* enantiomers are less cardiotoxic than their *R* antipodes. Commercial mepivacaine and bupivacaine comprise racemic, optically neutral, balanced mixtures of the respective *R*- and *S*- enantiomers. Ropivacaine and levobupivacaine, quite specifically, are purebred monomeric *S*-enantiomers.

Mepivacaine

Although mepivacaine (Carbocaine) has a cyclic (ringed) piperidine rather than a linear alkyl-amino hydrophilic tail, it resembles lidocaine in the key clinical respects of impulse-blocking potency and toxicity (see Fig. 16–6). Mepivacaine's duration of action may be slightly longer than that of lidocaine, though the difference is hardly sufficient to favor selection of one agent over the other. The 1.5% solution of mepivacaine has become a popular choice for major nerve blocks (e.g., brachial plexus) because of rapid onset of profound analgesia, predictable diffusion, moderate motor block, and a duration of action sufficient for outpatient surgery yet not so long as to require a prolonged recovery stay.

While marketing claims have been made for intrinsic vasoconstriction, in practice, epinephrine (5 μg/mL) commonly is added to mepivacaine to reduce absorption and prolong duration. Mepivacaine also lends itself well to mixing with a long-acting agent such as bupivacaine. The resultant "supercaine" combines the best features of both drugs to provide rapid onset of analgesia with long duration of block for postsurgical pain relief. Keep in mind, though, that the toxicity of local anesthetic mixtures such as supercaine equals, as a rough approximation, the sum of the toxicities of its component constituents.[2]

Mepivacaine's bi-cyclic structure (like that of bupivacaine and ropivacaine) guides it down a metabolic trail altogether different from that of lidocaine. A major product of hepatic mepivacaine metabolism in adult humans is obtained by *N*-demethylation of the piperidine nucleus to PPX which has proven stubbornly resistant to further degradation. An alternate metabolic route, far more productive with mepivacaine than with bupivacaine, is ring hydroxylation to meta-(2OH) and para-(3OH) hydroxymepivacaine prior to urinary excretion. Mepivacaine well illustrates the human body's successful attempts at lowering local anesthetic toxicity: whereas PPX is about two thirds as toxic as mepivacaine, para-hydroxy PPX is only a third as toxic. Subsequent oxidation or conjugation further lowers the toxicity of fragments. As mepivacaine stoutly resists linkage hydrolysis, conjugation to water-soluble renally excreted nontoxic glucuronides provides a safe alternate detoxification avenue.

Bupivacaine

Bupivacaine (Marcaine, Sensorcaine) is representative of the second generation of long-acting local anesthetics. Though very closely related to its mepivacaine and ropivacaine homologues (see Fig. 16–7), bupivacaine is an altogether different local anesthetic. Lengthening the one-carbon methyl tail of mepivacaine's piperidine ring to a four-carbon butyl chain imparts longer duration of action and enhances potency, although at the price of greater toxicity. Bupivacaine analgesia lasts two to three times longer than analgesia provided by lidocaine or mepivacaine. Repeated injection or continuous epidural infusion of bupivacaine could lead to accumulation of drug and metabolite as storage reservoirs become saturated over several days, creating the potential for rising bupivacaine blood levels and drug toxicity. Bupivacaine is highly lipid soluble and some 97% plasma protein bound.

By all appearances, bupivacaine was well on its way to stardom when, in the late 1970s, clinical and anecdotal reports appeared of sudden cardiac arrest after regional anesthesia with long-duration local anesthetics. Worse yet, the majority of adverse outcomes occurred in term-pregnant women.[25] Shortly, 0.75% bupivacaine was withdrawn from obstetric use. The potent 0.75% solution remains available, however, for nonobstetric use. It is a preferred local anesthetic for ophthalmic blocks and commonly is mixed with faster-onset shorter-duration local anesthetics such as lidocaine or mepivacaine.

For interventional pain management, 0.25% bupivacaine is the preferred concentration, as it provides more than adequate analgesia with minor to moderate motor block. The 0.5% solution is reserved for cases that call for profound muscle relaxation, such as joint manipulation. Whatever the concentration, it is the total drug mass of bupivacaine injected that sets limits on dosing. Manufacturer's recommendation is 1 to 2 mg/kg, or 150 to 200 mg for a fit adult. Judicious fractionated injection, while listening for the early warning signal of slurring speech, and constantly watching the electrocardiogram for rhythm changes, are readily adopted prudent precautions.

Firm tissue binding of injected bupivacaine ensures both buffering from too rapid blood level peaks and prolonged duration of action. Used for perineural analgesia, bupivacaine block may last 4 to 6 hours or longer. Duration of action in the epidural space is more on the order of 2 hours or less, so catheter placement is required for extended infusion periods. Not for lack of trying, epinephrine has been found wanting in either significantly reducing blood levels of absorbed bupivacaine or notably prolonging analgesia. Mostly, epinephrine side effects are produced without the proper payback of longer duration; experimentally, at least, epinephrine may even enhance bupivacaine's cardiotoxicity.[26]

PAIN MANAGEMENT

Bupivacaine is widely used in North America for prolonged pain relief by continuous catheter infusion. After an initial period of nerve tissue "soaking" with more concentrated bupivacaine, the infusate is diluted progressively down to 0.1% or even less. Highly useful in that respect is the synergy of analgesia when bupivacaine is added to an opioid infusion, permitting profound pain relief without the drawbacks of orthostatic hypotension or respiratory depression of either drug given alone.[27] Particularly gratifying is the effectiveness of the opioid-bupivacaine mixture in managing refractory neuropathic pain such as invasive plexopathies.[28] It is worth repeating that during continuous drug infusion the clinically effective local anesthetic concentration drops ever lower, eventually approaching the drug's theoretical C_m (see section on Tachyphylaxis).[2]

METABOLISM

Bupivacaine's amide linkage, well sheltered by piperidine at one end and by xylidine at the other end, is virtually impregnable to hydrolysis in humans. The initial metabolic thrust instead deflects to dealkylation of the piperidine nitrogen to yield PPX (Fig. 16–8). PPX, by the way, is also

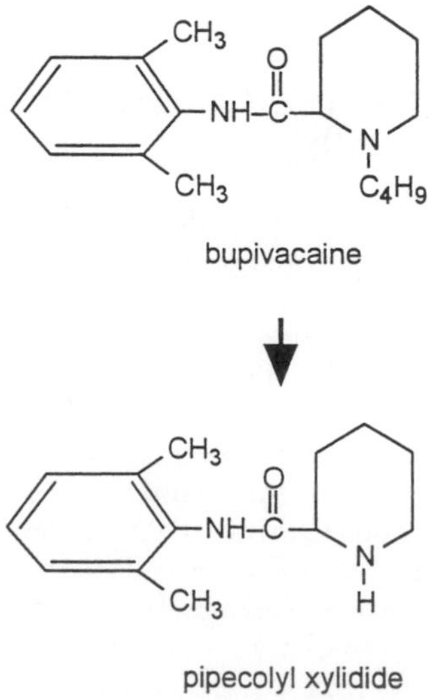

CH_3 / CH_3 / C_4H_9 / NH–C(=O)

bupivacaine

CH_3 / CH_3 / NH–C(=O) / N–H

pipecolyl xylidide

FIGURE 16–8 *Bupivacaine biotransformation. (From de Jong RH: Local Anesthetics. St. Louis, CV Mosby, 1994.)*

the dealkylation product of mepivacaine and ropivacaine metabolism, so that numerous similarities in eventual disposition of the three homologous local anesthetics may be noted. Debutylation is a remarkably effective detoxification process; PPX is only one eighth as lethal as its bupivacaine parent.[2]

Because bupivacaine is widely used for extended epidural or peripheral nerve infusion, metabolites, hitherto unknown after single dose administration, have been uncovered in humans, para-hydroxy (4-OH) bupivacaine being best characterized. PPX and 4-OH bupivacaine accumulate slowly when bupivacaine is infused at a rate sufficient to provide pain relief. As with the parent drug, buffer reservoir saturation may take from 1 to 2 days; after that initial equilibration period, plasma drug levels are wholly determined by hepatic and renal clearance rates.[29] Generally, plasma bupivacaine (and metabolite) concentrations tend to rise slowly during and after tissue buffer equilibration, counterbalanced by compensatory plasma protein production that tends to lower the free (unbound) drug fraction.[30]

CARDIOTOXICITY

Studies of the cardiac sodium channel have demonstrated threefold tighter affinity for *R*(+) than for *S*(−) bupivacaine.[9] The *R*(+) bupivacaine enantiomer thus appears to be the "fast-in, slow-out" member of the steric bupivacaine antipode pair, whereas the *S*(−) enantiomer is the less cardiotoxic of the two.[31] The issue is further complicated by the disparate effects of the two bupivacaine enantiomers on medullary control neurons, for *R* bupivacaine exerts severalfold greater cardiorespiratory depressant effect than the *S* enantiomer.[10] In short, bupivacaine cardiotoxicity is the net result of a summation of effects (largely attributable to the *R* enantiomer) of both *direct* myocardial and *indirect* brain stem components.

These far-reaching discoveries doubtlessly culminated in the introduction of ropivacaine, the *S* (levo) enantiomer of the propyl homologue of mepivacaine and bupivacaine, and subsequently of levobupivacaine, the purely monomeric *S* enantiomer of bupivacaine itself. Ropivacaine's channel association and dissociation constants may not be quite as favorable as those of lidocaine, but they are a considerable improvement over those of racemic (*RS*) bupivacaine.[32] Theory and in vitro analysis aside, ropivacaine represents a gratifying pharmacologic advance in patient safety, as we shall see next.

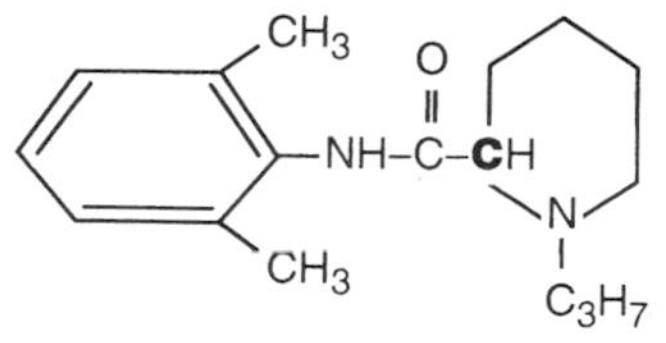

Ropivacaine

Ropivacaine, the third generation of the PPX amino amide series, is the propyl ($-C_3H_7$) homologue of PPX (see Fig. 16–7). Its pharmacologic properties thus fall between those of bupivacaine ($-C_4H_9$) and mepivacaine ($-CH_3$), leaning closer to the former than to the latter. Like its sisters, ropivacaine has an asymmetric chiral carbon atom at the join of the carboxy-amide linkage with the piperidine ring. This chiral carbon allows for two mirror-image steric twins of the molecule, the *S*(−) and the *R*(+) enantiomers (Fig. 16–9).[32] Whereas both mepivacaine and bupivacaine are dispensed as the optically inactive (left rotation nullifying right rotation) racemic *RS* mixture, ropivacaine is the optically active (left-rotating) pure *S*(−) monomer.

S-ropivacaine

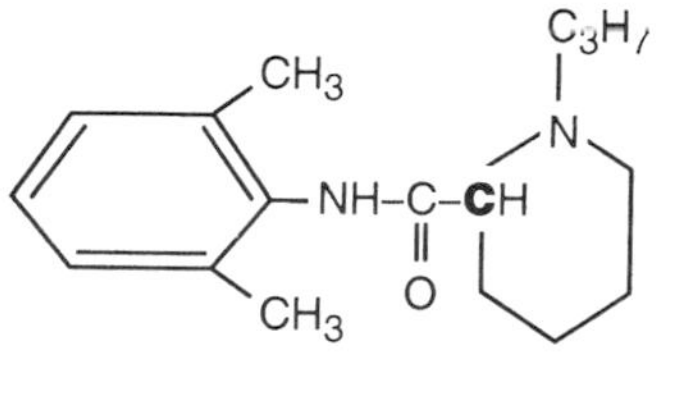

R-ropivacaine

FIGURE 16–9 *Ropivacaine. (P)ropivacaine is a homologue (propyl-PPX) of mepivacaine (methyl-PPX) and bupivacaine (butyl-PPX). All three have a* chiral *asymmetric carbon atom (boldface* **C***) where the aminoacyl linkage joins the piperidine ring. Two mirror-image optical isomers coexist: S-ropivacaine (top,* left*) and R-ropivacaine (bottom, right). Unlike its sister homologues, formulated as the racemic—RS(±); optically neutral—mixture, only the S(−) enantiomer of ropivacaine is used clinically; the R(+) enantiomer proved more cardiotoxic than the S(−) form. (From de Jong RH: Local Anesthetics. St. Louis, CV Mosby, 1994.)*

STEREOSPECIFICITY

Like mepivacaine and ropivacaine, bupivacaine has an asymmetric chiral carbon atom. The arcane concepts of chirality and stereospecificity may be clarified by an everyday example. The right hand (Fig. 16–10)—one of a left-right (mirror image) pair—slides only into the right glove, where it molds precisely to a specific fit. The right foot, conversely, fits nonspecifically into either one of a pair of socks.

Far from being a "me-too" drug, ropivacaine takes unique advantage of the high-potency, low-toxicity profile of the *S* enantiomer as compared with its *R* counterpart. In vitro studies comparing *S*(−) with *R*(+) ropivacaine show the former to be severalfold less arrhythmogenic than the latter. The former also is considerably less lethal than the latter, whereas nerve impulse–blocking potency and duration of blocking action compare favorably with those of racemic (*RS*) bupivacaine.[32] Of, as yet, uncertain clinical relevance is the dramatic 73-fold *R/S* stereoselectivity of an obscure potassium (flicker) channel discovered in the neural membrane of small myelinated nerve fibers.[11]

Clinically meaningful vasoconstriction, unlike the unsubstantiated claims made for mepivacaine, appears to accompany ropivacaine injection. Blanching and decreased cutaneous blood flow are observed when infiltrating ropivacaine subcutaneously, making it a good candidate for field block. Epidural blood flow, and thus drug absorption, likewise are reduced by ropivacaine.[32] Ropivacaine-induced vasoconstriction is borne out experimentally: human arte-

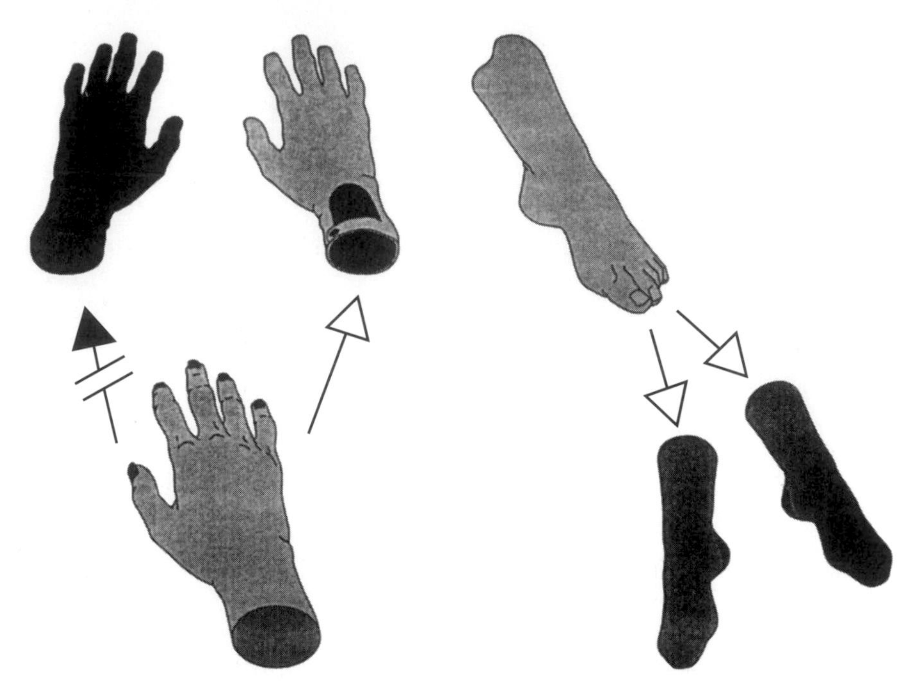

FIGURE 16–10 Stereospecificity. A stereoselective receptor accepts only the matching R or S configuration enantiomer; much as a right-hand glove fits only the right hand. The left-hand glove does not match at all with ("rejects") the right hand. A nonselective receptor, conversely, accepts either of the two steric antipodes; much as either of a pair of socks fits the right foot. (Drawing by David Factor, Medical Illustration, Mayo Clinic. Reproduced with artist's permission.)

rial rings constrict when bathed in ropivacaine, and, applied directly to spinal meninges, ropivacaine constricts pial blood vessels.[33] Yet, numerous virtues notwithstanding, ropivacaine should by no means be considered innocuous, for it can cause convulsions accompanied by life-threatening arrhythmias.[34] Further, uncertainties such as myotoxicity relative to bupivacaine (of concern in muscle trigger point injections) remain to be sorted out as yet.

METABOLISM

As with bupivacaine, PPX appears to be the main metabolic end product of hepatic dealkylation, the metabolite's toxicity being about one eighth that of parent ropivacaine (compare Fig. 16–8). In humans, the hepatic cytochrome P_{450} system accounts for the bulk of, if not all, metabolic activity.[35] Judging by the metabolism of mepivacaine and bupivacaine in humans, hydroxylated ropivacaine or PPX fragments, or both, may be expected, as well as water-soluble conjugation products. Renal excretion of intact ropivacaine is on the order of just a few percent of parent drug; excretion of PPX in humans, representing 50% or more of total metabolites, appears to be rate limited. Rate-limited renal excretion surfaces the possibility of metabolite accumulation during prolonged ropivacaine infusion.[36] Dose-ranging and pharmacokinetic studies in human subjects thus far support the claims of more rapid disposition and lesser systemic toxicity for ropivacaine relative to bupivacaine.[37]

Levobupivacaine

As noted, the *S* monomer of commercial racemic (*RS*) bupivacaine is considerably less cardiotoxic than its *R* antipode twin yet has nearly equipotent nerve-blocking capacity. Based on this stereoselectivity, ropivacaine was designed from the ground up as a brand new levomeric propyl-pipecolyl xylidide. A perhaps less circuitous path to have taken, so it seems, would be to refine the synthesis of bupivacaine itself so as to yield up solely the *S* monomer, in lieu of the present *RS* mixture of equal parts *R* and *S* enantiomers. Indeed, modern technology, using membrane separation synthesis, has made possible commercial quantity production of levobupivacaine (Chirocaine).

In human volunteer studies, intravenous levobupivacaine had significantly less adverse effect than *RS* bupivacaine on electrocardiogram and left ventricular contraction force.[38] When used for epidural anesthesia, levo (*S*) and racemic (*RS*) bupivacaine were essentially equipotent analgesics, and virtually indistinguishable in other clinical attributes as well.[39] Levobupivacaine already has been tested, and used with considerable acclaim, abroad[30]; it is awaiting FDA clearance for use in the United States. Although numerous reports attest to levobupivacaine's safety and efficacy as compared with racemic (*RS*) bupivacaine, critical evaluation still begs comparative human studies side-by-side with ropivacaine.

ADVERSE DRUG EFFECTS

While local anesthetics, by and large, have had a sterling record of safety and efficacy, familiarity with the various manifestations of drug reactions will provide early warning that something may be amiss—thus averting unpleasant or possibly life-threatening complications. Untoward responses to local anesthetics are categorized as systemic, local, global, or combinations of these.[2] Systemic reactions occur when organ systems distant to the injection site respond to bloodborne drug, whereas local reactions occur when local anesthetic injures the structures it contacts directly. Because local anesthetic is injected perineurally in concentrations manyfold greater than the experimental (C_m)—so as to offset gross inefficiencies of the transport and delivery system—cells or tissues in direct contact with, or close to, this strong solution could be harmed. Finally, buttressing the dividing line between systemic and localized reactions, are global reactions precipitated by minute quantities of drug in previously sensitized or genetically atopic persons.

Systemic Reactions

Systemic reactions, other than allergy, are dose-dependent. That is, the higher the local anesthetic concentration in the blood ("blood level" or "plasma level"), the more severe is the adverse reaction. Thus, measures aimed at lowering the local anesthetic blood level—such as using the lowest dose in the weakest solution, and minimizing absorption with a vasoconstrictor—go a long way toward reducing the incidence of systemic reactions. Said another way, systemic reactions to local anesthetics are the result of relative drug overdosing, whether from administering more than the recommended, or prudent, maximum dose, or from unintended intravascular injection of part or all of an otherwise unremarkable drug dose.

With that in mind, systemic reactions to local anesthetics follow a surprisingly predictable pattern, affecting the brain, the heart, or both, according to a blood level–dependent spectrum of intensities. Effects on the brain (cerebrotoxicity) range from mild but characteristic symptoms such as drowsiness to frank grand mal convulsions. In the heart (cardiotoxicity) the conducting and contractile systems are affected, site and virulence of effect varying with the particular local anesthetic. Before the introduction of second-generation long-acting local anesthetics (bupivacaine, etidocaine), classic local anesthetic reactions were confined largely to the central nervous system. Rarely, and then only in extreme instances (as with the infamous "Xylocaine murders"), was the cardiovascular system compromised. Bupivacaine (and etidocaine, now largely abandoned) changed all that, and refractory cardiac arrhythmias took precedence over the more readily treated traditional central nervous system symptoms.[2]

Overdose

The higher the blood (or plasma) local anesthetic level, and the faster it rises, the more likely is an adverse systemic response. The great majority of adverse systemic reactions to local anesthetics are straightforward time- and dose-dependent occurrences, and the more molecules attach to a receptor configuration, the more vigorous, precipitous, and refractory is the clinical response.

FDA-sanctioned field-tested dosing guidelines are set forth in Table 16–2, but the reader should note the term *manufacturer-suggested.* At best, these values represent conservative estimates for reasonably fit patients, derived in the main from postmarketing reports rather than from hard and fast evidence-based rules. The guidelines may be overly optimistic for the elderly or infirm patients and, conversely, too limiting for healthy ones. Note, too, that the assumption of perineural placement implicitly excludes unintended intravascular or intrathecal injection. That large a dose, unintentionally injected in the latter sites, has the potential for grave adverse effects on heart, brain, spinal cord, and circulation.

LIDOCAINE DOSING ANOMALY

A curious dichotomy in "safe dose" recommendation has sprung up in recent years with "tumescent anesthesia." In this technique, used extensively for liposuction, several liters of solution containing several thousand milligrams of very dilute lidocaine (0.05% to 0.10%) and epinephrine (1 : 1,000,000) are infiltrated subcutaneously.[40] The quantities of lidocaine so administered may seem staggering when compared with the 7 mg/kg dose limit for nerve block, yet lidocaine doses of 35 to 55 mg/kg are said to be safe in the sense that plasma levels remain well below toxic thresholds.[21] Limited clinical studies suggest one-compartment kinetics of late peaking and slow lidocaine absorption.

It may be that lidocaine, diluted close to its C_m, saturates the subcutaneous fat reservoir. Should that buffer hypothesis prove out, tumescent analgesia may offer an alternative for sustained drug delivery that is far simpler than perineural infusion. One application might be for sustained lumbar sympathetic blockade in ambulatory subjects. Meanwhile, the 35 mg/kg titanic dosing limit applies *specifically* and *only* to very dilute (not more than 0.1%) lidocaine. For all other applications, the recommended dose of undiluted lidocaine for nerve block procedures remains as shown in Table 16–2.

Cerebrotoxicity

Subtle early cerebral manifestations of a rising local anesthetic blood level are ringing in the ears, drowsiness, metallic taste in the mouth, and confusion. Convulsions occur when focal excitation of a subcortical limbic site (probably the amygdala) by bloodborne local anesthetic propagates beyond its initial bounds to spread globally throughout the brain. As local anesthetic blood levels rise further, limbic discharges fan out through the brain, precipitating synchronous epileptiform electroencephalographic bursts characteristic of a grand mal seizure.[41] (Paradoxically, local anesthetics are used in Europe as anticonvulsants.)

Although short-acting neuromuscular-blocking agents (e.g., succinylcholine) have been advocated for treating the convulsive muscle spasms of a seizure, paralyzing agents *do not stop* the brain's electrical seizure discharges; they merely stop the gross muscular manifestations of a convulsion. The one absolute indication for a paralyzing agent, prior to intubation, is inability to ventilate a convulsing patient with oxygen. Assisted ventilation not only satisfies the enormously increased oxygen demand of the convulsing brain and spasmodically contracting muscles but also lowers the arterial carbon dioxide tension, thus raising the brain's seizure threshold to local anesthetics.[2]

Benzodiazepines (e.g., midazolam) have proven to be both specific and effective in managing subcortical seizures. Thus, they have a leading role in preventing, and if necessary treating, local anesthetic–induced convulsions. By reducing limbic excitability, benzodiazepines suppress activation of the focal seizure generator and so are quite specific in preventing central local anesthetic toxicity.[2] If one anticipates a need for high doses of local anesthetic—close to presumed toxic limits, as in celiac plexus block—

TABLE 16–2 *Manufacturer's Suggested Perineural Local Anesthetic Dosages*

Local Anesthetic	Dose by Body Weight (mg/kg)	Maximum Adult Dose (mg)
Procaine (Novocain)	14	1000
Prilocaine (Citanest)	10	600
Lidocaine (Xylocaine)	7*	500*
Mepivacaine (Carbocaine)	7*	500*
Tetracaine (Pontocaine)	1½	100
Ropivacaine (Naropin)	2	200
Bupivacaine (Marcaine, Sensorcaine)	1–2	150

* With epinephrine 5 μg/ml (1 : 200,000).
Manufacturer-suggested dose limits for perineural (extravascular and extrathecal) use. This table in no way implies that these dosages are either "safe" or absolute maxima. Systemic reactions can be encountered with much smaller doses, whereas much larger doses, used judiciously, have been administered without ill effects.
(Updated from de Jong RH: Local Anesthetics, ed 2. St. Louis, CV Mosby, 1994.)

benzodiazepine premedication is advisable. If nothing else, the patient will be calmer thanks to the anxiolytic agent. Barbiturates such as thiopental once were used to treat local anesthetic–induced convulsions, but they have turned out to be nonspecific central nervous system depressants. Propofol, however, appears to have merit as a more specific and less systemically depressing anticonvulsant.[42]

Cardiotoxicity

Much as in nerve, local anesthetics limit the inward flow of cardiac sodium currents, so reducing the cardiac action potential. Cardiac tissue thus is rendered less excitable and more vulnerable to frequency dependence so that impulse propagation is slowed. In fact, lidocaine and congeners such as tocainide or mexiletine are widely used class I-B antiarrhythmics. Lidocaine is a fast-in fast-out sodium channel blocker that reaches steady state block in one or two heartbeats. Bupivacaine, to the contrary, is a fast-in slow-out local anesthetic whose blocking action increases with successive beats *and* with faster heart rates, thus opening the door for potentially malignant reentrant cardiac arrhythmias.[31] For reasons yet unclear, the heart is further sensitized to bupivacaine during pregnancy.

Local anesthetics with an asymmetric chiral carbon atom (e.g., mepivacaine and bupivacaine) exhibit pronounced stereoselectivity for the cardiac sodium channel–binding site, the *R* enantiomer having three- to fourfold greater receptor affinity than the *S* isopode. Ropivacaine and levobupivacaine, each pure *S* monomers, thus are inherently less cardiotoxic than racemic (*RS*) bupivacaine. As noted earlier, bloodborne bupivacaine exerts additional indirect cardiovascular effects by means of systemic excitation of medullary autonomic control sites.[10] Implicating a centrally propagated cardiovascular component in unanesthetized humans, too, is the fact that bupivacaine arrhythmias commonly precede convulsions. One isn't home scot-free entirely with either *S* monomer, however, as life-threatening arrhythmias may accompany or precede convulsions from a systemic reaction to either ropivacaine or levobupivacaine.[34, 43]

The clinical implications of experimental work with prevention or treatment of bupivacaine-induced cardiac arrhythmias remain murky, as work performed so far has studied either isolated hearts or surgically anesthetized animals. While experiments on isolated hearts may point the way, they eventually will need to be refined in the intact organism. Further, as nerve blocks are performed on conscious patients, experiments need to be conducted on previously instrumented unanesthetized animals. Thus, no single specific drug therapy for bupivacaine cardiotoxicity can yet be recommended (or condemned).

Although expectations run high that ropivacaine or levobupivacaine will eradicate the curse of racemic bupivacaine cardiotoxicity, uncertainty persists about whether the monomers will prove as hardy clinically. Levobupivacaine, the newly arrived *S* bupivacaine monomer, certainly bears watching as its longer four-carbon butyl side chain (as compared with ropivacaine's shorter three-carbon propyl tail) may yet produce greater potency and longer staying power. Whether these attributes will eventually be counterbalanced by greater toxicity will determine which of the two sisters will be the frontrunner, whether each will fill a different niche, or whether one will just drop out of the race.

Allergy (Global Reactions)

An exception to the rule equating the intensity of a toxic reaction with total drug mass is allergy, an adverse response to a substance that occurs after the subject has been sensitized to that drug or to a close chemical relative. Once a person is sensitized, minute quantities of the offending drug, now the *antigen*, can trigger a massive allergic response on encountering its immunoglobin (Ig) antibody. The mating of antigen and antibody initiates a swiftly cascading sequence of reactions. An immediate (systemic, anaphylactic) reaction occurs when humoral antibodies have been formed. If instead the antibody is tissue resident in lymphoid cells, a slower *delayed* (localized) reaction develops, the skin being a prominent target.[44]

The causative mechanism of an allergic reaction affects both speed of onset and severity of the reaction. The type I IgE-mediated antibody response is explosively progressive and pernicious; this is true *anaphylaxis*. Circulating bioamines, released by mast cell degranulation, trigger a massive systemic defense reaction: airway edema, bronchospasm, and hypotension each can be life threatening.[45] The slower-onset type IV allergic reaction follows non-

IgE–mediated release of histamine and other reactive products from sensitized lymphocytes. Depending on the quantity of mediator released, severity of the reaction can vary from rapid onset of anaphylactoid shock to slowly progressive contact dermatitis.

True allergy to amino amide local anesthetics (e.g., lidocaine, bupivacaine) is exceedingly rare, and most patients labeled allergic are *not* allergic to local anesthetic. The needle-shy dental patient, for instance, who responds with hyperventilation, sweating, or vasovagal reaction all too often is mislabeled allergic to the drug (rather than responsive to epinephrine). Even so, the physician cannot cavalierly ignore a patient history of allergy; prudence demands screening, if not actual testing.[44] There is little doubt that cross-sensitivity between amino esters (e.g., procaine, benzocaine, tetracaine) exists and extends to other PABA esters such as sunscreen lotions or preservatives of the paraben (e.g., methyl or propyl paraben) family.[45] Whether amino amide local anesthetics tend to cross-react within their class is far less conclusive. By and large, the vast majority (>90%) of so-called allergies to local anesthetic are adverse reactions to preservatives and additives in commercial bottled solutions.[46] True allergy to local anesthetic is best (and most safely) determined with progressive dilution intracutaneous testing, using freshly prepared agent in preservative-free saline.[44]

Local Reactions

Myotoxicity

High concentrations of local anesthetics can be toxic to muscle and irritating to subcutaneous tissue. Myotoxicity is attributable in part to calcium efflux from sarcoplasmic reticulum—a property intrinsic to all local anesthetics—but also appears to be drug species related: bupivacaine is the greatest offender, procaine the least.[47] In fact, pathologists choose 2% bupivacaine to model rhabdomyolysis and subsequent muscle regeneration.[2] Concern with myotoxicity would be greater were it not that the tissue matrix and essential neurovascular elements remain undamaged, ensuring rapid and complete structural regeneration.[48] Although 0.25% bupivacaine is widely used for muscle trigger point injections in North America, the reported incidence of clinical myotoxicity must be very low. Even densely innervated eye muscles, if they are at all affected by bupivacaine, quickly return to full functionality.[2]

Neurotoxicity

In the laboratory, local anesthetics are both effective sodium current blockers and destructive neurotoxins at concentrations severalfold lower than those used clinically. This may seem worrisome at first, until one notes the comfortable 50-fold therapeutic spread between median blocking and neurotoxic concentrations.[49] This is a considerably more generous operating window than attainable with most other therapeutics. For the time being, it appears that the controlled conditions of a laboratory environment magnify the more rugged real-life clinical situation; that is to say, a more concentrated local anesthetic solution is needed for regional block in humans but, by the same token, the neurotoxic concentration is commensurately higher.

RADICULOPATHY

The one clinical situation comparable to that of an isolated nerve stretched in a laboratory testing chamber is spinal analgesia where vulnerable bare spinal rootlets float enclosed in a sac of fluid. In years past, chloroprocaine or its stabilizers, perhaps both, exhibited demonstrable neurotoxicity. In the early 1990s, however, attention turned to continuous spinal anesthesia with concentrated (5%) hyperbaric lidocaine after several well-documented cases of cauda equina syndrome.[50] Although it was initially attributed to incomplete mixing secondary to low-flow release from fine-bore microcatheters, the lidocaine itself now has come under scrutiny, while the catheter delivery device has been recast in the lesser role of accessory.

RADICULAR IRRITATION

In the mid-1990s reports of a milder form of postspinal radiculopathy, presenting as delayed onset, transient, radiating pain in buttocks or thighs, began to appear. The pain syndrome is variously called (depending on the author's conviction) *transient radicular irritation* (TRI), *transient neurologic symptoms* (TNS), or simply *postspinal backache*. It starts hours to days after the patient has been discharged home, is radicular in distribution, does not impair motor function, vanishes without a trace within days, produces no hard neurologic findings, affects mostly fit ambulatory patients, and is more frequent after vigorous surgical manipulation than when the subject remains supine. Of concern to our readers is the higher incidence of TRI after lidocaine than after intrathecal bupivacaine or tetracaine.

The original thinking that 5% might be too concentrated a lidocaine solution and that dilution by half would solve the problem (as recommended by the FDA Advisory Committee) proved wishful. Even less than one third the dilution—to a 1.5% lidocaine solution—yielded about as high an incidence of TRI as the 2.5%, or even the original 5% concentration.[51] Furthermore, numerous studies have given dextrose (added to local anesthetic solution to render it denser than spinal fluid) a clean bill of health: for instance, TRI after intrathecal hyperbaric bupivacaine or tetracaine is quite uncommon.[50]

Crucial to interventional pain mangers is the obvious concern that TRI could be an early manifestation of low-grade local anesthetic radiculotoxicity. The question remains moot, although evidence of radiculo- and even myelotoxicity has been strengthened by the experimental finding that dorsal root axons *and* their ganglion cells are vulnerable to lidocaine.[52] Interpretation of the significance of TRI varies from benign myoskeletal backache to early-stage reversible neurotoxicity. However, the comforting idea that TRI is merely a severe but short-lived backache from unaccustomed stretching of relaxed muscle may be head-in-the-sand thinking, as even threefold diluted intrathecal lidocaine causes as severe TRI as the original 5% preparation.[51] The more prevalent, albeit grudging, perception is of a transient, reversible, and thus innocuous, chemical irritation of bare unprotected nerve roots. The author has taken the larger view of an exposure-dependent

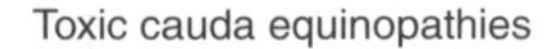

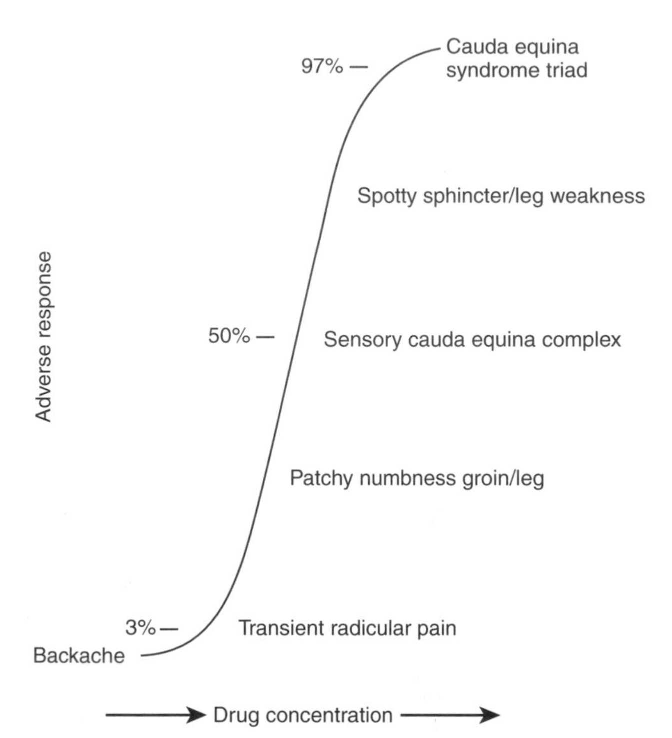

FIGURE 16–11 *Dose-effect plot. Proposed cumulative probability curve correlating adverse radiculotoxic response with periaxonal local anesthetic drug concentration. The vertical axis grades severity of postspinal neurologic sequelae on an ascending scale: from threshold transient irritation at the lower bound, to overt catastrophic cauda equina syndrome at the upper bound. A continuum of progressive neural injury unfolds between these scale-defining asymptotes. The horizontal axis (drug concentration) represents the toxicodynamic product of local anesthetic concentration at the drug-nerve interface and duration of drug-nerve contact in units of time. In short, the more concentrated the local anesthetic in the spinal fluid, and the longer cauda equina roots remain in contact with the dissolved drug mass, the more intense and the more lasting will be the chemical inflammatory reaction. (From de Jong RH: The intrathecal lidocaine enigma: On the brink of cauda equinopathy. Semin Anesth 17: 287–298, 1998.)*

dose-effect spectrum of neural injury ranging from reversible irritation (like a mild sunburn) at the low end, to irreversibly destructive neurolysis at the opposite end of the curve (Fig. 16–11).[53]

Whatever the outcome of the TRI controversy, the message is clear: spinal nerves are vulnerable to chemical agents injected into spinal fluid, including local anesthetics.[54] Practitioners beware: placing unproved medications in the spinal fluid is not as innocuous as we have been led to believe.

REFERENCES

1. Strichartz GR: Neural physiology and local anesthetic action. *In* Cousins MJ, Bridenbaugh PO (eds): Neural Blockade in Clinical Anesthesia and Management of Pain. Philadelphia, Lippincott-Raven, ed 3, 1998, pp 35–54.
2. de Jong RH: Local Anesthetics. St Louis, CV Mosby, ed 2, 1994.
3. Bernards CM, Hill HF: The spinal nerve root sleeve is not a preferred route for redistribution of drugs from the epidural space to the spinal cord. Anesthesiology 75:827–832, 1991.
4. Rosenberg PH: Intravenous regional anesthesia: Nerve block by multiple mechanisms. Reg Anesth 18:1–5, 1993.
5. Kuzma PJ, Kline MD, Calkins MD, Staats PS: Progress in the development of ultralong-acting local anesthetics. Reg Anesth 22:543–551, 1997.
6. Wang GK, Vladimirov M, Quan C, et al: *N*-butyl tetracaine as a neurolytic agent for ultralong sciatic nerve block. Anesthesiology 85:1386–1394, 1996.
7. Kohane DS, Yieh J, Lu NT, et al: A re-examination of tetrodotoxin for prolonged duration local anesthesia. Anesthesiology 89:119–131, 1998.
8. Nyström EUM, Buffington CW: Is there an anatomical explanation for tachyphylaxis in epidural anesthesia? Reg Anesth Pain Med 24:S16, 1999.
9. Valenzuela C, Snyders DJ, Bennett PB, et al: Stereoselective block of cardiac sodium channels by bupivacaine in guinea pig ventricular myocytes. Circulation 92:3014–3024, 1995.
10. Denson DD, Behbehani MM, Gregg RV: Enantiomer-specific effects of an intravenously administered arrhythmogenic dose of bupivacaine on neurons of the nucleus tractus solitarius and the cardiovascular system in the anesthetized rat. Reg Anesth 17:311–316, 1992.
11. Nau C, Vogel W, Hempelmann G, Brău ME: Stereoselectivity of bupivacaine in local anesthetic–sensitive ion channels of peripheral nerve. Anesthesiology 91:786–795, 1999.
12. de Jong RH: Ropivacaine: White knight or dark horse? The 1995 Gaston Labat Lecture. Reg Anesth 20:474–481, 1995.
13. Rowlingson JC: Toxicity of local anesthetic additives. Reg Anesth 18:453–460, 1993.
14. Krames ES: The chronic intraspinal use of opioid and local anesthetic mixtures for the relief of intractable pain: When all else fails! Pain 55:1–4, 1993.
15. Ostad A, Kageyama N, Moy RL: Tumescent anesthesia with a lidocaine dose of 55 mg/kg is safe for liposuction. Dermatol Surg 22:921–927, 1996.
16. Abram SE, Yaksh TL: Systemic lidocaine blocks nerve injury–induced hyperalgesia and nociceptor-driven spinal sensitization in the rat. Anesthesiology 80:383–391, 1994.
17. Ferrante FM, Paggioli J, Cherukuri S, Arthur GR: The analgesic response to intravenous lidocaine in the treatment of neuropathic pain. Anesth Analg 82:91–97, 1996.
18. Tanelian DL, Brose WG: Neuropathic pain can be relieved by drugs that are use-dependent sodium channel blockers: Lidocaine, carbamazepine, and mexilitine. Anesthesiology 74:949–951, 1991.
19. Sloan P, Basta M, Storey P, von Gunten C: Mexiletine as an adjuvant analgesic for the management of neuropathic cancer pain. Anesth Analg 89:760–761, 1999.
20. Bargetzi MJ, AoyamaT, Meyer UA: Lidocaine metabolism in human liver microsomes by cytochrome P450 IIIA4. Clin Pharmacol Ther 46:521–527, 1989.
21. Klein JA, Kassarjdian N: Lidocaine toxicity with tumescent liposuction: A case report of probable drug interactions. Dermatol Surg 23:1169–1174, 1997.
22. de Jong RH, Grazer FM: Titanic tumescent anesthesia. Dermatol Surg 24:689–692, 1998.
23. Riendeau LA, Bennett D, Black-Noller G, et al: Evaluation of the analgesic efficacy of EMLA cream in volunteers with differing skin pigmentation undergoing venipunture. Reg Anesth Pain Med 24:165–169, 1999.
24. Simon MAM, Gielen MJM, Alberink N, et al: Intravenous regional anesthesia with 0.5% articaine, 0.5% lidocaine, or 0.5% prilocaine. A double-blind randomized clinical study. Reg Anesth 22:29–34, 1997.
25. Albright GA: Cardiac arrest following regional anesthesia with etidocaine or bupivacaine. Anesthesiology 51:285–287, 1979.
26. Kinney WW, Kambam R, Wright W: Propranolol pretreatment reduces cardio-respiratory toxicity due to plain, but not epinephrine-containing, intravenous bupivacaine in rats. Can J Anaesth 38:533–536, 1991.
27. Solomon RE, Gebhart GF: Synergistic antinociceptive interactions among drugs administered to the spinal cord. Anesth Analg 78:1164–1172, 1994.
28. Krames ES: The chronic intraspinal use of opioid and local anesthetic mixtures for the relief of intractable pain: When all else fails! Pain 55:1–4, 1993.
29. Pere P, Tuominen M, Rosenberg PH: Cumulation of bupivacaine, desbutylbupivacaine and 4-hydroxybupivacaine during and after continuous interscalene brachial plexus block. Acta Anaesthesiol Scand 35:647–650, 1991.

30. Thomas JM, Schug SA: Recent advances in the pharmacokinetics of local anaesthetics. Long-acting amide enantiomers and continuous infusions. Clin Pharmacokinet 36:67–83, 1999.
31. Graf BM, Martin E, Bosnjak ZJ, Stowe DF: Stereospecific effect of bupivacaine isomers on atrioventricular conduction in the isolated perfused guinea pig heart. Anesthesiology 86:410–419, 1997.
32. de Jong RH: Ropivacaine. Anesth Clin North Am 2:109–130, 1998.
33. Iida H, Watanabe Y, Dohi S, Ishiyama T: Direct effects of ropivacaine and bupivacaine on spinal pial vessels in canine. Anesthesiology 87:75–81, 1997.
34. Ruetsch YA, Fattinger KE, Borgeat A: Ropivacaine-induced convulsions and severe cardiac dysrhythmia after sciatic block. Anesthesiology 90:1784–1786, 1999.
35. Oda Y, Furuichi K, Tanaka K, et al: Metabolism of a new local anesthetic, ropivacaine, by human hepatic cytochrome P_{450}. Anesthesiology 82:214–220, 1995.
36. Rosenberg PH, Heavner JE: Acute cardiovascular and central nervous system toxicity of bupivacaine and desbutylbupivacaine in the rat. Acta Anaesthesiol Scand 36:138–141, 1992.
37. Knudsen K, Beckman SM, Blomberg S, et al: Central nervous and cardiovascular effects of i.v. infusions of ropivacaine, bupivacaine and placebo in volunteers. Br J Anaesth 78:507–514, 1997.
38. Bardsley H, Gristwood R, Baker H, et al: A comparison of the cardiovascular effects of levobupivacaine and racbupivacaine following intravenous administration to healthy volunteers. Br J Pharmacol 46:245–249, 1998.
39. Lyons G, Columb M, Wilson RC, Johnson RV: Epidural pain relief in labour: Potencies of levobupivacaine and racemic bupivacaine. Br J Anaesth 81:899–901, 1998.
40. de Jong RH, Grazer FM: Tumescent liposuction alert: Deaths from lidocaine toxicity. Am J Forensic Med Pathol 20:101–102, 1999.
41. Baaijens PF, Gielen MJ, Vree TB, et al: Bupivacaine toxicity secondary to continuous cervical epidural infusion. Reg Anesth 20:163–168, 1995.
42. Momota Y, Artru AA, Powers KM, et al: Posttreatment with propofol terminates lidocaine-induced epileptiform electroencephalogram activity in rabbits: Effects on cerebrospinal fluid dynamics. Anesth Analg 87:900–906, 1998.
43. Huang YF, Pryor ME, Mather LE, Veering BT: Cardiovascular and central nervous system effects of intravenous levobupivacaine and bupivacaine in sheep. Anesth Analg 86:797–804, 1998.
44. Gall H, Kaufmann R, Kalveram CMK: Adverse reactions to local anesthetics: Analysis of 197 cases. J Allerg Clin Immunol 97:933–937, 1996.
45. Fisher MMcD, Bowey CJ: Alleged allergy to local anaesthetics. Anaesth Intensive Care 25:611–614, 1997.
46. Kajimoto Y, Rosenberg ME, Kyttä J, et al: Anaphylactoid skin reactions after intravenous regional anaesthesia using 0.5% prilocaine with or without preservative. Acta Anaesth Scand 39:782–784, 1995.
47. Hogan Q, Dotson R, Erickson S, et al: Local anesthetic myotoxicity: A case and review. Anesthesiology 80:942–947, 1994.
48. Komorowski TE, Shepard B, Okland S, Carlson BM: An electron microscopic study of local anesthetic–induced skeletal muscle fiber degeneration and regeneration in the monkey. J Orthopaed Res 8:495–503, 1990.
49. Bainton CT, Strichartz GR: Concentration dependence of lidocaine-induced irreversible conduction loss in frog nerve. Anesthesiology 81:657–667, 1994.
50. de Jong RH: Last round for a "heavyweight"? Anesth Analg 78: 3–4, 1994.
51. Pollock JE, Liu SS, Neal JM, Stephenson CA: Dilution of spinal lidocaine does not alter the incidence of transient neurologic symptoms. Anesthesiology 90:445–450, 1999.
52. Gold MS, Reichling DB, Hampl KF, et al: Lidocaine toxicity in primary afferent neurons from the rat. J Pharmacol Exp Ther 285:413–421, 1998.
53. de Jong RH: The intrathecal lidocaine enigma: On the brink of cauda equinopathy. Semin Anesth 17:287–298, 1998.
54. Brown DL, Ransom DM, Hall JA, et al: Regional anesthesia and local anesthetic–induced systemic toxicity: seizure frequency and accompanying cardiovascular changes. Anesth Analg 81:321–328, 1995.

CHAPTER • 17

Neurolytic Agents in Clinical Practice

Subhash Jain, MD • Rakesh Gupta, MD

Optimal use of a neurolytic agent requires that it be administered to produce effective analgesia without devastating side effects. Careful selection of patients, thorough knowledge of the pathophysiologic mechanisms of disease, and an understanding of the physiochemical properties of neurolytic agents and their effects on various body systems are necessary before they are used for neurolysis.

GENERAL CONSIDERATIONS

Chemical agents have been used for neurolysis since the turn of the twentieth century. Schloesser[1] reported using alcohol for trigeminal neuralgia in 1903 and noted the degeneration and subsequent absorption of most of the nerve. A neurolytic sympathetic block with alcohol was performed by Swetlow[2] in 1926 to relieve angina pectoris and abdominal pain. Dogliotti[3] employed alcohol for the first subarachnoid injection in 1930. Although a variety of agents have been used since then for neurolysis, only alcohol and phenol have withstood the test of time. Here we discuss all neurolytic agents used for the management of intractable pain. To understand their effects on the nerve fiber, it is important to review the anatomy and discuss the process of degeneration and regeneration of nerve fibers.

PHYSIOLOGIC CONSIDERATIONS IN NEUROLYTIC BLOCKADE

Peripheral nerve fibers are maintained in a specialized connective tissue called *peripheral gliocytes* or *Schwann cells*, which are responsible for myelination of these fibers. After an injury, Schwann cells help to sustain and guide the regeneration of the axon. *Epineurium*, the outer covering of the peripheral nerve, is rich in vascular supply and has an abundance of fat cells, fibroblasts, and mast cells that lend strength to the fiber and help to protect it against compression effects. Bundles or fascicles of nerve fiber are covered by a semipermeable membrane, *perineurium*, which helps to regulate the interstitial fluid exchange in and around the fascicles. *Endoneurium*, an extension of the perineurium, surrounds individual myelinated or unmyelinated nerve fibers and their Schwann cells. It also provides and maintains an environment suitable for nerve conduction. Endoneurium contains capillaries that provide a blood-nerve barrier similar to the blood-brain barrier, and the normal endoneurial fluid pressure as measured with micropipettes is between 1 and 3 cm H_2O.[4,5] The axon is covered by an *axolemma*, which encloses the axoplasm rich in neurofilaments, neuroblasts, vesicles, and other organelles.

NEUROPHYSIOLOGIC ASPECTS OF NERVE CONDUCTION

The process of myelination starts during the 16th to 20th week of gestation. In the peripheral nerve, a single Schwann cell is capable of myelinating only one part of the axon, whereas in the central nervous system, one Schwann cell can myelinate as many as three dozen axons. Along the length of the axon, a chain of Schwann cells encloses the axon completely, creating a mesentery or *mesaxon*. The successive cells interdigitate at nodes of Ranvier with a nodal gap of about 0.5 to 1 μ.[6] During impulse conduction, myelin acts as an insulating sheath, so that the underlying axoplasm is not depolarized and current travels from one node to the next (*saltatory conduction*).

The conduction velocity in peripheral nerve fibers is a function of the diameter of myelinated nerve fibers. A factor of 6 applies to fibers more than 5 μ in diameter, possibly because of longer internodal segments in thicker fibers. Although it is not necessary to have myelinated fibers for motor function in utero (as evidenced by movement at 10 weeks of intrauterine life), demyelination of adult nerve fibers seriously impairs nerve conduction. Regeneration of a nerve fiber is facilitated by the basal lamina of Schwann cells, which covers even the nodes of Ranvier and thus provides a continuous tube. When, however, a nerve is transected, the basal lamina is interrupted, making regeneration more difficult.

DEGENERATION AND REGENERATION

Wallerian degeneration is a process that follows an insult to the nerve fiber. Described first by Waller[7] in 1850, it starts at the distal stump almost immediately after the initial injury. The axon breaks down, and the axoplasm is enclosed within ellipsoids of myelin formed as a result of retraction of the myelin sheath. Lysosomal enzymes cause hydrolysis within these ellipsoids. Schwann cells start multiplying during the first week of injury, and macrophages continue to ingest debris. By the end of the first week, Schwann cells form a chain within the endoneurium. After about 2 weeks, macrophages disappear, leaving behind endoneurial tubes filled with Schwann cells.

Regeneration may start as early as 6 hours after a clean cut but may be delayed several weeks after a crush or tearing injury. Each axon produces several regenerating sprouts. Some of the sprouts succeed in making contact with the distal stump and begin growing distally at a rate of about 5 mm/day in the larger nerve trunks and 1 to 2 mm/day in the smaller ones. Functional recovery depends on the integrity of the endoneurium. Outcome is better with crush injuries than after a clean cut. Although sprouts of sensory fibers easily travel along motor neurons and vice versa, no functional contact is established. An accurate coaptation of the two severed ends is therefore essential to restore function in a clean-cut nerve.

Because the peripheral nerve lacks lymphatic innervation, any toxic, metabolic, or traumatic insult leads to an increase in endoneurial fluid pressure, probably secondary to mast cell degranulation and release of vasoactive substances, which increase the permeability of the blood-nerve barrier and thus lead to accumulation of fluid in the endoneurial space. This process peaks in 6 to 7 days and reverts to normal in about 30 days. Elevated endoneurial fluid pressure causes stretching of the perineurium and compression of perineurial vessels, thus producing ischemia of the nerve fiber.[8]

NEUROLYTIC BLOCKADE

Skillful performance of neurolytic blockade after very careful assessment and selection of patients has produced successful results for the last 90 years. Nevertheless, a thorough understanding of the actions, side effects, and possible complications of neurolytics, familiarity with various opioids, and knowledge of adjunctive pharmacologic agents are necessary before neurolysis is undertaken. Even among cancer patients with intractable pain, only about 30% require neurolysis as the ultimate means of producing effective analgesia.[9] Nevertheless, it remains an invaluable tool in the management of pain for certain patients with terminal cancer, certain neuralgias, vascular occlusive diseases, and hypophysectomy and when neurosurgical ablation is not an option.[10] Also, neurolytic blockade spares the basal lamina, facilitating regeneration of the axon, unlike surgical interruption, which has a higher incidence of neuroma formation. Thorough, informed patient consent must be obtained before the procedure. Although a diagnostic or prognostic block may not predict the exact outcome of the subsequent neurolysis, it can help to familiarize the patient with possible side effects. After neurolysis, the patient should be assessed for efficacy, side effects, and possible complications of the procedure. Opioid and adjuvant medications should be adjusted as necessary, precautions being taken to avoid opiate withdrawal.

Neurolytic Agents

Although a wide range of neurolytic agents may be used for the purpose of neurolysis, only a few are available as commercial preparations. Commonly used agents or procedures are absolute alcohol, phenol, cryoanalgesia, and radiofrequency lesions.

Ethyl Alcohol

Absolute alcohol is commercially available in the United States as a higher-than-95% concentration in 1-ml, single-dose ampules. A local irritant, alcohol can cause considerable pain during injection. The pain can be avoided by preinjection of small doses of a local anesthetic drug. Since the earliest reports on alcohol neurolysis, various concentrations and mixtures of alcohol have been used, with inconsistent results. One consensus was reached: a concentration stronger than 95% results in complete paralysis. Another study also concluded that a minimum concentration of 33% alcohol was necessary to obtain satisfactory analgesia without any motor paralysis (Table 17–1).[11-16]

Histopathologic studies have shown that alcohol extracts cholesterol, phospholipids, and cerebrosides from the nerve tissue and causes precipitation of lipoproteins and mucoproteins.[17] Topical application of alcohol to peripheral nerves produces changes typical of wallerian degeneration, as described earlier. A subarachnoid injection of absolute alcohol causes similar changes in the rootlets.[18] Mild focal inflammation of meninges and patchy areas of demyelination are seen in posterior columns, Lissauer's tract, and dorsal roots and rootlets. Later, wallerian degeneration is seen to extend into the dorsal horns. Injection of a larger volume can result in degeneration of the spinal cord. Owing to its hypobaric nature relative to CSF (specific gravity, 0.8 : 1.1, respectively), alcohol rises quickly to reach the

TABLE 17–1 ***Experimental Use of Ethanol Alcohol as a Neurolytic Agent in Peripheral Nerves: Summary***

Study (Year)	Concentration of Alcohol (%)	Result
Finkelberg (1907)[11]	60–80	Persistent paralysis
May (1912)[12]	76, 80, 90, 100	Motor paralysis
	50	No motor paralysis
Gordon (1914)[13]	80	Progressive motor paralysis
Nasaroff (1925)[14]	70	Incomplete and temporary paralysis
Labat (1933)[15]	48 (with 1% procaine), 95	No demonstrable difference in paralysis
Labat and Greene (1931)[16]*	33	No paresis or paralysis

* Study was undertaken for management of painful disorders.

top of the fluid level after intrathecal injection. Skillful positioning of the patient is thus of the utmost importance to avoid undesirable side effects from nonselective neurolysis by absolute alcohol (see Chapter 52).

After injection into the CSF, alcohol diffuses rapidly from the injection site. Only 10% of the initial dose remains at the site of the injection after 10 minutes, and about 4% remains after 30 minutes.[19] When injected near the sympathetic chain, alcohol destroys the ganglion cells and thus blocks all postganglionic fibers to all effector organs.[20] A temporary and incomplete block results if the injection affects only the rami communicantes of preganglionic and postganglionic fibers. Histopathologically, wallerian degeneration is evident in the sympathetic chain fibers.

Commonly, neurolytic blocks with alcohol are performed for cranial neuralgias (trigeminal and glossopharyngeal nerves), epidural and intrathecal interruption of neuraxial transmission, and lumbar sympathetic and celiac plexus lysis. The volume used is quite small, and, thus, none of the side effects of ingested ethanol are seen. Extreme care should be taken at the time of injection to avoid local tissue injury and cellulitis or necrosis of adjacent tissues. After the injection, the needle should be flushed with a local anesthetic or normal saline to avoid depositing residual alcohol along the needle track.

COMPLICATIONS OF ALCOHOL NEUROLYSIS

Use of alcohol for neurolysis is sometimes associated with very painful, annoying, and psychologically distressing neuralgias. Patients often complain bitterly about the neuralgia despite adequate and effective analgesia if they are not thoroughly oriented when their informed consent is obtained for the procedure. The pain is described as dull to severe, sometimes as burning, and occasionally as a sharp, shooting pain. Recovery from the pain may occur as soon as a few weeks after neurolysis or may take many months. The incidence of this complication is higher after a thoracic paravertebral sympatholytic injection, possibly because of the greater proximity of the somatic fibers to the sympathetic chain in the thoracic region, than in the lumbar region.

Hypesthesia or anesthesia of the dermatomal distribution of the nerve roots treated with neurolysis is another distressing complication. Sometimes the pain relief is overshadowed by this lack of sensation. Fortunately, this complication is rare and recovery is relatively quick.

Loss of bowel or bladder sphincter tone, leading to bowel or urinary incontinence, has also been seen with intrathecal alcohol neurolysis in the lower lumbar and sacral areas. Hypobaric alcohol should be used to advantage to avoid this complication. During sacral nerve root neurolysis, only one side should be blocked at a time. Genitofemoral neuralgia can cause severe groin pain in patients who undergo lumbar sympathetic neurolysis with alcohol. This is referred pain caused by degeneration of the rami communicantes from the L2 nerve root to the genitofemoral nerve.[21–23] Paraplegia can result if injection of alcohol causes spasm of the artery of Adamkiewicz.

Phenol

Phenol has been used extensively since the earliest published reports of its use on rabbit blood vessels (Table 17–2). It is not available commercially in the injectable form but can be prepared by the hospital pharmacy. Phenol acts as a local anesthetic in lower concentrations and as a neurolytic agent in higher concentrations and thus has the advantage of causing minimal discomfort on injection.

Phenol is available as a mixture with glycerine, in which it is highly soluble, and diffuses out slowly, resulting in pronounced localized tissue effects. This solution is hyperbaric relative to the cerebrospinal fluid and can be prepared in concentrations ranging from 4% to 10%. Another form is as an aqueous mixture, which is a far more potent neurolytic. Various concentrations between 3% and 10% have been studied in the past. Commonly concentrations between 6% and 8% are used (see Table 17–2). A concentration of 20% in glycerine has been reported for treatment of certain cases of spasticity.[34] Phenol may also be dissolved in a radiopaque dye to make a hyperbaric contrast solution.

Also called *carbolic acid*, phenol has a benzene ring with one hydroxyl group substituted for a hydrogen ion. In its pure state, phenol is colorless and poorly soluble, forming a 6.7% solution in water. Exposure to air causes oxidation and gives it a reddish tinge. Phenol is excreted by the kidneys as various conjugated derivatives.[35]

As compared with alcohol, phenol produces shorter-lived and less intense blockade. Moller and associates[36] compared various concentrations of alcohol and of phenol and concluded that 5% phenol equaled 40% alcohol in neurolytic potency.

Phenol spares posterior root ganglia while causing nonselective neurolysis by denaturing the proteins of axons and perineural blood vessels.[37] The process of degeneration takes about 14 days, and regeneration is completed in about 14 weeks. After an intrathecal injection of phenol, its concentration decreases rapidly—to 30% of the original concentration in 60 seconds and to 0.1% within 15 minutes.[38] High affinity of phenol for vascular tissues has been proposed by Wood[39] to be an important pathophysiologic factor in the observed neuropathy. This factor may raise concerns about the use of phenol for celiac plexus neurolysis, because major blood vessels lie very close to the plexus. Phenol causes concentration-dependent degeneration of

TABLE 17–2 Use of Phenol as a Neurolytic Agent: History

Study (Year)	Application
Nechaev (1933)[24]	Local anesthesia
Putnam and Hampton (1936)[25]	Gasserian ganglion neurolysis
Mandl (1947)[26]	Chemical sympathectomy
Haxton (1949)[27] and Boyd et al (1949)[28]	Paravertebral injection for intermittent claudication
Maher (1955)[29]	Intrathecal injection for cancer pain
Kelly and Gautier-Smith (1959)[30]	Intrathecal injection for spasticity of upper motor neuron disease
Nathan (1959)[31]	Intrathecal injection for spasticity of paraplegia
Nathan and Sears (1960)[32]	Effects on nerve conduction in cat spinal nerve roots
Iggo and Walsh (1960)[33]	Blockade of fibers in cat spinal nerve roots

the peripheral nerves as well. Given subcutaneously, however, it may cause ulceration of the overlying skin.

Glycerol

Earlier reports on the use of glycerol for relieving pain of trigeminal neuralgia[40] generated widespread interest in its use. Histopathologic examination revealed extensive myelin sheath swelling, axonolysis, and severe inflammatory response after intraneuronal injection. Electron microscopy confirmed wallerian degeneration, phagocytosis, and mast cell degranulation. The differential effects of various concentrations of glycerol have been studied in experimental models, but no histologic data are available to support these observations.

Ammonium Compounds

In 1942, Bates and Judovich[38] published their experience using ammonium salts for relief of intractable pain. They prepared an extract from a pitcher plant distillate (*Sarracenia purpurea*) and used it for various neuralgias. A selective action on the sensory fibers was noted, but motor function and cutaneous sensation were spared. Use of 6% ammonium salts (ammonium chloride and ammonium hydroxide) was reported in 5000 doses with favorable results. Subsequent clinical trials, however, have yielded unpredictable and unreliable results. Since then, a concentration of 10% has been used for intercostal blocks with acceptable analgesia and intact motor function.[41, 42] Histopathologically, injection of ammonium salts near a peripheral nerve causes acute degenerative neuropathy affecting all fibers.[43]

Hypertonic and Hypotonic Solutions

Use of hypertonic and hypotonic solutions in intrathecal injections for the treatment of pain[44] has been associated with changes of neuropathy[45–47] that have not been corroborated by histologic evidence.[48, 49] Osmotic swelling of the nerve bundle is proposed as the mechanism of nerve conduction blockade.[50] Later experiments demonstrated myelin degeneration and axonolysis after a nerve was soaked for at least 1 hour in distilled water or solutions of osmolality greater than 1000 mmol/L. Thus, earlier clinical observations were probably attributed to endoneurial edema rather than structural damage to the nerve fibers.

Hypothermia and Cryoanalgesia

Depending on the degree of hypothermia, a temporary or longer-lasting injury to nerve fibers can be produced. The effect of cold on A-delta and C fibers was studied by Denny-Brown and colleagues in 1945.[51] Physiologically, prolongation of action potential is seen when the nerve is cooled to 5° C.[43] All myelinated fibers can be blocked at a given temperature, whereas unmyelinated fibers require a lower temperature.[52, 53] Cytopathologic findings suggested acceleration of Schwann cell enzyme production as the possible cause of endoneurial capillary damage.[40]

Cryoanalgesia is the freezing of a small nerve segment with a 2-mm probe cooled to −60° C by rapid expansion of pressurized nitrous oxide from its tip. The probe is left in contact with the nerve tissue for 60 to 90 seconds and then allowed to "thaw" for another 45 to 60 seconds before being removed. An ice ball 2 to 4 mm in diameter is formed that freezes the nerve and completely damages the nerve fiber.[54] Endoneurial fluid pressure is elevated to 20 mm H_2O within 90 minutes. It drops over the next 24 hours and then increases again, to reach a plateau after 6 days, secondary to changes of wallerian degeneration. An acute injury is produced that lasts approximately 4 to 6 weeks. The basal lamina remains unharmed, thus acting as a conduit for the process of regeneration.

Selection of a Neurolytic Agent

Physical characteristics of the two more commonly used neurolytic agents make them suitable for two different subgroups of patients (Table 17–3). Alcohol, for example, is hypobaric and can be injected with the patient prone.

TABLE 17–3 *Comparison of Phenol and Alcohol as Neurolytic Agents*

Property	Phenol	Alcohol
Physical properties	Clear, colorless, pungent odor Poorly soluble in water Unstable at room temperature Hyperbaric relative to cerebrospinal fluid	Clear, colorless Absorbs water on exposure to air Stable at room temperature Hypobaric relative to cerebrospinal fluid
Chemical structure	Acid	Alcohol
Concentrations (%)	6–10	50–100
Equipotent neurolytic concentration (%)	5	40
Complications of use in neurolysis	Neuritis (uncommon) Toxicity at higher doses Hepatic and cardiac complications	Neuritis (common) Toxicity at commonly used doses
Sites of use (listed in order of preference)	Epidural Paravertebral Peripheral nerve roots Intrathecal Cranial nerves	Intrathecal Celiac ganglion Lumbar sympathetic chain Cranial nerves Paravertebral Epidural (low concentrations)

Thus, it is suitable for a patient who is unable to lie supine owing to pain. Hyperbaric phenol, on the other hand, can reach dorsal nerve roots of a supine patient after intrathecal injection. Jacob and Howland[55] found a higher incidence of sphincter impairment with alcohol than with phenol. In cases of intractable pain, however, analgesic efficacy was equal for the two agents.[56–58] Phenol in glycerine diffuses out very slowly. Therefore, its degenerative action can be well-controlled by adjusting patient position. Alcohol has a quicker onset of action, but its site of action can be controlled in the vertical neuraxis by tilting the table head to foot or to one side. Neuritis and burning pain on injection are seen with alcohol. For intrathecal use, Maher[59] advocates phenol over alcohol because of phenol's slow release and lower complication rate.

CONCLUSION

The use of neurolytic agents, such as alcohol, phenol, glycerol, and ammonium compounds, in various concentrations and at various sites in the body, has proved that the ideal of achieving adequate analgesia without attendant side effects is difficult. Enough damage needs to be done to the nerve to produce the changes of wallerian degeneration. Cautious use of neurolytic agents in carefully selected patients who have given fully informed consent is, therefore, warranted.

REFERENCES

1. Schloesser: Heilung peripherer Reizzustande sensibler und motorischer Nerven. Klin Monatsbl Augenheilkd 41:244, 1903.
2. Swetlow GI: Paravertebral alcohol block in cardiac pain. Am Heart J 1:393, 1926.
3. Dogliotti AM: A new method of block anesthesia: Segmental peridural spinal anesthesia. Am J Surg 20:107, 1933.
4. Low PA: Endoneurial fluid pressure and microenvironment of nerve. *In* Dyck PJ, Thomas PK, Lambert EH, Bunge R (eds): Peripheral Neuropathy. Philadelphia, WB Saunders, 1984, p 599.
5. Myers RR, Powell HC, Costello ML, et al: Endoneurial fluid pressure: Direct measurement with micropipettes. Brain Res 148:510, 1978.
6. Fitzgerald MJT: Degeneration and regeneration. *In* Neuroanatomy: Basic and Clinical. Philadelphia, WB Saunders, 1985, pp 16–19.
7. Waller A: Experiments on the section of the glossopharyngeal and hypoglossal nerves of the frog and observations of the alterations produced thereby in the structure of their primitive fibres. Philos Trans R Soc 140:423, 1850.
8. Myer RR, Powell HC: Galactose neuropathy: Impact of chronic endoneurial edema on nerve blood flow. Ann Neurol 16:587, 1984.
9. Ventafridda V, Narcello T, Augusto C, et al: A validation study of the WHO method for cancer pain relief. Cancer 59:850, 1987.
10. Cousins MJ, Dwyer B, Gibb D: Chronic pain and neurolytic neural blockade. *In* Cousins MJ, Bridenbaugh PO (eds): Neural Blockade in Clinical Anesthesia and Management of Pain, ed 2. Philadelphia, JB Lippincott, 1988, pp 1053–1084.
11. Finkelburg R: Experimentelle Untersuchungen über den Einfluss von Alkoholinjektionen und peripherische Nerven. Verh Dtsch Ges Inn Med 24:75, 1907.
12. May O: Functional and histological effects of intraneural and intraganglionic injection of alcohol. Br Med J 2:365, 1912.
13. Gordon A: Experimental study of intraneural injections of alcohol. J Nerv Ment Dis 41:81, 1914.
14. Nasaroff NN: Über Alkoholinjecktionen in Nervenstamine. Zentralbl Chir 52:2777, 1925.
15. Labat G: Action of alcohol on the living nerve. Curr Res Anesth Analg 12:190, 1933.
16. Labat G, Greene MB: Contribution to the modern method of diagnosis and treatment of so called sciatic neuralgias. Am J Surg 11:435, 1931.
17. Rumbsy MG, Finean JB: The action of organic solvents on the myelin sheath of peripheral nerve tissue—II (short-chain aliphatic alcohols). J Neurochem 13:1509, 1966.
18. Gallagher HS, Yonezawa T, Hoy RC, Derrick WS: Subarachnoid alcohol block. II: Histological changes in the central nervous system. Am J Pathol 35:679, 1961.
19. Matsuki M, Kato Y, Ichiyangi L: Progressive changes in the concentrations of ethyl alcohol in the human and canine subarachnoid space. Anesthesiology 36:617, 1972.
20. Merrick RL: Degeneration and recovery of autonomic neurones following alcoholic block. Ann Surg 113:298, 1941.
21. Rocco A: Radiofrequency lumbar sympatholysis: The evolution of a technique for managing sympathetically mediated pain. Reg Anesth 20:3–12, 1995.
22. Bogduk N, Tynan W, Wilson SS: The nerve supply to the human lumbar intervertebral discs. J Anat 132:39–56, 1981.
23. Edwards EA: Operative anatomy of the lumbar sympathetic chain. Angiology 12:184–198, 1951.
24. Nechaev VA: Solutions of phenol in local anesthesia. Soviet Khir 5:203, 1933.
25. Putnam TJ, Hampton OJ: A technique of injection into the gasserian ganglion under roentgenographic control. Arch Neurol Psychiatry 35:92–98, 1936.
26. Mandl F: Paravertebral Block. New York, Grune & Stratton, 1947.
27. Haxton HA: Chemical sympathectomy. Br Med J 1:1026, 1949.
28. Boyd AM, Ratcliff AH, Jepson RP, et al: Intermittent claudication. J Bone Joint Surg 3B:325, 1949.
29. Maher RM: Phenol for pain and spasticity. *In* Pain—Henry Ford Hospital International Symposium. Boston, Little, Brown, 1966, p 335.
30. Kelly RE, Gautier-Smith PC: Intrathecal phenol in the treatment of reflex spasms and spasticity. Lancet 2:1102–1105, 1959.
31. Nathan PW: Intrathecal phenol to relieve spasticity in paraplegia. Lancet 2:1099–1102, 1959.
32. Nathan PW, Sears TA: Effects of phenol on nervous conduction. J Physiol (Lond) 150:565–580, 1960.
33. Iggo A, Walsh EG: Selective block of small fibres in the spinal roots by phenol. Brain 83:701–708, 1960.
34. Pederson E, Juul-Jensen P: Treatment of spasticity by subarachnoid phenol glycerin. Neurology (Minneap) 15:256, 1965.
35. Felsenthal G: Pharmacology of phenol in peripheral nerve blocks: A review. Arch Phys Med Rehabil 55:13–16, 1974.
36. Moller JE, Helweg-Larson J, Jacobson E: Histopathological lesions in the sciatic nerve of the rat following perineural application of phenol and alcohol solutions. Dan Med Bull 16:116–119, 1969.
37. Smith MC: Histological findings following intrathecal injection of phenol solutions for the relief of pain. Anaesthesia 36:387, 1964.
38. Bates W, Judovich BD: Intractable pain. Anesthesiology 3:363, 1942.
39. Wood KM: The use of phenol as a neurolytic agent: A review. Pain 5:205, 1978.
40. Hakanson S: Trigeminal neuralgia treated by the injection of glycerol into the trigeminal cistern. Neurosurgery 9:638, 1981.
41. Miller RD, Johnston RR, Hosbuchi Y: Treatment of intercostal neuralgia with 10% ammonium sulfate. J Thorac Cardiovasc Surg 69:476, 1975.
42. Davies JJ, Stewart PB, Fink AP: Prolonged sensory block using ammonium salts. Anesthesiology 28:244, 1967.
43. Myers RR, Katz J: Neural pathology of neurolytic and semidestructive agents. *In* Cousins MJ, Bridenbaugh PO (eds): Neural Blockade in Clinical Anesthesia and Management of Pain, ed 2. Philadelphia, JB Lippincott, 1988, pp 1031–1051.
44. Hitchcock E: Osmolytic neurolysis for intractable facial pain. Lancet i:434, 1969.
45. Jewett DL, King JS: Conduction block of monkey dorsal rootlets by water and hypertonic saline solutions. Exp Neurol 33:225, 1971.
46. King JS, Jewett DL, Phil D, Sundberg HR: Differential blockade of cat dorsal root C fibers by various chloride solutions. J Neurosurg 36:569, 1972.
47. Robertson JD: Structural alterations in nerve fibers produced by hypotonic and hypertonic solutions. J Biophys Biochem Cytol 4:349, 1958.

48. Nicholson MF, Roberts FW: Relief of pain by intrathecal injection of hypothermic saline. Med J Aust 1:61, 1968.
49. Ochs S: Basic properties of axoplasmic transport. *In* Dyck PJ, Thomas PK, Lambert EH, Bunge R (eds): Peripheral Neuropathy. Philadelphia, WB Saunders, 1984, p 453.
50. Fink BR: Mechanism of hypo-osmotic conduction block. Reg Anesth 5:7, 1980.
51. Denny-Brown D, Adams R, Brenner C, Doherty MM: The pathology of injury to nerve induced by cold. J Neuropathol Exp Neurol 4:305, 1945.
52. Paintal AS: Block of conduction in mammalian myelinated nerve fibres by low temperatures. J Physiol 180:1, 1965.
53. Douglas WW, Malcolm JL: Effect of localized cooling on conduction in cat nerves. J Physiol (Lond) 130:63, 1955.
54. Myers RR, Powell HC, Costello ML, et al: Biophysical and pathologic effects of cryogenic nerve lesions. Ann Neurol 10:478, 1981.
55. Jacob RG, Howland WS: A comparison of intrathecal alcohol and phenol. J Ky Med Assoc 64:408, 1966.
56. Evans RJ, Mackay IM: Subarachnoid phenol nerve blocks for relief of pain in advanced malignancy. Can J Surg 15:50–53, 1972.
57. Wood KA: The use of phenol as a neurolytic agent: A review. Pain 5:205–229, 1978.
58. Gentil FF, Russo RP, Monti A, et al: Pain relief in cancerous patients by the use of phenol solution. Acta Univ Int Cancer 19:982–985, 1963.
59. Maher RM: Neurone selection in relief of pain: Further experiences with intrathecal injections. Lancet 1:16–19, 1957.

CHAPTER • 18

Cryoneurolysis in Clinical Practice

Lloyd R. Saberski, MD

Cryoanalgesic therapy has widespread and diverse application in the fields of pain management and neurosurgery. My purpose in this chapter is to sensitize the practitioner to the proper use and limitations of this relatively new technology, so that appropriate clinical decisions can be made. Examples of applications will be presented, but it is not my intent to address all potential uses of cryoanalgesia.

HISTORICAL CONSIDERATIONS

Cryoanalgesia is a technique in which cold is applied to produce pain relief. The analgesic effect of cold has been known to man for more than a millennium.[1] Hippocrates (460–377 BC) provided the first written record of the use of ice and snow packs applied before surgery as a local pain-relieving technique.[2] Early physicians such as Avicenna of Persia (980–1070 AD) and Severino of Naples (1580–1656) recorded using cold for preoperative analgesia.[3,4] In 1812, Napoleon's surgeon general, Baron Dominique Jean Larre, recognized that the limbs of soldiers frozen in the Prussian snow could be amputated relatively painlessly.[5] In 1851, Dr. James Arnott described using an ice-salt mixture to produce tumor regression as well as to obtain an anesthetic and hemostatic effect.[6] Richardson introduced ether spray in 1866 to produce local analgesia by refrigeration. This was superseded in 1890 by ethyl chloride spray.

Contemporary interest in cryoanalgesia was sparked in 1961, after Dr. Irvine Cooper described a cryotherapy unit in which liquid nitrogen was circulated through a hollow metal probe that was vacuum-insulated except at the tip. With this equipment it was possible to control the temperature of the tip by interrupting the flow of liquid nitrogen at temperatures within the range of room temperature and −196° C. Since it was a totally enclosed system, cold could be applied to any part of the body accessible to the probe. The first clinical application of this technique was in neurosurgery, for treatment of parkinsonism.[7,8] In 1967, Amoils developed a simpler hand-held unit that used either carbon dioxide or nitrous oxide. These devices were the prototypes for the current generation of cryoprobes used in cryoanalgesia (Figs. 18–1, 18–2).[9] The coldest temperature is approximately −70° C.

THE PHYSICS AND CELLULAR BASICS FOR CRYOANALGESIA

The working principle of a cryoprobe is that compressed gas (nitrous oxide or carbon dioxide) expands. The cryoprobe consists of an outer tube and a smaller inner tube that terminates in a fine nozzle (Fig. 18–3). High-pressure gas (650–800 lb/in^2) is passed between the two tubes and is released via a small orifice into a chamber at the tip of the probe. In the chamber, the gas expands, and the substantial reduction in pressure (80–100 lb/in^2) results in a rapid decrease in temperature, and, thus, cooling of the probe tip. (Absorption of heat from surrounding tissues accompanies expansion of any gas, according to the principles of the general gas law. This is the adiabatic principle of gas cooling and heat extraction, also known as the Joule-Thomson effect.) The low-pressure gas flows back through the center of the inner tube and back to the console, where it is vented. The sealed construction of the cryoprobe ensures that no gas escapes from the probe tip, handle, or hose.

The rapid cooling of the cryoprobe produces a tip surface temperature of approximately −70° C. Tissue in contact with the tip cools rapidly and forms an ice ball. The ice ball varies in size, depending on probe size, freeze time, tissue permeability to water, and presence of vascular structures (heat sink). The ice ball typically measures 3.5 to 5.5 mm in diameter. Further increase in size is prevented when thermal equilibrium is attained.

Precise levels of gas flow through the cryoprobe are essential for maximum efficiency. Inadequate gas flow will not freeze tissue. Excessive gas flow results in freezing down the stem of the probe and the associated risk of cold skin burns. The cryoprobe console is therefore fitted with a regulator and indicator that are adjusted for optimal performance.

The application of cold to peripheral nerves, whether by direct cooling of localized segments or complete immersion of tissue in a cold medium, induces reversible conduction block. The extent and duration of the effect are dependent on the temperature attained in the tissues and the duration of exposure.[1] When nerve fibers are progressively cooled a conduction block similar to that produced by local

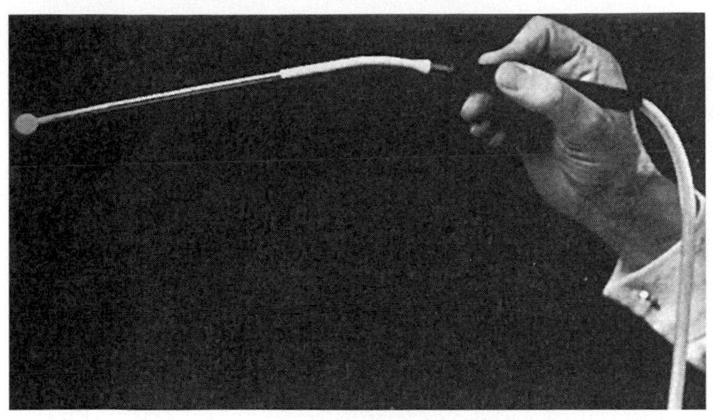

FIGURF 18–1 An early hand-held cryoprobe with Ice ball. (From Holden HB: Practical Cryosurgery. London, Pitman Medical, 1975.)

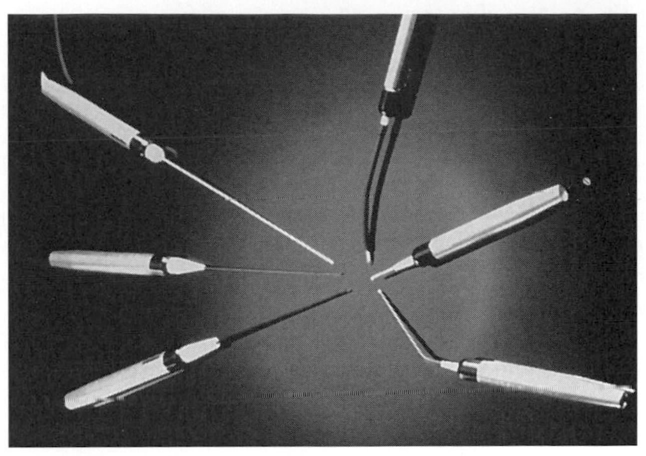

FIGURE 18–2 Contemporary hand-held Lloyd cryoprobes. (Courtesy of Westco Medical Corporation, San Diego, Calif.)

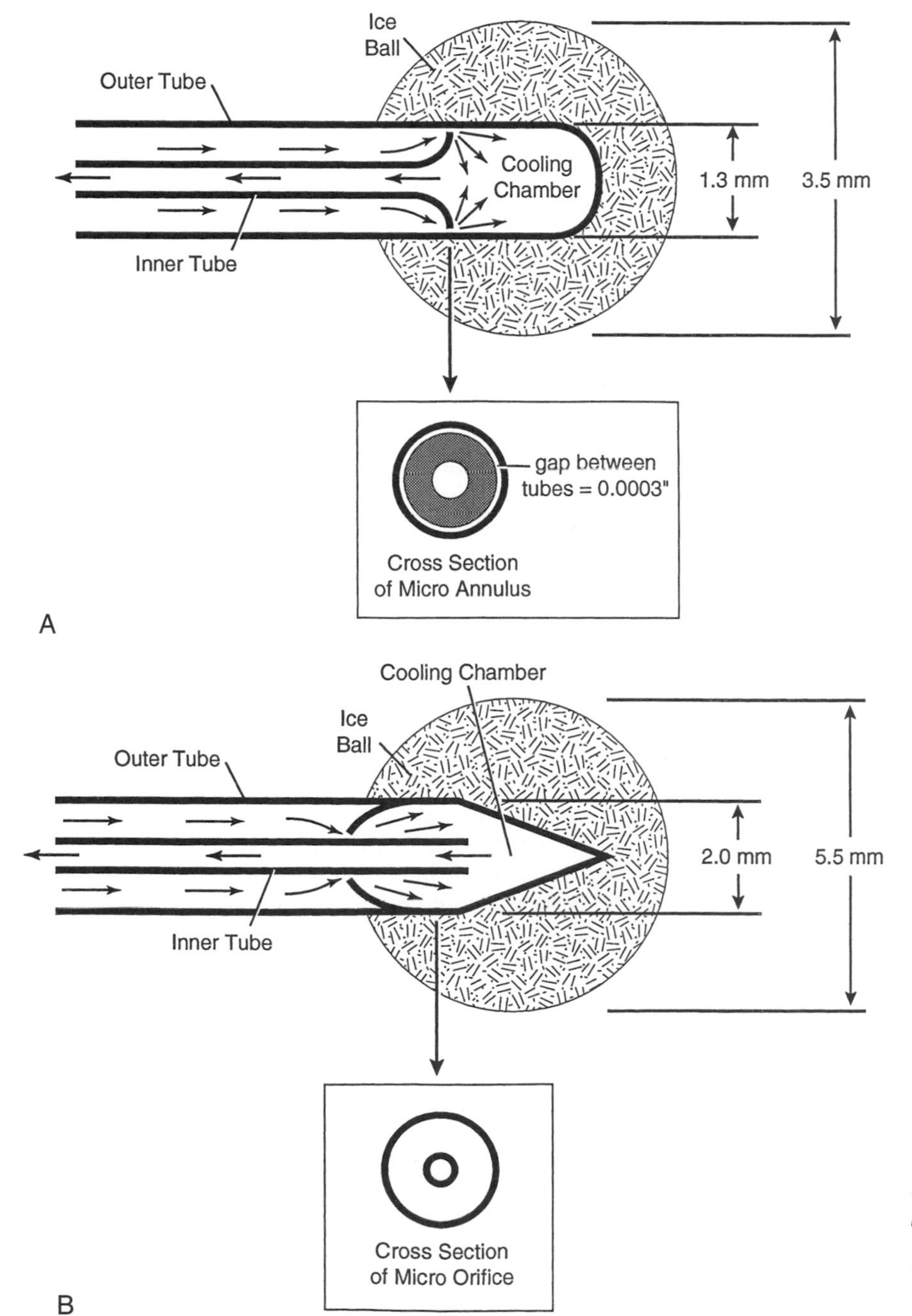

FIGURE 18–3 A, B. *Cross sections of two commonly used cryoprobe designs. High-pressure gas goes in through the outer tube at 650 to 800 psi. Low-pressure gas is vented out at 80 to 100 psi. Gas flow is at 7 to 9 L/min. Test conditions: Tip is inserted into water at 36° ± 1° C. An ice ball is formed within 60 sec.*

anesthetic develops. At 10° C, larger myelinated fibers cease conduction before unmyelinated fibers, but at 0° C all nerve fibers entrapped in the ice ball stop conduction. Some fibers resume conduction on rewarming. To obtain a prolonged effect from a cryolesion the intracellular contents of the nerve must be turned into ice crystals. There is little clinical difference as long as the temperature is below −20° C for 1 min.[10] When the nerve is frozen amidst other tissues, the duration of exposure becomes more important. Within the limitations of a specific cryoprobe and its steady state of thermal equilibrium, prolonging application of the cryoprobe increases the size of the ice ball and the likelihood of the nerve's being entrapped by a cryolesion. In practice, a freeze of 2 to 3 minutes' duration produces a good result. Prolonged exposure and repeated freeze-thaw cycles likely are beneficial with percutaneous techniques, especially when abundant surrounding soft tissue and nerve localization are poor.[1]

Histologically, the axons and myelin sheaths degenerate after cryolesioning (wallerian degeneration), but the epineurium and perineurium remain intact, thus allowing subsequent nerve regeneration. The duration of the block is a function of the rate of axonal regeneration after cryolesion, which is reported to be between 1 and 3 mm per day.[10] Since axonal regrowth is constant, the return of sensory and motor activity is a function of the distance between the cryolesion and the end organ.[1] The absence of external damage to the nerve and the minimal inflammatory reaction to freezing ensure that regeneration is exact. Thus, the regenerating axons are unlikely to form painful neuromas. (Surgical and thermal lesions interrupt perineurium and epineurium.) Other neurolytic techniques (alcohol, phenol) can potentially produce painful neuromas because the epineurium and perineurium are disrupted.

A cryolesion provides a temporary anesthetic block. Clinically, a cryoblock lasts weeks to months. The result depends on numerous variables, including operator technique and clinical circumstances. The analgesia often lasts longer than the time required for axons to regenerate.[16] The reasons for this are still a matter of speculation, but it is obvious that there is more to cryoanalgesia than just temporary disruption of axons. It is possible that sustained blockade of afferent input to the central nervous system (CNS) has an effect on CNS windup. A report suggests that cryolesions release sequestered tissue protein or facilitate changes in protein antigenic properties.[11] The result is an autoimmune response targeted at cryolesioned tissue. The first report of such a response was from Gander and Soanes,[12] who demonstrated tissue-specific autoantibodies after cryocoagulation of male rabbit accessory glands. This report was followed by a parallel clinical report of regression of metastatic deposits from prostatic adenocarcinoma after cryocoagulation of the primary tumor.[13] The significance of this for pain management is not clear; however, it does indicate that tumor growth and regression are affected by immune function. Perhaps immune mechanisms play a role in the analgesic response after cryoablation.

INDICATIONS AND CONTRAINDICATIONS

Cryoanalgesia is best suited for clinical situations when analgesia is required for weeks or months. Permanent blockade does not usually occur, since the cryoinjured axons regenerate. The median duration of pain relief is 2 weeks to 5 months.[14, 15] Cryoanalgesia is suited for painful conditions that originate from small, well-localized lesions of peripheral nerves; for example, neuromas, entrapment neuropathies, and postoperative pain.[16] Longer than expected periods of analgesia have been reported and may be from the patient's ability to more fully participate in physical therapy or from an effect of prolonged analgesia on central processing of pain (preemptive analgesic effect). Sustained blockade of afferent impulses[17–20] with cryoanalgesia may reduce plasticity (windup) in the CNS and decrease pain permanently.[21]

Cryoablative procedures can be performed open or closed (percutaneous), depending on the clinical setting. Most often, open procedures are performed as part of postoperative analgesia. Under direct visualization, the operator identifies the neural structure of concern, and the cryoprobe is applied for 1 to 4 minutes, depending on tissue heat, which is a function of blood supply and distance of the probe from the nerve. Care is taken not to freeze adjacent vascular structures. The cryoprobe is withdrawn only after the tissue thaws, as removing it earlier can tear tissue.

Percutaneous (closed) cryoablation is the technique of choice for outpatient chronic pain management. It has the advantage of easy application and few complications. Percutaneous (closed) cryoablative procedures have been used successfully for many benign and malignant pain syndromes, but, unfortunately, few scientific studies have been published, in part because there was little interest until recently in pain management techniques and because of lack of industry funding for advanced research.

Patients must give informed consent. The consent form should describe the risk-benefit ratios of cryoanalgesia and of regional anesthesia. Patients should be fully aware that, usually, a cryoanalgesia procedure is not a permanent solution. It can, however, ameliorate symptoms and allow the patient to participate better in physiotherapy. In some cases when there has been CNS windup, it may serve as a form of preemptive anesthetic and facilitate prolonged relief. Cryoanalgesia for chronic pain syndromes should always be preceded by diagnostic/prognostic local anesthetic injections. After a test block with local anesthetic, the examiner should inquire about the patient's tolerance to the numbness and the extent of pain reduction. If response to the test injections is inadequate, the patient will not have a good response to cryodenervation. Patients should also be aware that numbness can replace pain, and small areas of skin depigmentation can occur if the ice ball frosts skin because the probe is not deep enough or is inadequately insulated from tissues. All procedures are done with appropriate sterile preparation. As a general rule, infected areas are avoided.

CLINICALLY RELEVANT ANATOMY

For any given procedure, it is essential that the provider of cryoanalgesia be aware of the regional anatomy of interest. Since cryoanalgesia has widespread applications, thorough knowledge of neuroanatomy and regional anesthesia is required. In the next section, detailed descriptions and illustrations are provided for a number of procedures. The reader is referred to standard anatomy textbooks for more detailed discussion.

CLINICAL PEARLS AND TRICKS OF THE TRADE

Postoperative Pain Management

Postoperative use of cryoanalgesia should be widespread, but, unfortunately, in the United States, it is used routinely for postoperative analgesia in only a few centers. The reasons are several, among them a lack of controlled studies and physicians' reluctance to add time and costs to procedures, especially when they feel patients are already receiving adequate care. Interestingly, at many institutions, cryoanalgesia is reserved for patients with special analgesia needs and those at high risk who cannot receive standard postoperative treatment. Of the handful of studies that have been done,[22–26] most indicate significant reductions in pain and medication requirements. It is likely that use of postoperative cryoanalgesia will increase if it can be demonstrated that cost savings and improved long-term outcomes are the results.

Cryoanalgesia procedures are provided intraoperatively by surgeons who have access to involved peripheral nerve and pain management specialists participating in the operative procedure. At times, pain specialists are called upon to provide cryoanalgesia postoperatively, in which case they must decide whether some alternative is more suitable than open or closed cryodenervation.

Popular Cryodenervation Techniques for Postoperative Pain Management

POSTTHORACOTOMY PAIN

Intraoperative intercostal cryoneurolysis was first described by Nelson and associates in 1974.[27] Since that time, a large body of literature has been published that supports use of cryodeneravation as a component of a postoperative analgesia plan.[22–24, 28] Postthoracotomy cryoanalgesia is most effective for treating incisional pain, but it is not effective for pain from visceral pleura supplied by autonomic fibers or for ligament pain of the chest secondary to rib retraction. Postthoracotomy cryoanalgesia often has little effect on chest tube pain, for the same reasons. Patients treated with cryotherapy during thoracotomy have relatively less postoperative discomfort and opioid requirements both in the immediate postoperative period and over subsequent weeks. There has been only one documented report of neuritis as a complication of cryoneurolysis.[29] Sensory anesthesia lasts longer than 6 months along the sensory field of treated intercostal nerves.

For effective intraoperative cryoneurolysis, intercostal nerves on each side of the thoracotomy incision are lesioned. If a rib is removed, that intercostal nerve is also cryolesioned. The intercostal nerves are best cryoablated just lateral to the transverse process, before the collateral intercostal nerve branches (Fig. 18–4). Only a small area of skin innervated by the dorsal primary ramus will be missed. Care is taken to separate the intercostal nerves from the intercostal vessels, thereby removing a large heat sink that would be counterproductive to cryotherapy. The vessels are also protected from cold-induced thrombosis. A cryolesion sufficient to produce visible evidence of freezing is required. In general such a lesion takes 1 to 2 min. A second lesion can be placed after tissue thaws, but whether that is necessary when freezing of the first lesion is complete remains to be determined.

POSTHERNIORRHAPHY PAIN

Cryoneurolysis after herniorrhaphy was first described by Wood and coworkers in 1979.[30] A cryolesion of the ilioinguinal nerve reduces analgesic requirements during the postoperative period. The follow-up study in 1981 compared recovery from herniorrhaphy amongst three study groups: those treated, respectively, with oral analgesics, cryoanalgesia, and paravertebral blockade (the last two treatments supplemented with oral analgesics as needed). The study indicated that the cryoanalgesic group not only had less pain in the postoperative period but also used less opioid, resumed a regular diet earlier, were mobilized faster, and returned to work sooner.[25] Despite these successes, the technique is not widely used. Given its effectiveness and freedom of side effects, it is ideal for ambulatory surgery. After repair of the internal ring, posterior wall of the inguinal canal, and internal oblique muscle, the ilioinguinal nerve on the surface of the muscle is identified and mobilized. The surgeon elevates the nerve above the muscle, and an assistant performs the cryoablation.

Chronic Pain Management

For management of chronic pain, open cryoablation is avoided whenever the procedure can effectively be performed percutaneously. Before committing to cryoablation, the provider must perform a series of test blocks to determine presence of a consistent analgesic response. A favorable response prior to cryoablation is when the local anesthetic injection decreases pain and the numbness that replaces the pain is tolerated by the patient. Care must always be taken to ensure correct positioning of the needles. When necessary, fluoroscopic guidance should be used. The smallest amount of local anesthetic required to achieve blockade must be used. A tuberculin syringe that injects 0.1 mm at a time ensures that the anesthetic does not contaminate other structures, which would otherwise make interpretation of the block difficult. This contributes to accurate localization of the primary pain generator. If the block is successful, an appropriate dermatomal representation of the analgesia will be present. Subsequently, the patient is assessed for subjective changes in pain; however, this alone is insufficient to determine suitability for cryoablation. Many pain patients have suffered for a long time and are very hopeful that the next procedure is going to be the long-awaited successful treatment. Thus, they are responsive to suggestion and placebo effect. To identify those effects, the first test injection is done with lidocaine and the second with bupivacaine. In appropriate responders, a significantly longer duration of analgesia can be found with bupivacaine, assuming that all other variables remain the same. The effects of peripheral blockade on windup

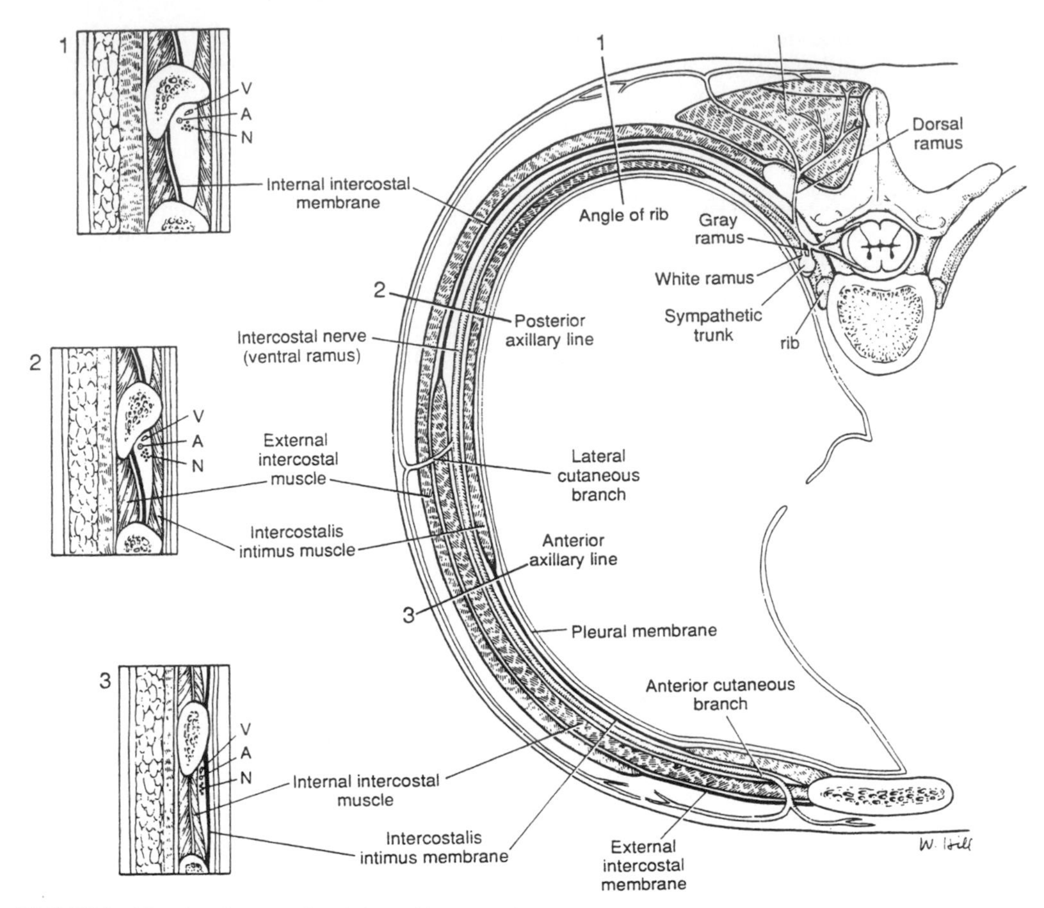

FIGURE 18–4 Cross-sectional view of intercostal nerve anatomy. (From Chung J: Thoracic pain. In *Sinatra RS, Hord AH, Ginsberg G, Preble L (eds): Acute Pain. St. Louis, CV Mosby, 1991.)*

and chronic pain are not clearly understood. To responsive patients a cryoablative procedure can be offered. For those patients who do not have the desired response to bupivacaine or lidocaine, further testing is necessary, including differential blockade with local anesthetics and normal saline and consideration of consultation with a clinical psychologist.

To successfully perform percutaneous cryoablation it is essential that the cryoprobe be properly placed. This is a disadvantage as compared with open cryoablative techniques used for postoperative pain management. The operator must ensure proper cryoprobe placement by using a combination of techniques (see later) that improve the chances that the ice ball will be made precisely on the pain generator. In addition, special care must be taken when using the cryoprobe for percutaneous procedures. Bending the probe during percutaneous introduction can distort the lumen of the low-pressure outer tube, increase the resistance pressure to the expanding nitrous oxide gas, and convert a low-pressure exhaust system to one of higher pressure. That eventuality would impede gas expansion, inhibit ice ball formation, and limit cooling of the probe. Therefore, to maintain the integrity of the cryoprobe, the probe should be placed through an introducer. The preferred introducers are large-bore intravenous catheters: 12-, 14-, or 16-gauge, depending on the size of the cryoprobe. The operator should always check to see that the cryoprobe fits through the lumen of the catheter. The depth at which the probe emerges from the distal tip of the catheter should be marked on the proximal shaft of the cryoprobe to ensure that the cryoprobe tip extends far enough beyond the catheter to create a full-sized ice ball.

Several techniques are utilized to enhance precise placement of the cryoprobe:

1. Careful palpation with a small blunt instrument such as a felt-tipped pen can help to localize a soft tissue neuroma or another palpable pain generator.
2. An image intensifier (fluoroscopy) can identify bony landmarks.
3. Contrast medium improves definition of tissue planes, capsules, and spaces. (Non-ionic contrast medium should be used in areas close to neural tissue.)
4. The nerve stimulator at the tip of the cryoprobe is used to produce a muscle twitch in a mixed nerve. The stimulator is set at 5 Hz for recruitment of motor fibers. The probe is closest to the nerve when the lowest output produces a twitch response. In general, we like to see twitches at 0.5 to 1.5 V. Small sensory branches contain no motor component and, thus, do not twitch with electrical stimulation. These fibers are localized by using higher-frequency (100 Hz) stimulation, which produces overlapping dysesthesia in the distribution of the small sensory nerve. This may reproduce the patient's pain. Again, use of low-output (<0.5–1.5 V) stimulation ensures closer placement of the cryoprobe to the nerve in question.

The operator freezes the nerve for 2 to 3 min. Often there is discomfort initially as cooling begins, but it should quickly dissipate. If significant pain persists beyond 30 secs, the operator should investigate whether the ice ball is in the proper position. (If the ice ball is not sufficiently close to the nerve and there is only partial freezing, mostly of larger myelinated fibers, then unchecked unmyelinated fiber input is left. This theoretically accounts for increased pain.) The brief cooling may already have altered nerve function, in which case, if positioning of the probe depends on feedback from the patient, it could be impeded. Before moving the probe, the operator must be sure to thaw the tip to prevent tissue damage from an ice ball sticking to the tissues. In general, with closed procedures, two freeze cycles of 2 min each, followed by thaw cycles are sufficient. In areas where there is a large vascular heat sink, longer periods of cryotherapy will be necessary. Pain relief should be immediate and should be assessed subjectively and by physical examination while the patient is on the procedure table. All relevant clinical information should be recorded in the medical record. A hard-copy radiograph should be obtained for most procedures when a fluoroscope is used.

Applied Cryoanalgesia for Chronic Pain

It is the goal of this section to give the reader the skills necessary to make proper clinical decisions regarding cryoanalgesia. Listing every procedure is beyond the scope of this chapter. In the following section I review many of the pain syndromes that are amenable to cryodenervation and describe in detail those that are requested most often. To perform cryolytic treatments correctly, the provider must be familiar with the regional anatomy and the principles of localizing pain generators described earlier.

Intercostal Neuralgia

Percutaneous cryolesions of the intercostal nerves can be offered for a variety of pain syndromes including postthoracotomy pain, traumatic intercostal neuralgia, rib fracture pain, and occasionally postherpetic neuropathy. For each of these conditions, a meticulous series of local anesthetic blocks is performed before consideration is given to cryoablation. The volume of local anesthetic should be kept to less than 3 to 4 mL to prevent tracking back into the epidural space. In addition, only two or three levels should be injected at any one time, since systemic absorption could confound interpretation of the patient's response. Since the intercostal nerve runs with a large arterial and venous heat source, two 4-min cryolesions at each level is suggested. The lesions should be made proximal to the pain at the inferior border of the rib (Fig. 18–5). After the procedure, a chest film is obtained to check for pneumothorax. Effective blockade of some patients with postherpetic neuropathy suggests that this pain is sometimes related to peripheral afferent input, as opposed to being strictly a central neuropathy.

Neuromas

Typically, painful neuromas are associated with lancinating or shooting pain that is aggravated by movement or deformation of nearby soft tissues. Neurophysiologically, this phenomenon is thought to reflect lower neural thresholds and ephatic transmission. First-line therapy should include empiric trials of anticonvulsants, tricyclic antidepressants, steroids, and local anesthetics, including topical local anesthetic cream or patch. These agents are thought to play a role in modulating neural thresholds. Cryoablation is considered only after careful mapping has isolated a very discrete pain generator (i.e., a neuroma). The initial injection can use a relatively larger volume of local anesthetic, but subsequent blocks should deliver small increments from a tuberculin syringe to ensure accurate interpretation. Cryoablation seems most effective when the volume of local anesthetic necessary to produce analgesia is 1 mL or less. Subsequent to the block with lidocaine, the patient's response and its duration are recorded. If initial blockade is successful in decreasing the patient's symptoms, it should be followed by at least one more injection with bupivacaine. A response of longer duration might be expected with the longer-acting local anesthetic.

Iliac Crest Bone Harvest

The pain associated with the harvest of iliac crest bone for fusion is often responsive to cryoablation when more conservative therapies have failed. Such pain is often associated with deep, lancinating pain and is often attributed to periosteal neuromas. The surface area is often quite large, and careful diagnostic mapping is required to localize the primary pain generator as precisely as possible. When no single pain generator is found and the periosteal surface that is the source of the pain remains large and unresponsive to other therapies (e.g., steroid injections and nonste-

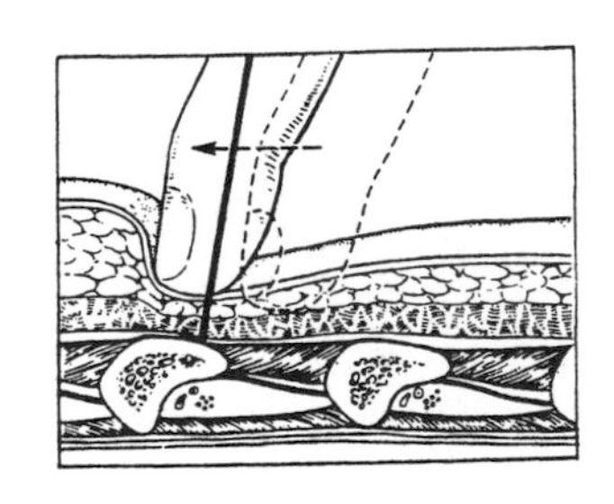

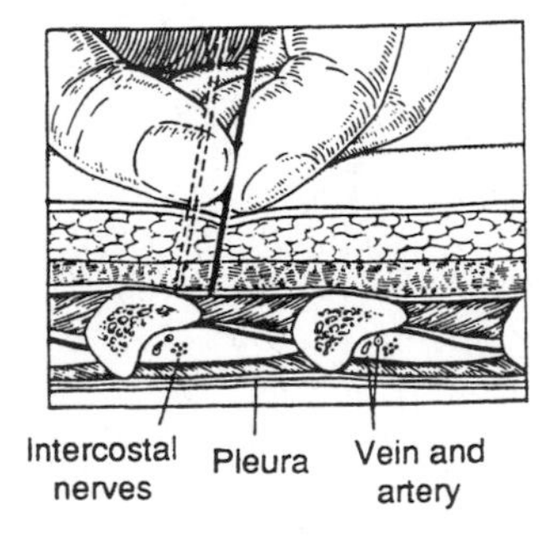

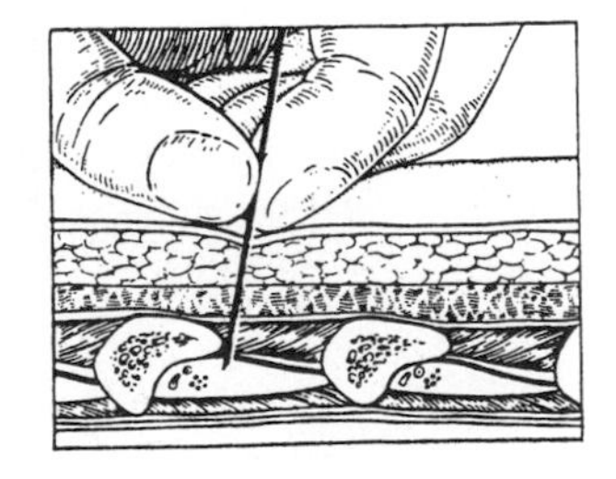

FIGURE 18–5 The percutaneous placement of a needle (introducer) onto an intercostal nerve at the inferior border of a rib. (From Chung J: Thoracic pain. In Sinatra RS, Hord AH, Ginsberg G, Preble L (eds): Acute Pain. St. Louis, CV Mosby, 1991.)

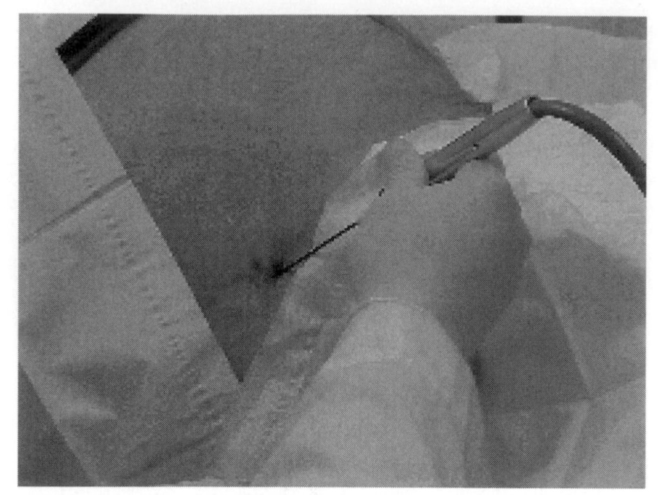

FIGURE 18–6 Cryoablation of an anterior iliac crest bone harvest site. (Also in color, see Color Plates.)

roidal antiinflammatory drugs), multiple cryoablations may be necessary during one session (Fig. 18–6; see also Case Report).

Biomechanical Spine Pain

Typically, biomechanical spine pain is exacerbated with movement, so physiotherapy often is futile. In general, there are no neurologic deficits and the pain is ascribed to a number of structures, including the articular facet nerves, the meningeal nerves, the anterior communicating ramus, and other branches of the posterior primary ramus (Figs. 18–7, 18–8). Cryolesions have been used effectively for cervical and lumbar facet syndromes[31] and for pain from the interspinous ligaments.[32] The success of cryolesioning is a function of patient selection, accurate probe placement,

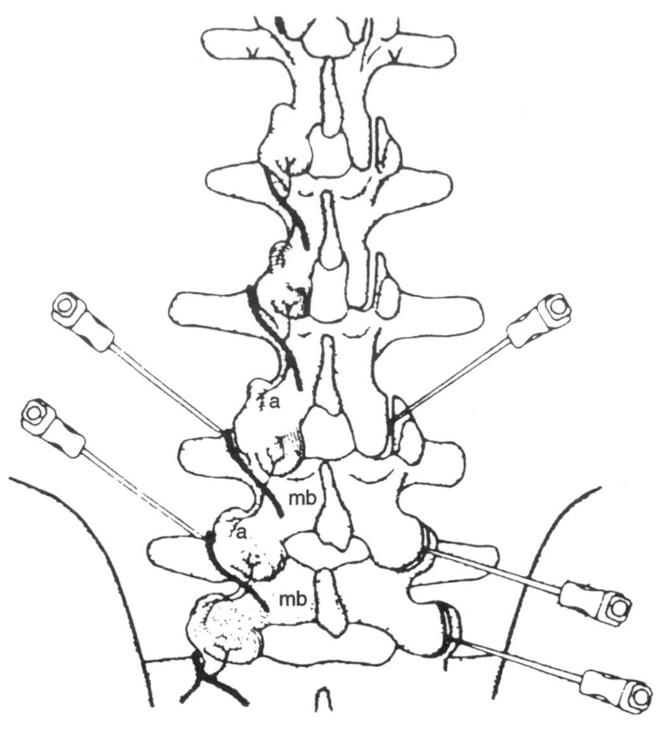

FIGURE 18–8 Dorsum of lumbar spine. a, Articular branch of facet; mb, medial branch of the posterior primary division. Needles placed into lumbar facet joints and onto medial branches. (From Cousins M, Bridenbaugh P (eds): Neural Blockade in Clinical Anesthesia and Management of Pain, ed 2 Philadelphia, JB Lippincott, 1994.)

and the follow-up rehabilitation program. For biomechanical pain of lumbar facet origin, the patient typically has pain that is exacerbated by hyperextension of the lumbar spine. The pain localizes to the lumbosacral junction and often radiates into the buttocks and the posterior aspect

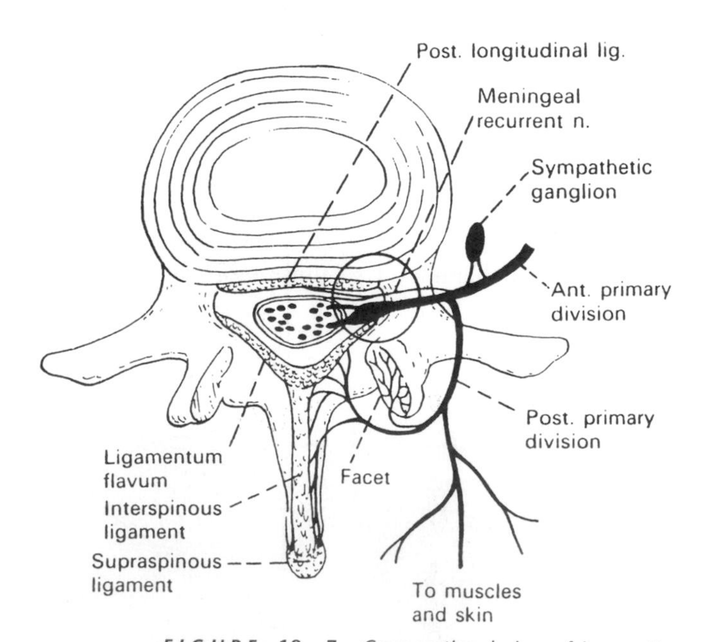

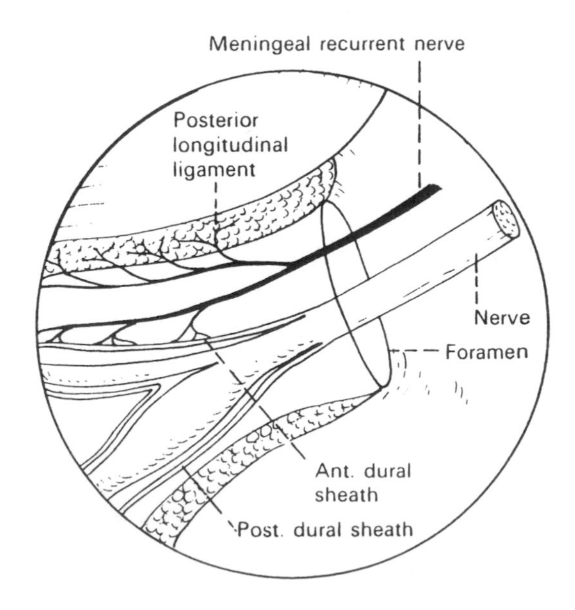

FIGURE 18–7 Cross-sectional view of innervation of the posterior motion segment, including the facet. (From Bonica J: The Management of Pain. Philadelphia, Lea & Febiger, 1990.)

of the thigh, generally never below the knee. These patients have significant muscle spasm, at times extending cephalad and caudad. They complain that movement is uncomfortable and are unable to participate in lumbar physiotherapy. Palpation reveals exquisite tenderness along the lumbar paravertebral margin. There are no significant neurologic changes, but, typically, other biomechanical problems are present, such as pelvic obliquity, functional leg length discrepancy, and sacroiliac joint dysfunction. Before an isolated facet arthropathy is addressed, attention should be directed to the associated biomechanical disorders. For instance, if a patient has a leg length discrepancy and pelvic shift, a shoe orthotic should be prescribed. When a patient has severe pain from the facet arthropathy, little is gained from prescribing physiotherapy. In such circumstances (which are not uncommon), denervation of the facet may enable the patient to participate in physiotherapy. A fluoroscopically guided diagnostic intraarticular facet block can be performed on those patients who fulfill the above criteria. The levels chosen for injection are determined by bone scan, CT, plain films, and, most important, the physical examination findings. Initial needle placement into the facet is guided by AP fluoroscopic visualization (Fig. 18–9A–C) after a small skin wheal is made. Correct intraarticular placement is confirmed with oblique imaging; the needle should be in the ear of the Scottie dog (Fig. 18–9D). (Often, as the needle enters the joint space, the operator feels as though the needle is being pushed through an orange peel; that is, he feels the loss of resistance.) Once the needle is within the joint, 1 mL of non-ionic contrast medium is injected. With facet arthropathy, this is often very painful. A fluoroscopic review of the area of interest of the contrast study shows the facet capsule filled with radiodense contrast medium. In some circumstances, the

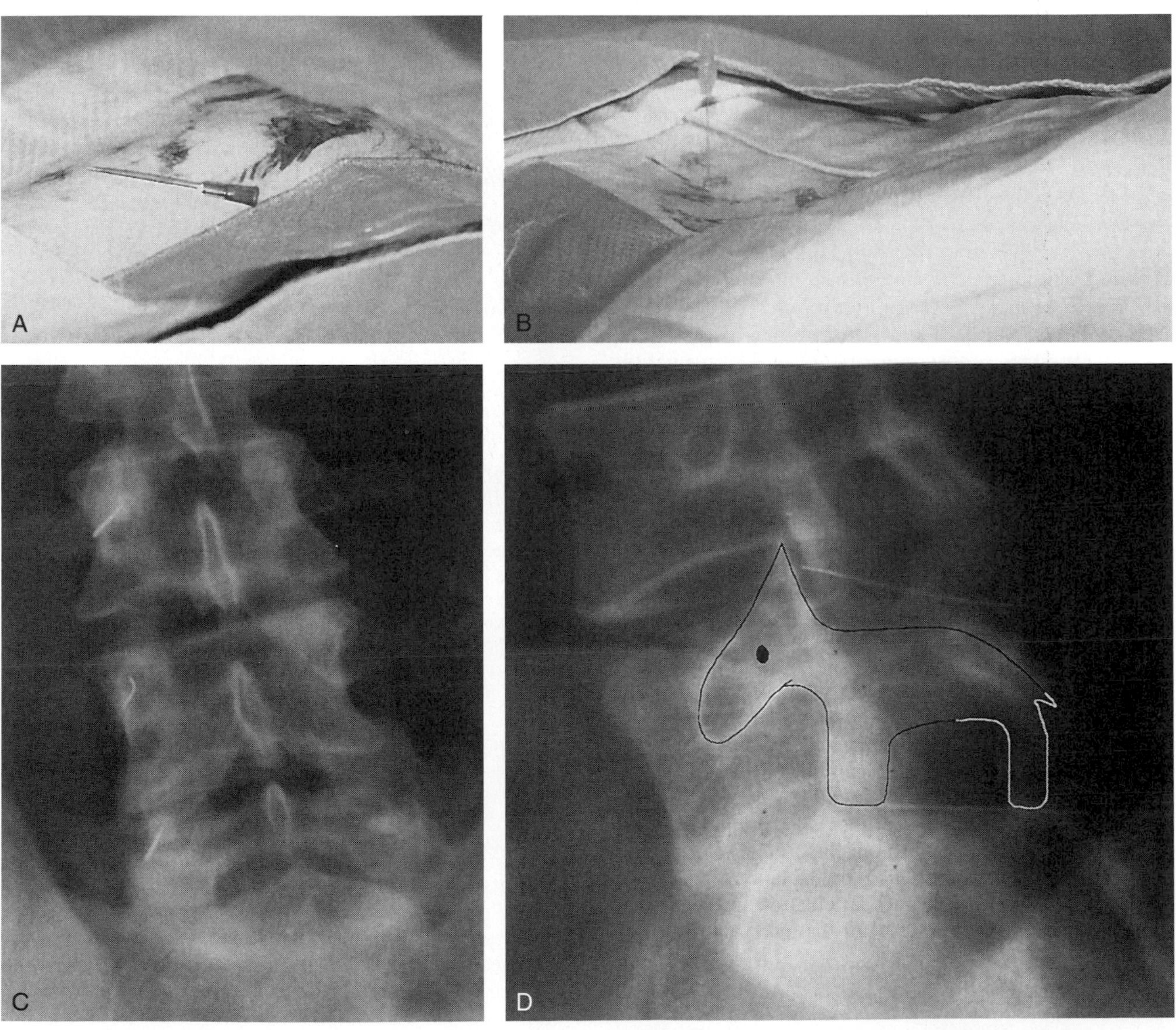

FIGURE 18–9 A, *Using fluoroscopy, the point of a needle is placed over the lumbar facet of interest. This corresponds to the junction of the transverse process and the pedicle.* B, *A 22-gauge finder (spinal) needle is then inserted through the skin at the point of the needle down to bone.* C, *AP x-ray projection shows the needle at the junction of the transverse process and the pedicle near the facet joint.* D, *Using an oblique projection, the needle is then manipulated into the Scotty dog's ear for intrarticular placement or into the Scotty dog's eye for the articular nerve (medial branch).*

capsule is deformed or leaky. At times, the capsule is large and cystic and projects into the canal. At this point, the patient is asked to carefully consider whether this is the usual pain or a different pain, and to rate it on the visual analogue scale. If the pain reproduced is representative of the usual pain, 1 mL of 1% lidocaine is injected. The needle is further manipulated, and the patient is asked how he or she feels and to arch the back. If the patient has a dramatic decrease in pain and improved movement, it is likely that a facet pain generator is present. If there is little change in symptoms, then up to an additional 4 mL of lidocaine can be injected incrementally. If there is no change in symptoms at the level under study, it is unlikely to be a primary pain generator. In patients who respond, a set of flexion-extension films should be made before discharge, since the analgesia provided by the block should allow better motion and help to reveal occult posterior elemental movement. If such is found, the patient would benefit from an orthopedic evaluation and consideration of fusion.

To confirm a facet pain generator repeat blockade of the facet nerves can be done next. If the result is similar, it is reasonable to consider ablation. Each facet has at least dual innervation and requires at least two local anesthetic injections. A needle is placed at the junction of the transverse process and the pedicle (the Scottie dog's eye on the oblique projection; Fig. 18–9D) at the level previously studied and the level above. A 100-Hz nerve stimulator is used to locate the sensory nerve. Subsequently, 2 mL of 0.25% bupivacaine is injected. Ten minutes later, the patient is reexamined. In patients who continue to be responsive, improvement is observed on physical examination, especially with lumbar hyperextension. For these patients a cryoablative procedure can be considered.

For the cryoablative procedure, the patient is positioned prone in the fluoroscopy suite. The lumbar spine is prepared and draped in standard sterile fashion. Superficial skin wheals are raised at the levels where cryoablations are to be performed. There is, however, a clinical suggestion that there are also contributions to facet innovation from the level below. For this reason, lumbar facet cryodenervations are often done at three levels, a technique popularized by Sebastian Thomas. A 12-gauge introducer catheter (Fig. 18–10A) is introduced to the junction of the transverse process and the pedicle, the Scottie dog's eye. At this point, the cryoprobe is inserted into the introducer catheter (Fig. 18–10B). The nerve stimulator is then used to locate the sensory branch. When pain is reproduced or the patient feels a dysesthesia overlapping the region of the pain, motor testing is in order, to ensure that the ice ball is not near a motor nerve. Two cryolesions are made, each of 2 min duration.

The patient is expected to have some postprocedure discomfort but should notice improvement. In the recovery room ice can be applied to the operative site for 30 min for local postoperative irritation and swelling. This may decrease swelling and facilitate mobilization. The patient should continue with lumbar strengthening programs as an outpatient. If the musculature is significantly deconditioned, it may be better to restart the program in water. After muscle condition improves, the patient should begin a supervised industrial rehabilitation program that offers vocational retraining and job placement.

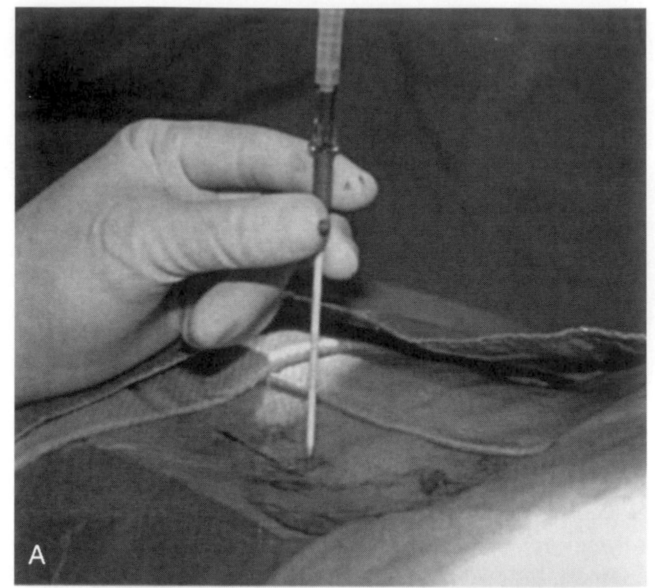

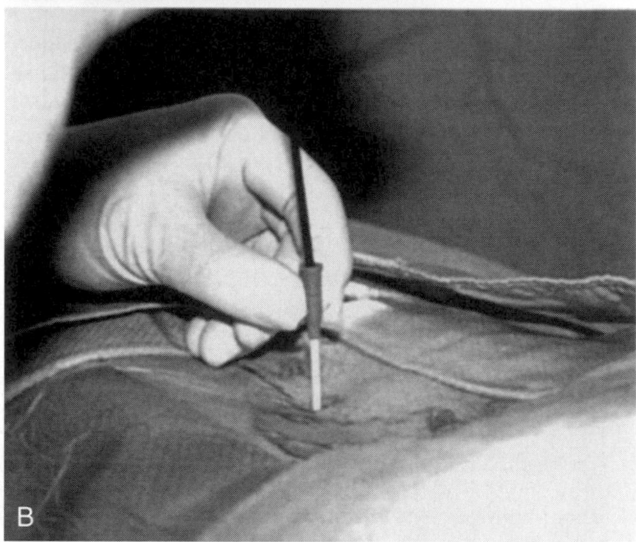

FIGURE 18–10 *A, For facet cryodenervation a 12-gauge introducer catheter is placed percutaneously along the tract of the finder needle. B, The cryoprobe is then placed through the introducer catheter. The final position of the probe is determined by the patient's response to 100 Hz stimulation. There should be no motor response to 5 Hz stimulation.*

Cervical Facet Syndrome

Patients with cervical facet syndrome typically present with severe posterior neck pain and muscle spasm. Palpation elicits pain over cervical facets and at the midline. The pain becomes considerably worse with hyperextension and loading of the cervical spine. Cervical facet syndromes generally are not associated with long track neurologic findings. A radionucleotide bone scan and a plain film may show evidence of posterior elemental arthritic disease. Spondylolisthesis should be sought with flexion-extension films. Significant movement might be better addressed with fusion.

If these patients fail to respond to conservative therapy, a diagnostic series of injections with fluoroscopic guidance is considered. To those who respond to local anesthetic injections with reduction in pain, cryodenervations can be offered as an adjunct to comprehensive physical therapy and rehabilitation. For those with apparent biomechanical neck pain that does not respond to local anesthetic injection, further workup is necessary to identify pain generators.

Interspinous Ligament Pain

Interspinous ligament pain is common after a spine operation (lumbar, thoracic, or cervical.) Pain impulses from interspinous ligaments are carried by the medial branch of the posterior ramus (see Fig. 18–8). Patients report severe movement-related spine pain, identified to midline, that is made worse with hyperextension and relieved by small volumes of local anesthetic injected into the intraspinous ligament. When cervical interspinous ligaments are involved, the patient frequently complains of posterior cervical headache. This headache is often mistaken for occipital neuralgia. Cryodenervation can be considered in local anesthetic–responsive patients. Again, the pain relief helps the patient to complete the necessary course of physical therapy.

Mechanical Spine Pain

Anterior mechanical (discogenic) spine pain is transmitted via different nerves, depending on the location of the injury—the sinuvertebral nerve (recurrent meningeal), small rami of the segmental nerve, rami of the communicating ramus, or sympathetic fibers.[33] Cryolesions have been placed successfully on rami communicantes after diagnostic local anesthetic injections have reduced the pain. Pain of sympathetic origin is not likely to respond to cryodenervation, since the heat carried by the major blood vessels interferes with ice ball formation. Percutaneous sympathectomy is best performed with radiofrequency thermal ablation or with phenol.

Coccydynia

When coccydynia has failed to respond to conservative therapy, including the patient's using a donut pillow, NSAID, and local steroid injections, consideration can be given to coccygeal neural blockade as the coccygeal nerve exits from the sacral canal at the level of the cornu. Bilateral test injections should produce short-term analgesia before cryoablation is considered. For cryoablation of the coccygeal nerve, the probe must be inserted into the canal to make contact with the nerve. Accurate placement of the ice ball is facilitated by using the 100-Hz stimulator and gauging the patient's response. Care should be taken to prevent bending the relatively large cryoprobe while inserting it into the canal.

Perineal Pain

Pain over the dorsal surface of the scrotum, perineum, and anus that has not responded to conservative management can at times be managed effectively with cryodenervation from inside the sacral canal with bilateral S4 lesions. Test local anesthetic injections should produce a positive response before cryoablations are performed bilaterally at the S4 level. Inserting the cryoprobe through the sacral hiatus up to the level of the fourth sacral foramen for placement of a series of cryolesions can give good analgesia. Bladder dysfunction is not usually encountered, and analgesia lasts 6 to 8 weeks.[34] Perineal pain is difficult to treat with intrathecal neurolytic agents without risking bladder and bowel dysfunction.

Ilioinguinal, Iliohypogastric, and Genitofemoral Neuropathies

Ilioinguinal, iliohypogastric, and genitofemoral neuropathies often complicate herniorrhapy, general abdominal surgery, and cesarean section. Patients present with sharp, lancinating to dull pain radiating into the lower abdomen or groin. The pain is exacerbated by lifting and defecating. If the patient proves responsive to a series of low-volume test injections, consideration can be given to cryodenervation of the appropriate nerve. Significant care and time must be spent localizing the nerve with the sensory nerve stimulator. The patient may help to localize the pain generator by pointing with one finger to the point of maximum tenderness. Unfortunately, these nerves are difficult to localize percutaneously, and that difficulty has led to frequent misdiagnosis of the pain generator. In an effort to improve accuracy of diagnosis, Saberski and Rosser developed the *conscious pain mapping* technique.[35] In a lightly sedated patient, a general surgeon working with a pain management specialist performs laparoscopic evaluation of the abdomen in an operating suite. The genitofemoral nerve, lateral femoral cutaneous nerve, and other structures are easily visualized (Fig. 18–11A–C). Blunt probing and patient feedback help to direct the physician to the area of pain. At times, objects such as ligatures and staples are found wrapped around the nerve, in which case they should be removed. If direct mechanical or electrical stimulation to the nerve reproduces the pain, cryoablation can be performed under direct vision. (Cryoablation is chosen as the appropriate test since duration of bupivicaine does not outlast discomfort of the perioperative period. The cryoblockade will provide weeks to months of reliable analgesia and help physicians and patient determine if that structure under surveillance carried the pain information.) Pain usually returns. A repeat cryoablation is possible when analgesia is long or an open surgical procedure with sectioning and burying can be performed.

Lower Extremity Pain

Many cutaneous nerve branches are responsive to cryodenervation. The clinician must always perform a complete physical examination, touching the painful area carefully. Once the primary pain generator is localized, a series of low-volume local anesthetic injections can be given. If the patient has a consistent response, cryodenervations, as outlined earlier, can be employed. Next I discuss some of the common lower extremity nerve pain syndromes that are often amenable to cryodenervation.

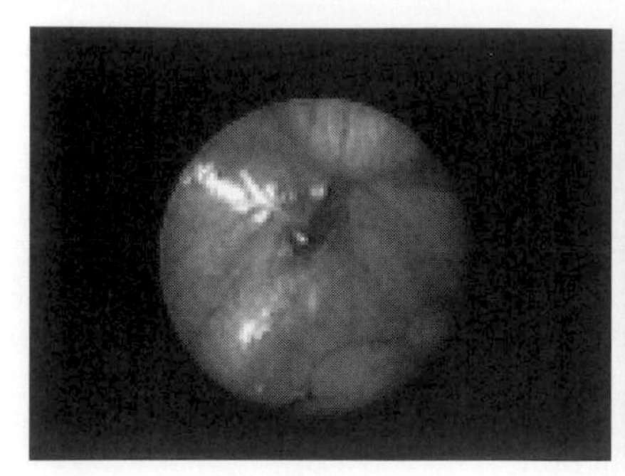
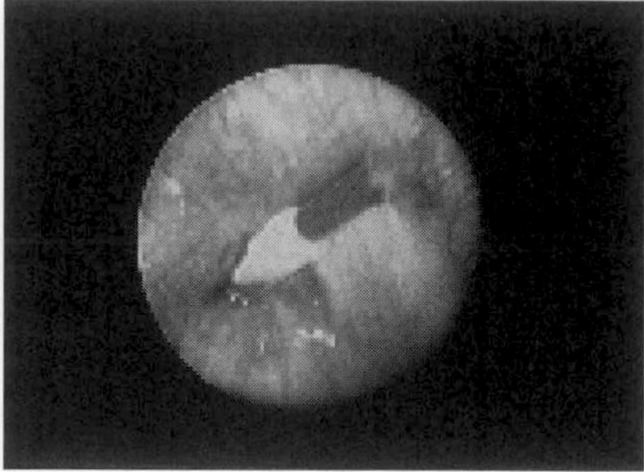
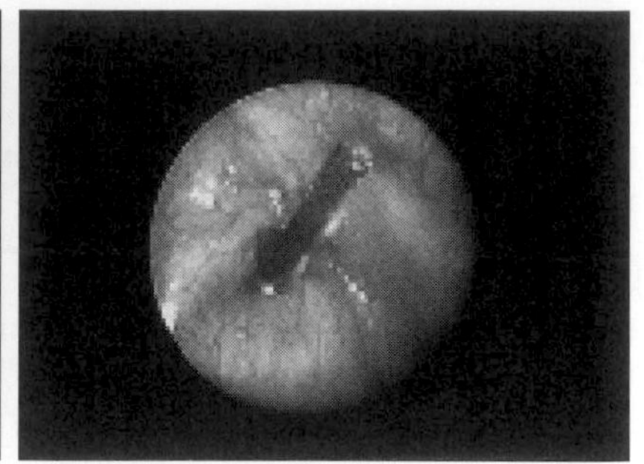

FIGURE 18–11 A, Insertion of the Lloyd cryoprobe through the abdominal wall and fascia onto the genitofemoral nerve. B, Ice-ball formation for cryodenervation of the genitofemoral nerve. C, Lloyd cryoprobe immediately after defrost. (Also in color; see Color Plates.)

Neuralgia due to irritation of the *infrapatellar branch of the saphenous nerve* develops weeks to years after blunt injury to the tibial plateau or after knee replacement. The nerve is vulnerable as it passes superficial to the tibial collateral ligament, piercing the sartorious tendon and fascia lata, and running inferior and medial to the tibial condyle. The clinical presentation consists of dull pain in the knee joint and achiness below the knee. Patients tend to adopt an antalgic gait. Pain with digital pressure is diagnostic. Patients are considered candidates for cryodenervation when they respond consistently to local anesthetic blocks. A 12-gauge intravenous catheter is used as the introducer, to prevent cold injury to the skin. Since prodding with the felt-tipped pen alone is sufficient to localize the pain generator, the sensory nerve stimulator does not have to be used.

Neuralgia due to irritation of the *deep and superficial peroneal and intermediate dorsal cutaneous nerves* can be seen weeks to years after injury to the foot and ankle. These superficial sensory nerves pass through strong ligamentous structures and are vulnerable to stretch injury with inversion of the ankle, compression injury due to edema, and penetrating trauma from bone fragments. The intermediate dorsal cutaneous nerve runs superficial and medial to the lateral malleolus and continues superficial to the inferior extensor retinaculum, terminating in the fourth and fifth toes. This nerve is particularly vulnerable to injury following sprains of the lateral ankle. The clinical presentation consists of dull ankle pain that is worse with passive inversion of the ankle. Disproportionate swelling, vasomotor instability, and allodynia are remarkably common. Patients tend to adjust their gait to minimize weight bearing on the lateral aspect of the foot. Pain with digital pressure in the area between the lateral malleolus and extensor retinaculum is diagnostic.

PERONEAL NERVE

Superficial and deep peroneal nerve injury often occurs in diabetics, who are vulnerable to compression injury from tight-fitting shoes and is less common after blunt injury to the dorsum of the foot. The clinical presentation consists of dull pain in the great toe that is often worse after prolonged standing. Again, patients tend to adjust their gait to minimize weight bearing on the anterior portion of the foot. Pain with digital pressure in the area between the first and second metatarsal heads is often diagnostic.

SUPERIOR GLUTEAL NERVE

Neuralgia due to irritation of the superior gluteal branch of the sciatic nerve is common after injury to the lower back and hip sustained while lifting. After exiting the sciatic notch, the superior gluteal nerve passes caudal to the inferior border of the gluteus minimus and penetrates the gluteus medius. Vulnerable as it passes in the fascial plane between the gluteus medius and gluteus minimus musculature, the superior gluteal nerve is injured as a result of shearing between the gluteal muscles on forced external rotation of the leg, and with extension of the hip under mechanical load. Rarely, it is injured by forced extension of the hip, an injury that might occur in a head-on automobile collision when the foot is pressed against the floorboards with the knee in extension as the patient braces for impact. The clinical presentation consists of sharp pain in the lower back, dull pain in the buttock, and vague pain to the popliteal fossa. Pain below the knee is unusual. Patients generally experience pain with prolonged sitting, leaning forward, or twisting to the contralateral side. Often, patients describe "giving way" of the leg. They usually sit with the weight on the contralateral buttock or cross their legs so as to minimize pressure on the involved side. With the patient in the prone position, the medial border of the ilium is palpated. The nerve is located 5 cm lateral and inferior to the attachment of the gluteus medius. The peripheral nerve stimulator is employed to ensure that motor units are not inadvertently blocked.

Craniofacial Pain

Craniofacial nerves can be cryolesioned with either percutaneous or open technique.[36] Entrapment neuropathies and neuromas are more responsive to local anesthetic and cryodenervations than are neuropathies of medical causes. Meticulous diagnostic injection ensures the best outcome with cryoablation.[15] If there is good analgesic response to a series of local anesthetic injections cryodenervation is an option. The technique of cryodenervations of cranial and facial nerves is the same as that for other peripheral nerves. A nerve stimulator is used to localize the nerve. Since these areas are relatively densely vascular, we suggest injecting a few milliliters of saline containing 1 : 100,000 epinephrine before inserting the cryoprobe introducer cannula. A postprocedural ice pack applied for 30 min reduces pain and swelling.

An irritative neuropathy of the *supraorbital nerve* (Fig. 18–12) often occurs at the supraorbital notch.[37] Vulnerable to blunt trauma, this nerve is often injured by deceleration against an automobile windshield. Commonly confused with migraine and frontal sinusitis, the pain of supraorbital neuralgia often manifests as a throbbing frontal headache. At times, many of the hallmarks of vascular headache are present, including blurred vision, nausea, and photophobia. This neuralgia often worsens over time, perhaps owing to scar formation around the nerve.

Neuropathic pain in the distribution of the supraorbital nerve can be addressed with an open or closed cryoablative procedure so long as appropriate conservative therapy has failed and the pain responds to a series of test local anesthetic injections. For an open procedure, the incision is buried beneath the eyebrow, so there is no obvious scar. For the percutaneous technique, the introducer catheter should be inserted at the eyebrow line to avoid damage to hair follicles.

The infraorbital nerve (see Fig. 18–12) is the termination of the second division of the trigeminal nerve. An irritative neuropathy can occur at the infraorbital foramen secondary to blunt trauma or fracture of the zygoma with entrapment of the nerve in the bony callus. Commonly confused with maxillary sinusitis, the pain of infraorbital neuralgia most often is exacerbated with smiling and laughing. Referred pain to teeth is common, and a history of dental pain and dental procedures is typical. Cryoablation can be accomplished via open or closed technique. The closed technique can be done from inside the mouth through the superior buccolabial fold. In both operations the probe is advanced until it lies over the infraorbital foramen. The intraoral approach has only cosmetic advantages.

The *mandibular nerve* can be irritated at many locations along its path. It is often injured as the result of hypertrophy of the pterygoids secondary to chronic bruxism, but it can also be irritated if the vertical dimension of the oral cavity is reduced owing to tooth loss or altered dentition. Pain is often referred to the lower teeth, and, again, patients frequently undergo dental evaluations and procedures.

Injury to the *mental nerve*, the terminal portion of the mandibular nerve, frequently occurs in edentulous patients. Pain can easily be reproduced with palpation.

The *auriculotemporal nerve* can be irritated at a number of sites, including immediately proximal to the parietal ridge at the attachment of the temporalis muscle, and, less commonly, at the ramus of the mandible. Patients often present with temporal pain associated with retroorbital pain. Pain is often referred to the teeth. Patients frequently awake at night with temporal headache. The pain, described as throbbing, aching, and pounding, can be bilateral, and it is commonly associated with bruxism and functional abnormalities of the temporomandibular joint, maxilla, and mandible. The clinician must rule out other medical causes for this form of headache, including temporal arteritis, before considering treatments for auriculo-

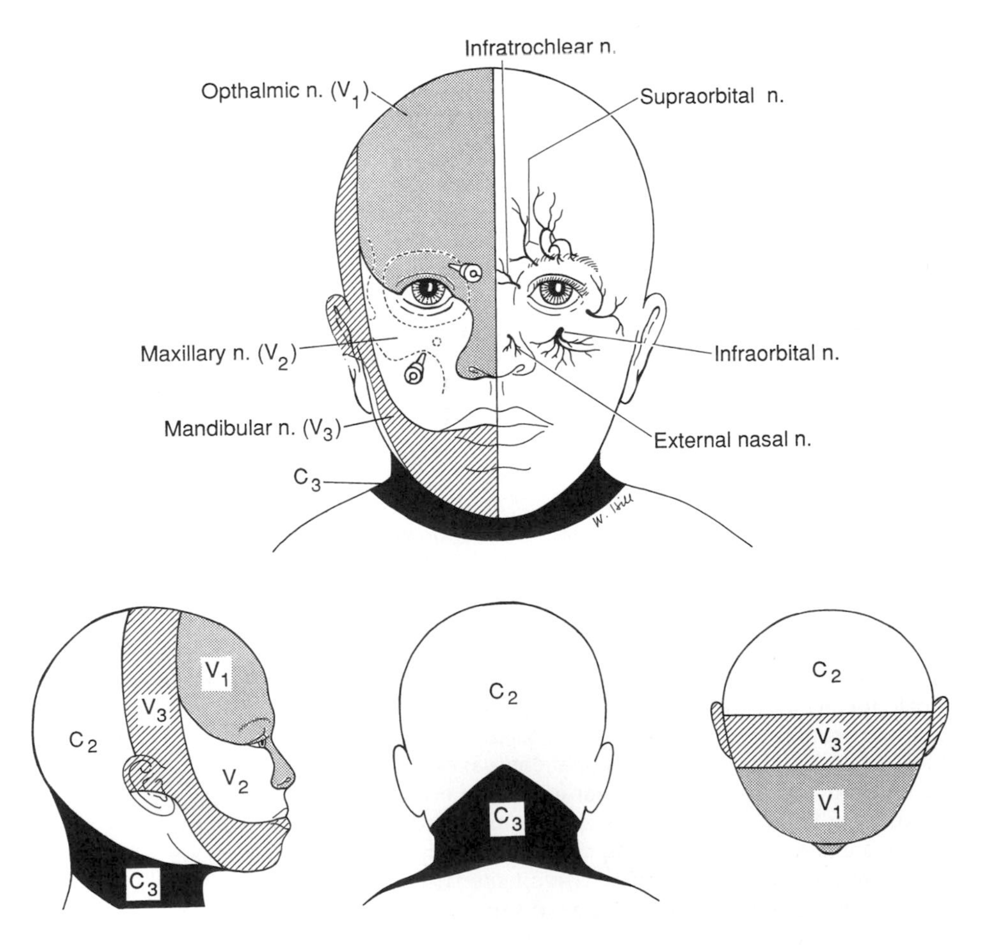

FIGURE 18–12 *Dermatome man showing commonly blocked cutaneous branches of the trigeminal nerve.*

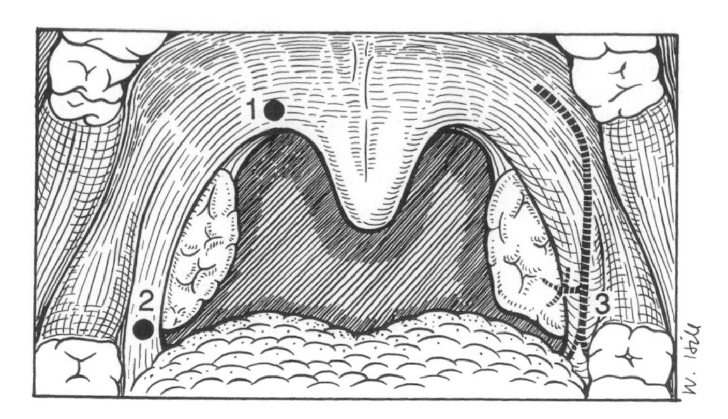

FIGURE 18–13 *The distal glossopharyngeal nerve subajcent to the tonsillar fossa. 1, 2, Locations for local anesthetic and cryodenervation. 3, The pathway of the glossopharyngeal nerve is quite superficial at this site. Care must be taken to avoid entering the artery.*

temporal neuralgia. Posterior auricular neuralgia often follows blunt injury to the mastoid area. It is common in abused women and usually involves the left side owing to the preponderance of right-handed abusers. The clinical presentation consists of pain in the ear associated with a feeling of "fullness" and tenderness. This syndrome is often misdiagnosed as a chronic ear infection. The posterior auricular nerve runs along the posterior border of the sternocleidomastoid muscle, superficially and immediately posterior to the mastoid.

The *glossopharyngeal nerve* lies immediately subjacent to the tonsillar fossa (Fig. 18–13). This painful condition can be treated by applying the cryoprobe for two cycles of 2 min each after local anesthetic injections have produced the appropriate responses. This is essentially a simple procedure, but it has distinct advantages over injection of this cranial nerve at the tip of the mastoid, where injection could block the vagus in addition to the spinal accessory nerves.[36]

Many other common peripheral nerve injuries are amenable to cryodenervation, including most cutaneous branches and the occipital, suprascapular, superficial radial, and anterior penetrating branches of the intercostal nerves. Applied carefully, the techniques outlined in this chapter will help to achieve a safe outcome and the best possible one.

CASE REPORT[38]

A 58-year-old woman sustained a traumatic spondylolisthesis at the L4–L5 level for which a spinal fusion was performed. Autogenous bone graft for the vertebral fusion was obtained from the left posterior iliac crest. Postoperatively, the patient continued to experience wrenching and searing pain at the iliac crest donor site (pain score 7 on the 10-point Verbal Analogue Scale [VAS]). Treatment with NSAID for 3 weeks and transcutaneous nerve stimulation for 2 weeks did not alleviate the pain (VAS = 5). The patient was then referred to the center for pain medicine for additional evaluation and treatment. The initial clinical assessment indicated the primary painful locus (7.5 cm by 5 cm) to be within the defect of the posterior iliac bone harvest site. The patient's symptoms—a constant, wrenching, and searing pain with radiation into the calf—were aggravated by walking and assuming the standing or sitting position and were partially relieved with rest. A diagnosis of postoperative iliac crest pain syndrome (a new name for this symptom complex) was made. Inflammation and a posttraumatic neuroexcitatory state induced by the surgical trauma were posited to be responsible for the pain. For these reasons, the iliac crest donor site was infiltrated with a series of local anesthetic injections (10 mL of 0.5% bupivacaine), NSAID (60 mg of ketorolac), and steroid (20 mg of triamcinolone) at 2- to 3-week intervals. The first four injections contained 10 mL of 0.5% bupivacaine and 60 mg of ketorolac. The first injection relieved the patient's pain completely (VAS = 0). The pain gradually returned to pretreatment levels (VAS = 7) during the next 2 weeks, with the notable difference that the locus of pain was reduced in size (5 cm by 2.5 cm). The pain locus corresponded to the center of the graft donor site. The three subsequent injections of bupivacaine and ketorolac had minimal effect on pain scores or size of the painful locus. For the fifth injection, therefore, 10 mL of 0.5% bupivacaine was mixed with 20 mg of triamcinolone. The response to this injection was dramatic: further shrinking of the painful locus (3 cm by 2 cm) and diminution in pain scores (VAS = 1). A sixth (and final) injection at week 12 produced further diminution of the painful locus to two discrete (1 cm by 1 cm) foci. The patient nevertheless described this pain as sharp and excruciating (VAS = 7). The relatively smaller size of the painful loci prompted selection of cryodenervation as a second step of treatment. A cryoprobe that produced 0.5-cm ice balls at thermal equilibrium was selected. A grid was then visualized over the area, and seven cryodenervations were performed, each of 3 minutes' duration. The patient experienced postprocedure discomfort, but it disappeared over the first week (VAS = 0; see Table 18–1), and the patient resumed all previous preoperative activities after 1 month. One year after the

TABLE 18–1 **Overview of Patient History**

Treatment Category	VAS* Reduction† (%)	Reduction in Area of Painful Locus‡,§ (%)
Pretreatment (Postoperative)	7 (N/A)	7.5 × 5 (N/A)
Symptomatic Treatment (NSAID and TENS)	5 (28.6)	7.5 × 5 (0)
Injection Therapy: Bupivacaine and Ketorolac		
• First Injection	0 (100)	0 (100)
• Second Injection	5 (28.6)	5 × 3 (60)
• Third Injection	4 (42.9)	5 × 2 (73.3)
• Fourth Injection	5 (28.6)	4.5 × 3 (64)
Bupivacaine and Triamcinolone		
• Fifth Injection	1 (85.7)	3 × 2 (84)
• Sixth Injection	6 (14.3)	1 × 1 & 1 × 1 (94.7)
Cryodenervation	1 (100)	0 (100)

* Verbal analogue pain scores.
† Reduction is expressed as % of baseline values at pretreatment (postoperative) stage.
‡ Measured by same physician using same amount of pressure for deep palpation, and recorded in centimeters.
§ One week after cryodenervation.

procedure, the patient continues to have complete mobility and activity.

DISCUSSION

The harvesting of bone has frequently been used in orthopedic surgery since 1901, when Von Eiselberg first reported autogenous cancellous bone transplantation.[39, 40] The sites frequently used to harvest donor bone include the iliac crests, ribs, and calvarium.[41–45] There is no consensus about one preferred site.[42–46] The posterior iliac crest is used for bone harvesting in a number of orthopedic and reconstructive procedures owing to its suitability as a donor site.[41, 46] The complications associated with bone graft harvesting from the posterior iliac crest include chronic pain, altered sensation at the harvest site, superior gluteal arteriovenous fistula, ureteral injury, sacroiliac joint dislocation, osteomyelitis, gluteal weakness, lumbar hernia, and injury to the sciatic and gluteal nerves.[47–52] Chronic pain is by far the most common postharvest complication (reported incidence 25%–38%).[47, 49, 52] The persistence of iliac crest donor site pain is thought to be a complication of total or partial injury to the cutaneous continuations of the lateral branches of the dorsal rami of L1–L3, collectively called the *superior cluneal nerves*.[48, 53] Modifying the surgical technique to avoid this complication has not significantly altered the incidence and characteristics of donor site pain.[47, 54–57] Findings of a few studies suggest the benefit of perioperative infiltration of the donor site with a local anesthetic (bupivacaine).[58–60] Others suggest giving bupivacaine via an indwelling epidural catheter for postharvest pain.[61, 62] Perioperative infiltration of the donor site with a local anesthetic may alleviate the acute pain, but, considering the incidence of chronic pain at donor site (25%–38%),[47, 49, 52] some 62% to 75% of patients will get local donor site anesthetic infiltration or intraoperative catheter treatment without any long-term benefit. Furthermore, it will increase direct and indirect hospital costs because of the additional procedure, longer hospital stay, and increased risk of complications.

The pathophysiologic mechanisms of persistent pain at the donor site are likely to be multiple and may involve various biochemical pathways. Injury, regeneration, and remodeling of cancellous bone are thought to be associated with marked increases in osteoclastic activity that is affected by prostaglandins (PG) via many different pathways.[63, 64] Harvey and coworkers used a dental model to show significant concentrations of PG in alveolar bone cysts.[65] Inflammatory cells, macrophages, lymphocytes, and monocytes initiate degradation of connective tissue,[66] presumably through increased PGE_2 production. Unfortunately, the plasma level of PG is of little clinical use, since there is 95% clearance by the pulmonary vascular bed within 3 to 6 sec.[67–69] Shindell and coworkers demonstrated that injections of steroid into bone cysts reduced PGE_2 concentrations by 52% to 93%.[70] The reduction in PGE_2 concentration has been proposed as one of the biochemical mechanisms responsible for the effectiveness of intralesional steroid therapy.[70] Also, ketorolac, a direct inhibitor of cyclooxygenase, decreases prostaglandin biosynthesis and likely raises neural threshold. PG, in addition to causing bone destruction, increase the sensitivity of peripheral nociceptors to pain mediators, including bradykinin.[71] The local anesthetic may affect the outcome by attenuating afferent input[72] and thus diminishing the plasticity of the central nervous system.

The reduction in the size of the patient's pain locus to only two discrete points most likely resulted from attenuation of afferent sensory input. This decrease in size of the painful locus made it possible to consider cryodenervation of the underlying periosteum. Cryodenervation has been used successfully for both postoperative and chronic pain relief. Unfortunately, few long-term outcome studies on the effectiveness of cryodenervation are available. A 10-year audit of cryodenervation for trigeminal neuralgia indicated a 6 months' median duration of relief, and comparable pain-free intervals after repeated cryodenervations.[73] Cryoanalgesia relieves pain by producing long-lasting neurolysis combined with axonal regeneration. Freezing of nerve results in axonal disintegration and degeneration of the myelin sheaths. The perineurium and epineurium are preserved, however, and regrowth of axons takes place in the original supporting structures at the rate of 1 to 3 mm/day.[74] This obviates growth of painful neuromas, a problem associated with other neurolytic and surgical techniques, but also limits the duration of effective analgesia.[73, 75, 76] At present, there is no conclusive physiologic explanation for the sometimes prolonged analgesic effect, since regeneration of axons appears to be completed in a matter of weeks after the procedure.[74, 77] It is possible that cryoanalgesia affects the plasticity of the CNS and diminishes pain overall. The complications associated with cryotherapy are relatively minor but include cold injury, skin discoloration, and numbness in the distribution of the treated peripheral nerve. An important limitation is that it can be applied only to sensory nerves, because ablation of mixed nerves would produce temporary paralysis of the corresponding muscles. Improvement can be attributed to additive analgesic effects of ketorolac, steroid, local anesthetic, and cryotherapy on several different nociceptive pathways. This combination may produce a balanced analgesia that is likely to be more effective and to have fewer side effects than any other approach. This two-step therapeutic approach may prove to be the treatment of choice for prolonged relief of chronic iliac crest harvest pain.

FUTURE DIRECTIONS

Cryotechnology offers promise for a wide variety of pain management needs. Its unparalleled track record for safety is remarkable. Its effective and safe use on sensory and mixed nerves contrasts with radiofrequency technology, which has the potential to produce deafferentation when applied to peripheral nerves. The lack of controlled studies, lack of uniform training, and poor communication between providers has impeded widespread use of the technology. To better address these issues, WESTCO Medical Corporation of San Diego, California, a major supplier of cryotechnology, has set up a cryotechnology users club whose primary objective is exchange of information and development of studies.

REFERENCES

1. Evans P: Cryo-analgesia: The application of low temperatures to nerves to produce anesthesia or analgesia. Anaesthesia 36:1003–1013, 1981.
2. Hippocrates: Aphorisms. vol 4, Heracleitus on the Universe. London, Heinemann, 1931; 5:165; 7:201.
3. Gruner O: A Treatise on the Canon of Medicine of Avicenna. London, Luzac, 1930.
4. Bartholini T: De Nivis usu Medico Observationes Variae, Hafniae. Copenhagen, P. Haubold, 1661.
5. Larre D: Surgical Memoirs of the Campaigns of Russia, Germany and France. Philadelphia, Carey & Lea, 1832.
6. Arnott J: On severe cold or congelation as a remedy of disease. London, Medical Gazette, 1848, pp 936–938.
7. Holden HB: Practical Cryosurgery. London, Pitman, 1975, pp 2–3.
8. Cooper IS: Cryosurgery in modern medicine. J Neurol Sci, 2:493, 1965.
9. Amoils SP: The Joule-Thomson cryoprobe. Arch Ophthalmol 78:201–207, 1978.
10. Evans P, Lloyd J, Green C: Cryo-analgesia: The response to alterations in freeze cycle temperature. Br J Anaesth 53:1121, 1981.
11. Holden HB: Practical Cryosurgery. London, Pitman, 1975, p 9.
12. Gander MJ, Soanes WA, Smith V: Experimental prostate surgery. Invest Urol 1:610, 1964.
13. Soanes WA, Ablin RJ, Gander MJ: Remission of metastatic lesions following cryosurgery in prostatic cancer: Immunologic considerations. J Urol 104:154, 1970.
14. Lloyd J, Barnard J, Glynn C: Cryo-analgesia: A new approach to pain relief. Lancet 2:932–934, 1976.
15. Barnard J, Lloyd J, Glynn C: Cryosurgery in the management of intractable facial pain. Br J Oral Surg 16:135, 1978.
16. Peuria M, Krmpotic-Nemanic J, Markiewitz A: Tunnel Syndromes. Boca Raton, Fla, CRC Press, 1991.
17. Wall PD: The prevention of postoperative pain. Pain 33:289–290, 1988.
18. Armitage EN: Postoperative pain—prevention or relief? Br J Anaesth 63:136–137, 1989.
19. Cousins MJ: Acute pain and injury response, immediate and prolonged effects, Reg Anesth 14:162–179, 1989.
20. McQuay HJ, Carroll D, Moore RA: Postoperative orthopedic pain—the effect of opiate premedication and local anesthetic blocks. Pain 33:291–296, 1988.
21. Woolf CJ, Wall PD: Morphine sensitive and insensitive actions of C-fibre input on the rat spinal cords. Neurosci Lett 64:221–225, 1986.
22. Glynn C, Lloyd J, Barnard J: Cryo-analgesia in the management of pain after thoracotomy, Thorax 35:325–327, 1980.
23. Katz J, Nelson W, Forest R, Bruce D: Cryo-analgesia for postthoracotomy pain. Lancet i:512–513, 1980.
24. Orr I, Keenan D, Dundee J: Improved pain relief after thoracotomy: Use of cryoprobe and morphine infusion. Br Med J 283:88–90, 1981.
25. Wood G, Lloyd J, Bullingham R, et al: Postoperative analgesia for day case herniorrhaphy patients. A comparison of cryo-analgesia, paravertebral blockade and oral analgesia. Anesthesia Volume 36:603–610, 1981.
26. Gough JD, Williams AB, Vaughan RS: The control of post-thoracotomy pain: A comparative evaluation of thoracic epidural fentanyl infusions and cryo-analgesia, Anesthesia 43:780–783, 1988.
27. Nelson K, Vincent R, Bourke R: Interoperative intercostal nerve freezing to prevent postthoracotomy pain. Ann Thorac Surg 18(3):280–285, 1974.
28. Maiwand O, Makey AR: Cryo-analgesia for relief of pain after thoracotomy. B Med J 282:49–50, 1981.
29. Conacher ID, Locke T, Hilton ML: Neuralgia after cryo-analgesia for thoracotomy. Lancet 1:277, 1986.
30. Wood G, Lloyd J, Evans P, et al: Cryo-analgesia and day case herniorrhaphy (Letter). Lancet ii:479, 1979.
31. Brechner T: Percutaneous cryogenic neurolysis of the articular nerve of Lushka. Regl Anesthesiol 6:18–22, 1981.
32. Trescott A: Workshop for Cryotherapy. 6th International Congress on Pain, Atlanta, Ga, April 20, 1994.
33. Sluijter ME: Radiofrequency lesions of the communicating ramus in the treatment of low back pain. *In* Racz G (ed): Techniques of Neurolysis. Boston, Kluwer, 1989.
34. Raj P: Practical Management of Pain. Chicago, Year Book, 1986, p 779.
35. Saberski L, Rosser J: Laparoscopic concious pain mapping. (Submitted for publication, 2000).
36. Raj P: Practical Management of Pain. Chicago, Year Book, 1986, p 777.
37. Klein DS, Schmidt RE: Chronic headache resulting from postoperative supraorbital neuralgia. Anesth Analg 73:490–491, 1991.
38. Saberski LR, Ahmad M, Munir A, Brull S: Management of iliac crest bone harvest site pain. (Submitted for publication, 2000).
39. Witsenburg B: The reconstruction of anterior residual bone defects in patients with cleft lip, alveolus and palate. A review. J Maxillofac Surg 13:197–208, 1985.
40. Canady JW, Zeitler DP, Thompson SA, Nicholas CD: Suitability of the iliac crest as a site for harvest of autogenous bone grafts. Cleft Palate-Craniofac 30:579–581, 1993.
41. Citardi MJ, Friedman CD: Nonvascularized autogenous bone grafts for craniofacial skeletal augmentation and replacement. Otolaryngol Clin North Am 27:891–910, 1994.
42. Laurie SW, Kaban LB, Mulliken JB, Murray JE: Donor-site morbidity after harvesting rib and iliac bone. Plast Reconstr Surg 73:933–938, 1984.
43. Raulo Y, Baruch J: Utilisation de la voute cranienne comme site de greffes osseuses en chirurgie cranio-maxillo-faciale. Chirurgie 116:359–362, 1990.
44. Motoki DS, Mulliken JB: The healing of bone and cartilage. Clin Plast Surg 17:527–544, 1990.
45. Gerbino G, Berrone S, De Gioanni PP, Appendino P: Valutazione clinica degli esiti di prelievo osseo da cresta iliaca. Minerva Stomatol 41:57–61, 1992.
46. Fernyhough JC, Schimandle JJ, Weigel MC, et al: Chronic donor site pain complicating bone graft harvesting from the posterior iliac crest for spinal fusion. Spine 17:1474–1480, 1992.
47. Kurz LT, Garfin SR, Booth RE Jr: Harvesting autogenous iliac bone grafts. A review of complications and techniques. Spine 14:1324–1331, 1989.
48. Goulet JA, Senunas LE, DeSilva GL, Greenfield ML: Autogenous iliac crest bone graft. Complications and functional assessment. Clin Orthop 83:76–81, 1997.
49. Arrington ED, Smith WJ, Chambers HG, et al: Complications of iliac crest bone graft harvesting. Clin Orthop 82:300–309, 1996.
50. Younger EM, Chapman MW: Morbidity at bone graft donor sites. J Orthop Trauma 3:192–195, 1989.
51. Summers BN, Eisenstein SM: Donor site pain from the ilium. A complication of lumbar spine fusion. J Bone Joint Surg 71B:677–680, 1989.
52. Kurz LT, Garfin SR, Booth RE: Iliac bone grafting: Techniques and complications of harvesting. *In* (ed): Complications of Spine Surgery, Baltimore, Williams & Wilkins, 1989, pp 323–334.
53. Tanishima T, Yoshimasu N, Ogai M: A technique for prevention of donor site pain associated with harvesting iliac bone grafts. Surg Neurol 44:131–132, 1995.
54. Schnee CL, Freese A, Weil RJ, Marcotte PJ: Analysis of harvest morbidity and radiographic outcome using autograft for anterior cervical fusion. Spine 22:2222–2227, 1997.
55. Fernandes HM, Mendelow AD, Choksey MS: Anterior cervical discectomy: An improvement in donor site operative technique. Br J Neurosurg 8:201–203, 1994.
56. David DJ, Tan E, Katsaros J, Sheen R: Mandibular reconstruction with vascularized iliac crest: A 10-year experience. Plast Reconstr Surg 82:792–803, 1988.
57. Brull SJ, Lieponis JV, Murphy MJ, et al: Acute and long-term benefits of iliac crest donor site perfusion with local anesthetics. Anesth Analg 74:145–147, 1992.
58. Hahn M, Dover MS, Whear NM, Moule I: Local bupivacaine infusion following bone graft harvest from the iliac crest. Int J Oral Maxillofac Surg 25:400–401, 1996.
59. Wilkes RA, Thomas WG: Bupivacaine infusion for iliac crest donor sites. J Bone Joint Surg 76B:503, 1994.

60. Dunstan SP, Korczak PK: Use of epidural catheter for postoperative pain relief for bone harvesting from iliac crest. Br J Oral Maxillofac Surg 34:436–437, 1996.
61. Kennedy BD, Hiranaka DK: Use of a modified epidural catheter for analgesia after iliac crest bone procurement. J Oral Maxillofac Surg 53:342–343, 1995.
62. Dietrich JW, Goodson JM, Raisz LG: Stimulation of bone resorption by various prostaglandins in organ culture. Prostaglandins 10:231–240, 1975.
63. Vaes G: Cell-to-cell interactions in the secretion of enzymes of connective tissue breakdown, collagenase and proteoglycan-degrading neutral proteases. A review. Agents Actions 10:474–485, 1980.
64. Harvey W, Guat-Chen F, Gordon D, et al: Evidence for fibroblasts as the major source of prostacyclin and prostaglandin synthesis in dental cysts in man. Arch Oral Biol 29:223–229, 1984.
65. Vaes G, Huybrechts-Godin G, Hauser P: Lymphocyte-macrophage-fibroblast co-operation in the inflammatory degradation of cartilage and connective tissue. Agents Actions Suppl 7:100–108, 1980.
66. Clyman RI, Mauray F, Heymann MA, Roman C: Effect of gestational age on pulmonary metabolism of prostaglandin E1 & E2. Prostaglandins 21:505–513, 1981.
67. Weiss M, Forster W: Pharmacokinetics of prostaglandins: prediction of steady-state concentrations during intravenous infusion. Int J Clin Pharmacol Ther Toxicol 18:344–347, 1980.
68. Vane JR: The release and fate of vaso-active hormones in the circulation. Br J Pharmacol 35:209–242, 1969.
69. Shindell R, Huurman WW, Lippiello L, Connolly JF: Prostaglandin levels in unicameral bone cysts treated by intralesional steroid injection. J Pediatr Orthop 9:516–519, 1989.
70. Buckley MM, Brogden RN: Ketorolac. A review of its pharmacodynamic and pharmacokinetic properties, and therapeutic potential. Drugs 39:86–109, 1990.
71. Young ER, MacKenzie TA: The pharmacology of local anesthetics—a review of the literature. J Can Dent Assoc 58:34–42, 1992.
72. Zakrzewska JM: Cryotherapy for trigeminal neuralgia: A 10-year audit. Br J Oral Maxillofac Surg 29:1–4, 1991.
73. Evans PJ: Cryo-analgesia. The application of low temperatures to nerves to produce anaesthesia or analgesia. Anaesthesia 36:1003–1013, 1981.
74. Lloyd JW, Barnard JD, Glynn CJ: Cryo-analgesia. A new approach to pain relief. Lancet 2:932–934, 1976.
75. Barnard D, Lloyd J, Evans J: Cryo-analgesia in the management of chronic facial pain. J Maxillofac Surg 9:101–102, 1981.
76. Saberski L: Cryo-neurolysis in clinical practice. *In* Waldman S, Winnie A (eds): The Textbook of Interventional Pain Management. Philadelphia, WB Saunders, 1994.

CHAPTER • 19

Radiofrequency Techniques in Clinical Practice

Matthew T. Kline, MD • Way Yin, MD

RADIOFREQUENCY LESION GENERATION IN THE NERVOUS SYSTEM

The application of radiofrequency (RF) lesions generated in the nervous system for a variety of therapeutic purposes has had excellent success. In comparison to other selective lesioning techniques, modern RF methods afford several clinical and practical advantages.

METHODS OF CREATING NERVOUS SYSTEM LESIONS

Historically, numerous techniques have been used to selectively destroy nerve tissue in the brain and elsewhere in the body; the most important of these techniques include cryogenic surgery, focused ultrasound, chemical destruction, ionizing radiation, mechanical methods, lasers, radiofrequency heating method, and direct current heating method. A brief critique of these methods is given here, with a view of their relative merits as compared with the RF heating method. The RF and direct current (DC) heating methods involve the passage of current from an electrode placed in the target zone through the surrounding tissue, thus heating and destroying the tissue in the vicinity of the electrode.

Cryogenic Surgery

Cryogenic surgery has typically involved inserting a probe into the brain or other body tissue and cooling the tip of the probe to extremely low temperatures to freeze a region of tissue around the tip. Technically, this has been accomplished with ingenious cryogenic devices, usually cannulas with internal channels to circulate very cold liquids such as liquid nitrogen, or rapid expansion of gas, creating extremely low temperatures at the probe tip, but not along its shaft. The cryogenic surgery technique has been applied extensively for intracranial stereotaxy in the past decades, but its use has declined in recent years. Cryofreezing techniques using similar modern instrumentation have become popular for freezing tumors elsewhere in the body, as in the liver and prostate.[1, 2] Several difficulties in using the cryogenic technique in the brain—and, for that matter, elsewhere in the body—have become apparent. Cryogenic probes usually have diameters of 3 mm or larger, a size that tends to be unacceptable for many procedures in the brain and the peripheral nervous system. There is also the potential for the frozen tissue to stick to the tip of the probe as it is being withdrawn from the brain or other tissue if defreezing is not done carefully and completely. Cryogenic probes, which have had a prominent place in neurosurgery, are not easily adapted to percutaneous procedures owing to their intrinsic construction.

Focused Ultrasound

Focused ultrasound has the advantage of making a trackless lesion and, thus, has the potential to be totally noninvasive. Ultrasound was used in the 1950s for neurosurgical functional lesions made in the brain. Significant mechanical disadvantages of ultrasound technique include (1) the scatter of ultrasound from surrounding bony structures, making it difficult to fully control; (2) the necessity, for achieving trackless lesions in the brain, of making a large craniotomy so as to properly couple the ultrasonic transducer to the brain tissue; and (3) the inability to quantify the temperature distribution at the ultrasonic focal site, leaving the technique without adequate monitoring.

Our thanks to William Rittman III and Eric Cosman, PhD, for technical and historical data provided.

Our thanks to Wolfram Klawitter from Ziehm International for his technical support and assistance in the capture and reproduction of the fluoroscopic images contained herein.

Our thanks to Don Garlotta and Beverly Sanchez for their technical assistance in the operating rooms in the capture and reproduction of the fluoroscopic images contained herein.

Our thanks to Barbara Urmston for her support and preparation of this manuscript.

Induction Heating

Induction heating, using either implanted pellets of metal or highly intense electromagnetic fields, suffers from the lack of knowledge about the thermal distribution near the lesion site and from the inability to reproducibly and quantitatively control lesion size. Induction heating, like ultrasound, seems to have more applicability in hyperthermia therapy, in which more diffuse, nonlethal thermal elevations of tissue temperature are the desired objective.

Chemical Destruction

Chemical destruction, as by injection of alcohol, phenol, or glycerol, has often been used primarily for peripheral nerve denervation. Spirited controversy compares the merits of chemical injection techniques and the RF heating method. The obvious advantage of chemical injection is its simplicity, an attribute illustrated by the widespread use of nerve blocks and of glycerol injections in the treatment of trigeminal neuralgia. The most obvious and commonly reported disadvantage is that the spread of the injected material in the target tissue region is impossible to control, leading to lesions that are irregular and variable in size and shape and inconsistent in therapeutic effects.

Ionizing Radiation

The use of ionizing radiation, internally implanted and external beam arrays, has played a major role in the treatment of tumors. This modality has also been used for destruction of smaller functional targets. External-beam radiation has the advantage of being noninvasive.

Brachytherapy

Brachytherapy—the implantation of radioactive seeds, such as iodine 125 (^{125}I) or iridium 192 (^{192}Ir)—is widely practiced in neurosurgery.[3–11] Furthermore, focal external beam irradiation employing radioactive sources such as cobalt 60 (^{60}Co) and linear accelerators (LINAC) in techniques called *stereotactic radiosurgery* and *stereotactic radiotherapy* respectively, has become very popular. Radiosurgery using linear accelerators is able to ablate targets as small as a few millimeters in diameter with precision that is submillimeter. Sophisticated computer graphic workstations and three-dimensional treatment planning systems enable highly controlled planning so that the external photon beams will avoid critical structures.[12–14] It is possible, therefore, to make very small therapeutic lesions noninvasively by stereotactic radiosurgery methods. Time fractionation may further augment effectiveness and safety. The difficulties with these methods, as compared with the RF technique, are that they do not afford interactive target identification by means of stimulation and other methods and that the extent of circumscription of the radiation, and the uncertainty about radiation to normal surrounding tissues, may be problematic.

Mechanical Methods

Mechanical methods for making lesions in the nervous system, including the use of the lucotome and other tools, have been effective in some settings. It is clear that very small lesions can be made in this way. The dangers of these techniques are primarily hemorrhage and the lack of quantitative controls. Focused electromagnetic radiation with large, external arrays of microwaves has not been widely used to date. This technology has potential but suffers from the same disadvantages as induction heating and focused ultrasound, namely, the inability to monitor the temperature distribution as the lesions are being made without the direct implantation of temperature sensors.

Lasers

Lasers have been used to make lesions in the brain, spinal cord, and elsewhere in the body. Although much work has been done comparing laser and RF heating methods, it is difficult to quantify the extent and rapidity of tissue destruction using the laser, because it is not amenable to adequate temperature monitoring and produces varying effects, depending on tissue parameters such as blood flow and thermoconductivity. Laser light of different wavelengths and differing photon delivery systems may also significantly affect the size and controlability of a laser-generated lesion. Thus, the use of lasers for making therapeutic lesions, for example, in the dorsal root entry zone (DREZ) lesion procedure, has come under some criticism in comparison with the RF technique, because of the lack of quantification and consistency and the production of defects.[15]

BRAIN LESIONING WITH ELECTRIC CURRENT

The Direct Current Electrolytic Lesion

Many 19th-century workers experimented with making lesions in neural tissue using direct current (DC). Because the brain is composed largely of electrolytes, it was natural to place electrodes in it and to see what happens when current is passed between them. In this way, Beaunis (1868), Fournie (1873), and others made the first electrolytic brain lesions in animals using bipolar DC electrodes. Golsinger (1895) did the same with monopolar brain electrodes. Horsley and Clarke (1905), who carefully studied the quality of lesions as a function of electrode polarity and material, concluded that the anodal (positive electrode) lesion was superior because it generated less gas. They put forward empirical rules for "incrementing" anodal lesion size on the basis of current and time parameters. The first stereotactic DC brain lesions were described in 1947.

DC lesions can be variable in size, up to a factor of 4 to 1 for a fixed electrode geometry, lesion current, and lesion time.[16] The reason for the erratic nature of DC lesions is that they depend strongly on electrolysis, with its inherent polarization and gas formation, and on the specific anatomy of tissue planes and vascular interruptions. These factors make DC electrolytic lesions both ragged at the circumference and variable in size and thus unacceptable for accurate lesion making.

The Radiofrequency Electrolytic Lesion

The first practical and commercially available RF lesion generators were built in the early 1950s using continuous-wave RF in the 1-MHz range. The brain lesions made with these machines using the controls of current and power level had smooth borders, an immediate improvement over DC lesions.[17, 18]

Advantages of the Radiofrequency Heating Method

RF lesion technology has certain advantages over other techniques for making discrete therapeutic or functional lesions in the brain and elsewhere in the body. With the advent of temperature control, *quantifiable lesions* could be made consistently from one patient to another, with the added safety factor of *avoiding unwanted and uncontrolled side effects*, such as sticking, charring, and formation of explosive gas. The concept of *differential selection of pain fibers* (versus other neural fibers) has been suggested, and there is some indication from a clinical experience that it is achievable using the RF method. Because of the very nature of the RF electrode, it is directly amenable to *stimulation, impedance monitoring,* and *recording,* all of which greatly enhance the surgeon's ability to know that the electrode is at the appropriate target for making the lesion. Because the RF lesion electrode is, in fact, an electrical connection, it automatically provides these secondary target benefits. RF electrodes adapt to stereotactic technique and to other fixation devices because of their *convenient, cylindrical, narrow* geometry. They can be made in a variety of elaborate shapes with extremely small tips ranging as small as 0.25 mm, or with side-issue tips for searching space near the target volume for the appropriate target point. The electrodes can be made very robust and in a nearly endless variation of shapes and configurations. This is another of the decisive advantages that are available with the RF lesioning technique. Perhaps, overall, the most telling attributes of the RF lesion method are that it has been safe, effective, and simple to use.

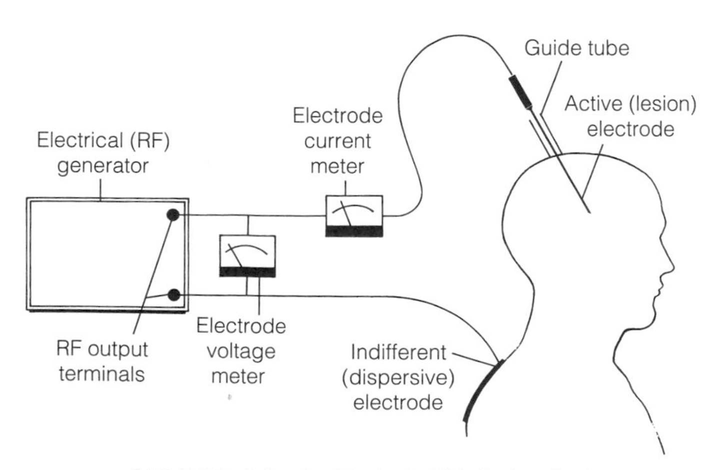

FIGURE 19–1 The basic RF lesioning circuit.

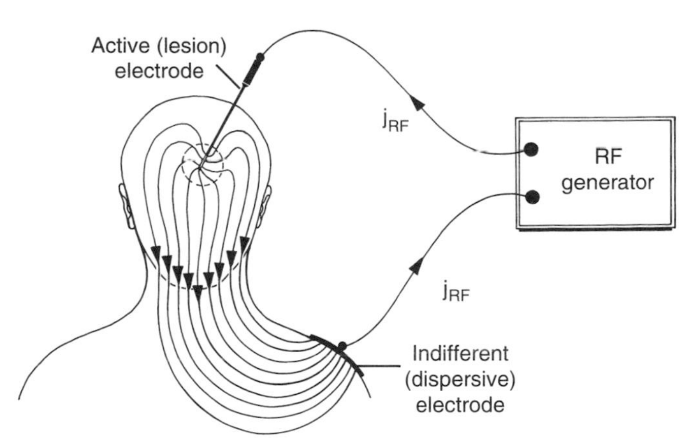

FIGURE 19–2 The spread of the RF current density (j_{RF}) in the tissue between the active and dispersive electrodes.

PHYSICAL PRINCIPLES OF LESION GENERATION

Basic Concepts of Heat Lesioning and Monitoring

The basic RF lesioning circuit is shown schematically in Figure 19–1. The RF generator is the source of RF voltage across its output terminals. When it is connected to electrodes placed on the body, current flows between them through the tissue. Thus, the body becomes an element of the complete electric circuit. The *active* electrode is positioned where the heat lesion is to be made, and the *dispersive* or *indifferent* electrode is a larger-area electrode that usually is not intended to produce tissue heating. The path of the electric current lines in the body between the active and dispersive electrodes is illustrated in Figure 19–2.

Field patterns near a straight-tipped active electrode are shown in Figure 19–3. The mechanism for tissue heating in the 1-MHz range is primarily ionic, rather than dielectric, and is qualitatively simple to understand. The RF voltage on the tip sets up electric field lines in space around

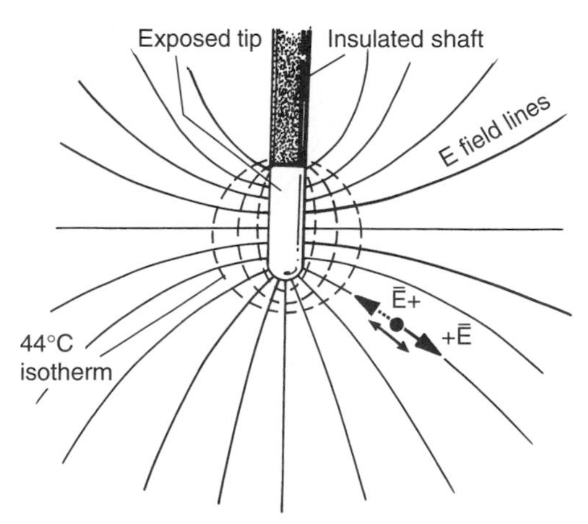

*FIGURE 19–3 A typical electric field line pattern (*solid lines*) around the exposed tip of an RF lesion electrode in a uniform medium, with typical isotherms (*dashed lines*). The 44° C isotherm is at the outer limits of the permanent lesion zone.*

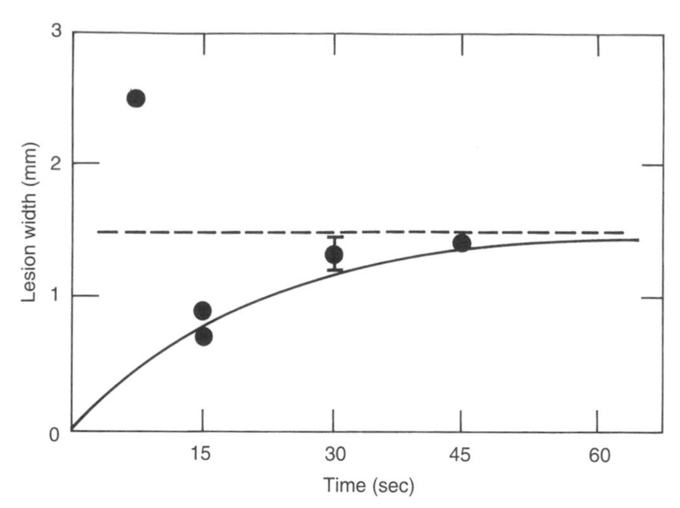

FIGURE 19–4 A plot of DREZ lesion width over time. In this experiment, the temperature was 75° C.

the exposed electrode tip according to the basic laws of electrostatics. The heat is generated in the tissue, not in the electrode tip. Because the tip is lying in the heated tissue, the tip absorbs heat from the tissue. If the electrode is designed properly, it will not absorb much heat at equilibrium, and thus the tip temperature is approximately equal to that of the hottest tissue adjacent to it. Because temperature is the fundamental lesion parameter, it must be measured; and monitoring tip temperature makes it possible to control the lesion's size. For consistent prediction of lesion size, the correct electrode tip size and lesion temperature at the tip must be selected.

Consistency of lesion size also depends on eliminating the time dependence of the lesion's size. This is easily done by letting the lesion come to thermal equilibrium. Lesion size in relation to time for a given tip temperature or RF current is illustrated in Figure 19–4, based on experimental data.[19] The nominal radius of the lesion approaches a maximum value as equilibrium between the RF heat into and the heat conduction away from the tissue around the tip is established. Equilibrium size is reached in about 60 sec, and very nearly so in 30 sec. During that first 30 sec, the lesion size is increasing. One can make a "time-dependent" lesion, whose size increases nearly linearly over time for about the first 15 sec. In this way, the lesion volume can be increased gradually. The current needed to achieve a given tip temperature, however, depends on variables such as resistance, heat conduction, and tip geometry. Moreover, the time versus lesion size curve shown in Figure 19–4 depends on other variables such as vascularity and proximity to cerebrospinal fluid (CSF), bone, and other heat sinks. Thus, it is preferable to eliminate uncertainties of the time-current prescription by choosing an appropriate tip size and temperature and then allowing the lesion size to reach its equilibrium value by means of a 30- to 60-sec exposure.

There is a narrow zone of reversibility for lesions in the brain. Brain tissue can withstand temperatures up to about 42.5° C without injury for minutes. Temporary cessation of certain neural functions may occur between 42.5° and 44° C, whereas temperatures above 45°C result in some form of permanent damage.[20] Thus, there should be a thin zone of reversibility on the perimeter of the zone of permanent destruction (Fig. 19–5). Practical use of this zone has not yet been exploited in clinical lesion making, but anyone performing RF stereotaxy must be aware of how critical these temperatures are in the brain.

In the peripheral nervous system, one of the more promising aspects of RF lesion making is the possibility of accurate and highly selective destruction of pain-carrying nerve fibers. An apparent example of this is in the trigeminal ganglion, where, at temperatures near 60° to 70° C, the highly myelinated A-beta fibers seem to survive better than the unmyelinated A-delta and C fibers. This observation derives from clinical experience: trigeminal neuralgia can be specifically eliminated but tactile and motor innervation

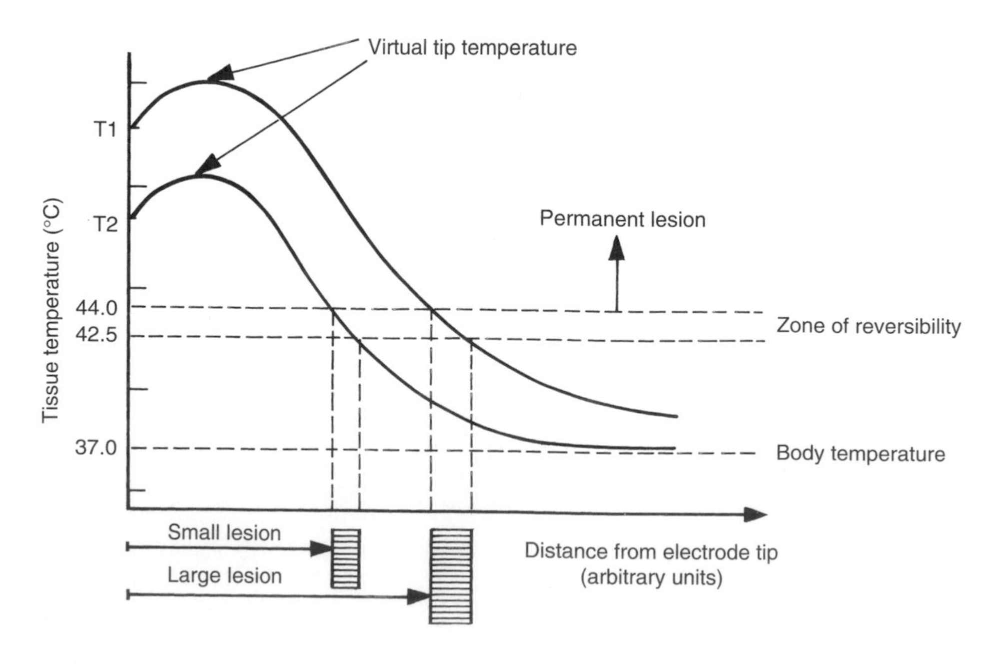

FIGURE 19–5 The distribution of tissue temperature as a function of distance from the active electrode tip. The actual function depends on the shape of the tip and the point on the tip from which the distance is measured.

are preserved. Here again, the importance of temperature as the fundamental lesion parameter is underscored.

The "Golden Rules" for Lesion Generation (for Homogeneous Conductive Medium)

Temperature is the fundamental lesion parameter (Fig. 19–6). Measurement of temperature not only ensures quantification and consistency of lesion size but is also essential for safety, to avoid the boiling point and to ensure that the lesion is, indeed, being made at the electrode tip and not elsewhere. Other aspects of temperature monitoring, such as dynamic response and automatic overheating control, are addressed later in this chapter.

The RF current heats the tissue, and the tissue heats the electrode tip. This fundamental concept enables accurate monitoring of tissue temperature. A common misconception is that the electrode tip itself becomes hot because power dissipates through it. The converse is actually true: The tissue becomes hot because of power dissipation in the tissue itself; the heat flows *back* to the electrode tip and heats it. Thus, an accurate representation of tissue temperature can be gained by monitoring the temperature at the electrode tip. There are engineering subtleties to proper temperature monitoring of an RF lesion electrode tip, however. If the electrode tip has a high thermal mass or if the temperature sensor is not located in intimate thermal conduction connection to the surface of the electrode, time delays and inaccuracies can result that can lead to serious adverse effects in the lesioning process. Thus, properly designing an RF electrode so that it adequately measures the temperature of the tissue is essential.

Consistent lesion size is determined by proper choice of electrode tip size and temperature. This is an important concept. Selection of the proper tip size, shape, and configuration and the achievement of a desired electrode tip temperature are the key factors in achieving consistent RF lesioning for any given procedure in a given anatomic area. Prescriptions of lesion making based on power, time, current, voltage, or other parameters have variable results, are unpredictable, and often produce uncontrolled effects and unsatisfactory clinical results. Although temperature is the most important *observable* parameter in the clinical process, it is wise clinical practice to monitor and record other parameters, such as power, current, voltage, and impedance. If these other parameters are in acceptable ranges of normal, the lesioning process is going satisfactorily; if they are not in acceptable ranges, something is grossly wrong with the setup, such as a short circuit, open circuit, or misplaced electrode tip.

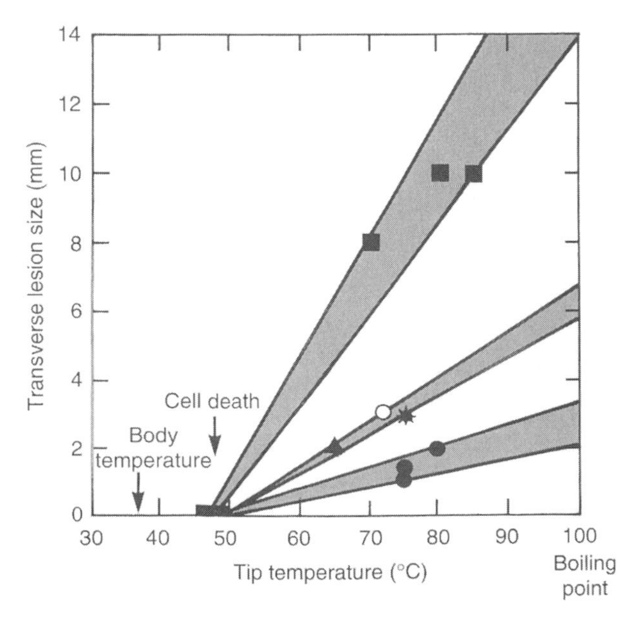

FIGURE 19–6 Plot of lesion width versus electrode tip diameter and temperature. Area bounding squares *represents tip diameter of 1.6 mm; area bounding* solid circles *represents tip diameter of 0.25 mm; area bounding* triangle *represents tip diameter of 1.1 to 1.2 mm. (*Open circle *and* asterisk *are the same values as the triangle.)*

Equilibrium lesions should be made by sustaining the proper tip temperature for 30 to 60 sec. This rule embodies the process of the equilibrium or asymptotic lesion and circumvents variability secondary to the lesion-time buildup curve, which can be a function of other parameters in the environment. The time constant for any given tip geometry or physical location can differ, but in most settings, in homogeneous tissue, 30 to 60 sec is adequate to approximate the maximum of the exponential asymptotic curve.

Unpredictable Factors in the Lesioning Process

Although the general rules just described have given excellent results, some are difficult to predict or quantify and can cause deviations in the RF lesion process. Most important among them is the nonhomogeneous tissue in the medium itself (Fig. 19–7). Proximity of the electrode to a CSF cistern or ventricle can present a low-impedance shunt pathway for RF current and thus draw the lesion heat to *it* rather than to neighboring tissue. Such an effect is commonly seen during lesion making in the trigeminal ganglion. Even more dramatic might be the effect of a large nearby blood vessel, which can sink heat away from the surrounding tissue and produce asymmetry in lesion shape.

Proximity to bone is another significant environmental variable. Bone has a lower conductivity for heat and current and thus creates discontinuity, especially in procedures such as facet denervation and ganglion RF procedures, in which the nerves to be heated lie next to large bones. In this situation, there is a complex of slower heating of the bone itself and a tendency for thermal insulation against the bone mass. The RF heating most likely is shunted to the tissue and away from bone. As the bone warms up, however, it becomes a reservoir of heat, and affects the time constants (see Fig. 19–4).

Empirical Lesion Sizes and Recommended Electrode Geometries and Lesion Parameters in the Brain and Spinal Cord

Overall, the experience with RF lesioning using acceptable lesion parameters has yielded excellent and consistent results (see Fig. 19–6). It is not known how lesion size changes

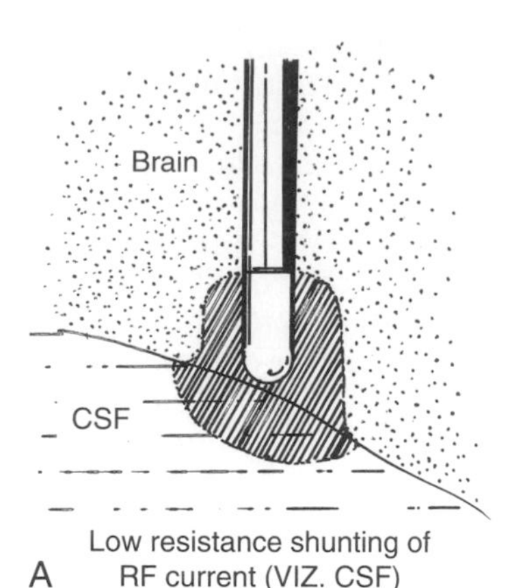

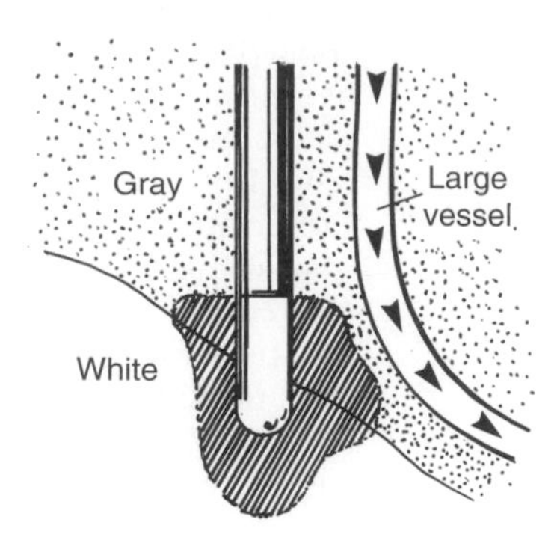

FIGURE 19–7 Conditions affecting the size and shape of an RF lesion. A, Low-resistance shunting of RF current. B, Nonuniform impedances, large blood vessels. (See text for discussion.)

between the first few weeks after lesioning and death. It appears that thalamotomies electrode tips of about 1.1 mm in diameter and 3 to 5 mm in length at temperatures of 65° to 75° C produce lesions about 3 mm in circumference or diameter and 4 to 7 mm in length. Lesion shapes are typically prolate ellipsoids of revolution for simple cylindrical electrodes. Lesions made in the cingulum with electrodes of 1.6-mm tip diameter and 10-mm tip length at 80° to 90° C are typically 10 mm in diameter and 12 mm long.

Information has also been accumulated on very small lesions in the spinal cord using very-fine-gauge electrodes.[21] Empirical information on DREZ-type electrodes, which are 0.25 mm in diameter with 2-mm tips, was gathered from experiments in the spinal cords of cats. Lesioning at 75° C for 15 seconds gave rise to lesion sizes of the order of 0.7 to 0.9 mm in diameter and 1.8 to 2.2 mm in length. Increasing the lesioning time to 45 seconds increased the lesion's size to 1.4 mm in diameter and 2.3 mm in length. Lesioning at 80° C for 15 seconds produced lesions of 2 mm in diameter and approximately 2 mm long. These data are consistent with indirect information on similar-sized electrodes used in percutaneous cordotomy. Lesions on the order of 2 to 3 mm in diameter by 2 to 3 mm in length were seen to occur when an electrode of the order of 0.5 mm in diameter by 2 to 2.5 mm in length was placed in the lateral spinal thalamic tract.[19, 22–24] This electrode size appears to be satisfactory when properly placed for percutaneous cordotomy procedures with the objective of pain relief in cancer patients. Unfortunately, these measurements were made at a time when current and time lesion parameter prescriptions were used, but not temperature monitoring. It is also known, however, that using the Type LCE Levin Cordotomy Electrode with tip dimensions of 0.25 mm in diameter and 2 mm in length produces adequate percutaneous cordotomy lesions at 80° to 85° C for 30 sec.[25]

A summary of empirical lesion size data gathered in this way is shown in Figure 19–6. These graphs may serve as "cononical curves" for estimating the lesion size of a given tip size and tip temperature. In Figure 19–6, the transverse lesion diameter (the width or girth of the lesion) is plotted as a function of the tip temperature of the electrode measured in degrees centigrade. Each of the graphs is drawn for different tip diameters, based on the data cited. The long axis of the lesion can be assumed to be approximately 1 to 3 mm longer than the tip of the electrode for an axially symmetric and approximately cylindrical electrode geometry. These curves are based on lesion data in the brain and spinal cord and may not apply in extremely inhomogeneous tissues or in close proximity to large bony masses.

Practical Aspects of Radiofrequency Lesion Making

The modern RF lesion generator system includes not only the means to make the lesion and display the temperature of the electrode tip but also auxiliary electronic aids to improve target determination, safety, and ease of operation.

A modern RF lesion generator system is a sophisticated microprocessor-based apparatus with multiple functions to enhance the lesion generation process. It has a built-in advanced impedance monitor, a wide parameter stimulator, a lesion generator, and digital readout of all relevant parameters—impedance, stimulation parameters, power, voltage, current, time, and device function status. Its advanced temperature-monitoring system has not only thermistor and thermocouple readouts but also analogue and digital display of temperature (both important, for reasons discussed later) and an automatic overheating control system, which enables automatic locking onto a lesion temperature once the desired electrode tip temperature has been achieved. Because the system is based on a microprocessor, many functions can be monitored simultaneously, and an alphanumeric status display on the front panel gives the operator an instant report of the status of the generator and problems, should they arise, such as short circuit or open circuit.

Recording Parameters

It is good practice to record voltage, current power, temperature, time, and electrode type for each lesion. Such data are very useful in analyzing any problem that might arise and in evaluating the operator's awareness of what these values should be under normal conditions. Erratic behavior of temperature, voltage, or current readings (a too rapid or too slow response for a given RF-power increase) should be regarded as a warning of possible trouble.

Temperature Readings

The operator should always ensure, before lesioning, that the temperature meter reads body temperature at about 37° C. This is the simplest check to ensure that the electrode, thermistor, and temperature monitoring circuitry are functioning properly. The RF power should be raised slowly, and the operator should make sure that the temperature increase is normal; if it is not, the operator should not continue to raise the power and should check the system carefully. With any reading over 80° C, close attention must be paid, because in that range a rapid "runaway" to boiling (100° C) is possible.

Electrode tip temperature may be controlled by a direct temperature control mechanism. The operator manually increases the RF voltage on the electrode. Output should always be increased gradually and carefully while the operator observes the increase in tip temperature reading as the tissue begins to heat up. As the desired tip temperature is approached, the RF control knob should be attended to and the temperature meter watched to prevent drift of tip temperature from the desired lesion temperature.

Cables

By far, the greatest proportion of all equipment problems in RF lesioning arises from faulty cables. The cable is vulnerable to damage during handling and sterilizing. Thus, it is advisable to have sterilized spare cables on hand during the operation. The operator should remember that switching to the impedance monitor can allow an instant check of cable and electrode continuity during the procedure.

Electrode Insulation

Insulation on the electrode should be checked for cracks or breaks before each procedure. Broken insulation can cause current to flow elsewhere than to the target region and to cause unwanted tissue damage.

Dispersive Electrodes

Skin burns at the dispersive electrode arise because it has too small an area relative to that of the active electrode tip. Thus, to be maximally safe, a large-area dispersive electrode is recommended rather than spinal needles placed in muscle or fatty tissue. A stainless steel, large-area dispersive electrode with area of at least 150 cm^2 is recommended, and an ample coating of conductor gel for good electrical conductivity. Such an electrode can be taped onto the arm, hip, or another area near muscle for an adequate, low-impedance dispersive connection.

CLINICAL APPLICATIONS OF LESIONING

Only modern, thermally coupled electrode systems should be used, and it is recommended that disposable cannulas be used whenever possible. The electrode systems and the associated wires should be gas sterilized before each operative procedure. Heat sterilization is not recommended, because it decreases the life expectancy of the reusable electrode systems. The safest way to maintain the long-term integrity of the electrode systems is to allow for adequate sterilization using a cool-gas sterilization cycle. This means that multiple wires and electrode systems need to be kept on hand if RF procedures are to be performed on a regular basis.

Regardless of the RF unit chosen, the lesion generator must be able to stimulate at multiple frequencies, monitor impedance, voltage, amperage, and temperature, allow for gradual increases in lesion temperature, and use modern, thermally coupled electrodes. For component maintenance, it is recommended that at least two electrode systems with lengths of 50, 100, and 150 mm be kept in sterile packages. It is also recommended that cannula systems in the 50-mm, 100-mm, and 150-mm lengths with both 5-mm and 2-mm active tip exposures be kept in stock. These are the electrode and cannula systems most often used for the majority of spinal rhizotomy procedures. The 150-mm cannula with both 10- and 15-mm active tip exposures is useful for lumbar disc, sacroiliac joint, and lumbar sympathectomy procedures. Other specialized electrodes worthy of general consideration are blunt, curved-tipped electrodes in 100- and 150-mm lengths with 10-mm active tips.

Lumbar Spine Disorders

Lumbar spinal disease is a common problem and often difficult to treat. To properly understand the use of RF lesions in the treatment of chronic pain of the low back, one must be familiar with the anatomy and pathophysiology of the lumbar spine (see also Chapter 5).

Spinal Anatomy and Pain Procedures

The lumbar spine has many potential pain generators. Some areas that have been identified by neuroanatomic dissections are the annulus of the disc, the posterior longitudinal ligament, portions of the dural lining, the facet joints and capsules, the spinal nerve roots and their associated dorsal root ganglia, the sacroiliac joint, its capsule and ligaments, and the associated musculature.[26–32] Specific RF techniques have been devised for the treatment of pain emanating from the facet joints, nerve roots, annulus fibrosus, and sacroiliac joint.[33–38] No specific RF techniques have been devised for the treatment of pain emanating from the dural lining, the posterior longitudinal ligament, or myofascial trigger points.

The lumbar facet joints receive innervation from multiple levels of the lumbar spine. To properly denervate a lumbar facet joint, two levels must be lesioned (Fig. 19–8).[26, 35, 38]

Lumbar Facet Joint Pain

The role of the facet joint in the production of chronic pain has been known since 1911,[39–41] although Ghormely[42] was the first clinician to use the term *facet syndrome*. Many authors have reported on facet joint pain[43] and its treatment

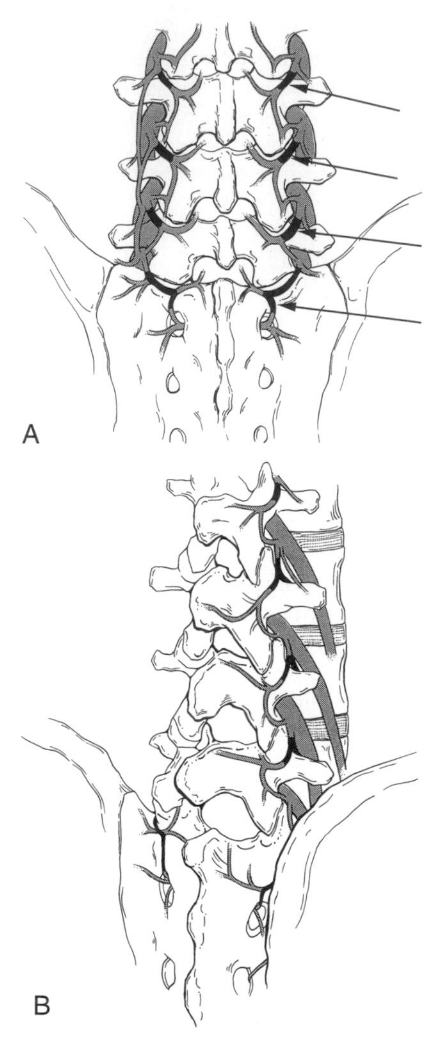

FIGURE 19–8 *Drawings of the nerve supply to the lumbar facet joints (arrows). A, Anteroposterior and B, oblique views.*

with selective RF lesions.[34, 35, 37, 44–73] Approximately 50% to 67% of properly selected patients with chronic, mechanical low back pain realize moderate to significant reduction in pain or improvement in range of motion after RF facet rhizotomy.[34, 36, 38, 44–73] In one controlled, meticulously performed clinical study, 87% of patients reported greater than 60% pain relief (60% reported >90% relief) 1 year after RF lumbar facet denervation.[74]

Lumbar facet joint pain can be manifested as an acute or chronic problem. It can be secondary either to long-term degenerative changes or to acute trauma, as in a motor vehicle accident.[75, 76] Imaging studies frequently show a normal-looking facet joint, and the x-ray status of the joint bears no relationship to the joint's pain status.[77]

Patients with facet joint pain commonly present with deep, aching pain in the paravertebral regions of the low back. They often have a somatic referral pattern of pain into the buttocks, posterior or anterior thigh, or knee region, and aching in the area of the hip.[48, 77]

On physical examination there is usually palpable tenderness over the facet joints. This is often associated with back pain when the lumbosacral junction is extended or flexed to the side. In patients who suffer from facet joint pain alone, the neurologic examination is normal. Straight leg raising may not be painful, and the deflexion maneuver is uniphasic. The diagnosis of facet joint pain cannot be made on the basis of history and manual examination alone. Relief from intraarticular or medial branch local anesthetic blockade is an important indicator of the diagnosis of facet joint pain, but results can be false-positive and blockade is not a substitute for careful history taking and a detailed and focused manual examination.[78]

Lumbar Facet Joint Rhizotomy

A patient suffering from facet joint pain (emanating from the L5–S1 and L4–L5 joints) is first placed prone on the fluoroscopy table. A small amount of intravenous sedation is given. The patient needs to remain awake enough to cooperate throughout the procedure, because it is critical that he or she respond properly to electrical stimulation. It is the stimulation process that allows for accurate electrode placement with a high level of safety.

After the patient's back is antiseptically prepared, the C-arm fluoroscopic device is used to identify the junction of the sacral ala with the superior articulating process of S1. The groove formed by this junction is the site of the L5 dorsal ramus. The second and third targets are the superior and medial aspects of the transverse processes at L5 and L4 (junction of transverse process with superior articulating process).

The skin and subcutaneous tissues are anesthetized with 0.5% lidocaine prior to placement of the RF cannulas. The first cannula is placed so that it just touches the target point for the L5 dorsal ramus (in the groove between the sacral ala and the superior articulating process of S1). The remaining cannulas are placed so that they just touch the superomedial aspects of the transverse processes at L5 and L4. At the level of the sacral ala and the transverse processes, the cannula is slipped over the leading edge of the periosteum and advanced approximately 2 mm. This allows more precise alignment of the RF cannula with the long axis of the facet joint nerve.

Correct use of the fluoroscopy unit enables the clinician to adequately image the periosteal target points. At the level of the sacral ala, a direct posterior view with 5 to 10 degrees of angulation usually shows the anatomy accurately. At the level of the transverse processes of L5 and L4, an oblique view (5–15 degrees) is usually necessary to show the most mediad aspect of the transverse process. Sometimes craniad or caudad movement of the fluoroscopy tube is necessary to sharpen the image of the edge of the transverse process, especially to avoid superimposed osteophytes that can block the correct view (Fig. 19–9).

The RF cannulas should lie parallel to the nerve to be lesioned whenever possible. Because the length of the lesion corresponds to the length of the bare metal tip exposed, a larger portion of the nerve is lesioned when the cannula is placed parallel to the nerve.

After the cannulas have been placed, it is wise to check the electrical impedance, which is usually between 300 and 700Ω when the cannulas are positioned correctly. Checking the impedance is a good method for measuring the overall integrity of the RF system. After the impedance has been

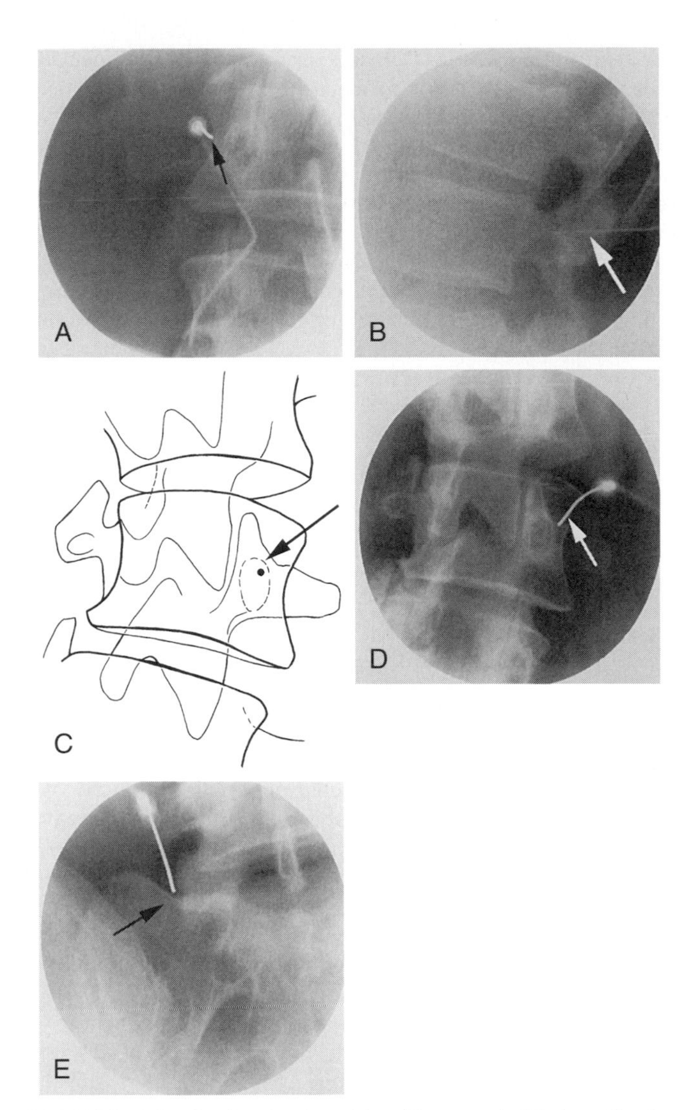

FIGURE 19–9 *Lumbar facet joint rhizotomy.* A, *PA view of lumbar medial branch lesion;* B, *lateral view of lumbar medial branch lesion;* C, *lumbar medial branch target point, oblique view;* D, *lumbar medial branch target point, oblique view;* E, *lesion point for L5 dorsal ramus.*

checked, a lateral view further confirms correct placement of the cannulas, with the tips posterior to the respective foramina. The next step involves electrical stimulation at 50 Hz. Stimulation in the paravertebral and hip areas should be noted when the medial branches are stimulated at this frequency. Strong stimulation should be noted at less than 1.0 V at 50 Hz when the cannula is in correct alignment with the facet joint nerve. Next, stimulation is performed at 2 Hz, and lower-extremity motor fasciculations should be absent at 2.5 V. Multifidus muscle stimulation is usually noted at the 2-Hz point. After confirmation of correct placement with both fluoroscopy and stimulation, 1 mL of 2% lidocaine is injected through each of the cannulas. Thirty seconds is allowed to pass; then lesions are created at a temperature of 80° C applied for 60 sec. After the lesions are completed, the cannulas are removed and sterile bandages are placed at the puncture sites.

The risks of the lumbar facet rhizotomy include numbness and weakness in the lower extremities, although long-term sensory or motor deficits are quite uncommon. Accurate stimulation during the operative procedure prevents nerve root injury. Occasionally, patients develop mild dysesthesia or short-term motor and sensory changes; this is unusual, however, and the vast majority have no complications involving neurologic changes.

Some patients notice motor extremity weakness immediately after the procedure, which is usually due to extravasation of local anesthetic onto the main nerve root during the procedure. This phenomenon usually resolves within 1 to 2 hours postoperatively. Most patients are fit to go home 2 hours after the procedure. Patients can expect to have 1 to 2 weeks of perioperative discomfort—pain in the paravertebral regions and the upper buttock. Hip pain can be bothersome after this procedure. It usually begins on the 3rd postoperative day and can last as long as 10 days. If the pain is severe enough, appropriate analgesics, and even a short course of oral steroids, can be helpful. The cause of the hip pain is unclear but might be related to spasm of the quadratus lumborum.

It is important to bear in mind that mechanical low back pain is frequently associated with multiple pain generators. More than one facet joint can be involved, or the problem may involve discs and facets. A careful physical examination is critical to exploring for signs of combined involvement of any of the previously mentioned pain generators.

Functional Stereotactic Identification of Symptomatic Levels and Subsequent Radiofrequency Lesioning

As advances are made in the techniques of lesion-specific therapies for chronic pain, the opportunity to definitively ascertain, in real time, the relative contribution of any purported and identifiable pain generator becomes extremely attractive. A functional stereotactic approach, where electrode proximity to the target nerve tissue may be objectively assessed with patient-blinded sensory and/or motor stimulation, has broad application in percutaneous RF techniques. Maximizing the proximity of the electrode to the target nerve tissue increases the likelihood that a therapeutic lesion will encompass the structures that are causing symptoms.

Sensory and motor stereotaxy guides several RF procedures currently performed (most notably dorsal root ganglion partial rhizotomy, gasserian rhizotomy, and sphenopalatine ganglionolysis), but may be applied to virtually any radiofrequency procedure currently performed. The adoption of a functional stereotactic approach minimizes the risk that "innocent" structures will be lesioned and may give the physician a more objective assessment of the relative contributions of any particular pain generator to the patient's overall pain picture. Sensory stereotaxy may also be used to confirm clinical suspicions that a given structure may, or may not, be involved in the primary pain complaint.

We recommend that the functional RF lesioning procedure be guided by precise fluoroscopic imaging in conjunction with a sound functional stereotactic approach. Functional stereotaxy has become invaluable in determining the symptomatic levels of involvement in facet-related pain and ganglion rhizotomy and reliably reproduces sympathetic ganglion–mediated and splanchnic pain. Indeed, if concordant symptoms are not reproduced with low-voltage sensory stimulation, either the electrode is positioned improperly or the target structure is not involved in the patient's symptom complex. In either of these cases, no lesioning should be performed. With few exceptions, patients undergoing functional stereotactic RF procedures should be *awake. Minimal supplemental reversible analgesic medication* (e.g., alfentanil, fentanyl) may be administered judiciously, but only when absolutely required. Any alteration in the patients' ability to differentiate their responses to stereotactic stimulation can compromise the efficacy and safety of the procedure.

EXAMPLE 1

If, on the basis of a careful history and physical examination, facet joint pain is suspected, confirmation of the clinical diagnosis is mandatory before RF denervation is considered. Despite the most carefully performed physical examination, the presence of other active lumbar pain generators may confound definitive diagnosis that relies on clinical examination findings alone. Selective medial branch or intraarticular facet joint injections are invaluable in determining the *presumptive* levels of facet involvement and in identifying the relative contribution of facet-related pain to the patient's overall pain picture. The use of corticosteroid medications (e.g., triamcinolone, concentration 4–8 mg/mL) in conjunction with small (diagnostic) doses of local anesthesia (0.5–0.7 mL total volume) may prolong the benefit experienced by the patient (and, in a reasonable percentage of patients, be sufficiently therapeutic as to provide long-term relief), and a reproducible response with high-grade improvement of pain must be documented before consideration of RF denervation.

Despite the most carefully performed physical examination and meticulous injection technique, however, the precise distribution of medial branch–mediated pain is impossible to determine by diagnostic injection alone. If the patient's pain is dramatically or completely reduced after diagnostic or confirmatory local anesthetic or steroid injection, the physician can only surmise that an adequate number of levels has been injected, without knowing if asymptomatic levels have also been injected.

Utilizing sensory stereotaxy during the RF facet denervation procedure ensures that only—and all—symptomatic levels are denervated and avoids unnecessary lesioning of asymptomatic levels. Because the medial branch of the posterior primary rami provides primary facet capsular sensory innervation (along with segmental ipsilateral multifidus motor innervation), sensory stereotaxy may be utilized to verify proximity of the RF electrode to the symptom-producing nerves, maximizing the likelihood that the target nerve will lie within the 45° C isotherm, or "kill zone," of the lesion.

Once the electrodes have been placed in the approximate location of the medial branch nerves under fluoroscopic guidance, precise final electrode positioning may be guided by the patient's subjective and objective responses to low-voltage sensory stimulation. Low-voltage sensory stimulation between 0.2 and 0.5 V (1 msec pulse duration, frequency 50 Hz) should reproduce concordant pain, in conjunction with simultaneous segmental ipsilateral multifidus contraction. Stimulation of non-symptomatic levels will produce segmental multifidus contraction *without* reproducing concordant pain, generally described by patients as a sensation of light paresthesia, or "tightness," in the back and areas of sensory referral.

Before RF denervation is undertaken, attempts should be made to selectively reproduce concordant pain at the lowest stimulation voltage possible (0.15–0.3 V). This correlates with proximity of the electrode to the target nerve, which maximizes the likelihood of successful denervation. No radiating paresthesias should be experienced in the distribution of the anatomically related spinal nerve root. Stimulation should be performed with the patient blinded, to eliminate observational bias.

EXAMPLE 2

Sensory stereotaxy may play a vital role in the diagnosis of complex pain problems. In the case of a 29-year-old woman with a history of iatrogenic chronic celiac plexopathy secondary to pancreatic duct outlet obstruction after an exploratory laparotomy, an alcohol celiac plexus block was performed at another institution. After the lytic block, the patient suffered intractable diarrhea and had been managed by another practitioner with steroid and local anesthetic celiac plexus blocks. After 9 months, the local anesthetic/steroid injections were no longer effective, and the patient was referred to one of the authors (WY) for further evaluation and management. A stereotactic RF splanchnic denervation procedure was performed, which reduced the patient's symptoms approximately 50%. The patient still required a significant opioid analgesic supplement. Stereotactic thoracic sympathetic stimulation was subsequently performed. Findings were significant thoracic sympathetic involvement and reproduction of concordant pain with bilateral sympathetic ganglionic stimulation up to the level T8. Stereotaxy-guided RF lesions were made over the symptomatic sympathetic ganglia, and the patient remained completely pain-free for 9 weeks (i.e., she needed absolutely no prescription or over-the-counter analgesics). The patient's pain began to return 10 weeks after the RF procedure. The patient was then referred for bilateral thoracoscopic surgical thoracic sympathectomy at the levels of T8–T12. Fortunately, the patient experienced complete relief of her pain after her surgical sympathectomy and has remained completely pain-free and without medication for more than 2 years.

Caudal Approach to Lumbar Medial Branch Denervation

To maximize the success of any RF procedure, every effort must be made to place the active tip of the electrode as close to the target nerve as possible. The effective size of the nerve lesion will also be increased if the cannula is

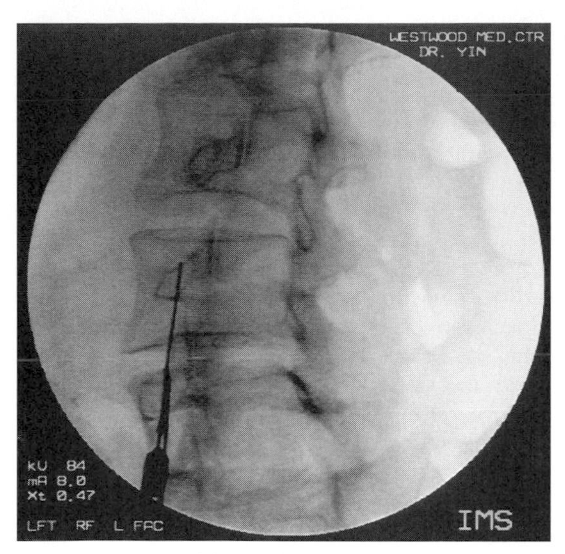

FIGURE 19–10 Oblique images of caudal posterolateral lumbar medial branch RF denervation. Note electrodes overlapping Burton's point at L3 and L4.

placed as nearly parallel to the nerve as possible. Commercially available blunt-tipped RF cannulas (Radionics, Inc., Burlington, Mass.) combined with a slight curve (10–15 degrees) involving the active distal tip have augmented the safety and technical efficacy of many RF procedures. For many lumbar facet denervation procedures, especially in larger patients or those who have undergone previous surgical interventions, 20-gauge, 100-mm long blunt, curved-tip RF cannulas with a 10-mm active tip may be used to great effect. These 20-gauge cannulas produce quantitatively larger thermal lesions than 22-gauge electrodes, the diameter of the lesion being roughly related to the square of the radius of the electrode, and linearly related to the length of the active tip.

The caudal approach using a blunt-tipped electrode differs from the posterolateral approach in several ways. The patient is positioned in the prone position, and anteroposterior fluoroscopic images are obtained to identify lumbar levels. The caudal posterior oblique approach may be used for the lumbar medial branches of T12–L5, as it most closely parallels the course of the medial branch nerve as it wraps around the superomedial aspect of the transverse process beneath the mamilloaccessory ligament before it divides into separate articular branches. It is important to remember that any given lumbar medial branch crosses over the superomedial aspect of the transverse process of the next level *below* (i.e., the L2 medial branch will be found crossing over the superomedial aspect of the L3 transverse process). Posterior oblique fluoroscopic projections are obtained (30–40 degrees) to identify the junction of the superomedial aspect of the transverse process with the superior articulating process (Burton's point), and the skin is marked over this radiographic landmark. The electrode entry sites for the caudal posterior oblique approach start at the skin markings *one level below* each respective level. The entry sites are anesthetized with a small volume of local anesthetic, and short (1.25-inch) 16-gauge intravenous cannulas are placed through the skin and subcutaneous fascia to facilitate passage of the blunt-tipped electrodes.

The electrodes are then advanced in a posterolateral and cephalad approach toward Burton's point one level above the skin entry site under posterior oblique fluoroscopic guidance (Fig. 19–10). Once bony contact is made with the transverse process, the cannula tip is rotated to overlie the superomedial aspect of the transverse process under anteroposterior fluoroscopic imaging (Fig. 19–11). Lateral images are taken to verify that the cannula tips do not approach the intervertebral neural foraminal apertures (Fig. 19–12).

The caudal approach to the L5 posterior primary ramus differs from the approach to T12–L4, in that it is a posterior parasagittal approach (the iliac wing obstructs a posterolateral approach). Under anteroposterior fluoroscopic

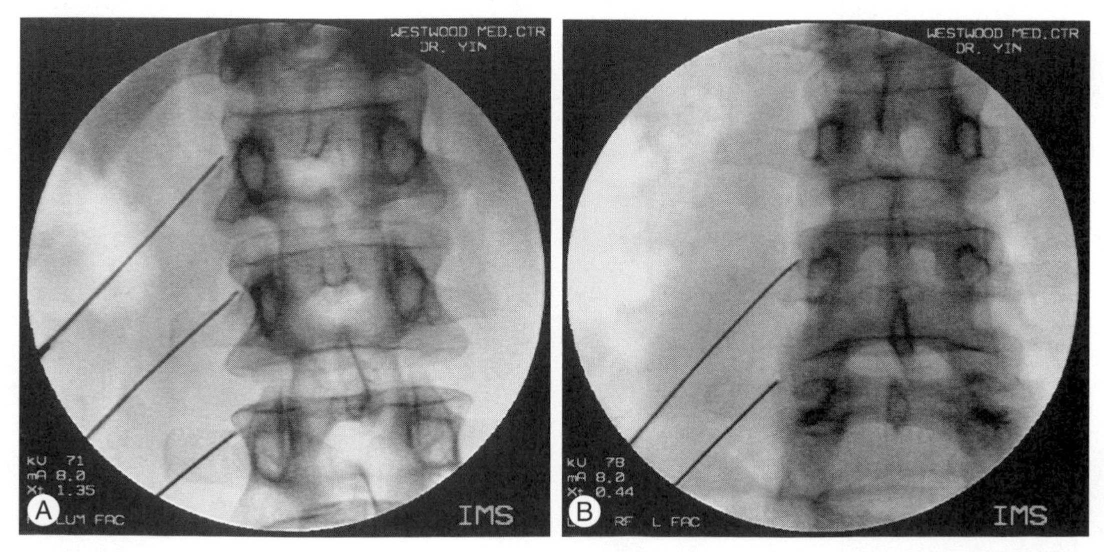

FIGURE 19–11 A, *AP projection of caudal posterolateral lumbar medial branch RF denervation using curved blunt electrode, left T12, L1, L2 medial branch nerves.* B, *AP projection of caudal posterolateral lumbar medial branch RF denervation, left L3, L4 medial branch nerves.*

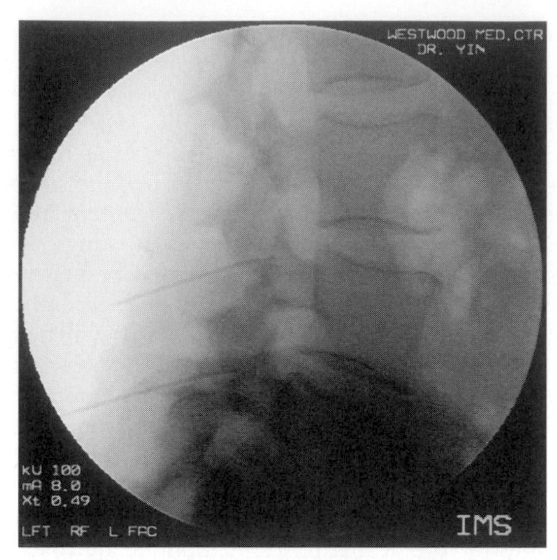

FIGURE 19–12 *Lateral radiographs of caudal posterolateral lumbar facet RF denervation using curved blunt electrodes, L4 medial branch and L5 posterior primary ramus. Note electrode tip position relative to intervertebral neural foramina.*

imaging, the superomedial aspect of the sacral ala (which corresponds developmentally to the transverse process of S1) is identified, and a skin entry site marked and anesthetized approximately 2–3 cm caudal. The blunt-tipped electrode is then advanced toward the superomedial aspect of the sacral ala, the tip of the electrode overlapping this structure as it is at other levels (Fig. 19–13).

Sensory stereotactic localization of the medial branch nerves is then performed (as described earlier). No segmental multifidus contraction is generally observed on stimulation of the L5 posterior primary ramus. Before RF denervation, 1 mL of 2% lidocaine is injected, and thermal lesioning is performed (at 80°–85° C for 60 sec).

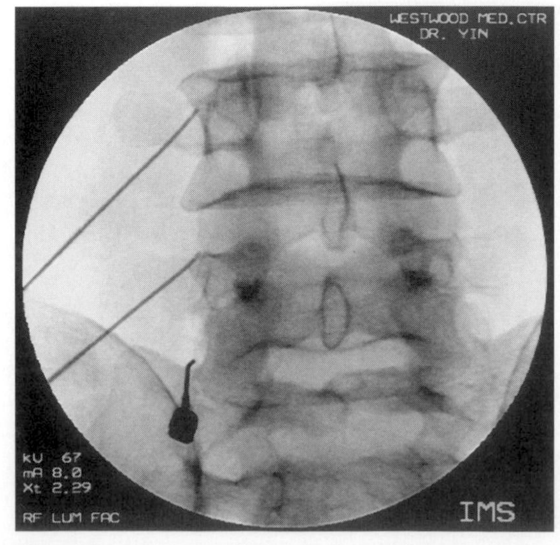

FIGURE 19–13 *AP radiograph of caudal posterolateral lumbar medial branch RF denervation of left L3, L4 and left L5 posterior primary ramus.*

Thoracic Facet Joint Pain

Thoracic facet joint pain can also be treated with RF neurotomy. The course of the medial branch differs from that in the lumbar region, but the technique can be similar. Detailed dissections of the medial branches of the dorsal rami were performed by Chua.[79, 85] The typical courses of the medial branches in the upper (T1–T4) and lower thoracic levels (T9–T10) exited the intertransverse space in a mediolateral direction, crossing the superolateral corners of the transverse process at their inflection point. From the inflection point, the nerve moved mediad and downward across the posterior surface of the transverse process. Exceptions were noted at the midthoracic levels (T5–T8), where the nerve follows a parallel course but at times is displaced superiorly and may not contact the inflection point of the transverse process. At the T11–T12 levels, the nerve follows a course analogous to that of the lumbar region. Stimulation can be achieved both at the inflection point and at the more traditional "medial position" described for the lumbar medial branches. Good results have been noted after RF lesioning in either position, which indicates that the fibers of the medial branch may find their way back to the superomedial position, as it crosses medially from the inflection point.[79, 80, 85] The fluoroscopy tube may need to be angled craniad or caudad to show separation of the transverse process from its associated rib. If the medial approach is chosen, the facet rhizotomy in the thoracic region is similar to that of the lumbar region. Otherwise, the nerve can be lesioned at the inflection point. Among other potential complications in the thoracic region is a small risk of pneumothorax (Fig. 19–14).

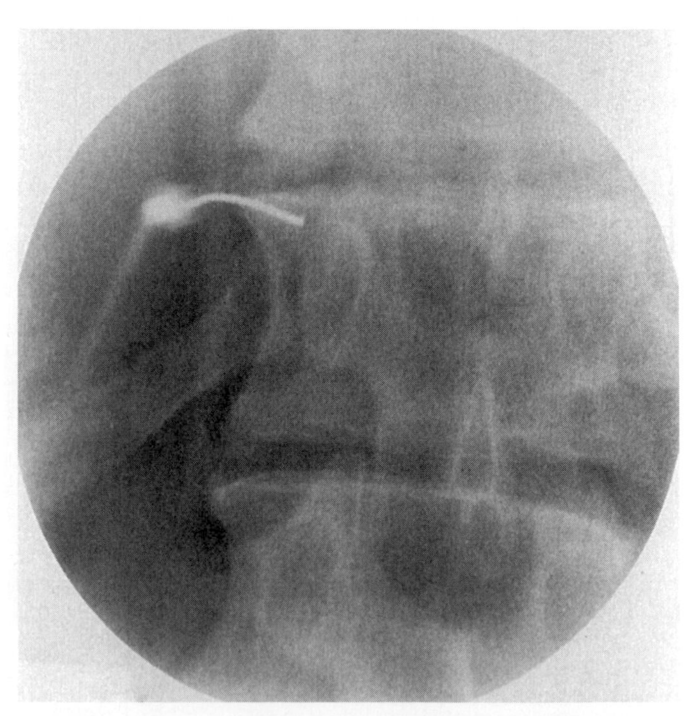

FIGURE 19–14 *Posterior view of a thoracic facet RF rhizotomy procedure demonstrates the correct cannula position for a lesion of the T11 facet joint nerve.*

Sacroiliac Joint Pain

Biomechanical analysis reveals the principal function of the sacroiliac joint complex to be stress reduction, as opposed to active movement.[81] The deep and superficial sacroiliac joint ligaments serve a vital function in maintaining the integrity of the joint complex, binding the sacrum to the ilia. Unusual stress on the ligaments because of abnormalities in axial loading may result in the development of chronic sacroiliac joint complex pain.

Sacroiliac joint can produce symptoms quite similar to facet joint abnormalities. Pain emanating from the sacroiliac joint usually causes buttock pain and referred mechanical symptoms. Areas of referral include the hip, groin, anterior thigh, and calf. Examination usually detects distinct tenderness over the middle and lower sacroiliac joint. Compression tests are frequently painful and distraction tests often reveal a poor joint mobility. Patients with sacroiliac joint pain frequently report that their pain is at its worst when they first arise in the morning and abates over the next several hours. Typically, sacroiliac joint pain is exacerbated with prolonged sitting or standing, is relieved with lumbosacral flexion, and is accompanied by findings of reproducible tenderness directly over the posterior ligamentous structures. Details of the examination of a painful sacroiliac joint have been reviewed in the literature.[82] The clinical suspicion of sacroiliac joint intraarticular or ligament pain may be confirmed by differential, fluoroscopically guided interosseous ligament or intraarticular injection of local anesthetic, with or without steroid. The reported prevalence of sacroiliac joint pain (15%)[83] may underestimate the true prevalence in the population of chronic back pain sufferers.[84] Overlapping patterns of referred mechanical or somatic pain of discogenic origin (especially in the L4–L5 and L5–S1 intervertebral discs) further confound the clinical diagnosis.

The sensory innervation of the sacroiliac joint complex remains to be described definitively. The need to distinguish posterior from anterior sacroiliac pain and intraarticular pain from ligamentous pain further complicates the issue. Approximately 50% to 60% of patients with intractable posterior ligamentous or intraarticular pain will experience prolonged high-grade relief from sensory stereotactic sacral posterior primary ramus rhizotomy.

Rhizotomy of the Sacroiliac Joint

The patient is placed in the prone position on the fluoroscopy table. The fluoroscopy unit is angled in so that the lines of the posterior aspects of the joint are seen. The tube is angled caudad and obliquely from the side opposite the joint to be lesioned; that is, an oblique view at 15 to 20 degrees from the opposite side of the body is used to correctly visualize the posterior joint lines.

One technique used to denervate the sacroiliac joint involves the formation of bipolar lesions using two electrode systems, the first being the active electrode and the second being a ground system. Bipolar electrode wires can be obtained from the manufacturer of the RF generator so that the second cannula can attach directly to the ground plug. Lesioning can be performed between points A and B to produce a linear lesion. As long as the distance between the two cannulas does not exceed five times the diameter of an individual cannula, a linear lesion is produced between the two electrodes. Multiple linear lesions can be produced along the entire length of the sacroiliac joint to effectively denervate the posterior aspect of the joint and its capsule. Because the bipolar method produces multiple, overlapping, linear lesions, stimulation prior to lesioning is not necessary with this technique (Fig. 19–15).

This allows the clinician to anesthetize the skin, subcutaneous tissues, and joint before performing the procedure. Thus, this rhizotomy technique is almost painless. Usually, 15 to 20 connecting linear lesions are produced along the posterior sacroiliac joint. Each bipolar lesion is created at a temperature of 80° C for 60 sec (using two cannulas, each

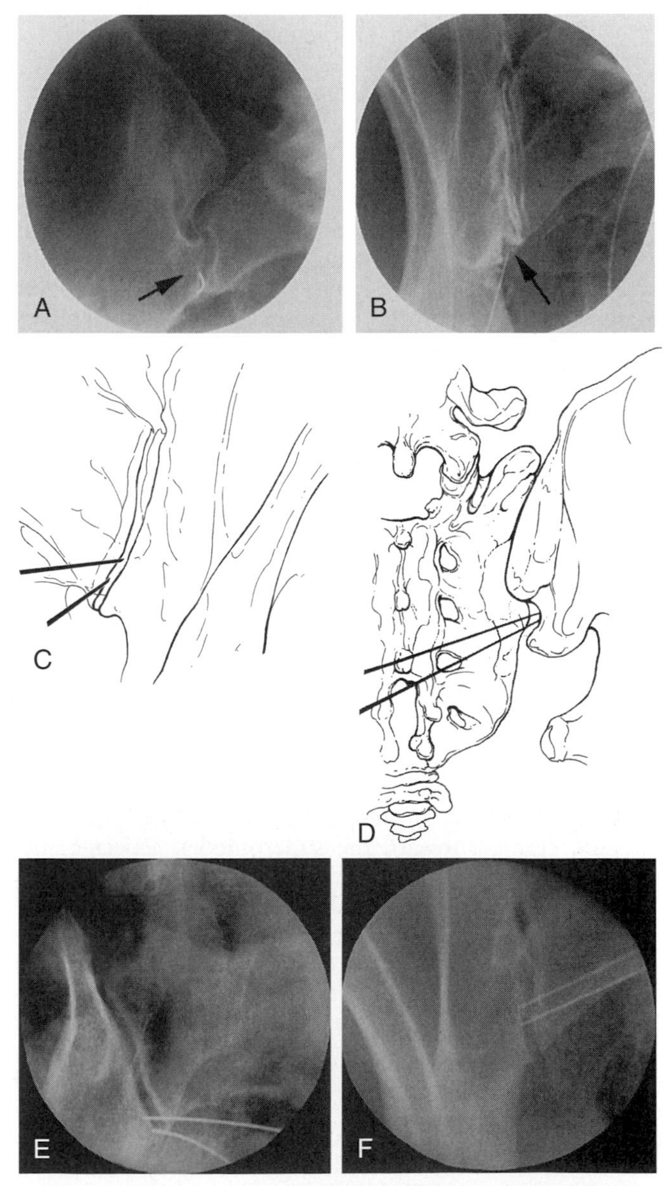

FIGURE 19–15 A, *Radiograph demonstrates the needle position* (arrow) *for entry into the posteroinferior aspect of the sacroiliac joint.* B, *Arthrogram of the sacroiliac joint; note the needle entry into the inferior aspect of the joint* (arrow). C, D, *Drawing of two RF cannulas in parallel alignment for a bipolar lesion at the posteroinferior aspect of the sacroiliac joint.* E, F, *Radiographs demonstrate the RF cannula positions for bipolar lesions at the inferoposterior aspect of the sacroiliac joint.*

150 mm long with 10-mm active tips). It is important to make certain that the lesions overlap slightly, so that a complete linear lesion is produced along the entire posterior joint line. As one moves farther craniad, the cannula's entry must be farther medial to be positioned beneath the posterior iliac crest.

The S2 level contributes much to the innervation of the sacroiliac joint. An S2 ganglionotomy can be an important adjunct to the sacroiliac joint rhizotomy (if the S2 analgesic test block gives good relief). Some patients have residual buttock, referred posterior thigh, or hip pain after sacroiliac joint rhizotomy, and, if the S2 test block temporarily relieves the residual pain, an S2 ganglionotomy often ameliorates the residual symptoms. Patients usually experience 2 weeks of buttock discomfort after sacroiliac joint rhizotomy. Patchy decreased skin sensation in the buttock is sometimes seen and it usually resolves in 2 to 6 weeks.

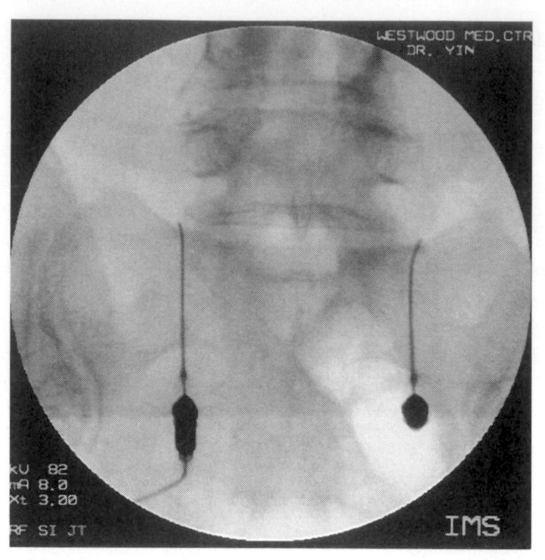

FIGURE 19–16 AP image illustrates electrode placement for bilateral L5 posterior primary ramus stereotactic lesion for sacroiliac joint denervation.

Sacroiliac Joint Stereotactic Posterior Primary Ramus Rhizotomy

The stereotactic sacroiliac denervation procedure differs from the bipolar technique in that individual posterior primary rami are localized near their decussation at the level of the dorsal sacral foraminal apertures. Reproduction of concordant pain guides the rhizotomy procedure. The preferred technique uses a 20-gauge, 100-mm blunt-tipped, 10-mm active tip, curved-tip RF electrode.

As with the bipolar technique, the patient is placed prone on the fluoroscopy table. The fluoroscopy unit is angled so that the sacrum is seen *en face* (i.e., the L5-S1 disc space is seem "crisply"), the objectives being maximal visualization of the lateral border of the dorsal foraminal apertures of S1 and S2 and clear delineation of the superomedial aspect of the sacral ala.

A skin entry site is marked and anesthetized over the approximate position of the second sacral dorsal foraminal aperture, and a 1.25-inch 16-gauge intravenous catheter is inserted to facilitate placement of the blunt-tipped electrode. Through this single skin entry site, the electrode may be serially repositioned to approach the posterior primary rami of L5, S1, S2, and, if necessary, S3.

Under anteroposterior fluoroscopic guidance, the electrode is introduced through the intravenous catheter and directed craniad, toward the superomedial aspect of the ipsilateral sacra ala. The electrode tip is rotated to slightly overlap the cranial and dorsal aspect of the sacral ala, and sensory stereotactic localization of the L5 posterior primary ramus is performed as described previously. Unlike L5 posterior primary ramus denervation of the L5-S1 lumbar facet joint, the sensory branch innervating the proximal sacroiliac joint may lie 0.5 to 1.5 cm lateral to the most medial aspect of the sacral ala. The electrode is repositioned until the sacral contribution of the L5 posterior primary ramus is identified. If concordant pain is elicited with sensory stimulation, the electrode is gently manipulated until the minimum patient-blinded sensory stimulation voltage is obtained. Ideally, this should be in the 0.2- to 0.3-V range (Fig. 19–16). Care is taken during the sacral posterior rhizotomy procedure to make sure that the elicited stimulation covers only the areas of concordant pain; unintentional lesioning of closely related cutaneous branches often leads to the discomfort of postrhizotomy dysesthesias, cutaneous hyperalgesia, or numbness. The elicitation of paresthesia covering areas of pain, but not reproducing concordant pain, indicates localization of asymptomatic sensory branches at the anatomic level examined. Only branches that cause symptoms should be denervated.

Once the localization of any symptomatic branch has been confirmed with patient-blinded sensory stimulation, motor stimulation should be performed at 2 Hz at 0.8 to 1.0 V to minimize the likelihood that nearby motor branches to the gluteal musculature will be involved in the RF lesion. Before an RF lesion is generated, 1 mL of 2% lidocaine should be injected through the RF cannula to provide adequate local anesthesia during the lesioning process. Typically, RF lesioning applies 80° to 85° C for 60 sec.

The sensory branches at the levels of S1 (Fig. 19–17), S2 (Fig. 19–18), and S3 (Fig. 19–19) are approached in the following fashion. Under anteroposterior fluoroscopic imaging, the lateral aspect of the dorsal sacral foraminal apertures is visualized. Occasionally, slight oblique projections with cranial angulation of the imaging system may be required to visualize these faint structures. Initially, the blunt-tipped RF cannulas should be placed along the lateral aspect of the dorsal sacral foraminal aperture of interest, with the tip of the electrode just barely sliding into the foramen itself. Sensory stereotactic localization of the posterior primary rami branches innervating the posterior sacroiliac structures is then performed, the tip of the electrode being manipulated along the lateral arc of the dorsal sacral foraminal aperture until regional paresthesias are elicited or concordant pain is reproduced. The electrode is further manipulated until the sensory stimulation voltage required to reproduce concordant pain is at its minimum (0.2–0.4 V). The stimulation is then performed with the patient blinded, to eliminate bias. Motor stimulation is kept within the range of 0.8 and 1 V to make sure that no motor branches to the gluteal musculature will be involved in the lesion. The electrode *must not* rest within the dorsal

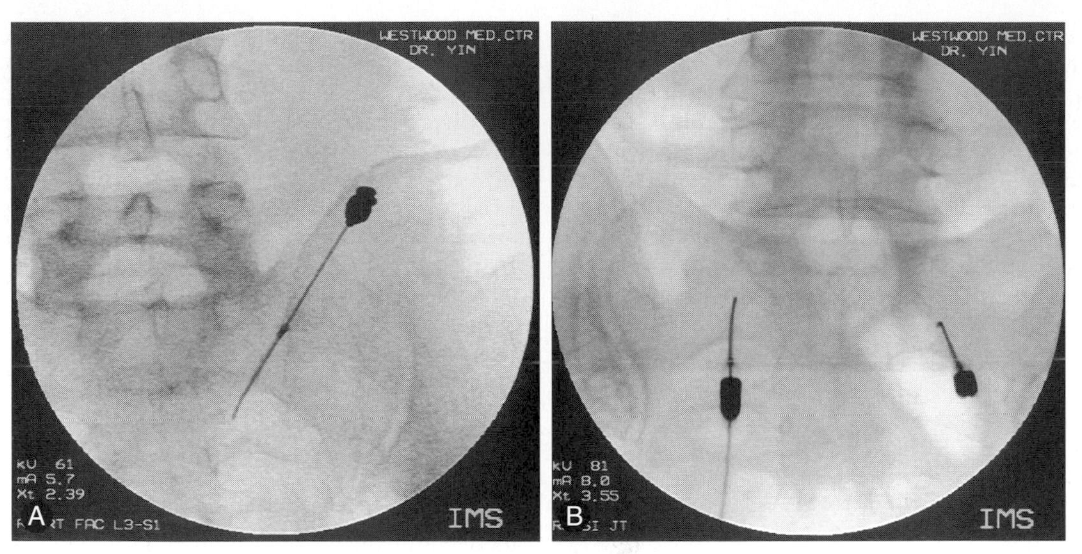

FIGURE 19–17 A, *AP image illustrates position of electrode for right S1 posterior primary ramus stereotactic lesion.* B, *AP image of different positions of S1 posterior primary ramus determined by sensory stereotaxy in bilateral sacroiliac joint denervation.*

foraminal apertures proper, lest unintentional lesioning of the sacral nerve roots or branches to the perineal, genital, or perianal regions results. When performing bilateral procedures, it is important to realize that the location of symptomatic posterior primary rami branches often is not symmetric, a finding that has been implicated in the wide variety of referred somatic pain patterns that accompany sacroiliac joint pain.[86] The posterior primary rami branches of S2 and S3 are similarly examined. The overwhelming majority of patients (90%–100%) with symptomatic sacroiliac joint complex pain will have identifiable symptomatic L5 and S1 posterior primary rami contributions. Approximately 60% to 70% have an identifiable contribution from S2, and approximately 30% to 40% have a significant S3 contribution.

Lumbar Discogenic Pain

Discogenic pain can occur in the absence of disc herniation or even obvious disc injury. Internal disruptions of a disc can appear entirely normal when studied by imaging methods.[87–89] Electromyographic studies frequently do not provide any specific diagnosis for an internally disrupted disc. In fact, persons with an internally disrupted disc can present with low back pain and referred lower extremity symptoms and may have normal findings on neurologic examination. Patients with lumbar discogenic pain frequently have a painful and biphasic deflexion maneuver, and the sitting, straight leg–raising examination produces low back pain. Sometimes, the only way to accurately identify a discogenic pain syndrome is with diagnostic disc injections. The sources of innervation within the disc annulus include the

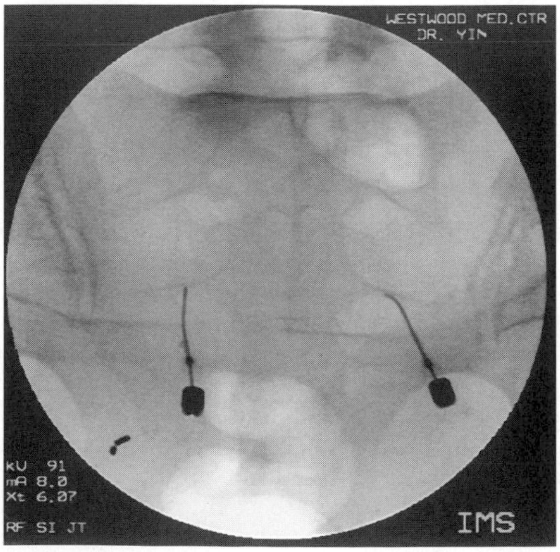

FIGURE 19–18 *AP radiograph illustrates bilateral electrode placement for S2 posterior primary ramus stereotactic lesion.*

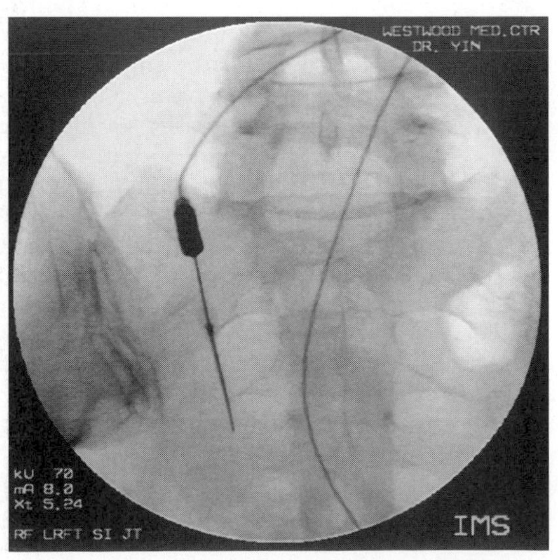

FIGURE 19–19 *AP radiograph illustrates electrode placement for S3 posterior primary ramus stereotactic lesion.*

sinuvertebral nerves, branches of the lumbar ventral rami, the gray ramus communicans, and branches of the sympathetic chain. The gray ramus communicans (ramus communicans nerve) is one of the targets for RF lesions. RF lesions of the ramus communicans nerve are particularly useful for treating pain emanating from the anterior and lateral aspects of the disc annulus.

Currently, RF techniques developed for the treatment of lumbar discogenic pain include RF lesions of the ramus communicans nerves as well as intradiscal RF lesions.[37, 90] More recently, the Intradiscal Electrothermal Annuloplasty (IDET) procedure has been developed as a specific means for treating lumbar discogenic pain.

Lesioning of the Ramus Communicans Nerve

Anatomic studies suggest that the ramus communicans nerve sends fibers to more than one level. Thus, if discography has shown that the L4–L5 disc is the painful level, then lesions of the ramus communicans nerves should be performed at L4 and L5.

The patient is first placed prone on the fluoroscopy table. The newer "curved-blunt" RF cannula should be considered for this procedure. It allows easier and more precise placement with less chance for trauma to the segmental nerves. Electrodes 150 mm long with 10-mm active tips are used. Alternatively, 22-gauge 150-mm SMK electrodes with 5-mm active tips may be used if the blunt electrodes are not available. The patient is monitored and given intravenous sedation but is kept awake enough to provide accurate verbal responses during the stimulation portion of the procedure.

At each level to be lesioned, the fluoroscopy unit should be directed craniad or caudad so that the disc is clearly visualized. That is, the end plates of the disc and the vertebral body should be clearly visualized. Oblique angulation at 15 to 25 degrees is used so that the body of the vertebra just covers the lateral tip of the transverse process. The ramus communicans nerve tends to run at the lower third of the vertebral body.

The skin and subcutaneous tissues overlying the entry points are anesthetized with 0.5% lidocaine. The RF cannula is introduced parallel to the fluoroscopy beam and is advanced until the periosteum at the lower third of the vertebral body is contacted. At this point, a lateral fluoroscopic view is taken, and the cannula is advanced until it is halfway between the anterior and posterior borders of the vertebral body. Direct contact with the periosteum should be maintained at all times. Once the cannula is properly positioned, electrical stimulation is applied; proper stimulation of the ramus communicans nerve produces a deep aching sensation in the back with 50-Hz stimulation at 1.0 V. Stimulation with 2 Hz at 2.5 V should fail to produce lower-extremity motor stimulation. If motor stimulation is seen, the tip of the RF cannula is too close to the lumbar nerve roots. A lesion should not be produced when the cannula tip is in such a position. The cannula should be moved slightly craniad, caudad, anteriorly, or posteriorly, until stimulation of the ramus communicans nerve can be made without stimulating the motor portion of the lumbar nerves. This usually requires only a small change in position. A 1-mL dose of 2% lidocaine is passed through the RF cannula, and a 60-sec delay is allowed for it to take effect. A thermal lesion is then created for 60 sec at 80° C. Lesions at the L4 and L5 ramus communicans nerves are made in similar fashion. Angulation of the fluoroscopy tube differs according to what level is being lesioned. The same theory, however, applies at all levels.

If the discogenic pain is unilateral, the ramus communicans lesions should be made only on the symptomatic side. If the pain is bilateral, ramus communicans lesions need to be made on both sides.

Lumbar Disc Procedure

Because the nerves within the disc annulus serve as the messengers for the pain signal leaving the disc, interruption of these fibers can lessen the symptoms of discogenic pain. Selective provocational or analgesic discography is critical for accurate diagnosis of lumbar discogenic pain. Discography must be done as a staging procedure before lesioning of the ramus communicans or the RF lumbar disc procedure. The RF lumbar disc procedure calls for the placement of a 150-mm cannula with a 10-mm active tip into the nucleus of the affected disc. A 6-min 85° C lesion is performed.

The patient is given preoperative antibiotics as prophylaxis against disc infection. The patient is placed prone on the fluoroscopy table, and the fluoroscopy unit is angled at 15 to 20 degrees from an oblique approach to correctly image the painful disc. The skin and subcutaneous tissues are anesthetized with lidocaine, and the RF cannula is advanced in a percutaneous manner until it contacts the disc annulus (just lateral to the inferior aspect of the superior articulating process). The cannula is passed into the disc and advanced until it enters the central aspect of the nucleus as seen by posteroanterior and lateral views. Electrical stimulation is checked at 2 Hz. If lower extremity motor fasciculations are negative at 2.5 V, it is safe to perform the lesion. No intradiscal local anesthetic is used. Reproduction of pain is usually noted but does not begin until 90 sec has passed. It will peak between the third and fourth minutes of the lesion process. Thermal equilibrium for this lesion requires at least 4 min, in distinct contrast to other types of RF lesions (Fig. 19–20).[91]

SEQUELAE AND COMPLICATIONS

Patients tend to have postoperative pain for 1 to 2 weeks after RF lesioning of the ramus communicans nerve or intradiscal RF lesioning. It is not unusual to develop mild dysesthesias that last 7 to 10 days. The vast majority of such dysesthesias resolve without complication within 3 weeks. In most patients, 2 to 4 weeks must pass before the full efficacy of the procedure can be determined.

Risks of the procedure include injury to the lumbar nerve roots with sensory or motor changes. The intradiscal RF lesion has the potential complication of postoperative disc infection; thus the use of prophylactic antibiotics. Occasionally, patients have significant postoperative pain and dysesthesias, and, once disc space infection has been ruled out, a 5- to 7-day course of oral steroid therapy is required. Disc infection is uncommon, but strict aseptic technique, including surgical scrub before the surgical skin prepara-

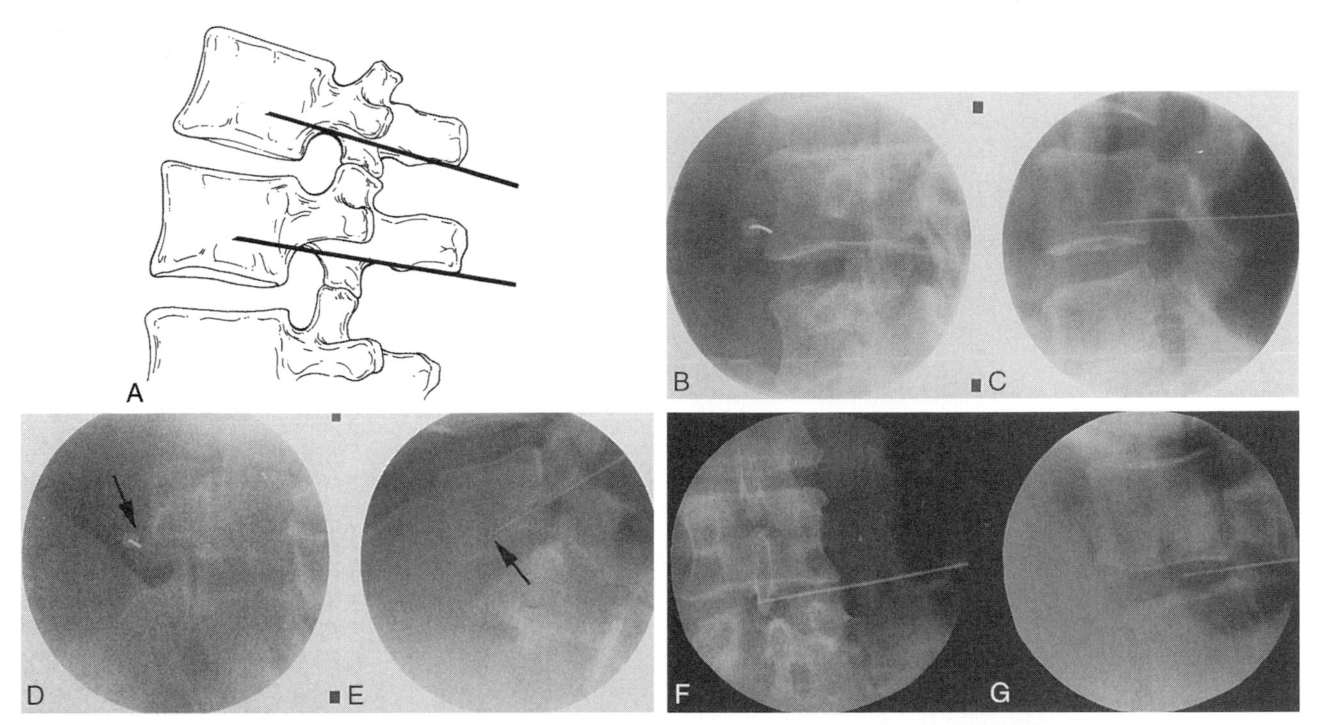

FIGURE 19–20 A, *Drawing of the cannula positions for lesions of the ramus communicans nerves.* B, *Oblique and* C, *lateral radiographs demonstrate RF cannula position for lesioning of the L4 ramus communicans nerve.* D, *Oblique and* E, *lateral views show the RF cannula position* (arrows) *for lesioning the L5 ramus communicans nerve.* F, *Posteroanterior and* G, *lateral radiographs show the RF cannula position for an intradiscal RF lesion.*

tion, plus preoperative antibiotic therapy, should be part of any intradiscal procedure.

Intradiscal Electrothermal Annuloplasty

A novel application of RF technology has been developed specifically for lumbar intradiscal lesioning. This system (SpineCATH Intradiscal Catheter, Oratec Interventions, Menlo Park, Calif.) differs significantly from existing intradiscal RF technologies. The length of the active lesioning thermocouple is nearly 6 cm and the diameter nearly 18 gauge. The system does not rely on ionic heating of the surrounding tissue; RF energy is used to generate heat through a resistive coil, in turn heating an insulating coating covering the thermocouple. Transfer of heat to surrounding tissue occurs through conduction rather than ionic heating. This mechanism of tissue heating is fundamentally different from traditional RF lesioning, where the electrode actually absorbs heat from the surrounding tissue. The heat lesion is controlled through a feedback bimetal thermistor at the end of the thermocouple. The thermocouple is also flexible, and to a certain extent "steerable" within the nucleus of the disc. The thermocouple is introduced into the disc through an introducer needle, which is not insulated. The advantages of this system over a rigid electrode include a significantly larger thermal lesion (the combination of larger thermocouple radius and length), the ability to direct the flexible thermocouple over a relatively large portion of the nuclear-annular boundary, and more consistent transannular heating.[32] Conductive intradiscal thermal lesioning may also be less dependent on the homogeneity of disc nuclear water content.

The Oratec SpineCATH system also differs fundamentally from traditional RF methods in that it has been designed for the single purpose of intradiscal heating. No sensory or motor stimulation is possible, as the system is internally grounded. The impedance measured by the system (120–200 ohms) is independent of surrounding tissue properties and is used to verify the electrical integrity of the resistive coil and surrounding insulation. The SpineCATH may be used only with an Oratec lesion generator and is not cross-compatible with other RF generators.

Mechanism of Action

In vitro and in vivo studies have demonstrated that outer annular temperatures of 40° to 45° C can be produced with the SpineCATH system. This temperature range should be sufficient to denervate annular nociceptive fibers, although permanent cell death may not follow axonal injury. Exposure of collagen to temperatures between 60° and 75° C results in disruption of intermolecular hydrogen bonds; this finding has been correlated with demonstrable shrinking of collagen molecules on electron microscopy. Intradiscal heating has been demonstrated in vitro to result in a 7% reduction in overall disc volume, although no in vivo studies have validated a long-term reduction in disc volume after IDET.

Theoretically, reduction in chronic discogenic pain by IDET may result from thermal denervation of annular nociceptive fibers (including chemically sensitized fibers), thermal remodeling of annular collagen, and, possibly, reduction in disc volume. The precise mechanism of action remains unclear, however. Maximum reduction in pain following IDET may not occur until 3 to 4 months after the procedure. A combination of varied physiologic processes in response to intradiscal thermal injury is most likely involved, including the inflammatory, proliferative, and fibrotic phases of normal wound healing.

Efficacy

Several clinical studies examining the IDET procedure have demonstrated promising results in patients suffering discogenic pain without radiculopathy. As with other interventional or surgical procedures, proper patient selection appears to be critical for success, in conjunction with a methodical, prolonged, graduated, postprocedure home-based rehabilitation and back exercise program. Patients with preserved intradiscal height appear more likely to benefit than patients with severe degenerative disease, and patients with previously operated discs and discogenic pain in levels adjacent to previous fusion may have poorer prognoses.[92] In one controlled study, 32 of 36 patients reported improvement in pain after IDET. Significant mean reductions in visual analogue pain scores were reported in this group (8/10 to 2.7/10), with concomitant reductions in supplemental opioid analgesic requirements and improvements in disability scores as compared with conservative care.[93] Long-term follow-up studies are in progress, and the duration of benefit in early-phase long-term follow-up studies is promising.[94]

For patients with discogenic pain without radiculopathy, IDET may present a very attractive, less invasive alternative to lumbar discectomy and fusion.

Lumbar

The patient is placed in the prone position on the fluoroscopy table. The back is prepared with antiseptic solution as for discography; it is recommended that a formal surgical "prep" be performed. Preoperative antibiotics may be administered intravenously. The patient may be lightly sedated but must be easily aroused, responsive to voice, and able to report pain during the procedure. The physician dons sterile gown and gloves, and meticulous aseptic technique is observed throughout.

Posterior lateral oblique fluoroscopic images are obtained, and the target disc is identified. Oblique projections, with cephalad angulation as required, are obtained so that the lateral border of the superior articular process overlaps the middle of the target disc in anteroposterior and lateral dimensions (35–50 degrees), and the inferior and superior end plates of the adjoining vertebral bodies are distinct. A skin entry site is marked over the lateral aspect of the superior articular process overlying the target disc and anesthetized with buffered lidocaine. A 1.25-inch 14-gauge intravenous catheter introduced through the skin and Scarpa's fascia greatly facilitates the subsequent introduction of the styleted SpineCATH 17-gauge introducer needle and preserves a modified two-needle approach to the disc. Before the 17-gauge needle is introduced, a 22-gauge, 5-inch spinal needle may be used to inject a small amount (0.5 mL) of lidocaine over the sensitive periosteum of the superior articular process.

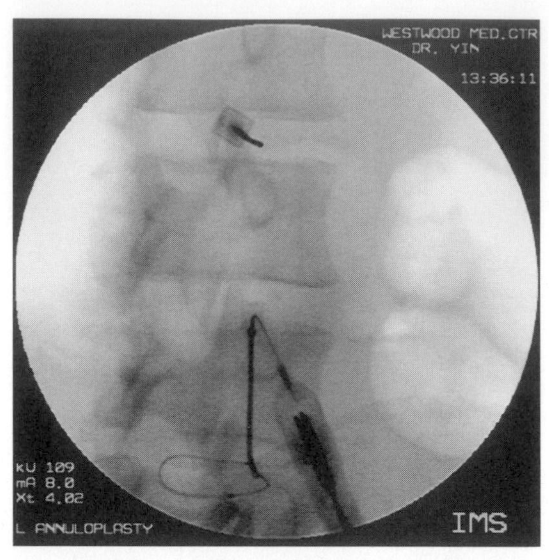

FIGURE 19–21 Oblique radiograph demonstrates intradiscal placement of introducer needle in L2–L3 disc. Note presence of SpineCATH in L4–L5 disc, ready for intradiscal lesion.

The 17-gauge introducer needle may be gently curved to facilitate steering, although this may be necessary only at the L5–S1 level in most patients. The introducer needle is advanced through the 14-gauge intravenous catheter under posterior oblique fluoroscopic guidance toward the lateral aspect of the superior articular process overlapping the target disc. Care is taken to remain close to the lateral aspect of the superior articular process, medial to the ipsilateral exiting nerve root at that level (Fig. 19–21). The disc is entered along its posterolateral margin, and the needle is advanced slightly ventrally. In contrast to discography, the ideal introducer needle position is not in the center of the disc. The introducer needle should lie in the posterolateral quadrant of the disc, ipsilateral to the annular entry site (Fig. 19–22). Multiplanar fluoroscopic images are taken throughout the needle insertion process. The

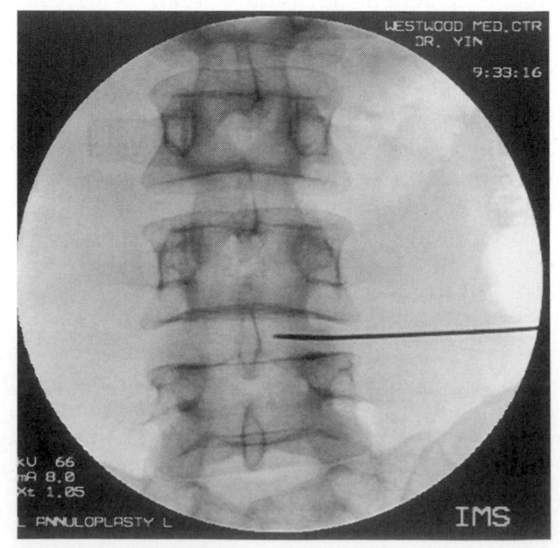

FIGURE 19–22 AP radiograph illustrates introducer needle placed in superolateral quadrant of L4–L5 disc.

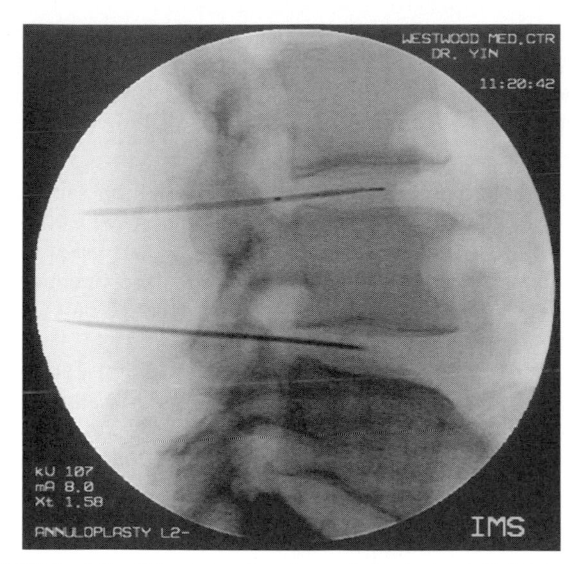

FIGURE 19–23 *Lateral radiograph illustrates initial SpineCATH insertion. Note that proximal heating element marker is visible within the introducer needle.*

bevel of the introducer needle is then turned toward the center of the disc, and the stylet removed. The Spine CATH heating element is then introduced through the introducer needle; placing a gentle curve in the catheter may facilitate intradiscal placement along the nuclear-annular boundary. A small volume of local anesthetic with antibiotic may be injected into the nucleus of the disc before placing the heating element (e.g., 0.5 mL of 0.5% bupivacaine with 4–30 mg/mL of cefazolin).

Under anteroposterior and lateral fluoroscopic imaging, the heating element is carefully directed across the midline of the disc, and around the periphery of the posterior lateral and posterior inner annulus (Figure 19–23). Care is taken to make sure that the heating element does not penetrate the disc annulus; extradiscal positioning of the element may result in thermal lesioning or other injury to the spinal cord or nerve roots, with catastrophic consequences. In severely disrupted discs, the heating element may be passed through the annulus without significant resistance, underscoring the importance of obtaining frequent multiplanar fluoroscopic views during catheter advancement (Fig. 19–24A). Ideally positioned, the active portion of the heating element spans the posterolateral disc from pedicle to pedicle (Fig. 19–24B).

Once proper placement of the intradiscal heating element has been verified with multiplanar fluoroscopy, the radiopaque markers denoting the length of active tip of the heating element should span the target lesion zone, ideally from pedicle to pedicle. Incomplete coverage of the posterior disc annulus has prompted some clinicians to advocate a bilateral approach with a second lesion performed if necessary. Repositioning of the catheter has been associated with kinking of the catheter and with damage to its insulation; either situation requires that the catheter be removed and replaced. Before heat lesioning, the proximal portion of the active heating element must *not* be in contact with the distal end of the introducer needle.

Once the SpineCATH is acceptably positioned and correct system impedence and thermistor function are verified, intradiscal heating is performed. Temperature guidelines have been recommended by the manufacturer, and involve incremental (1° C) increases from 65° to 80° or 90° C over a period of 14 to 17 min. The procedure is generally tolerated well; complaints of severe back pain or lower extremity pain should prompt cessation of heating and reevaluation of catheter position and catheter integrity. Occasional complaints of leg pain, sometimes extending below the knee, may reflect referred pain of disc origin (as

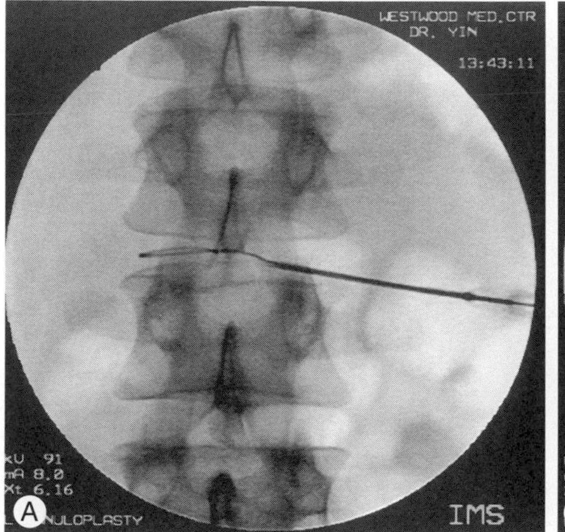

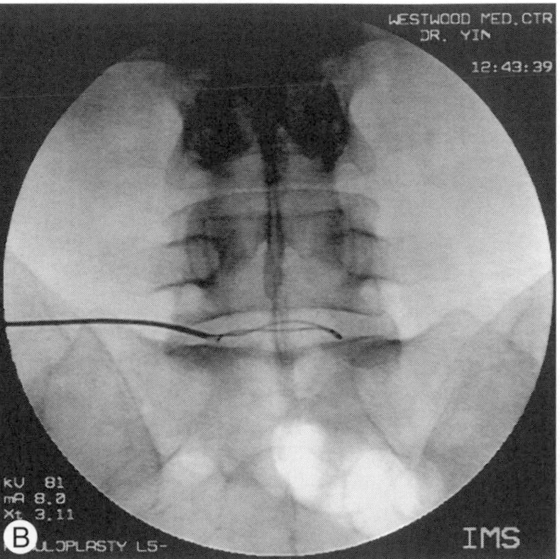

FIGURE 19–24 *A, AP radiograph illustrates nearly complete intradiscal placement of L3–L4 SpineCATH. Note distal heating element marker is only at midline; in its final position, the active portion of heating element will extend from pedicle to pedicle. B, Final positioning of SpineCATH heating element within L5–S1 disc. Note pedicle-to-pedicle placement of active element of catheter spanning the posterior nuclear-annular boundary.*

opposed to direct thermal stimulation of the nerve root), and have been correlated with increasing intradiscal thermal stimulation intensity.[93] Before intradiscal catheter placement, 0.5 mL of 0.5% bupivacaine may be injected through the introducer needle into the disc to enhance the patient's comfort.

SEQUELAE AND COMPLICATIONS

Reported complications from IDET have been rare. In skilled hands, complications will likely remain few, but the number of technical and infectious complications may increase as the technology is more variously applied. Many patients experience exacerbation of back pain, and some may experience radicular symptoms after IDET. Putatively, this pain corresponds with the inflammatory phase of thermal injury and may represent sterile discitis. Most cases respond to activity limitations, NSAID therapy, and opioid analgesia. With severe exacerbations of back or leg pain after the procedure, careful evaluation should be performed for epidural hematoma, abscess, and infectious discitis. If no infectious cause is suspected and no other complication is evident, intravenous or oral "pulse dose" steroid therapy may be effective. Persistent pain may be treated with lesion-specific epidural or transforaminal steroid injection.

Thoracic

Treatment of thoracic discogenic pain remains problematic. Results of open or thoracoscopic video-assisted thoracic discectomy and fusion are less than encouraging. Intradiscal thermal lesioning may be a tantalizing, minimally invasive alternative to surgical thoracic discectomy and fusion. Although no clinical studies have addressed the efficacy or safety of IDET or other intradiscal RF lesioning techniques for the treatment of thoracic discogenic pain, a case report is presented in the hope of stimulating further research in this area.

CASE REPORT: THORACIC INTRADISCAL ELECTROTHERMAL LESION FOR INTRACTABLE THORACIC DISCOGENIC PAIN WITH THORACIC RADICULOPATHY (WY).

A 49-year-old man with a 20-year history of intractable and progressively disabling midthoracic pain radiating to the left flank with torsional movement of the trunk had failed to derive benefit from a comprehensive array of conventional, noninterventional modalities of therapy over the past 2 decades. An exhaustive evaluation revealed no intraabdominal or thoracic visceral abnormalities. Cardiology and gastroenterology evaluations revealed no disease. Plain films of his thoracic spine were unremarkable, and magnetic resonance imaging (MRI) of the dorsal spine revealed central and right-sided disc protrusion without extruded fragment at the T7–T8 level. Two separate sets of thoracic epidural and foraminal low-volume steroid injections provided reproducible, nearly complete (85%–90%) relief of his midthoracic and radiating flank pain but of limited duration (3 weeks), without incremental improvement. Selective provocative thoracic discography revealed multiple morphologic derangements of the thoracic discs at all levels from T6 to T10. Left-sided contrast extravasation through an annular tear outlining the left T6 nerve root was visualized at T6–T7, but no pain was reproduced with contrast injection (peak 60 psi). The disc protrusion at the T7–T8 level seen on MRI was not observed on discography, and no symptoms were reproduced with intradiscal injection, although a left lateral annular tear was present with extravasation of contrast outlining the left T7 nerve root (peak 120 psi). At the T8–T9 level, a clear posterior lateral annular tear was visualized during injection (120 peak psi), with extravasation of contrast circumferentially outlining the left-sided nerve roots of T8 and T9 (Fig. 19–25). Precise reproduction of the patient's concordant pain was reproduced despite the lack of clear disc protrusion or herniation. Epidural extravasation

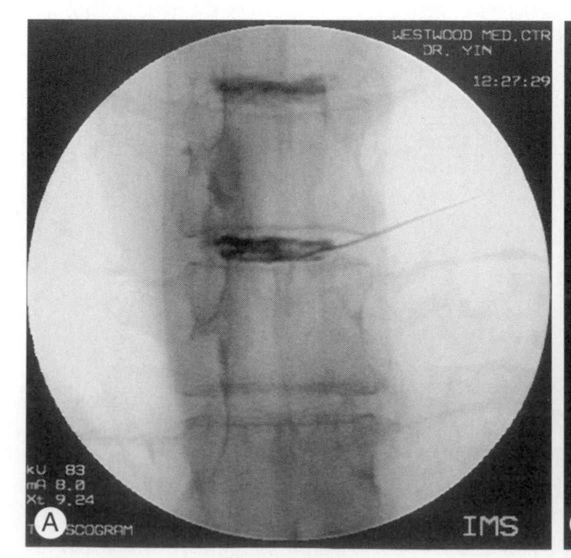

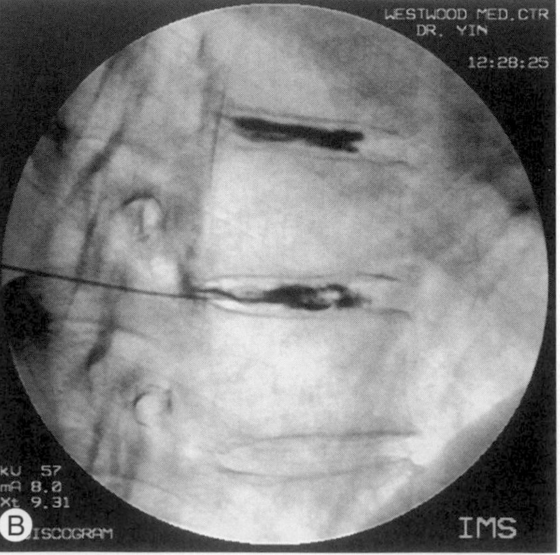

FIGURE 19–25 *A, Anteroposterior radiograph of T8–T9 provocative discography. B, Lateral radiographs of T8–T9 provocative discography. Note clearly visible left posterior lateral annular fissure and extravasation of contrast outlining left T8 and T9 nerve roots and lateral epidural space.*

of contrast through a clearly defined right posterolateral disc bulge was visualized on injection of the T9–T10 disc (peak 60 psi); however, this injection did not elicit any pain.

The patient was referred for surgical consultation. After discussing the risks and potential benefits of open and thoracoscopic thoracic discectomy and fusion with the surgeon, the patient declined surgical intervention. He continued to work full time as the president of his own oil exploration services company.

Alternative options were discussed in detail with the patient. The possibility of performing a thoracic intradiscal annuloplasty procedure was discussed, along with the experimental nature of this particular application of the technology. A detailed discussion of the potential risks associated with the procedure, both known and unknown, ensued. After thorough consideration of his available options, the patient elected to proceed with IDET at the T8–T9 level.

A right-sided modified posterior parasagittal curved cannula technique was employed and entry gained into the target disc without pain or technical difficulty. A precurved SpineCATH catheter was inserted into the T8–T9 disc without difficulty, and the active tip was oriented to completely cover the area of the annular tear. A 90° C intradiscal lesion was created without intraoperative complications (Fig. 19–26). (Owing to the smaller size of the thoracic disc, the needle was withdrawn 3 mm to gain adequate clearance from the active proximal portion of the heating element.) The patient tolerated the procedure well, had no evidence of pneumothorax or other complication on postoperative chest films, and was discharged home the same day.

In postoperative follow-up, the patient reported mild worsening of his pain after the procedure. Two weeks after the procedure he felt that his pain had been reduced approximately 50% and reported complete resolution of his

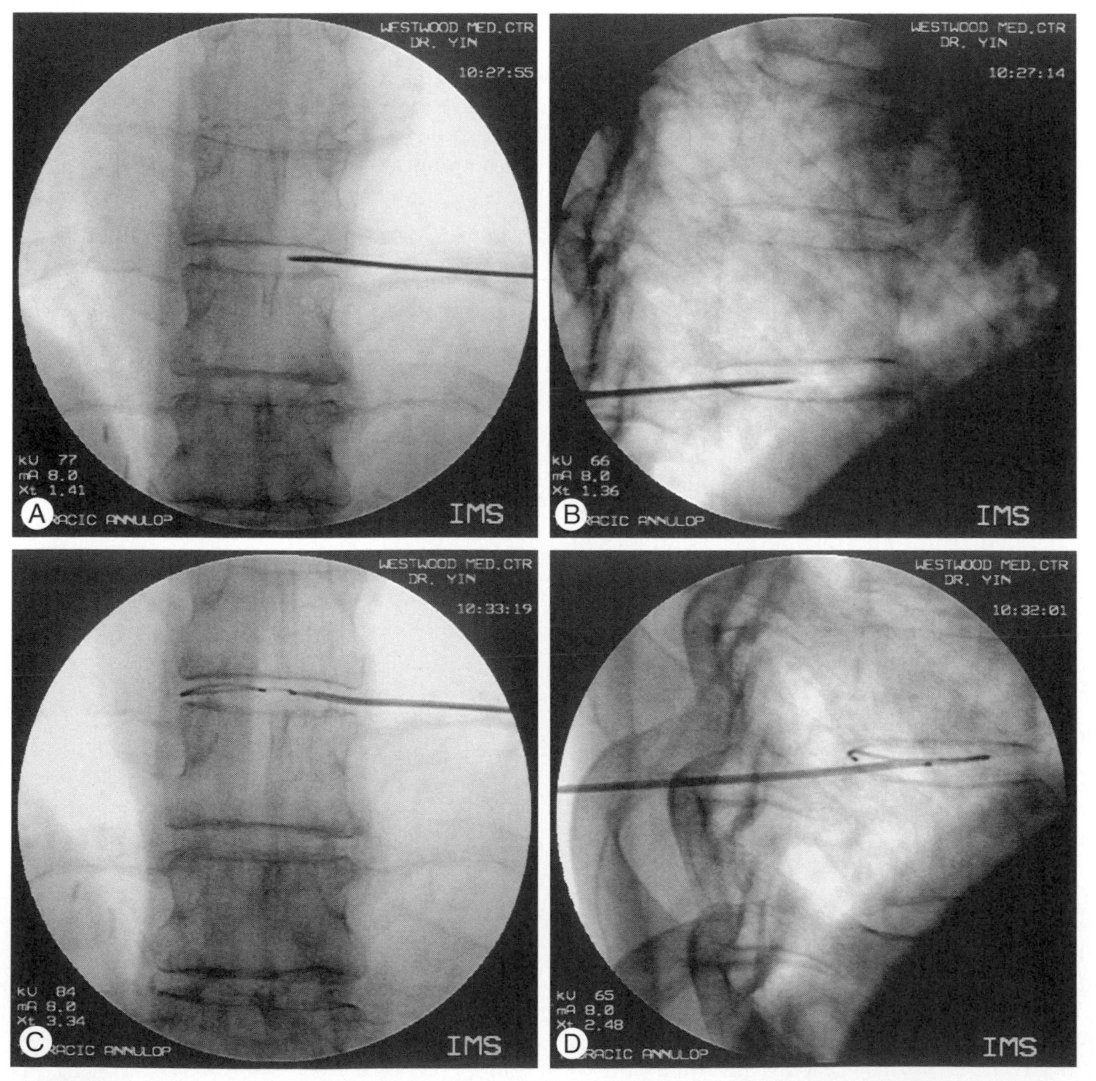

FIGURE 19–26 *A, Anteroposterior radiograph of T8–T9 IDET introducer needle placement. B, Lateral radiographs of T8–T9 IDET introducer needle placement. C, Anteroposterior radiograph illustrates SpineCATH placement for T8–T9 intradiscal thermal lesion. D, Lateral radiograph illustrates final SpineCATH placement for thermal lesion of left posterior lateral T8–9 annular fissure. Note that introducer needle has been withdrawn 3 mm to clear proximal marker of heating electrode.*

thoracic radicular symptoms. He complained of mild burning pain in the midback region. His subsequent recovery was unremarkable, with incremental improvement reported at 6 week postprocedure follow-up. Four months after thoracic IDET, the patient reported greater than 75% subjective improvement in his thoracic pain, with a corresponding decrease in his VAS from 8/10 to 2/10. Although not completely eliminated, the patient's back pain was markedly improved, and he was extremely pleased with the outcome.

Dorsal Root Ganglionotomy

RF dorsal root ganglion lesioning is useful for pain emanating from the lumbar spinal nerves.[33,37,38,58,95] This procedure is reserved for patients who have failed more conservative interventional treatments and for whom open surgical intervention is not an option. If prognostic blocks of the posterior column (facet joints) and the anterior column (disc) are negative and if the pain predominantly involves the lower extremity, diagnostic sleeve blocks of the segmental nerve roots are indicated. Although disease of the segmental lumbar nerves does not cause back pain *per se*, injuries to the segmental nerves are commonly associated with other injuries in the lumbar spine. Back pain is usually a direct result of mechanical abnormalities of the lumbar spine, but it is not uncommon for a patient to suffer from combined mechanical symptoms and radiculopathy. Under these circumstances, it is important to determine whether the practitioner is dealing with a problem that represents mechanical pain with referred mechanical symptoms or lower extremity symptoms due to disease of the spinal nerves.

Once the diagnosis of referred mechanical pain in the lower extremities has been excluded, the practitioner needs to explore the role of the segmental spinal nerves and the sympathetic nervous system. Diagnostic blocks of the spinal nerves and the sympathetic nerves must be performed to distinguish between radiculopathy and sympathetically maintained pain. The distinction is important because the treatments differ. Once the appropriate diagnostic blocks have been performed, however, the practitioner is in a position to treat the segmental nerve problems with a dorsal root ganglion lesion.

Lumbar Ganglionotomy

Lumbar ganglionotomy is usually performed using a 150-mm cannula with a 5-mm active tip. The cannula is passed percutaneously toward the vertebral body (just inferior to the transverse process). As the cannula approaches the vertebral body, a lateral fluoroscopic view is taken to ensure that the foramen is clearly visualized. The cannula is directed toward the dorsal and superior quadrant of the foramen and is advanced until it passes beneath the transverse process into the superior, dorsal quadrant of the foramen. A direct posteroanterior view is taken, and the cannula is advanced until it reaches the midpoint of the respective facet joint line. A repeat lateral view is taken to make certain that the cannula still resides within the superior, dorsal quadrant of the foramen. With the cannula in this position, stimulation is performed, and satisfactory paresthesia into the leg (along the dermatome that is affected) should be noted at less than 1.0 V with 50-Hz stimulation. If stimulation is noted at less than 0.3 V, the cannula should be repositioned, because it is too close to the ganglion and postoperative neuritis could result. Ideal stimulation is between 0.4 and 0.7 V at 50-Hz stimulation. Sensory stimulation should be done in increments of 0.1 V to avoid unnecessary pain. Stimulation is then performed at 2 Hz. There should be a clear dissociation between motor and sensory stimulation; that is, the voltage required to see motor fasciculations in the lower extremity at 2 Hz should be at least two times the voltage that produces sensory stimulation in the lower extremity at 50 Hz. Thus, if good sensory stimulation at 50 Hz was noted at 0.5 V, motor fasciculations at 2 Hz should not be seen at voltages less than 1.0 V. The point of dissociation defines the position of the dorsal root ganglion. If dissociation between sensory and motor stimulation cannot be obtained, the cannula is not aligned with the dorsal root ganglion and lesioning is not advisable.

Once correct dissociation has been obtained, 1 mL of 2% lidocaine is passed onto the ganglion. A 10-min delay is allowed for the anesthetic to work, and a thermal lesion is created at a temperature between 60° and 65° C, depending on the stimulation threshold. The lower the stimulation threshold, the lower the temperature should be. The lesion is maintained for 60 sec (Fig. 19–27).

Sacral Dorsal Root Ganglionotomy

Once the prognostic blocks have been performed and the painful level has been identified, the patient is brought back for a dorsal root ganglion lesion. It is useful to give the patient a bowel preparation the day before, because bowel gas sometimes obscures the sacral foraminal openings. This practice is particularly useful for clinicians who are relatively new at performing these procedures.

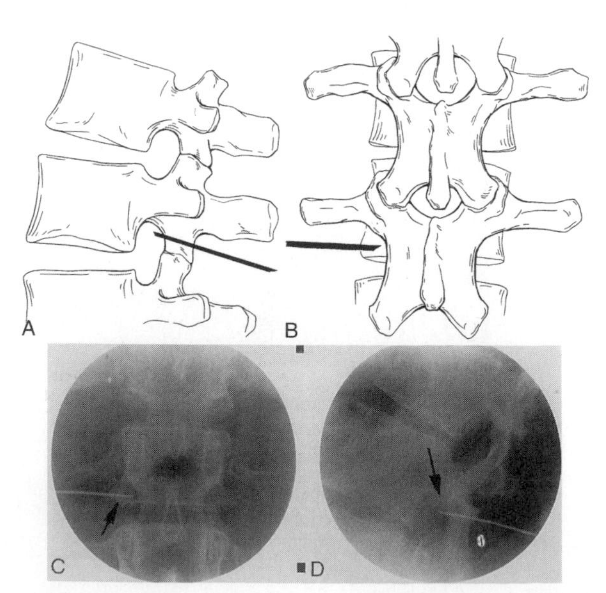

FIGURE 19–27 *Lumbar ganglionotomy.* A, *Lateral and* B, *posteroanterior views of the cannula position for a lumbar ganglionotomy procedure.* C, *Posteroanterior and* D, *lateral views demonstrate the RF cannula position* (arrows) *for a lumbar ganglionotomy procedure.*

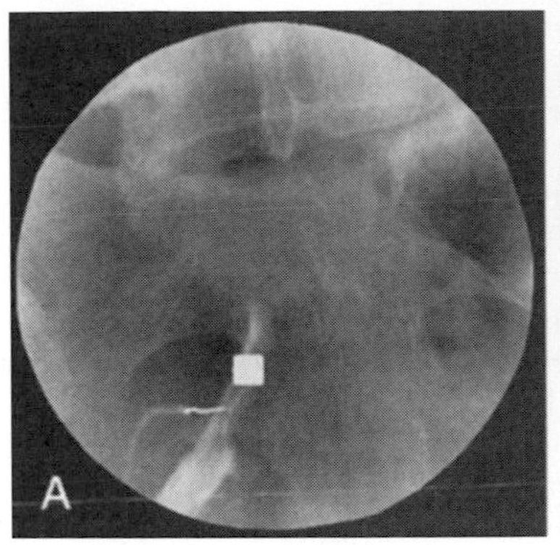

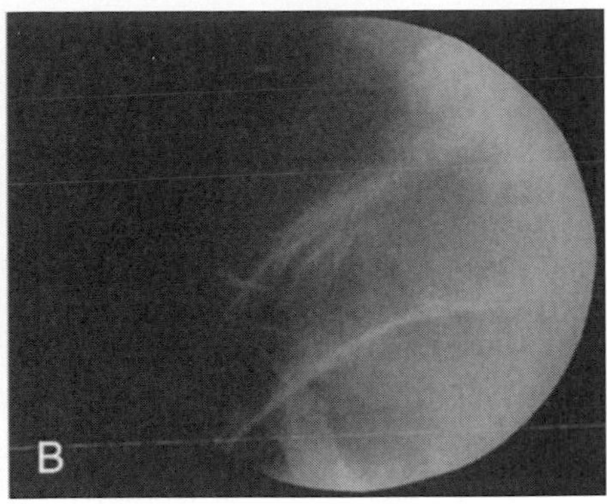

FIGURE 19–28 S2 ganglionotomy procedure. A, Posteroanterior radiograph. The introducer cannula overlies the outline of the S2 root sleeve. The introducer cannula is seen in the middle of the root sleeve. The fine needle is the introducer needle used to inject the root sleeve with contrast material. B, Lateral view through the sacrum. The lower needle has been passed through the sacral foramina onto the peripheral aspect of the nerve for injection of contrast material. The upper needle is the RF cannula, which has been passed through the burr hole to rest over the S2 ganglion.

The S1 and S2 nerves are commonly affected. The S5 ganglionotomy is very useful for the treatment of chronic coccygeal pain.

The S1 and S2 ganglionotomy procedures are performed in a similar fashion. The S1 technique is performed by passing a needle through the S1 foraminal opening adjacent to the nerve. Contrast material is injected to outline the S1 root sleeve. The authors prefer to use Omnipaque 240 water-soluble contrast material for all procedures. A point halfway between the S1 foraminal opening and the craniad border of the sacrum, which intersects the sacral root sleeve, is chosen, and a burr hole is made through the plates of the posterior sacrum. The burr hole is created with a K wire and a small pneumatic drill.

The S2 dorsal root ganglion resides halfway between the S1 and S2 foraminal openings, where the halfway point intersects the S2 nerve. It is mandatory that an accurate outline of the respective root sleeve be seen, so that the K wire can be passed through the sacrum directly over the dorsal root ganglion.

Once the burr hole has been created and the RF cannula has been passed into the sacral canal (directly over the dorsal root ganglion), stimulation can be performed. The cannula should have a 5-mm active tip. Dissociation between sensory and motor stimulation should be obtained. The stimulation and dissociation parameters are identical to those described earlier for lumbar ganglionotomy. It is desirable to have good stimulation at 50 Hz between 0.4 and 0.7 V. Lesioning temperatures are between 60° and 65° C, and the duration is 60 sec. After lesioning, 40 mg of triamcinolone is injected through the cannula to lessen the postoperative pain (Fig. 19–28).

S5 DORSAL ROOT GANGLIONOTOMY

Dorsal root ganglion lesioning of the S5 nerves can be useful in the management of coccydynia. Coccydynia may or may not be associated with trauma and is commonly difficult to treat. Many patients continue to experience pain even if the coccyx is removed. Because the coccyx is innervated by the S5 nerves, lesions of the S5 ganglia can be useful in treating this difficult problem. If a patient is experiencing pain on both sides of the coccyx, bilateral S5 lesions must be made. The S5 ganglion lies behind the sacrum at a level 1 cm inferior to the S2 foraminal opening, along the *midline* of the sacrum. A point approximately 1 cm caudal to the S2 foraminal opening and approximately 2 mm lateral to the midline of the sacrum is chosen as the entry site. No contrast material is used for this procedure.

The skin and subcutaneous tissues are anesthetized over the entry point. An introducer is passed through the tissues until it touches the periosteum 1 cm caudal to the S2 foraminal opening and 2 mm lateral to the midline of the sacrum. A K wire is passed through the introducer, and a burr hole is created through the posterior sacrum under direct fluoroscopic guidance. An RF cannula with a 5-mm active tip is passed through the introducer into the canal over the S5 ganglion (Fig. 19–29). Stimulation is performed, and response should be noted between 0.4 and 1.0 V at 50 Hz. It should be felt *directly* in the area of the coccyx. To check for motor fasciculations, the clinician

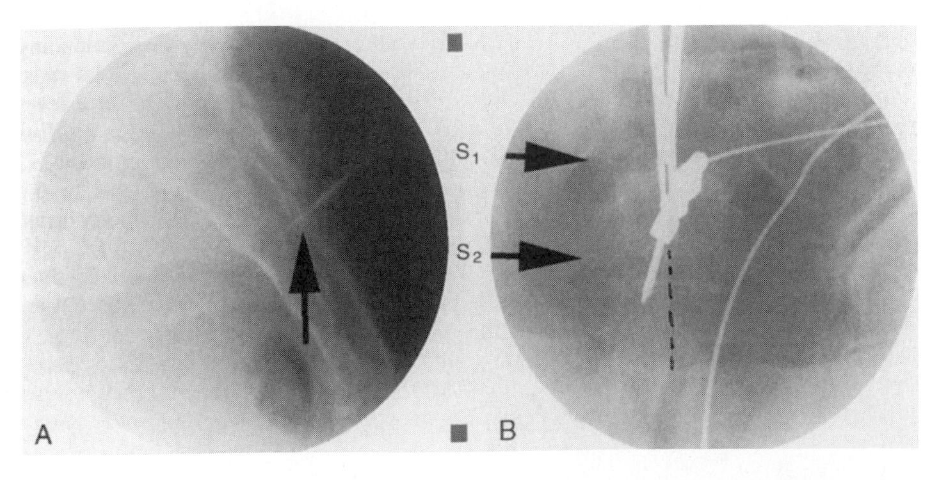

FIGURE 19–29 Radiographs of S5 ganglionotomy procedure. A, Lateral view through the sacrum. The tip of the radiofrequency cannula (arrow) has been passed through the posterior aspect of the sacrum via a burr hole. B, Posteroanterior view. Note that the introducer cannula is just lateral to the medial border of the sacrum (dashed line) and 1 cm inferior to the S2 foraminal opening. (Note that the foramina are marked S1 and S2.)

should gently place a finger in the external sphincter of the patient's anus. When motor stimulation is performed at 2 Hz, contractions of the external sphincter of the anus should not be noted at twice the sensory stimulation. If motor stimulation of the external sphincter is noted at lower thresholds, the cannula is too close to the S4 ganglion and needs to be repositioned in a more *medial* direction, since the S4 ganglion is just a few millimeters lateral to the S5 ganglion. After proper dissociation between S5 and S4 stimulation has been demonstrated, 1 mL of 2% lidocaine is passed onto the ganglion, and 5 min is allowed to pass. A thermal lesion is then created at a temperature between 60° and 65° C, depending on the level of stimulation. The duration of the lesion is 60 sec. After the lesion has been created, 40 mg of triamcinolone is passed onto the lesion site. If the patient has bilateral coccygeal pain, the contralateral S5 dorsal root ganglion lesion should be performed 4 weeks later, if no complications are apparent after the initial lesion.

Sacral Dorsal Root Ganglion Lesion, Curved Cannula Approach

A curved electrode approach toward RF sacral dorsal root ganglion lesion may be performed as an alternative to the burr hole rhizotomy. The curved cannula technique is more technically demanding than the burr hole approach but is particularly applicable to the S1 and S2 levels. A theoretical advantage of the curved cannula technique is that it places a relatively larger section of the active electrode (2–5 mm) adjacent to the target nerve tissue. The curved electrode approach is also associated with less postoperative discomfort than the burr hole approach. A more pronounced continuous curve is placed over the distal 2 to 2.5 cm of the electrode at an angle of approximately 20 to 30 degrees. The patient is placed in the prone position on the fluoroscopic table. A posterior oblique approach is made under fluoroscopic guidance through the dorsal sacral foraminal aperture, with the electrode guided along the dorsal aspect of the foramen until the tip lies over the region of the dorsal root ganglion. A high-quality contrast study is mandatory to outline the silhouette of the selected nerve root and the swelling of the dorsal root ganglion utilizing nonionic contrast medium (e.g., iohexol, 240 mg/mL). Visualization of the dorsal root ganglion is essential to facilitate placement of the electrode adjacent to it. Sensory stereotactic stimulation at 0.15 to 0.2 V is performed until concordant pain or paresthesias are reproduced over the target somatic region. At these sensory stimulation thresholds, motor stimulation should be absent at 0.5 to 0.7 V (2 Hz, 1 msec pulse duration). It is important to maintain sensory and motor dissociation to minimize the risk of motor nerve injury.

Recent developments in RF generator design have permitted the delivery of RF energy with a high concentration of heat. These design modifications allow the delivery of lower temperature RF lesions while maintaining relatively high current and voltage. The precise relationships between these variables and their effects on the ultimate clinical outcome remain unclear. However, in the authors' experience, the creation of lower-temperature lesions for sensitive procedures such as dorsal root ganglion and gasserian rhizotomy appears to significantly decrease the risk of postprocedure neuritis while preserving the desired beneficial clinical outcome.

For selective partial dorsal root ganglion rhizotomy, a high verniation lesion at a temperature of 50° to 54° C is performed for 120 to 240 sec. Selective sensory stereotaxy and subsequent sacral dorsal root ganglion lesioning has been invaluable for the treatment of rare intractable buttock region pain (S2) and the elimination of acetabular pain after total hip arthroplasty (S1; Fig. 19–30).

Risks of this procedure include postoperative neuritis, motor dysfunction, and sensory loss over the superficial cutaneous distributions of the targeted nerve root. Owing to the potential for these sequelae, meticulous attention must be paid to radiologic, stereotactic stimulation, and technical parameters.

Thoracic Dorsal Root Ganglionotomy

In the thoracic region, a dorsal root ganglionotomy can be performed in a manner similar to that for the ganglionotomy technique in the lumbar region. The dorsal root ganglion in the thoracic region lies in the superior dorsal quadrant of the foramina (at a point halfway across the line

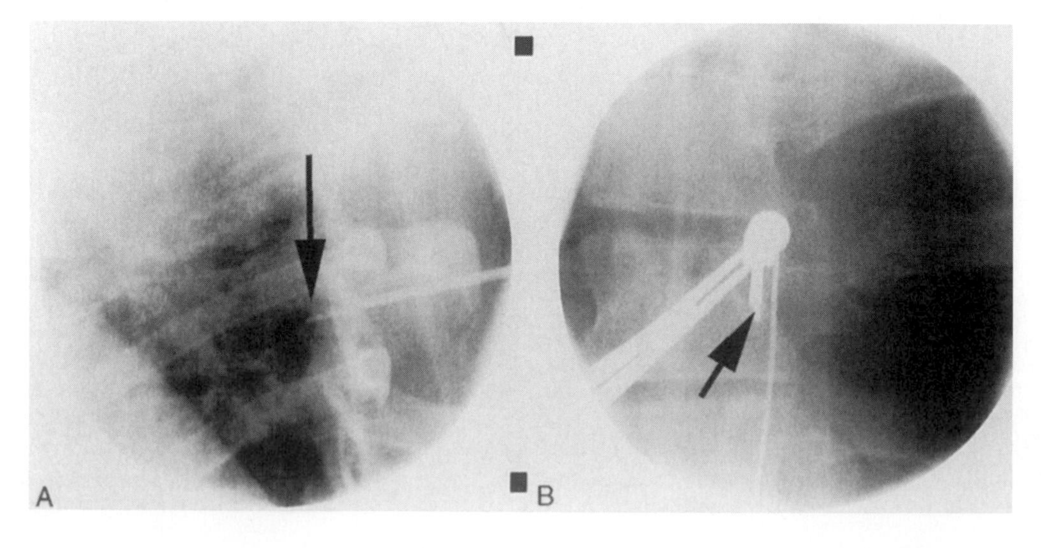

FIGURE 19–30 A, Oblique imaging of right S1 curved electrode approach for dorsal root ganglion lesion. B, Right S1 contrast study outlining distal DRG at initiation of sensory stereotaxy.

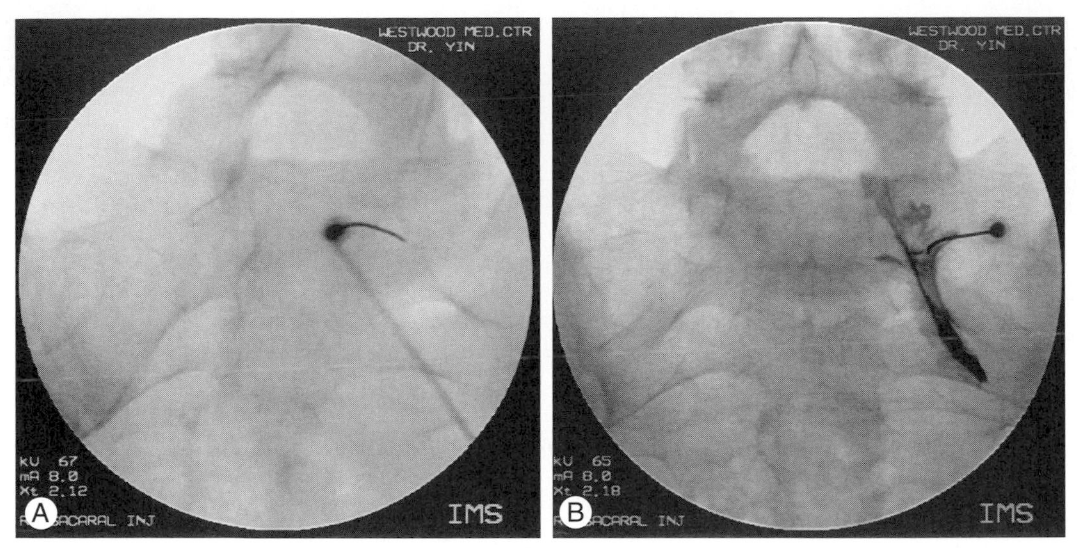

FIGURE 19–31 A, *Lateral radiograph shows cannula position* (arrow) *for a thoracic ganglionotomy.* B, *A burr hole through the thoracic lamina* (arrow) *allows the RF cannula to be passed into the thoracic foramen.*

of the pedicle). At the lower levels, it is possible to utilize an approach identical to that described for the lumbar region. The cannula position, stimulation, and lesion parameters are the same.

In the higher thoracic regions, the pleura can be injured when an oblique approach is used. Thus, in the upper thoracic regions, it is recommended that a burr hole be placed through the lamina at a point directly over the midpoint of the pedicle as seen on a posteroanterior view and over the dorsal and superior foramina as seen on a lateral view. Proper mediolateral orientation is rechecked with a posteroanterior view. This approach allows access through the burr hole to the dorsal and superior foraminal quadrant where the ganglion resides.

A repeat lateral fluoroscopic view is checked to make certain that the cannula lies within the superior dorsal quadrant of the foramina. An RF cannula with a 5-mm active tip is used and is passed through the burr hole into proper position. Stimulation is identical to that for the lumbar ganglionotomy procedure. Once appropriate stimulation with dissociation between sensory and motor function has been obtained, the dorsal root ganglion is anesthetized and a lesion is made in a manner identical to that described for the lumbar ganglionotomy (Fig. 19–31).

Thoracic Dorsal Root Ganglionotomy: Parasagittal Approach

A modification of a posterior parasagittal curved-electrode approach may be utilized as an alternative to the burr hole technique for thoracic dorsal root ganglion lesion. *It must be emphasized that both approaches, like other procedures outlined in this chapter, carry significant potential for morbidity in inexperienced hands. The risks of the burr hole laminotomy approach parallel those of an open procedure performed with an operating microscope, without allowing direct visualization of relevant anatomic structures, and the curved-electrode approach carries the additional potential for pneumothorax and other visceral, vascular, or neural injuries.*

As for the sacral curved-electrode approach, the patient is placed in the prone position on the fluoroscopy table. A pronounced curve is placed over the distal 2 to 2.5 cm of the electrode; typically a 100-mm, 2-mm active tip SMK electrode is chosen.

A skin entry site is marked approximately 2 cm lateral to the junction between the inferior medial aspect of the thoracic transverse process and the lamina of the target spinal level. Under anteroposterior fluoroscopic imaging, the electrode is advanced in such a manner that the tip contacts the lateral aspect of the lamina at its junction with the inferior medial border of the transverse process. The electrode is then carefully advanced just deep to the lateral border of the lamina, toward the region overlying the exiting thoracic nerve root, making sure that the tip of the electrode remains dorsal to the exiting nerve root (Fig. 19–32). Once the electrode has been advanced into the

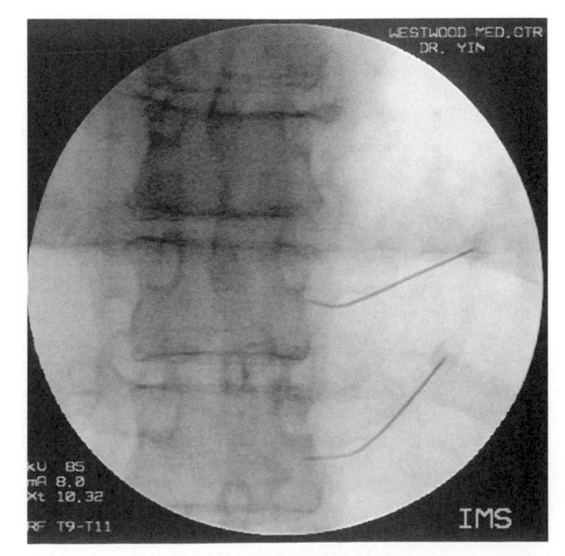

FIGURE 19–32 AP image illustrates posterior parasagittal curved electrode approach toward right T8 and T9 dorsal root ganglia.

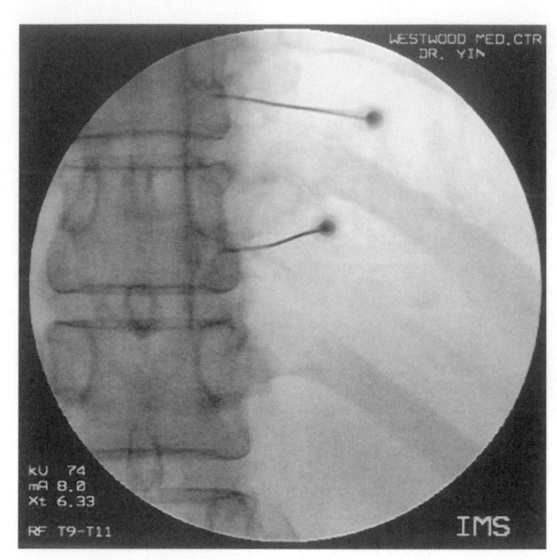

FIGURE 19–33 *AP image of contrast study outlining the right thoracic dorsal root ganglion and adjacent electrode placement.*

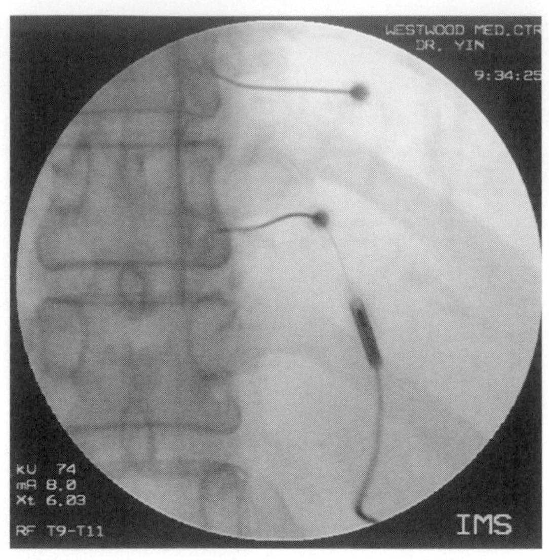

FIGURE 19–35 *AP image of sensory stereotactic localization of right T8 and T9 dorsal root ganglia.*

mid–superior dorsal aspect of the intervertebral neural foramen, a contrast study is performed to outline the exiting nerve root (Fig. 19–33). A lateral fluoroscopic image is taken to confirm proper electrode tip position (Fig. 19–34).

Sensory stereotactic localization of the dorsal root ganglion is then performed utilizing sensory stimulation at 0.15 to 0.2 V (50 Hz, 1 msec pulse duration; Fig. 19–35). Motor dissociation is confirmed with 2 Hz stimulation at 0.5 to 0.7 V. When patient-blinded precise reproduction of concordant pain or paresthetic coverage of the desired somatic region is obtained, a small amount of local anesthetic (0.5 mL 2% lidocaine) is injected before lesioning. For this type of selective thoracic dorsal root ganglion lesion, a high verniation lesion at a temperature of 50° to 54° C is performed for 120 to 240 sec.

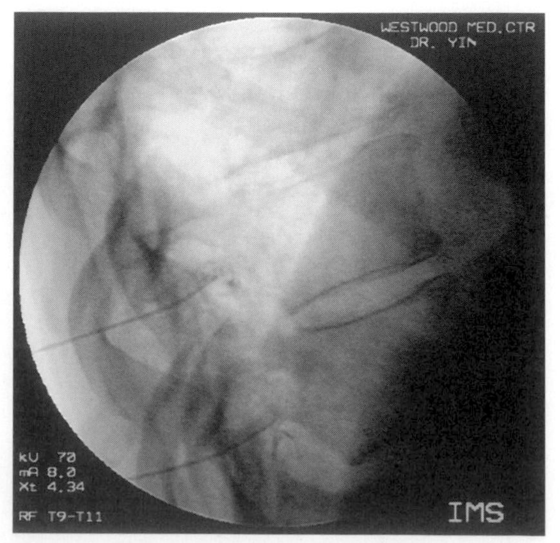

FIGURE 19–34 *Lateral image, contrast study shows initial placement of RF electrodes before dorsal root ganglion sensory stereotaxy T8, T9.*

GENERAL USE OF SACRAL, LUMBAR, AND THORACIC GANGLIONOTOMY PROCEDURES

In general, ganglionotomies should *not* be used to treat deafferentation pain. The dorsal root ganglion lesion should usually be reserved for either radiculopathy or pain related to a specific and well-defined dermatome. Deafferentation pain (such as postherpetic neuralgia, poststroke syndromes, and multiple sclerosis) and sympathetically maintained pain are not commonly treated with a dorsal root ganglion lesion, owing to the risk of exacerbating the deafferentation pain. The purpose of this technique is to produce a well-defined lesion in the dorsal root ganglion while maintaining an adequate afferent input. It is *not* desirable to produce numbness in the area that is lesioned. A lesion that produces numbness on a long-term basis can be associated with deafferentation pain as a postoperative complication. Because the dorsal root ganglion cells are more sensitive to heat than other structures within the mixed nerve, the clinician is using a differential heat lesion to preferentially affect pain pathways while leaving the motor, proprioceptive, and afferent pathways relatively intact. It would be unwise to use higher temperatures in an attempt to produce longer-acting pain relief, because higher temperatures have a greater chance of decreasing afferent input and, thus, of producing deafferentation pain as a postoperative complication. If more than one level is involved, it is best to wait 4 weeks between lesions. The greater the number of levels lesioned, the greater is the chance of producing deafferentation pain as a complication.

LESIONS IN THE CERVICAL REGION

RF lesions can be useful to treat pain in the cervical spine, but the operator must appreciate the complex anatomic relationships.[33, 38, 58, 68–70, 95–99] Distinct structures that are dense with pain receptors can cause both localized and

TABLE 19–1 *Cervical Pain Generators*

Structure	Implications
Cervical discs	May cause neck pain, chronic headaches, and symptoms referred into facial region. Facial pain requires exploration of relationship between cervical discs and facial pathways. Arm or hand pain may be radiculopathy or referred mechanical symptom from abnormal cervical disc.
Cervical facet joints	Can cause chronic mechanical symptoms in neck, shoulder, and intracapsular region. Upper and midcervical facet joint abnormalities may cause headaches. Do not usually cause referred facial pain. C0–C1 and C1–C2 joints are included here and are associated with occipital headaches.
Cervical nerve roots	Can cause upper extremity pain, especially if isolated; such isolated pain may also be sympathetically maintained.
Myofascial tissues in neck and suboccipital region	May cause mechanical symptoms in neck, referred symptoms in shoulders, and chronic headaches. May also cause facial pain. Should be examined for increased muscle tension, trigger points, and tight bands. Myofascial abnormalities due to underlying mechanical trauma are also common.

referred pain (Table 19–1). Like lumbar discs, cervical discs have nerve fibers in the outer portion of the annulus.[100] Discogenic irritation in the cervical spine can produce neck pain with headaches and symptoms referred to the shoulder and upper extremities. The cervical disc is a joint that maintains a distinct relationship with its associated facet joints. In the cervical region, the disc and the associated facet joints at each level form a three-joint complex (as they do in the lumbar spine). It is not unusual for combined discogenic and facet joint pain to develop.[101]

Pain related to these areas can be associated with degenerative disease or acute injury, as from whiplash or other trauma.[102–110] There is often poor correlation between imaging findings and the actual site of the mechanical pain pathway.[89] A normal-looking cervical disc can be disrupted and painful, and an abnormal-looking one can be asymptomatic.[88] Facet joints may appear normal yet still be painful. As in the lumbar spine, it is important to perform prognostic blocks of the suspect structures to determine whether they are painful. The most common sources of symptoms are the cervical discs, facet joints, nerve roots, and the supporting cervical musculature. The importance of cervical myofascial symptoms (tight bands, trigger points, and asymmetric muscle tissues) should not be underestimated. RF lesions in the neck can be useful in the treatment of discogenic pain, facet joint problems, and irritated nerve roots.

Disease of the cervical spine can produce referred symptoms into the face and chronic headaches. For patients suffering from headaches or facial pain, it is important to thoroughly evaluate the cervical spine as a potential source of the problem. The upper cervical nerve roots (C2–C4) have connections with the superior cervical ganglion. The superior cervical ganglion has connections with the deep petrosal nerve, which in turn has connections with the vidian nerve. The vidian nerve leads directly to the sphenopalatine ganglion, which has connections with branches of the trigeminal nerve. Pain from the upper cervical spine can cause symptoms referred into the frontal and maxillary region. The caudal nucleus of the trigeminal nerve can descend to the C3, or even C4, level. Constant stimuli in the upper cervical region from irritated pathways can cause stimulation of the lower portion of the caudal nucleus of the trigeminal nerve; this phenomenon can produce referred facial pain. The sphenopalatine ganglion, which may act as a central pathway between the cervical spine and the facial region, is a complicated structure with multiple types of afferent fibers and ganglion cells (Figs. 19–36, 19–37).

The Cervical Facet Joints

When a patient presents with well-circumscribed pain overlying the cervical facet joints, there is a good possibility that the joints are involved in the problem.[110] Affected patients commonly report pain in the neck and shoulder girdle with associated headaches, and even ear pain.[111, 112] Diagnostic injections of the facet joints are important and can help to make the diagnosis, but false-positive results sometimes occur.[113] A careful history and detailed manual examination should be done.[110]

Anatomy

The medial branch wraps around the posterior aspect and sends branches along the waist of the cervical facet column at two levels for each joint. The C2–C3 facet joint is supplied by part of the third occipital nerve as it crosses the midportion of the C2–C3 joint and a communicating branch of C2 just adjacent and craniad to the midportion of the C2–C3 joint, on the arch of C2.

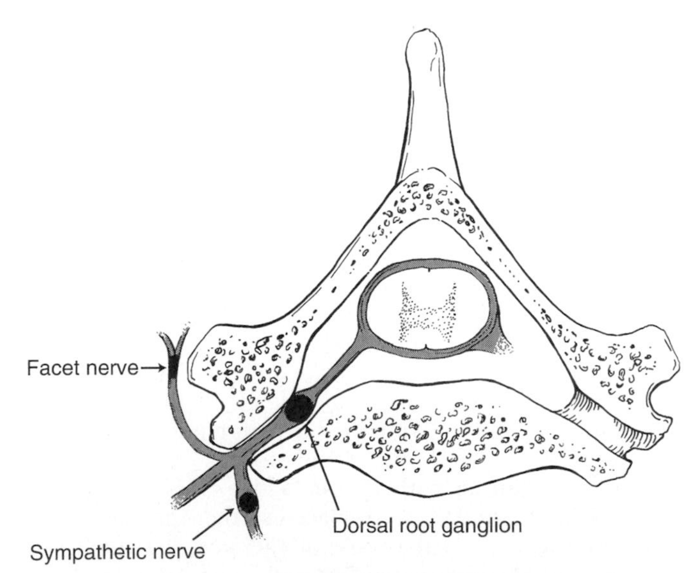

FIGURE 19–36 A cross section through the cervical spine. The relationships among the facet joint nerves, sympathetic nerves, and dorsal root ganglion are shown. Each of these nerves can be lesioned with an RF procedure.

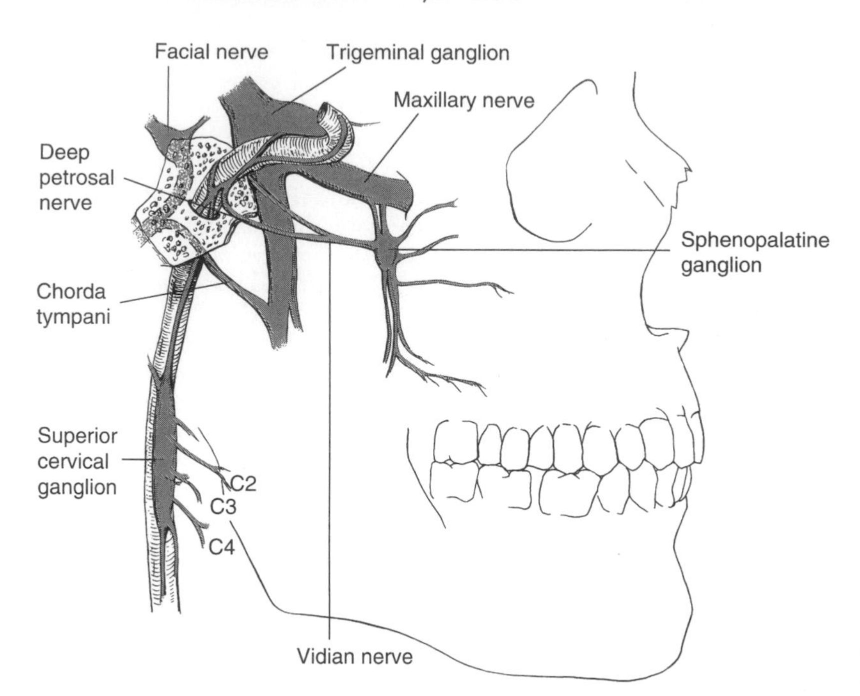

FIGURE 19–37 Drawing shows the complex anatomic relationship between the cervical nerves and the trigeminal system.

Lesions

To denervate the facet joints at any level from C2 to C6, the patient is placed in a supine position and an oblique approach is used.[38, 68, 69, 98] For the C7 medial branch, the patient is placed in the prone position, and an approach similar to that for the lumbar facet joint denervation is used; that is, the cannula is passed onto the superomedial aspect of the transverse process of C7 and "walked off" the leading edge (approximately 2 mm anteriorly) until the facet joint nerve can be stimulated. For the C8 medial branch, a similar approach may be taken at the superomedial aspect of the T1 transverse process for the articular branches of this nerve; however, the main trunk of the C8 medial branch is located at the inflection point of (superior lateral) the T1 transverse process.[79, 85] Sometimes the C5–C6 joint requires a posterior approach when the patient has a short, thick neck. Position for the C2 communicating nerve contribution is different. The posterior primary ramus of C2, which is larger than the anterior ramus, continues as the greater occipital nerve. It is not prudent to lesion that nerve. There are, however, communicating branches from the posterior primary ramus of C2 that supply the C2–C3 facet joint. To denervate these branches, the cannula is placed on the C2 arch at a point 3 to 5 mm craniad to the midportion of the C2–C3 facet joint. The C3 contribution (third occipital nerve) to the C2–C3 facet joint is lesioned as it crosses the midpoint of the joint. Lesions are first made at the middle of the joint and then 3 to 5 mm craniad to lesion the C2 communicating branch (exact distances depend on stimulation).

A 50-mm cannula with a 4-mm active tip is used for the lesions. The cannulas are all placed so that the bare metal tip comes to rest on the waist of the facet joint column. An oblique approach is used at first. The cannula enters from a point posterior to the spine and is moved anteriorly until it is aligned with the waist of the facet joint column. This point is just posterior to the associated transverse process and is well posterior to the associated foraminal opening. It is important to avoid the segmental nerve. On a lateral view, the electrode is seen at the "centroid" of the articular pillar. Stimulation at 50 Hz should be felt in the neck and shoulder region at 1.0 V (or less). Absence of upper extremity motor fasciculations should be noted with 2 V at 2 Hz stimulation. Motor fasciculations in the paracervical musculature are common. After proper stimulation, 0.5 mL of 2% lidocaine is passed through each cannula to anesthetize the lesion site. Lesioning is performed at 80° C for 60 sec (Fig. 19–38).

Lesions of the lower facet joint nerves are made through a posterior approach with the patient in the prone position. For the medial branch of C7 and the articular branches of C8 and T1, the fluoroscopy unit is set up for a posterior view with some craniad angulation so that the appropriate transverse process can be distinguished. Either a 50-mm or 100-mm cannula with a 5-mm active tip is passed until it touches the superomedial border of the transverse process. The cannula is advanced 2 mm over the leading edge of the transverse process. Stimulation is performed as previously described, and absence of upper extremity motor fasciculations should be noted. Lesion parameters are the same as those described for the upper cervical spine. For cervical facet lesioning, it is prudent to take at least two different views (anteroposterior, lateral, and when necessary, oblique) to confirm correct needle placement. Anteroposterior views should show the cannula lying next to the lateral aspect of the midportion (waist) of the lamina. Lateral views should show that the cannula tip is posterior to the foraminal opening and level with the "centroid" of the articular pillar. The C8 and T1 lateral views are not seen clearly because of the overlying scapula. The most important criterion for the facet joint lesion is to *combine* correct stimulation parameters with correct radiographic placement whenever possible. If the cannula appears to have correct anatomic alignment but the proper stimulation pa-

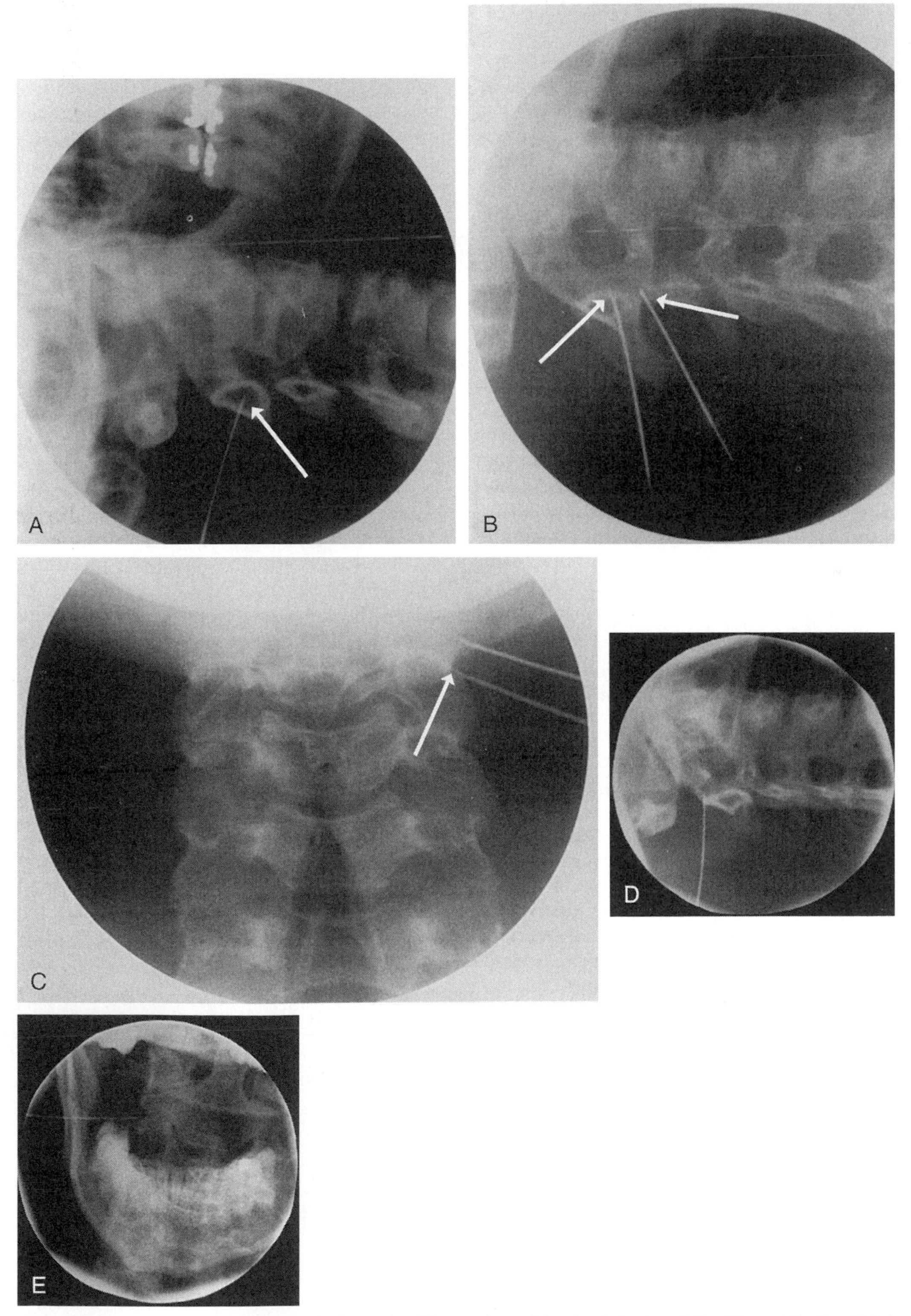

FIGURE 19–38 A, *Radiograph shows the RF cannula position for lesioning of the C3 contribution (third occipital nerve) to the C2–3 facet joint.* B, *Oblique and* C, *posteroanterior radiographs show RF cannula position* (arrows) *for lesioning of the C3 facet joint nerves to the C2–3 joint (left cannula in* B*) and the C3–4 joint (right cannula in* B*). Note in* C *that the lower C3 cannula is resting directly along the waist of the cervical facet joint line* (arrow). D, *RF cannula position for lesion of the C2 communicating branch, oblique view. E, Anteroposterior view (through the mouth) of the RF cannula position for lesioning of the C2 communicating branch.*

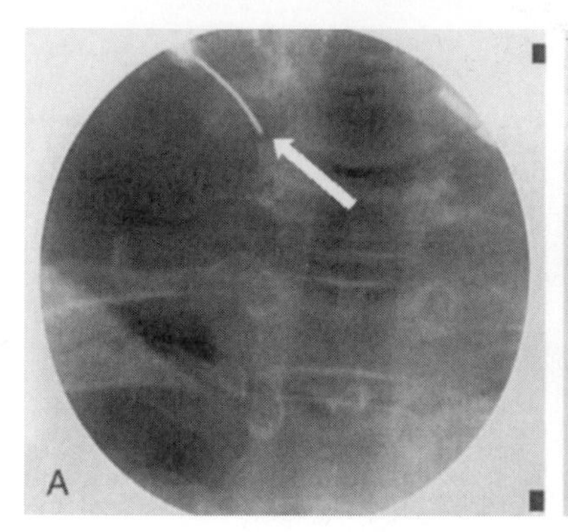

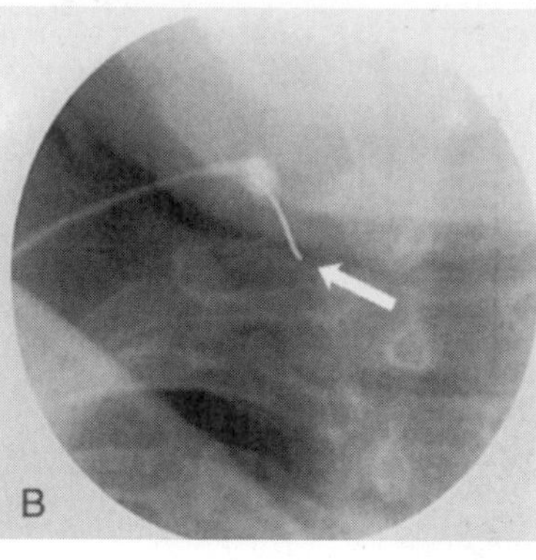

FIGURE 19–39 Radiographs representing the RF cannula position for lesioning of the lower cervical facet joints through a posterior approach. Note that the cannula rests at the superomedial aspect of the transverse process. The cannula is "walked" over the leading edge, and the lesion is performed much as in the lumbar facet joint rhizotomy. A, The cannula rests on the superomedial aspect of the transverse process of C7. B, The cannula rests on the transverse process of T1.

rameters are not obtained, RF lesioning should not be performed. When parameters are in doubt, it is best to abandon the procedure (Fig. 19–39).

Recovery from a cervical facet joint denervation is fairly rapid, and most patients show signs of good relief within 10 days. Minor dysesthesias and patchy numbness can occur but are not dangerous complications. Occasionally painful hypersensitivity of the neck or shoulder necessitates a brief course of steroids. Lesions of a C2–C3 joint sometimes produce short-term vertigo, which is treated with meclizine for a few days. Such complications usually resolve within 2 to 4 weeks after the procedure.

The Cervical Facet Joints: Alternate Posterior Parasagittal Approach with Curved Tip Electrodes

An alternative to the oblique approach that facilitates access to the lower cervical medial branch nerves is posterior parasagittal entry. The patient is placed in the prone position with the neck flexed slightly forward. The region from the nuchal crest to the upper dorsal spine is cleansed with antiseptic solution. The fluoroscopy unit is brought in from the head of the table.

Anteroposterior images are obtained to visualize the waist of the lamina (medial indentations of the cervical lamina just caudal to the superior articulating processes) from C3 through C6. At the level of C7 and T1, the transverse processes are identified. At C2, the lateral aspect of the lamina just cephalad to the inferior articular process of C2 is identified.

The aforementioned bony landmarks are identified, and skin entry sites are marked directly overlying the bony targets, coaxial with the x-ray beam. 100-mm active tip 22-gauge electrodes are used, with a slight (10–15 degrees) smooth curve placed in the distal 5 to 7 mm. The C2 communicating branch of the posterior primary ramus supplying the superior portion of the C2–C3 joint is approached under anteroposterior fluoroscopic imaging. The electrode is guided down to the C2 dorsal lamina in a posterior parasagittal plane, coaxial with the x-ray image. Once bony contact is made (generally near the midpoint of the junction of the caudal and middle thirds of the C2 lamina, 3 to 5 mm craniad to the lesion point of the third occipital nerve at the level of the C2–C3 facet joint), the electrode is rotated laterally and advanced 1–2 mm around the lateral aspect of the C2 lamina, then redirected medially so that the electrode tip hugs the lateral lamina (Fig. 19–40). Lateral images are then taken, verifying placement of the electrode's active tip overlying the midportion of the C2 lamina but well dorsal of the exiting C3 nerve root (Fig. 19–41).

The C3–C6 medial branch nerves are approached at the level of the waist of the lamina, again in a posterior parasagittal plane, under anteroposterior imaging. The goal of the posterior approach is to approximate the active electrode tips parallel and adjacent to the medial branch nerves as they wrap around the waist of the lamina before decussating into individual superior and inferior articular branches. The electrodes are advanced to contact the dorsal lateral cervical lamina, then rotated so that the curve of the electrode tip is directed laterally. The electrode is then advanced fractionally around the lateral border of the lamina. The electrode tip is redirected medially, and lateral fluoroscopic images are used to guide further advancement of the electrode (approaching the "centroid" of the articular pillar). The electrode is held close to the lateral lamina, parallel to the dorsally directed medial branch nerves (Fig. 19–42).

At the levels of C7, C8, and T1, the transverse processes of C7 and T1 are used as radiographic landmarks. The C7 medial branch nerve is approached at the level of the superior medial aspect of the transverse process of C7; the

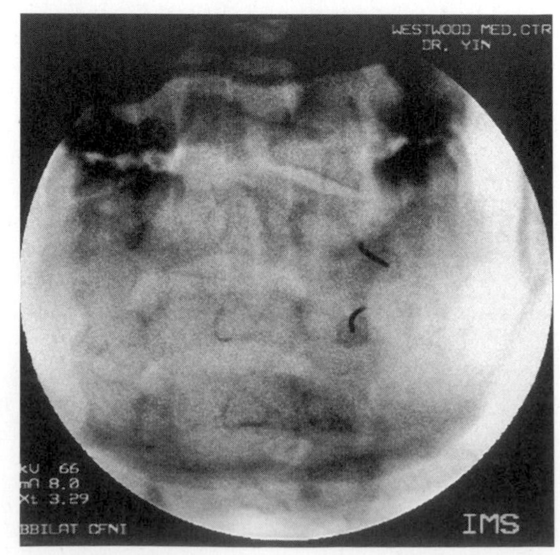

FIGURE 19–40 AP image illustrates placement of C2 and C3 medial branch electrodes.

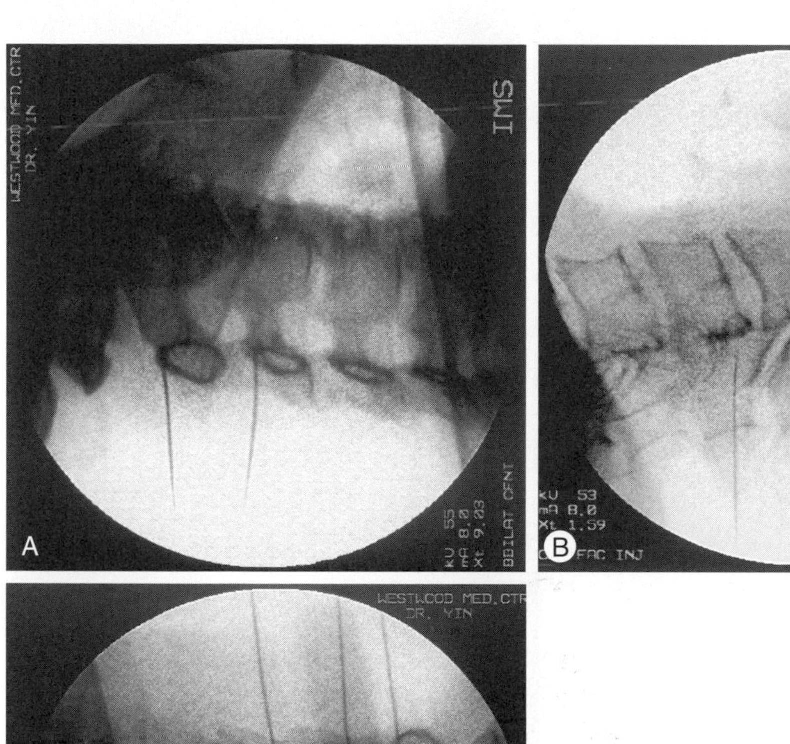

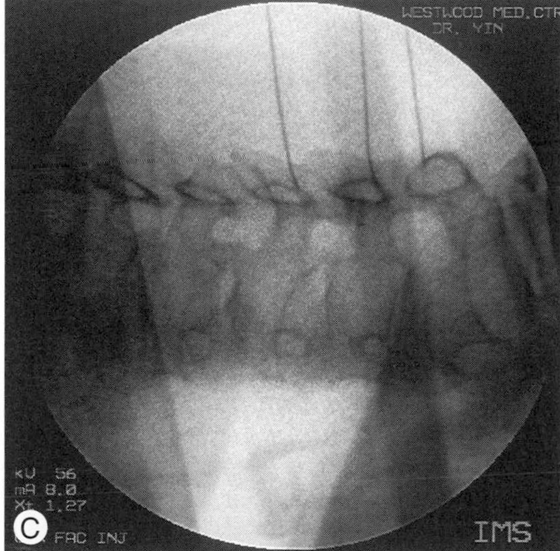

FIGURE 19–41 A, *Oblique radiograph of electrode placement for C2 and C3 medial branch lesion.* B, *Lateral radiograph illustrates electrode placement for C3, C3, C4 medial branch denervation.* C, *Oblique radiograph shows electrode positioning for third occipital nerve denervation.*

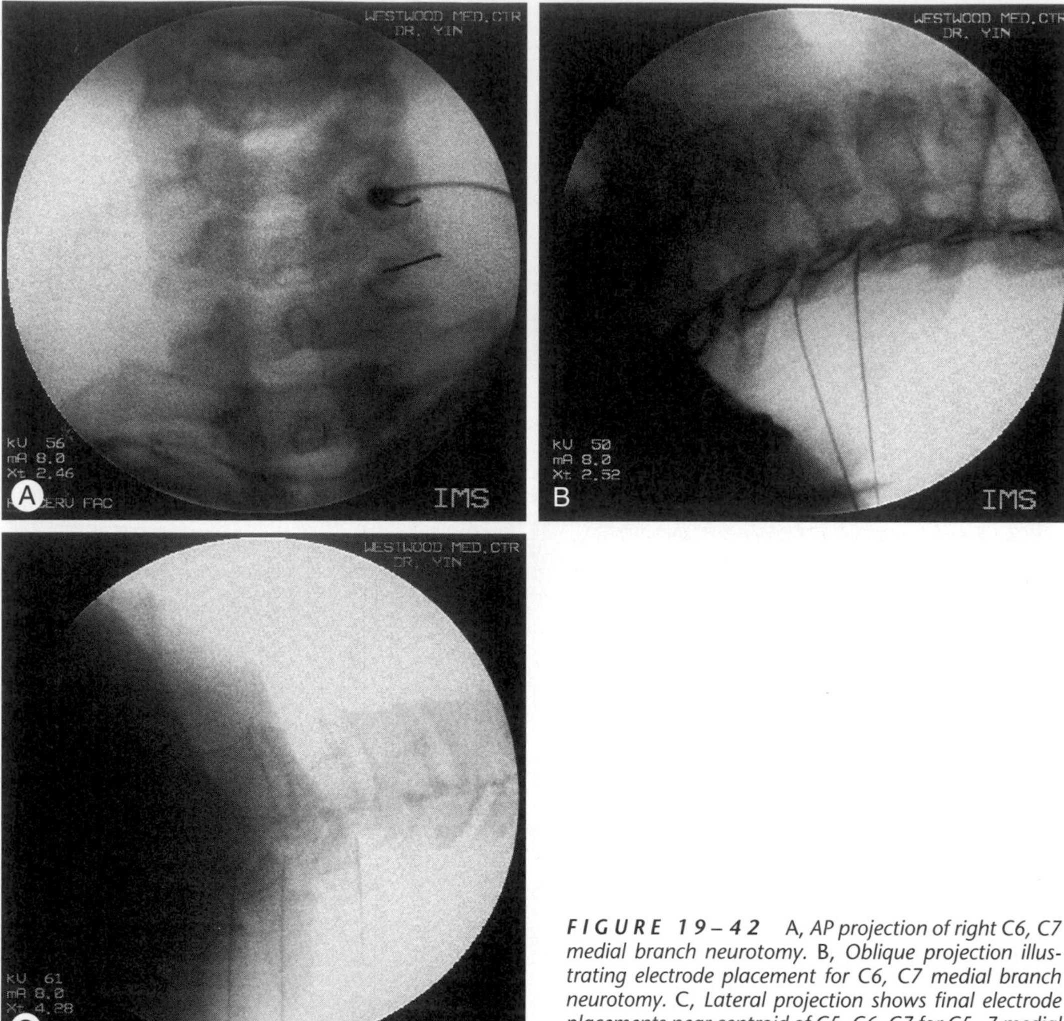

FIGURE 19–42 A, *AP projection of right C6, C7 medial branch neurotomy.* B, *Oblique projection illustrating electrode placement for C6, C7 medial branch neurotomy.* C, *Lateral projection shows final electrode placements near centroid of C5, C6, C7 for C5–7 medial branch neurotomy.*

electrode tip is maneuvered to slightly overlap this portion of the process. The C8 medial branch nerve is approached at the superior lateral aspect of the T1 transverse process, but articular branches are often found at the superior medial aspect of the T1 transverse process (Fig. 19–43). The T1 medial branch nerve crosses the superior lateral aspect of the T2 transverse process,[79] although specific articular branches may be found medially along the dorsal aspect of the lamina adjacent to the superior and inferior articular processes.

Once the RF electrodes have been placed in positions approximating the location of the medial branch nerves or their articular branches, sensory and motor stereotaxy is performed to guide or "fine tune" final electrode placement. Patient-blinded sensory stimulation that reproduces concordant pain (at 0.2–0.3 V, 50 Hz), in conjunction with segmental multifidus contraction, verifies placement of the electrode tip over symptomatic levels. Observed multifidus contraction without concordant pain or the development of nonpainful paresthesias indicates localization of an asymptomatic branch. Only the symptomatic levels are lesioned, as with the oblique approach.

Diagnosis and Treatment of Cervical Symptoms

Lesions of the cervical dorsal root ganglion can be useful for discogenic pain or segmental pain related to disease of the spinal nerve.[33, 34, 56] C2 and C3 ganglion lesions can be useful for treating "resistant" C2–C3 facet pain. Prognostic blocks are important for correctly isolating the painful segment before lesioning. Lesions of the dorsal root ganglion have the potential to produce deafferentation pain; thus, careful prognostic blocks should be performed as a staging procedure. If cervical discogenic pain is suspected, discography can be performed to isolate the specific segment causing the problems. If a radiculopathy is considered the source of the upper extremity pain, both EMG studies and prognostic sleeve blocks are helpful for determining the involved level.

Cervical Ganglionotomy

RF lesions of the cervical dorsal root ganglion are made in a similar manner at the levels C3 through C7. C8 should

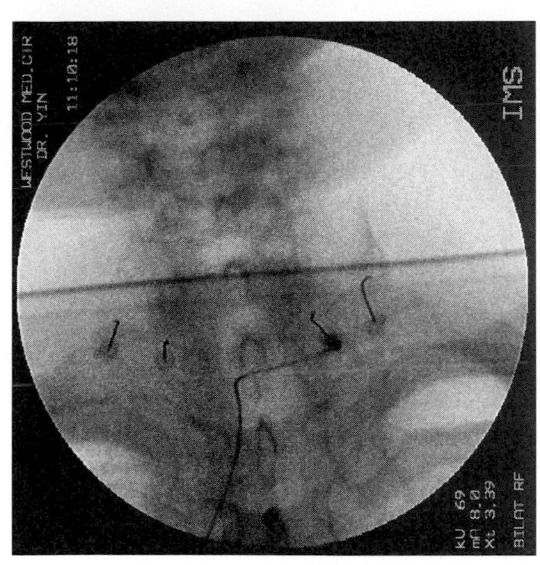

FIGURE 19–43 *AP radiograph illustrates placement of electrodes for bilateral C8 medial branch denervation. Note placement of electrode for C8 medial branch at superolateral aspect of T1 transverse process and placement of electrode at superomedial aspect of T1 transverse process for C8 articular branch localized with sensory stereotaxy.*

be avoided, owing to its tendency to develop neuritis and even deafferentation pain. The RF cannula is advanced from an oblique approach until it touches the 6 o'clock position of the posterior foraminal canal. The cannula is then advanced along the floor of the canal and halfway across the facet joint line. It is closely applied to the floor (posterior aspect) of the foraminal canal to maintain a safe distance from the vertebral artery.

Stimulation parameters are quite similar to those described for the lumbar ganglionotomy. At 50 Hz, good paresthesia in the upper extremity should be noted between 0.4 and 0.7 V. At 2 Hz, motor fasciculations should be seen at twice the voltage needed for the sensory stimulation. Then, 1 mL of 2% lidocaine is passed through the cannula and a 10-min delay is allowed for it to take effect. Thermal lesions are made between 60° and 65° C, depending on the stimulation threshold, for 60 sec. The correct cannula to use for this lesion is either the SMK 50 mm with a 4-mm active tip or the SMK 100 mm with a 5-mm active tip. The goal of this procedure is to produce a discrete injury to the pain pathways while preserving normal proprioception, touch, and motor function. Numbness is not a desirable outcome. Some sensory changes may be noted during the first days to weeks after the procedure. The vast majority of patients have normal sensory function after 4 weeks. It takes 4 weeks to determine the full effects of the procedure, because inflammation of the ganglion follows lesioning. Patients commonly experience increasing pain for days to weeks, until all postoperative pain resolves.

Ganglionotomy at the C2 level is different. Under lateral fluoroscopic guidance, a 50-mm electrode with a 4-mm active tip is advanced perpendicular to a point at the upper two thirds of the arch of C2 (junction of posterior two thirds with the ventral third of the arch). The cannula is advanced (under anteroposterior fluoroscopic viewing) halfway across (and posterior to) the C1–C2 joint using a through-the-mouth view. Because motor function from the C2 level is not a significant concern, sensory stimulation is the only parameter that needs to be checked. At 50 Hz stimulation, paresthesia to the suboccipital region should be noted between 0.4 and 0.7 V. Then, 1 mL of 2% lidocaine is passed onto the ganglion to anesthetize the lesion site. A thermal lesion is created between 55° and 60° C, depending on the stimulation threshold. Lesions at the C2 level tend more often to be associated with postoperative neuritis. The authors recommend performing cooler, high-verniation lesions at C2. Ganglionotomy at the C2 and C3 levels can be very helpful in the treatment of C2 and C3 "pattern" headaches. Mechanical problems of *any* aspect of the motion segment anywhere from C0 through C4 can cause occipital neck pain with associated headaches, and cervical disc lesions even farther caudad can also cause headaches (Fig. 19–44). Indications for cervical ganglionotomy include pain from the cervical disc, radiculopathy, and headaches. Patients are generally discharged 2 hours after the procedure has been performed.

Cervical Disc Procedure

Cervical discogenic pain is an important and underdiagnosed cause of chronic headaches and neck pain. Injury to *any* cervical disc can be associated with headaches. Provocational and/or analgesic discography is the key for diagnosing a painful cervical disc. If a painful level is discovered, the clinician should consider the RF cervical disc procedure.

The patient is placed in the supine position. An oblique approach from the *right* side is used for the procedure. The patient is given preoperative antibiotics 45 min beforehand. After sterile preparation, fluoroscopy is used to visualize the painful disc.

A 100-mm cannula with a 5-mm active tip is used. The cannula is placed into the disc from a right oblique approach, just anterior to the uncovertebral joint. A curved cannula is advanced into the center of the disc as seen by lateral and anteroposterior views. Stimulation with 2 V at 50 Hz and 2 Hz should be negative. No local anesthetic is used for the lesion. Pain is common during the lesion process, beginning at about 90 sec and peaking at 3.5 min. The lesion temperature is increased over 20 to 30 sec to 80° C and maintained for 4 min.

Pain relief is sometimes immediate. Other patients achieve maximal relief some 2 to 4 weeks after the procedure.

Disc infection is a risk, but it is minimized with preoperative antibiotics and a right-sided approach (to avoid the esophagus). Nerve root injury is another potential risk but should be quite rare when proper technique is used. If clear-cut radicular symptoms occur during the lesion process, the procedure should be stopped immediately (see Fig. 19–44 I, J).

Lesions of the Stellate Ganglion

The stellate ganglion is a combination of the inferior cervical and the first thoracic sympathetic ganglia. RF lesions of the stellate ganglion can be useful in managing sympathetically maintained pain.[114] The ganglion lies just anterior to the longus colli muscle at the anterior and lateral borders of the C7 vertebral body. It is a rather diffuse structure.

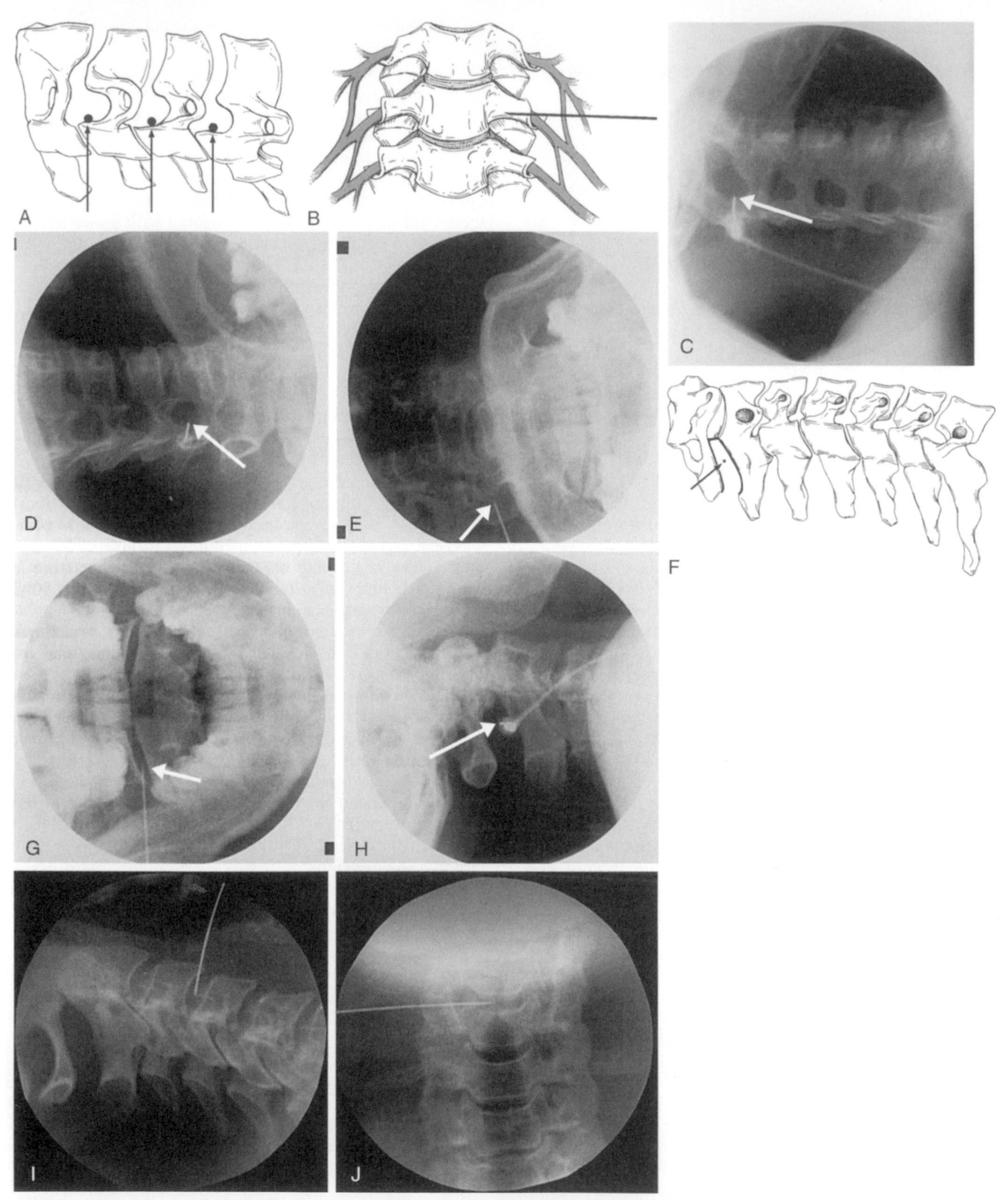

FIGURE 19–44 A, *Drawing of the entry points* (solid circles) *for a cervical dorsal root ganglionotomy procedure. Each point is on the floor of the foraminal canal at the 6 o'clock position* (arrows). B, *Posteroanterior view of the cervical spine. The RF cannula tip* (arrow) *is in the correct position for a cervical dorsal root ganglionotomy procedure. Note that the tip of the cannula has passed halfway across the cervical facet joint line.* C, *Oblique radiograph of a cervical spine. Note that the RF cannula has entered the 6 o'clock position along the floor of the C3 foraminal canal* (arrow). D, *Oblique radiograph shows the RF cannula position* (arrow) *for a C4 ganglionotomy.* E, *Posteroanterior radiograph shows the cannula position for a C4 dorsal root ganglionotomy procedure. Note that the RF cannula tip has passed halfway across the cervical facet joint line* (arrow). F, *Drawing of a lateral view of the cervical spine. The dot in the arch of the C2* (arrow) *represents the entry point for a C2 dorsal root ganglionotomy procedure.* G, H, *The correct cannula position for a C2 dorsal root ganglionotomy. The lateral view through the arch of C2.* H, *An RF cannula* (arrow) *is entering the arch of C2. On the posteroanterior view through the mouth,* G, *the RF cannula is passing halfway across the C1–C2 joint* (arrow). I, *RF cannula position for a C3–C4 disc procedure, lateral view.* J, *RF cannula position for a C3–C4 disc procedure, anteroposterior view.*

Partial lesions of the stellate ganglion can produce long-term, high-quality pain relief.

Under fluoroscopic guidance, an RF cannula with a 5-mm active tip is advanced from an anterior approach until the superolateral aspect of C7 is encountered. The cannula is pulled back anteriorly approximately 2 mm to make sure that the active tip is anterior to the longus colli. The final position is on the vertebral body at its junction with the transverse process. Proper stimulation technique is crucial to avoid injury to the phrenic or recurrent laryngeal nerves. Both AP and lateral views are checked prior to each lesion. A total of three lesions are made. These include the point just described, a point just lateral and caudal (on the medial aspect of the transverse process), and a point 5 mm caudal (on the anterolateral aspect of the vertebral body). These three lesions create a triangular zone of thermal interruption to the cervical sympathetic fibers.

Before each lesion, the following stimulation technique should be used. At 2 Hz, the patient is asked to say "E" while stimulation is applied at 2.5 V. The patient's ability to articulate should be not at all impaired. If it is, the cannula is too close to the recurrent laryngeal nerve (which is anterior and medial to the proper lesion zone). At the same time, the operator's hand is placed just under the rib cage to feel for movement of the diaphragm. Although the phrenic nerve should be well lateral to the lesion site, any movement of the diaphragm with 2.5 V at 2 Hz warrants immediate investigation of the cannula position. After proper stimulation parameters have been met, 0.5 mL of 0.25% bupivacaine is passed through the cannula and a lesion is made at 80° C for 30 sec. The cannula is immediately moved, and the entire process is repeated for the second and third lesions. Bupivacaine is chosen for its slow onset, which makes inadvertent anesthetizing of the phrenic or recurrent laryngeal nerves less likely before the lesion process.

If a cannula with a 7-mm active tip is used, the cannula can be applied directly to bone and does not need to be pulled back in an anterior fashion. The longus colli muscle is approximately 5 mm thick at its thickest point. The lesion, at least 2 mm, will be made anterior to the muscle while using this variation. It is preferable to have the cannula firmly anchored; thus the appeal of this approach.

Careful stimulation technique is crucial for safe performance of this procedure. The operator must bear in mind that the lesion on the medial aspect of the transverse process must be made with extreme care. The anterior portion of the transverse process is quite narrow at this point, and the RF cannula *must* stay in the same plane as for the ventral aspect of the vertebral body, to prevent injury to the segmental nerves or vertebral artery (Fig. 19–45).

Last, the clinician may wish to direct the RF cannula caudad, to the "groove" where the head of the first rib meets the ventrolateral aspect of the body of T1. At this ventrolateral position, a fourth lesion can be done to interrupt some of the thoracic sympathetic fibers. Care must be taken to stay on the ventral aspect of the vertebral body at the junction of the rib and vertebral body.

Alternatively, one may wish to proceed instead to the T2 and T3 sympathectomy (described later). If hand pain is the predominant symptom, the T2–T3 technique should be considered, since a significant amount of sympathetic outflow to the hand comes from these two levels.

This is a discrete lesion that does not interrupt the entire ganglion. Impressive results can be seen, however, and the technique can be repeated if necessary. Lesions of the stellate ganglion can be useful for the treatment of sympathetically maintained pain, including reflex sympathetic dystrophy, causalgia, posttraumatic dystrophies, and Raynaud's phenomenon. This technique does not usually produce Horner's syndrome (superior cervical ganglion) as can other sympatholytic procedures.

Lesions Used to Treat Chronic Headaches

The use of RF procedures to manage chronic occipital pain and headaches has been reported by several authors.[97, 115–118] It is important to determine whether the mechanical components of the cervical spine are contributing to the headache. Obviously, a thorough neurologic evaluation of any patient suffering from chronic headaches is mandatory. Appropriate studies, as indicated by the clinical history, are important. Even if a patient does have mechanical findings in the cervical spine, other more serious problems that could be contributing to the headache must be ruled out. A careful neurologic evaluation is needed to rule out such problems as chronic inflammatory disease, vasculitis, vascular anomalies, and even neoplasms. Migraine headaches, although considered a vascular phenomenon, can be trig-

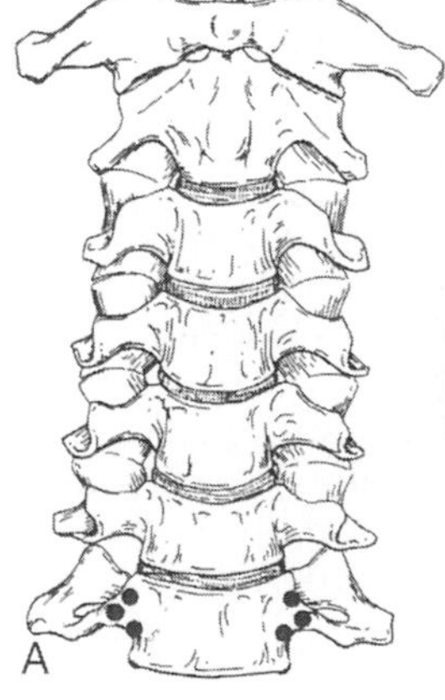

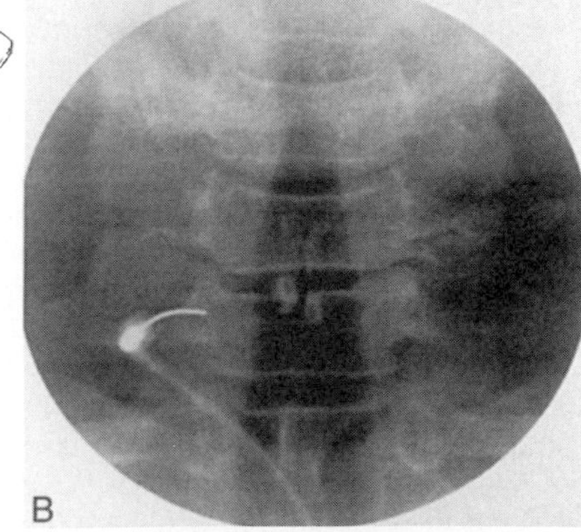

FIGURE 19–45 A, *Drawing of a posteroanterior view of the cervical spine. Dots mark the target points for RF lesioning of the cervical sympathetic nerves. Note that these are at the junction of the medial aspect of the transverse process with the lateral aspect of its respective vertebral body.* B, *Posteroanterior radiograph of the cervical spine. Note that, at the C7 level, the RF cannula rests at the junction of the lateral aspect of the vertebral body with the medial aspect of the transverse process. This represents the correct cannula position for lesioning of the C7 sympathetic fibers.*

gered by abnormalities in the cervical spine. Even a patient with a true migraine headache may respond to appropriate RF lesions in the cervical spine. Although the headache may not be cured, the frequency and even duration of the headache can be improved if the mechanical problem is treated. Some persons who have been diagnosed with migraine headaches are suffering from pure mechanical problems. They demonstrate significant decreases in both frequency and intensity of their headaches when the cervical abnormalities are treated.

Cluster headaches can also respond favorably to RF lesions. Some persons with cluster headaches have concomitant mechanical problems in the cervical spine. Many of these patients have evidence of cervical disease on physical examination, and many have functional abnormalities.

If prognostic blocks show that the facet joints are causing or contributing to the headaches, RF cervical facet rhizotomy should be performed. If diagnostic root sleeve injections or cervical discography shows that the headaches are related to an abnormal disc, an RF cervical disc procedure or ganglionotomy should be considered, but only after careful prognostic blocks have been performed.

Upper Cervicogenic Headache

Cervicogenic headaches involving the upper cervical and suboccipital region are quite common and can be caused by any number of bony, articular, and soft tissue lesions. Secondary myofascial tension may make definitive clinical diagnosis, based solely on detailed history and careful physical examination, even more difficult, and a methodical, systematic diagnostic approach is imperative for success in dealing with these frequently challenging cases.

The general evaluation of suboccipital, occipital, and upper cervical headaches begins with a careful history and meticulous physical examination. A history of cervical or cranial trauma may be relevant, and symptoms suggestive of nerve root involvement (greater or lesser occipital neuralgia, cervical radicular pain) may steer the investigation toward evaluation of the cervical discs and related nerve root structures. Before consideration of interventional diagnostic or therapeutic procedures, conservative and pharmacologic modalities must be exhausted, and diagnostic evaluations performed, including plain films and MRI studies of the cervical and cranial regions. Identifying treatable sources of cervicogenic or suboccipital headache is often complex and time-consuming, and most patients have seen several specialists. Nonetheless, more often than not, treatable sources of cervicogenic and suboccipital headache are identifiable with a careful and methodical approach.

A history of radiating scalp pain in the distribution of the occipital nerves, coupled with exacerbation and reproduction of pain on palpation of these structures at or proximal to the nuchal crest, should prompt consideration of occipital neuralgia. Differential diagnostic injections of the greater and lesser occipital nerves definitively diagnose primary occipital neuralgia (C3 and/or C3 dorsal root ganglion involvement). Affected patients generally respond well to steroid injections over the dorsal root ganglia of C2 and/or C3, and in refractory cases, excellent results have been obtained with percutaneous functional stereotactic RF dorsal root ganglion lesion with high verniation at 50° to 54° C, 45 to 55 V, for 120 to 240 sec. Severe, refractory cases have also been managed with open exploration of the occipital nerve just proximal to the nuchal crest and cryolesioning of the greater occipital nerve and its branches under direct vision. Implanted quadripolar occipital nerve stimulation devices have also been effective as a rescue intervention.

Suboccipital pain without nerve root involvement may be secondary to upper cervical facet capsular pain or degenerative disease, upper cervical discogenic pain (most commonly C2–C3, and C3–C4), pain due to bony lesions, including metastases, rare ligamentous instability of the C1–C2 or C2–C3 vertebral joint complexes, atlantooccipital (AO) joint/capsular pain, and atlantoaxial (AA) joint/capsular pain. Advanced diagnostic procedures such as C2, C3, and/or C4 medial branch injection, provocative cervical discography, and AO and AA joint injection may provide definitive diagnosis of the predominant source of pain in the suboccipital and upper cervical regions. Definitive therapeutic interventions exist for medial branch–mediated pain (see section on Cervical Facet Rhizotomy), and many patients with cervical discogenic pain of C2–C3 or C3–C4 origin respond to intradiscal steroid or intradiscal RF lesion.

C2 Rami Communicans Lesion

Pain of AA and AO joint origin is more difficult to treat, as the sensory innervation of these joints and joint capsules is poorly understood. Sluijter has advocated a lower-temperature high-verniation lesioning of the C1 nerve as effective treatment for suboccipital headaches presumed to be of AO or AA joint origin.[119]

One of the authors (WY) has developed an approach targeting the ramus communicans nerves at the C2 level, located adjacent to the ventral lateral aspect of the vertebral body of C2 at its junction with the ventral inferior medial transverse process. A small sulcus, or groove, exists in this region of the C2 vertebra, directed lateral to medial at an angle of approximately 45 to 60 degrees from horizontal, pointing to the dens.

Although a comparative study examining the possible correlation of AA and AO joint pain with C1 dorsal root ganglion or C2 ramus communicans origin has yet to be performed, the authors feel that, based on sensory stereotactic findings, the C2 ramus communicans may provide a source for some treatable AA, and possibly AO, joint–mediated pain. Deep suboccipital pain without occipital radiation and unresponsive to diagnostic occipital nerve block, exacerbated by palpation over the C1–C2 arch, seems to correlate well with C2 ramus communicans–mediated pain. Patients also occasionally complain of coexisting nonradiating pain over the crown or vertex. This clinical impression has led one of the authors (WY) to virtually abandon diagnostic AO and AA joint injections in favor of C2 ramus communicans injection, and, if required, RF lesion.

The confirmation of C2 gray rami–mediated suboccipital headache is made with fluoroscopically confirmed small volume injection of local anesthetic and depot corticosteroid (0.5 to 0.7 mL bupivacaine with triamcinolone, 8 mg/mL). Approximately 20% to 25% of patients will benefit dramatically from local anesthetic with steroid injection alone, obviating more aggressive therapy. Patients with recurrent, refractory pain who have experienced reproducible high-grade temporary improvement with local anesthetic and steroid injection over the C2 ramus communicans may benefit from a percutaneous sensory stereotactic RF C2 communicans lesion. The long-term results are frequently stunning.

Technique

It must be emphasized that, like C2 cervical dorsal root ganglion lesioning and percutaneous cordotomy, the technique of C2 ramus communicans lesion is technically demanding. Considerable potential for patient morbidity exists if performed by inexperienced practitioners unfamiliar with advanced fluoroscopy-guided procedures and upper cervical bony and soft tissue anatomy.

The patient is placed supine on the fluoroscopy table with the head and neck slightly extended. The neck, submandibular, and retroauricular regions are prepared. The fluoroscopic unit is brought in from the head. Lateral fluoroscopic images are obtained, and the "lateral mass" of C2 (including the C2 transverse process and inferior articular pillar) and the ventral aspect of the C2 vertebral body are identified. Parallax is eliminated with rotation and cephalad or caudad angulation of the x-ray beam as needed. A skin entry site is marked and anesthetized below the angle of the mandible, lateral to the carotid sheath, similar to that that would be used for C3 or C4 ganglionotomy. (Anterior oblique angulation of the fluoroscopic unit is used initially; after the electrode has been introduced through the skin, lateral images are used to guide placement, as no clear radiographic landmarks are present on anterior oblique fluoroscopic images. A coaxial, or "tunnel vision" approach is not feasible.) A 100-mm, 2-mm active tip 22-gauge RF electrode with a small distal curve (10–15 degrees) is introduced under lateral fluoroscopic guidance and directed medially and cephalad under lateral fluoroscopic imaging toward the ventral lateral aspect of the C2 vertebral body at its junction with the ipsilateral ventral inferior medial C2 transverse process. The path of the electrode passes lateral and dorsal to the carotid sheath. Care is taken to stay ventral to the exiting C3 nerve root and ventral to the vertebral artery yet dorsal to the pharyngeal structures. Bony contact may be made at the ventrolateral aspect of the lateral inferior end plate of the C2 vertebral body at its junction with the C2–C3 intervertebral disc. The electrode is then rotated and directed cephalad, hugging bone, into the sulcus along the ventral lateral aspect of the C2 vertebral body, medial to the ventral aspect of the C2 transverse process (Fig. 19–46).

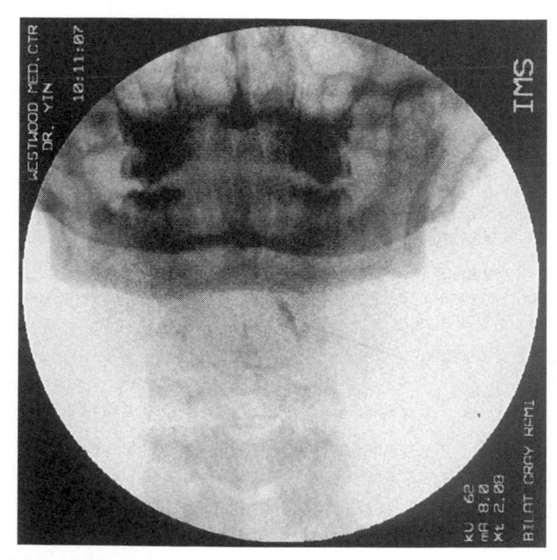

FIGURE 19–46 *AP radiograph demonstrates the ventral sulcus (filled with contrast) at C2 with the electrode positioned for ramus communicans RF lesion.*

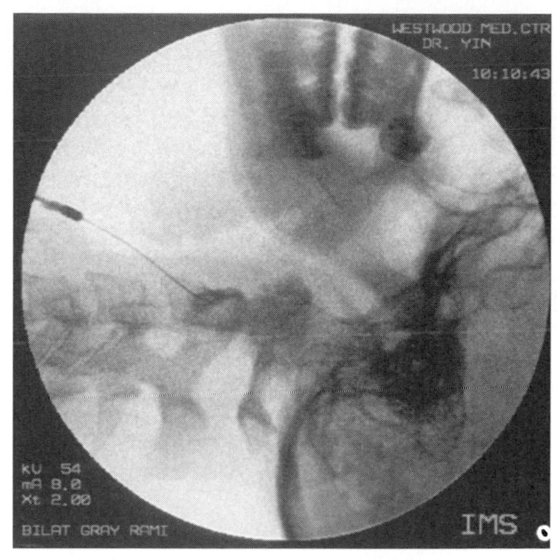

FIGURE 19–47 *Lateral radiograph demonstrates contrast medium ventral to C2 "lateral mass" and electrode positioned for ramus communicans RF lesion.*

Careful aspiration is performed; no blood or other body fluid should be aspirated. A small-volume contrast study is then performed, using 0.2 to 0.4 mL of nonionic contrast, such as iohexol, 240 mg/mL. Contrast spread should be limited to the immediate perivertebral region, outlining the sulcus on anteroposterior fluoroscopic imaging. In lateral radiographs, the contrast should appear to silhouette the ventral aspect of the transverse process of C2 (Fig. 19–47).

Sensory stereotaxy is performed next, utilizing 0.15 to 0.2 V at 50 Hz, 1 msec pulse duration. The electrode is manipulated with very small movements along the ventral sulcus of C2 until concordant suboccipital pain is reproduced in a patient-blinded fashion. Elicitation of sharp radiating infraauricular/neck pain indicates stimulation of the ventral C3 nerve root and is unacceptable. Elicitation of deep or superficial infraauricular pain or anterior cervical/submandibular pain may indicate possible stimulation of the chorda tympani and is unacceptable. There are no motor branches associated with the ramus communicans nerve; motor stimulation generally is not performed. Once concordant suboccipital pain has been elicited in a reproducible, patient-blinded fashion, 0.5–1 mL 2% lidocaine is injected before RF lesioning.

The RF lesion is performed at 80° C for a period of 60 sec and repeated once the electrode tip has returned to ambient body temperature. The size of the lesion created by the 2-mm active tip is small, but this approach reduces the risk of inadvertent C3 or chorda tympani lesion that could occur with a 5-mm active tip. After the lesioning, a small amount of corticosteroid, with or without local anesthetic, may be injected and the electrode removed. The patient may be discharged after a 1- to 2-hour post-procedure observation period. Patients frequently complain of some deep neck soreness, which may last 2 to 3 days and occasionally of pain with swallowing, which is similarly self-limited. Occasionally, despite negative stimulation, patients may complain of some temporary radiating pain in the infraauricular region radiating down the ipsilateral neck. This may be a result of localized inflammation irritating the chorda tympani or ventral C3 nerve root after the thermal lesion and is generally self-limited.

Lesions of the Sphenopalatine Ganglion

Lesions of the sphenopalatine ganglion can be useful in the treatment of patients with cluster headaches, certain types of migraine headaches, and neuritis of the sphenopalatine ganglion. On lateral fluoroscopic view, the sphenopalatine fossa sits at the tip of the petrous bone, just beneath the sphenoid sinus. This ganglion lies in the sphenopalatine "groove," which connects the fossa with the nasal cavity. The sphenopalatine ganglion lies medial to the maxillary nerve, and its fossa can be recognized on a lateral radiograph as a wedge-shaped structure situated at the tip of the petrous mass and just inferior to the anterior aspect of the sphenoid sinus.

If a prognostic block provides good relief, then an RF lesion of the sphenopalatine ganglion is performed, as follows. The patient is placed in the supine position on the fluoroscopy table. Preoperative antibiotics are given 45 min beforehand. The head should be fixed in neutral position with a strip of tape. The fluoroscopy unit is set up to produce a lateral projection. An opaque marker is held over the sphenopalatine fossa, and a mark is placed on the skin at that point. After the patient has been prepared and draped, the skin and subcutaneous tissues are anesthetized with local anesthetic. The entry point is usually just superior to the mandibular arch. A 100-mm cannula with 2-mm active tip is used for the procedure. The cannula is advanced perpendicular to and between the prominences of the mandible, usually in the center of the sphenopalatine fossa as seen on fluoroscopy. A curved cannula tip facilitates movement around the bony structures. The cannula is slowly advanced medially until it enters the sphenopalatine fossa. Intermittent anteroposterior views are taken to make certain that the cannula is on course and well caudal of the orbit. As the cannula is advanced farther, it makes contact with the maxillary nerve. A paresthesia to the maxilla is noted at that point. The fluoroscopy unit is then changed to an anteroposterior projection. The cannula is advanced farther medially until it is just adjacent to the lateral wall of the nasal cavity. It is then advanced 1 to 2 mm at a time until it slips into the groove in the nasal cavity. If the cannula contacts bone and not the groove, its position should be changed slightly until it is felt to move into the groove.

As the cannula slips into proper position, stimulation should begin at 50 Hz. If the cannula is in correct position, a tingling sensation in the nose is noted at approximately 1.0 V. Frequently, tingling is noted in the soft palate, in which case the cannula should be advanced in a slightly more medial direction. Stimulation should be performed again, and, if the cannula is in correct position, the majority of the stimulation is noted in the nasal region. If only a small amount of paresthesia is felt in the soft palate and the majority in the nasal cavity, the cannula is in correct position, and 1.0 mL of 2% lidocaine can be injected through the cannula to anesthetize the sphenopalatine ganglion.

The thermal lesion is created for 60 sec at 80° C, and the cannula is advanced 1 mm medially. A second lesion is made in an identical manner, and the cannula is again advanced 1 mm, where the third and final lesion is then created.

The cannula is withdrawn after the third lesion, and the patient is observed for 2 hours. Some 10% to 20% of patients experience epistaxis after the procedure. This is not a dangerous problem, but the patient should not be discharged until it has fully resolved. Postoperative discomfort can last as long as 2 weeks. A small percentage of patients develop some sensory loss in the soft palate after this procedure (Fig. 19–48).

Lesions of the Trigeminal Ganglion

The first descriptions of RF thermal lesions of the trigeminal ganglion were published by Sweet and Wepsic,[120] who confirmed its efficacy. Reports of trigeminal thermal lesions in more than 1000 cases over a 10-year period were published in 1990 by Broggi and colleagues.[121] The value of RF procedures in the treatment of trigeminal neuralgia has been confirmed by numerous series over the past 15 years. Initially, analgesia or hypalgesia was believed to be a normal component of the procedure. Over time, it has been shown that use of lower temperatures can control the paroxysmal pain while minimizing sensory loss.

Other techniques, such as glycerol rhizolysis and microcompression injury to the gasserian ganglion, have been used to treat trigeminal neuralgia. RF procedures, however, have the most long-term follow-up data. Interventional treatment should be reserved for patients whose disease is not controlled by medications and for those who are unable to use medications because of intolerable side effects.

In one large study, almost 95% of patients had dramatic reductions in paroxysmal pain after RF lesion of the trigeminal ganglion.[121] The mortality rate in this series was zero, and the morbidity was approximately 35%. Complications included masseter weakness (10.5%), parasthesias requiring medical management (5.2%), painful anesthesia (1.5%), ocular palsies (0.5%), corneal reflex impairment without keratitis (19.7%), corneal reflex impairment with keratitis (0.6%), and vasomotor rhinorrhea (0.1%). In spite of a fairly high incidence of manageable complications, the vast majority of patients were satisfied with the procedure; that is, the relief of pain was so significant that the morbidity was considered relatively minor in comparison.

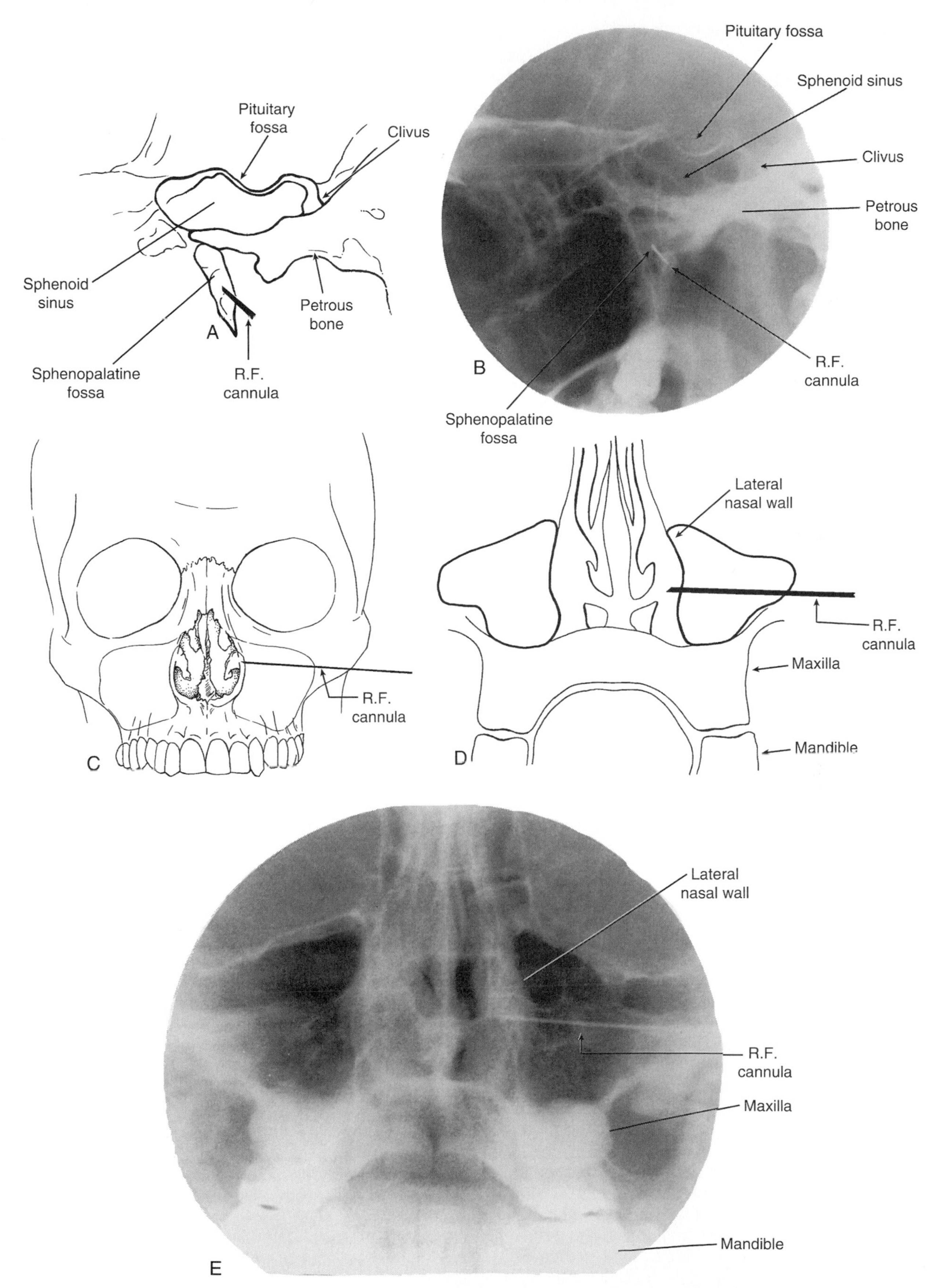

FIGURE 19–48 A, B, *Drawing and radiograph are lateral views of the base of the skull as it is seen on the fluoroscopy screen as the RF cannula passes through the sphenopalatine fossa toward the sphenopalatine ganglion. Note the relative positions of the identified structures.* C, *Drawing of a posteroanterior view through the nasal and maxillary region. The RF cannula is shown entering the lateral wall of the nasal cavity. It is within the lateral wall of the nasal cavity (middle turbinate) that the sphenopalatine ganglion resides.* D, E, *Drawing and radiograph show a closer view of the lateral walls of the nasal cavity and the maxilla. Note the relative positions of the lateral wall of the nasal cavity and the RF cannula.*

No long-term prospective studies have compared the efficacy, morbidity, and mortality of RF thermal lesions of the trigeminal ganglion and open decompression of the posterior fossa. Percutaneous procedures might be safer in elders and in patients with serious underlying medical problems. For young, healthy patients with trigeminal neuralgia, many neurosurgeons believe that open decompression is the treatment of choice.

The advantage of the RF procedure is that the lesion can be well-controlled. Disadvantages of techniques that use liquid neurolytic agents include possible spread into the subarachnoid space with harm to the central nervous system. A higher incidence of neuropathy is associated with the use of liquid neurolytic agents. Whether or not glycerol produces the same incidence of neuropathy as phenol or alcohol has yet to be shown. Even with glycerol, control of the solution is not as precise as control of a thermal lesion. With a thin, insulated RF cannula and 2-mm active tip, it is possible to produce lesions to individual branches of the trigeminal ganglion without affecting the remaining branches. It is not possible to do this with neurolytic solutions. The technique of percutaneous microcompression of the trigeminal ganglion shows some early promising results, but, as yet, no long-term follow-up has been performed with a sufficient number of patients.

Trigeminal Neuralgia: Symptom Complex

Trigeminal neuralgia is a disease of intermittent facial pain seen commonly in middle-aged and older patients. The pain is usually unilateral and is most commonly associated with the lower divisions of the trigeminal nerve. There are usually pain-free intervals between attacks, and the pain tends to come in paroxysms. It is not unusual for the pain to be provoked by stimulation of trigger points, points on the face, jaw, or neck where the pain can actually be triggered. Usually, no sensory loss is associated with this disease. The disorder can be associated with other diseases, such as multiple sclerosis, posterior fossa tumors, posterior fossa vascular anomalies, and herpes zoster. For most cases, the cause is not known.

Patients with trigeminal neuralgia demand a comprehensive neurologic evaluation. Appropriate evoked potential and spinal fluid analyses are necessary to rule out the possibility of multiple sclerosis (prevalence 2%–3%). The majority of patients with trigeminal neuralgia can be managed medically, most often with carbamazepine. Some who are unable to tolerate therapeutic doses of these medications or whose symptoms do not respond could be candidates for interventional management (Fig. 19–49).

Located in the medial aspect of the middle cranial fossa, the gasserian ganglion is surrounded by dura within Meckel's cavern. On the medial aspect of the gasserian ganglion lie the cavernous sinus and internal carotid artery. The ganglion sits posterior and superior to the foramen ovale. Entrance to it is via the foramen ovale, which measures 5 to 10 mm in diameter and 5 to 7 mm in depth. The most important part of the technique of RF ablation of the gasserian ganglion is proper fluoroscopic imaging of the foramen ovale. The most medial aspect of the foramen ovale leads to the first division, the central portion to the second

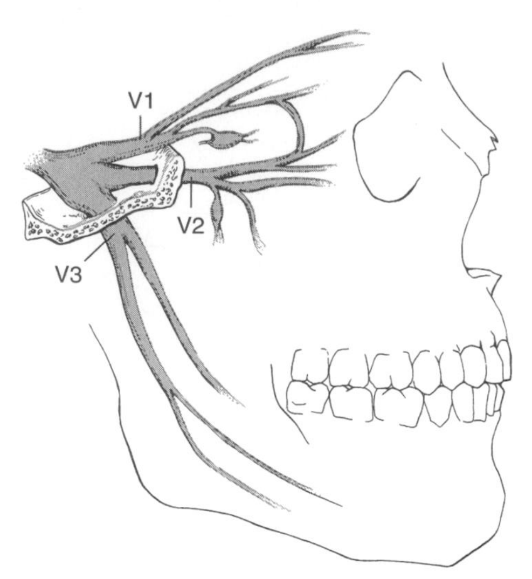

FIGURE 19–49 Drawing of the distribution of the trigeminal nerves. V1 is the first division, V2 the second, and V3 the third division of the trigeminal system.

division, and the lateral aspect to the third division of the gasserian ganglion. The third division is most superficial, the second intermediate, and the first the deepest.

Technique of Gasserian Ganglionotomy

Prophylactic antibiotics should be given 1 hour before the operative procedure. The patient is placed in the supine position with the neck extended. A steep subzygomatic fluoroscopic view is taken with 10 to 15 degrees of lateral rotation. The foramen ovale can be directly visualized "just medial" to the mandibular arch. To perform this technique smoothly, the needle should be passed in a line parallel to the fluoroscopic beam. Doing this enables the electrode to follow the beam directly into the foramen ovale, eliminating all guesswork and allowing precise positioning of the cannula. With this technique, superficial landmarks are no longer needed, because the operator simply follows the beam directly to the target site.

The technique of RF lesioning of the gasserian ganglion is described here as it is performed in a patient with trigeminal neuralgia of the first division. The patient is positioned as previously described. The x-ray beam should be directly beneath the zygoma with 10 to 15 degrees of lateral rotation, to bring the foramen ovale clearly into view. A mark is placed on the skin overlying the foramen ovale as seen under fluoroscopy (usually 1–2 cm lateral and 1 cm inferior to the corner of the mouth). In this example, the electrode tip is directed toward the most medial aspect of the foramen ovale.

After the patient's face has been prepared and draped, an anesthetic dose of propofol (isopropyl phenol) is given intravenously by the monitoring anesthesiologist. The physician performing the procedure should not be involved in giving the anesthetic. After the patient has lost consciousness but is breathing spontaneously, the physician places one finger in the patient's mouth and advances the RF cannula percutaneously. The finger is in the mouth to detect penetration of the oral cavity. If this occurs, the cannula should be removed and a new cannula should be used. As the cannula is advanced subcutaneously beneath the zygoma, it is directed parallel to the fluoroscopic beam and toward the foramen ovale. The cannula is advanced to the medial aspect of the foramen ovale, and then approximately 2 mm farther once it has entered the canal (Fig. 19–50). A lateral view is obtained through the region of the petrous bone and clivus. The cannula is advanced farther, until it reaches the junction of the petrous mass and the clivus. At this point, the stylet of the cannula is removed, and slow leakage of cerebrospinal fluid should be seen, indicating that the dura within Meckel's cavern has been punctured.

After the patient has emerged from the anesthetic, stimulation is performed. At 50-Hz stimulation, good paresthesia along the first division of the fifth nerve should be noted at less than 0.5 V. At 2-Hz stimulation, one should fail to see masseter muscle contraction with 0.7 to 1.0 V. For lesioning of the third division, it may not be possible to avoid masseter stimulation, and some mild masseter weakness may be an unavoidable result. It is best to give additional doses of propofol if the cannula is advanced or withdrawn, because such maneuvers can be quite painful. Once proper paresthesia has been obtained, the first lesion can be created.

The physician can never go wrong choosing a thermal lesion that is too cool. Significant perioperative problems, however, can result from a needle that is too hot. Thus, it is best to start with thermal lesions at 60° C for 60 sec. If the patient has multiple sclerosis, using less heat should be considered. Excessively hot lesioning temperatures can cause deafferentation pain after the procedure.

After appropriate stimulation parameters are identified, the patient is given an additional dose of propofol until consciousness is again lost. At that point, a lesion is made. *Profound anesthesia should be avoided.* Such a lesion can lead to deafferentation pain and loss of the corneal reflex. Done properly, however, most patients will achieve excellent pain relief and maintain an adequate corneal reflex. This technique need not be painful or unpleasant for the patient. With modern short-acting intravenous anesthetics, patients can be fully anesthetized for the placement of the cannula and the creation of the lesion.

Thermal lesions of the gasserian ganglion can also be useful in the management of intractable cluster headaches that fail to respond to the sphenopalatine lesion. This technique is also useful for treating pain secondary to cancer.

Patients are admitted for overnight observation after the procedure. Dexamethasone should be given immediately after the procedure and for the first 48 hours. This regimen will decrease edema and the chances of corneal insensitivity. If there is any drying of the cornea, saline eye drops should be used to lubricate it. Discomfort can last 2 to 4 weeks after the procedure, and appropriate analgesics may be necessary during this period. Some patients also have unpleasant dysesthesias. If patients were taking medications such as Tegretol preoperatively, the therapy should not be stopped abruptly. All such medications should be tapered in dose over 2 weeks after the procedure. It can be anticipated that at least 80% of patients experience high-grade pain relief. In the first year, approximately 15% to 20% of patients have a partial recurrence of pain; for these patients, a second ganglionotomy can be done.

SYMPATHECTOMY IN THE LUMBAR AND THORACIC REGIONS

The use of neurodestructive techniques in the sympathetic nervous system was first described in 1924.[122] The technique was later refined and used to promote improved blood flow in persons suffering from peripheral vascular disease.[123] Over the years, lumbar sympathectomy has been shown to be useful in the treatment of certain patients with reflex sympathetic dystrophy, vascular occlusive diseases, vasospastic diseases (Raynaud's syndrome), and other types of sympathetically maintained pain.

Sympathectomy, with resultant vasodilatation, improved blood flow, and higher temperatures in both the arm and leg can be readily and safely performed with percutaneous RF lesions of the thoracic or lumbar sympathetic chain. The technique of RF lumbar sympathectomy has been well described in the literature.[124–126]

Anatomy of the Lumbar Sympathetic Chain

In the lumbar region, the sympathetic chain and ganglia extend from L1 to L5. These chains are continuous with the thoracic sympathetic chain above and the pelvic sympathetic fibers below. In the lumbar region, the sympathetic chain and its ganglia lie near the anterolateral surface of the vertebral body. There is variability in the position, but the chain always lies anterior to the psoas sheath. The sympathetic chain and ganglia are separated from the somatic nerves, and if the RF cannula is properly placed, precise lesions of the sympathetic chain and ganglia can be performed without producing injury to the somatic nerves. RF lesioning of the sympathetic nerves should not be performed until fluoroscopy-directed test blocks with local anesthetic have shown a desired clinical effect.

The aorta and inferior vena cava sit just anterior to the body of the vertebra, and puncture of these structures should be avoided. The ureters and somatic nerves are close to the sympathetic chain, and injury to these structures must also be avoided. At the L2 and L3 levels, the genitofemoral nerve lies close to the sympathetic chain, and injury to this structure can cause severe postoperative groin pain.

The test block should be performed using only 2 mL of combination local anesthetic with a final concentration of 1% lidocaine and 0.25% bupivacaine at each level. The test block should be done at the levels of L2, L3, and L4, or, if the foot is involved, at L3, L4, and L5. The purpose of a small volume of local anesthetic is to avoid extravasation onto the somatic nerves (which would invalidate the test block). A proper sympathetic test block is one that produces sympathetic blockade with no loss of sensory or motor function. If sensory or motor dysfunction is noted after the test block, the results are invalid, and the test must be repeated. If possible, sedation should not be used during sympathetic test blocks, because it can prevent proper interpretation of the clinical results. If it is abso-

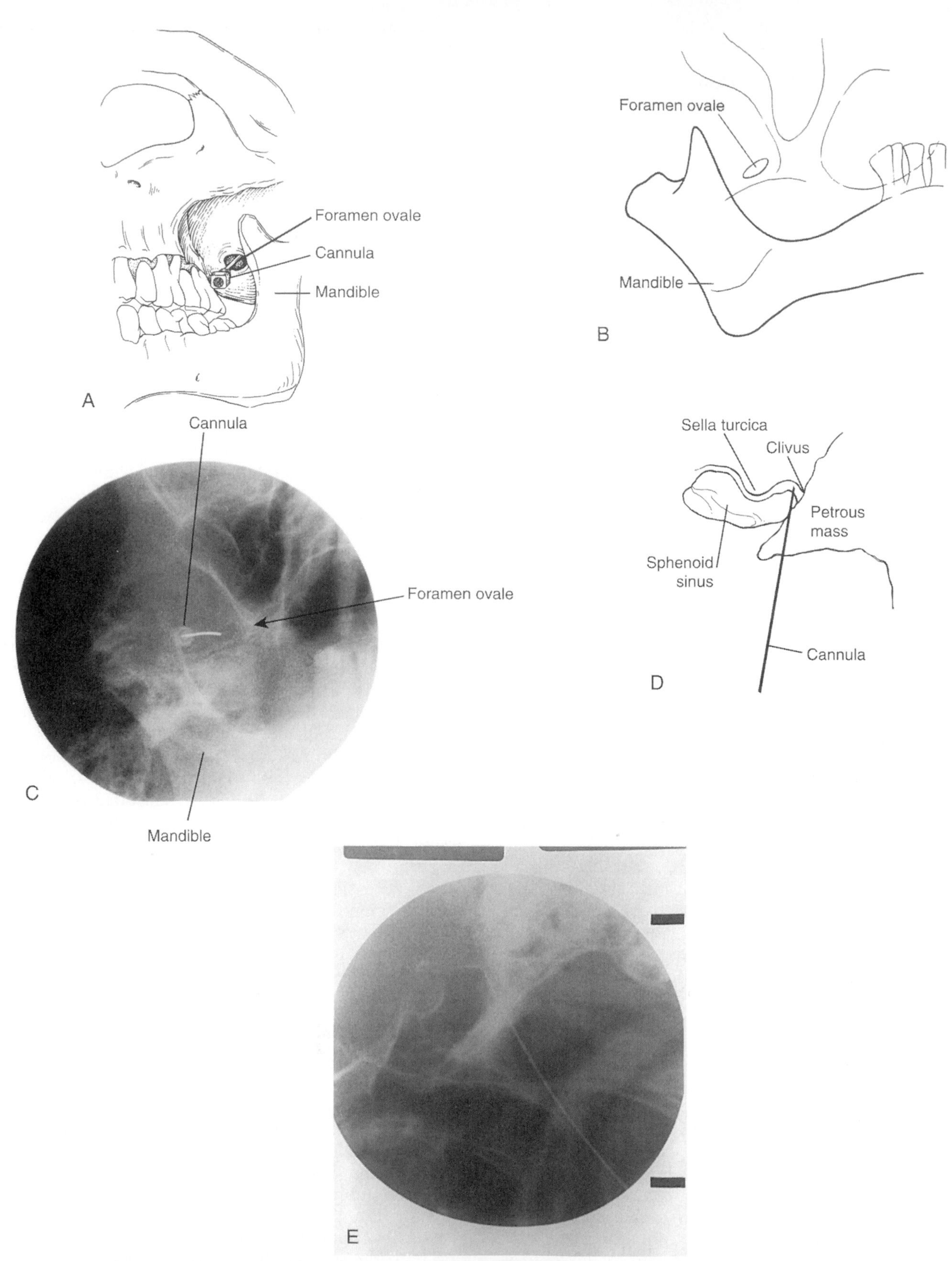

FIGURE 19–50 A, *Drawing shows the entry of an RF cannula into the foramen ovale. Note that the cannula passes beneath the zygoma to enter the foramen ovale at the base of the skull.* B, C, *Drawing and radiograph of the steep subzygomatic view as seen on the fluoroscopy screen. With approximately 15 degrees of lateral angulation, the foramen ovale is seen just inside the upper aspect of the mandible.* C, *The radiofrequency cannula has entered the most lateral aspect of the foramen ovale.* D, *Drawing of the lateral view through the base of the skull as it appears during placement of an RF cannula through the foramen ovale. Note the relationships between the identified structures. The RF cannula tip is just at the junction of the clivus with the sphenoid sinus.* E, *Lateral radiograph through the base of the skull shows the RF cannula passing through the junction of the sphenoid sinus and the clivus.*

lutely necessary, only short-acting agents such as propofol should be given.

Technique of Lesioning of the Lumbar Sympathetic Chain and Ganglia

The patient is placed in the prone position on the fluoroscopy table and is sedated and monitored. A C-arm fluoroscopic device is used to identify the vertebral bodies at L2, L3, and L4. If the foot is involved, the L5 level needs to be lesioned as well. The sympathetic ganglia at L2 and L3 can be variable, sometimes being as much as 15 mm posterior to the anterior aspect of the vertebral body (depending on the level). The ganglion at L2 rests near the junction of the lower third with the upper two thirds of the vertebral body. The ganglion at L3 lies near the junction of the upper third with the lower two thirds of the vertebral body. It is preferable to lesion these levels to include the sympathetic chain and its associated ganglia to produce a longer-lasting lesion. The position of the L4 ganglion is more variable than that of the L2 and L3 ganglia.

The new curved-blunt RF cannula (discussed earlier) should be considered for the RF lumbar sympathectomy procedures. An electrode 150 mm in length with a curved 10-mm active tip is used. A posterior view under fluoroscopic guidance is used to identify the second, third, and fourth vertebral bodies. An oblique view is taken with craniad or caudad rotation so that the disc space is sharply visualized. With the fluoroscopic device obliquely rotated to approximately 20 degrees (so that the vertebral bodies "cover" the transverse processes), the cannulas are inserted and directed toward the target points described earlier. The cannulas should be directed parallel to the fluoroscopy beam until the lateral aspect of the vertebra is contacted.

Small amounts of intravenous sedation are given to enable the patient to lie comfortably during placement of the RF cannulas. After contact with the vertebral bodies has been made, a lateral view is taken. The cannulas are advanced so they touch the periosteum of the vertebral body, and they are moved anteriorly until they contact the anterior aspect. The fluoroscopy unit is then moved to produce a posteroanterior view. The cannulas are in correct position when their tips are directly behind the middle of the facet joint line while in contact with the vertebral body.

At 50 Hz stimulation, the patient should develop a deep pain in the back at approximately 1.0 V. Lower extremity motor fasciculations should be negative with 3.0 V at 2 Hz stimulation. If sensory stimulation at the L2 or L3 level provokes parasthesias in the groin, the cannula should be repositioned, because it is too close to the genitofemoral nerve. When the radiologic criteria have been met and the stimulation parameters are correct, the lesions can be made.

The lesions are made after 1 mL of 2% lidocaine is injected through the cannula. A thermal lesion is created for 60 sec at 80° C. At the L2 level, one lesion is adequate to produce a 10-mm lesion from the anterior aspect of the vertebral body posteriorly. The cannulas at the L3 and L4 levels should be positioned initially at a point 5 mm posterior to the anterior aspect of the vertebral body. Stimulation and lesioning should be done at this position. The cannulas should then be moved 5 mm anterior for the second stimulation and lesion at each of these levels. With this technique, the cannulas are moved away from the segmental nerves when the second lesion is done.

Thus, a 15-mm "strip" lesion is made at the L3 and L4 levels and a 10-mm lesion at the L2 level. If the foot is involved, another 15-mm lesion must be made at the L5 level as well. The lesions at each level are made between the anterior aspect of the vertebral body and the anteromedial aspect of the psoas sheath (Fig.19–51).

Potential complications include injury to the genitofemoral nerve (which could produce neuropathic pain in the groin). Injury to the somatic nerves, with subsequent sen-

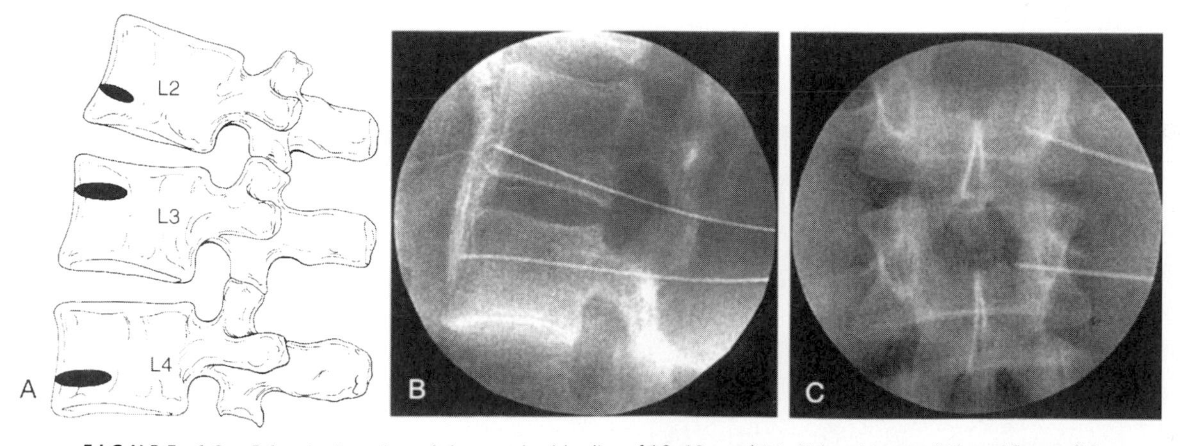

FIGURE 19–51 *A, Drawing of the vertebral bodies of L2, L3, and L4. Either 10-mm (L2) or 15-mm (L3 and L4) lesion strips (solid ovals) are used to interrupt the lumbar sympathetic chain. Note the positions of the lesion strips relative to the anterior aspect of the vertebral bodies. It is important to keep in mind that the lumbar sympathetic chain is always anterior to the psosas muscle but that the relative positions of the sympathetic chain with the anterior aspect of the vertebral body can vary. Thus, using lesion strips increases the probability of interrupting the sympathetic chain with an RF lesion. B, Lateral radiograph shows the RF cannula positions at the L2 and L3 levels for lesioning of the lumbar sympathetic chain. C, Posteroanterior radiograph shows the RF cannula positions during lesioning of the lumbar sympathetic chain. Note that the tips of the RF cannulas are directly behind the facet joint line.*

sory or motor loss is possible but can be avoided with proper stimulation. Retrograde ejaculation can occur in men and is seen more often after bilateral lumbar sympathectomy. Postoperative discomfort lasts approximately 5 days, but pain relief should be immediate if the lesions have been correctly targeted.

The incidence of injury to the lumbar spinal and genitofemoral nerves is higher with liquid neurolytic techniques than with the RF procedure, which also produces a better-controlled lesion. Vascular uptake of neurolytic solutions can lead to complications. Ureteral injuries may also occur with neurolytic agents.

The low morbidity and almost zero mortality with the RF technique speak well for its safety. The technique can be repeated if necessary, and the repeat procedure carries no higher risk of morbidity than the first one. The RF technique is an outpatient procedure and is safer and more cost-effective than open surgical sympathectomy.

Given the low morbidity, almost zero mortality, cost-effectiveness, and ability to repeat the technique, if necessary, RF ablation of the lumbar sympathetic chain appears to be the procedure of choice for producing long-term lumbar sympatholysis.

Lesioning of the Thoracic Sympathetic Structures

Anatomy and Test Blocks

The upper thoracic sympathetic chain is an extension of the cervical sympathetic chain and continues caudad. It lies along the periosteum of the vertebral body farther posterior than the lumbar sympathetic chain (Fig. 19–52A).[127] The technique of upper thoracic RF sympathectomy has been thoroughly discussed in the literature.[128–131]

The technique of thoracic sympathectomy usually involves lesions of the sympathetic chain at the T2 and T3 levels. These levels have significant outflow to the upper extremity and can be involved in sympathetically maintained upper extremity pain. A small amount of local anesthetic placed on the stellate ganglion tends to produce physiologic effects similar to those seen when a small amount of local anesthetic is placed on the thoracic sympathetic chain at the T2 and T3 levels; that is, a warm, dry, vasodilated upper extremity. The T2 and T3 levels probably have even more outflow to the hand than does the C7 level, however. Test blocks should be performed with local anesthetic before the RF procedure and should

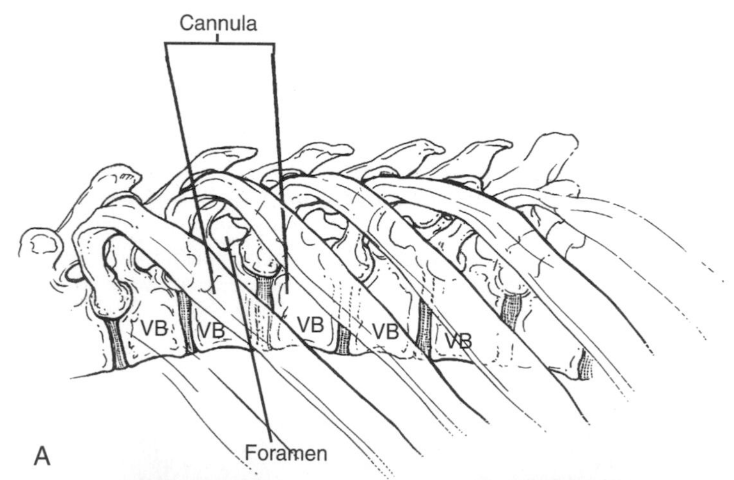

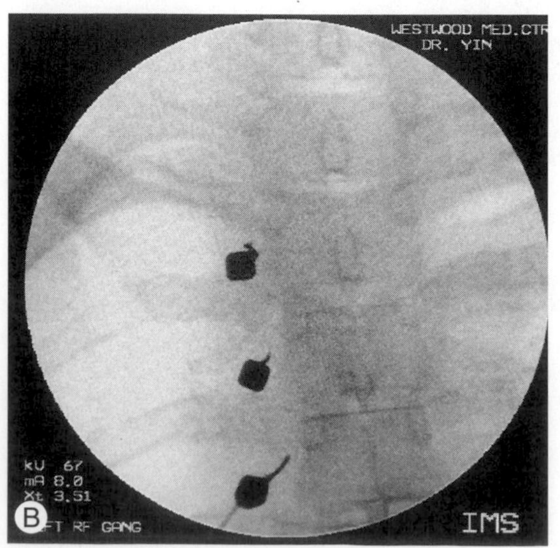

FIGURE 19–52 A, *Drawing of a lateral view through the thoracic spine. Note the relative positions of the thoracic foramina, the vertebral bodies (VB), and the tips of the RF cannulas. This is the correct position for RF lesions of the thoracic sympathetic chain at the T2 and T3 levels.* B, *AP image of electrode placement for left T2, T3, T4 posterior parasagittal sympathetic ganglia RF lesion. Note medial orientation of electrode tips toward costovertebral junction approaching posterolateral aspect of vertebral bodies, beneath lamina.*

be performed under direct fluoroscopic guidance. The volume of local anesthetic solution should be limited to 2 mL to produce precise and highly reproducible results. If the patient obtains greater relief when the cervical sympathetic fibers are anesthetized, it is prudent to perform an RF lesion of those fibers (see section on Lesioning of the Stellate Ganglion). If test blocks of the T2 and T3 sympathetic chain show more favorable results, an RF lesion of the T2 and T3 sympathetic fibers should be performed. In some instances, lesions to both the cervical and thoracic outflow are needed to control symptoms.

Posterior Parasagittal Approach

The thoracic nerve root, dorsal root ganglia, sympathetic ganglia, and splanchnic structures may be reached by a novel posterior parasagittal approach utilizing curved electrodes. This approach provides access to the thoracic paravertebral sympathetic structures at any level from T2 through T12, decreases the risk of inadvertent pneumothorax, and allows access to the midthoracic levels, which were previously difficult to approach safely using a traditional posterolateral approach. The use of blunt tipped electrodes greatly improves the safety of thoracic posterior parasagittal techniques, especially when applied toward lesions of the thoracic sympathetic and splanchnic structures. This "posterior parasagittal curved-needle" approach developed by one of the authors (WY) has been used in more than 500 individual thoracic segmental procedures, with no pneumothorax to date.

The technique takes advantage of the fact that the thoracic paravertebral ganglionic structures generally lie directly ventral and medial to the junction of the inferior medial border of the transverse processes with the superior lateral thoracic lamina at the same level when viewed in the anteroposterior fluoroscopic plane. This bony landmark is constant throughout the thoracic region from T1 to T11; at the level of T12, radiographically, the transverse process is essentially vestigial. The necessity to steer the tip of the electrode during fluoroscopically guided placement demands a curved-tip electrode. Blunt-tipped and cutting-tip 20-gauge RF electrodes with 10-mm active tips are commercially available (Radionics, Inc., Burlington, Mass.) in 100-mm lengths. The blunt-tipped ones are recommended for thoracic paravertebral sympathetic ganglionic and splanchnic RF procedures. For discrete selective thoracic dorsal root ganglion RF procedures, 22-gauge 100-mm short-beveled electrodes with 2- to 5-mm active tips are preferred (see earlier sections).

It must be emphasized that all percutaneous thoracic procedures carry the risk of pneumothorax, even in skilled hands. Paravertebral procedures carry the risk of vascular, visceral (e.g., esophagus, bronchi), and nerve (spinal cord, vagus, phrenic, intercostal) injury, and the potential to injure other anatomically juxtaposed structures (e.g., lymphatic vessels). These procedures should be performed only by skilled physicians expert in percutaneous stereotactic RF interventions under fluoroscopic guidance.

In the upper thoracic region (T1–T6), the thoracic sympathetic ganglia lie just ventral to the level of the heads of the ribs, approximately at the junction of the dorsal and middle third of the vertebral body as visualized in lateral projections and just deep to the thoracic parietal pleura. In the lower thoracic region (T7–T12), the sympathetic ganglia may lie slightly more ventral, approaching the midpoint of the vertebral body in lateral projections. Unlike the corresponding ganglia in the lumbar regions, the thoracic sympathetic ganglia *do not* lie along the anterolateral aspect of the vertebral bodies.

A common posterior parasagittal fluoroscopically guided approach may be made toward the thoracic nerve root, dorsal root ganglia, sympathetic ganglia, and, in the lower thoracic region, splanchnic nerves. The patient is placed prone on the fluoroscopy table, and the skin of the back prepared in the standard fashion. Anteroposterior fluoroscopic images are obtained, and the imaging system tilted cephalad or caudad to "square off" the vertebral end plates of the area of interest. The inferomedial border of the transverse process at its junction with the superior lateral lamina of the level desired is identified, and a skin entry site is marked and anesthetized directly overlying this mark. If the recommended blunt-tipped electrodes are utilized, a 1.25-inch 16-gauge intravenous catheter is introduced percutaneously at a depth just sufficient to penetrate the dermis and underlying thoracic paravertebral fascia. (Overvigorous insertion of this introducer cannula may result in inadvertent lung injury.)

The blunt, curved-tip electrode is then inserted through the introducer cannula and directed under anteroposterior fluoroscopic guidance to contact the bony landmark previously described. Once contact is made with bone, the electrode tip is rotated laterally and the electrode advanced just past the lateral lamina. Once past the lamina, the electrode tip is immediately rotated medially and directed toward the superior lateral vertebral body (Fig. 19–52B). Lateral fluoroscopic images are then obtained to ascertain the depth of electrode placement. Maintaining medial electrode tip direction, the electrode may be advanced to the desired level before sensory stereotactic localization of the target structure. In the upper thoracic spine, levels T1–T4, the transverse processes are relatively prominent, and care must be taken to ensure that the tip of the electrode is directed quite medially once it is past the level of the lateral lamina.

Once past the lamina, the electrodes are advanced until contact is made with the superolateral aspect of the vertebral body. (The operator takes care to avoid transfixing the exiting thoracic nerve root; if radiating paresthesias are encountered at this stage, the electrode is withdrawn and redirected, with the approach adjusted slightly caudal, aiming to traverse medial and caudal to the exiting nerve root.) The blunt-tipped electrodes are then advanced along the periosteum of the thoracic vertebral body, with the depth of placement guided by lateral fluoroscopic imaging. Once the active tip of the electrode has bisected the imaginary junction between the dorsal and middle thirds of the vertebral body, further advance is halted and anteroposterior images are obtained to verify electrode placement directly adjacent to the vertebral body. As there may be as little as 2 to 3 mm of potential space between the lateral thoracic vertebral periosteum and the pleura, meticulous attention to multiplanar fluoroscopic technique and use of blunt-tipped RF cannulas are imperative to minimize risk of pneumothorax or collateral tissue injury. The distal tips of

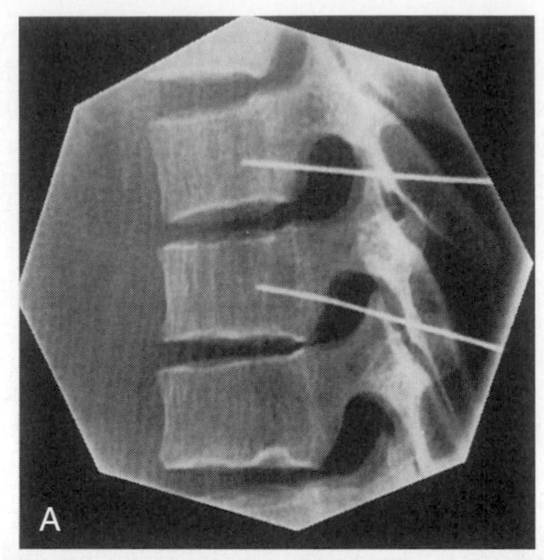

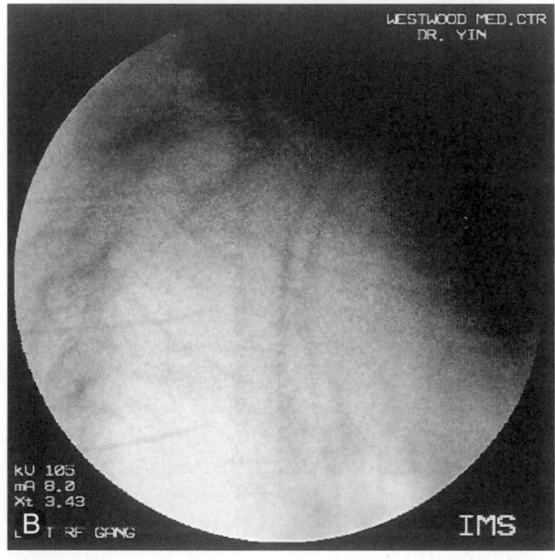

FIGURE 19–53 A, *Lateral view through skeleton shows T2, T3 sympathetic lesion.* B, *Lateral radiograph of electrode placement for T2, T3, T4 sympathetic ganglion RF lesion. Note active tips of electrodes overlapping junction of posterior and middle thirds of vertebral bodies.*

the electrodes are oriented cephalad. Lateral fluoroscopic images are obtained to verify that the electrode tip does not venture near the ventral aspect of the vertebral body; thermal lesioning of the esophagus might result, with disastrous consequence (Fig. 19–53). Anteroposterior fluoroscopic images are again obtained to verify juxtaposition of the electrode to the vertebral body. Careful aspiration is performed, and confirmatory contrast study performed to verify electrode placement in the paravertebral potential space. In the upper thoracic region, oblique fluoroscopic projections may be useful if the scapulas and humerus compromise adequate visualization (Fig. 19–54).

Sensory stereotactic stimulation is then performed at 0.5 to 0.7 V at 50 Hz, 1 msec pulse duration. Reproduction of concordant pain is sought with sequential sensory stimulation of the sympathetic ganglia. Elicitation of radiating somatic dermatomal pain indicates stimulation of the thoracic nerve roots, and the electrodes must be repositioned ventrally, or angled more cephalad and ventral to the exiting nerve root. Once concordant pain is reproduced, signifying successful stereotactic localization of symptomatic sympathetic ganglia, fine manipulation of the electrode tip is performed under real-time fluoroscopic imaging to maximize stimulation, while the stimulation threshold is decreased to 0.3 to 0.5 V. It is the authors' experience that

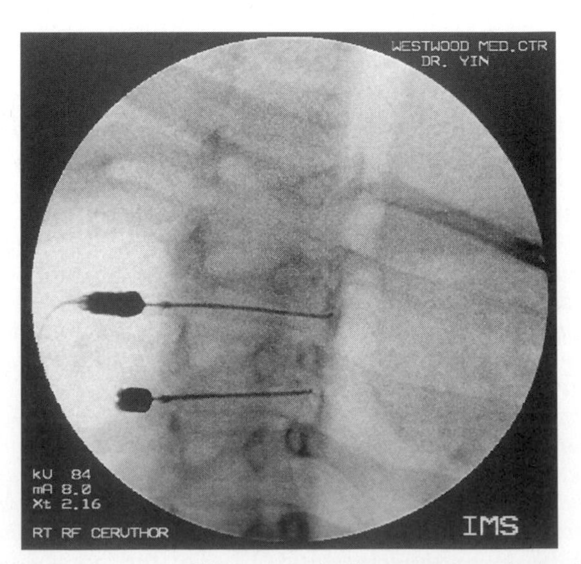

FIGURE 19–54 Oblique projection illustrates electrode placement and contrast study for right T2 and T3 sympathetic ganglia RF lesion. Note that contrast is limited to the paravertebral region at the junction of rib heads and vertebral bodies.

reproduction of sympathetic-mediated pain with ganglionic stimulation may require higher stimulation voltages than reproduction of somatic pain.

Once the symptomatic sympathetic ganglia levels have been localized with sensory stereotaxy, motor stimulation is performed, again to verify adequate electrode distance from the exiting thoracic nerve roots and to verify that other motor nerves (e.g., phrenic nerve) will not be involved in the ensuing thermal lesion. Before RF lesioning, 1 to 1.5 mL of 2% lidocaine is injected. The lesion is generally made at 80° C for a period of 60 sec.

The positioning of even blunt-tipped electrodes in the thoracic paravertebral region is often accompanied by significant patient discomfort. The judicious application of small amounts of reversible intravenous benzodiazepine and opioid analgesia may be required. The services of a qualified anesthesiologist administering intravenous analgesia may be invaluable. Bolus infusions of short-acting induction agents (e.g., isopropyl phenol or thiopental) are discouraged due to concerns of involuntary patient movement, and concerns of providing adequate airway management should overzealous sedation result in respiratory depression or airway obstruction.

As with other functional stereotactic procedures, the patient must be fully awake and capable of fine sensory discrimination before sensory stereotactic localization of the sympathetic ganglia is undertaken.

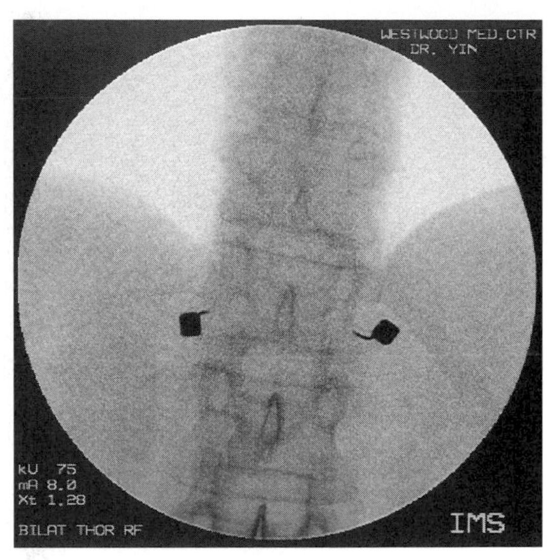

FIGURE 19–55 AP image of RF electrode placement for bilateral thoracic stereotactic splanchnic lesion. Note position of electrodes close to the lateral aspect of T12 vertebral body.

Thoracic Splanchnic Denervation

Thoracic splanchnic denervation provides a lesion-specific alternative to lytic celiac plexus injection and chemical splanchnectomy for the management of chronic celiac plexus–mediated pain. The thoracic splanchnic nerves provide afferent and efferent autonomic (primarily sympathetic) and sensory innervation to many of the retroperitoneal viscera of the upper abdominal area. Afferent sensory fibers may conduct sensation from the capsule of the spleen, liver (Glisson's capsule), biliary tree, kidneys, and pancreas[132] and they have been surgically ablated for the treatment of suprarenal and essential hypertension (Pende's and Peet's procedures, respectively).[133] Chemical splanchnectomy has been demonstrated to equal lytic celiac plexus injection in efficacy.[134] Percutaneous stereotactic RF thoracic splanchnic lesions may be used for the control of celiac plexus–mediated retroperitoneal visceral pain, and unlike other techniques of neurolysis, provide advantages of definitive identification of pain-conducting structures and generation of a controlled neurolytic lesion of predictable size. Before consideration of thoracic RF splanchnic lesioning, confirmatory low-volume thoracic splanchnic injections must be performed.

Three splanchnic nerves have been identified in adult humans. The greater splanchnic nerve, composed of myelinated preganglionic and visceral afferent fibers, is typically thought to provide primary sensory innervation to the pancreas and proximal retroperitoneal visceral structures and generally arises from the thoracic sympathetic ganglia of T5–T9. The lesser splanchnic nerve (approximately 95% of adults have one) arises from filaments from the sympathetic ganglia of T9–T12, and the least splanchnic nerve (55% of adults) may be related to the thoracic splanchnic ganglion at T12.[135] The splanchnic nerves course over the anterior lateral and lateral thoracic vertebral bodies ventral to the thoracic sympathetic chain.

A common stereotactic RF lesion of the splanchnic nerves is made with a posterior parasagittal approach at the level of T12. Because of the relative proximity of the individual splanchnic nerves (greater, lesser, least), it may be impossible to definitively and differentially lesion any one of these particular nerves. Sensory stereotaxy is thus invaluable in establishing the location of symptomatic splanchnic fibers before RF lesioning.

Unlike other thoracic levels, the transverse process of T12 is generally small and may not be visible on antero-

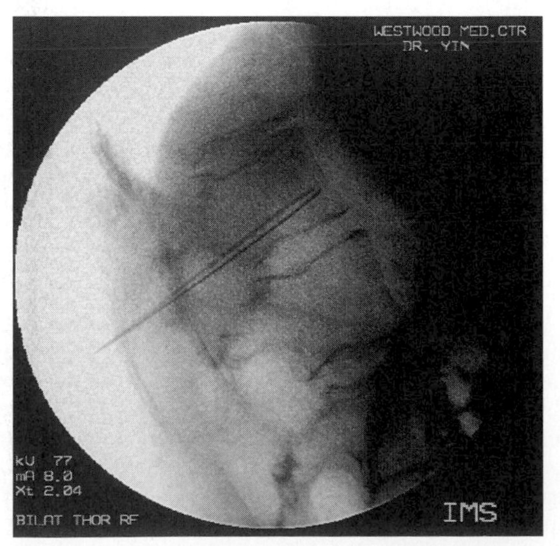

FIGURE 19–56 Lateral image illustrates absolutely farthest ventral placement of RF electrodes for thoracic stereotactic splanchnic lesion.

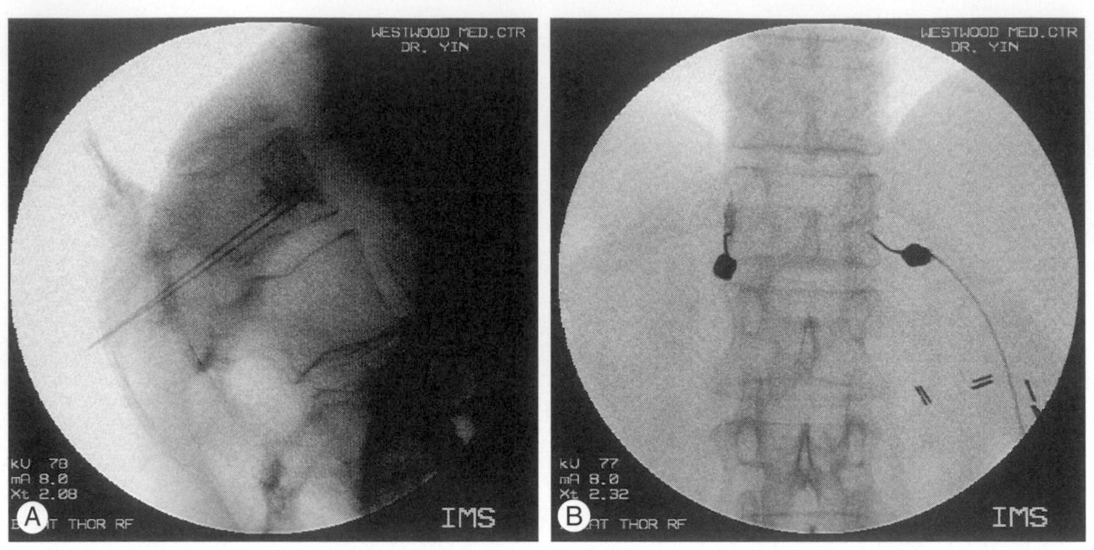

FIGURE 19–57 A, *Lateral contrast study before stereotactic localization of thoracic splanchnic nerves.* B, *AP contrast study during stereotactic splanchnic lesion.*

posterior radiographs. The skin entry site is marked over the lateral aspect of the vertebral body at T12, at the junction of the caudal (inferior) and middle thirds of the vertebral body, caudad to the exiting T12 nerve root (Fig. 19–55). A 16-gauge intravenous introducer catheter is introduced as previously described, and a 100-mm, 10-mm active tip, blunt, curved tip electrode is inserted through the introducer cannulas. The electrodes are directed under anteroposterior fluoroscopic imaging to contact the posterolateral aspect of the T12 vertebral body. Lateral images are then obtained to guide initial depth of electrode placement. The electrodes are advanced along the periosteum of the lateral aspect of the T12 vertebral body until the distal tip of the electrode approaches the junction of the middle and ventral (anterior) thirds of the vertebral body on lateral radiographs (Fig. 19–56). The procedure is repeated on the contralateral side. It is imperative that the distal extent of the electrodes does not approach the ventral aspect of the vertebral body; esophageal injury might result, with devastating consequences. Careful aspiration test and contrast studies are performed, and confirmatory anteroposterior and lateral radiographs are taken. The spread of contrast should remain in the immediate paravertebral region; some caudal spread of contrast may be seen if the electrodes rest ventral and medial to the crus of the diaphragm (Fig. 19–57).

Sensory stereotactic localization of the splanchnic nerves is then performed; initial stimulation may require 0.7 to 1.0 V. Subjective localized back pain is common in the higher range of stimulating voltages. The electrodes are maneuvered incrementally along the lateral aspect of the T12 vertebral body until the patient's visceral pain is reproduced. The stimulating voltage is decreased to the target range of 0.3 to 0.5 V with further fine manipulation of the electrode. As with thoracic sympathetic stereotaxy, radiating paresthesias along the flank indicate stimulation of the T12 nerve root. Should they occur, the electrode must be repositioned before RF lesioning, to avoid unintentional thermal injury to the nerve root. Motor stimulation is performed at 2 Hz, 1.0 to 1.5 V to verify that the distal electrode is not in the immediate vicinity of the phrenic nerve. If sensory stereotaxy does not reproduce concordant pain, lesions may be performed, though with a correspondingly lower expectation of success. RF lesions are performed at 80° C for a period of 60 sec. Secondary and tertiary lesions are performed overlapping the 50° to 55° C isotherm of previous lesions to ensure adequate splanchnic denervation.

As with all thoracic percutaneous paravertebral procedures, the patient is observed in the recovery area for signs of respiratory compromise or other complication, and postprocedure chest films are mandatory before discharge. Typically, splanchnic denervation is tolerated well, and predominant complaints being acting back pain that subsides within the first several postoperative days and generally responds to mild opioid analgesics or NSAID. The relief of visceral pain is typically immediate when the procedure is successful. Postoperative complaints of worsening abdominal pain or chest pain must be evaluated promptly, as potential complications could include visceral (pancreatic, esophageal, pulmonary) or major vascular injury (hemorrhagic complications).

REFERENCES

1. Onik GM, Porterfield B, Rubinsky B, Cohen J: Percutaneous transperineal prostate cryosurgery using transrectal ultrasound guidance: Animal model. Urology 37:277–281, 1991.
2. Onik GM, Cohen JK, Reyes GD, et al: Transrectal ultrasound-guided percutaneous radical cryosurgical ablation of the prostate. Cancer 72:1291–1299, 1993.
3. Mundinger F, Weigel K: Long-term results of stereotactic interstitial curietherapy. Acta Neurochir Suppl (Wien) 33:367–371, 1984.
4. Ostertag CB, Groothius D, Kleihue P: Experimental data on early and late morphologic effects on permanently implanted gamma and beta sources (iridium 192, iodine 125, and yttrium 90) in the brain. Acta Neurochir Suppl (Wien) 33:271–280, 1984.

5. Ostertag CB, Weigel K, Birg W: CT after long-standing implantation of cerebral gliomas. *In* Szikla G (ed): Stereotactic Cerebral Irradiation. Amsterdam, Elsevier/North Holland, 1979.
6. Gutin PH, Bernstein M, Sanyo Y, et al: Combination therapy with BCNU and low dose rate radiation in the 9L rat brain tumor and spheroid models: Implications for brain tumor brachytherapy. Neurosurgery 15:781–786, 1984.
7. Gutin PH, Dormandy RH: A coaxial catheter system for afterloading radioactive sources for the interstitial irradiation of brain tumors. J Neurosurg 56:734–735, 1982.
8. Gutin PH, Phillips TL, Hosobuchi Y, et al: Permanent and removable sources for the brachytherapy of brain tumors. Int J Radiat Oncol Biol Phys 7: 1371–1381, 1981.
9. Gutin PH, Phillips TL, Wara WM, et al: Brachytherapy of recurrent malignant brain tumors with removable high-activity iodine-125 sources. J Neurosurg 60:61–68, 1984.
10. Gutin PH, Phillips TL, Wara WM, et al: Brachytherapy with removable ^{125}I sources for the treatment of recurrent malignant brain tumors. Acta Neurochir Suppl (Wien) 33:363–366, 1984.
11. Gutin PH, Leibel SA, Wara WM, et al: Recurrent malignant gliomas: Survival following interstitial brachytherapy with high-activity iodine-125 sources. J Neurosurg 67:864–873, 1987.
12. Kooy HM, Nedzi LA, Loeffler JS, et al: Treatment planning for stereotactic radiosurgery of intracranial lesions. Int J Radiat Oncol Biol Phys 21:683–693, 1991.
13. Tsai JS, Buck BA, Svensson GK, et al: Quality assurance in stereotactic radiosurgery using a standard linear accelerator. Int J Radiat Oncol Biol Phys 21:737–748, 1991.
14. Alexander E III, Loeffler JS, Lunsford LD: Stereotactic Radiosurgery. New York, McGraw-Hill, 1993.
15. Young RF: Clinical experience with radiofrequency and laser DREZ lesions. J Neurosurg 72:715–720, 1990.
16. Sweet WH, Mark VH: Unipolar anodal electrolyte lesions in the brain of man and cat. Report of five human cases with electrically produced bulbar or mesencephalic tractotomies. AMA Arch Neurol Psychiatry 70:224–234, 1953.
17. Hunsperger RW, Wyss OAM: Production of localized lesions in nervous tissue by coagulation with high frequency current. Helveti Physiol Pharmacol Acta 11:283–304, 1953.
18. Mundinger F, Reichert T, Gabriel E: Untersuchungen zu den physikalischen und technischen Voranssetzungeneiner dosierten Hochfrequenzkoagulation bei stereptaktischen Hirnoperation. Zeitsch Chir 19:1051–1063, 1960.
19. Rosomoff HL, Carroll F, Brown J, Sheptak T: Percutaneous radiofrequency cervical cordotomy: Technique. J Neurosurg 23:639–644, 1965.
20. Brodkey J, Miyazaki Y, et al: Reversible heat lesions: A method of stereotactic localization. J Neurosurg 21:49, 1964.
21. Cosman ER, Nashold BS, Ovelan-Levitt J: Theoretical aspects of radiofrequency lesions in the dorsal root entry zone. Neurosurgery 156:945–950, 1984.
22. Fox JL: Experimental relationship of radio-frequency electrical current and lesion size for application to percutaneous cordotomy. J Neurosurg 33:415–421, 1970.
23. Lin PM, Gildenberg PL, Polakoff PP: An anterior approach to percutaneous lower cervical cordotomy. J Neurosurg 25:553–560, 1966.
24. Mullan S: Percutaneous cordotomy. J Neurosurg 35:360–366, 1971.
25. Levin AB, Cosman ER: Thermocouple-monitored cordotomy electrode: Technical note. J Neurosurg 53:266–268, 1980.
26. Bogduk N, Twomey LT: Clinical Anatomy of the Lumbar Spine. Edinburgh, Churchill Livingstone, 1987.
27. Bogduk N: The innervation of the lumbar spine. Spine 8(3):286–293, 1983.
28. Schwarzer AC, Aprill CN, Derby R, et al: The relative contributions of the disc and zygapophysial joint in chronic low back pain. Spine 19(7):801–806, 1994.
29. Schwarzer AC, Aprill CN, Derby R, et al: The roles of the zygapophysial joint and intervertebral disc in chronic low back pain: Results of a multicenter study. ISIS Newsletter 2(2):59–84, 1994.
30. Travel JG, Simons DG: Myofascial Pain and Dysfunction—The Trigger Point Manual. Baltimore, Williams & Wilkins, 1983.
31. Schwarzer AC, Aprill CN, Bogduk N: The sacroiliac joint in chronic low back pain. Spine 20(1):31–37, 1995.
32. Gharpuray V, Clemson S, et al: Intervertebral disc temperature distribution comparison: Radiofrequency needle versus thermal catheter. North American Spine Society, 14th Annual Meeting, Chicago, Ill., 1999.
33. Nash TP: Clinical note percutaneous radiofrequency lesioning of dorsal root ganglia for intractable pain. Pain 24:67–73, 1986.
34. North RB, Kidd DH, Campbell JN, Long DM: Dorsal root ganglionectomy for failed back surgery syndrome: A 5-year follow-up study. J Neurosurg 74:236–242, 1991.
35. North RB, Zahurak M, Kidd D: Radiofrequency lumbar facet denervation: Analysis of prognostic factors. Pain 57:77-83, 1994.
36. Ray CD: Percutaneous Radiofrequency Facet Nerve Block. Radionics Procedure Technique Series. Burlington, Mass., Radionics Corp, 1982.
37. Sluijter ME: The use of radiofrequency lesions for pain relief in failed back patients. Int Disabil Studies 10:37–42, 1988.
38. Kline MT: Stereotactic Radiofrequency Lesions as Part of the Management of Chronic Pain. Orlando, Fla., Paul M Deutsch, 1992.
39. Goldthwait JE: The lumbosacral articulation: An explanation of many cases of "lumbago," "sciatica" and paraplegia. Boston Med Surg J 64:365–372, 1911.
40. Putti V: New conceptions in the pathogenesis of sciatic pain. Lancet 2:53–60, 1927.
41. Williams PC, Yglesias L: Lumbosacral facetectomy for post fusion persistent sciatica. J Bone Joint Surg 15:579, 1933.
42. Ghormely RK: Low back pain with special reference to articular facet with presentation of an operative procedure. JAMA 101:1773–1777, 1933.
43. Helbig T, Lee CK: The lumbar facet syndrome. Spine 13(1):61–64, 1988.
44. Anderson KH, Mosel C, Varnet K: Percutaneous facet denervation in low-back and extremity pain. Acta Neurochir (Wien) 87:48–51, 1987.
45. Arbit E, Krol G: Percutaneous radiofrequency neurolysis guided by computed tomography for the treatment. Neurosurgery 29:580–582, 1991.
46. Banerjee T, Pittman HH: Facet rhizotomy: Another armamentarium for treatment of low backache. NC Med J 37:354–360, 1976.
47. Bogduk N, Long DM: Lumbar medical branch neurotomy: A modification of facet denervation. Spine 5:193–201, 1980.
48. Burton CV: Percutaneous radiofrequency facet denervation. Appl Neurophysiol 39:80–86, 1977.
49. Hickey RFJ, Tregonning GD: Denervation of spinal facet joints for treatment of chronic low back pain. NZ Med J 85:96–99, 1976.
50. Ignelzi RJ, Cummings TW: A statistical analysis of percutaneous radiofrequency lesions in the treatment of chronic low back pain and sciatica. Pain 8:181–187, 1980.
51. Ignelzi RJ: Radiofrequency lesions in the treatment of lumbar spinal pain. Contemp Neurosurg 12:1–5, 1990.
52. McCulloch JA: Percutaneous radiofrequency lumbar rhizolysis (rhizotomy). Appl Neurophysiol 39:87–96, 1976.
53. McCulloch JA, Organ LW: Percutaneous radiofrequency lumbar rhizolysis. Can Med Assoc J 116:300–311, 1977.
54. Mehta M, Sluijter ME: The treatment of chronic back pain: A preliminary survey of the effect of radiofrequency denervation of the posterior vertebral joints. Anaesthesia 34:768–775, 1979.
55. Ogbury JS, Simons H, Lehrman RAW: Facet "denervation" in treatment of low back syndrome. Pain 2:257–263, 1977.
56. Oudenhoven RC: Articular rhizotomy. Surg Neurol 2:275–278, 1974.
57. Oudenhoven RC: Results of facet denervation. Presented at the International Society for the Study of the Lumbar Spine, Paris, 1981.
58. Pagura JR: Percutaneous radiofrequency spinal rhizotomy: Proceedings of the American Society of Stereotactic and Functional Neurosurgery, Durham, NC. Appl Neurophysiol 46:138–146, 1983.
59. Pawl RP: Results in the treatment of low back syndrome from sensory neurolysis of the lumbar facets (facet rhizotomy) by thermal coagulation. Proc Inst Med Chgo 30:150–151, 1974.
60. Pierron D, Robine D, Cornejo M, Dubeaux P: Chronic low back pain and lumbar rhizotomy. Agressologie 32:263–265, 1991.
61. Rashbaum RF: Radiofrequency facet denervation. Orthop Clin North Am 14:569–575, 1983.
62. Savitz MH: Percutaneous radiofrequency rhizotomy of the lumbar facets: Ten years' experience. Mt Sinai J Med 58:177–178, 1991.

63. Schaerer JP: Radiofrequency facet rhizotomy in the treatment of chronic neck and low back pain. Int Surg 63:53–59, 1978.
64. Schaerer JP: Treatment of prolonged neck pain by radiofrequency facet rhizotomy. Neurol Orthop Med Surg 72:74-76, 1988.
65. Shealy CN: Percutaneous radiofrequency denervation of spinal facets: Treatment for chronic back pain of sciatica. Neurosurgery 43:448–451, 1975.
66. Shealy CN: Technique for Percutaneous Spinal Facet Rhizotomy. Radionics Procedure Technique Series. Burlington, Mass., Radionics Corp, 1975.
67. Shealy N: Facet denervations in the management of back and sciatic pain. Clin Orthop 115:157–164, 1976.
68. Sluijiter ME, Mehta M: Recent developments in radiofrequency denervation for chronic back and neck pain (Abstract). Pain Suppl 1:290, 1981.
69. Sluijiter ME, Mehta M: Treatment of chronic back and neck pain by percutaneous thermal lesions. *In* Lipton S, Miles J (eds): Modern Methods of Treatment, vol 3: Persistent Pain. London, Academic Press, 1981, pp 141–179.
70. Sluijter ME: Percutaneous Thermal Lesions in the Treatment of Back and Neck Pain. Radionics Procedure Techniques Series. Burlington, Mass., Radionics Corp, 1981.
71. Stolker RJ, Vervest ACM, Groen GJ: Percutaneous facet denervation in chronic thoracic spinal pain. Acta Neurochir (Wien) 122: 82–90, 1993.
72. Gallagher J, Vadi PLP, Wedley JR, et al: Radiofrequency facet joint denervation in the treatment of low back pain: A prospective controlled double-blind study to assess its efficacy. Pain Clinic 7(3):193–198, 1994.
73. Koning HM, Mackie DP: Percutaneous radiofrequency facet denervation in low back pain. Pain Clinic 7(3):199–204, 1994.
74. Dreyfuss P, Halbrook B, Pauza K, et al: Lumbar radiofrequency neurotomy for chronic zygaphophysial joint pain. North American Spine Society, 14th Annual Meeting, Chicago, Ill., 1999.
75. Taylor JR, Twomey LT, Corker M: Bone and soft tissue injuries in post-mortem lumbar spines. Paraplegia 28:119–129, 1990.
76. Twomey LT, Taylor JR, Taylor MM: Unsuspected damage to lumbar zygapophysial joints after motor-vehicle accidents. Med J Aust 151:210–217, 1989.
77. Schwarzer AC, Wang S-C, O'Driscoll D, et al: The ability of computed tomography to identify a painful zygapophysial joint in patients with chronic low back pain. Spine 20(8): 907–912, 1991.
78. Schwarzer AC, April CN, Derby R, et al: The false-positive rate of uncontrolled diagnostic blocks of the lumbar zygapophysial joints. Pain 58:195–200, 1994.
79. Chua W, Bogduk N: The surgical anatomy of thoracic facet denervation. Acta Neurochir 136:140–144, 1995.
80. Stolker RJ, Vervest ACM, Ramos LMP, Groen GJ: Electrode positioning in thoracic percutaneous partial rhizotomy: An anatomical study. Pain 57:241–251, 1994.
81. Bogduk, N: Clinical Anatomy of the Lumbar Spine and Sacrum. New York, Churchill Livingstone. 1997.
82. Laslett M, Williams M: The reliability of selected pain provocation tests for sacroiliac joint pathology. Spine 19:1243–1249, 1994.
83. Schwarzer A, Aprill C, et al: The sacroiliac joint in chronic low back pain. Spine 20:31–37. 1995.
84. Dreyfuss P, Cole A, et al: Sacroiliac joint injection techniques. *In* Injection Techniques: Principles and Practice. Philadelphia, WB Saunders, 1995, pp 785–813.
85. Chua WH: Clinical anatomy of the thoracic dorsal rami. Presented at The Second Annual Scientific Meeting of the International Spinal Injection Society (ISIS), Minneapolis, Minn., 1994.
86. Bernard T, Cassidy J: The sacroiliac joint syndrome: pathophysiology, diagnosis, and management. *In* Frymoyer J (ed): The Adult Spine: Principles and Practice. New York, Raven, 1991, pp 2017–2130.
86a. van Kleef M, Barendse G, Dingemans W, et al: Effects of producing a radiofrequency lesion adjacent to the dorsal root ganglion in patients with thoracic segmental pain. Clin J Pain 11:325–332, 1995.
87. Bernard TN JR: Lumbar discography followed by computed tomography—refining the diagnosis of low-back pain. Spine 15:690–707, 1990.
88. Kornberg M: Discography and magnetic resonance imaging in the diagnosis of lumbar disc disruption. Spine 14:1363–1372, 1989.
88a. Sluijter ME, Koesveld-Baart CC: Interruption of pain pathways in the treatment of the cervical syndrome. Anaesthesia 35:302–307, 1980.
89. Aprill C: Diagnostic disc injection. *In* Frymoyer JW (ed): The Adult Spine: Principles and Practice. New York, Raven, 1991, pp 403–442.
90. Sluijter ME: The use of radiofrequency lesions of the communicating ramus in the treatment of low back pain. *In* Gabor R (ed): Techniques of Neurolysis. Boston; Kluwer, 1989.
91. Troussier B, Lebus JF, Chirossel JP, et al: Percutaneous intradiscal radio-frequency thermocoagulation—A cadaveric study. Spine (20):1713–1718, 1995.
92. Maurer P: Thermal lumbar disc annuloplasty: Initial clinical results. North American Spine Society, 14th Annual Meeting, Chicago, Ill., 1999.
93. Karasek M, Karasek D, et al: A controlled trial of the efficacy of intra-discal electrothermal treatment for internal disc disruption. North American Spine Society, 14th Annual Meeting, Chicago, Ill, 1999.
94. Saal J, Saal J: Intradiscal electrothermal annuloplasty (IDET) for chronic disc disease: Outcome assessment with minimum one year follow-up. North American Spine Society, 14th Annual Meeting, Chicago, Ill., 1999.
95. Sluijter ME: Interruption of nerve pathways in the treatment of nonmalignant pain. Appl Neurophysiol 47:195–200, 1984.
96. Bogduk N, Barnsely L: Radiofrequency neurotomy of the medial branches of the cervical dorsal rami (abstract). Aust NZ J Med 22:736, 1992.
97. Sluijter ME, Vercruysse PR: Radiofrequency Lesions in the Treatment of Cervical Headache. Pain Relief Clinic, Lutherse Diakoneesen Ziekenhuis, Amsterdam, 1987.
98. Sluijter ME: Radiofrequency Lesions in the Treatment of Cervical Pain Syndromes. Radionics Procedure Technique Series. Burlington, Mass., Radionics, 1990.
99. Lord SM, Barnsley L, Wallis BJ, et al: Percutaneous radio-frequency neurotomy for chronic cervical zygapophysial-joint pain. N Engl J Med 335 (23);1721–1726, 1996.
100. Bogduk N, Windsor M, Inglis A: The innervation of the cervical intervertebral discs. Spine 13(1):2–8, 1988.
101. Bogduk N, Aprill C: On the nature of neck pain, discography and cervical zygapophysial joint blocks. Pain 54:213–217, 1993.
102. Taylor J, Twomey L: Disc injuries in cervical trauma. Lancet 44(24):1318, 1990.
103. Taylor JP, Twomey LT: Acute injuries to cervical joints: An autopsy study of neck sprain. Spine 18(9):1115–1122, 1993.
104. Taylor JR, Finch P: Acute injury of the neck: Anatomical and pathological basis of pain. Ann Acad Med 22(2):187–192, 1993.
105. Aprill C, Bogduk N: The prevalance of cervical zygapophysial joint pain. Spine 17:744–747, 1991.
106. Barnsley L, Lord SM, Wallis BJ, Bogduk N: The prevalence of chronic cervical zygapophysial joint pain after whiplash. Spine 20(1):20–26, 1995.
107. Bogduk N: Mechanisms of neck injuries. Aust Dr Weekly 24:38–40, 42–43, 1989.
108. Bogduk N: The anatomy and pathophysiology of whiplash. Clin Biomechan 1:92–101, 1986.
109. Bogduk N, Marsland A: The cervical zygapophysial joints as a source of neck pain. Spine 13(6):610–617, 1986.
110. Jull G, Bogduk N, Marshall A: The accuracy of manual diagnosis for cervical zygapophysial joint pain syndromes. Med J Aust 148:233–236, 1988.
111. Bovim G, Berg R, Dale LG: Cervicogenic headache: Anesthetic blockades of cervical nerves (C2–C5) and facet joint (C2–C3). Pain 49:315–320, 1992.
112. Lamer TJ: Ear pain due to cervical spine arthritis: Treatment with cervical facet injection. Headache 31:682–683, 1991.
113. Barnsley L, Lord S, Wallis B, Bogduk N: False-positive rates of cervical zygapophysial joint blocks. Clin J Pain 9:124–130, 1993.
114. Geurts JWM, Stolker RJ: Percutaneous radiofrequency lesion of the stellate ganglion in the treatment of pain in upper extremity reflex sympathetic dystrophy. Pain Clin 6:17–25, 1993.
115. Chambers WR: Posterior rhizotomy of the second and third cervical nerves for occipital pain. JAMA 155:431–432, 1954.
116. Blume H, Kakolewski J, Richardson R, Rojas C: Radiofrequency denaturation in occipital pain: Results in 450 cases. Appl Neurophysiol 45:541–548, 1981.

117. Kleef MV, et al: Effects and side effects of a percutaneous thermal lesion of the dorsal root ganglion in patients with cervical pain syndrome. Pain 52:49–53, 1993.
118. Koch D, Wakhloo AK: CT-guided chemical rhizotomy of the C1 root for occipital neuralgia. Neuroradiology 34:451–452, 1992.
119. Sluijter M: C1 Dorsal nerve root lesion in the treatment of suboccipital headache. Personal communication, 1998.
120. Sweet WH, Wepsic JG: Controlled thermocoagulation of trigeminal ganglion and rootlets for differential destruction of pain fibers. J Neurosurg 40:143–156, 1974.
121. Broggi G, Franzini A, Lasio G, et al: Long-term results of percutaneous retrogasserian thermorhizotomy for "essential" trigeminal neuralgia: considerations in 1000 consecutive patients. Neurosurgery 26:783–786, 1990.
122. Adson AW, Brown GE: Treatment of Raynaud's disease by lumbar ramisection and ganglionostomy and perivascular sympathetic neurectomy of the common iliac. JAMA 84:1908–1910, 1924.
123. DeBakey ME, Creech O, Woodhall JP: Evaluation of sympathectomy in arteriosclerotic peripheral vascular disease. JAMA 144:1227–1331, 1950.
124. Pernak J: Percutaneous radiofrequency thermal lumbar sympathectomy. Pain Clinic (80)1:99–106, 1995.
125. Noe CE, Haynesworth RF: Lumbar radiofrequency sympatholysis. J Vasc Surg 17:801–806, 1993.
126. Haynesworth RF, Noe CE: Percutaneous lumbar sympathectomy: A comparison of radiofrequency denervation versus phenol neurolysis. Anaesthesiology 74:459–463, 1991.
127. Yarzebski JL, Wilkinson HA: T2 and T3 sympathetic ganglia in the adult human: A cadaver and clinical-radiologic study and its clinical application. Neurosurgery 21:339–341, 1987.
128. Wilkinson HA: Radiofrequency percutaneous upper thoracic sympathectomy. N Engl J Med 311:34–36, 1984.
129. Wilkinson HA: Percutaneous radiofrequency upper thoracic sympathectomy: A new technique. Neurosurgery 15:811–814, 1984.
130. Wilkinson HA: Percutaneous radiofrequency upper thoracic sympathectomy. Neurosurgery 38(4): 715–725, 1996.
131. Wilkinson HA: Stereotactic radiofrequency sympathectomy. Pain Clinic (8)1:107–115.
132. Raj P. Visceral pain (tutorial review). Pain Digest 9:197–208, 1999.
133. Banerjee T, Domingues da Silva A: Signs, Syndromes and Eponyms: Our Legacy. Lebanon, NH, American Association of Neurological Surgeons, 1999.
134. Ischia S, Ischia A, Polati E, Finco, G: Three posterior celiac plexus block techniques. A prospective, randomized study in 61 patients with pancreatic cancer pain. Anesthesiology 76:4, 1992.
135. Williams P, Warwick R, (eds): Gray's Anatomy. Philadelphia, WB Saunders, 1980.

CHAPTER • 20

Atlantooccipital and Atlantoaxial Injections in the Treatment of Headache and Neck Pain

Gabor B. Racz, MD, ChB • Susan R. Anderson, MD • Phillip S. Sizer, Jr, MEd, PT • Valerie Phelps, PT

Clinicians face many challenges when attempting to treat patients with pain-producing afflictions of the upper cervical spine. Local cervical pain and cervicogenic headaches[1,2] arising from the upper cervical spine are as common as simple treatments for these conditions are rare. Upper cervical conditions are linked to the structural and functional complexities of these segments. Diagnosis is confounded by contributions from the autonomic nervous system, dura mater, adjacent vertebral arterial system, and activity in cervical cranial nerve ganglia to upper cervical symptoms.[3,4] It is also important to remember that the vertebral arteries and upper cervical dura are innervated by the first three cervical nerves. Painful lesions that originate in these structures (such as vertebral artery aneurysm and inflammation of the dura by infection or blood) can be mistaken for cervical headache syndromes.[2,5] Clearly, intracranial causes of headache (tumors, hemorrhage, and arteriovenous malformations) as well as systemic diseases (temporal arteritis, the arthritides, hypertension, migraine, infections, and so forth) must also be sought.

PATHOANATOMY

The articulations of the upper cervical spine are considered the most intricate of all articulations in the body.[6] The remarkable mobility of the upper cervical spine is well-known. Because of the great relative weight of the cranium and its contents, the muscles, tendons, ligaments, and joints in the cervical area are all subject to damage by trauma at multiple levels. The bones and their facets are also subject to arthritic changes. In pathologic states, neck movement is commonly painful and range of motion is restricted on examination. This so-called hypomobility lesion may be secondary to intraarticular adhesions, capsular scarring, or local muscle hypertonicity.[2]

The upper cervical spine is distinctly different, on several accounts, from segments in the lower cervical spine. Anatomically, C0–C1, C1–C2 (atlantooccipital and atlantoaxial segments, respectively) differ from the cervical disc segments (C2–C3 to C6–C7) in their architecture: they lack both intervertebral discs and uncinate processes. While the biomechanical coupling behaviors are greatest in the upper cervical segments, the contralateral coupling behaviors of C0–C1, C1–C2 segments contrast the ipsilateral coupling behaviors observed in the cervical disc segments. Functionally, the upper cervical spine demonstrates several distinctive utilities that confirm its importance. The muscle and joint receptors from these segments play a vital role in providing information on the orientation of the body in space, as this information is integrated into the afferent symphony provided by the statolyths, semicircular canals, eyes, and ears. Furthermore, C0–C3 acts as a relay station, where the information on head position is harmonized with afference from positions and movements of the trunk and extremities. These afferent interactions become vital to maintaining balance and improving coordination between head, trunk, and limbs. Disturbances in motion and control of the upper cervical spine may not only produce pain and dysfunction but may also alter balance and coordination.

Each architectural component of the upper cervical spine contributes to the structural distinctions observed in this region. The orientation of the occipital condyles differs in each anatomic plane. The cartilage covering the articular facets is 2.0 to 3.0 mm thick and is biconvex, but this convexity can be appreciated only from a lateral view, where the cartilage surfaces appear to be relatively flat from a ventral view. These biconvexities allow for rapid head movements. Additionally, the articular condyles of the occiput are not always completely covered by cartilage, potentially demonstrating two articular facets on each side.[7]

The atlas (C1) is unique in that it lacks a vertebral body and, instead, functions as a disc, or "relay center," between the occiput and C2. The cranial articular surfaces for the occiput are large and biconcave, complementing the occipital articular surfaces. The posterior arch is very deep, so palpation is very challenging. The anterior and posterior arches form the triangular spinal foramen that accommodates the brain stem. The transverse processes are long and perforated, accommodating the passage of the vertebral arteries through the transverse foramina. After exiting these transverse foramina, they course through grooves that can be observed posterior to the lateral masses. These grooves, or occasional tunnels, accommodate the vertebral arteries as they loop for a second time in the upper cervical region (Fig. 20–1). Bone changes can occur here that have the potential to compromise vertebral artery function and promote symptoms associated with vertebral basilar insufficiency.[8] The architecture at these grooves is different in males and in females; as a consequence women may be more susceptible to arterial compromise.[9]

The resulting oval, bean-shaped joints of C0–C1 course ventromedial to dorsolateral in the transverse plane, 50 to 60 degrees from the frontal plane (see Fig. 20–1). In the frontal view these articulations course caudomedial to craniolateral (Fig. 20–2). The C0–C1 joints are ellipsoid, allowing flexion and extension and lateral (sidewise) bending and accounting for the great mobility the head requires.

The axis, or C2, is most characterized by the dens, which looks like an asparagus spear projecting craniad from the front of the bony segment. With the dens, or odontoid process, C2 forms a pivot around which C1 and the head turn (Fig. 20–3).[7] The dens is highly susceptible to deformity, so the clinician must be acutely aware of the architectural configuration before implementing manual techniques to the upper cervical spine. The dens may vary in

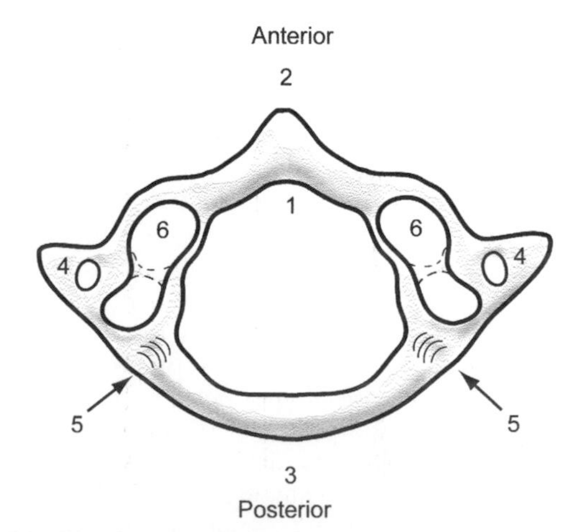

FIGURE 20–1 *The atlas (C1). 1, facet for the dens; 2, anterior tubercle; 3, posterior tubercle; 4, transverse foramen; 5, groove for the vertebral artery; 6, cartilage over superior articular facet. (Reprinted with permission from the International Academy of Orthopaedic Medicine-US.)*

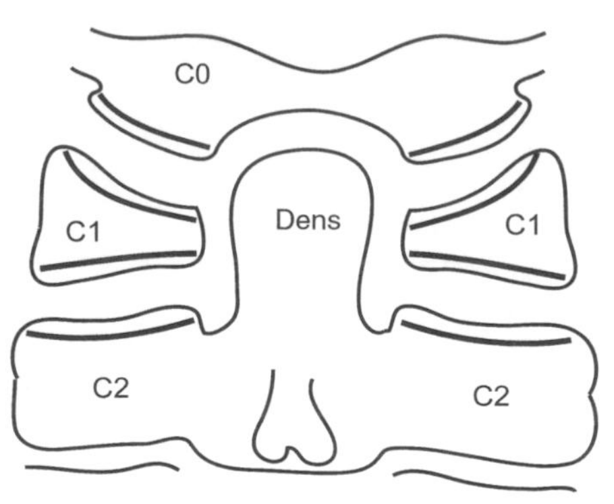

FIGURE 20–2 *Upper cervical spine (C0–C1, C1–C2). Joint orientations in the frontal plane. (Reprinted with permission from the International Academy of Orthopaedic Medicine-US.)*

its orientation in the cervical space (i.e., straight, or directed backward and/or sideways). Thus, a gap on sagittal x-ray films between the dens and the anterior arch of C1 is not necessarily abnormal. This gap, which is full of cartilage, is normally 2 to 3 mm wide and should not exceed 3 mm, even during flexion or extension. Any deviation from these normative values indirectly indicates atlantodental dislocation or lesions of the ligaments, articular capsules, or facet joints.[10]

Four articular systems can be observed between C1 and C2: two central joints and two lateral joints. All are synovial

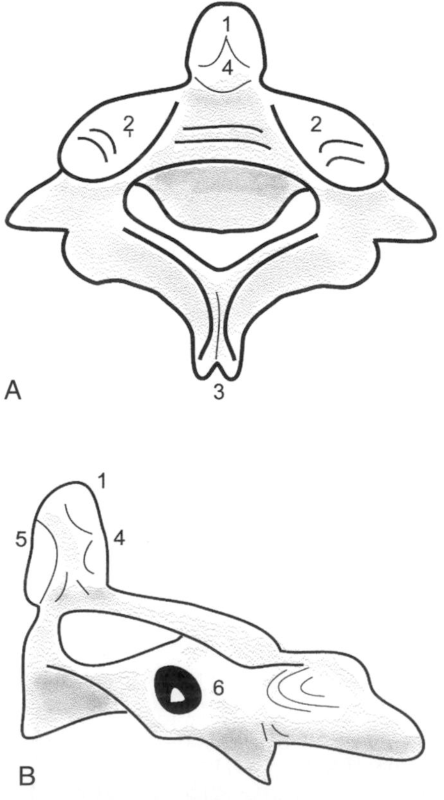

FIGURE 20–3 *The axis (C2). A, Cranial view; B, sagittal view. 1, Dens or odontoid process; 2, superior articular facet; 3, spinous process; 4, groove for transverse ligament of atlas (TLA); 5, facet for anterior arch of the atlas; 6, transverse foramen. (Reprinted with permission from the International Academy of Orthopaedic Medicine-US.)*

joints and therefore can be the site of inflammation or articular damage and degradation. The two central joints comprise the median atlantoaxial joint and surround the dens. The anterior atlantoaxial (or atlantodental) joint is interposed between the dens and the anterior arch of the atlas. Posterior to the dens is the joint between the dens and the transverse ligament of the atlas (TLA), the lower component of the cruciform ligament, which can also be interpreted as the bursa atlantodentalis.[7] From a sagittal view, the lateral atlantoaxial joint is biconvex on both the left and the right side (Fig. 20–4), and its convexities are accentuated by increased thickness in articular cartilage (1.4–3.2 mm). These incongruencies are accommodated by large, intraarticular menisci that emerge from flaccid, roomy joint capsules. The menisci are subject to degradation, producing interposition with rotation between C1 and C2 and resulting in sharp, local, catching pain. These four joint systems allow for flexion, extension, and rotation, but afford very little lateral bending. Virtually no axial separation is allowed between C1 and C2, owing to the strong stabilizing influence of the TLA on a normally configured dens. Any deformity to the dens (such as that associated with Down syndrome[11]) might possibly compromise this stabilizing feature, produce excessive separation, and merit avoiding any therapeutic traction maneuvers to the neck altogether.

Because of the proximity of the brain stem and spinal cord to the segments of the upper cervical spine, the ligaments in this region must afford strong intersegmental support. The TLA courses between lateral masses of C2 behind the dens, precluding any separation between C1 and C2 (Fig. 20–5). Additionally, this ligament prevents posterior tipping of the dens into the brain stem and spinal cord during forward flexion of the head, which could cause the patient to have a "drop attack." Compromise to this ligament, for example after a whiplash injury, puts the brain stem and cord at risk for compression by the dens during normal flexion.

The TLA accompanies the alar ligaments in keeping the dens centralized within its boundaries (Fig. 20–6). In all humans, right and left occipital branches of the alar ligament course from the posterior tip of the dens to the occiput. These branches are 11 to 13 mm long and are composed of type I collagen, producing only a 5% to 6% length deformation potential. Fewer people demonstrate right and left atlantal branches, which course only 3 to 4 mm from the anterior dens to the posterior internal surface of the anterior arch of C1. The alar ligaments are tight during extension, side bending, and ipsilateral rotation. In addition to functioning as the "ligaments of life," the alar ligaments relegate the upper cervical spine to very powerful coupling behaviors. Because of them, any kinetic side-bending activity is accompanied by significant synkinetic rotational motion and vice versa. This coupling behavior is accentuated when the patient is sitting, owing to gravity loading of the facets.[12] When there is a lesion to these ligaments, rotation, side bending, and extension can in-

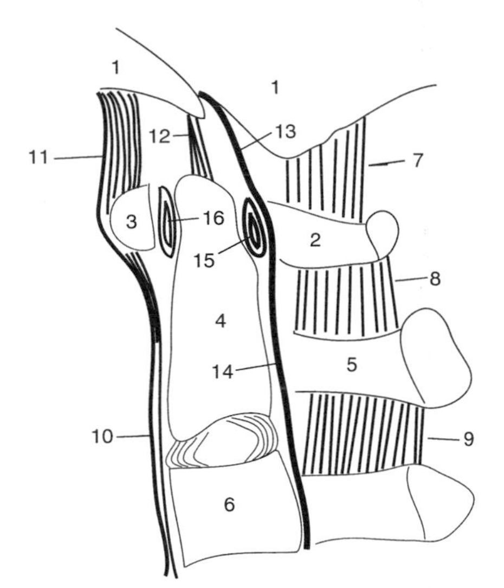

FIGURE 20–5 The ligaments of the upper cervical spine. 1, Occiput; 2, posterior arch of the atlas; 3, anterior arch of the atlas; 4, dens of the axis; 5, posterior arch of C2; 6, vertebral body of C3; 7, posterior atlantooccipital membrane; 8, ligamentum flavum, C1–C2; 9, ligamentum flavum, C2–C3; 10, anterior longitudinal ligament; 11, anterior atlantooccipital membrane; 12, apical ligament of the atlas; 13, tectorial membrane; 14, posterior longitudinal ligament; 15, transverse ligament of atlas (TLA); 16, synovial compartment between the dens and the anterior arch of the atlas. (Reprinted with permission from the International Academy of Orthopaedic Medicine-US.)

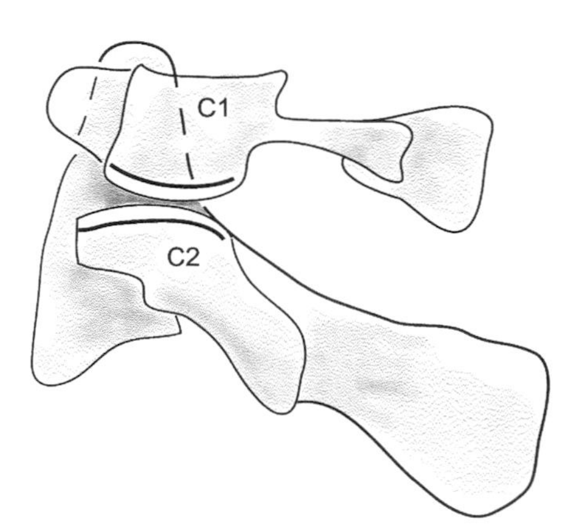

FIGURE 20–4 Lateral atlantoaxial joint (C1–C2). Biconvexity in the sagittal plane. (Reprinted with permission from the International Academy of Orthopaedic Medicine-US.)

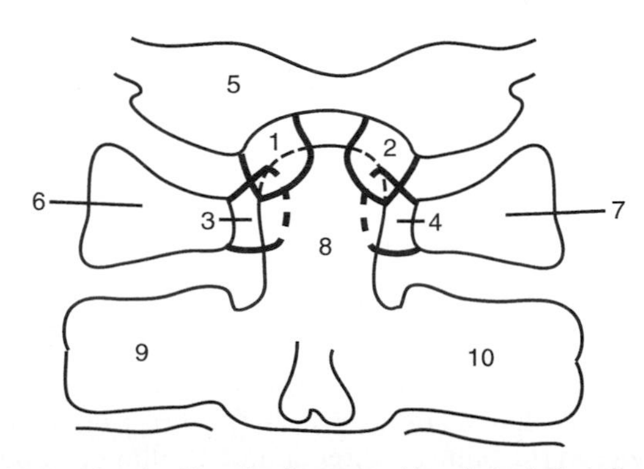

FIGURE 20–6 The alar ligaments (dorsal view). 1, Left occipital alar ligament; 2, right occipital alar ligament; 3, left atlantal alar ligament; 4, right atlantal alar ligament; 5, occiput; 6, left C1; 7, right C1; 8, dens; 9, left C2; 10, right C2. (Reprinted with permission from the International Academy of Orthopaedic Medicine-US.)

crease in the C1–C2 segment,[13] placing the vertebral artery at greater risk for stretching injuries or sympathetic plexus irritation.[14]

The anterior longitudinal ligament of the lower cervical spine becomes the anterior atlantooccipital and atlantoaxial membranes. The ligamentum flavum becomes the posterior atlantoaxial and atlantooccipital membranes. Whereas the ligament contains much elastin, these membranes are stiff and inelastic (see Fig. 20–5). The nuchal ligament is peculiar to this region of the spine as a continuation of the interspinous and supraspinous ligaments. This system demonstrates two different components: a funicular component continuing from the supraspinous ligament and a lamellar component coursing ventrally from the funicular component to the spinous processes.[15] This ligament imposes a powerful influence on the upper cervical spine during full cervical flexion and extension. With full cervical flexion, paradoxically, the C0–C1 segment extends.[16] This paradoxical motion merits testing upper cervical flexion with full cervical retraction and upper cervical extension with full cervical protraction.[17]

When discussing the pathologic anatomy of the upper cervical spine, certain neural structures must be mentioned. The sympathetic innervation to the head, upper cervical spine, and throat comes primarily from C8 and T1–T4. The supply to the middle and lower cervical spine, upper back, and arm arises from T4–T9. These arrangements are important when discussing management options for patients who suffer from chronic headache and neck pain, as the autonomic nervous system contributes to these conditions.

Also noteworthy is the location of the accessory nerve nuclei, found in the spinal cord between C1 and C4.[18] Patients who suffer from chronic upper cervical conditions may experience increased tone in their upper trapezius muscles ("tight traps") secondary to sensitization and reorganization of interneurons at those same levels. This reorganization sensitizes the cranial nerve nuclei, increasing the efferent signals to the trapezius. A similar condition can arise from the trigeminal nuclei in the spinal cord between C1 and C4.[18] Chronic afference from the cervical spine can also sensitize these cranial nerve nuclei, resulting in chronic headache in the cutaneous trigeminal distribution.[3]

BIOMECHANICS OF THE UPPER CERVICAL SPINE

The principal motions allowed at C0–C1 are flexion and extension to a maximum of approximately 30 to 35 degrees from a fully flexed to a fully extended position. The axis for these motions courses through both external auditory meati of the ears, with isolated flexion approaching 10 degrees and isolated extension measuring approximately 25 degrees.[19, 20] During these motions, the occipital joint partner arthrokinematically rolls in the direction of motion and slides in the opposite direction, the rolling component being greater than the sliding component. This segment also demonstrates a small amount of side bending. During right side bending (with the axis coursing through the nose), the occiput rolls to the right and slides to the left. Thus, the atlas slides relatively to the right, which can easily be palpated. Additionally, any loss of these sliding movements impedes flexion and extension or side bending in the upper cervical spine, limitations that warrant therapeutic manual techniques aimed at restoring motion.

The atlantoaxial joint has the widest range of motion of all articulations in the neck. Motion at C1–C2 is limited to anterior and posterior rocking (20 degrees[17]) and rotation, without allowing any side bending. Rotation around an axis coursing through the dens is limited to 40 to 45 degrees to each side.[6, 19–22] The odontoid process permits stable rotation and allows 5 to 10 degrees of flexion and 10 degrees of extension.[6, 18] With rightward rotation, the right facet of C1 translates posterior to the right facet of C2 and the left C1 facet anterior to left C2. Additionally, C1 demonstrates slight caudal translation on C1, owing to the convex-convex relationships of the C1–C2 zygapophyseal joints.

A chin tuck motion is possible at C0–C1 in isolation from other movements in the cervical spine and imposes a very heavy load on the TLA. Used as an exercise, this motion can induce headaches because of these imposed stresses. Otherwise, it is impossible for the segments in the cervical spine to make solitary movements, owing in part to the powerful influence of the alar ligaments on kinetic coupling. When an individual bends the entire cervical spine laterally, the upper cervical spine must rotate contralateral to the direction of bending to keep the eyes directed forward. Otherwise, the coupling pattern of the lower cervical spine would force the head to rotate in the same direction as the bending. Additionally, lateral bending requires the upper cervical spine to flex, to keep the eyes level. Otherwise, a person with a flexion limitation in the upper cervical spine would look up when attempting a cervical side-bending motion.[23–25]

Lateral bending at C0–C1 and C1–C2 directly influences motion at C2–C3. Bending to the right at C0 recruits rightward rotation of C2 on C3, by virtue of tension loading in the right occipital and left atlantal branches of the alar ligament system (Figs. 20–7, 20–8). This same rightward rotation of C2 on C3 produces relative leftward rotation of C1 on C2, lending to the contralateral coupling produced in the upper cervical spine.[13] Additionally, if C2

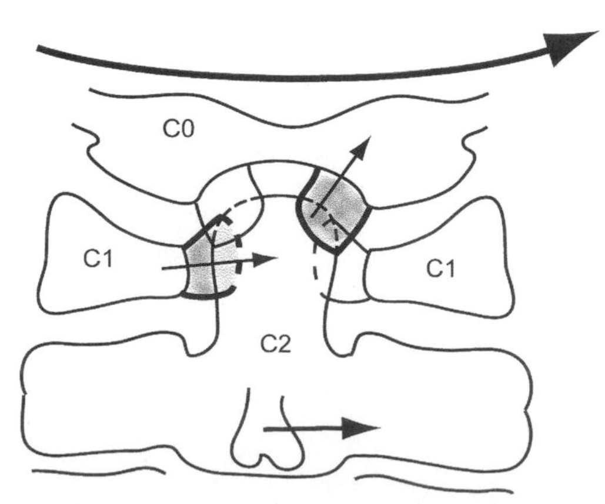

FIGURE 20–7 Influence of the alar ligaments on coupled motion in the upper cervical spine (C0–C3, dorsal view). Leftward occipital side bending is accompanied by rightward occipital translation. Rightward translation tension-loads the right occipital and left atlantal alar ligaments. (Reprinted with permission from the International Academy of Orthopaedic Medicine-US.)

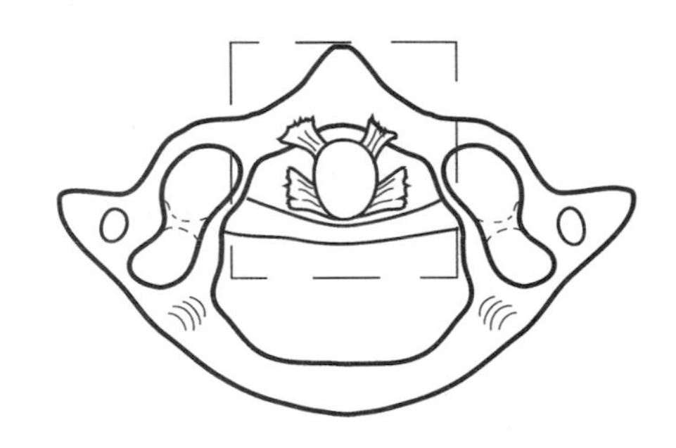

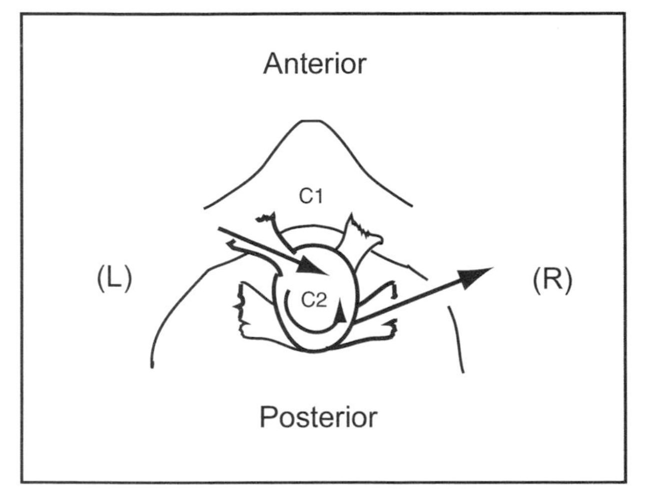

FIGURE 20–8 Influence of the alar ligaments on coupled motion in the upper cervical spine (C0–C3, cranial view). Leftward occipital side bending is accompanied by rightward occipital translation. Rightward translation tension-loads the right occipital and left atlantal alar ligaments. This tension behavior induces leftward rotation of C2 on C3, and subsequent right rotation of C1 on C2. (Reprinted with permission from the International Academy of Orthopaedic Medicine-US.)

cannot rotate on C3, then C0 will not be capable of bending to the side, creating the appearance of motion limitation in segments C0–C2. Therefore, the C2–C3 motion segment can be considered a functional component of the upper cervical spine, as normal C2–C3 motion is biomechanically crucial for upper cervical function. This relationship should inspire clinicians to observe first for C2–C3 motion limitations when patients present with upper cervical dysfunction.

Cervical axial rotation also requires additional motions at the upper cervical spine. With rotation, the alar ligaments once again induce contralateral upper cervical coupling by forcing the occiput to bend toward the side opposite the direction of rotation.[13] The lower cervical spine bends the same direction as the rotation to keep the head erect and the eyes level and to counter the side bending in the upper cervical spine.[26] Additionally, the cervical spine extends above C3 and flexes below C3 to keep the eyes level and the head erect. Otherwise the person would look down when attempting rotation.

INTRODUCTION TO THE CLINICAL EXAMINATION

Several characteristic clinical signs and symptoms can be indicative of contribution of the upper cervical spine joints to pain in the upper neck or occipital region.[27, 28] When investigating the upper cervical spine as a cause of headache, several other pathologic lesions should be considered or ruled out.

DIFFERENTIAL DIAGNOSIS

Cervicotrigeminal relay has been cited by several authors to explain patients' experiencing, not only occipital pain, but also frontoocular pain from an affliction of the upper cervical spine.[29–36] Nociceptive afferent input to the C1 to C4 neurologic levels can be somatotopically transmitted to the lower part of the spinal trigeminal tract, resulting in pain projected to the area of the trigeminal ophthalmic branch. As a result of central sensitization in this area, the trigeminal nerve is triggered and the patient can experience an occipital headache with pain that "pulls" from the occiput to the forehead.[37] Other authors attribute a central role in headache to the trigeminal vascular system.[3, 38–42]

The three most common complaints in *functional vertebrobasilar insufficiency*,[18, 43–45] as described by Oostendorp, are headache, dizziness, and neck pain. Symptoms are precipitated by spasm of the vertebral arteries. Mechanical triggering alone (as by stretching[13]) is not enough to close off an artery or bring about a spasm; however, it can damage the outer layer of the vessel, setting up local inflammation. In the chemical component of this pathologic lesion, inflammatory products are released both from the vessel wall and the free nerve endings in the perivascular plexus. This release lowers the membrane threshold, both in the periphery and centrally. As a result, the vessel wall becomes more sensitive to mechanical triggers; increased stressors with chronic increased activity of the sympathetic nervous system lead to massive reactions to the smallest of triggers. This condition leads to angiospasm, resulting in general dysregulation in the vascularity of the vertebral arteries and their branches. Consequently, fibrosis of the arterial wall develops, which increases the chance of damaging the wall, especially during cervical spine movements. All imaging studies for vertebrobasilar insufficiency are typically negative. According to Oostendorp, extension is the most provocative position during clinical testing for functional vertebrobasilar insufficiency.[18] This is interesting to note, because investigators have demonstrated that the position of extension does not have an effect on the vertebral artery blood flow. Instead, true vertebrobasilar insufficiency testing shows the disruption to blood flow to be greatest in positions of flexion with rotation or extension with rotation.[46, 47]

Discogenic lesions associated with annular tears at the C3–C4 to C5–C6 segments were found to refer pain to a variety of sites, including the upper cervical and occipital regions.[48] In a population of 5000 headache patients, Jenkner found that 40% demonstrated cervicogenic pain. Two thirds of the latter group exhibited a kyphotic disc segment on x-ray examination. This entire group experienced pain relief from a specific ventral manipulative technique; 82% actually showed restoration of cervical motion on radiographs.[49]

Dwyer and coworkers[50] observed nonradicular pain referral patterns to the upper cervical spine and occipital region upon injection of their patients' C2–C3 and C3–C4 zygapophyseal joints. In addition, Bogduk reported that at least 27% of the headaches after whiplash could be traced to the C2–C3 zygapophyseal joints.[51] Radicular symptoms have been observed with an inflamed C3 root, as the result of a rare laterally prolapsed C2–C3 disc. This condition has been reported to cause numbness in the C3 dermatome and tenderness of the occipital nerve points.[52]

Other afflictions that could cause pain in the region of the upper cervical spine and head include vertebral artery aneurysm and inflammation of the dura by infection or blood.[2, 5] Intracranial causes of headache (tumors, hemorrhage, arteriovenous malformations) as well as systemic diseases (temporal arteritis, arthritides, hypertension, migraine, infections) should also be considered. Anomalies of the craniovertebral junction, including basilar invagination, congenital atlantoaxial dislocation, separated odontoid process, and occipitalization of the atlas, can cause pain in the occipital region. Finally, acquired craniovertebral junction lesions, such as tumor (primary or metastatic), osteomyelitis, Pott's or Paget's disease, rheumatoid arthritis, and ankylosing spondylitis, can produce similar findings.[53]

CLINICAL HISTORY

Upper cervical joint lesions are several, including (1) segmental hypermobility or laxity as a result of a systemic disease,[54–57] aging,[58] or trauma,[59–62] and (2) segmental hypomobility as a result of aging,[58, 63, 64] or trauma (e.g., whiplash[65–67]). Clinicians must look for historical cues and patterns that suggest these conditions. For example, a patient's age can affect the onset of cervicogenic headache. Upper cervical, suboccipital, and occipital symptoms that result from upper cervical afflictions have been described in children as young as 6 years[68] and in adults to age 89.[69]

Gender sometimes plays a role. Women working in managerial and professional occupations are at significantly higher risk of cervicogenic headache as compared with women in clerical or blue-collar jobs, whereas there are no similar findings for men.[70] Additionally, painful upper cervical osteoarthritis is more prevalent in women than in men.[71]

The symptoms associated with upper cervical disease are distinctive. The chief complaint with occipitoatlantal or atlantoaxial joint lesions is pain, generally produced with certain movements or positions of the head. The pain is usually very local, either intermittent or constant. Pain can be unilateral or bilateral.[72, 73] Dreyfuss and coworkers reported that the C1–C2 joint pain referral pattern is small and rather localized in the suboccipital region.[74] In contrast, C0–C1 joints were found to provoke diffuse unilateral suboccipital and occipital pain. In addition, atlantoaxial arthritis is present in 4% of all patients with degenerative arthritis of the peripheral joints or spine.[75]

Referred sensations associated with cervicocephalic syndrome are observed in chronic cases.[71, 76] Symptoms of numbness and tingling help clinicians to distinguish between joint lesions and lesions of the C1–C3 roots. Especially in instances of chronic or severe pain, the patient might also complain of blurred vision or dizziness.[77–81] Less common symptoms are nausea, vomiting, photophobia, and phonophobia.[82, 83]

When differentiating between painful migraine and cervicogenic headache, Sjaastad and associates[72] found that 90% of migraine patients initially experienced pain in the forehead and temporal regions that then was referred to the rest of the head. On the other hand, 73% of cervicogenic headache patients first felt pain in the neck, which then was referred to the head. Often, cervicogenic headache symptoms are not relieved by salicylates or medications typically prescribed for the treatment of migraine[72, 82]; however, a full-blown attack of either could mimic the other.

Symptoms can be elicited by certain activities or postures. In addition to occurring spontaneously, symptoms can often be precipitated by prolonged awkward positioning of the head, as when backing a car, turning the head toward someone during conversation, or sleeping the entire night with the head turned to one side.[77, 82] Once established, cervicogenic headache symptoms can persist. Fredriksen and colleagues discussed clinical manifestation of upper cervical symptoms and occipital pain in a relatively small study group.[82] Their patient population had been experiencing symptoms a mean of 13 years. Exacerbation of symptoms ranged from a period of 3 hours to 3 weeks, with intervals between these flare-ups of from 2 days to 2 months.

Onset of symptoms varies from spontaneous to traumatic. Lesions can develop in the upper cervical segments as a result of whiplash trauma. Penning reported that the primary mechanism of whiplash injury is hypertranslation of the head, not hyperextension. He found that rotation of the C0–C2 junction was greater with simple head translations than during head flexion or extension and thus concluded that upper cervical rotational injuries would be more common.[65] Trauma deceleration rates also appear to affect injury patterns, as more violent decelerations tend to produce injuries at higher levels of the cervical spine.[66]

CLINICAL EXAMINATION

Decreases or increases in ranges of general cervical motion may not be observable in cases of unilateral or unisegmental hypomobility or hypermobility, because the kinetic chain of other cervical joints can mask such a disturbance. Often, however, specific cervical testing can determine the local loss or gain in motion,[84, 85] and often, the examiner can recognize patterns of movement during general testing that indicate loss of motion in the upper cervical spine.

Although loss of motion can be subtle in patients with severe atlantoaxial osteoarthritis, Star and colleagues[71] reported severe limitations (>50%) of axial rotation and lateral bending of the cervical spine. Radiography demonstrated lateral mass degeneration in all of their patients.

Active range of motion of the cervical spine is generally performed to provoke the patient's symptoms and to assess limitation of motion. Pain provocation can be isolated to, or emphasized in, the upper cervical spine by means of testing rotation or lateral bending from a position of protraction and retraction. The flexion and extension of the C0–C2 segments are greatest during retraction and protraction, respectively.[17] Thus, an affliction of these seg-

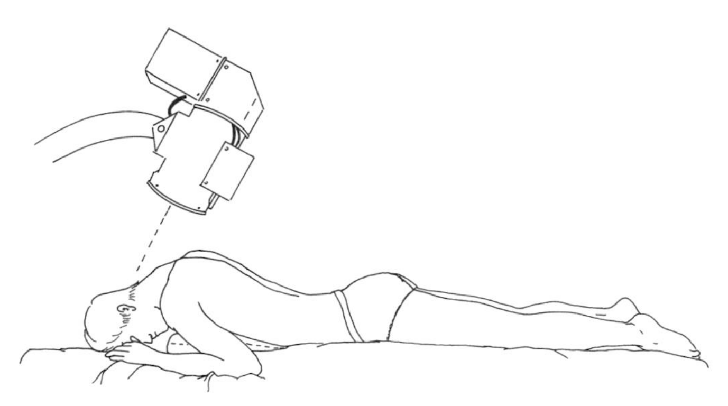

FIGURE 20–9 Positioning of patient and C arm for atlantooccipital and atlantoaxial blocks: The "Grashey view."

ments will be more accurately elicited by protraction or retraction rather than by general extension or flexion of the entire cervical spine. It follows that, when rotation is performed at the end of the range of protraction or retraction is determined to be most painful, the segment most likely affected is C1–C2. On the other hand, when side-bending is performed at the end of the range of protraction or retraction, the joint most likely affected is C0–C1.

A limitation of motion at the C0–C1 or C1–C2 segments renders the upper cervical spine incapable of compensating for coupling at the cervical disc segments. This can manifest itself in a number of "deviated" patterns during active cervical motions.[23]

- *Upper cervical flexion.* Nodding the head from a position of end-range cervical axial rotation allows assessment of the range of upper cervical spine flexion. It is primarily the Co to Cy segments that perform this movement; thus a lesion at this level could cause pain or limitation of motion during this test.
- *Upper cervical extension.* Loss of upper cervical extension can be suspected when the patient's head is positioned in upper cervical flexion at the end of the range of axial rotation.
- *C1–C2 rotation.* A patient with C1–C2 hypomobility is often unable to perform a pure lateral bending motion, in one or both directions. For instance, if leftward rotation is limited at the C1–C2 segment, the patient cannot bend the cervical spine to the right side while keeping the eyes in the frontal plane. Instead, rightward bending is coupled with rightward rotation.
- *Upper cervical lateral bending.* When a patient has compromised lateral bending in the upper cervical spine, especially in the segments from C0–C3, he or she will be unable to incorporate a "side nod" into the total cervical sidewise bending motion. Side bending appears to come only from the lower cervical spine as the patient seems to "lay the head down on the shoulder."

Resisted testing of the cervical spine is generally negative, although, in cases of severe osteoarthritis, the tests can be painful because of the increase in joint compression associated with accentuated muscle forces. Tests against resistance may also be painful if the patient has upper cervical fractures or another serious lesion.

TECHNIQUE[86]

We utilize the posterior approach to the atlantooccipital and atlantoaxial joints because of the safety it affords. A lateral approach has been described by Dreyfuss and associates,[74, 87] who appear to utilize it with safety and facility.

Each of our patients is taken to the fluoroscopy suite and placed in the prone position with several blankets positioned under the chest to allow the head to be slightly flexed. The fluoroscopy C arm approaches the table from the head in an anteroposterior direction. It is then rotated in the sagittal plane so that the beam passes from the anterosuperior aspect to the posteroinferior aspect (Fig. 20–9).[88] This rotation is done under fluoroscopic visualization until the foramen magnum and the atlantooccipital joint are visualized. A pointer, and later a marking pen, is utilized to mark the needle insertion site, which is lateral to the foramen magnum toward the confluence of bone shadows that describe the atlantooccipital joint. This skin is prepared and draped in the usual sterile fashion, and a skin wheal is raised with local anesthetic at the insertion site. We use a 25-gauge spinal needle to perform this procedure, for reasons of safety, and therefore utilize an introducer needle to break the skin and direct the thinner block needle. A through-the-eye-of-the-needle technique is used, allowing the x-ray beam to define the course of the needle. The introducer needle, appearing as a small point on the screen (thus the name *through-the-eye-of-the-needle* technique), is placed and directed toward the posterolateral aspect of the atlantooccipital joint. The vertebral artery lies medial to this facet, having passed from lateral to medial below it (Figs. 20–10, 20–11). Generally speaking, the introducer needle's limited length prevents its entering the foramen magnum. The 25-gauge needle with the stylet in place is then carefully passed through the introducer until bone contact is made. If the atlantooccipital joint is entered, a distinctive "pop" almost always is felt. The C arm can then be rotated to the horizontal plane, and the needle can be seen to have entered the joint. The atlantooccipital joint

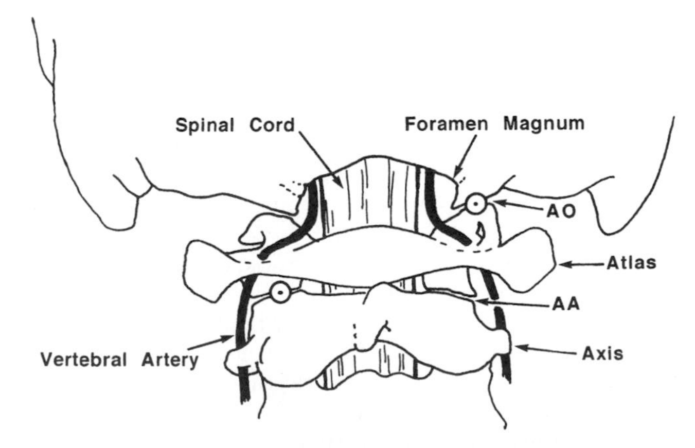

FIGURE 20–10 Diagram of the placement of 25-gauge spinal needle into the anterior axial joint on the left (AA) and the anterior occipital joint on the right (AO) as seen by "through the eye of the needle" technique. The spatial relationships of these needles with the vertebral arteries, foramen magnum, and spinal cord are shown. The circled dot is equivalent to "through the eye of the needle."

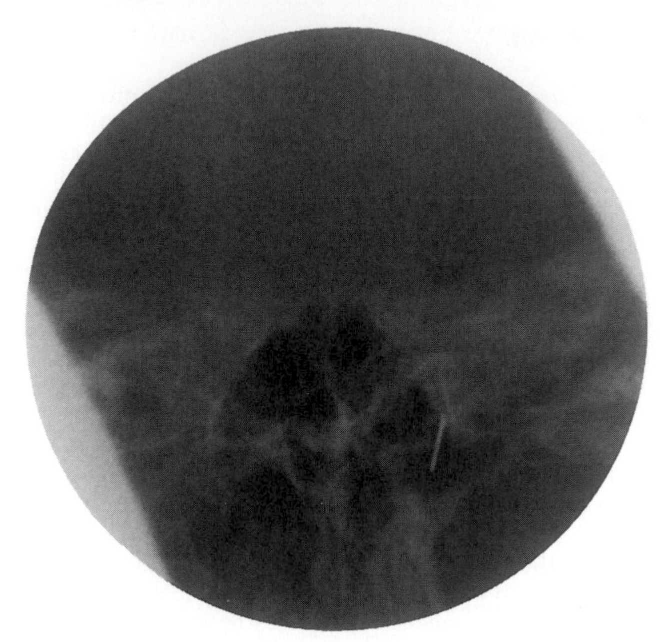

FIGURE 20–11 Placement of introducer needle on anteroposterior fluoroscopic view.

is anterior to the posterolateral columns of the spinal cord. The previously described anteroposterior fluoroscopic view with sagittal plane rotation is essential to avoid placing the needle in the spinal cord.[86]

If, after removal of the stylet, aspiration results prove negative, 1 mL of Omnipaque 240 is injected under fluoroscopy using a flexible T piece connected to the spinal needle. With good placement, the classic bilateral concave dye pattern is seen on lateral fluoroscopic view, representing the dye's lining of the joint capsule (Fig. 20–12). It is not uncommon, in the presence of trauma, for the dye to penetrate the torn capsule and enter the cervical epidural space. Venous runoff of dye almost always heralds placement of the needle outside the joint, which is surrounded by a rich venous plexus. In the presence of venous runoff or spread of dye into the epidural space, the injection is stopped, and either the needle is redirected (in the case of venous runoff) or the block is abandoned (when dye is seen to invade the epidural space). Biplanar views are again checked before injection of local anesthetic, to ensure safe and appropriate placement of the needle. If the dye spread remains circumscribed and the joint is outlined as described earlier, 1 to 1.5 mL of 0.2% ropivacaine with 20 mg of triamcinolone is slowly injected.[86]

Working from the same fluoroscopic view, the atlantoaxial joint is likewise injected. The vertebral artery at this level lies *lateral* to the atlantoaxial articulation as it courses through the C1 and C2 foramina (see Fig. 20–10). The beam is placed for an anteroposterior view to identify the foramen magnum and the atlas. The introducer needle is directed at the posterolateral aspect of the atlantoaxial joint, as the C2 ganglion lies at the midpoint of the space. The needle is advanced in the anterior and medial direction until it enters the joint cavity, when a distinctive "pop" is felt. The lateral view demonstrates the tip of the needle in the middle of the joint (Fig. 20–13).[90, 91] One milliliter of nonionic, water-soluble contrast (Omnipaque 240) is injected after negative aspiration for blood or cerebrospinal fluid. The film should demonstrate the bilateral concavity of the joint, and the dye should remain confined to the joint space (Fig. 20–14). If the dye remains circumscribed, 1 to 1.5 mL of 0.2% ropivacaine with 20 mg of triamcinolone is slowly injected. It is not uncommon for the patient to experience an exacerbation of the occipital headache during the injection.[74, 86]

Brief periods of ataxia in the immediate postblock period have been noted by us and others.[86, 91] This ataxia may be secondary to the reproduction of pain by joint distension or by absorption of local anesthetic into either the vertebral arteries or the valveless venous plexus that is posterior to

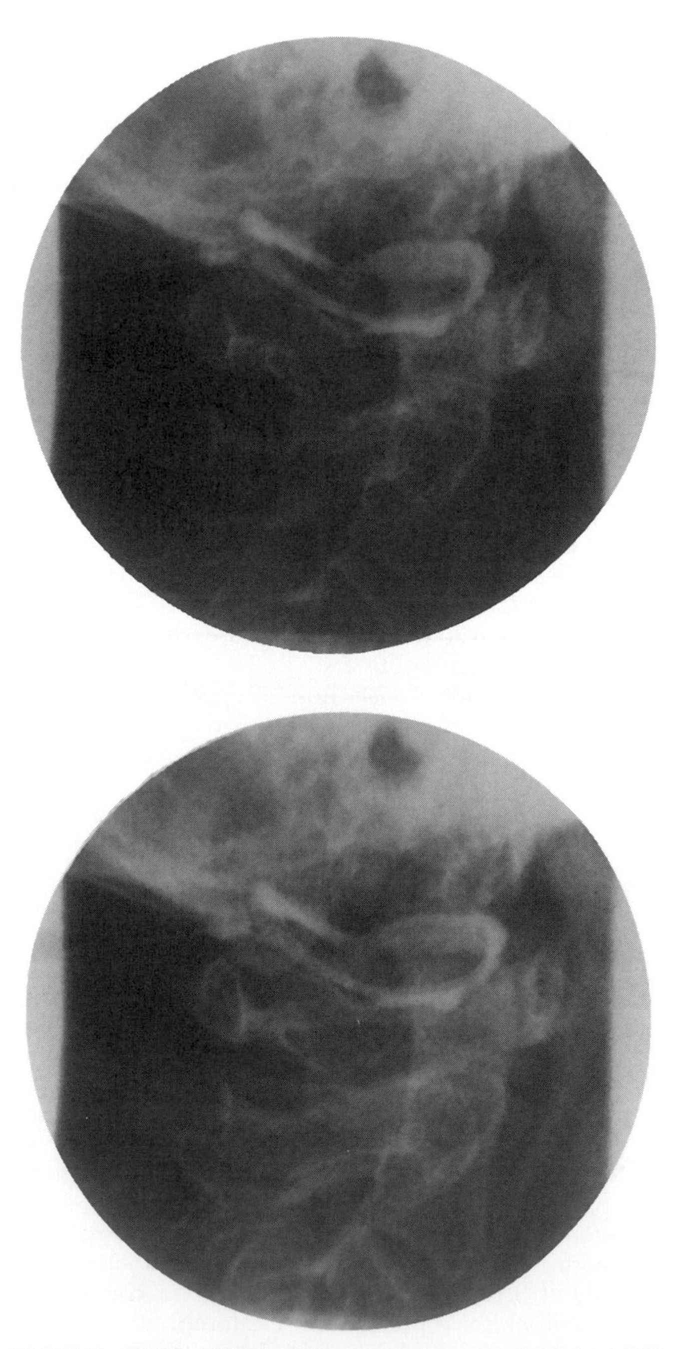

FIGURE 20–12 Slightly oblique lateral views revealing "classic" filling of atlantooccipital joint after injection of Omnipaque.

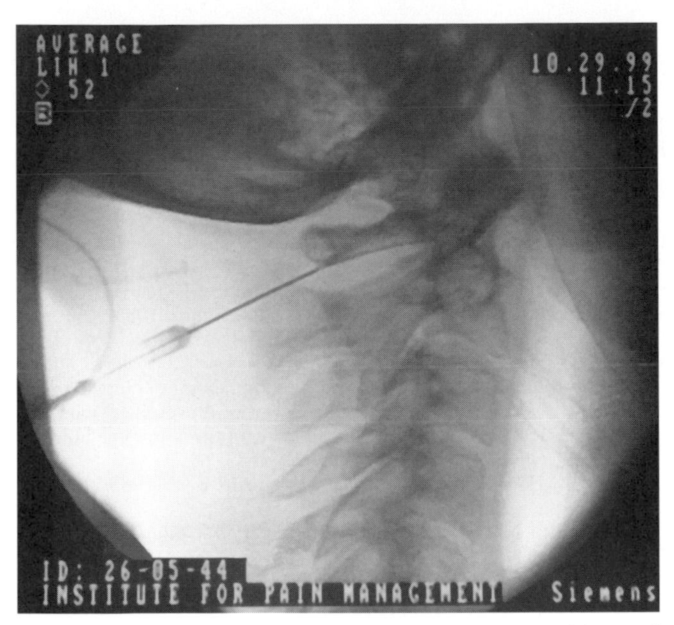

FIGURE 20–13 Lateral view demonstrates placement of the needle in the middle of the atlantoaxial joint.

the facets. Our patients are therefore observed for approximately 30 min before discharge.[86]

Complications of atlantooccipital and atlantoaxial blocks include epidural and intrathecal injections and intravascular injections into the adjacent venous plexus, vertebral artery, and possibly the carotid artery. Although only a small amount of local anesthetic is injected, its proximity to the brain ensures a higher intracranial concentration than would be anticipated, and it is possible for symptoms common to local anesthetic central nervous system toxicity to result.[86]

Although we have rarely seen pain caused by isolated injury to the atlantooccipital and atlantoaxial joints, injecting them may have a place in the treatment of some patients' headaches. This is especially true when the pain is occipital or suboccipital and is exacerbated by the neck movements typically associated with these joints.[86]

TECHNIQUE FOR PULSED RADIOFREQUENCY

Pulsed radiofrequency (RF) is being studied as a neuromodulatory technique. The advantages of pulsed RF over RF include these: It is a painless procedure (and, so, does not require local anesthetic) because no depolarization takes place. No neuritis-like reactions result. It has not produced side effects. Clinically, it is not neuroablative.[92] These advantages make it an excellent option for treatment of referred pain involving the medial branches of the C1 and C2 dorsal rami.

The technique for pulsed RF of the C1 dorsal ramus is very similar to the approach for atlantooccipital joint injection. Instead of a 25-gauge spinal needle, however, a 16-gauge angiocatheter is used as the introducer. The C1 dorsal ramus (suboccipital nerve) courses cephalad from the posterior arch of the atlas. This posterolateral aspect is the target. A 20-gauge, 10-cm, curved, blunt-tipped RF needle with a 10-mm active tip is directed through the angiocatheter to the target until bone contact is made with the posterior arch of the atlas. The tip is then directed cephalad. Proximity to the C1 dorsal ramus is then determined by sensory testing at 50 Hz, and a paresthesia in the nerve root distribution between 0.3 and 0.7 V indicates satisfactory placement. Stimulation at 0.5 V is optimal. Stimulation at less than 0.3 V indicates possible intraneural placement and the needle must be retracted and redirected. Stimulation at more than 0.7 V signifies approximate placement near the desired dorsal rami, and minimal advancement or redirection will achieve optimal placement. After proper needle placement is confirmed, the dorsal ramus is subjected to pulsed RF at 42° C for 120 sec. The procedure is repeated twice, for a total of three applications. The needles are then withdrawn and the site is covered with antibiotic and a Band-Aid.

The technique for pulsed RF of the C2 dorsal ramus is also very similar to the approach for atlantoaxial joint injection. The C2 dorsal ramus arises just below the lateral atlantoaxial joint and its branches supply the atlantooccipital and the atlantoaxial synovial spaces. Instead of the 25-gauge spinal needle, a 16-gauge angiocatheter is used as the introducer needle. This angiocatheter is directed toward the posterior aspect of the atlantoaxial joint. A 20-gauge, 10-cm, curved, blunt-tipped, RF needle with a 10-mm active tip is directed through the angiocatheter and advanced until contact is made with the lamina of C2. The needle is then angulated slightly toward the inferior aspect of the posterior mass of the atlas.[93] Proximity to the C2 dorsal ramus is then determined by sensory testing, as described earlier. Again, after confirmation of needle placement, the dorsal ramus is treated with pulsed RF at 42° C for a total of three applications of 120 sec each.

DISCUSSION[86]

Deep suboccipital pain that is movement related can be one of the most elusive pains to diagnose and to treat. One

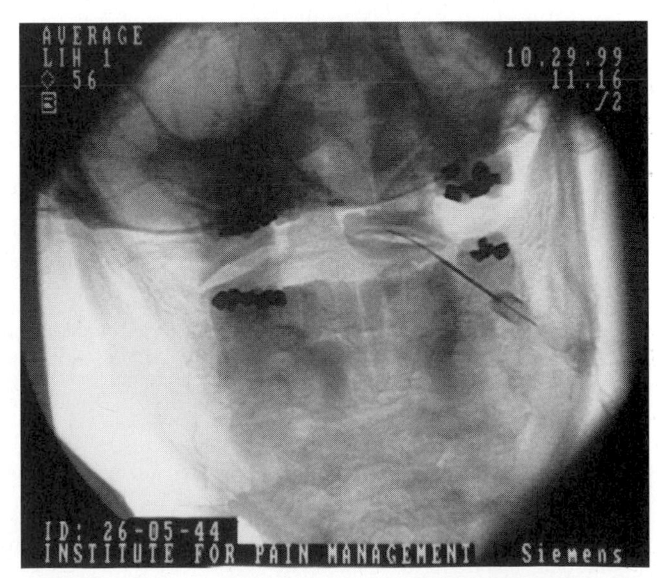

FIGURE 20–14 Anteroposterior view demonstrates filling of the atlantoaxial joint with contrast. Note the bilateral concavity.

of the interesting aspects of the series of Busch and Wilson[91] was the use of intracapsular injection of local anesthetic and steroid instead of putting the patient's head in a neurosurgical frame to immobilize it entirely.[94] Theoretically, once the motion ceases, the pain responds favorably to the stabilization of the fusion. The majority of patients choose the route of repeat injections in the hope that the anti-inflammatory effect of injections will "settle the disease down" and limit pain from the swollen joint.[86] Pulsed RF is a neuromodulatory technique for referred pain involving the medial branches of the C1 and C2 dorsal rami. The patient must follow a multidisciplinary program of continuing physical therapy, functional restoration, psychotherapy, and drug management. Because frequent emergency room visits for pain crisis are common, detoxification may be in order. Owing to the rarity of the disease, (1) the diagnosis is often missed and (2) conducting single-center, prospective double-blind studies is difficult. Neural blockade at the atlantooccipital and atlantoaxial joints is a very technically demanding technique. The physician doing the procedure must avoid placing a needle into the brain stem or the vertebral artery and injecting either air or particulate matter such as precipitated steroids. Therefore, it is strongly urged that the procedure be carried out by clinicians who are very experienced in working under fluoroscopic guidance and who recognize the three-dimensional hazards of placing a needle so close to the foramen magnum and the brain stem. The procedure is most gratifying when carried out properly. The patient reports pain relief for the first time and demonstrates the ability to perform nodding and rotating movements that previously were the cause of severe suboccipital pain.[86]

REFERENCES

1. Bogduk N, Marsland A: The cervical zygapophyseal joints as a source of neck pain. Spine 13:610–617, 1988.
2. Bogduk N, Corrigan B, Kelly P, et al: Cervical headache. Med J Austr 143:202–207, 1985.
3. Gawel MJ, Rothbart PJ: Occipital nerve block in the management of headache and cervical pain. Cephalalgia 12(1):9–13, 1992.
4. Jansen J, Vadokas V, Vogelsang JP: Cervical peridural anaesthesia: An essential aid for the indication of surgical treatment of cervicogenic headache triggered by degenerative diseases of the cervical spine. Functional Neurol 13:79–81, 1998.
5. Bogduk N: The anatomy and mechanism of cervical headaches. *In* Proceedings of Cervical Headaches Symposium. Sydney, Manipulative Therapists Association of Australia, 1983.
6. Bogduk N: The clinical anatomy of the cervical dorsal rami. Spine 7:319–330, 1982.
7. Winkel D, Aufdemkampe G, Matthijs O, et al: Cervical spine functional anatomy. *In* Diagnosis and Treatment of the Spine. Gaithersburg, Md., Aspen, 1996, pp 546–558.
8. Aboumadawi A, Solanki G, Casey ATH, Crockard HA: Variation of the groove in the axis vertebra for the vertebral artery—implications for instrumentation. J Bone Joint Surg 79B:820–823, 1997.
9. Ebraheim NA, Xu RM, Ahmad M, Heck B: The quantitative anatomy of the vertebral artery groove of the atlas and its relation to the posterior atlantoaxial approach. Spine 23:320–323, 1998.
10. Panjabi MM, Dvorak J, Sandler A, et al: Cervical spine kinematics and clinical instability. *In* Clark CR (ed): The Cervical Spine. Philadelphia: Lippincott-Raven, 1998.
11. Karol LA, Sheffield EG, Crawford K, et al: Reproducibility in the measurement of atlantooccipital instability in children with Down syndrome. Spine 21:2463–2467, 1996.
12. Lewit K, Krausova L: Beitrag zur flexion der Halswirbelsaule. Fortschr Roentgenstr 97:38, 1962.
13. Dvorak J, Dvorak J: [Manual Medicine. Diagnosis]. Stuttgart, Thieme, 1991, pp 10–11.
14. Wilauschus WG, Kladny B, Beyer WF, et al: Lesions of the alar ligaments. In vivo and in vitro studies with magnetic resonance imaging. Spine 20(23):2493–2498, 1995.
15. Van der EI: Wervelkolom. Manuele Diagnostiek. Rotterdam, Manthel, 1992, p 453.
16. Arlen A: Die paradoxale Keppbewegung der Atlas in der Funktionsdiagnostik der Halswirbelsaule. Manual Med 1:16, 1977.
17. Ordvay NR, et al: Cervical flexion, extension, protrusion, and retraction: A radiographic segmental analysis. Spine 24:240–247, 1999.
18. Oostendorp R: [Functional Vertebrobasilar Insufficiency.] Doctoral Thesis, University of Nijmegen, The Netherlands, 1988.
19. Jofe M, White A, Panjabi M: Clinically relevant kinematics of the cervical spine. *In* Sherk H, Dunn E, Eismont F, et al (eds): The Cervical Spine, ed 2. Philadelphia, JB Lippincott, 1989, pp 57–69.
20. Worth DR, Selvik G: Movements of the craniovertebral joints. *In* Grieve GP (ed): Modern Manual Therapy of the Vertebral Column. London, Churchill Livingstone, 1987, pp 53–63.
21. Panjabi MM: Three-dimensional movements of the upper cervical spine. Spine 13:726–728, 1988.
22. Penning L: Normal movements of the cervical spine. Am J Roentgenol 130:317–326, 1979.
23. Jirout J: Funktionelle Pathologie und Klinik der Wirbelsaule. Stuttgart, Gustav Fischer, 1990.
24. White AA, Panjabi M: Clinical Biomechanics of the Spine, ed 2. Philadelphia, JB Lippincott, 1990, p 92.
25. Von Guttman G: X-ray diagnosis of spinal dysfunction. Manuelle Medizin 5:73, 1982.
26. Penning L, Wilmink JT: Rotation of the cervical spine. A CT study in normal subjects. Spine 12:732–738, 1987.
27. International Headache Society: Headache classification and diagnostic criteria for headache disorders, cranial neuralgias, and facial pain. Cephalalgia 8(Suppl) 71–I72:19–22, 1988.
28. Friedman MM, Nelson AJ: Head and neck pain review: Traditional and new perspectives. Journal of Orthopaedic and Sports Physical Therapy 24:268–278, 1996.
29. Jansen J, Bardosi A, Hildebrandt J, Lücke A: Cervicogenic hemicranial attacks associated with vascular irritation or compression of the cervical nerve root C2. Clinical manifestations and morphological findings. Pain 39:203–212, 1989.
30. Escolar J: The efferent connections of the 1st, 2nd, and 3rd cervical nerves in the cat. An analysis by Marchi and Radolsky methods. J Comp Neurol 89:79–92, 1948.
31. Van Valkenburg CT: Über die anatomischen und funktionellen Beziehungen der Radix descendens trigemini zum oberen Halsmark. Arch Neurol Psychiatry 14:238–254, 1924.
32. Kerr FWL: Atypical facial neuralgias: Their mechanism as inferred from anatomic and physiologic data. Proc Staff Meet Mayo Clin 36:254–260, 1961.
33. Kerr FWL: Structural relation of the trigeminal spinal tract to upper cervical roots and the solitary nucleus in the cat. Exp Neurol 4:134–148, 1961.
34. Kerr FWL, Olafson RA: Trigeminal and cervical volleys. Arch Neurol 5:171–178, 1961.
35. Eder M, Tilscher H: Pathophysiologie unk Klinik gestörter Kopfgelenke. Manuelle Medizin 34:241–244, 1996.
36. Mark BM: Cervicogenic headache differential diagnosis and clinical management: Literature review. J Craniomandibular Pract 8:332–338, 1990.
37. Shigenaga Y, Okamoto T, Nishimori T, et al: Oral and facial representation in the trigeminal principal and rostral spinal nuclei of the cat. J Comp Neurol 244:1–18, 1986.
38. Keller JT, Beduk A, Saunders MC: Origin of fibres innervating the basilar artery of the cat. Neurosci Lett 58:263–268, 1985.
39. Moskowitz MA: The neurobiology of vascular head pain. Ann Neurol 16:157–168, 1984.
40. Drummond PD, Gonski A, Lance JW: Facial flushing after thermocoagulation of the gasserian ganglion. J Neurol Neurosurg Psychiatry 46:611–616, 1983.
41. Samnegard H, Thulin L, Tyden G, et al: Effect of substance P on internal carotid artery blood flow in man. Acta Physiol Scand 104:491–495, 1978.
42. Owman C, Anderson J, Hauko J, Hardebo JE: Neurotransmitter amines and peptides in the cerebrovascular bed. *In* MacKenzie ET,

Seylaz J, Bes A (eds): Neurotransmitters and the Cerebral Circulation. New York, Raven, 1984, pp 11–38.
43. Gutmann G: Zum Problem des Vasospasmus im A. vertebralis-basilaris-Gefässbereich. *In* Gutmann G (ed): Arteria Vertebralis. Berlin, Springer-Verlag, 1985.
44. Lewit K: Kopfgelenke und Gleichgweichtsstörun. Manuelle Medizin 24:26–29, 1986.
45. Lewit K, Berger M: Zervikales Störungsmuster bei Schwindelpatiën-ten. Manuelle Medizin 21:15–19, 1983.
46. Gutmann G, Biedermann H: Funktionelle Pathologie und Klinik der Wirbelsäule, Band 1: Die Halswirbelsäule (Teil 2). Stuttgart, Gustav Fischer, 1984.
47. Krueger BR, Okazaki H: Vertebral-basilar distribution, infarction following chiropractic cervical manipulation. Mayo Clinic Proc 55:322–332, 1980.
48. Schellhas KP, Smith MD, Gundry CR, Pollei SR: Cervical discogenic pain. Spine 21:300–311, 1996.
49. Jenkner FL: [An old remedy newly evaluated: the cervical syndrome]. Wien Med Wochenschr 144:102–108, 1994.
50. Dwyer A, Aprill C, Bogduk N: Cervical zygapophyseal joint pain patterns I: A study in normal volunteers. Spine 15: 453–461, 1990.
51. Spitzer WO, Skovoron ML, Salmi LR, et al: Scientific monograph of the Quebec Task Force on Whiplash-Associated Disorders: Redefining whiplash and its management. Spine 20 (Suppl): 1S–73S, 1995.
52. Jansen J, Bardosi A, Hildebrandt J, Lücke A: Cervicogenic, hemicranial attacks associated with vascular irritation or compression of the cervical nerve root C2. Pain 39:203–212, 1989.
53. Wilson PR: Chronic neck pain and cervicogenic headache. Clin J Pain 7:5–11, 1991.
54. Babini SM, Cocco JA, Babini JC, et al: Atlantoaxial subluxation in systemic lupus erythematosus: Further evidence of tendinous alterations. J Rheumatol 17:173–177, 1990.
55. Collacott RA, Ellsion D, Harper W, et al: Atlanto-occipital instability in Down's syndrome. J Ment Defic Res 33:499–505, 1989.
56. Jagjivan B, Spencer PAS, Hosking G: Radiological screening for atlanto-axial instability in Down's syndrome. Clin Radiol 39:661–663, 1988.
57. Wetzel FT, La Rocca H: Griesel's syndrome. Clin Orthop 240:141–152, 1989.
58. Ghanayem AJ, Leventhal M, Bohlman H: Osteoarthrosis of the atlanto-axial joints. J Bone Joint Surg 78A:1300–1307, 1996.
59. Derrick LJ, Chesworth BM: Post–motor vehicle accident alar ligament laxity. Journal of Orthopaedic and Sports Physical Therapy 16:6–11, 1992.
60. Fielding JW, Cochran GVB, Lasing III JF, Hohl M: Tears of the transverse ligament of the atlas. J Bone Joint Surg 56A:1683–1691, 1974.
61. Kennedy JC: Ligamentous injuries in the adolescent. *In* Kennedy JC (ed): The Injured Adolescent Knee. Baltimore, Williams & Wilkins, 1979, pp 1–42.
62. Levine AM, Edwards CC: Traumatic lesions of the occipitoatlantoaxial complex. Clin Orthop 239:53–68, 1989.
63. Zapletal J, de Valois C: Radiologic prevalence of advanced lateral C1–2 osteoarthritis. Spine 22:2511–2513, 1997.
64. Star MJ, Curd JG, Thorne RP: Atlantoaxial lateral mass osteoarthritis. Spine 17:S71–S76, 1992.
65. Penning L: Acceleration injury of the cervical spine by hypertranslation of the head: Part 1. Effect of normal translation of the head on cervical spine motion: A radiological study. Eur Spine J 1:7–12, 1992.
66. Panjabi MM, Cholewicki J, Nibu K, et al: Biomechanics of whiplash injury. Orthopade 27:813–819, 1998.
67. Grifka J, Hedtmann A, Pape HG, et al: Biomechanics of injury of the cervical spine. Orthopade 27:802–812, 1998.
68. Fredriksen TA, Hovdal H, Sjaastad O: "Cervicogenic headache": Clinical manifestation. Cephalalgia 7(2):147–160, 1987.
69. Zapletal J, de Valois JC: Radiologic prevalence of advanced lateral C1–C2 osteoarthritis. Spine 22:2511–2513, 1997.
70. Grimmer K: Relationship between occupation and episodes of headache that match cervical origin pain patterns. J Occup Med 35:929–935, 1993.
71. Star MJ, Curd JG, Thorne RP: Atlantoaxial lateral mass osteoarthritis: A frequently overlooked cause of severe occipitocervical pain. Spine 17(S):71–76, 1992.
72. Sjaastad O, Fredriksen TA, Sand T: The localization of the initial pain of attack. A comparison between classic migraine and cervicogenic headache. Funct Neurol 4:73–78, 1989.
73. Leone M, D'Amico D, Moschiano F, et al: Possible identification of cervicogenic headache among patients with migraine: An analysis of 374 headaches. Headache 35:461–464, 1995.
74. Dreyfuss P, Michaelsen M, Fletcher D: Atlanto-occipital and lateral atlanto-axial joint pain patterns. Spine 19:1125–1131, 1994.
75. Halla JT, Hardin JG: Atlantoaxial (C1–C2) facet joint osteoarthritis: A distinctive clinical syndrome. Arthritis Rheum 30:577–582, 1987.
76. Simeone FA, Rothman RH: Cervical disc disease. *In* Simeone FA, Rothman RH, (eds): The Spine. Philadelphia, WB Saunders, 1982, p 453.
77. Friedman MM, Nelson AJ: Head and neck pain review: Traditional and new perspectives. Journal of Orthopaedic and Sports Physical Therapy 24:268–278, 1996.
78. Hassenstein B: [The region of the occipital joints in relation to the orientation in space: system theory related respectively biokybermetic stand points.] *In* Wolff H-D (ed): [The Special Position of the Cervicooccipital Region]. Berlin, Springer, 1988, pp 1–17.
79. Bogduk N: Cervical causes of headache and dizziness. *In* Grieve GP (ed): Modern Manual Therapy of the Vertebral Column. New York, Churchill Livingstone, 1987, pp 289–302.
80. Pfaffenrath V, Dandekar R, Pollman W: Cervicogenic headache—the clinical picture, radiological findings and hypothesis on its pathophysiology. Headache 27:495–499, 1987.
81. Pfaffenrath V, Kaube H: Diagnostics of cervicogenic headache. Functional Neurol 5:159–164, 1990.
82. Fredriksen TA, et al: "Cervicogenic headache": Clinical manifestation. Cephalalgia 7(2):147–160, 1987.
83. Pfaffenrath V, Dandekar R, Pollman W: Cervicogenic headache—the clinical picture, radiological findings and hypothesis on its pathophysiology. Headache 27:495–499, 1987.
84. Pfaffenrath V, Dandekar R, Mayer ET, et al: Cervicogenic headache: Results of computer-based measurements of cervical spine mobility in 15 patients. Cephalalgia 8:45–48, 1988.
85. Vernon H, et al: Cervicogenic dysfunction in muscle contraction headache and migraine: A descriptive study. J Manipulative Physiol Ther 15:418–429, 1992.
86. Racz GB, Sanel H, Diede JH: Atlanto-occipital and atlantoaxial injections in the treatment of headache and neck pain. *In* Waldman S, Winnie A (eds): Interventional Pain Management. Philadelphia, WB Saunders, 1996, pp 220–222.
87. Dreyfuss P, Rogers J, Dreyer S, Fletcher D: Atlanto-occipital joint pain: A report of three cases and description of an intra-articular joint block technique (Abstract). Reg Anesth 19(5):344–351, 1994.
88. Ballinger P (ed): Merrill's Atlas of Radiographic Positions and Radiographic Procedures, ed 6. St Louis, CV Mosby, 1986, pp 238–243.
89. Manning DC, Rowlingson JC: Back pain and the role of neural blockade. *In* Cousins MJ, Bridenbaugh PO (eds): Neural Blockade in Clinical Anesthesia and Management of Pain, ed 3. Philadelphia, Lippincott-Raven, 1998, pp 897–900.
90. Waldman SD: Atiantoaxial block technique. *In* Waldman SD (ed): Atlas of Interventional Pain Management. Philadelphia, WB Saunders, 1998, pp 6–9.
91. Busch E, Wilson P: Atlanto-occipital and atlanto-axial injections in the treatment of headache and neck pain. Reg Anesth 14:45, 1989.
92. Sluijter ME, Van Kleef M: Characteristics and mode of action of radiofrequency lesions. Curr Rev Pain 2:143–150, 1998.
93. Chevrot A, Cermakova E, Vallee C, et al: C1-2 arthrography. Skel Radiol 24:425–429, 1995.
94. Taylor JR, Finch P: Acute injury of the neck: Anatomical and pathological basis of pain. Ann Acad Med Singapore 22:187–192, 1993.

CHAPTER • 21

Sphenopalatine Ganglion Blockade

Miles Day, MD • Gabor Racz, MD

The sphenopalatine ganglion (SPG) has been involved in the pathogenesis of pain since Sluder first described sphenopalatine neuralgia in 1908, and treated it with the sphenopalatine ganglion block (SPGB).[1] Over the past century, physicians have performed SPGB for pain syndromes ranging from headache and facial pain to sciatica and dysmenorrhea.[1] In the medical literature on SPGB, large gaps—spanning decades—reflect physicians' varying interest in and skepticism about the efficacy of SPGB in ablating the cause of pain. Currently, SPGB is used for relief of facial pain and headache. It has provided pain relief in patients when conventional pharmacologic therapy has become less effective or altogether ineffective.

INDICATIONS

SPGB has been utilized to treat many painful medical syndromes. Sluder, who is credited as the first physician to describe SPGB for the treatment of sphenopalatine neuralgia, described a unilateral facial pain at the root of the nose that sometimes spread toward the zygoma and extended back to the mastoid and occiput.[1] This pain is typically associated with parasympathetic features such as lacrimation, rhinorrhea, or mucosal congestion.[2] Sluder believed the cause of this pain was the spread of infection from the paranasal sinuses that irritated the SPG. This was initially accepted as a possible cause but came into question when other syndromes, such as low back pain, sciatica, and dysmenorrhea, were attributed to irritation of the SPG. Eagle, in the early 1940s, sought to revive interest in sphenopalatine neuralgia when he presented his thesis to the American Laryngological, Rhinological, and Otological Society. He agreed with Sluder on the existence of sphenopalatine neuralgia but disagreed on its cause.[3] Eagle believed that intranasal deformities, such as deviated septum, septal spurs or ledges, and prominent turbinates, were responsible for irritation of the ganglion, which caused the pain. Others attribute it to a reflex vasomotor change or possibly a vasomotor syndrome.[4] Regardless of the cause, sphenopalatine neuralgia is an indication for SPGB.

Trigeminal neuralgia is also an indication for SPGB. In 1925, Ruskin disagreed with Sluder on the indication for SPGB and suggested involvement of the SPG in the pathogenesis of trigeminal neuralgia.[5] The SPG is directly connected to the maxillary branch of the trigeminal nerve via the pterygopalatine nerves (see later). He believed that blockade of the SPG would in turn relieve the symptoms associated with trigeminal neuralgia. Few case reports in the current literature support this theory.[6]

Although new medications for the treatment of migraine and cluster headache are introduced every year, a certain small subset of patients fail to respond to oral and parenteral dosing and are forced to seek alternative methods for pain control. In recent years, blockade of the SPG has been utilized in such cases, with varying success.[7–9]

Another indication for SPGB is atypical facial pain. Such pain is usually unilateral, is described as constant, aching, and burning, and is not confined to the distribution of a cranial nerve.[10] It may involve the entire face, scalp, and neck. The pain may have a sympathetic component, which makes the SPGB ideal, because the postganglionic sympathetic nerves pass through the ganglion.

Other reported indications for SPGB include back pain, sciatica, angina, arthritis, herpes zoster ophthalmicus, and pain from cancer of the tongue and floor of the mouth.[11–13] These are not "true" indications for SPGB; instead, they reveal its broad applications in situations when conventional therapies are ineffective.

ANATOMY AND PHYSIOLOGY

The SPG is the largest group of neurons outside the cranial cavity. It lies in the pterygopalatine fossa, which is approximately 1 cm wide and 2 cm high and resembles a "vase" on a lateral fluoroscopic view. The pterygopalatine fossa is bordered anteriorly by the posterior wall of the maxillary sinus, posteriorly by the medial plate of the pterygoid process, medially by the perpendicular plate of the palatine bone, and superiorly by the sphenoid sinus, and laterally it communicates with the infratemporal fossa.[14] The foramen

This chapter was previously published as an article titled "Sphenopalatine, Ganglion Analgesia" in *Current Review of Pain* 3(5), pp. 342–347, 1999.

rotundum, through which the maxillary branch of the trigeminal nerve passes, is located on the superolateral aspect of the pterygopalatine fossa; the opening to the pterygoid canal, which houses the vidian nerve, is located on the inferomedial portion of the fossa. The ganglion within the fossa is located posterior to the middle turbinate of the nose and lies a few millimeters deep to the lateral nasal mucosa. Also contained in the fossa is the maxillary artery and its multiple branches. The maxillary branch of the trigeminal nerve exits the cranial vault through the foramen rotundum and is located cephalad and slightly lateral to the pterygopalatine fossa.

The SPG has a complex neural center and has multiple connections. It is "suspended" from the maxillary branch of the trigeminal nerve at the pterygopalatine fossa via the pterygopalatine nerves and lies medial to the maxillary branch when viewed in the sagittal plane. Posteriorly, it is connected to the vidian nerve, also known as the nerve of the pterygoid canal, which is formed by the greater petrosal and the deep petrosal nerves. The ganglion itself has efferent branches and forms the superior posterior lateral nasal and pharyngeal nerves. Caudally, the ganglion is in direct connection with the greater and lesser palatine nerves.

As a neural center, the ganglion has sensory, motor, and autonomic components. The sensory fibers arise from the maxillary nerve, pass through the SPG, and are distributed to the nasal membranes, the soft palate, and some parts of the pharynx.[3] A few motor nerves are also believed to be carried with the sensory trunks. The autonomic innervation is more complex. The sympathetic component begins with preganglionic sympathetic fibers originating in the upper thoracic spinal cord, forming the white rami communicantes, coursing through the sympathetic chain, and ending in the superior cervical sympathetic ganglion, where the preganglionic fibers synapse with the postganglionic ones. The postganglionic fibers then join the carotid nerves before branching off and traveling through the deep petrosal and vidian nerves. The postganglionic sympathetic nerves continue their path through the SPG on their way to the lacrimal gland and the nasal and palatine mucosa. The parasympathetic component has its preganglionic origin in the superior salivatory nucleus then travels through a portion of the facial nerve (VII) before forming the greater petrosal nerve. The greater petrosal nerve in turn joins the deep petrosal nerve to form the vidian nerve, which ends in the SPG. Within the ganglion, the preganglionic fibers synapse with their postganglionic cells and continue on to the nasal mucosa, and one branch travels with the maxillary nerve to the lacrimal gland.

PATHOPHYSIOLOGY

The role of the SPG in the pathogenesis of pain still remains controversial. Sluder believed that paranasal sinus infections caused irritation of the ganglion resulting in pain, whereas Eagle felt that nasal deformities were responsible for the irritation of the ganglion, and thus the pain.[2, 3] Ruskin proposed involvement of the SPG in the pathogenesis of trigeminal neuralgia, but the exact cause of this disorder is indeterminate even today.[5] Another hypothesis posits a dysequilibrium between sympathetic and parasympathetic tone in the ganglion that results in release of substance P or blockade of local enkephalins.[15] Still another hypothesis revolves around the belief that focal demyelination in the ganglion produces abnormal impulses in the afferent nociceptive C fibers and leads to pain.[15] General consensus on the role and pathogenesis of the SPG remains elusive.

TECHNIQUES

The SPG can be blocked by several techniques. The drugs frequently used are local anesthetics (4% cocaine, 2% to 4% lidocaine, or 0.5% bupivacaine), depot steroids, and/or 6% phenol. To prolong the blockade, radiofrequency thermocoagulation (RFTC) can be employed, and more recently at our institution, electromagnetic field (EMF) pulsed radiofrequency lesioning has been used. The current hypothesis on the mechanism of action of EMF is that the membranes of nerves have a capacitor function and that EMF creates a high electric field that punches holes in the capacitor, thus blocking transmission of stimuli through A-delta and C fibers.[16] Informed consent must be obtained and complications must be explained before the blockade.

Technique One: Intranasal Topical Application of Local Anesthetic[17]

Intranasal application of local anesthetic is relatively easy to perform and if efficacious can be taught to the patient. The operator dips a 3.5-inch cotton-tipped applicator in the anesthetic solution (cocaine or lidocaine) and inserts it through the naris on the affected side while holding the applicator parallel to the zygomatic arch, which corresponds to the middle turbinate. The applicator is advanced slowly and directed laterally toward the back of the nasal pharynx. The ganglion lies a few millimeters beneath the lateral nasal mucosa. Once the applicator is in place, a second one is inserted in the same fashion but slightly superior and posterior to the first. The applicators are left in place for approximately 30 to 45 minutes. Because of the connections with the lacrimal gland, SPGB produces ipsilateral tearing secondary to parasympathetic activity. If it is efficacious, this block can be repeated or an RFTC or EMF procedure can be performed for prolonged analgesia. We do not recommend use of phenol for neurolysis with this technique.

Technique Two: Greater Palatine Foramen Approach[18]

The patient lies supine with the neck slightly extended. The greater palatine foramen is located just medial to the gumline of the third molar. Sometimes a dimple marks the foramen. A dental needle is inserted at a 120-degree angle through the mucosa and into the foramen. It is advanced approximately 2.5 cm in a superior and slightly posterior direction. Paresthesia may be elicited, since the maxillary nerve is just cephalad to the ganglion. A 2-ml dose of cocaine or lidocaine is injected after negative aspirate and confirms the SPGB as before. No data are available on standard RFTC or EMF lesioning or phenol injection of the SPG via this approach.

Technique Three: Infrazygomatic Arch Approach[17]

Many use this approach "blind," without C-arm fluoroscopy, but at our institution we recommend using fluoroscopy. The patient lies supine with the head inside the C arm. A lateral view of the upper cervical spine and the mandible is obtained and the head rotated until the rami of the mandible are superimposed one on the other. The C arm is moved slightly cephalad until the pterygopalatine fossa is visualized. It should resemble a "vase" when the two pterygopalatine plates are superimposed upon one another and is located just posterior to the posterior aspect of the maxillary sinus (Fig. 21–1A). The needle is inserted under the zygoma and anterior to the ramus of the mandible. A curved, blunt-tipped needle is less traumatic to the underlying structures than a sharp needle. When a blunt needle is used, a 1.25-in angiocatheter two sizes larger than the blunt needle must be inserted first. The needle is directed medial, cephalad, and slightly posterior toward the pterygopalatine fossa (Fig. 21–1B). An anteroposterior view confirms the proper direction and positioning of the needle (Fig. 21–1C). The tip of the needle should be advanced until it is adjacent to the lateral nasal mucosa. If resistance is felt at any time, the needle must be slightly withdrawn and redirected. The operator takes care to avoid advancing the needle through the lateral nasal mucosa. If a stimulating needle is used, sensory stimulation is applied on a 1-V scale at 75 pulses per second and 0.25- to 0.5-msec pulse width.[17] A paresthesia should be felt at 0.5 to 0.7 V. When the stimulator is correctly situated on the ganglion, the paresthesia should be felt at the root of the nose. If the paresthesia is felt in the upper teeth, the maxillary branch of the trigeminal nerve is being stimulated and the needle must be redirected more caudad. Stimulation of the greater and lesser palatine nerves results in paresthesias of the hard palate. In this case, the needle is anterior and lateral and should be redirected in a more posterior and medial direction. Once it is properly positioned, 1 to 2 ml of local

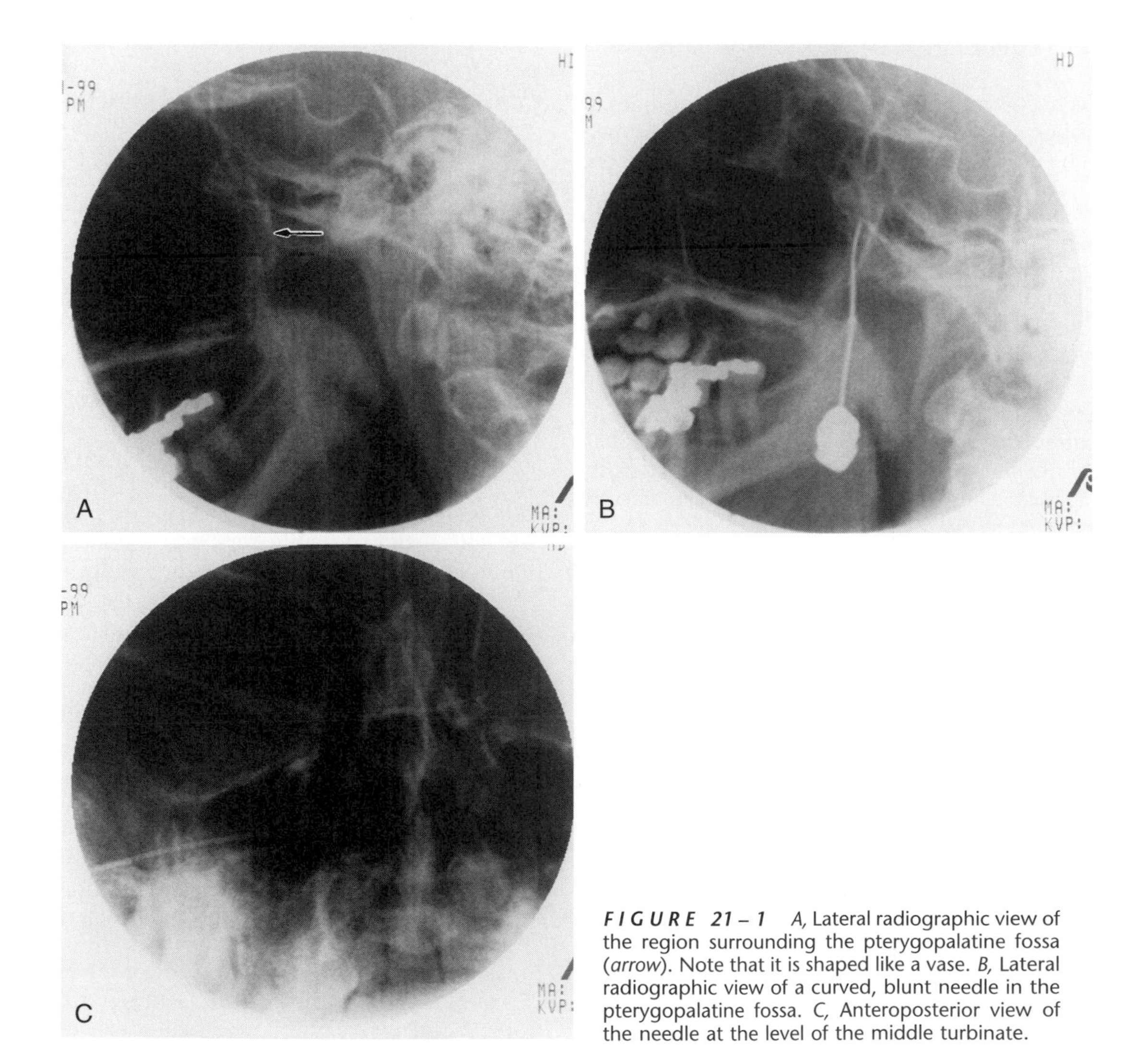

FIGURE 21–1 *A,* Lateral radiographic view of the region surrounding the pterygopalatine fossa (*arrow*). Note that it is shaped like a vase. *B,* Lateral radiographic view of a curved, blunt needle in the pterygopalatine fossa. *C,* Anteroposterior view of the needle at the level of the middle turbinate.

anesthetic is injected, with or without steroid. If pain relief is obtained, RFTC or EMF pulsed radiofrequency lesioning can be planned.

Technique Four: RFTC and EMF Pulsed Radiofrequency Lesioning[17]

Lesioning of the SPG can be performed with either RFTC or EMF after a successful block has been produced with local anesthetic. An insulated 20- or 22-gauge, 10-cm, curved, blunt-tipped RFK (Racz-Finch Kit; Radionics, Burlington, VT) needle with a 5- to 10-mm active tip is used. After proper placement and stimulation as described in technique three, radiofrequency lesioning is performed for 70 to 90 seconds at 80° C. Two lesions are usually made. Before lesioning, 1 to 2 ml of local anesthetic is injected. EMF pulsed radiofrequency lesioning is performed at 42° C for 120 seconds. Two or three lesions (120 seconds) can be made without local anesthetic, since the temperature of the lesioning is barely above normal body temperature.

THE TEXAS TECH EXPERIENCE

At Texas Tech we routinely employ all of the techniques of SPGB described so far except the greater palatine foramen approach. The indications for blockade include all of those mentioned previously. Our routine is to start with the intranasal technique, using two applicators soaked with 4% cocaine. Occasionally, a third applicator is placed if the nasal passage is large enough. Depending on the efficacy of the block, we either repeat the block, when the pain relief lasts longer than 1 month or, when relief is shorter-lived, we proceed to RFTC or EMF. If the patient is reliable and receives extended relief with the intranasal block, we prescribe 2% lidocaine in a nasal spray and instruct the patient to inhale two squirts through the ipsilateral naris, as needed for headache or pain. The patient is cautioned against using the lidocaine more than two or three times per day, to avoid local anesthetic toxicity. Occasionally, the intranasal technique is ineffective owing to incorrect placement of the applicator, failure of the local anesthetic to reach the SPG, or incorrect clinical diagnosis. In this situation, we perform the infrazygomatic arch approach under fluoroscopic guidance. If that is efficacious, we proceed to RFTC or EMF. To our knowledge, no prospective study comparing RFTC and EMF of the SPG has been performed, but such investigation is warranted. We have also attempted—unsuccessfully—electrical stimulation of the SPG in a patient with neuropathic pain in the mandibular division of the trigeminal nerve.

On average, the intranasal approach has served us only as a diagnostic block: very few patients have enjoyed more than a few days' to a couple of weeks' relief. After RFTC, our patients report partial to complete relief for 1 to 3 months (unpublished data). EMF has been performed a handful of times with one patient reporting 13 days of complete pain relief with gradual return of her facial pain over a month's time.

EFFICACY

Current literature on the efficacy of SPGB for various medical conditions is scant and patient populations rather small. One study by Sanders and Zuurmond examined the efficacy of SPGB in 66 patients suffering from episodic and chronic cluster headaches.[8] All had previously been treated with various pharmacologic and/or surgical therapy, without significant pain relief. The patients were divided into two groups, those with episodic and those with chronic pain, with sample sizes of 56 and 10 patients, respectively. All received three radiofrequency lesions at 70° C for 60 seconds. Thirty-four (60.7%) of 56 patients with episodic cluster headaches and 3 (30%) of the 10 with the chronic type received complete pain relief during a mean follow-up period of 29 months. Salar, Iob, and Fiore reported using percutaneous RFTC of the SPG for sphenopalatine neuralgia in seven patients.[14] Each received two lesions, at 60° and 65° C, respectively, for 60 seconds. One patient required repeat lesioning, and two underwent two additional RF procedures. All of the patients were pain free over a follow-up period ranging from 6 to 34 months. One case report in the *Nebraska Medical Journal* reported complete pain relief of trigeminal neuralgia over 30 months in a woman who received 10 intranasal SPGB.[6] Prasanna and Murthy reported complete pain relief for at least 12 months in a patient suffering from herpes zoster ophthalmicus who was treated with SPGB for residual ear pain that had not been alleviated with previous stellate ganglion blocks.[12] The same authors also reported immediate short-term pain relief with intranasal blockade of the SPG in 10 patients suffering intractable pain from cancer of the tongue and the floor of the mouth.[13] Further studies are needed—and eagerly awaited.

SIDE EFFECTS AND COMPLICATIONS

Blockade of the SPG is not a benign procedure. Infection can occur if proper aseptic technique is breached. Epistaxis can occur if the practitioner is not careful when placing the cotton-tipped applicators into the nasal passage or if too much pressure is applied to the needle and it is pushed through the lateral nasal wall when using the infrazygomatic arch approach. Hematoma formation is possible if the large venous plexus overlying the pterygopalatine fossa or the maxillary artery is punctured. Use of a blunt-tipped needle virtually eliminates this complication. Radiofrequency lesioning of the SPG can result in hypesthesia of the palate, but that is usually transient.[8, 14] Accurate needle placement with fluoroscopic guidance and the use of electrical stimulation can considerably decrease the incidence of hypesthesia.

Recently we noted bradycardia in some patients during radiofrequency and EMF lesioning of the SPG. When the lesioning was halted, the bradycardia resolved. Atropine was given to a couple of patients to complete the lesioning. To our knowledge, this has not been reported in the literature. A reflex resembling the oculocardiac reflex may be the cause.

CONCLUSION

Although blockade of the SPG has been performed for the past 90 years, the role of the SPG in the pathogenesis of pain remains in debate. Indications supported by current literature include sphenopalatine and trigeminal neuralgia, cluster and migraine headaches, and atypical facial pain. Various techniques have been described and are effective if performed properly.

Can a precise technique be developed for blocking the sphenopalatine ganglion? The techniques previously described are quite effective if the anatomy of the patient is "normal." They become more difficult to perform when the anatomy has been altered secondary to surgery, infection, or expected genetic variations. Electrical stimulation of the SPG along with fluoroscopy enables us to pinpoint the location of the SPG, but this requires placing a needle, which can cause bleeding. There is a case report of the stereotactic radiosurgical treatment of sphenopalatine neuralgia in a patient who after two high-dose radiation treatments of the SPG was pain free at 2-year follow-up.[15] This technique requires no needles but does require placement of a stereotactic headframe, and the radiobiologic effect of high-dose radiation on the SPG remains unknown. Currently, a precise technique does not exist, but the search continues.

REFERENCES

1. Waldman S: Sphenopalatine ganglion block—80 years later. Regional Anesth 18:274–276, 1993.
2. Sluder G: Etiology, diagnosis, prognosis and treatment of sphenopalatine neuralgia. JAMA 61:1201–1216, 1913.
3. Eagle W: Sphenopalatine neuralgia. Arch Otolaryngol 35:66–84, 1942.
4. Bonica JJ: Pain caused by cancer of the head and neck and other specific syndromes. *In* The Management of Pain, ed 2, vol I. Malvern, PA, Lea & Febiger, 1990.
5. Ruskin S: Contributions to the study of the sphenopalatine ganglion. Laryngoscope 35(2):87–108, 1925.
6. Manahan A, Maleska M, Malone P: Sphenopalatine ganglion block relieves symptoms of trigeminal neuralgia: A case report. Nebraska Med J 81(9):306–309, 1996.
7. Cepero R, Miller R, Bressler K: Long-term results of sphenopalatine ganglioneurectomy for facial pain. Am J Otolaryngol 8(3):171–174, 1987.
8. Sanders M, Zuurmond W: Efficacy of sphenopalatine ganglion blockade in 66 patients suffering from cluster headaches: A 12- to 70-month follow-up evaluation. J Neurosurg 87(6):876–880, 1997.
9. Ryan R, Facer G: Sphenopalatine ganglion neuralgia and cluster headache: Comparisons, contrasts, and treatment. Headache 17(1):7–8, 1977.
10. Phero J, McDonald J, Green D, Robins G: Orofacial pain and other related syndromes. *In* Raj P (ed): Practical Management of Pain. St. Louis, CV Mosby, 1992.
11. Lebovits A, Alfred H, Lefkowitz M: Sphenopalatine ganglion block: Clinical use in the pain management clinic. Clin J Pain 6(2):131–136, 1990.
12. Prasanna A, Murthy P: Combined stellate ganglion and sphenopalatine ganglion block in acute herpes infection. Clin J Pain 9(2):135–137, 1993.
13. Prasanna A, Murthy S: Sphenopalatine ganglion block and pain of cancer. J Pain 8:125, 1993.
14. Salar G, Ori C, Iob I: Percutaneous thermocoagulation for sphenopalatine ganglion neuralgia. Acta Neurochir (Wien) 84:24–28, 1987.
15. Pollock B, Kondziolka D: Stereotactic radiosurgical treatment of sphenopalatine neuralgia. J Neurosurg 87:450–453, 1997.
16. Sluijter M, van Kleef M: Characteristics and mode of action of radiofrequency lesioning. Curr Rev Pain 2:143–150, 1998.
17. Raj P, Rauck R, Racz G: Autonomic nerve blocks. *In* Raj P (ed): Pain Medicine: A Comprehensive Review. St. Louis, CV Mosby, 1996.

RECOMMENDED READING

18. Waldman S: Sphenopalatine ganglion block. *In* Hahn MB, McQuillan PM, Sheplock GJ (eds): Regional Anesthesia: An Atlas of Anatomy and Technique. St. Louis, CV Mosby, 1996.
19. Waldman S: Evaluation and treatment of common headache and facial pain syndromes. *In* Raj P (ed): Practical Management of Pain. St. Louis, CV Mosby, 1992.

CHAPTER • 22

Occipital Nerve Block

David L. Brown, MD • Gilbert Y. Wong, MD

HISTORICAL CONSIDERATIONS

Occipital nerve block is most often used to diagnose or treat occipital pain. There are many causes of occipital pain, and they are frequently grouped together as *occipital neuralgia.* This categorization was first used in 1821, when Beruto y Lentijo and Ramos made reference to an occipital neuralgic syndrome.[1] Early in this century, Luff[2] and Osler and McRae[3] reemphasized the importance of attempting to identify the causes of occipital pain. Other investigators suggested that, in addition to the neuropathic changes that lead to occipital headaches, the pain characteristic of occipital neuralgia may also be related to arthritis of the cervical spine (cervicogenic headache) and other rarer but serious conditions (Table 22–1).[4–8] After the development of safe injectable local anesthetics, occipital nerve block was commonly used in the diagnosis and treatment of pain originating in the occipital region. Occipital nerve block also provides scalp anesthesia for surgical procedures when local infiltration techniques alone do not suffice.

INDICATIONS AND CONTRAINDICATIONS

Occipital nerve block is most often used to diagnose and treat pain in the occipital region. When it is used for diagnosis, a careful history and thorough physical examination are necessary to minimize the chance that serious causes of occipital pain will be missed or diagnosis delayed (see Table 22–1). By International Headache Society definition, occipital neuralgia is relieved by local anesthetic blockade of the involved occipital nerve; thus, the principal indication for occipital block is diagnosis.[9] Another indication is the treatment of chronic occipital neuralgia, often with a series of therapeutic blocks combining local anesthetic and depot corticosteroid. Because of the preservatives included in depot corticosteroid preparations, it is suggested that a minor degree of neurolysis may result and contribute to prolonging pain relief.[10]

If occipital nerve block is used to differentiate occipital neuralgia from pain of other causes, one must remember that potential interneuronal connections within the upper spinal cord may allow occipital nerve (C2) pain to be referred to the trigeminal distribution (Fig. 22–1).[11] This referred pain is due to the proximity of the C2 root to the trigeminal spinal nucleus. Thus, block of the occipital nerve may relieve pain outside the typical C2 distribution but within the trigeminal distribution.[12]

CLINICALLY RELEVANT ANATOMY

The cutaneous innervation of the posterior head and neck comes from the cervical spinal nerves. The dorsal rami of C2 end in the greater occipital nerve, which provides cutaneous innervation to the major portion of the posterior scalp (Fig. 22–2). Based on cadaver studies, the topographic anatomy of the occipital nerve can vary.[13] After following a winding course as the medial branch of the dorsal ramus of C2, the greater occipital nerve ascends in the posterior neck from its origin lateral to the lateral atlantoaxial joint and deep to the oblique inferior muscle. At this point, a communicating branch from C3 may join the greater occipital nerve (Fig 22–3).[14, 15] The greater occipital nerve ascends in the posterior neck over the dorsal surface of the rectus capitis posterior major muscle, and, approximately at the midpoint of this muscle, the greater occipital nerve turns dorsally to pierce the fleshy fibers of the semispinalis capitis, after which it runs a short distance rostrolaterally, lying deep to the trapezius. The nerve becomes subcutaneous slightly inferior to the superior nuchal line, not by piercing the trapezius, as is often suggested, but by passing above an aponeurotic sling. This sling is composed of a blending of the aponeurotic insertions of the trapezius and sternocleidomastoid muscles medially and laterally, respectively.[15]

As the occipital nerve emerges via this aponeurotic sling, it is close to the occipital artery. At this point, the greater occipital nerve is immediately medial to the occipital artery, and the artery is lateral to the inion (Fig. 22–4A). Again, the ventral rami of C2 through C4 provide the majority of cutaneous innervation to the anterior and lateral portions of the neck, with C2 providing innervation to the scalp through both the lesser occipital and posterior auricular nerves (see Fig. 22–2).

TABLE 22–1 ***Possible Causes of Occipital Pain Syndrome***

Relatively Common	Relatively Rare
Headache	Arnold-Chiari malformation
Tension	Tumor
Vascular	Primary
Cervicogenic	Secondary
Occipital neuralgia	Infection
Cervical arthritis	Mastoid
Myofascial pain	Intraspinal

CLINICAL PEARLS AND TRICKS OF THE TRADE

The most effective patient position for the greater or lesser occipital block is sitting with the neck in a flexed position. The selection of the nerve(s) to be blocked may depend, in part, on the pain distribution and the ability to reproduce the pain with palpation. The occipital artery is the most useful landmark for locating the greater occipital nerve, which lies immediately medial to the artery. A short (1- to 1.5-in), 25-gauge needle is inserted through the skin at the level of the superior nuchal line. The artery is commonly found at a point approximately a third of the distance from the external occipital protuberance to the mastoid process on the superior nuchal line. The lesser occipital nerve is commonly found at a point two thirds the distance from the external occipital protuberance on the superior nuchal line. Injection of 3 to 5 mL of local anesthetic produces satisfactory greater or lesser occipital nerve anesthesia in the corresponding area. If a diagnostic block is planned, the dose should be limited to 1 to 2 mL to minimize confusion with relief of myofascial pain when larger volumes are injected (Fig. 22–4B). Bovim and Sand[16] reported that greater occipital nerve block reduced pain in 19 of 22 patients with cervicogenic headache (Fig. 22–5). Cervical epidural nerve block with local anesthetic and corticoste-

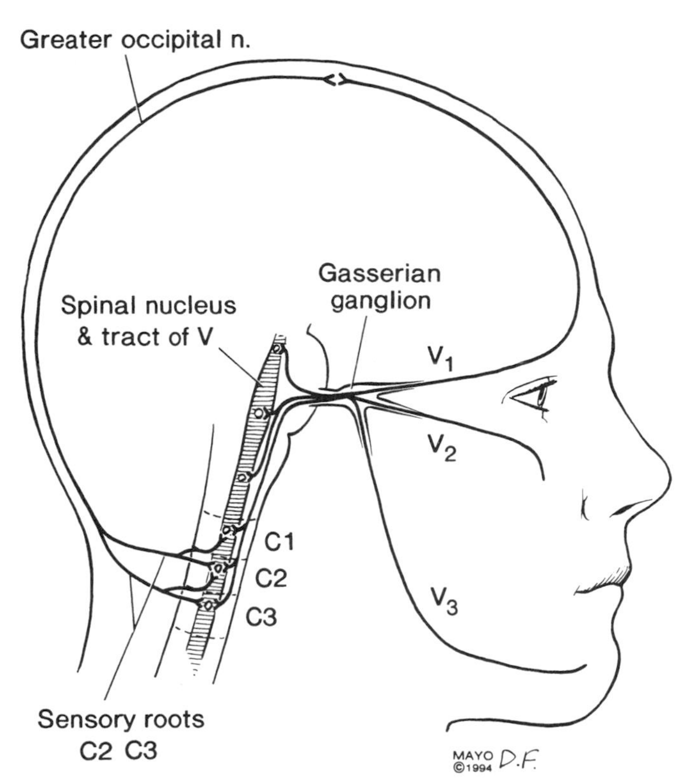

FIGURE 22–1 The cervicotrigeminal interneuronal relay. A potential overlap of central neuronal connections occurs between the spinal nucleus of the trigeminal nerve and the upper cervical cord neurons. The trigeminal nucleus develops from the pyramidal decussation and descends to the level of C2, and perhaps as far caudad as C4, as the nucleus caudalis, which principally subserves pain and temperature information to the head and neck. This trigeminal nucleus is associated, both morphologically and functionally, with the upper cervical segments, and its cells form a column continuous with the column of cells forming the posterior horn in the cervical cord. (Modified from Anthony M: Headache and the greater occipital nerve. Clin Neurol Neurosurg 94:297–301, 1992.)

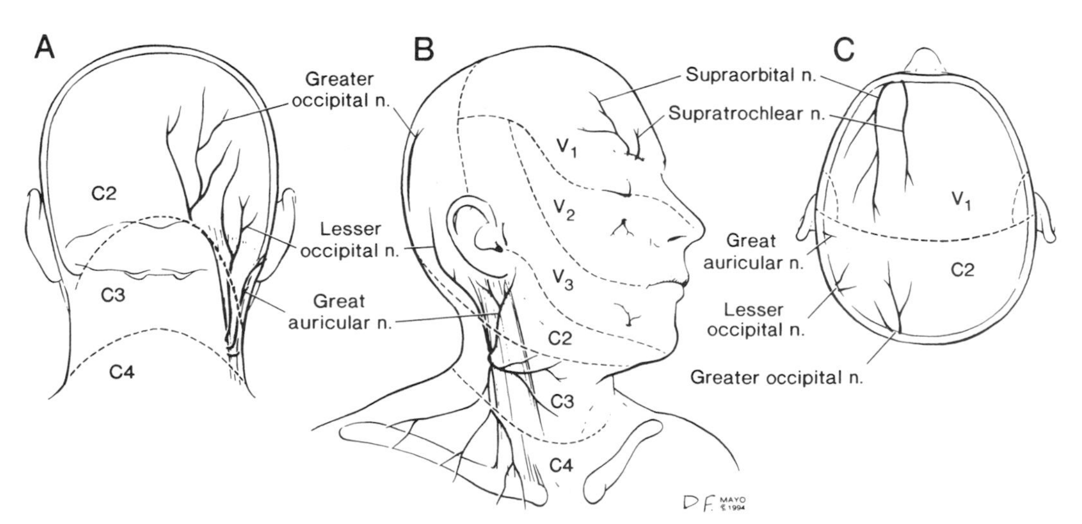

FIGURE 22–2 Peripheral sensory and dermatomal innervation of greater and lesser occipital nerves and of other head and neck nerves. A, posterior view; B, anterolateral view; C, top, cephalocaudad view.

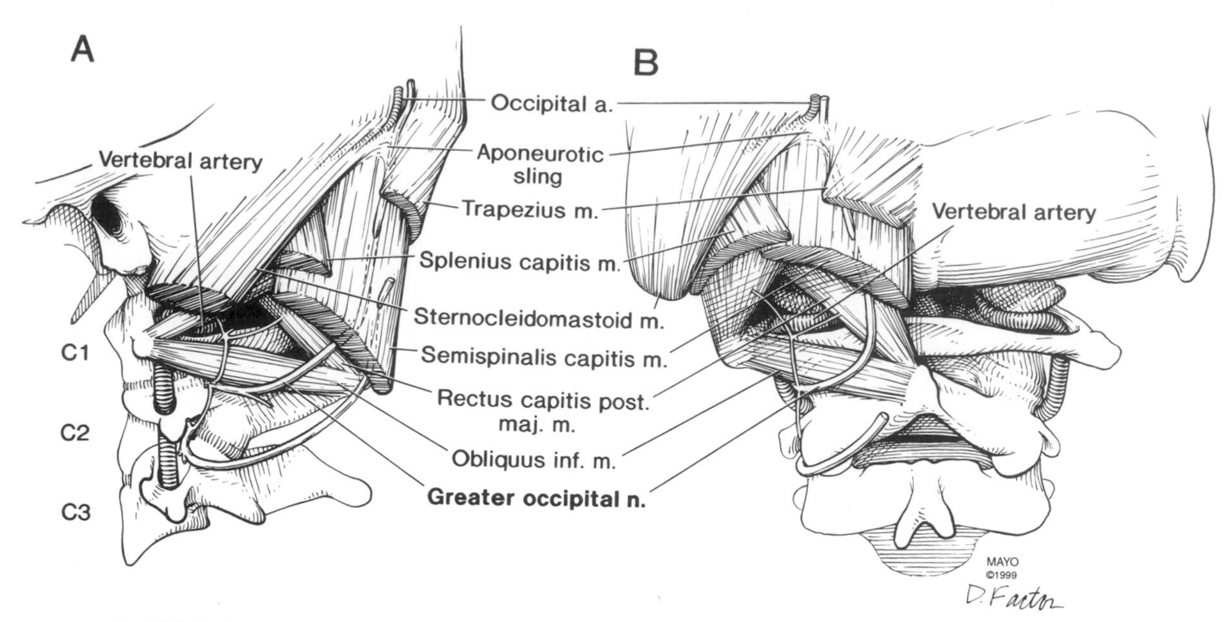

FIGURE 22–3 *Anatomic schematic of the* greater occipital nerve *in the neutral position as it arises from the medial branch of the dorsal ramus of the second cervical nerve, on its way to its eventual subcutaneous position, lateral to the inion (external occipital protuberance).* A, *lateral view;* B, *posterior view. (Modified from Vital JM, Grenier F, Dautheribes M, et al: An anatomic and dynamic study of the greater occipital nerve [n. of Arnold]: Applications to the treatment of Arnold's neuralgia. Surg Radiol Anat 11:205–210, 1989.)*

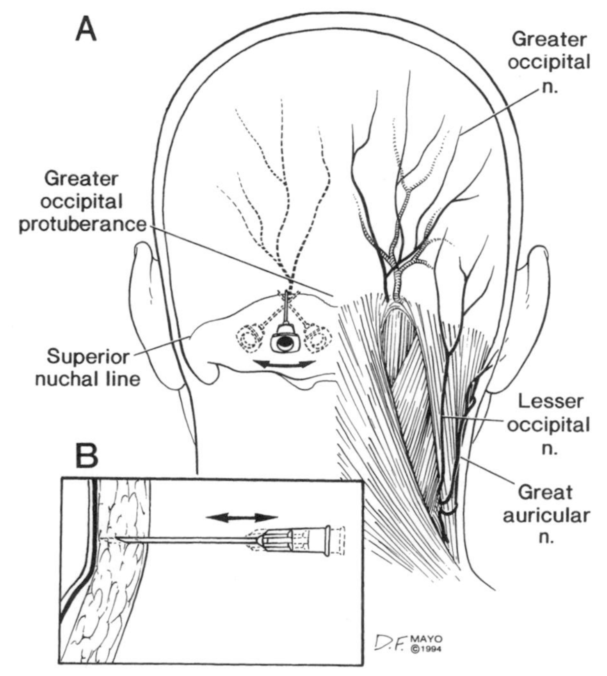

FIGURE 22–4 A, *Posterior view of the course of the greater occipital nerve and artery as they course cephalad in the neck, via the aponeurotic sling on their way to the posterior scalp.* B, *Method of blocking the greater occipital nerve on the superior nuchal line. Note the "wall" of local anesthetic developed in a mediolateral sequence to ensure adequate block of the greater occipital nerve.*

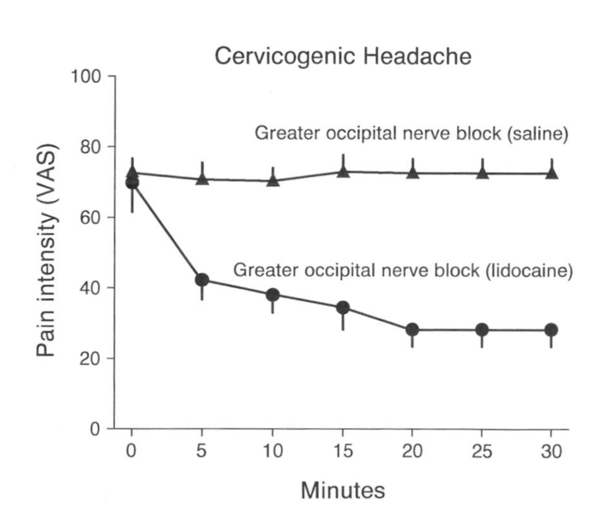

FIGURE 22–5 *Pain relief measured by Visual Analog Scale (VAS) in patients with cervicogenic headache when 1.5 to 2.0 ml of saline or lidocaine was used during greater occipital nerve block. Measurements were made every 5 minutes for 70 minutes. There were no major changes from 30 to 70 minutes. The bars indicate standard error of the mean (SEM). $P < .05$ from the 5th minute onward. (Modified from Bovim G, Sand T: Cervicogenic headache, migraine without aura and tension-type headache: Diagnostic blockade of greater occipital and supraorbital nerves. Pain 51:43–48, 1992. Copyright 1992, with permission from Elsevier Science.)*

roid could be considered for cervicogenic headache that is refractory to occipital nerve block.

PITFALLS

When a diagnostic block is planned, it is important to keep the dose of local anesthetic small, to avoid confounding results with relief of myofascial pain. Likewise, relief of ipsilateral retroorbital or temporal pain does not rule out occipital neuralgia as the cause of an occipital pain syndrome, because pain relief is produced outside the "typical" sensory distribution of the occipital nerve.[12] Rather, owing to the brain stem and spinal cord interneuronal connections between the trigeminal nucleus and C2, it is common to find retroorbital pain relieved by greater occipital nerve block.[12] Patients whose occipital pain is complicated by confounding economic variables, especially those who have sustained flexion-extension neck injuries in motor vehicle accidents and are involved in litigation for compensation, are difficult for us to manage until the confounding economic variables are resolved or removed. Failure to obtain successful occipital nerve block can be due to an anatomic variation.

COMPLICATIONS

The superficial location of this block should make complications uncommon. In spite of the close relationship between the occipital artery and nerve, intravascular injection is uncommon. The small volume of local anesthetic and corticosteroid injected makes systemic toxicity a rare event. Some patients who have undergone posterior suboccipital cranial surgery are referred for evaluation of an occipital pain syndrome. One needs to be cautious about the occipital nerve block in such patients, because subcranial injections producing total spinal anesthesia have been reported.

FUTURE DIRECTIONS

The development of long-acting local anesthetics may allow prolonged relief of occipital neuralgia. Depot formulations of local anesthetics may, indeed, be more useful than intermittent blocks. Nevertheless, proof of such a theory needs further study.

REFERENCES

1. Perelson HN: Occipital nerve tenderness: A sign of headache. South Med J 40:653–656, 1947.
2. Luff AP: The various forms of fibrositis and their treatment. Br Med J 1:756–760, 1913.
3. Osler W, McRae T: The Principles and Practice of Medicine, ed 10. New York, D Appleton, 1925, p 1117.
4. Horton BT, Macy D Jr: Treatment of headache. Med Clin North Am 30:811–831, 1946.
5. Nielsen JM: Textbook of Clinical Neurology. New York, Paul B. Hoeber, 1941, p 509.
6. Pollock LJ: Head pain: Differential diagnosis and treatment. Med Clin North Am 25:3–31, 1941.
7. Echni G, Benner B: Occipital neuralgia and the C1–2 arthrosis syndrome. J Neurosurg 61:961–965, 1984.
8. Sjaastad O, Federiksen JA, Pfaffenrath V: Cervicogenic headache: Diagnostic criteria. Headache 30:725–726, 1990.
9. Headache Classification Committee of the International Headache Society: Classification and diagnostic criteria for headache disorders, cranial neuralgias and facial pain. Cephalgia 9 (Suppl 7):1–96, 1988.
10. Selby R: Complications of Depo-Medrol. Surg Neurol 19:393–394, 1983.
11. Kerr FWL: A mechanism to account for frontal headache in cases of posterior fossa tumour. J Neurosurg 18:605–609, 1961.
12. Anthony M: Headache and the greater occipital nerve. Clin Neurol Neurosurg 94:297–301, 1992.
13. Becser N, Bovim G, Sjaastad O: Extramural nerves in the posterior part of the head. Anatomic variations and their possible clinical significance. Spine 23(13):1435–1441, 1998.
14. Vital JM, Grenier F, Dautheribes M, et al: An anatomic and dynamic study of the greater occipital nerve (n. of Arnold): Applications to the treatment of Arnold's neuralgia. Surg Radiol Anat 11:205–210, 1989.
15. Bogduk N: The clinical anatomy of the cervical dorsal rami. Spine 4:319–330, 1982.
16. Bovim G, Sand T: Cervicogenic headache, migraine without aura and tension-type headache: Diagnostic blockade of greater occipital and supra-orbital nerves. Pain 51:43–48, 1992.

CHAPTER • 23

Blockade of the Gasserian Ganglion

Steven D. Waldman, MD, JD

HISTORICAL CONSIDERATIONS

On December 6, 1884, Halstead and Hall reported their success in blocking the branches of the trigeminal nerve with local anesthetic in the *New York Medical Journal.*[1] Shortly after this landmark publication, these distinguished New York surgeons demonstrated the utility of "nerve blocks" when Hall had Halstead remove a lipoma from his forehead under "painless" nerve block anesthesia.[2] One can only imagine the tremendous benefit that this clinical discovery afforded surgeons and their patients at a time when, in the absence of endotracheal intubation, muscle relaxants, and sophisticated monitoring, head and neck surgery was, at best, an extremely risky undertaking.

The effectiveness of nerve blocks was rapidly exploited for pain management. Blockade of the gasserian ganglion and distal trigeminal nerve were among the first applications of nerve blocking for pain. By 1900, blockade of these neural structures was considered one of the primary means of alleviating the pain of trigeminal neuralgia and pain secondary to cancers of the face and head.[3] These techniques remained the mainstays of the nonsurgical treatment of trigeminal neuralgia until the introduction of carbamazepine in 1960.

The shift to the managed care paradigm has led pain management specialists to seek the most efficacious, safe, and cost-effective treatments for headache and facial pain.[4,5] This paradigm shift has led to renewed interest in gasserian ganglion block for the management of a variety of painful conditions. This chapter reviews the current indications, contraindications, and technique for blockade of the gasserian ganglion.

INDICATIONS AND CONTRAINDICATIONS

Blockade of the gasserian ganglion with local anesthetics and steroids and destruction of this neural structure by freezing, radiofrequency lesioning, neurolytic agents, compression, and other means have many applications in contemporary pain management.[6] Advances in radiographic imaging, electronics, and needle technology have improved the efficacy and reduced the cost, complications, and adverse side effects of these useful pain management procedures.

Gasserian Ganglion Block

Indications for gasserian ganglion block are summarized in Table 23–1. In addition to applications for surgical anesthesia, gasserian ganglion block with local anesthetics can be utilized as a diagnostic tool when performing differential neural blockade on an anatomic basis for evaluation of head and facial pain.[7] This technique is also useful as a prognostic indicator of the degree of motor and sensory impairment that the patient might experience when destruction of the gasserian ganglion is being considered.[3]

Gasserian ganglion block with local anesthetic may be utilized to palliate acute pain emergencies, including trigeminal neuralgia and cancer pain, while waiting for pharmacologic, surgical, and antiblastic methods to become effective.[8]

Destruction of the gasserian ganglion is indicated for palliation of cancer pain, including the pain of invasive tumors of the orbit, maxillary sinus, and mandible.[9] This technique is also useful in the management of the pain of trigeminal neuralgia that has been refractory to medical management or for patients who are not candidates for surgical microvascular decompression.[10] Gasserian ganglion destruction has also been utilized successfully in the management of intractable cluster headache and in the palliation of ocular pain secondary to persistent glaucoma.[3,11,12]

Contraindications to blockade of the gasserian ganglion are these:

- Local infection
- Sepsis
- Coagulopathy
- Significantly increased intracranial pressure
- Disulfiram therapy (if alcohol is used)
- Significant behavioral abnormalities

Local infection and sepsis are absolute contraindications to gasserian ganglion block,[13] and coagulopathy and markedly increased intracranial pressure strong contraindications. Owing to the desperation of many patients suffering from

TABLE 23–1 *Indications for Gasserian Ganglion Block*

Local Anesthetic Block	Neurolytic Block or Neurodestructive Procedure
Surgical anesthesia	Palliation of cancer pain
Anatomic differential neural blockade	Management of trigeminal neuralgia
Prognostic nerve block prior to neurodestructive procedures	Management of cluster headache
Palliation in acute pain emergencies	Management of intractable ocular pain

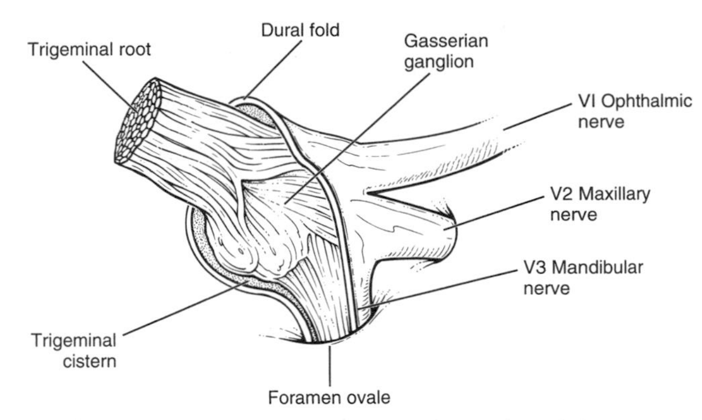

FIGURE 23–1 *Gasserian ganglion and Meckel's cave.*

aggressively invasive head and face malignancies, however, ethical and humanitarian considerations dictate use of this procedure despite the increased risks of bleeding or spinal fluid leak secondary to coagulopathy or increased intracranial pressure, respectively.

CLINICALLY RELEVANT ANATOMY

The Role of the Trigeminal System

The trigeminal nerve is the largest and the most complex of the cranial nerves, containing both sensory and motor fibers.[14] Somatic afferent impulses carried by the trigeminal nerve transmit pain, light touch, and temperature sensation. Information is transmitted to the central nervous system via the trigeminal nerve from the skin of the face, the mucosal lining of the nose and mouth, the teeth, and the anterior two thirds of the tongue.[15] The trigeminal nerve also carries both proprioceptive impulses and afferent impulses from stretch receptors of the teeth, oral mucosa, muscles of mastication, and temporomandibular joint to aid in mastication.

In addition to the sensory innervation just described, visceral efferent fibers help to innervate a variety of muscles of facial expression, the tensor tympani, and some muscles of mastication. Communications exist between the trigeminal nerve and the autonomic nervous system, including the ciliary, sphenopalatine, otic, and submaxillary ganglia and the oculomotor, facial, and glossopharyngeal nerves. Because of the complex structure of the trigeminal nerve, a thorough understanding of the clinically relevant anatomy is crucial to obtaining optimal results with neural blockade.

The Gasserian Ganglion

The gasserian ganglion is formed from two roots that exit the ventral surface of the brain stem at the midpontine level (Fig. 23–1).[16] These roots pass forward and lateral in the posterior cranial fossa across the border of the petrous temporal bone. They then enter a recess called Meckel's cave, which is formed by an invagination of the surrounding dura mater into the middle cranial fossa. The dural pouch that lies just behind the ganglion, called the trigeminal cistern, contains cerebrospinal fluid. The gasserian ganglion is canoe-shaped and has three sensory divisions, the ophthalmic (V_1), maxillary (V_2), and mandibular (V_3), that exit on the anterior convex aspect. A smaller motor root joins the mandibular division as it exits the cranial cavity via the foramen ovale.

The Ophthalmic Division

The ophthalmic branch, the smallest division of the trigeminal nerve, is purely sensory in function (Fig. 23–2).[17] It enters the orbit via the superior orbital fissure. The branch is divided into the frontal, nasociliary, and lacrimal nerves. The terminal cutaneous branches of the frontal nerve consist of the supraorbital and supratrochlear nerves. These terminal branches exit the orbital cavity anteriorly and provide innervation to the upper eyelid, forehead, and the anterior scalp. The terminal cutaneous branches of the nasociliary nerve consist of the infratrochlear and external nasal branches, which provide cutaneous and mucosal in-

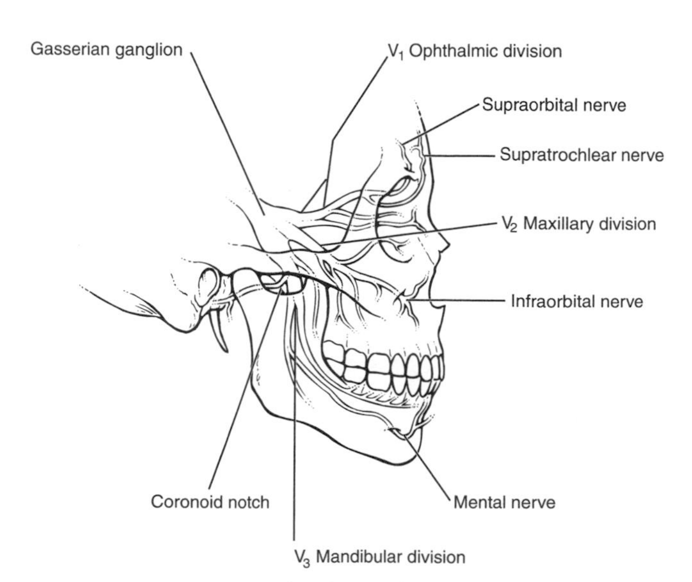

FIGURE 23–2 *The trigeminal nerve and its branches.*

nervation to the apex and ala of the nose and anterior nasal cavity. The lacrimal nerve continues, without any additional major branches, to innervate the lacrimal gland and outer canthus of the eye.

The Maxillary Division

The maxillary division is a pure sensory nerve. It exits the middle cranial fossa via the foramen rotundum and crosses the pterygopalatine fossa (Fig. 23–3).[17] Passing through the inferior orbital fissure, it enters the orbit, emerging on the face via the infraorbital foramen.

The branches of the maxillary nerve are divided into four regional groups: (1) the intracranial group, including the middle meningeal nerve, which innervates the dura mater of the medial cranial fossa; (2) the pterygopalatine group, including the zygomatic nerve, which provides sensory innervation to the temporal and lateral zygomatic region, and the sphenopalatine branches, which help to innervate the mucosa of the maxillary sinus, upper gums, upper molars, and mucous membranes of the cheek; (3) the infraorbital canal group, comprising the anterosuperior alveolar branch, which innervates the incisors and canines, the anterior wall of the maxillary antrum, and the floor of the nasal cavity, and the middle superior branch, which supplies the premolars; and (4) the infraorbital facial group, consisting of the inferior palpebral branch, which innervates the conjunctiva and skin of the lower eyelid; the external nasal branch, which supplies the side of the nose; and the superior labial branch, which supplies the skin of the upper lip and part of the oral mucosa (see Fig. 23–2).

The Mandibular Division

The large sensory root and smaller motor root of the mandibular division leave the middle cranial fossa together via the foramen ovale.[17] Then they join to form the mandibular nerve (see Fig. 23–3). This combined trunk gives off two branches: (1) the nervus spinosus, which runs superiorly with the middle meningeal artery through the foramen spinosum to supply the dura mater and the mucosal lining of the mastoid sinus, and (2) the internal pterygoid, which supplies the internal pterygoid muscle and gives off branches to the otic ganglion. The mandibular nerve then divides into a small anterior and a large posterior trunk (see Fig. 23–2).

Branches from the small anterior trunk are the buccinator nerve, which is purely sensory and innervates the skin and mucous membrane overlying the anterior portion of the buccinator muscle; the masseteric nerve, which provides motor innervation to the masseter muscle; the deep temporal nerves, which provide motor innervation to the temporalis muscle; and the external pterygoid nerve, which provides motor innervation to the external pterygoid muscle.

The large posterior trunk comprises primarily sensory fibers but a small number of motor fibers as well. Branches of the posterior trunk are (1) the auriculotemporal nerve, which provides innervation to skin anterior to the tragus and helix, the lining of the acoustic meatus, the tympanic membrane, the posterior temporomandibular joint, the parotid gland, and the skin of the temporal region; (2) the lingual nerve, which provides sensory innervation to the dorsum and lateral aspects of the anterior two thirds of the tongue and the lateral mucous membranes of the mouth as well as the sublingual gland; and (3) the inferior alveolar nerve, which provides sensory innervation to the lower teeth and mandible. The terminal branch of the inferior alveolar nerve is the mental nerve, which exits the mandible via the mental foramen and provides sensory innervation to the chin and to the skin and mucous membrane of the lower lip.

TECHNIQUE

The patient lies supine with the cervical spine extended over a rolled towel. Approximately 2.5 cm lateral to the corner of the mouth, the skin is carefully prepared with povidone iodine solution, and sterile drapes are placed.[7] The skin and subcutaneous tissues are then anesthetized

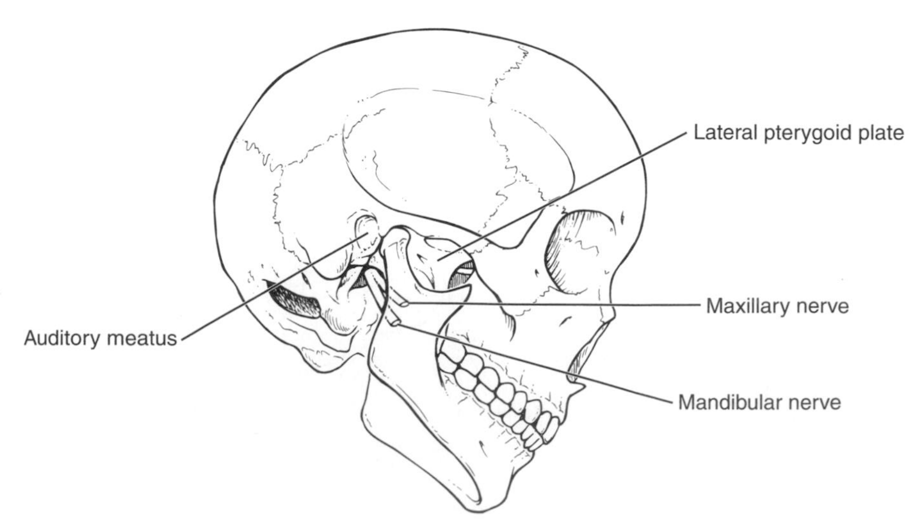

FIGURE 23–3 Major branches of the trigeminal nerve.

with 1% lidocaine with epinephrine. A 20-gauge, 13-cm Hinck needle is advanced through the anesthetized area, traveling perpendicular to the pupil of the eye (when the eye is in midposition) in a cephalad trajectory toward the auditory meatus (Fig. 23–4).[13] The needle is advanced until contact is made with the base of the skull (Fig. 23–5). The needle tip is withdrawn slightly and "walked" posteriorly into the foramen ovale (Fig. 23–6). Paresthesia of the mandibular nerve may occur as the needle enters the foramen ovale.[7]

After the foramen ovale is entered, the stylet of the Hinck needle is removed. The operator carefully aspirates for blood. Free flow of cerebrospinal fluid (CSF) is typical. Failure to observe free flow of CSF does not necessarily mean that the needle tip does not lie within the central nervous system close to the gasserian ganglion but simply that the needle tip rests, not within the trigeminal cistern, but more anteriorly, within Meckel's cave.[13]

The needle position should be confirmed by radiography before any local anesthetic or neurolytic substance is injected (Figs. 23–7, 23–8). After needle position is confirmed, 0.1-mL aliquots of a preservative-free local anesthetic, such as 1.0% lidocaine for diagnostic blocks and 0.5% bupivacaine for therapeutic blocks, or of sterile glycerol, 6.5% phenol in glycerin, or absolute alcohol may be injected.[7] An average volume of 0.4 mL of neurolytic solution is usually adequate to provide long-lasting pain relief. Owing to significant interpatient variability in the size of Meckel's cave, however, careful titration of the total injected volume is indicated.

If hyperbaric neurolytic agents are utilized, the patient should assume a sitting position with the chin on the chest before the injection, to ensure that the solution is placed primarily around the maxillary and mandibular divisions (Fig. 23–9) and avoids the ophthalmic division. The patient should remain in the supine position when absolute alcohol is used. This approach to the gasserian ganglion may be utilized to place radiofrequency needles, cryoprobes, and stimulating electrodes.

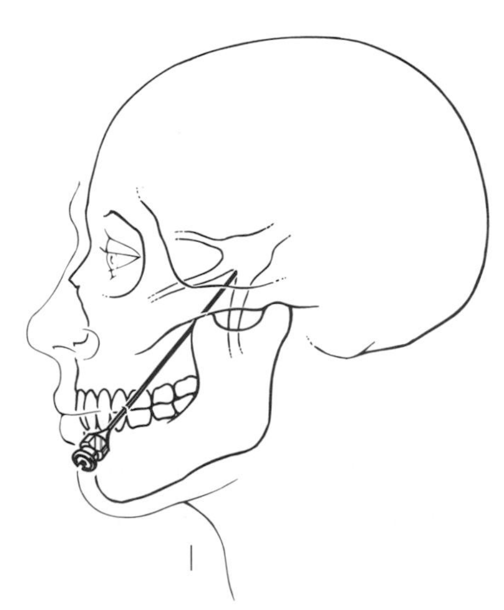

FIGURE 23–4 Needle trajectory for gasserian ganglion block.

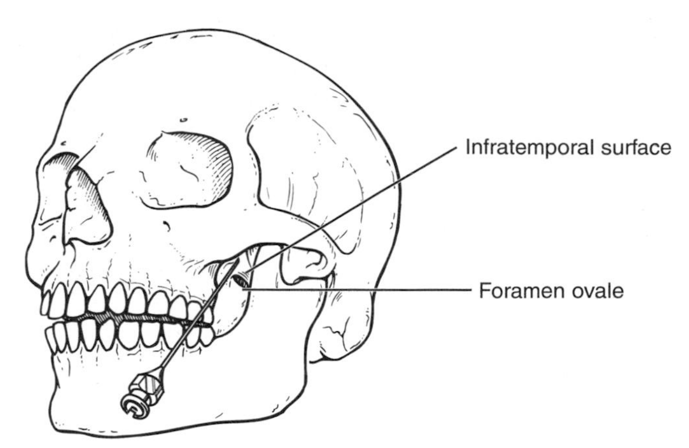

FIGURE 23–5 Needle against roof of infratemporal surface.

Practical Considerations

Because of the densely vascular nature of the pterygopalatine and its proximity to the middle meningeal artery, significant hematoma of the face and subscleral hematoma of the eye are not uncommon sequelae. The patient should be warned of the probability of these complications before institution of the block. Because the ganglion lies within the CSF small amounts of local anesthetic injected through the needle may produce total spinal anesthesia.[13] For this reason, it is imperative that small doses of local anesthetic be injected incrementally, allowing time after each dose to observe its effect.[3] Chemical neurolysis and neuroablative procedures on the gasserian ganglion should be performed only by persons familiar with the anatomy and the technique of gasserian ganglion block, and only under radiographic guidance.

CONCLUSION

Gasserian ganglion block is a straightforward technique with a favorable risk-to-benefit ratio when careful attention is paid to the functional anatomy, indications, and contraindications. Given the cost-effective nature of this technique,

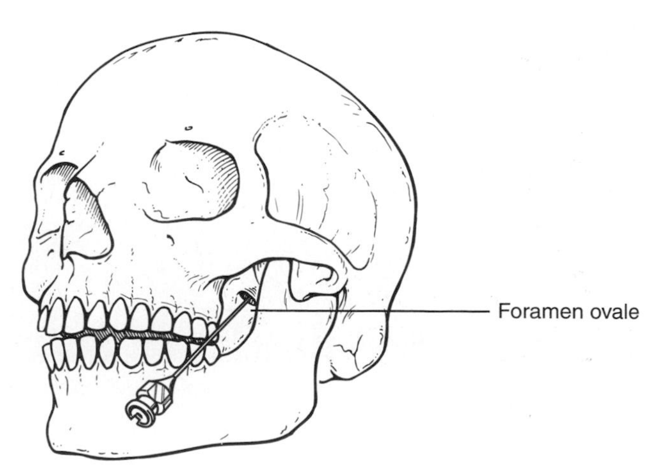

FIGURE 23–6 Needle "walked" into foramen ovale.

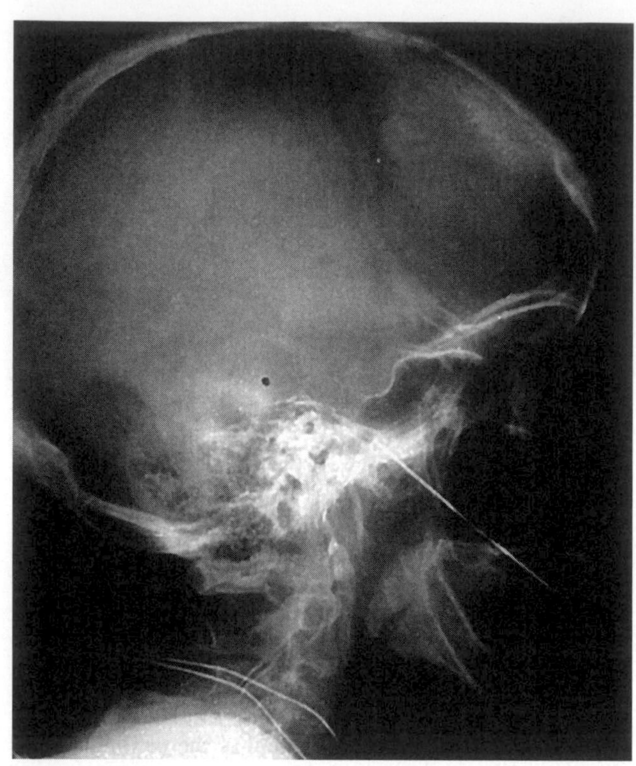

FIGURE 23–7 *Lateral view of the needle placed through the foramen ovale.*

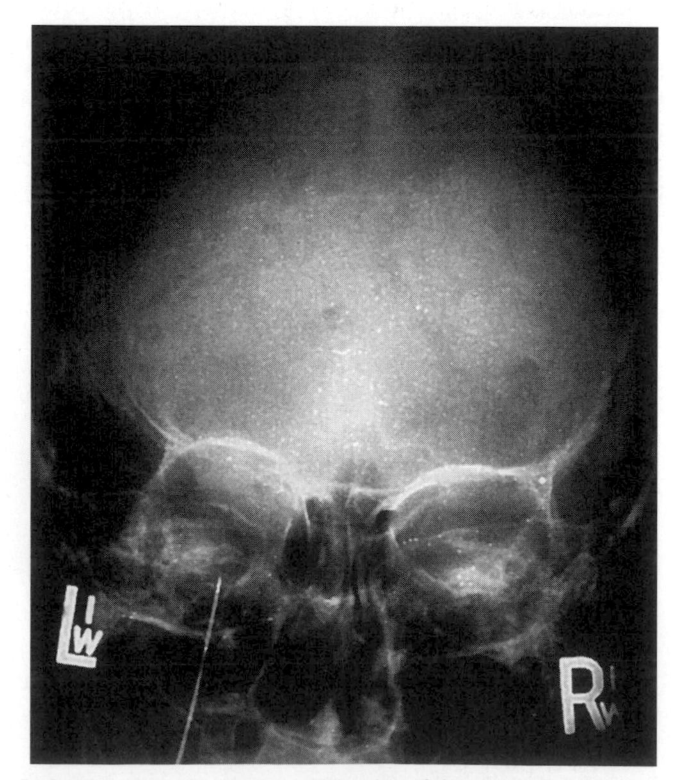

FIGURE 23–8 *Anteroposterior view of the needle placed through the foramen ovale.*

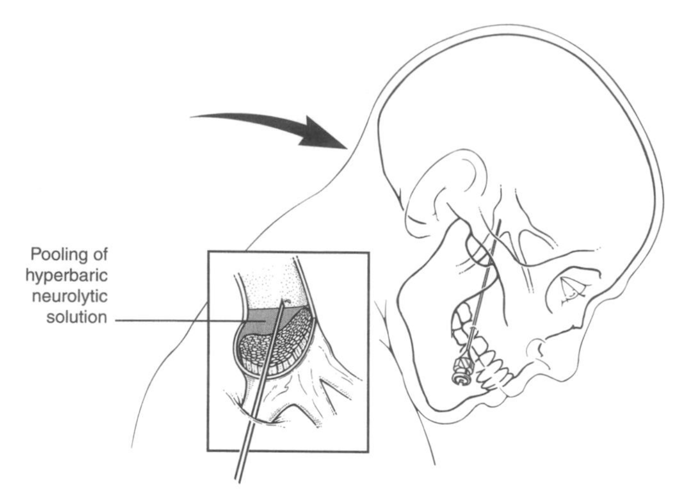

FIGURE 23–9 *Patient positioning for gasserian ganglion block with hyperbaric solution.*

gasserian ganglion block is a reasonable next step for patients suffering from facial pain and cluster headache who have not responded to more conservative therapy.

REFERENCES

1. Hall RJ: Hydrochlorate of cocaine. NY Med J 40:643–644, 1886.
2. Winnie AP: The early history of regional anesthesia in the United States. *In* Scott DB, McClure J (eds): Regional Anesthesia, 1884–1984. Sodertalje, Sweden, ICM Press, 1984, p 35.
3. Bonica JJ: Neurolytic blockade and hypophysectomy. *In* Bonica JJ (ed): The Management of Pain. Philadelphia, Lea & Febiger, 1990.
4. Waldman SD: Medical Staff Credentialing-Physician Constitutional Rights & Remedies-Part I: The Law and Public Policy of Medical Staff Credentialing. Am J Pain Manage 7:100–104, 1997.
5. Waldman SD: Medical staff credentialing—physician constitutional rights & remedies—Part II: The law and public policy of medical staff credentialing. Am J Pain Manage 7:146–150, 1997.
6. Waldman SD: Gasserian ganglion block. *In* Hahn MB, McQuillan PM, Sheplock GJ (eds): Regional Anesthesia. St. Louis, CV Mosby, 1996, pp 41–44.
7. Waldman SD: Gasserian ganglion block. *In* Waldman SD: Atlas of Interventional Pain Management Techniques. Philadelphia, WB Saunders, 1998, pp 23–29.
8. Waldman SD: Management of acute pain. Postgrad Med 87:15–17, 1992.
9. Lipton S: Neurolysis: Pharmacology and drug selection. *In* Patt RB (ed): Cancer Pain. Philadelphia, JB Lippincott 1993, pp 354–355.
10. Waldman SD: Trigeminal neuralgia. Intern Med 13:45–53, 1992.
11. Waldman SD: Cluster headache. Intern Med 13:31–32, 1992.
12. Waldman SD: Evaluation and treatment of common headache and facial pain syndromes. *In* Raj PP (ed): Practical Management of Pain. St. Louis, CV Mosby, 1992, p 217.
13. Feldstein G: Percutaneous retrogasserian glycerol rhizotomy. *In* Racz G (ed): Techniques of Neurolysis. Boston, Kluwer, 1989, pp 126–128.
14. Brown DL: Trigeminal (gasserian) ganglion block. *In* Brown DL (ed): Atlas of Regional Anesthesia, ed 2. Philadelphia, WB Saunders, 1999, p 137–141.
15. Raj PP, Gesund P, Phero J: Rationale and choice for surgical procedures. *In* Raj PP (ed): Clinical Practice of Regional Anesthesia. New York, Churchill Livingstone, 1991, pp 200–209.
16. Katz J: Gasserian ganglion. *In* Katz J (ed): Atlas of Regional Anesthesia. Norwalk, Conn, Appleton & Lange, 1994, pp 4–5.
17. Neill RS: Head, neck and airway. *In* Wildsmith JAW, Armitage EN (eds): Principles and Practice of Regional Anesthesia. New York, Churchill Livingstone, 1987.

CHAPTER • 24

Blockade of the Trigeminal Nerve and Its Branches

Steven D. Waldman, MD, JD

INDICATIONS AND CONTRAINDICATIONS

Blockade of the trigeminal nerve and its branches with local anesthetics, steroids, or neurolytic agents and destruction of these structures by freezing, radiofrequency lesioning, and other means have many applications in contemporary pain management. Technologic advances in radiographic imaging, electronics, and needle technology have improved the efficacy and decreased the cost, complications, and adverse side effects of these procedures.

The indications for blockade of the trigeminal nerve and its branches are summarized in Table 24–1. In addition to applications for surgical anesthesia, trigeminal nerve block with local anesthetic can be utilized as a diagnostic and prognostic maneuver when performing differential neural blockade on an anatomic basis.[1] This technique can be utilized to treat trismus secondary to tetanus and as an aid in awake endotracheal intubation.[2] Trigeminal nerve block with local anesthetic or steroids is an excellent adjunct to the pharmacologic treatment of trigeminal neuralgia.[3] The use of this technique allows rapid palliation of pain while oral medications are being titrated to effective levels; it may also be of value in patients with atypical facial pain.[4] Other indications for trigeminal nerve block with local anesthetic or steroids are acute pain secondary to trauma, neoplasms of the head and face, cluster headaches refractory to sphenopalatine ganglion block, and the pain of acute herpes zoster in the distribution of the trigeminal nerve that is not controlled by stellate ganglion block.[5, 6]

Indications for destruction of the distal trigeminal nerve and its branches are similar to those for gasserian ganglion block.[2] Because more peripheral destruction of the trigeminal nerve results in lower incidences of unwanted motor and sensory disturbance than destruction of the gasserian ganglion (especially corneal anesthesia), this approach may be the preferred course when it is efficacious for the pain syndrome being treated.

Contraindications to blockade of the trigeminal nerve and its branches are as follows:

- Local infection
- Sepsis
- Disulfiram therapy (if alcohol is used)
- Significant behavioral abnormalities

Local infection and sepsis are absolute contraindications to all procedures.[2,7] Coagulopathy is a relative contraindication to blockade of the trigeminal nerve and its branches; however, owing to the desperation of many patients suffering from aggressively invasive head and face malignancies, ethical and humanitarian considerations dictate the use of this procedure despite the increased risk of bleeding. If there are strong clinical indications, blockade of the distal trigeminal nerve and its branches utilizing a 25-gauge needle may be carried out in the presence of coagulopathy, albeit with increased risk of ecchymosis and hematoma formation.

CLINICALLY RELEVANT ANATOMY

The Role of the Trigeminal System

The trigeminal nerve, the largest and the most complex of the cranial nerves, contains both sensory and motor fibers.[8, 9] Somatic afferent impulses carried by the trigeminal nerve transmit pain, light touch, and temperature sensation. Information is transmitted to the central nervous system via the trigeminal nerve from the skin of the face, the mucosal lining of the nose and mouth, the teeth, and the anterior two thirds of the tongue.[8] The trigeminal nerve also carries both proprioceptive impulses and afferent impulses from stretch receptors of the teeth, oral mucosa, muscles of mastication, and temporomandibular joint to aid in mastication.

In addition to the sensory innervation just described, visceral efferent fibers help to innervate a variety of muscles of facial expression, the tensor tympani, and some muscles of mastication. Communications exist between the trigeminal nerve and the autonomic nervous system, including the ciliary, sphenopalatine, otic, and submaxillary ganglia and the oculomotor, facial, and glossopharyngeal nerves. Because of the complex nature of the trigeminal nerve, a thorough understanding of the clinically relevant anatomy

TABLE 24–1 **Indications for Blockade of the Trigeminal Nerve and Its Branches**

Local Anesthetic Block	Neurolytic Block or Neurodestructive Procedures
Surgical anesthesia	Palliation of cancer pain
Anatomic differential neural blockade	Management of trigeminal neuralgia
Prognostic nerve block before neurodestructive procedures	Management of cluster headache
Treatment of trismus	
Aid to awake endotracheal intubation	
Palliation in acute pain emergencies	
Palliation of acute herpes zoster	

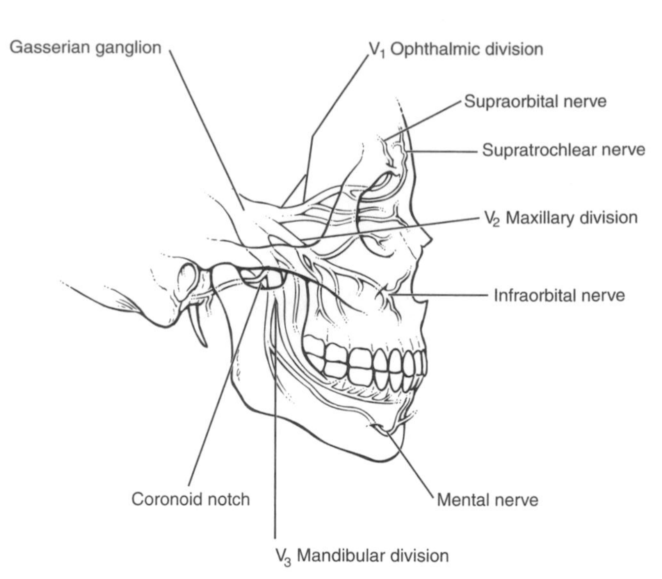

FIGURE 24–2 The trigeminal nerve and its branches.

is crucial to obtaining optimal results of neural blockade of these structures.

The Gasserian Ganglion

The gasserian ganglion is formed from two roots that exit the ventral surface of the brain stem at the midpontine level (Fig. 24–1).[10] These roots pass in a forward and lateral direction in the posterior cranial fossa across the border of the petrous temporal bone. They then enter a recess called *Meckel's cave*, which is formed by an invagination of the surrounding dura mater into the middle cranial fossa. The dural pouch that lies just behind the ganglion, called the trigeminal cistern, contains cerebrospinal fluid.

The gasserian ganglion is canoe shaped. Its three sensory divisions, the ophthalmic (V_1), maxillary (V_2), and mandibular (V_3), exit the anterior convex aspect of the ganglion. A smaller motor root joins the mandibular division as it exits the cranial cavity via the foramen ovale.

The Ophthalmic Division

The ophthalmic branch, the smallest division of the trigeminal nerve, is purely sensory in function (Fig. 24–2).[11] It enters the orbit via the superior orbital fissure. The branch is divided into the frontal, nasociliary, and lacrimal nerves. The terminal cutaneous branches of the frontal nerve consist of the supraorbital and supratrochlear nerves. These terminal branches exit the orbital cavity anteriorly and provide innervation to the upper eyelid, forehead, and anterior scalp. The terminal cutaneous branches of the nasociliary nerve consist of the infratrochlear and external nasal branches, which provide cutaneous and mucosal innervation to the apex and ala of the nose and anterior nasal cavity. The lacrimal nerve continues, without additional major branches, to innervate the lacrimal gland and outer canthus of the eye.

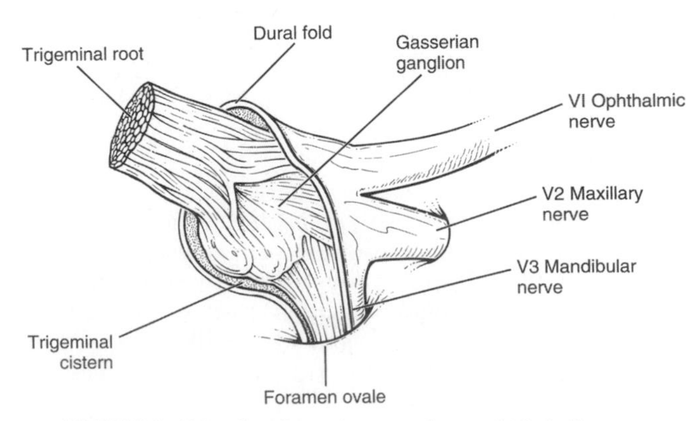

FIGURE 24–1 Gasserian ganglion and Meckel's cave.

The Maxillary Division

The maxillary division is a pure sensory nerve. It exits the middle cranial fossa via the foramen rotundum and crosses the pterygopalatine fossa (Fig. 24–3).[8] Passing through the inferior orbital fissure, it enters the orbit, emerging on the face via the infraorbital foramen.

The branches of the maxillary nerve are divided into four regional groups: (1) the intracranial group, including the middle meningeal nerve, which innervates the dura mater of the medial cranial fossa; (2) the pterygopalatine group, including the zygomatic nerve, which provides sensory innervation to the temporal and lateral zygomatic region, and the sphenopalatine branches, which help to innervate the mucosa of the maxillary sinus, upper gums, upper molars, and mucous membranes of the cheek; (3) the infraorbital canal group, composing the anterosuperior alveolar branch, which innervates the incisors and canines, the anterior wall of the maxillary antrum, and the floor of the nasal cavity, and the middle superior branch, which supplies the premolars; and (4) the infraorbital facial group, consisting of the inferior palpebral branch, which innervates the conjunctiva and skin of the lower eyelid; the external nasal branch, which supplies the side of the nose;

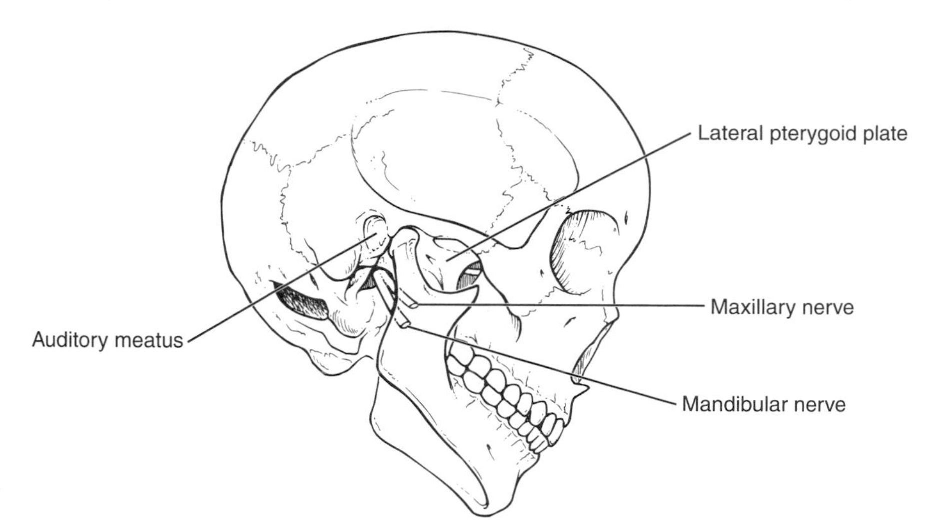

FIGURE 24–3 *Major branches of the trigeminal nerve.*

and the superior labial branch, which supplies the skin of the upper lip and part of the oral mucosa (see Fig. 24–2).

The Mandibular Division

The large sensory root and smaller motor root of the mandibular division leave the middle cranial fossa together via the foramen ovale.[8] They then join to form the mandibular nerve (see Fig. 24–3). This combined trunk gives off two branches: the nervus spinosus, which runs superiorly with the middle meningeal artery through the foramen spinosum to supply the dura mater and the mucosal lining of the mastoid sinus; and the internal pterygoid, which supplies the internal pterygoid and gives off branches to the otic ganglion. The mandibular nerve then divides into a small anterior and a large posterior trunk (see Fig. 24–2).

Branches from the small anterior trunk are the buccinator nerve, which is purely sensory and innervates the skin and mucous membrane overlying the anterior portion of the buccinator muscle; the masseteric nerve, which provides motor innervation to the masseter muscle; the deep temporal nerves, which provide motor innervation to the temporalis muscle; and the external pterygoid nerve, which provides motor innervation to the external pterygoid muscle.

The large posterior trunk comprises primarily sensory fibers but contains a small number of motor fibers as well. Branches of the posterior trunk are the auriculotemporal nerve, which provides innervation to skin anterior to the tragus and helix, the lining of the acoustic meatus, the tympanic membrane, the posterior temporomandibular joint, the parotid gland, and the skin of the temporal region; the lingual nerve, which provides sensory innervation to the dorsum and lateral aspects of the anterior two thirds of the tongue and the lateral mucous membranes of the mouth as well as the sublingual gland; and the inferior alveolar nerve, which provides sensory innervation to the lower teeth and mandible. The terminal branch of the inferior alveolar nerve, the mental nerve, exits the mandible via the mental foramen and provides sensory innervation to the chin and to the skin and mucous membrane of the lower lip.

TECHNIQUE OF BLOCKADE OF THE MAXILLARY AND MANDIBULAR DIVISIONS OF THE TRIGEMINAL NERVE VIA THE CORONOID APPROACH

The patient is placed in the supine position. The coronoid notch is palpated by asking the patient to open and close the mouth several times. The level of the coronoid notch is at the external auditory meatus (Figs. 24–4, 24–5). After the notch is identified, the patient is asked to hold the mouth in the neutral position.[2, 8]

A 22-gauge, 3.5-inch styletted spinal needle is inserted just beneath the zygomatic arch, at the midpoint of the coronoid notch (Fig. 24–6). The needle is advanced approximately 1.5 to 2 inches perpendicular to the base of the skull, until the lateral pterygoid plate is encountered

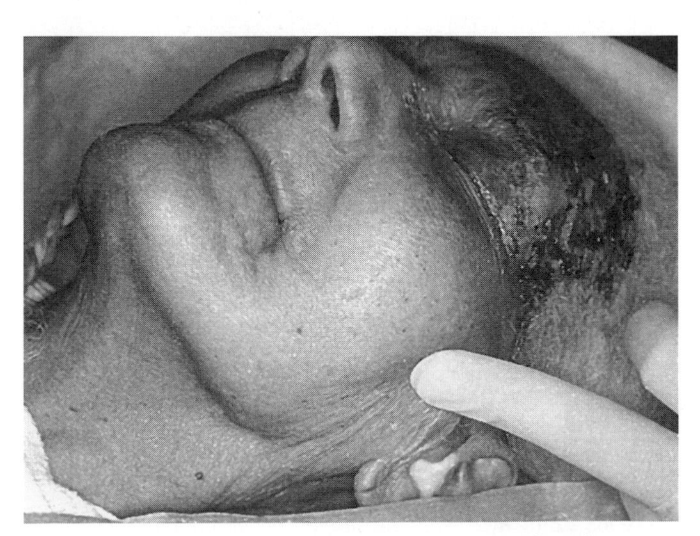

FIGURE 24–4 *Palpation of the coronoid notch.*

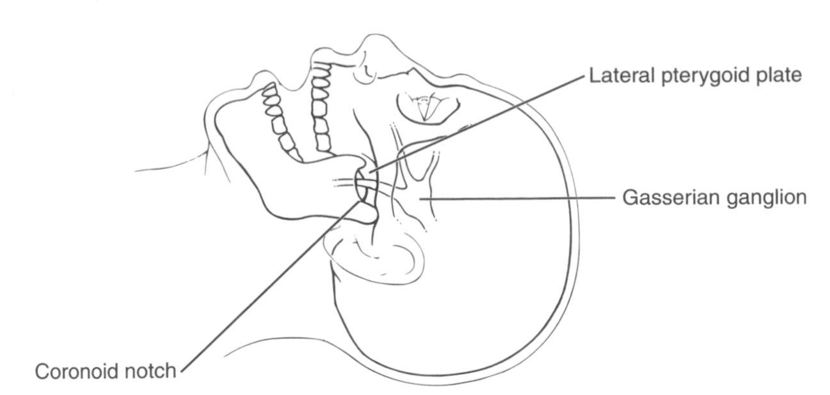

FIGURE 24–5 Patient position for maxillary and mandibular nerve block.

(Fig. 24–7). At this point, if both maxillary and mandibular nerve blocks are desired, the needle is withdrawn approximately 1 mm. After careful aspiration for blood, 7 to 10 mL of preservative-free local anesthetic is injected in small increments (Fig. 24–8).[2] During the injection procedure, the patient must be observed carefully for signs of local anesthetic toxicity. For selective maxillary nerve block, the styletted spinal needle is withdrawn and reinserted to slip just above the anterior margin of the lateral pterygoid plate (Fig. 24–9).[2] A maxillary paresthesia is generally produced approximately 1 cm deeper than the level at which the pterygoid plate was first encountered. After careful aspiration, 3 to 5 mL of preservative-free local anesthetic may be injected in increments.

If selective blockade of the mandibular division of the trigeminal nerve is desired, the lateral pterygoid plate is identified and the needle is withdrawn and directed slightly farther posteriorly and inferiorly. A paresthesia in the mandibular distribution is elicited in most cases (Fig. 24–10).[2] After careful aspiration, 3 to 5 mL of preservative-free local anesthetic is injected in incremental doses.

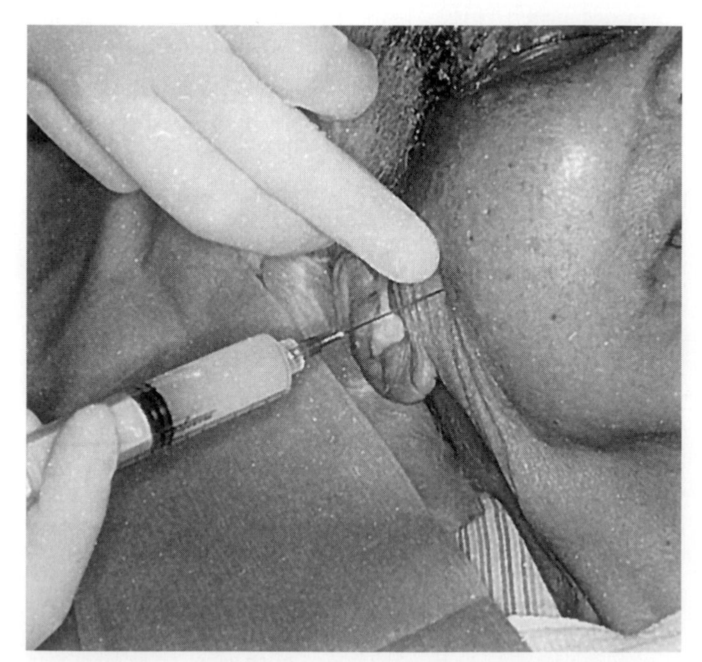

FIGURE 24–6 Correct needle position for the trigeminal nerve block via the coronoid notch.

For diagnostic and prognostic blocks, 1.0% preservative-free lidocaine is a suitable local anesthetic.[12] For therapeutic blocks, 0.5% preservative-free bupivacaine in combination with 80 mg of depot methylprednisolone (Depo-Medrol) is injected.[2] Subsequent daily nerve blocks are carried out in a similar manner, substituting 40 mg of methylprednisolone for the initial 80-mg dose. Five to six trigeminal nerve blocks daily may be required to treat the painful conditions listed earlier.[4] If selective neurolytic block of the mandibular or maxillary nerve is desired, incremental 0.1-mL injections of sterile glycerol, 6.5% phenol in glycerin, or alcohol to a total volume of 1.0 mL may be utilized after adequate pain relief with local anesthetic blocks is confirmed.[13]

Practical Considerations

The pterygopalatine space is densely vascular. The possibility of intravascular uptake of local anesthetic is significant with this nerve block. Careful aspiration of blood and incremental dosage with local anesthetic are important to allow early detection of local anesthetic toxicity. Careful observation of the patient during and after the nerve block is mandatory.[2]

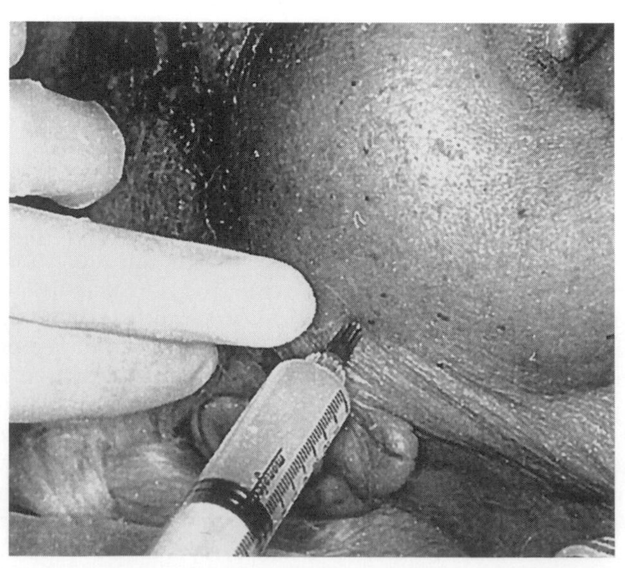

FIGURE 24–7 Needle tip positioned in the pterygopalatine fossa.

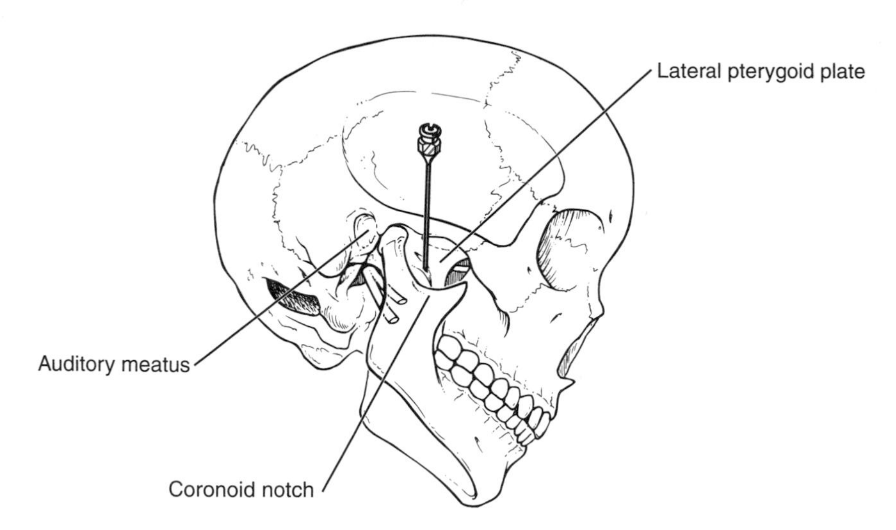

FIGURE 24–8 *Nonselective trigeminal nerve block.*

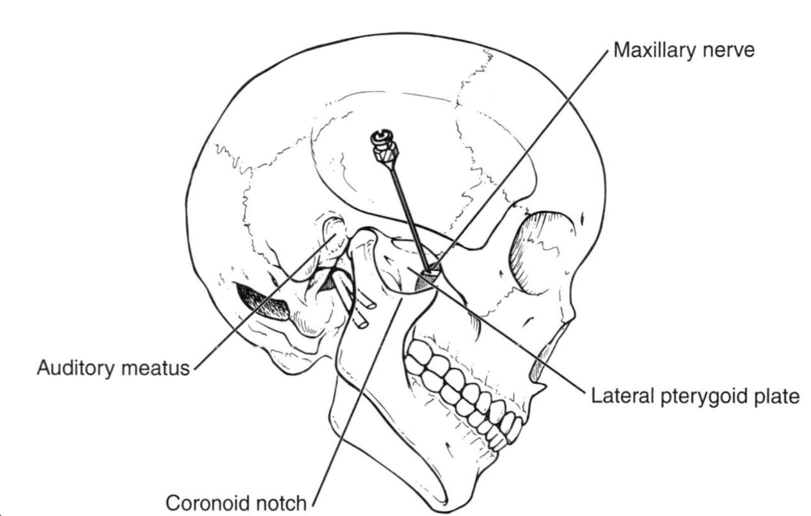

FIGURE 24–9 *Selective maxillary nerve block.*

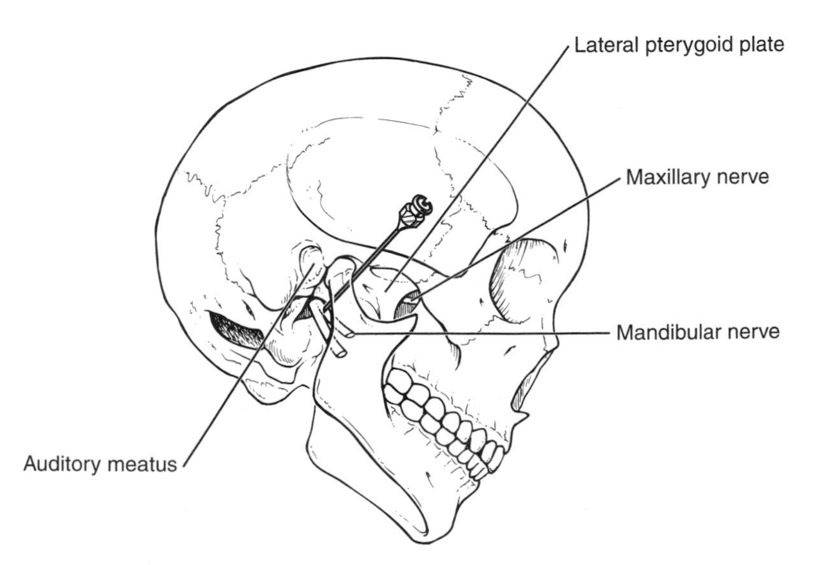

FIGURE 24–10 *Selective mandibular nerve block.*

TECHNIQUE OF NEURAL BLOCKADE OF THE SUPRAORBITAL AND SUPRATROCHLEAR BRANCHES OF THE OPHTHALMIC DIVISION OF THE TRIGEMINAL NERVE

The patient is placed supine with the head in neutral position. The supraorbital notch is identified by palpation. The skin is prepared with povidone iodine solution, care being taken to avoid spilling solution into the eye.

A 25-gauge, 1.5-inch needle is advanced perpendicularly to the skin at the level of the supraorbital notch. Three to 4 mL of preservative-free local anesthetic is injected in a fan configuration to anesthetize the peripheral branches of the nerve (Fig. 24–11).[14] To block the supratrochlear nerve, the needle is then directed medially from the supraorbital notch toward the apex of the nose.[8] Paresthesias are occasionally elicited.[7] If neurolytic block of the supraorbital and supratrochlear branches is desired, incremental 0.1-mL injections of sterile glycerol or 6.5% phenol in glycerin, up to total volume of 0.5 mL, may be utilized after adequate pain relief with local anesthetic blocks is confirmed.[13]

Practical Considerations

Because of the loose alveolar tissue of the eyelid, a gauze sponge should be used to apply gentle pressure on the eyelids and supraorbital tissues to keep the local anesthetic from dissecting into the eyelid and supraorbital tissues. This pressure is maintained after the nerve block to avoid periorbital hematoma and ecchymosis.

TECHNIQUE OF NEURAL BLOCKADE OF THE INFRAORBITAL BRANCH OF THE MAXILLARY NERVE

The Intraoral Approach

The upper lip is folded backward, and a cotton ball soaked with 10% cocaine solution or 2% viscous lidocaine is placed in the alveolar ridge, just inferior to the intraorbital foramen (Fig. 24–12). After adequate topical anesthesia is obtained, a 25-gauge, 1.5-inch needle is advanced through the anesthetized area superiorly toward the infraorbital foramen.[2] A paresthesia may be elicited.[2] After careful aspiration, 2 to 3 mL of preservative-free local anesthetic is injected.[3] If neurolytic block of the infraorbital nerve is desired, incremental 0.1-mL injections of sterile glycerol or 6.5% phenol in glycerin may be utilized after adequate pain relief with local anesthetic block is confirmed.[3]

Practical Considerations

As with the supraorbital nerve block, pressure over the inferior periorbital tissues limits dissection of the local anesthetic superiorly into the periorbital region and avoids ecchymosis and hematoma formation. The intraoral route is particularly suited to pediatric patients.

The Extraoral Approach

The infraorbital ridge of the maxillary bone is identified, and the infraorbital foramen is then palpated. The skin is prepared with povidone-iodine solution, care being taken to avoid spillage of the solution into the eye. A 25-gauge, 0.5-inch needle is then advanced at a 45-degree angle toward the foramen (see Fig. 24–12).[15] A paresthesia may be elicited. After careful aspiration of blood, 2 to 3 mL of preservative-free local anesthetic is injected. Percutaneous neurolytic block of the infraorbital nerve is performed much as for the intraoral route.

Practical Considerations

As with the intraoral approach, pressure must be applied to the infraorbital tissues to avoid dissection of local anesthetic. When the infraorbital branch is blocked utilizing the extraoral approach, if the needle enters the infraorbital foramen it should be withdrawn to avoid hematoma, injection-induced compressive neuropathy, and damage to the contents of the orbit.

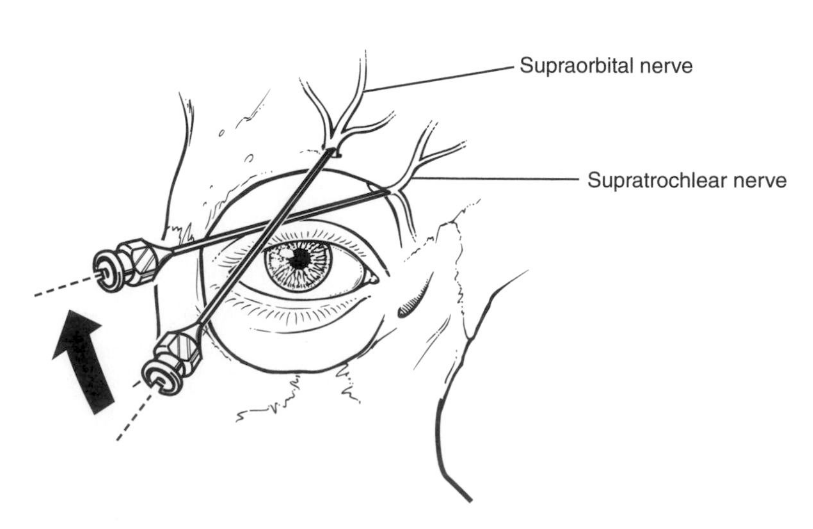

FIGURE 24–11 Supraorbital and supratrochlear block.

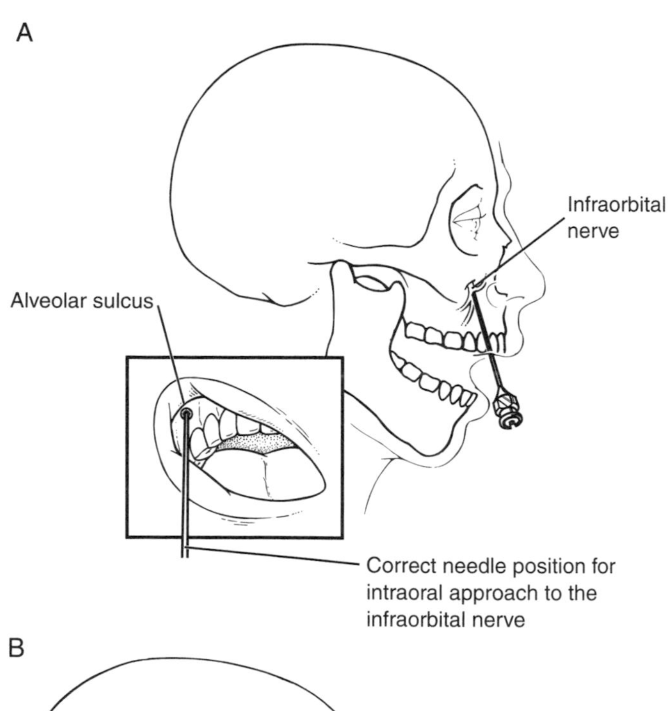

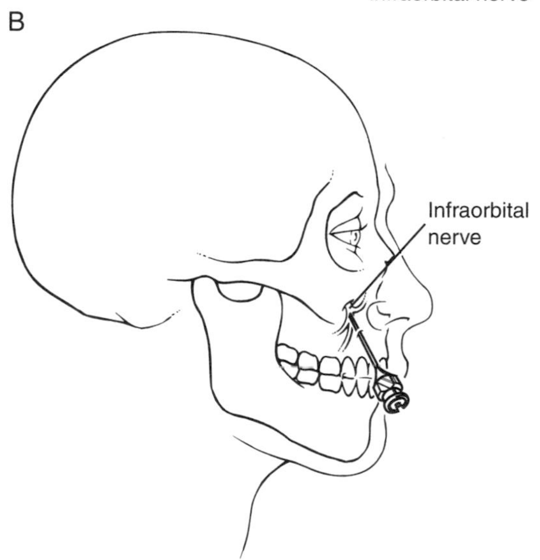

FIGURE 24–12 *Intraoral,* A, *and extraoral,* B, *approaches to infraorbital nerve block.*

TECHNIQUE OF NEURAL BLOCKADE OF THE MENTAL BRANCH OF THE MANDIBULAR NERVE

The Intraoral Approach

The lower lip is pulled downward and away from the face. A cotton ball soaked in 10% cocaine or 2% viscous lidocaine is then placed in the alveolar ridge against the mucosa, just superior to the mental foramen.[2] After topical anesthesia is obtained, a 25-gauge, 1.5–inch needle is advanced via the anesthetized area in a perpendicular plane (Fig. 24–13). Paresthesia occasionally develops. After careful aspiration of blood, 2 to 3 mL of preservative-free bupivacaine is injected.[2] If neurolytic block of the mental nerve is desired, successive 0.1-mL injections of sterile glycerol or 6.5% phenol in glycerin may be utilized after adequate pain relief with local anesthetic blocks is confirmed.

The Extraoral Approach

An area approximately 2 cm from the midline in a plane parallel with the supraorbital and infraorbital foramina is identified. Careful palpation generally allows identification of the mental foramen. The skin is prepared with povidone-iodine solution. A 25-gauge, 1.5-inch needle is advanced

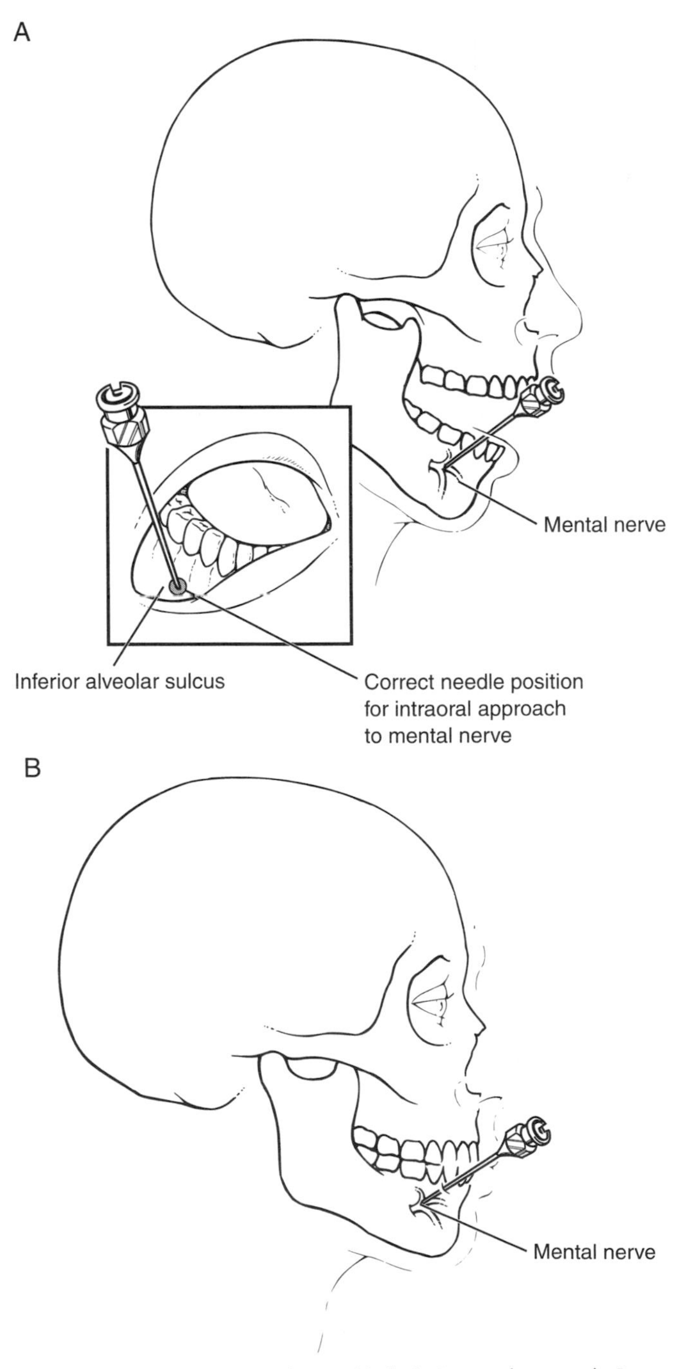

FIGURE 24–13 *Mental nerve block.* A, *Intraoral approach;* B, *extraoral approach.*

toward the foramen (see Fig. 24–13).[16] If the needle enters the mental foramen, it should be withdrawn to avoid injection-induced compressive neuropathy. After careful aspiration of blood, 2 to 3 mL of preservative-free local anesthetic is injected. If neurolytic block of the mental nerve is desired, incremental 0.1-mL injections of sterile glycerol or 6.5% phenol in glycerin, to a total volume of 0.5 mL, may be given after adequate pain relief with local anesthetic blocks is confirmed.

Practical Considerations

Because of the acute angle at which the mental branch exits the mental foramen, it is susceptible to compression neuropathy. For this reason, it is advisable to avoid advancing the needle into the canal, because theoretically hematoma formation or increased pressure during injection can cause compression neuropathy.

COMPLICATIONS AND UNWANTED SIDE EFFECTS

The potential complications and unwanted side effects of blockade of the trigeminal nerve and its branches are as follows:

- Activation of herpes labialis and herpes zoster
- Postprocedure dysesthesias, including anesthesia dolorosa
- Abnormal motor function, including weakness
- Facial asymmetry
- Horner's syndrome
- Facial ecchymosis and hematoma
- Ocular subscleral hematoma
- Local anesthetic toxicity
- Trauma to nerves
- Infection
- Sloughing of skin and subcutaneous tissue

Although it is more often associated with procedures involving the gasserian ganglion, blockade of the trigeminal nerve and its branches may activate herpes labialis and, occasionally, herpes zoster in the distribution of the trigeminal nerve.

A small number of patients who undergo chemical neurolysis or neurodestructive procedures of the trigeminal nerve and its branches have postprocedure dysesthesias in the area of anesthesia.[17] These symptoms range from mild, uncomfortable burning or pulling sensations to severe pain. Severe postprocedure pain, called anesthesia dolorosa, may be worse than the patient's original pain complaint and often is harder to treat. Sloughing of skin and subcutaneous tissue has been associated with anesthesia dolorosa.

In addition to disturbances of sensation, neurolytic block or neurodestructive procedures of the trigeminal nerve and its branches may result in abnormal motor function, including weakness of the muscles of mastication and facial asymmetry secondary to weakness and altered proprioception.[13] Horner's syndrome may also occur from block of the paratrigeminal sympathetic fibers.

Owing to the vascular nature of the pterygopalatine space, facial ecchymosis, and hematoma, including ocular subscleral hematoma, are common.[8, 18] Although generally not harmful, these unwanted side effects are quite distressing to the patient, so each patient should be forewarned of the possibility before the procedure. The vascularity of this anatomic region also increases the potential for local anesthetic toxicity.[18]

The terminal branches of the trigeminal nerve are susceptible to trauma from needle, hematoma, and compression during injection procedures.[2] These complications, although usually transitory, can be quite upsetting to the patient. Infection, although also uncommon, is always a possibility, especially in immunocompromised cancer patients. Early detection of infection is crucial to avoiding potentially life-threatening sequelae.

FUTURE DIRECTIONS

There is no doubt that continuing advances in the understanding of the basic science of pain will improve management of the patient suffering pain. Research on the serotoninergic system and its role in the pathogenesis of headache, for example, has led to the development of a whole new class of drugs that have revolutionized the way clinicians manage acute migraine and cluster headache.[19] The search for safer local anesthetic has yielded ropivacaine, which appears to have less cardiac toxicity than bupivacaine.[20] In view of the relatively high incidence of local anesthetic toxicity associated with this technique, such a characteristic would obviously offer a great advantage for neural blockade of the trigeminal system. Microencapsulation of local anesthetics with lecithin appears to increase the duration of action fourfold; this advance would be beneficial for trigeminal nerve block when the lesion responsible for the pain is self-limited.

REFERENCES

1. Waldman SD: Trigeminal nerve block. *In* Weiner RS (ed): Innovations in Pain Management, vol I. Orlando, Fla, PMD Press, 1990, pp 10–15.
2. Waldman SD. Trigeminal block. *In* Waldman SD: Atlas of Interventional Pain Management Techniques. Philadelphia, WB Saunders, 1998, pp 30–39.
3. Waldman SD: Trigeminal neuralgia. Intern Med 13:45–53, 1992.
4. Waldman SD: The role of neural blockade in the management of headaches and facial pain. Curr Rev Pain 1:346–352, 1997.
5. Waldman SD: Cluster headache. Intern Med 13:31–33, 1992.
6. Waldman SD: Evaluation and treatment of common headache and facial pain syndromes. *In* Raj PP (ed): Practical Management of Pain. St. Louis, CV Mosby, 1992, p 217.
7. Feldstein G: Percutaneous retrogasserian glycerol rhizotomy. *In* Racz G (ed): Techniques of Neurolysis. Boston, Kluwer, 1989, pp 126–128.
8. Hahn MB: Trigeminal nerve block. *In* Hahn MB, McQuillan PM, Sheplock GJ (eds): Regional Anesthesia. St. Louis, CV Mosby, 1996, pp 41–44.
9. Brown DL: Trigeminal (gasserian) ganglion block. *In* Brown DL (ed): Atlas of Regional Anesthesia. Philadelphia, WB Saunders, 1999, pp 149–166.
10. Katz J: Gasserian ganglion. *In* Katz J (ed): Atlas of Regional Anesthesia. Norwalk, Conn, Appleton & Lange, 1994, pp 4–5.
11. Neill RS: Head, neck and airway. *In* Wildsmith JAW, Armitage EN (eds): Principles and Practice of Regional Anesthesia. New York, Churchill Livingstone, 1987.
12. Raj PP: Prognostic and therapeutic local anesthetic blocks. *In* Cousins MJ, Bridenbaugh DO (eds): Neural Blockade. Philadelphia, JB Lippincott, 1988, pp 900–901.

13. Bonica JJ: Neurolytic blockade and hypophysectomy. *In* Bonica JJ (ed): The Management of Pain. Philadelphia, Lea & Febiger, 1990.
14. Katz J: Supraorbital nerve. *In* Katz J (ed). Atlas of Regional Anesthesia. Norwalk, Conn, Appleton & Lange, 1994, pp 25–26.
15. Katz J: Infraorbital nerve. *In* Katz J (ed): Atlas of Regional Anesthesia. Norwalk, Conn, Appleton & Lange, 1994, pp 14–15.
16. Katz J: Mental nerve. *In* Katz J (ed): Atlas of Regional Anesthesia. Norwalk, Conn, Appleton & Lange, 1994, pp 27–28.
17. Lipton S: Neurolysis: Pharmacology and drug selection. *In* Patt RB (ed): Cancer Pain. Philadelphia, JB Lippincott, 1993, pp 354–355.
18. Waldman SD: Complication of trigeminal nerve block. Pain Clin 7:211–215, 1994.
19. Waldman SD: Recent advances in analgesic therapy: Sumatriptan. Pain Digest 3:260–263, 1993.
20. Waldman SD: Recent advances in analgesic therapy: Ropivacaine. Pain Digest 4:42–45, 1994.

CHAPTER • 25

Glossopharyngeal Nerve Block

Steven D. Waldman, MD, JD

HISTORICAL CONSIDERATIONS

The early use of glossopharyngeal nerve block in pain management centered around two applications: (1) the treatment of glosspharyngeal neuralgia and (2) the palliation of pain secondary to head and neck malignancies. In the late 1950s, the clinical utility of glossopharyngeal nerve block as an adjunct to awake endotracheal intubation was documented.

Weisenburg first described pain in the distribution of the glossopharyngeal nerve in a patient with a cerebellopontine angle tumor in 1910.[1] In 1921, Harris reported the first idiopathic case and coined the term *glossopharyngeal neuralgia*.[2] He suggested that blockade of the glossopharyngeal nerve might be useful in palliating this painful condition.

Early attempts at permanent treatment of glossopharyngeal neuralgia and cancer pain in the distribution of the glossopharyngeal nerve consisted principally of extracranial surgical section or alcohol neurolysis of the glossopharyngeal nerve.[3] These approaches met with limited success in the treatment of glosspharyngeal neuralgia but were useful in some patients suffering from cancer pain mediated via the glossopharyngeal nerve. Intracranial section of the glossopharyngeal nerve was first performed by Adson in 1925 and was subsequently refined by Dandy. The intracranial approach to section of the glosspharyngeal nerve appeared to yield better results for both glossopharyngeal neuralgia and cancer pain but was a much riskier procedure.[4] Recently interest in extracranial destruction of the glossopharyngeal nerve by glycerol or by creation of a radiofrequency lesion has been renewed.

INDICATIONS AND CONTRAINDICATIONS

Indications for glossopharyngeal nerve block are summarized in Table 25–1. In addition to applications for surgical anesthesia, glossopharyngeal nerve block with local anesthetics can be utilized as a diagnostic tool when performing differential neural blockade on an anatomic basis in the evaluation of head and facial pain.[5] Glossopharyngeal nerve block is used to help differentiate geniculate ganglion neuralgia from glossopharyngeal neuralgia. If destruction of the glossopharyngeal nerve is being considered, this technique is useful as an indicator of the extent of motor and sensory impairment that the patient will likely experience.[6] Glossopharyngeal nerve block with local anesthetic may be utilized to palliate acute pain emergencies, including glossopharyngeal neuralgia and cancer pain until pharmacologic, surgical, and antiblastic methods take effect.[7] This technique is also useful for atypical facial pain in the distribution of the glossopharyngeal nerve[8] and as an adjunct for awake endotracheal intubation.[9]

Destruction of the glossopharyngeal nerve is indicated in the palliation of cancer pain, including invasive tumors of the posterior tongue, hypopharynx, and tonsils.[10] This technique is useful in the management of the pain of glossopharyngeal neuralgia for those patients who have failed to respond to medical management or who are not candidates for surgical microvascular decompression.[11]

Contraindications to blockade of the glossopharyngeal nerve, are summarized in Table 25–2. Local infection and sepsis are absolute contraindications to all procedures. Coagulopathy is a strong contraindication to glossopharyngeal nerve block, but owing to the desperate nature of many patients' suffering from invasive head and face malignancies, ethical and humanitarian considerations dictate its use, despite the risk of bleeding.

When clinical indications are compelling, blockade of the glossopharyngeal nerve utilizing a 25-gauge needle may be carried out in the presence of coagulopathy, albeit with increased risk of eccymosis and hematoma formation.

CLINICALLY RELEVANT ANATOMY

The glossopharyngeal nerve contains both motor and sensory fibers.[10] The motor fibers innervate the stylopharyngeus muscle. The sensory portion of the nerve innervates the posterior third of the tongue, palatine tonsil, and the mucous membranes of the mouth and pharynx. Special visceral afferent sensory fibers transmit information from the taste buds of the posterior third of the tongue. Information from the carotid sinus and body, which help to control blood pressure, pulse, and respiration are carried via the carotid sinus nerve, a branch of the glossopharyngeal

TABLE 25–1 Indications for Glossopharyngeal Nerve Block

Local anesthetic block
- Surgical anesthesia
- Anatomic differential neural blockade
- Prognostic nerve block prior to neurodestructive procedures
- Acute pain emergencies (palliation)
- Adjunct to awake intubation

Neurolytic block or neurodestructive procedure
- Cancer pain (palliation)
- Management of glossopharyngeal neuralgia

TABLE 25–2 Contraindications to Glossopharyngeal Nerve Block

Local infection
Sepsis
Coagulopathy
Disulfiram therapy (if alcohol is used)
Significant behavioral abnormalities

nerve.[10] Parasympathetic fibers pass via the glossopharyngeal nerve to the otic ganglion. Postganglionic fibers from the ganglion carry secretory information to the parotid gland.[12]

The glossopharyngeal nerve exits the jugular foramen near the vagus and accessory nerves and the internal jugular vein.[13] All three nerves lie in the groove between the internal jugular vein and internal carotid artery (Fig. 25–1). Inadvertent puncture of either vessel during glossopharyngeal nerve block can result in intravascular injection or hematoma formation. Even small amounts of local anesthetic injected into the carotid artery at this site can produce profound local anesthetic toxicity.[11]

One landmark for glossopharyngeal nerve block is the styloid process of the temporal bone. This structure is the calcification of the cephalad end of the stylohyoid ligament. Although usually easy to identify, when ossification is limited, it may be difficult to locate with the exploring needle.

TECHNIQUE

The Extraoral Approach

The patient is placed in the supine position. An imaginary line is visualized running from the mastoid process to the angle of the mandible (Fig. 25–2).[14] The styloid process should lie just below the midpoint of this line. The skin is "prepped" with antiseptic solution. A 22-gauge, 1.5-inch needle attached to a 10-ml syringe is advanced at this midpoint location in a plane perpendicular to the skin (Fig. 25–3). The styloid process should be encountered within 3 cm. After contact is made, the needle is withdrawn and walked off the styloid process posteriorly. As soon as bony contact is lost and careful aspiration reveals no blood or cerebrospinal fluid, 7 ml of 0.5% preservative-free lidocaine combined with 80 mg of methylprednisolone is injected in incremental doses. Subsequently, daily nerve blocks are performed in the same manner but substituting 40 mg of methylprednisolone for the first 80-mg dose. This approach may also be utilized for breakthrough pain in patients who previously experienced adequate pain control with oral medications.[11]

The Intraoral Approach

The tongue is anesthetized with 2.0% viscous lidocaine. The patient opens his mouth wide, and the tongue is retracted downward with a tongue depressor or laryngoscope blade (Fig. 25–4). A 22-gauge, 3.5-inch spinal needle that has been bent approximately 25 degrees is inserted through the mucosa at the lower lateral portion of the posterior tonsillar pillar. The needle is advanced approximately

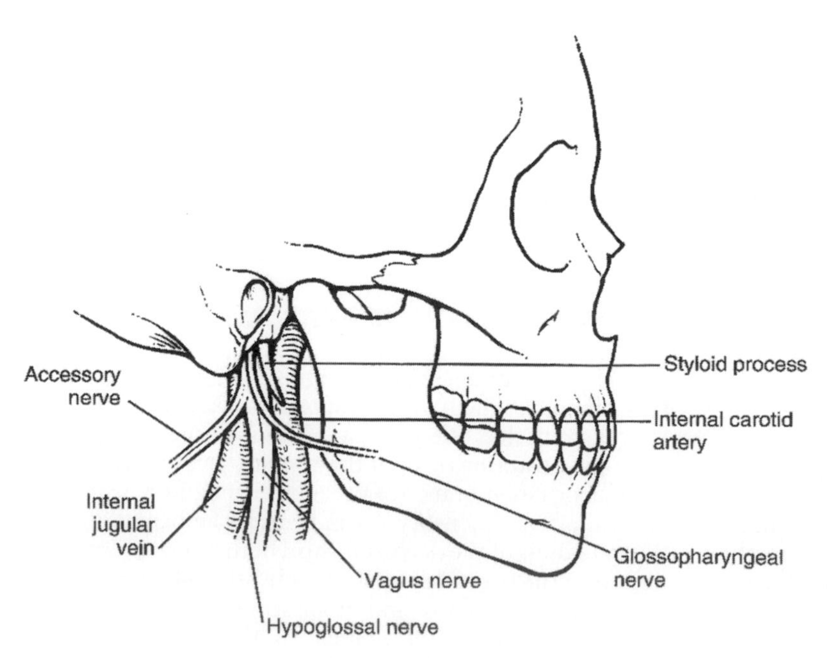

FIGURE 25–1 Relationship of glossopharyngeal, vagus, and hypoglossal nerves to artery and vein in context with skull and mandible.

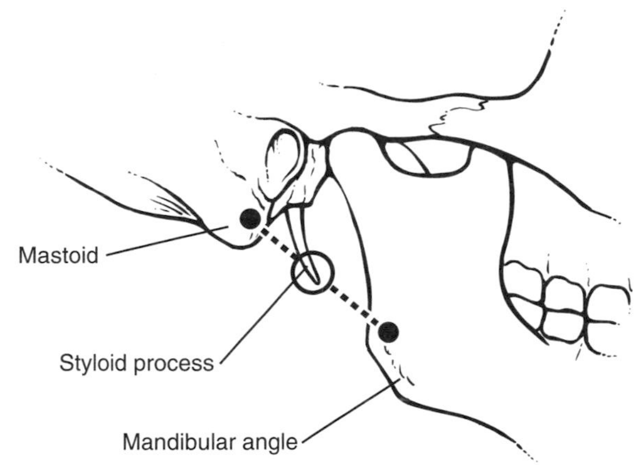

FIGURE 25–2 Close-up view of the line from mastoid to styloid.

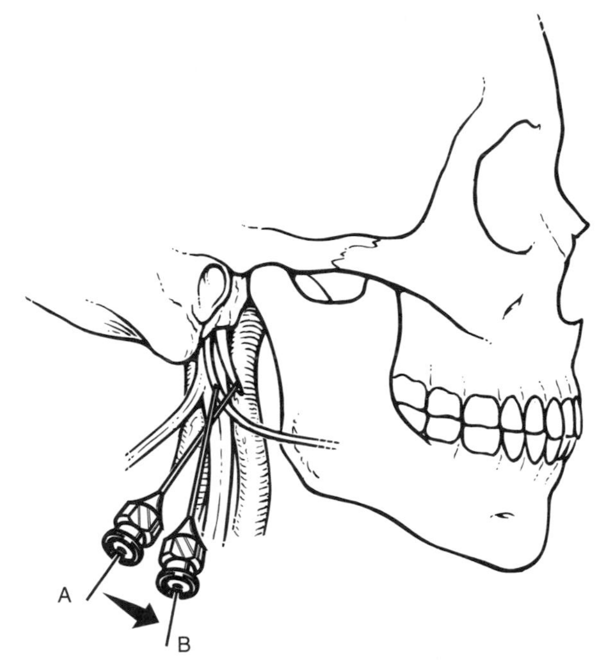

FIGURE 25–3 Needle placement for glossopharyngeal nerve block. A, Needle is in contact with styloid process. B, Needle is redirected posteriorly to the glossopharyngeal nerve.

0.5 cm. After careful aspiration for blood and cerebrospinal fluid, local anesthetic or steroid or both are injected in a manner like that for the extraoral approach to glossopharyngeal nerve block.

POTENTIAL COMPLICATIONS OF GLOSSOPHARYNGEAL NERVE BLOCK

The major complications associated with glossopharyngeal nerve block (Table 25–3) are related to trauma to the internal jugular and carotid artery.[10] Hematoma formation and intravascular injection of local anesthetic with subsequent toxicity are significant problems for the patient. Blockade of the motor portion of the glossopharyngeal nerve can result in dysphagia secondary to weakness of the stylopharyngeus muscle.[9] If the vagus nerve is inadvertently blocked, as it often is during glossopharyngeal nerve block, dysphonia secondary to paralysis of the ipsilateral vocal cord may occur. Reflex tachycardia secondary to vagal nerve block is also observed in some patients.[10] Inadvertent block of the hypoglossal and spinal accessory nerves during glossopharyngeal nerve block will result in weakness of the tongue and trapezius muscle.[15]

A small percentage of patients who undergo chemical neurolysis or neurodestructive procedures of the glossopharyngeal nerve experience postprocedure dyesthesias in the area of anesthesia.[16] These symptoms range from a mildly uncomfortable burning or pulling sensation to severe pain. Such severe postprocedure pain is called *anesthesia dolorosa*. Anesthesia dolorosa can be worse than the

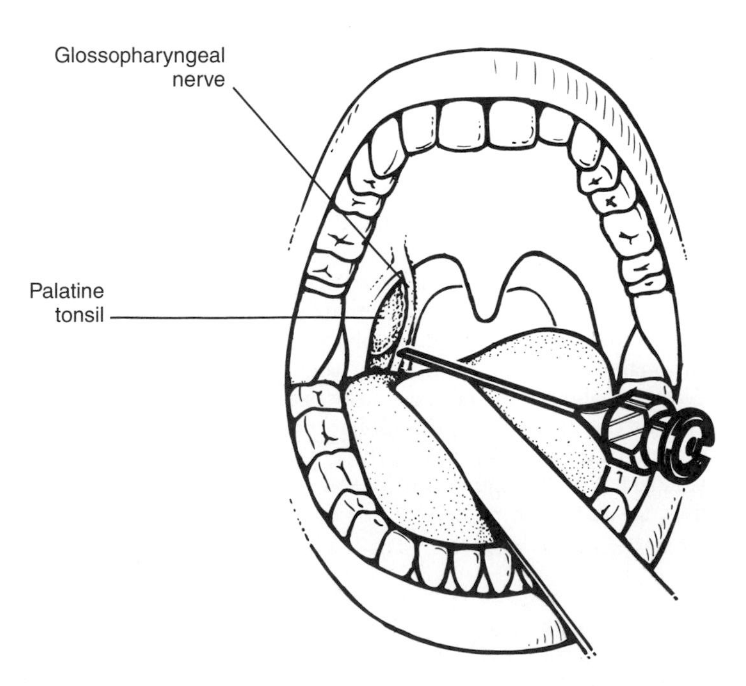

FIGURE 25–4 Intraoral approach to glossopharyngeal nerve block.

TABLE 25–3 Complications and Unwanted Side Effects of Blockade of the Glossopharyngeal Nerve Block

Dysphagia
Ecchymosis and hematoma
Postprocedure dysesthesias
Anesthesia dolorosa
Weakness of trapezius muscle
Weakness of tongue
Hoarsness
Infection
Tachycardia
Local anesthetic toxicity
Trauma to nerves
Sloughing of skin and subcutaneous tissue

patient's original pain and is oftentimes harder to treat. Sloughing of skin and subcutaneous tissue has been associated with anesthesia dolorosa.

The glossopharyngeal nerve is susceptible to trauma from needle, hematoma, or compression during injection procedures. Such complications, while usually transitory, can be quite upsetting to the patient.

Although uncommon, risk of infection is ever present, especially in immunocompromised cancer patients.[6] Early detection of infection is crucial to avoiding potentially life-threatening sequelae.

NEURODESTRUCTIVE PROCEDURES

The injection of small quantities of alcohol, phenol, and glycerol into the area of the glossopharyngeal nerve often provide long-term relief from glossopharyngeal neuralgia and cancer-related pain that has been refractory to optimal trials of the therapies discussed earlier.[10, 13] Destruction of the glossopharyngeal nerve can be also carried out by creating a radiofrequency lesion under biplanar fluoroscopic guidance.[17] This procedure is reserved for patients in whom all the treatments discussed here for intractable glossopharyngeal neuralgia have failed and whose physical status precludes more invasive neurosurgical treatments.

MICROVASCULAR DECOMPRESSION OF THE GLOSSOPHARYNGEAL ROOT

Microvascular decompression of the glossopharyngeal root (Jannetta's procedure) is the neurosurgical procedure of choice for intractable glossopharyngeal neuralgia.[18] The rationale for this operation is the theory that glossopharyngeal neuralgia is, in fact, a compressive mononeuropathy. In this operation, the glossopharyngeal root is identified close to the brain stem and the compressing blood vessel is isolated. A sponge is interposed between the vessel and nerve, effecting a cure.

Intracranial section of the glossopharyngeal nerve is indicated for intractable cancer pain in the distribution of the glossopharyngeal nerve that does not respond to more conservative treatment approaches.[10]

CONCLUSION

The pain specialist should be aware of the clinical utility of glossopharyngeal nerve block. Correctly used, pharmacologic therapy combined with glossopharyngeal nerve block should control the pain of glossopharyngeal neuralgia and cancer-related pain in the distribution of the glossopharyngeal nerve in the vast majority of cases. Surgical therapy should be considered when conservative therapy fails to provide long-lasting relief from pain mediated via the glossopharyngeal nerve.

REFERENCES

1. Weisenburg TH: Cerebello-pontine tumour diagnosed for six years as tic douloureux. JAMA 54:1600–1604, 1910.
2. Harris W: Persistent pain in lesions of the peripheral and central nervous system. Brain 44:557–571, 1921.
3. Doyle JB: A study of four cases of glossopharyngeal neuralgia. Arch Neurol Psychiatr 9:34–36, 1923.
4. Dandy WE: Glossopharyngeal neuralgia: Its diagnosis and treatment. Arch Surg 15:198–215, 1927.
5. Waldman SD: The role of neural blockade in the management of headaches and facial pain. Curr Rev Pain 1:346–352, 1997.
6. Waldman SD: The role of nerve blocks in pain management. *In* Weiner R (ed): Comprehensive Guide to Pain Management. Orlando, Fla, PMD Press, 1990, pp 10-1–10-33.
7. Waldman SD: Management of acute pain. Postgrad Med 87:15–17, 1992.
8. Waldman SD. The role of nerve blocks in the management of headache and facial pain. *In* Diamond S (ed): Practical Headache Management. Boston, Kluwer, 1993, pp 99–118.
9. Brown DL: Glossopharyngeal nerve block. *In* Brown DL (ed): Atlas of Regional Anesthesia, pp 203–208. Philadelphia, WB Saunders, 1999.
10. Bonica JJ: Neurolytic blockade and hypophysectomy. *In* Bonica JJ (ed): The Management of Pain. Philadelphia, Lea & Febiger, 1990, pp 1996–1999.
11. Waldman SD, Waldman KA: The diagnosis and treatment of glossopharyngeal neuralgia. Am J Pain Manage 5:19–24, 1995.
12. Pitkin GP: The glossopharyngeal nerve. *In* Southworth JL, Hingson RA (eds): Conduction Anesthesia, Philadelphia, JB Lippincott, 1946, pp 46–49.
13. Bajaj P, Gemavat M, Singh DP: Ninth cranial nerve block in the management of malignant pain in its territory. Pain Clin 6:153–208, 1993.
14. Murphy TM: Somatic blockade of the head and neck. *In* Cousins MJ, Bridenbaugh PO (eds): Neural Blockade, ed 2. Philadelphia, JB Lippincott, 1988, pp 546–548.
15. Katz J: Glossopharyngeal nerve block. In Katz J (ed): Atlas of Regional Anesthesia. Norwalk, Conn, Appleton & Lange, 1994, p 52.
16. Brisman R: Retrogasserian glycerol injection. *In* Brisman R (ed): Neurosurgical and Medical Management of Pain. Boston, Kluwer, 1989, pp 51–56.
17. Arbit E, Krol G: Percutaneous radiofrequency neurolysis guided by computerized tomography for the treatment of glossopharyngeal neuralgia. Neurosurgery 29:580–583, 1991.
18. Fraioloi B, Esposito V, Ferrante L, et al: Microsurgical treatment of glossopharyngeal neuralgia. Neurosurgery 25:630–633, 1989.

CHAPTER • 26

Vagus Nerve Block

Steven D. Waldman, MD, JD

HISTORICAL CONSIDERATIONS

Early in the history of regional anesthesia, vagus nerve block was utilized to treat a variety of conditions that included both pain as well as cardiac arrythmias. Often combined with stellate ganglion block, blockade of the vagus nerve was a mainstay in the treatment of intractable angina and pain emanating from the esophagus, trachea, and other mediastinal structures.[1] Many of the early indications for vagus nerve block now are treated medically or surgically, but vagus nerve block remains useful for management of cancer pain in structures innervated by this nerve.

INDICATIONS

Vagus nerve block with local anesthetics can be utilized as a diagnostic tool when performing differential neural blockade on an anatomic basis to evaluate head and facial pain.[2] When destruction of the vagus nerve is being considered, this technique is a useful indicator of the degree of motor and sensory impairment the patient may experience. Vagus nerve block with local anesthetic can be utilized to palliate acute pain emergencies, including vagal neuralgia and cancer pain, while waiting for pharmacologic, surgical, or antiblastic methods to take effect.[3] Vagus nerve block is utilized as a diagnostic and therapeutic maneuver when vagal neuralgia is suspected. Destruction of the vagus nerve is indicated for palliation of cancer pain, including that associated with invasive tumors of the larynx, hypopharynx, and pyriform sinus, and occasionally intrathoracic malignancies.[3,4]

Owing to the desperate situation of many patients suffering from aggressive head and neck malignancies, blockade of the vagus nerve utilizing a 25-gauge needle may be carried out in the presence of coagulopathy or anticoagulation, albeit with increased risks of ecchymosis and hematoma formation.

CLINICALLY RELEVANT ANATOMY

The vagus nerve contains both motor and sensory fibers.[5] The motor fibers innervate the pharyngeal muscle and provide fibers for the superior and recurrent laryngeal nerves. The sensory portion of the nerve innervates the dura mater of the posterior fossa, the posterior aspect of the external auditory meatus and inferior aspect of the tympanic membrane, and the mucosa of the larynx below the vocal cords. The vagus nerve also provides fibers to the thoracic contents, including the heart, lungs, and major vessels.

The vagus nerve exits from the jugular foramen close to the spinal accessory nerve (Fig. 26–1). The vagus lies just caudad to the glossopharyngeal nerve and is superficial to the internal jugular vein. The vagus courses downward from the jugular foramen within the carotid sheath along with the internal jugular vein and internal carotid artery.

The technique of blockade of the vagus nerve is much like that of glossopharyngeal nerve block.[3] The key landmark for vagus nerve block is the styloid process of the temporal bone. This osseous process represents the calcification of the cephalad end of the stylohyoid ligament. Although usually easy to identify, if ossification is limited, the styloid process may be difficult to locate with the exploring needle.

TECHNIQUE

The patient is placed in the supine position. An imaginary line is visualized running from the mastoid process to the angle of the mandible. The styloid process should lie just below the midpoint of this line. The skin is "prepped" with antiseptic solution. A 22-gauge, 1.5-inch needle attached to a 10-ml syringe is advanced at this midpoint in a plane perpendicular to the skin. The styloid process should be encountered within 3 cm (Fig. 26–2). After contact is made, the needle is withdrawn and walked off the styloid process posteriorly and slightly downward. The needle is advanced approximately 0.5 cm past the depth at which the styloid process was identified. If careful aspiration reveals no blood or cerebrospinal fluid, 5 mL of 0.5% preservative-free lidocaine combined with 80 mg of methylprednisolone is injected in incremental doses. Subsequent daily nerve blocks are carried out in a similar manner, substituting 40 mg of methylprednisolone for the initial 80-mg dose. This approach may also be utilized for breakthrough pain in patients who previously experienced adequate pain control with oral medications.

SIDE EFFECTS AND COMPLICATIONS

The major complications of vagus nerve block are related to trauma to the internal jugular and carotid arteries.[2, 3] Hematoma formation and intravascular injection of local anesthetic (with subsequent toxicity) are not uncommon after vagus nerve block. Blockade of the motor portion of the vagus nerve can result in dysphonia and difficulty coughing secondary to blockade of the superior and recurrent laryngeal nerves. Reflex tachycardia secondary to vagal nerve block is also observed in some patients. Inadvertent block of the glossopharyngeal, hypoglossal, and spinal accessory nerves during vagus nerve block will result in weakness of the tongue and trapezius muscle and numbness in the distribution of the glossopharyngeal nerve.

Although uncommon, the risk of infection is ever present, especially in immunocompromised cancer patients. Early detection of infection is crucial to avoiding potentially life-threatening sequelae.

CLINICAL PEARLS

Vagus nerve block should be considered in two clinical situations: (1) for vagal neuralgia and (2) for persistent, ill-defined pain related to the cancers discussed earlier that fails to respond to conservative measures. Vagal neuralgia is clinically analogous to trigeminal and glossopharyngeal neuralgia. It is characterized by paroxysms of shocklike pain into the thyroid and laryngeal areas. Pain occasionally radiates into the jaw and upper thorax. Attacks of vagal neuralgia may be precipitated by coughing, yawning, or swallowing. Excessive salivation may be present. This is a rare pain syndrome and should be considered a diagnosis of exclusion.

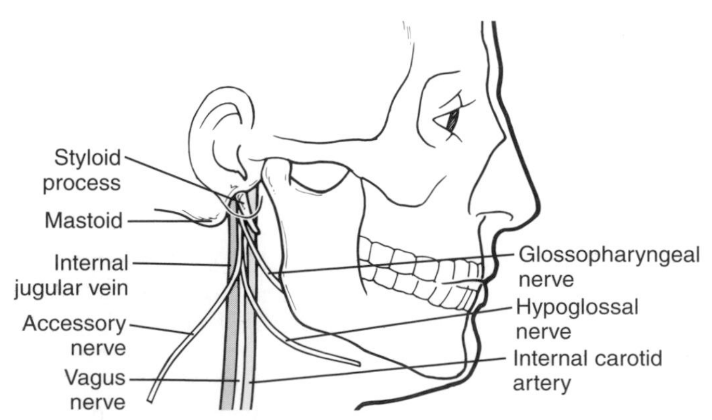

FIGURE 26–1 *The vagus nerve and surrounding structures.*

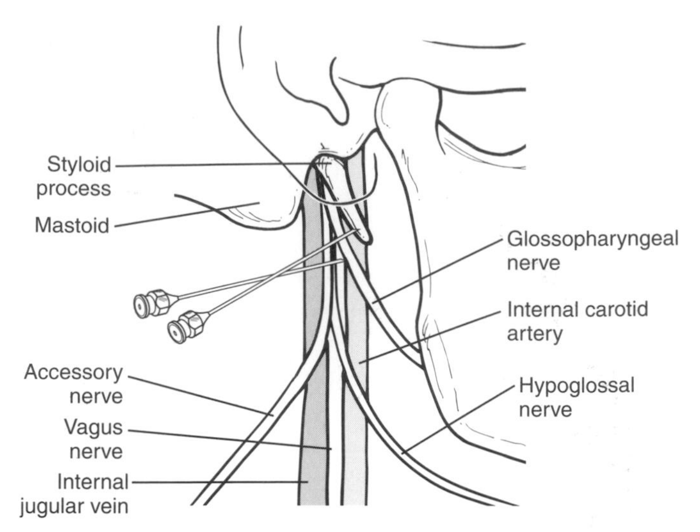

FIGURE 26–2 *Positioning of needle for vagus nerve block.*

Neurolytic block with small quantities of alcohol, phenol, or glycerol has been shown to provide long-term relief for patients suffering from vagus neuralgia and cancer-related pain that does not respond to more conservative treatments. The vagus nerve can also be destroyed by creating a radiofrequency lesion under biplanar fluoroscopic guidance.

The proximity of the vagus nerve to major vessels makes postblock hematoma and ecchymosis distinct possibilities. While these complications are usually transitory, they can be quite upsetting to the patient. Therefore, the patient should be warned of these possibilities before the procedure. The dense vascularity of this region also increases the likelihood of inadvertent intravascular injection. Even small amounts of local anesthetic injected into the carotid artery at this level will result in local anesthetic toxicity and seizures. Incremental dosing and careful monitoring of the patient for signs of local anesthetic toxicity help to avoid these complications.

REFERENCES

1. Harris W: Peripheral pain in lesions of the peripheral and central nervous systems. Brain 44:557–571, 1921.
2. Katz J: Vagus nerve block. *In* Katz J (ed): Atlas of Regional Anesthesia. Norwalk, Conn, Appleton-Century-Crofts, 1995, pp 52–53.
3. Waldman SD: Vagus nerve block. *In* Waldman SD (ed): Atlas of Interventional Pain Management Techniques. Philadelphia, WB Saunders, 1998, pp 76–79.
4. Bonica JJ: Neurolytic blockade. *In* Bonica JJ (ed): The Management of Pain, ed 2. Philadelphia, Lea & Febiger, 1990, pp 1996–1999.
5. Bonica JJ: General considerations of pain in the head. *In* Bonica JJ (ed): The Management of Pain, ed 2. Philadelphia, Lea & Febiger, 1990, pp 660–665.

CHAPTER • 27

Phrenic Nerve Block

Mark A. Greenfield, MD

The pain management consultant may be asked to evaluate a patient for phrenic nerve block. Blockade of the phrenic nerve, like other nerve blocks, is but one component of a multifaceted approach to the patient with acute or chronic pain syndromes. It may become a very useful treatment modality for patients who do not respond to other therapeutic interventions.

CLINICAL ANATOMY

The phrenic nerve, the most important branch of the cervical plexus, comprises the ventral roots of C3–C5, the principal component being the anterior primary ramus of C4. The three nerve roots join at the lateral border of the scalenus anterior muscle, and the phrenic nerve passes inferiorly between the omohyoid and sternocleidomastoid muscles. In 20% to 84% of patients, an accessory phrenic nerve arises from C5 and contributes to the phrenic nerve, joining the main nerve in the root of the neck or behind the clavicle.[1] In the phrenic nerve's course distally, it lies close to the internal mammary artery, the root of the lung, the pericardium, and the peritoneum. The superior and inferior sympathetic ganglia, the spinal accessory nerve, and the hypoglossal nerve also have communications with the phrenic nerve as it courses through the chest.

INDICATIONS

Phrenic nerve block can be useful in the diagnosis and treatment of intractable singultus (Latin for *sob* or *speech broken by sobbing*), or hiccups. Hiccups, while ubiquitous, serve no known physiologic function. *Persistent* hiccups are defined as an episode that lasts less than 1 month; *intractable* hiccups last longer than a month. Table 27–1 describes some of the complications of intractable hiccups.[2] Benign and persistent or intractable hiccups have different causes (Table 27–2).[3] Chronic idiopathic hiccups are believed to be attributable to central and peripheral mechanisms. It has been suggested that chronic hiccups may result from chronic stimulation of a central nervous system "hiccup center." The afferent limb of the hiccup reflex includes not only the phrenic nerve but also the vagus nerve and the sympathetic chain from T6 to T12.[4] This hiccup center is believed to comprise a complex association between several areas of the central nervous system. This includes the phrenic nerve nuclei, the brain stem, the respiratory center, the hypothalamus, and the medullary reticular formation. The primary efferent limb of this reflex is mediated by motor fibers of the phrenic nerve. Interestingly, the majority of hiccup spasms are unilateral and usually confined to the left hemidiaphragm.[5]

The ill-defined supraclavicular or scapular pain of diaphragmatic or subdiaphragmatic cancers may be elucidated or ameliorated by phrenic nerve block. This referred pain is known as *Kerr's sign* and often does not respond to direct tumor treatments.[6]

The pain management specialist must try to establish an underlying cause to guide therapeutic intervention. A targeted history and physical examination are essential first steps, followed by laboratory studies. The workup would also be expected to include magnetic resonance imaging (MRI) studies of the head, especially the posterior fossa and brain stem.[2, 7, 8] Imaging of the diaphragmatic and subdiaphragmatic regions should also be performed.

After identification and treatment of underlying causes, different therapies may be entertained. In 1932, Dr. C. W. Mayo said, in reference to the myriad of remedies and treatments for hiccups, "The amount of knowledge on any subject such as this can be considered as being in inverse proportion to the number of different treatments suggested and tried for it."[9] After nonpharmacologic, noninvasive therapies have been tried and found unsuccessful, drug therapy may be used. Table 27–3 lists several medications that have been utilized to treat hiccups.[7, 10–12]

PROCEDURE

The patient is placed supine with the head turned away from the side being blocked and is then asked to lift his or her head against resistance to identify the sternocleidomastoid muscle. The groove between the posterior border of the sternocleidomastoid muscle and the anterior scalene muscle then becomes palpable (Fig. 27–1).[13, 14] At a level

TABLE 27–1 Complications of Intractable Hiccups

Malnutrition
Cardiac dysrhythmias
Insomnia
Fatigue/exhaustion/dehydration
Gastroesophageal reflux
Weight loss
Death

1 inch above the clavicle, sterile preparation is performed. A 22-gauge, 1.5-inch block needle is inserted parallel to the scalene muscle with a slightly anterior trajectory (Fig. 27–2). At a depth of approximately 1 inch, and after gentle aspiration to identify blood or cerebrospinal fluid, 8 to 10 mL of local anesthetic is incrementally injected (infiltrated) along the anterior surface of the anterior scalene muscle. This nerve block is often done in a fanlike manner. Phrenic nerve block with local anesthetic may be used in a prognostic manner to evaluate the possibility of neurodestruction of the phrenic nerve by chemical neurolysis, cryoneurolysis, radiofrequency lesioning, phrenic nerve stimulation (diaphragmatic pacing), or surgical crushing of the nerve.[15] A depot steroid may be added to the local anesthetic for inflammation-associated pain that is mediated via the phrenic nerve.[6] A nerve stimulator with stimulation as low as 0.75 mA may be useful in this block to observe diaphragmatic contraction (via fluoroscopy or ultrasound).[16] The patient is then monitored closely for changes in vital signs (especially signs of respiratory compromise) and signs of local anesthetic toxicity and of inadvertent subarachnoid injection.

TABLE 27–2 Causes of Persistent or Intractable Hiccups

Idiopathic
Psychogenic
- Conversion reaction
- Malingering
- Hysterical neurosis
- Personality disorder

Organic
- Central nervous system
  - Neoplasm
  - Multiple sclerosis
  - Cerebrovascular accident
  - Trauma
- Peripheral nervous system (secondary to phrenic or vagus nerve irritation)
  - Renal (uremia) or hepatic disorders
  - Cancer (gastric, pancreatic, pulmonary)
  - Pericarditis
  - Intestinal obstruction/gastric distension
  - Tumors or cysts of neck
  - Hiatal hernia
- Drug-induced/metabolic
  - Intravenous steroids
  - Benzodiazepines, barbiturates
  - General anesthesia
  - Infection (sepsis, malaria, tuberculosis, influenza)
  - Electrolyte disturbances (hypocalcemia, hyponatremia)

TABLE 27–3 Pharmacologic Management of Hiccups

Drug	Class	Action
Chlorpromazine	Phenothiazine	Central
Haloperidol	Phenothiazine	Central
Amitriptyline	Tricyclic antidepressant	Central
Diphenylhydantoin	Anticonvulsant	Central
Valproic acid	Anticonvulsant	Central
Carbamazepine	Anticonvulsant	Central
Baclofen	GABAmimetic	Central
Gabapentin	Anticonvulsant	Central
Nifedipine	Calcium channel blocker	Central, peripheral
Nimodipine	Calcium channel blocker	Central, peripheral
Metoclopramide	Dopamine antagonist	Gastric emptying
Midazolam	Benzodiazepine	Central
Omperazole	Proton pump inhibitor	Suppress Gastric acid
Cisapride	Myenteric plexus activity	Facilitate gastric emptying

For further discussion, see references 13 and 14.

SIDE EFFECTS AND COMPLICATIONS

The proximity of several major blood vessels to the phrenic nerve may produce local anesthetic toxicity from intravascular uptake or inadvertent intravascular injection.[17] In addition, this region's vascularity may result in hematoma and/or ecchymosis. While many of these vessels may be available to direct pressure to control bleeding, bleeding

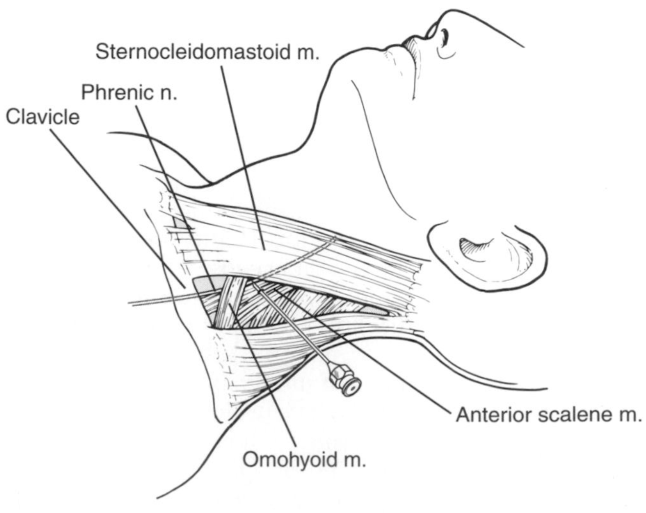

FIGURE 27–1 Relationship of the phrenic nerve to the muscles of the neck.

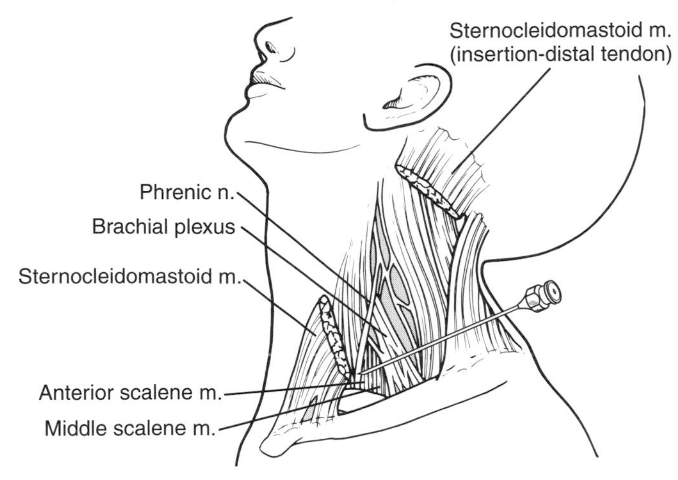

FIGURE 27–2 *Needle placement for phrenic nerve block.*

of the subclavian vessels may be difficult to control. Manual pressure to the area blocked and application of ice packs after the nerve block is performed decrease bleeding or ecchymosis. Ice packs applied at 20-minute intervals may also be useful in limiting these side effects or complications.

With injection of the phrenic nerve, unilateral diaphragmatic paralysis is expected. Unilateral paralysis of the diaphragm may lead to a 37% reduction in total lung capacity. Maximal voluntary ventilation and vital capacity may be decreased by 20%.[18] This reduction in lung function may be exacerbated by spread of the local anesthetic solution to the recurrent laryngeal nerve and associated hoarseness secondary to vocal cord paralysis and difficulty clearing secretions.

The phrenic nerve also lies close to central neuraxial structures. Should the needle be placed too deep, unintended subarachnoid or epidural block could result. The consequences of either block could be significant sensory and motor block and marked respiratory compromise, or even cardiopulmonary arrest.

Other possible complications of phrenic nerve block are infection and pneumothorax. Horner's syndrome may be produced by spread of local anesthetic to the sympathetic ganglia. Left phrenic nerve block carries a risk of injury to the thoracic duct and, possibly, formation of a chylothorax.

CONCLUSIONS

Phrenic nerve block is a useful diagnostic and therapeutic tool. The primary indications are chronic hiccups refractory to other nonpharmacologic and pharmacologic interventions. Phrenic nerve block may provide the pain management physician with useful information for the diagnosis and treatment of chronic shoulder or supraclavicular pain mediated by diaphragmatic or subdiaphragmatic processes. Careful attention to the clinically relevant anatomy should minimize side effects and complications and promote symptomatic relief.

REFERENCES

1. Fodstad H, Nilsson S: Intractable singultus: A diagnostic and therapeutic challenge. Br J Neurosurg 7:255–260, 1993.
2. Rousseau P: Hiccups. South Med J 2:175–181, 1995.
3. Petroianu G: Idiopathic chronic hiccup (ICH): Phrenic nerve block is not the way to go. Anesthesiology 5:1284–1285, 1998.
4. Lewis JH: Hiccups: Causes and cures. J Clin Gastroenterol 7:539–552, 1985.
5. Kolodzik PW, Eilers MA: Hiccups: Review and approach to management. Ann Emerg Med 20:565–573, 1991.
6. Waldman SD: *In* Waldman SD (ed): Atlas of Interventional Pain Management. Philadelphia, WB Saunders, 1998, pp 83–85.
7. Petroianu G, Hein G, Petroianu A, et al: ETICS study: Empirical therapy of idiopathic chronic singultus. Z Gastroenterol 36:559–566, 1998.
8. Williamson BW: Management of intractable hiccup. Br Med J 2:501–503, 1977.
9. Mayo CW: Hiccup. Surg Gynecol Obstet 55:700–708, 1932.
10. Friedman NL: Hiccups: A treatment review. Pharmacotherapy 6:986–995, 1996.
11. Hernandez JL, Fernandez-Miera MF, Sampedro I, et al: Nimodipine treatment for intractable hiccups. Am J Med 106:600, 1999.
12. Quigley C: Nifedipine for hiccups. J Pain Symptom Manage 13:313, 1997.
13. Walker P, Watanabe S, Bruera E: Baclofen, a treatment for chronic hiccup. J Pain Symptom Manage 16:125–132, 1998.
14. Wilcock A, Twycross R: Midazolam for intractable hiccup. J Pain Symptom Manage 12:59–61, 1996.
15. Fodstad H, Blom S: Phrenic nerve stimulation (diaphragm pacing) in chronic singultus. Neurochirurgia (Stuttg) 27:115–116, 1984.
16. Okuda Y, Kitajima T, Asai T: Use of a nerve stimulator for phrenic nerve block in treatment of hiccups. Anesthesiology 88:525–527, 1998.
17. Bonica JJ: Regional analgesia with local anesthetics. *In* Bonica JJ (ed): The Management of Pain. Philadelphia, Lea & Febiger, 1990, pp 1903–1904.
18. Baum GL: Neurologic diseases. *In* Baum GL, Wolinsky PMD (eds): Textbook of Pulmonary Diseases. Orlando, 1994, pp 1673–1674.

CHAPTER • 28

Spinal Accessory Nerve Block

Steven D. Waldman, MD, JD

HISTORICAL CONSIDERATIONS

Historically, spinal accessory nerve block was utilized primarily to treat the cervical dystonias. A mainstay in the treatment of spasmodic torticollis, blockade of the spinal accessory nerve has in large part been replaced by botulinum toxin, favored for its long duration of action and safety. Electromyographic guidance has further increased the efficacy and safety of the botulinum toxin technique.[1]

INDICATIONS

Spinal accessory nerve block is useful in the diagnosis and treatment of spasm of the sternocleidomastoid and trapezius muscles.[2] It is occasionally useful diagnostically to determine whether such spasms are mediated via the spinal accessory nerve[1] and is utilized prognostically with local anesthetic before destruction of the spinal accessory nerve for the palliation of spastic conditions of the sternocleidomastoid or trapezius.[3] Neurodestruction of the spinal accessory nerve may be achieved by chemical or cryoneurolysis, radiofrequency lesioning, or surgical crushing or resection of the nerve.[2,3]

CLINICALLY RELEVANT ANATOMY

The spinal accessory nerve arises from the nucleus ambiguus. The nerve has two roots, which leave the cranium together along with the vagus nerve via the jugular foramen.[4] The fibers of the spinal root pass inferiorly and posteriorly to provide motor innervation to the superior portion of the sternocleidomastoid muscle. The spinal accessory exits the posterior border of the sternocleidomastoid in the upper third of the muscle. The nerve, in combination with the cervical plexus provides innervation to the trapezius muscle.

TECHNIQUE

The patient is placed supine with the head turned away from the side to be blocked. A total of 10 mL of local anesthetic is drawn up into a 20-mL sterile syringe. For conditions mediated via the spinal accessory nerve that are thought to have an inflammatory component, a total of 80 mg of depot steroid is added to the local anesthetic with the first block and 40 mg with subsequent blocks.[2]

The patient is then asked to raise his or her head against the resistance of the pain specialist's hand to help to identify the posterior border of the sternocleidomastoid muscle. The posterior border of the upper third of the muscle is then identified. At a point just behind the posterior border of the upper third, after preparation of the skin with antiseptic solution, a 1.5-inch needle is inserted with a slightly anterior trajectory (Fig. 28–1). When the needle has been inserted to a depth of approximately 3/4 inch, gentle aspiration is applied to identify blood or cerebrospinal fluid. If the aspiration test is negative and no paresthesia into the brachial plexus is elicited, 10 mL of solution is slowly injected in a fan configuration while the patient is monitored closely for signs of local anesthetic toxicity or inadvertent subarachnoid injection.

SIDE EFFECTS AND COMPLICATIONS

The proximity of the spinal accessory nerve to the external jugular vein and other large vessels creates the potential for inadvertent intravascular injection or local anesthetic toxicity from intravascular absorption.[2,3] The pain specialist should carefully calculate the total (milligram) dose of local anesthetic that may safely be given. This vascularity also gives rise to an increased incidence of postblock ecchymosis and hematoma formation. In spite of the vascularity of this anatomic region, the technique can safely be performed in patients taking anticoagulants by utilizing a 25- or 27-gauge needle, albeit with increased risk of hematoma, if the clinical situation dictates a favorable risk-benefit ratio. The risk of these complications can be decreased by applying manual pressure to the area of the block immediately after the injection. Cold packs applied for 20-minute periods after the block also reduce postprocedure pain and bleeding.

In addition to the potential for complications involving the vasculature, the proximity of the spinal accessory nerve

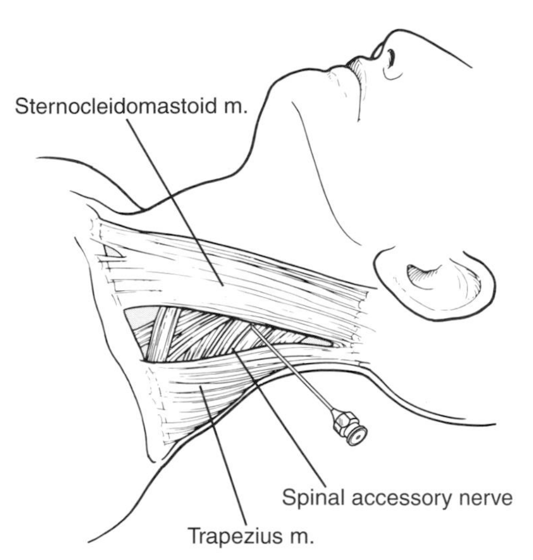

FIGURE 28–1 *Needle placement for spinal accessory nerve block.*

to the central neuroaxial structures and the phrenic nerve carries risk of side effects and complications. If the needle is placed too deep, inadvertent epidural, subdural, or subarachnoid injection is a possibility. If the local anesthetic utilized for this block is accidentally placed in any of these spaces, significant motor and sensory block results. Unrecognized, these complications could be fatal. Blockade of the phrenic nerve may occur during blockade of the spinal accessory nerve. In the absence of significant pulmonary disease, unilateral phrenic nerve block should rarely create respiratory embarrassment; although, blockade of the recurrent laryngeal nerve with the attendant vocal cord paralysis, combined with paralysis of the diaphragm, may make clearing of pulmonary and upper airway secretions difficult. Blockade of the vagus and glossopharyngeal nerves can also occur during spinal accessory nerve block.[1]

CLINICAL PEARLS

The cause of a spastic condition of the cervical musculature should be ascertained before spinal accessory nerve block is performed. Demyelinating disease and cervical dystonias (including spasmodic torticollis and posterior fossa and brain stem tumors) must be ruled out. The workup should include magnetic resonance studies of the head, with special attention to the posterior fossa and brain stem, electromyography, and, if indicated, trimodal evoked potentials. Laboratory testing for the inflammatory myopathies and the collagen vascular diseases should be considered, as the clinical situation dictates.

Botulinum toxin administered under electromyographic guidance may allow better control of the amount of muscle weakness produced when treating spasticity of the cervical musculature (as compared with neurodestructive procedures to the spinal accessory nerve).

REFERENCES

1. Waldman SD: Vagus nerve block. *In* Waldman SD (ed): Atlas of Interventional Pain Management Techniques. Philadelphia, WB Saunders, 1998, pp 76–79.
2. Katz J: Vagus nerve block. *In* Katz J (ed): Atlas of Regional Anesthesia. Norwalk, Conn, Appleton-Century-Crofts, 1995, pp 52–53.
3. Bonica JJ: Neurolytic blockade. *In* Bonica JJ (ed): The Management of Pain, ed 2. Philadelphia, Lea & Febiger, 1990, pp 1996–1999.
4. Pitkin GP: Anatomy of the cranial nerves. *In* Pitkin GP (ed): Conduction Anesthesia. Philadelphia, JB Lippincott, 1946, pp 56–57.

CHAPTER • 29

Cervical Plexus Blockade

John L. Pappas, MD • Carol A. Warfield, MD

HISTORY

Cervical plexus blocks were first performed by Halsted at Bellevue Hospital in New York in 1884.[1–3] He performed many experiments with the new anesthetic cocaine, including one that demonstrated that excellent surgical anesthesia could be obtained by injecting the nerve trunks in the neck. The first description of cervical plexus blockade for surgical anesthesia was published in Germany in 1912 by Kappis,[4] who advocated a posterior approach. Two years later, Heidenhein[5] introduced the lateral approach to cervical plexus blockade. These techniques were popularized in France by Pauchet and in America by Labat.[1]

The posterior approach has never achieved widespread acceptance except as an alternative to the lateral approach. Through the years, many modifications of the lateral approach have been described. Most have altered the position of the primary line that connects the tip of the mastoid process to the anterior tubercle of C6. The change in position is intended to place the primary line more precisely over the tips of the cervical transverse processes.[2] Other methods of cervical plexus blockade have included a single-injection technique and a technique that uses the angle of the mandible and the thyroid notch as topographic landmarks to improve the success rate of the block.[1, 3, 6–8] Both the lateral and the posterior approach to cervical plexus blockade are described here.

INDICATIONS

Cervical plexus blockade has a variety of indications. Because it can be performed easily in a supine patient, almost any patient is a candidate. Surgical procedures in the anterior and lateral neck and supraclavicular fossa can be performed using either superficial or deep cervical plexus blocks.[3, 7]

Superficial cervical plexus blockade provides surface anesthesia of the neck but not muscle relaxation. It is important to realize that superficial blockade provides the same sensory (dermatome) anesthesia as deep cervical plexus block, which simply incorporates the motor component of the cervical plexus at the nerve roots before the sensory and motor aspects separate.[9] It is therefore useful in procedures in which retraction of the major muscles of the neck is not required, such as cervical fat pad biopsy, lymph node biopsy, plastic procedures, and superficial surgical procedures in the neck.[8, 9] Some have even advocated superficial cervical plexus blocks for carotid artery surgery to avoid the potential complications of deep cervical plexus blockade.[10–12] For adequate anesthesia, however, it may also be necessary to inject local anesthetic under the carotid sheath, under the adventitia of the carotid bifurcation, and into the superior angle of the incision.

Deep cervical plexus blockade provides anesthesia of the deep and superficial branches of the cervical plexus, because the nerve roots are anesthetized before the motor and sensory components separate. Thus, the deep block anesthetizes not only all the sensory components of the cervical plexus but also the muscles that arise and insert on the corresponding cervical vertebrae and transverse processes of C2–C4.[9]

Practically any procedure involving the anterior or lateral aspect of the neck may be performed with this technique: dissections of the neck; excision of masses, tumors, thyroglossal cysts, or branchial cysts; operations on the thyroid, parathyroid, or lymph glands; operations on the trachea and larynx; and operations on the blood vessels, including ligations of the carotid and lingual arteries and carotid endarterectomy.[1, 6]

Most of these procedures require only unilateral blockade of the deep cervical plexus. Bilateral blockade is advocated, however, for any operative procedure that extends to within 0.5 inch of the midline of the neck.[1] Such procedures include thyroidectomy and excision of the lymphatic glands of the neck. During thyroidectomy, in spite of the depth of anesthesia after bilateral blockade, traction on the gland is felt as choking, so intravenous sedation is required.[6] In addition, bilateral blockade causes bilateral phrenic nerve paresis and carries the potential for respiratory compromise.

Carotid endarterectomies are perhaps the most common procedures performed with cervical plexus blockade. Most clinicians who use regional anesthetic techniques for these procedures advocate performing both superficial and deep cervical plexus blockade to ensure a high success rate, owing to the difficulties of establishing general anesthesia and endotracheal intubation with an open wound in the neck.

Several studies have compared general anesthesia with regional anesthesia for carotid endarterectomy. Most cited the value of direct assessment of central nervous system function in the awake patient and the ability to assess the need for vascular shunting as the major advantages of regional anesthesia.[13–19]

Cervical plexus blocks are also performed for relief of pain in the neck and occiput secondary to pharyngeal cancer and metastatic lesions and for occipital and posterior auricular neuralgias associated with acute inflammation or compression of the cervical plexus by tumors or aneurysms.[3, 17–21]

Deep cervical plexus blockade, especially bilateral blockade of the fourth cervical nerve, is quite useful for relief of hiccups. The success of the block may be determined during fluoroscopy, which should demonstrate bilateral diaphragmatic paresis. Although the paresis is temporary, permanent relief may be afforded by breaking the hiccup cycle.[3, 6]

CONTRAINDICATIONS

There are no specific contraindications to cervical plexus blockade aside from those to regional blocks in general, such as coagulopathy, infection at the site of the block, a history of allergy to local anesthetics, and patient refusal.[7] Significant respiratory disease is a relative contraindication, especially to bilateral cervical plexus block, because of the potential for blockade of the phrenic nerve, which can cause diaphragmatic paralysis.

ANATOMY OF THE CERVICAL PLEXUS

The cervical plexus is formed by the anterior primary division of the first four cervical nerves. The anterior and posterior roots of cervical nerves C2–C4 emerge from the spinal canal through their respective intervertebral foramina. The first cervical nerve, the suboccipital nerve, emerges between the occipital bone and the posterior arch of the atlas. The posterior sensory root of this nerve is much smaller than the anterior motor root and may be entirely absent (Fig. 29–1).[1]

After the mixed nerves are formed by the union of the anterior and posterior roots, they divide into anterior and posterior primary divisions. The exception is the first cervi-

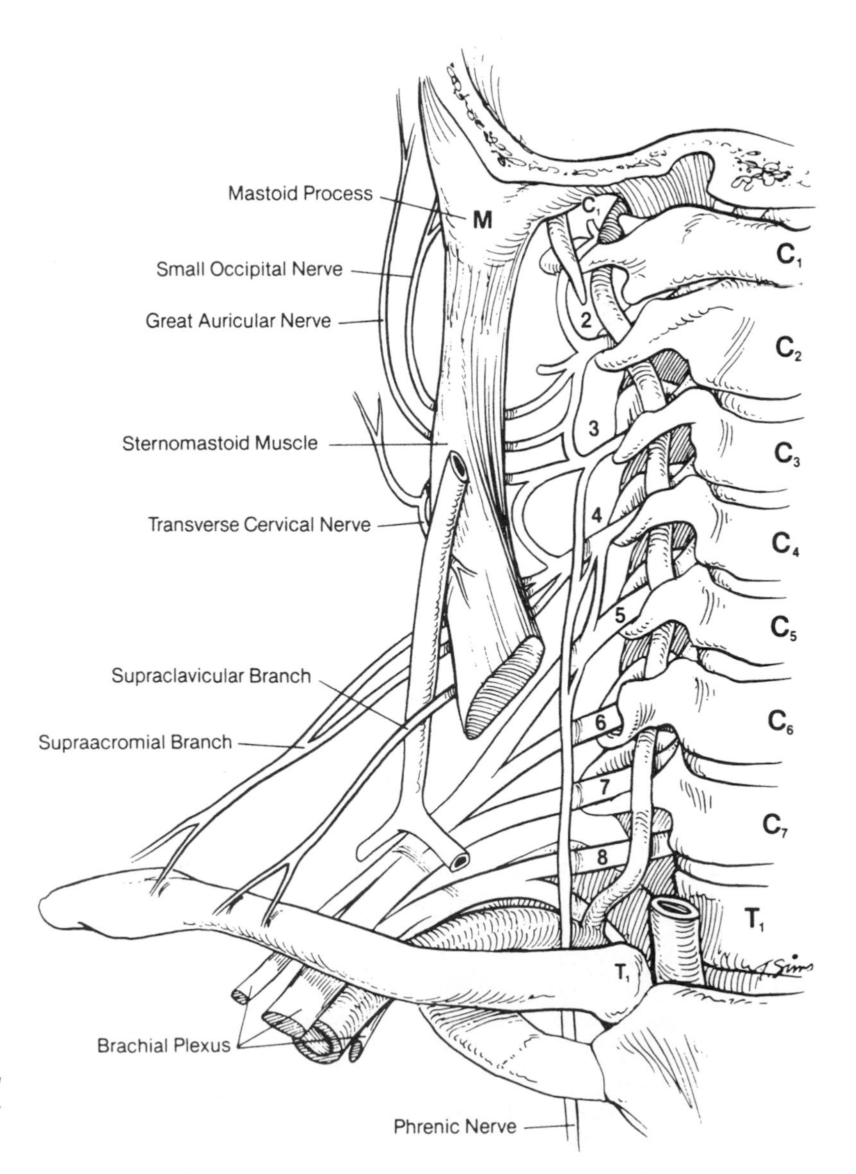

FIGURE 29–1 Formation of the cervical plexus and its branches (From Pai U, Raj P: Peripheral nerve blocks: Cervical plexus. In *Raj P (ed): Handbook of Regional Anesthesia. New York, Churchill Livingstone, 1985, pp 163–167.)*

cal nerve, which seldom has an anterior division. Because the first cervical nerve is composed almost exclusively of motor fibers to the muscles of the suboccipital triangle and only rarely has any significant sensory component, it is usually unnecessary to block this nerve.

After exiting the intervertebral foramina, the anterior primary rami of C2–C4 pass in an anterocaudolateral direction behind the vertebral artery and vein, in the gutter formed by the anterior and posterior tubercles of the corresponding transverse processes of the cervical vertebrae (Fig. 29–2).[3, 22] The tubercles of the transverse processes lie 0.5 inch (1.3 cm) to 1.25 inches (3.2 cm) below the skin, depending on the size of the patient and the cervical level. The lower cervical tubercles are more superficial than the tubercles of the upper cervical transverse processes.[23] The anterior tubercles are located farther cephalad and medial than the posterior tubercles.[1]

The first cervical nerve passes under the vertebral artery in its relationship to the posterior arch of the atlas and is held in place by a fibrous tunnel.[1] The anterior primary rami of C2–C4 are also held firmly on the transverse process by a fibrous tunnel. After leaving the transverse processes, these nerves are enclosed in a perineural space formed by the muscles and tendons attached to the anterior and posterior tubercles of their respective cervical vertebrae. The muscles and tendons of the anterior tubercles are the longus colli, the longus capitis, and the scalenus anterior. Those attached to the posterior tubercles are the scalenus medius, the scalenus cervicis, and the longissimus cervicis.[1, 2] As the prevertebral fascia moves laterally and splits to invest these muscles and tendons, it forms a closed fascial space that is a superior extension of the interscalene space (Fig. 29–3).[2] The fascia investing the muscles and tendons that lie anterior and posterior to the cervical plexus provides an envelope around the plexus, which can serve as a perineural sheath and provides the basis for a single-injection technique to block the cervical plexus.[2]

Within the perineural sheath, the anterior primary rami of C2–C4 divide into ascending and descending branches forming a series of three loops known as the *cervical plexus* (Fig. 29–4).[2, 3, 23, 24] The cervical plexus, which lies lateral to the upper four cervical vertebrae and anterior to the levator scapulae muscle and the middle scalene muscle, is covered by the sternocleidomastoid muscle. Each loop gives rise to a superficial and a deep branch. It is this anatomic separation that enables the sensory branches of the cervical plexus, via the superficial branches, to be blocked selectively without any motor blockade in the neck.

The superficial branches of the cervical plexus pierce the deep fascia of the neck approximately at the middle of the posterior margin of the sternocleidomastoid muscle, just below the emergence of the accessory nerve. Then they

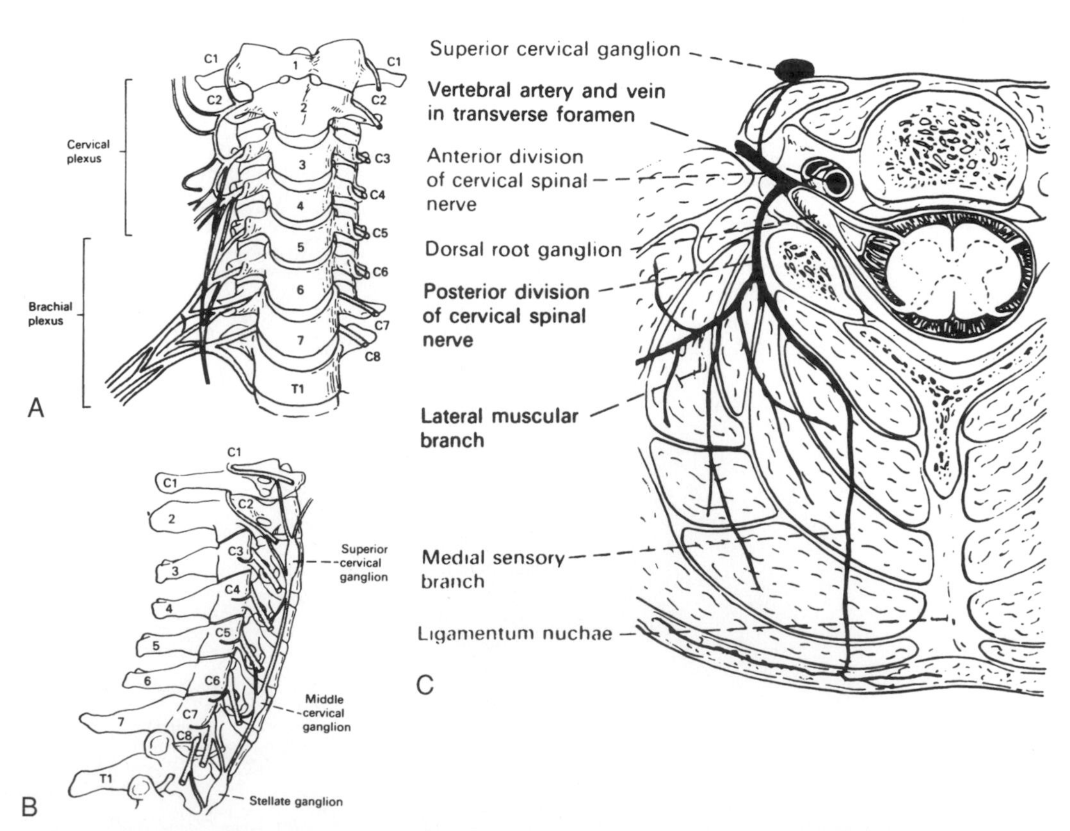

FIGURE 29–2 Cervical and first thoracic spinal nerves. A, Anterior view showing the formation of the cervical and brachial plexus. B, Lateral view showing the course and relation of the cervical nerves and the cervical sympathetic chain. C, Cross section of the third cervical segment showing the course and distribution of the posterior primary division with its medial branch passing posteriorly to supply the skin and subcutaneous structures and the lateral branch supplying the muscles. Also shown is a cross section of the superior cervical ganglion and its connection to the nerve by the white ramus communicans. Note the vertebral vessels just anterior to the nerves. (From Bonica JJ: The Management of Pain, ed 2. Philadelphia, Lea & Febiger, 1990, pp 823–825.)

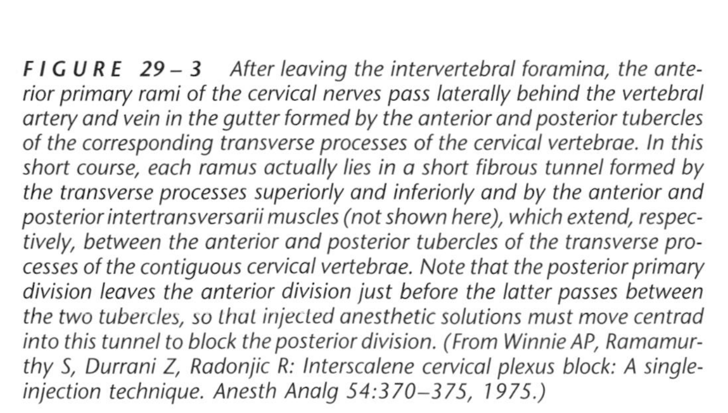
FIGURE 29–3 After leaving the intervertebral foramina, the anterior primary rami of the cervical nerves pass laterally behind the vertebral artery and vein in the gutter formed by the anterior and posterior tubercles of the corresponding transverse processes of the cervical vertebrae. In this short course, each ramus actually lies in a short fibrous tunnel formed by the transverse processes superiorly and inferiorly and by the anterior and posterior intertransversarii muscles (not shown here), which extend, respectively, between the anterior and posterior tubercles of the transverse processes of the contiguous cervical vertebrae. Note that the posterior primary division leaves the anterior division just before the latter passes between the two tubercles, so that injected anesthetic solutions must move centrad into this tunnel to block the posterior division. (From Winnie AP, Ramamurthy S, Durrani Z, Radonjic R: Interscalene cervical plexus block: A single-injection technique. Anesth Analg 54:370–375, 1975.)

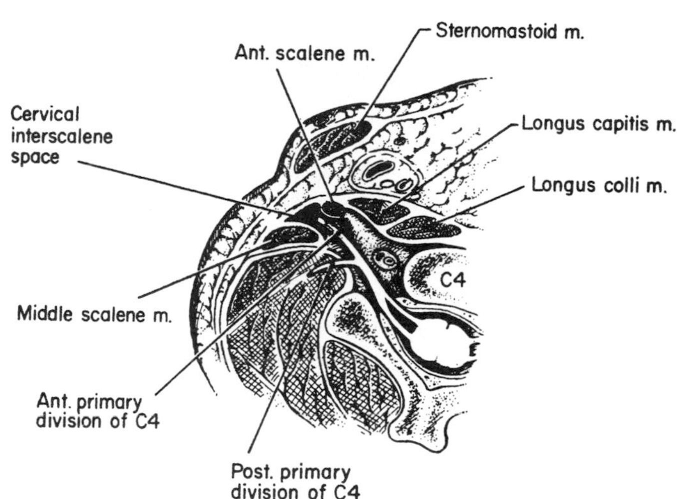

curve around the posterior border of the muscle and proceed to supply the skin and superficial fascia of the head, neck, and shoulder (Figs. 29–5, 29–6). The ascending branches (small occipital and great auricular nerves) supply the occipitomastoid region of the head, the auricle of the ear, and the parotid gland; the transverse branch (superficial cervical) innervates the anterior part of the neck between the lower border of the jaw and the sterum; and the descending branches (suprasternal, supraclavicular, and supraacromial) supply the shoulder and upper pectoral region (Fig. 29–7).[6, 7, 21, 24]

The deep cervical plexus supplies mainly the deep structures of the anterior and lateral neck and sends branches to the phrenic nerve (Fig. 29–8). It also contributes to the hypoglossal loop.[3, 6] One group of nerve branches, the lateral (external) group, proceeds from beneath the sternocleidomastoid muscle in a posterolateral direction toward the posterior triangle. This group provides muscular branches to the scalenus medius, sternocleidomastoid, trapezius, and levator scapulae muscles. The medial (ventral) group runs medially and forward to the anterior triangle. It provides muscular branches to the rectus capitis lateralis and rectus capitis anterior, longus capitis, and longus colli muscles, and to the diaphragm via the phrenic nerve. By means of the ansa hypoglossi, it also innervates the thyrohyoid, geniohyoid, omohyoid, sternothyroid, and sternohyoid muscles (Fig. 29–9).[3, 6, 24]

The cervical plexus communicates with the sympathetic chain in the neck by means of rami communicantes. Sympathetic fibers do not accompany the spinal nerves from their origin in the cord. Instead, they are derived from the superior, middle, and inferior (stellate) cervical

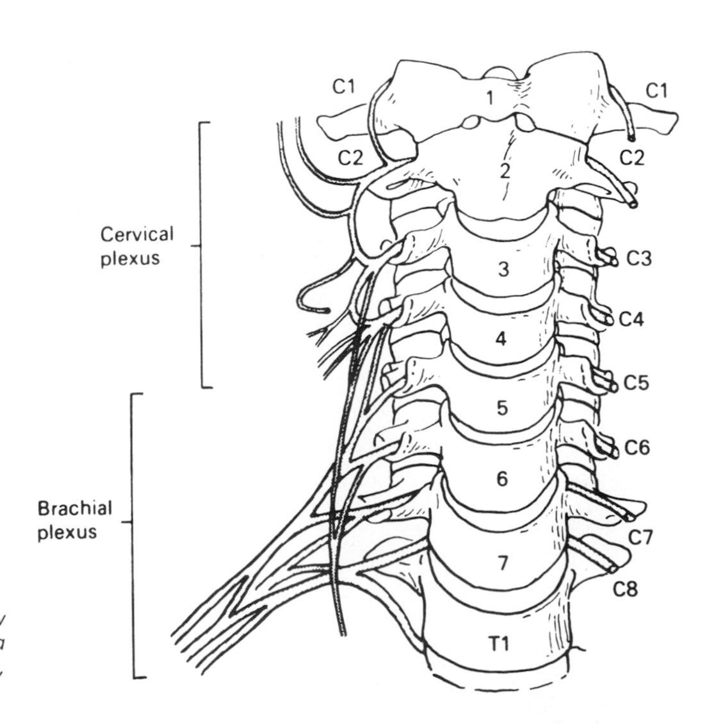

FIGURE 29–4 Cervical and first thoracic spinal nerves. Anterior view showing the formation of the cervical and brachial plexus. (From Bonica JJ: The Management of Pain, ed 2. Philadelphia, Lea & Febiger, 1990, pp 823–825.)

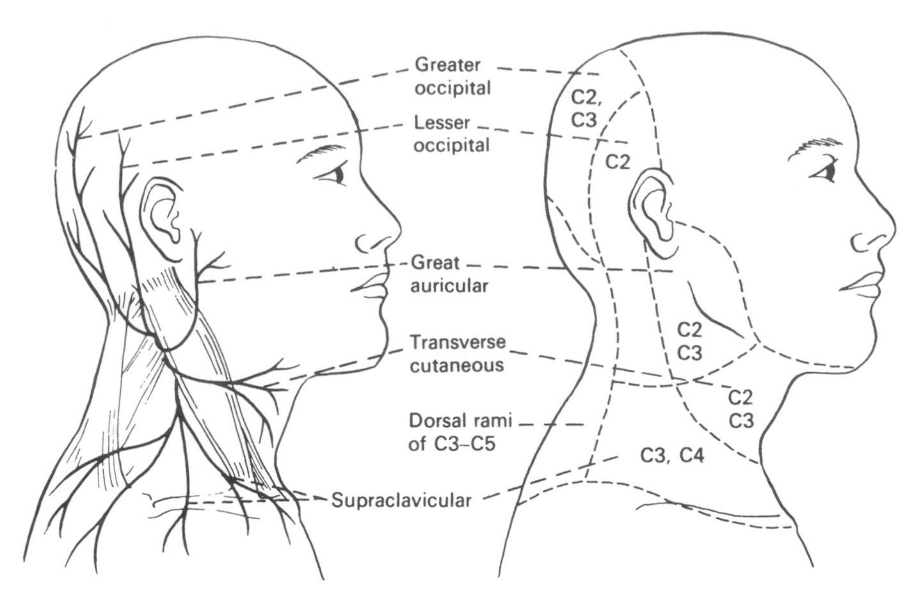

FIGURE 29–5 *Cutaneous nerves derived from the cervical plexus. (From Bonica JJ: The Management of Pain, ed 2. Philadelphia, Lea & Febiger, 1990, pp 823–825.)*

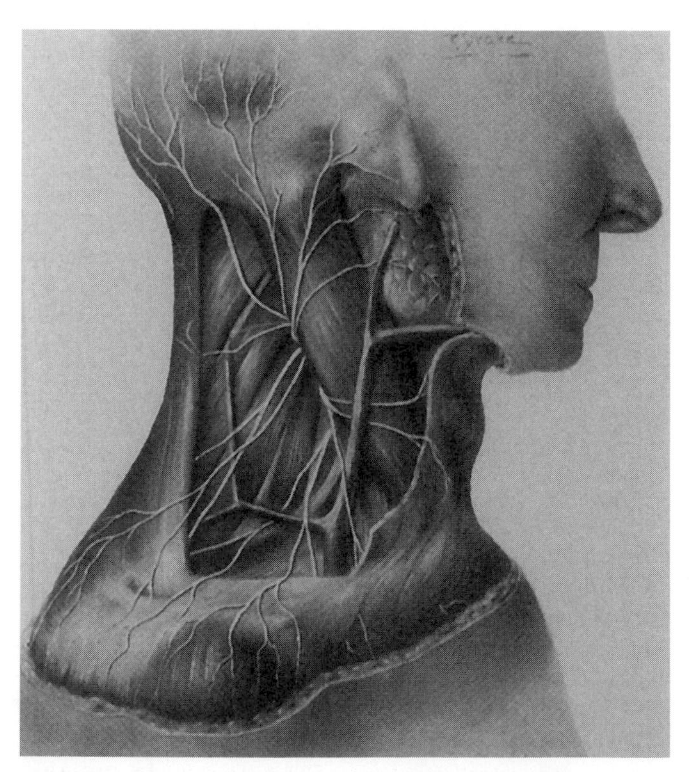

FIGURE 29–6 *Superficial branches of the cervical plexus at their points of emergence on the posterior margin of the sternocleidomastoid muscle. (From Adriani J: Labat's Regional Anesthesia: Techniques and Clinical Applications, ed 3. Philadelphia: WB Saunders, 1967, pp 180–195.)*

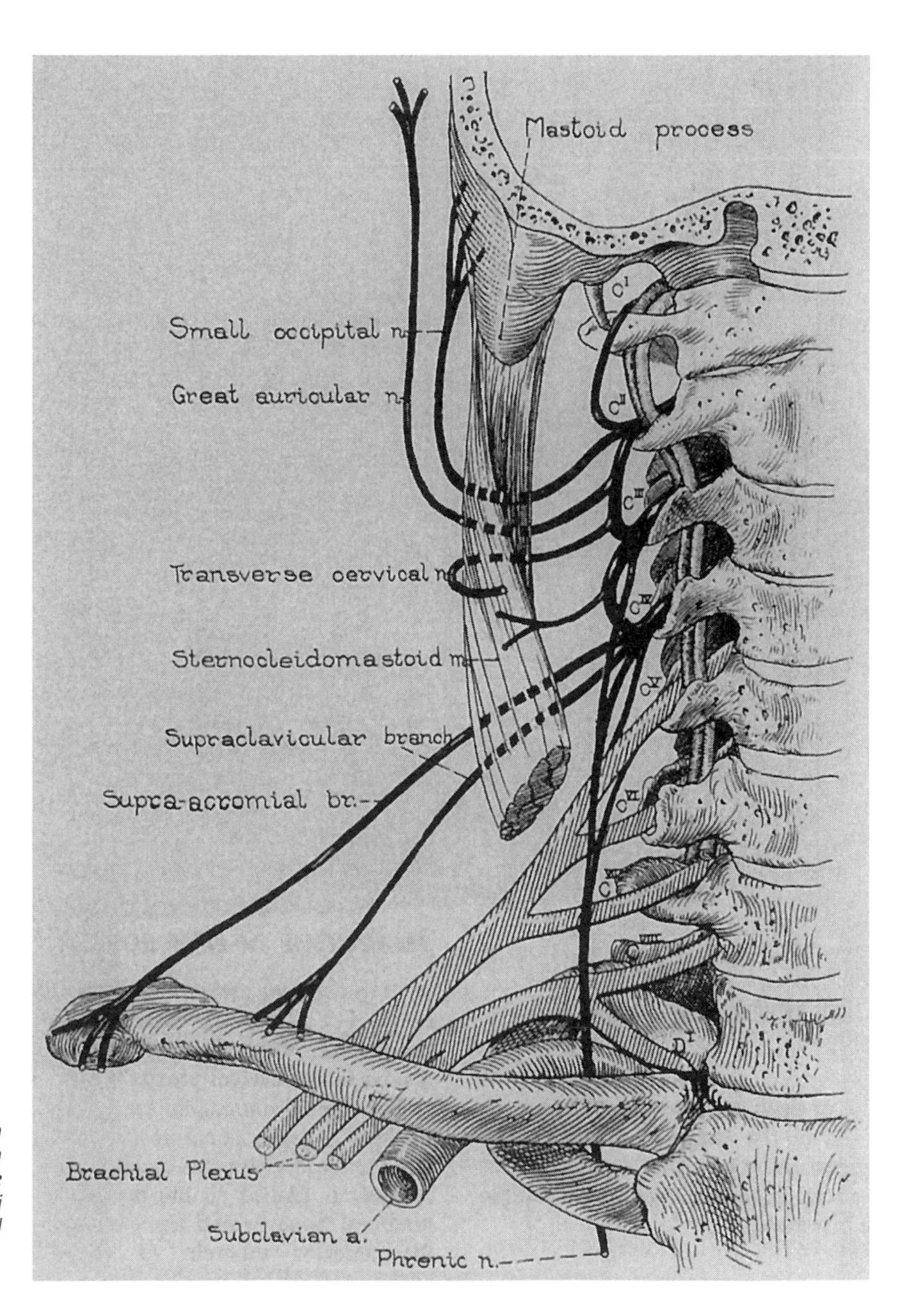

FIGURE 29–7 *Semischematic representation of the cervical plexus and the phrenic nerve shown in relation to the transverse processes, which are threaded by the vertebral blood vessels. (From Adriani J: Labat's Regional Anesthesia: Techniques and Clinical Applications, ed 3. Philadelphia, WB Saunders, 1967, pp 180–195.)*

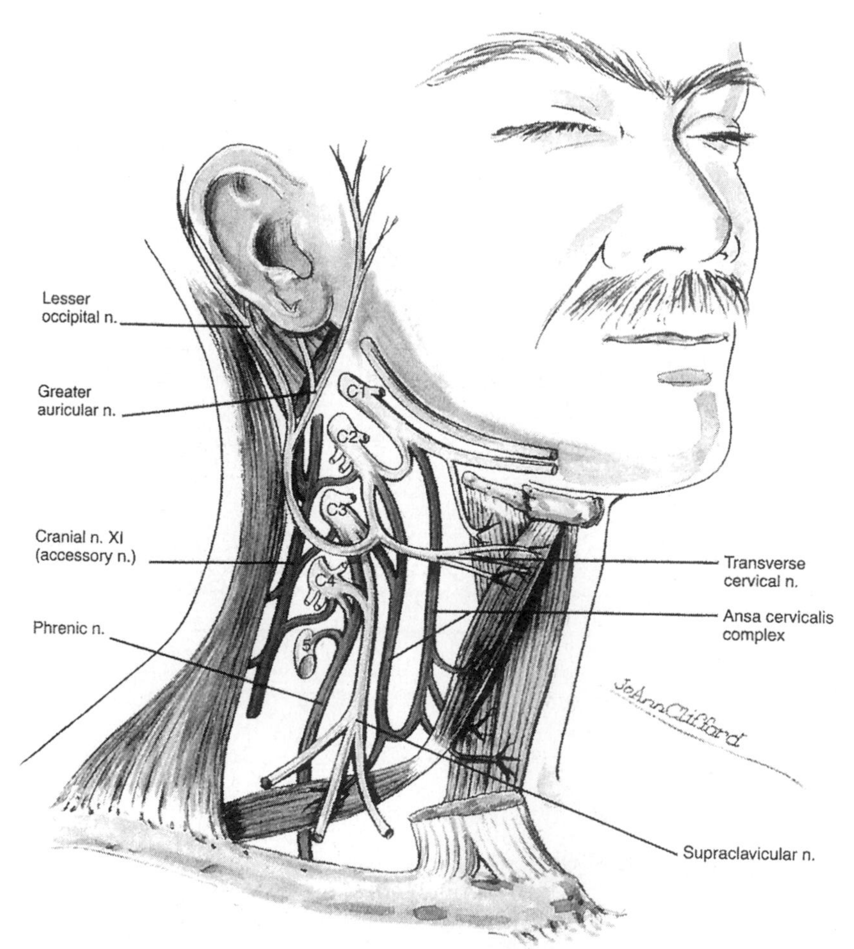

FIGURE 29–8 *Cervical plexus functional anatomy—ventral rami of C1, 2, 3, 4. (From Brown DL: Atlas of Regional Anesthesia. Philadelphia, WB Saunders, 1992, pp 165–170.)*

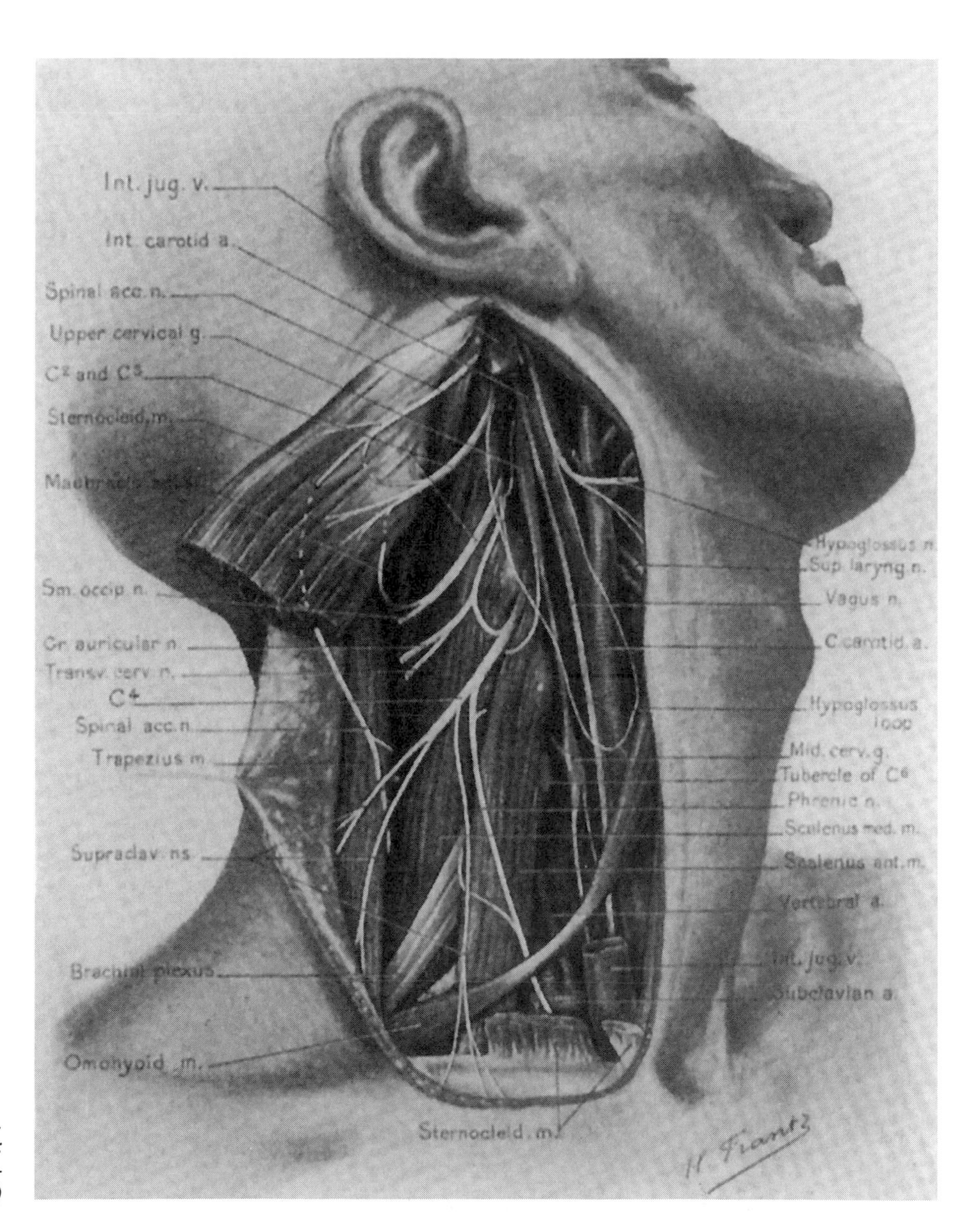

FIGURE 29–9 *The cervical plexus. (From Adriani J: Labat's Regional Anesthesia: Techniques and Clinical Applications, ed 3. Philadelphia, WB Saunders, 1967, pp 180–195.)*

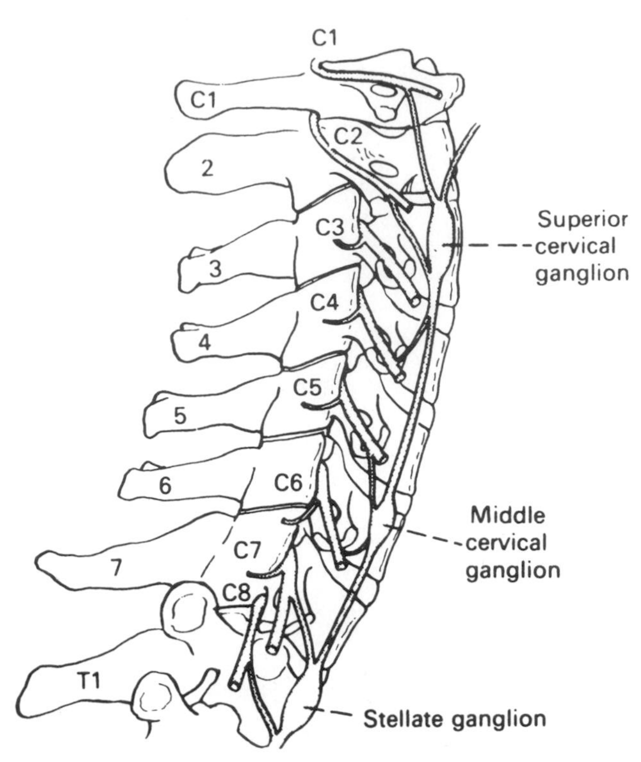

FIGURE 29–10 Cervical and first thoracic spinal nerves. Lateral view showing the course and relation of the cervical nerves and the cervical sympathetic chain. (From Bonica JJ: The Management of Pain, ed 2. Philadelphia, Lea & Febiger, 1990, pp 823–825.)

ganglia (Fig. 29–10).[6,24] The cervical plexus also communicates with the vagus, hypoglossal, and accessory cervical nerves.[24] These communications may explain some of the side effects often seen with cervical plexus blockade.

CLINICAL PEARLS AND TRICKS OF THE TRADE

The choice of a superficial or deep cervical plexus block, or both, is based on the surgical procedure and the desired extent of anesthesia. Only one technique has been described for superficial blockade, whereas multiple techniques are available for deep blockade.

Technique of Superficial Block

Superficial cervical plexus blockade provides the same sensory (dermatome) anesthesia as the deep cervical plexus block, which also incorporates the motor component of the cervical plexus at the nerve roots before the sensory and motor branches separate.[9] The patient is placed in the supine position with the head turned away from the side to be blocked. The patient may be asked to raise the head slightly to better outline the border of the sternocleidomastoid muscle midway between its origin on the clavicle and its insertion on the mastoid. This is also the point where the external jugular vein crosses the posterior border of the sternocleidomastoid muscle (Fig. 29–11).

Superficial cervical plexus blockade requires a sufficient volume of local anesthetic to be effective. A 22-gauge, 4-cm or a 25-gauge, 1-inch needle is inserted subcutane-

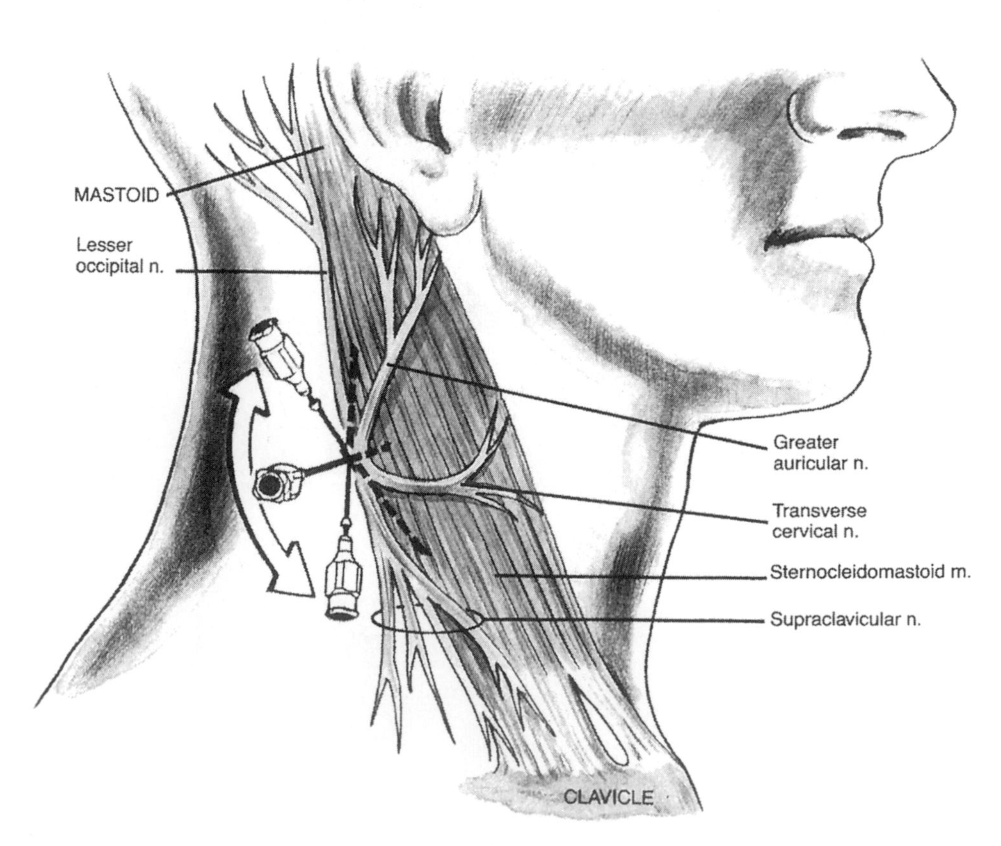

FIGURE 29–11 Superficial cervical plexus block—anatomy and technique. (From Brown DL: Atlas of Regional Anesthesia. Philadelphia: WB Saunders, 1992, pp 165–170.)

ously immediately posterior and deep to the midpoint of the sternocleidomastoid muscle. Then, approximately 5 mL of local anesthetic is injected at this midpoint. The needle is redirected both superiorly and inferiorly along the posterior border of the sternocleidomastoid muscle, and approximately 5 mL of local anesthetic is injected along each of these sites for a total of 15 mL of local anesthetic (Fig. 29–12).[8,21,22,25] Paresthesias are not sought. This injection produces cutaneous analgesia of the neck from the mandible to the clavicle anteriorly and laterally (Fig. 29–13).[21]

Technique of Deep Block

Deep cervical plexus blockade anesthetizes all of the sensory components of the cervical plexus and the muscles that arise and insert on the corresponding cervical vertebrae and transverse processes of C2–C4. If this deep cervical plexus is blocked close to the lateral edges of the transverse processes, the nerve roots are anesthetized before the motor and sensory components separate. This is one of the primary differences between deep and superficial cervical plexus blocks.[9] A deep cervical plexus block is a paravertebral nerve block of C2–C4 as the nerves emerge from the foramina in the cervical vertebrae. The patient is in the same position as for superficial cervical plexus block.

The lateral route, also known as the Heidenhein or Labat method, is the most often described, because the superficial landmarks for this technique are numerous and reliable. A mark is placed on the tip of the mastoid process of the temporal bone behind the ear. A second mark is placed on the anterior tubercle of the C6 transverse process, Chassaignac's tubercle, at the level of the cricoid cartilage. The most prominent cervical transverse process, C6, may be felt by deep palpation between the trachea and carotid sheath at the level of the cricoid cartilage. A straight line, known as the primary line, is drawn between these two marks to indicate the position of the cervical transverse processes. Some advocate drawing this line parallel and

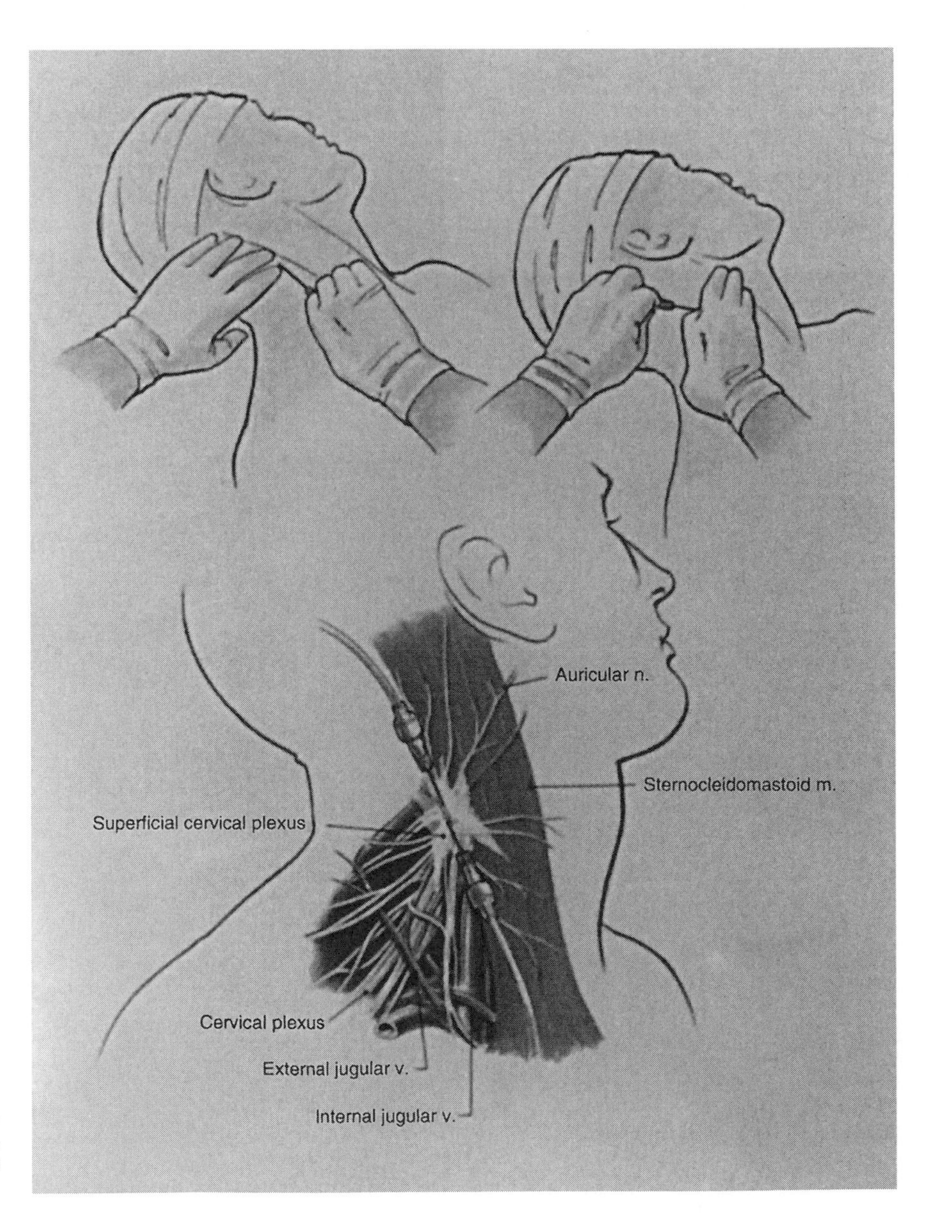

FIGURE 29–12 Superficial cervical plexus. (From Katz J: Atlas of Regional Anesthesia, ed 2. Norwalk, Conn: Appleton and Lange, 1994, pp 40–43.)

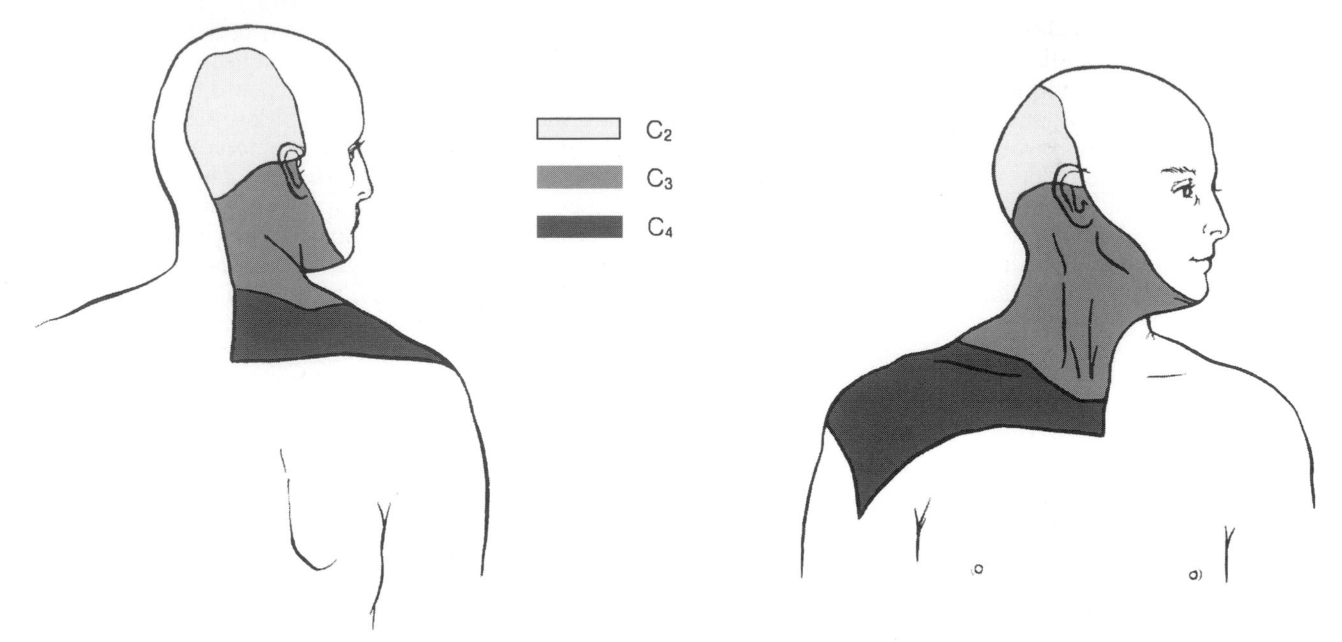

FIGURE 29–13 *Superficial cervical plexus block—distribution of cutaneous anesthesia. (From Carron H: Cervical plexus blocks.* In *Regional Anesthesia: Techniques and Clinical Applications. New York, Grune and Stratton, 1984, pp 10–15.)*

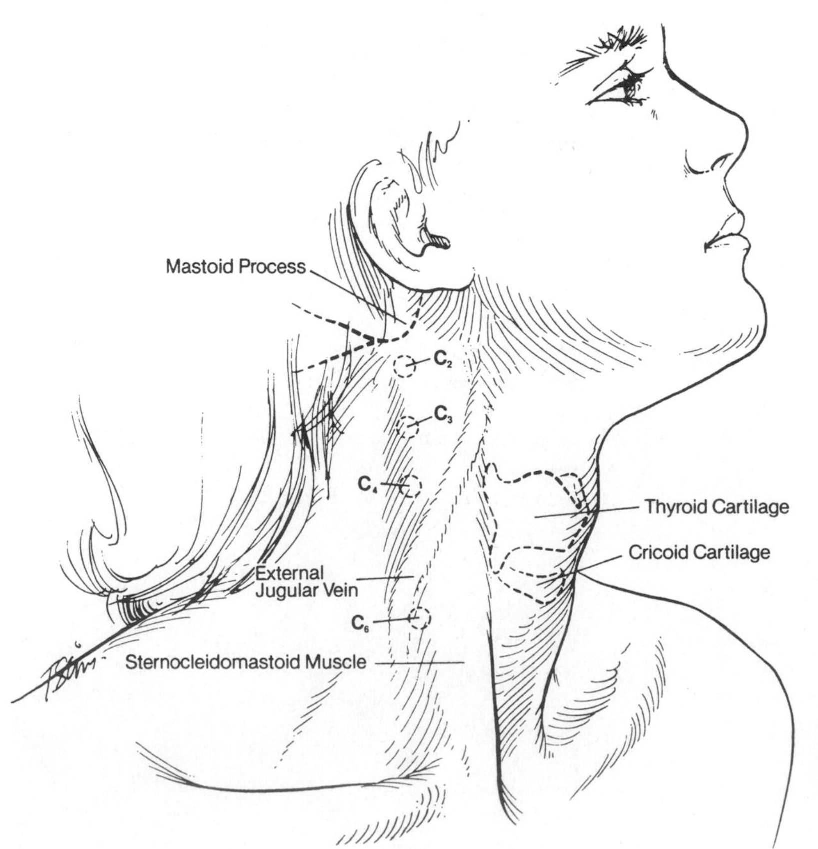

FIGURE 29–14 *Position and surface landmarks for performing cervical plexus block. (From Pai U, Raj P: Peripheral nerve blocks: Cervical plexus.* In *Raj P (ed): Handbook of Regional Anesthesia. New York, Churchill Livingstone, 1985, pp 163–167.)*

1 cm posterior to the first line to produce a more accurate superficial indicator of the cervical transverse processes below.[22] Still others construct the primary line by connecting the mastoid process with the suprasternal notch.[25]

On this line, the transverse processes of C2–C4 are palpated. The transverse process of C2 is approximately 1.5 cm caudad to the tip of the mastoid process. Points marked 1.5 and 3.0 cm below this first point on the primary line indicate the transverse processes of C3 and C4, respectively. The transverse process of C3 can be found at the level of the body of the hyoid bone, and the C4 transverse process is located at the level of the upper border of the thyroid cartilage (Figs. 29–14, 29–15).

Skin wheals are raised at these three points with a 27-gauge needle. A 22-gauge, 5-cm or a 25-gauge, 1-inch, short beveled block needle is inserted medially and caudad to a depth of 1.5 to 2.0 cm, until the tip of the transverse process is contacted at the three designated points. The needle is walked laterally until it slips off the most lateral aspect of the bone, and the tip is then reidentified. It is important to locate the transverse processes as far laterally as possible to avoid injection into the vertebral artery.[26] It is important to maintain a caudad direction to avoid unintentional entry into the intervertebral foramen, which would result in epidural or subarachnoid injection. Paresthesias may or may not be elicited. Then, 3 to 5 mL of local anesthetic is injected through each needle after careful aspiration for blood and cerebrospinal fluid. If the needles are properly placed, the onset of analgesia occurs within 5 min, regardless of what agent is used. The area of cutaneous anesthesia is the same as for superficial cervical plexus blockade, but deeper structures are also anesthetized (Fig. 29–16).[3, 6–8, 21–23, 25]

Alternative Techniques for Deep Block

Because the cervical plexus is invested in the prevertebral fascia between the anterior and middle scalene muscles, Winnie has advocated a single-injection technique for neural blockade.[2] The positioning of the patient and identification of bony landmarks are as noted previously. The posterior border of the sternocleidomastoid muscle at the level of C4 is identified, and the clinician's fingers are rolled laterally until the groove between the scalenus anterior and scalenus medius muscles is palpated. A 22-gauge, 5-cm or 25-gauge, 1-inch short, beveled block needle is inserted medially and caudally at this point until either paresthesia is elicited or the transverse process of C4 is encountered. Local anesthetic, 10 to 25 mL, is injected after aspiration to check for blood and cerebrospinal fluid.[2, 11, 27] Fortunately, the perineural sheath provides a space that communicates freely in the cervical region, so the local anesthetic solution can spread easily to adjacent levels.[21] Finger pressure at the C5 transverse process can be used to prevent caudad spread of the anesthetic toward the brachial plexus (Figs. 29–17, 29–18).

The single-injection technique can also be performed using a nerve stimulator to produce twitches of the neck muscles and paresthesias over the shoulder and upper arm

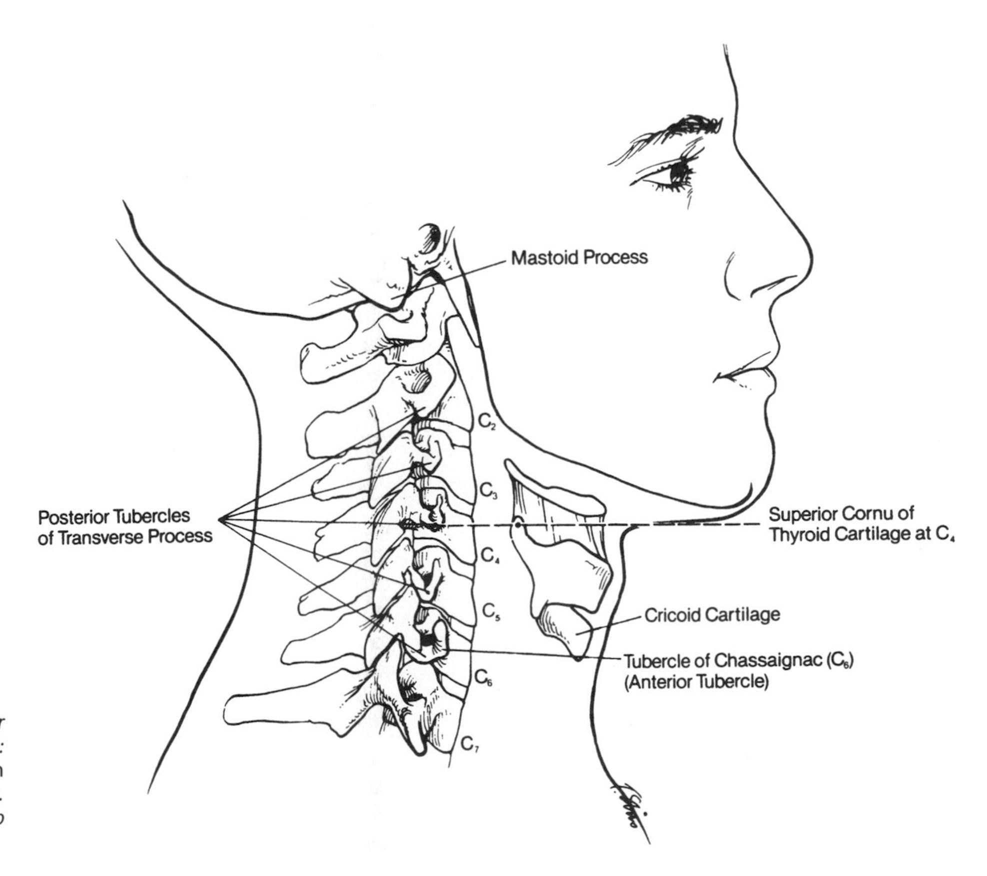

FIGURE 29–15 Bony landmarks for the cervical plexus block. (From Pai U, Raj P: Peripheral nerve blocks: Cervical plexus. In *Raj P (ed): Handbook of Regional Anesthesia. New York, Churchill Livingstone, 1985, pp 163–167.)*

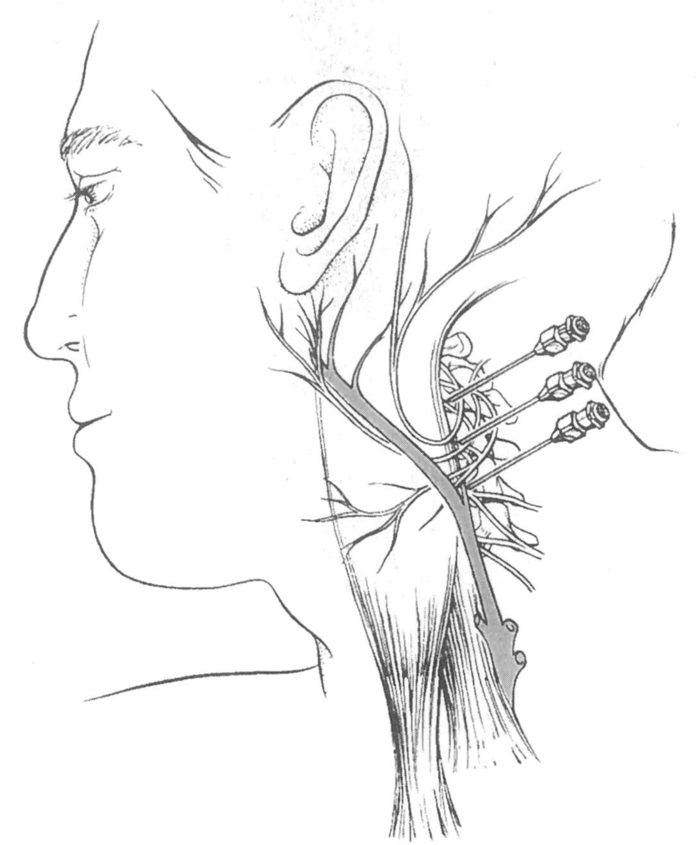

FIGURE 29–16 *Deep cervical plexus block—anatomic drawing.* Right to left, *The needles are noted at the sulci of the transverse processes of C2, C3, and C4. (From Carron H: Cervical plexus blocks.* In *Regional Anesthesia: Techniques and Clinical Applications. New York, Grune and Stratton, 1984, pp 10–15.)*

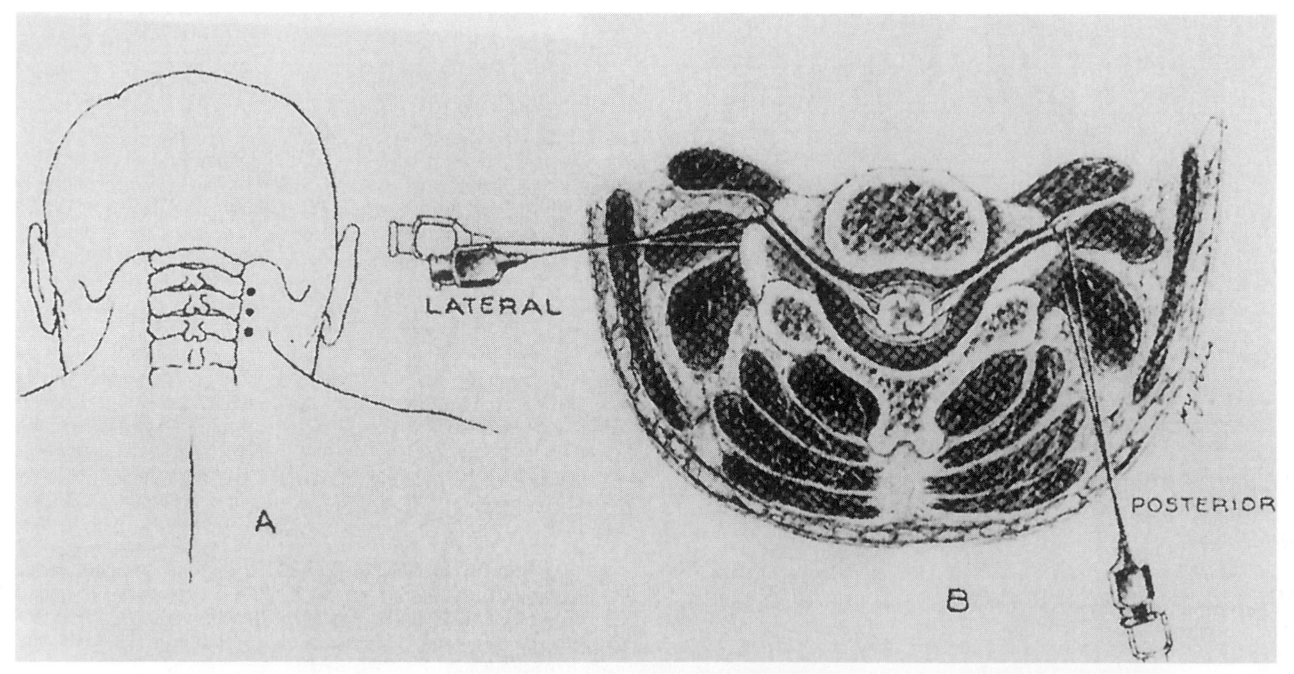

FIGURE 29–17 *"Deep cervical block" by the original posterior (Kappis) and lateral (Heidenhein) routes.* A, *With the posterior approach, the needles are inserted 3 cm from the midline and advanced until the articular pillar is contacted, whereupon the needles are withdrawn and reinserted farther laterally until they "walk off" the lateral margin of the transverse processes. At that point the local anesthetic is injected. With the lateral approach, a line is drawn from the mastoid process above to the transverse process of C6 below, indicating the location of the cervical transverse processes.* B, *Then, using either two or three needles, the lateral margins of the second, third, and fourth cervical transverse processes are contacted, whereupon the anesthetic solution is injected. (From Winnie AP, Ramamurthy S, Durrani Z, Radonjic R: Interscalene cervical plexus block: A single-injection technique. Anesth Analg 54:370–375, 1975.)*

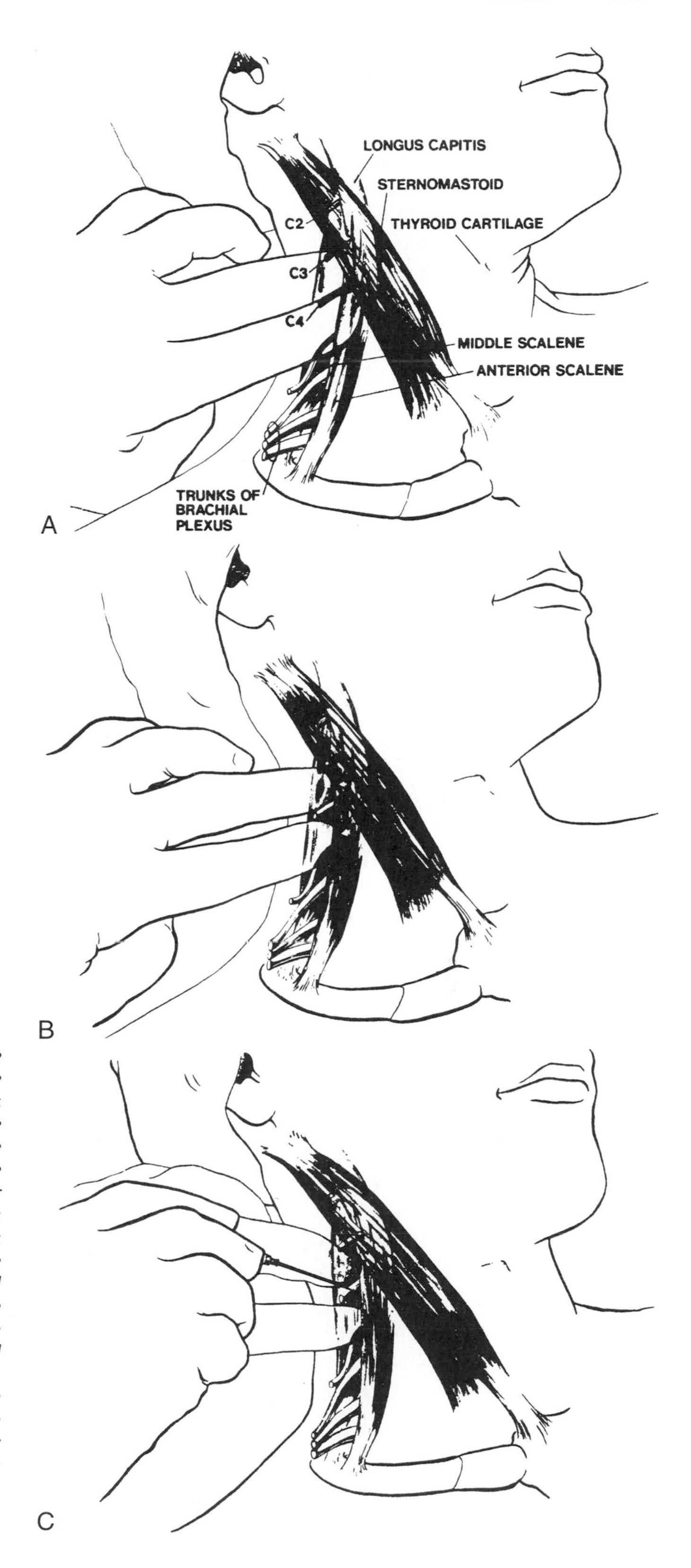

FIGURE 29–18 *The technique of interscalene cervical plexus block.* A, *In step 1, the patient is supine with the head turned slightly to the side opposite that to be blocked. The level of C4 is determined by noting the level of the upper margin of the thyroid cartilage. While the patient elevates the head to bring the sternocleidomastoid muscle into prominence, the anesthetist places the index and middle fingers behind (posterior to) the latter muscle at the level of C4, and the patient is asked to relax. The palpating fingers now lie upon the anterior surface of the belly of the anterior scalene muscle.* B, *In step 2, the anesthetist now carefully rolls the fingers laterally until the groove between the anterior and middle scalene muscles is palpated. When two fingers are utilized for palpation, digital pressure indents the skin and decreases the distance between the skin and cervical transverse processes.* C, *In step 3, an immobile needle is inserted at the level of C4 between the palpating fingers as they depress the skin over the interscalene groove. The needle is advanced perpendicular to the skin in all planes; that is, the direction is mostly mesiad but slightly dorsad and caudad. The caudal direction is critical to the safety of the technique, because the advancing needle, properly directed, encounters the next cervical transverse process if parasthesias are not produced. A horizontal direction would allow a needle that has missed the cervical roots to enter the vertebral vessels or the epidural or subarachnoid space. (From Winnie AP, Ramamurthy S, Durrani Z, Radonjic R: Interscalene cervical plexus block: A single-injection technique. Anesth Analg 54: 370–375, 1975.)*

before the blockade.[28] An 18-gauge Venflon needle connected to an electrode of the nerve stimulator is inserted as above; the other electrode is placed on the shoulder of interest. Once appropriate twitches are obtained, 10 to 15 mL of local anesthetic is injected after aspiration to check for blood and cerebrospinal fluid.

Another method of using a nerve stimulator with the single-injection technique was recently described.[29] A short, beveled needle (Stimuplex cannulas; Braun, Melsungen, Germany) is connected to a nerve stimulator and directed in the interscalene groove at the level of the upper margin of the thyroid cartilage (C4–C5). The needle is then directed caudad and medially until elevation and internal rotation of the scapula is elicited (Fig. 29–19). This muscle-evoked response occurs because of stimulation of the levator muscle of the scapula. The tip of the needle is positioned correctly when a current intensity of less than 0.5 mA elicits this muscle response. Forty milliliters of local anesthetic is then injected slowly while digital pressure is applied below the needle. The use of a nerve stimulator may increase the success rate of the block and improve the quality of anesthesia.

Another alternative route of deep cervical plexus blockade was described by Rovenstine and Wertheim.[1, 6] The patient is placed supine with the head midline and the chin pointing upward. The landmarks are the condyle of the mandible, the surface of the second lower molar, and the transverse processes of the cervical vertebrae. A vertical line is drawn through the condyle of the mandible, perpendicular to the operating table. The transverse processes of the cervical vertebrae are palpated, and a horizontal line is drawn along them, making right angles with the vertical line. A second perpendicular line is drawn that passes over the surface of the second molar. The point of intersection of this line with the horizontal line is marked, as is a point 1 cm caudad to the first point on the horizontal line. This latter point corresponds to the top of the transverse process of the second cervical vertebra. Points 2.5 and 3.5 cm caudad to the first point are marked on the skin. These correspond to the tips of the transverse processes of C3 and C4, respectively. Four points are thus drawn on the horizontal line, the upper point serves only as a reference point, and the three lower points indicate sites of injection. Injection of local anesthetic for deep cervical plexus blockade is carried out as described for the lateral approach (Figs. 29–20, 29–21).

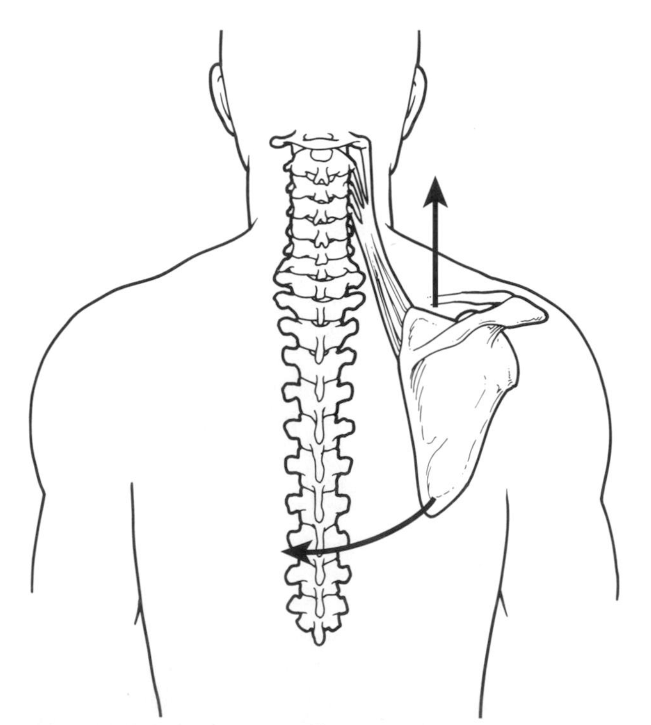

FIGURE 29–19 Movement of the scapula elicited by stimulation of the cervical plexus. (Redrawn from Merle JC, Mazoit JX, Desgranges P, et al: A comparison of two techniques for cervical plexus blockade: evaluation of efficacy and systemic toxicity. Anesth Analg 89:1360–1370, 1999.)

Posterior Approach

A posterior approach for deep cervical plexus blockade has also been described. The patient lies in the lateral position with the side to be blocked superior. The head is supported with cushions to prevent distortion of the structures of the neck and to render the landmarks more accessible. The cervical spinous processes are identified, C7 being most prominent. If they are difficult to palpate, the spinous process of C6 can be identified by drawing a line from the cricoid cartilage to the back of the neck. The transverse processes of C5–C2 are located 1.5, 3.0, 4.5, and 6.0 cm above C6, respectively.

Skin wheals are raised opposite the spinous processes of C2–C4 approximately 2 cm from the midline (Fig. 29–22). A 22-gauge, 8-cm needle is passed through these points parallel to the sagittal plane of the neck, until its point reaches the lateral transverse processes of the vertebrae. The needle is then withdrawn into the subcutaneous tissue and redirected obliquely and outward. When the needle point rests along the lateral aspect of the vertebral arch, it is advanced 1 cm farther, and local anesthetic is injected as for the lateral approach.[6]

The posterior approach is technically difficult, and results of blockade using it have been poor. The landmarks are difficult to identify accurately, and the depth of needle insertion is greater with this technique, it is therefore used only in cases in which the lateral approach is technically impossible (e.g., because of a tumor in the neck at the site of injection).[2]

Anesthetic Agents

A variety of local anesthetic agents have been used for surgical procedures under cervical plexus blockade.[29–35] For short-duration procedures, 1% to 2% lidocaine or mepivacaine can be used.[32, 34] For prolonged blockade, a 50:50 mixture of 1% to 2% lidocaine and 0.5% to 0.75% bupivacaine can be used.[35–38] Others use various concentrations of plain bupivacaine, 0.375% to 0.5%, for both the deep and superficial block.[11, 27, 30] The newer local anesthetics, such as ropivacaine and levobupivacaine, are used in similar volume and concentrations and offer similar anesthesia, perhaps with a better safety profile.

Epinephrine, 1:200,000 solution, can also be used to prolong blockade. Since this block is most often used for carotid endarterectomies in a high-risk group of patients, however, addition of epinephrine may produce undesirable cardiovascular effects.[9, 39]

A total volume of 10 to 15 mL of local anesthetic is usually used for superficial cervical plexus blockade, and a total volume of 9 to 25 mL for deep cervical plexus blockade. The single-injection deep cervical plexus block usually requires 10 to 25 mL of local anesthetic, although greater volumes have been used.[2, 11, 27, 29, 31]

In addition to local anesthetic alone, neurolytic blockade using equal parts of 0.5% bupivacaine with absolute alcohol

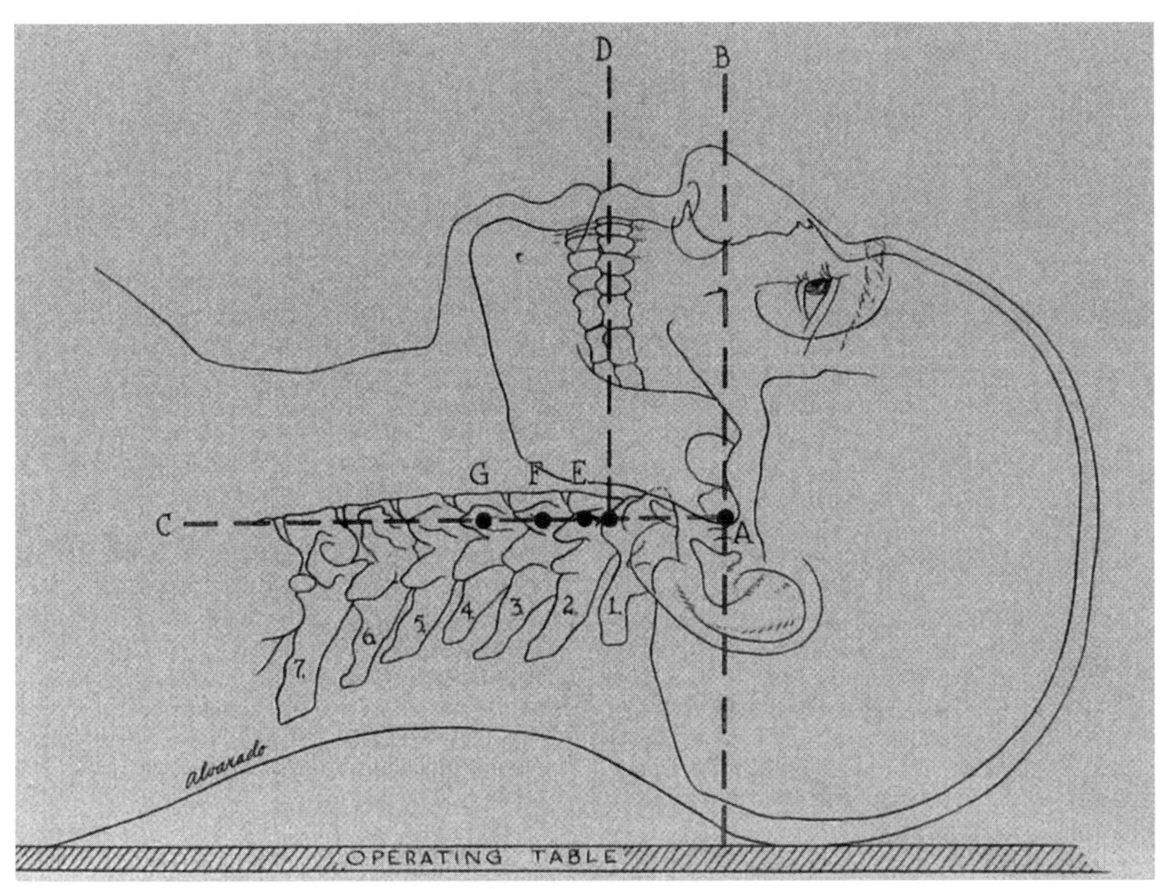

FIGURE 29-20 *Cervical plexus block by alternate route (Rovenstine and Wertheim). A, Condyle; B, line through condyle perpendicular to surface of the operating table; C, line forming a right angle with line B, passing through the condyle and parallel to surface of the operating table; D, tip of mastoid; E, point 0.5 cm below tip of mastoid and site of injection of C2; F, point 1 cm below E and site of injection of C3; G, point 1.5 cm below F and site of injection of C4. (From Adriani J: Labat's Regional Anesthesia: Techniques and Clinical Applications, ed 3. Philadelphia, WB Saunders, 1967, pp 180–195.)*

have been used to block the cervical plexus for neck pain secondary to metastatic lesions. Depo-Medrol, 40 mg, has also been added to local anesthetics for its antiinflammatory actions.[20]

Several studies have measured the blood levels of local anesthetic and monitored side effects after cervical plexus blockade and found no significant degree of toxicity. One study using lidocaine 1.5% with epinephrine 1:200,000 at 6 mg/kg found that symptoms of lidocaine toxicity did not occur.[41] Another study using a mixture of lidocaine and bupivacaine for cervical plexus blockade at commonly used concentrations and volumes also failed to elicit toxic systemic effects.[33] Bupivacaine levels were also measured in a study in which patients received a combination of general anesthesia and cervical plexus blockade. The mean total bupivacaine dose was 3.4 mg/kg, higher than the manufacturer's recommendation of 2 mg/kg. Nevertheless, there were no signs of systemic bupivacaine toxicity during the procedure or in the postoperative period.[42] Although cervical plexus blockade is safe, the usual recommendations of multiple aspirations, slow injection, and careful needle placement must be observed.

PITFALLS

Cervical plexus blockade fails for many reasons. Once the landmarks have been located, care should be taken to ensure that the patient does not move; otherwise, the landmarks may be misleading and the block may fail.[23] The needle should not be inserted too deep. The depth of the tips of the transverse processes from the skin varies from approximately 1.3 to 3.2 cm, depending on the pressure of palpation, the build of the patient, and the location of the injection. The transverse processes become more superficial as they descend.[22, 23]

The needle should also be directed slightly caudad to avoid entry into the epidural or subarachnoid space. The neck is a densely vascular area, so aspiration before injection is mandatory. Injection of a 1-mL test dose of anesthetic is prudent to detect any systemic effect. Placement of the needle should be at the lateral surface of the transverse processes before injection. If the needle lies too far posteriorly, analgesia will be poor. If the needle tip is placed too far anteriorly, puncture of the carotid artery, internal jugular vein, or vertebral vessels may occur, with subse-

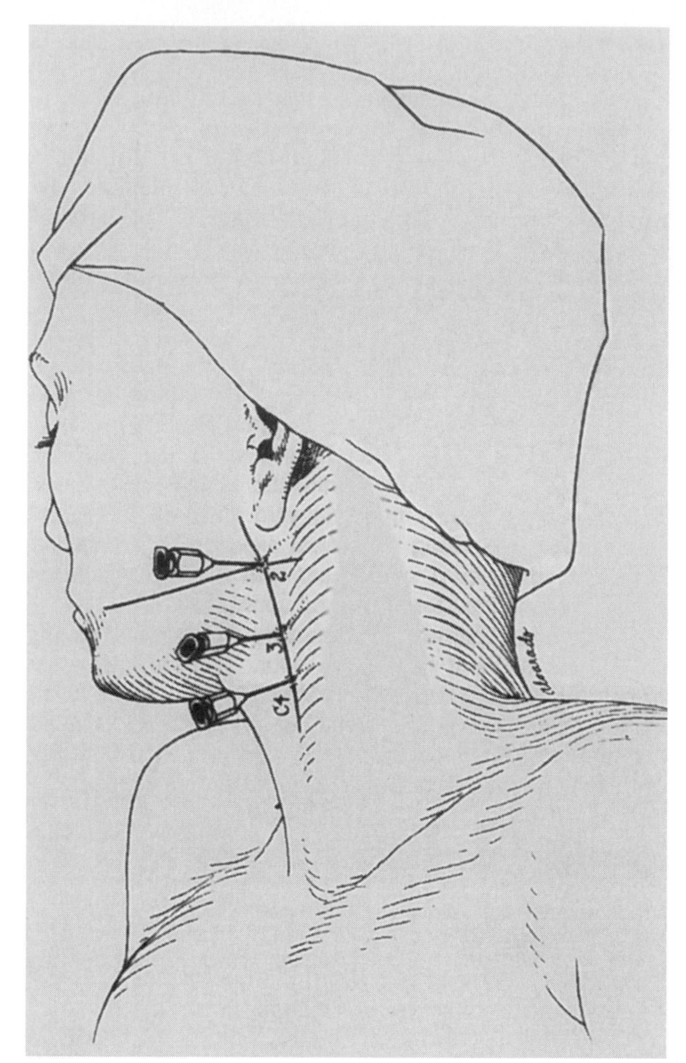

FIGURE 29–21 Cervical plexus block; site of injection by alternate route. (From Adriani J: Labat's Regional Anesthesia: Techniques and Clinical Applications, ed 3. Philadelphia, WB Saunders, 1967, pp 180–195.)

quent hematoma formation. This may make operating conditions difficult. Injection too far anteriorly may also cause sympathetic ganglion blockade, resulting in Horner's syndrome.[6]

If the cervical plexus block is unsuccessful and if time permits, the block may be repeated. The total dose of local anesthetic should be calculated to avoid injection of a toxic dose.[40] If partial blockade is obtained, supplementation with intravenous agents can be considered. If these techniques fail, a means providing general anesthesia should be used.[7]

COMPLICATIONS

A variety of complications can occur with cervical plexus blockade. The block is occasionally inadequate and has to be supplemented by infiltration of additional local anesthetic. This is more common when the site of operation extends beyond the midline of the neck during unilateral blockade.[16] Surgical traction high in the neck wound, where glossopharyngeal innervation occurs, commonly requires supplementation of anesthesia.[14] Discomfort can also occur because of retraction onto the mandibular periosteum, which is innervated by branches of the mandibular division of the trigeminal nerve. Supplementation of anesthesia may also be necessary in this area.[35]

Because the neck is richly vascular, intravascular injections of local anesthetic may occur. Accidental injection into the internal and external jugular veins during superficial cervical plexus blockade may result in systemic toxicity, tears in the wall of the vein leading to hematoma formation, and, possibly, air embolism if the needle is not attached to the syringe. Accidental injection of even 0.2 mL of local anesthetic into the vertebral artery, which travels through the foramina transversaria in each transverse process, can produce profound toxic effects, including convulsions, apnea, total reversible blindness, and unconsciousness. This is due to the direct flow of the artery to the brain stem.[27, 40] If colloidal materials such as depot steroids are added to local anesthetics for pain management, injection of this material into the vertebral artery can result in Wallenberg's syndrome or occlusion of the posterior inferior cerebellar artery (Fig. 29–23).[21–23, 25, 39]

In addition, injecting a large volume of local anesthetic anterior to the transverse processes during deep cervical plexus blockade may compress the carotid sheath. This could impair blood flow to the brain, which would be

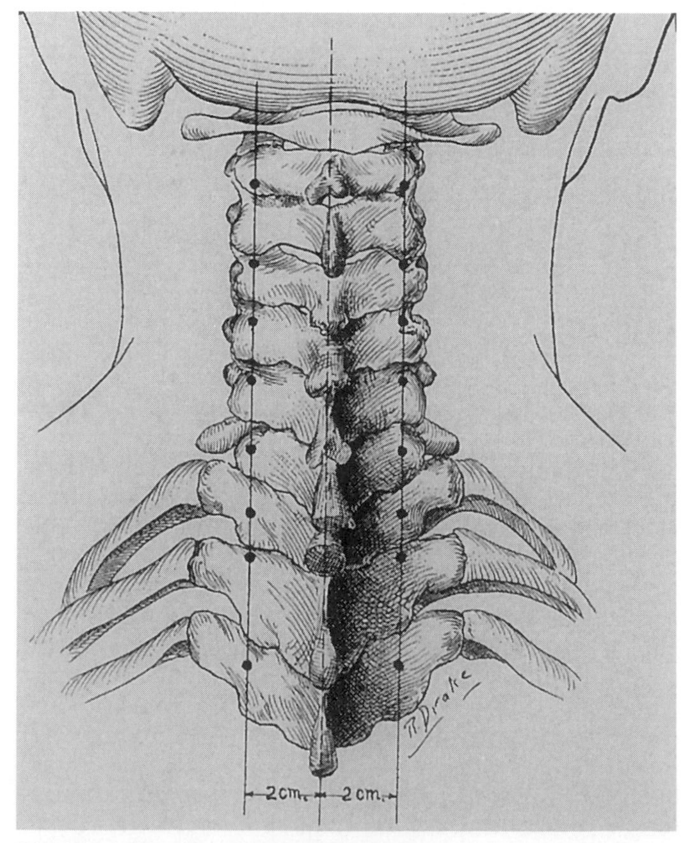

FIGURE 29–22 Cervical plexus block by the posterior route. Superficial landmarks as viewed on the skeleton. The wheals are raised opposite the spinous processes, at a distance of 2 cm from the midline. These landmarks apply to the cervical area only. (From Adriani J: Labat's Regional Anesthesia: Techniques and Clinical Applications, ed 3. Philadelphia, WB Saunders, 1967, pp 180–195.)

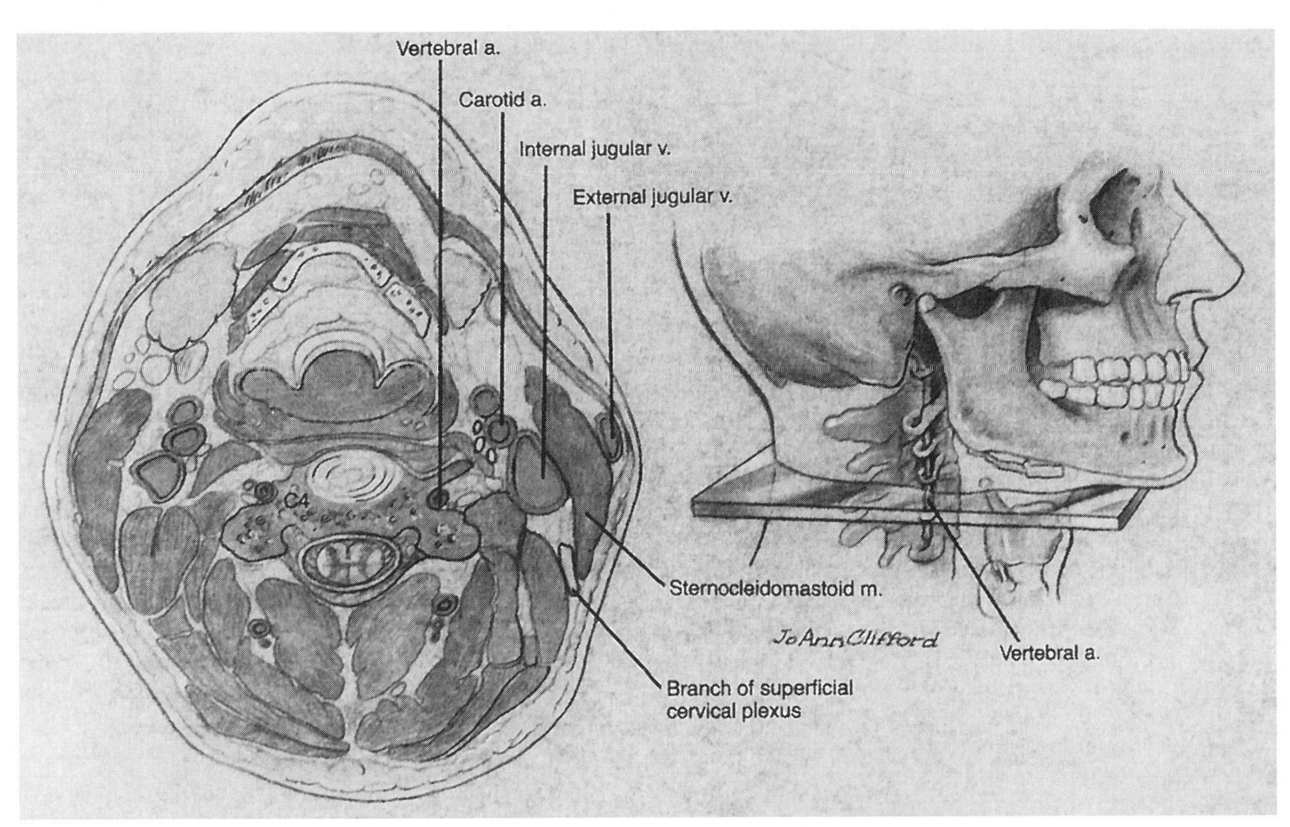

FIGURE 29–23 Cervical plexus cross-sectional anatomy—midpoint of sternocleidomastoid muscle. (From Brown DL: Atlas of Regional Anesthesia. Philadelphia, WB Saunders, 1992, pp 165–170.)

especially deleterious to patients with preexisting carotid artery disease.

Local anesthetic injection into the epidural or subarachnoid spaces is also possible through penetration into dural sleeves or through the intervertebral foramina.[21, 23, 25, 39, 43, 44] There is also the potential complication of injury to the spinal cord. Careful aspiration is required for any evidence of cerebrospinal fluid. Epidural injection, unlike subarachnoid injection, cannot spread into the cranium. An epidural block at the cervical level results in anesthesia of the upper limbs and thorax and can cause bilateral phrenic nerve block with subsequent bilateral diaphragmatic paralysis.[9]

The recurrent laryngeal nerve is blocked in 2% to 3% of cases during unilateral cervical plexus blockade. It occurs when local anesthetic is injected too deep along the posterior border of the sternocleidomastoid muscle. Sequelae are hoarseness, aphonia, and difficulty breathing. Blockade of the vagus nerve also may occur, which causes increased heart rate and loss of phonation. Bilateral hypoglossal nerve denervation with resultant total upper airway obstruction has been described.[37]

The phrenic nerve, arising mainly from C4 with small branches from C3 and C5, can be blocked (50% of cases) during deep cervical plexus blockade, causing transient diaphragmatic paresis and mild hypercapnia.[45, 46] If only one hemidiaphragm is paralyzed, only patients with chronic obstructive pulmonary disease seem to be at risk for significant changes in carbon dioxide concentration. Most patients describe only a "heavy chest" sensation.[9] This is usually treated by providing reassurance, administering supplemental oxygen, and elevating the patient's head.

Bilateral phrenic nerve blockade can be a serious hazard, especially in patients with concurrent respiratory compromise, and endotracheal intubation may be required.[31] If respiratory compromise from a paralyzed diaphragm could be a risk to a given patient, bilateral cervical plexus blocks should be avoided. If such blocks are carried out, dilute concentrations and small volumes of local anesthetic agents should be used.[21]

Blockade of the ninth and tenth cranial nerves or a combination of both through the pharyngeal plexus can also occur during deep cervical plexus blockade. This can cause dysphagia, and patients usually complain of a sensation of fullness in the back of the throat, which dissipates with time.[9]

Because the deep cervical plexus lies below the deep cervical fascia, spread of anesthetic to the cervical sympathetic chain, including the stellate ganglion, should not occur. If infiltration has spread anterior to the prevertebral fascia, the cervical sympathetic chain can be blocked, with resultant Horner's syndrome. This can be manifested as ptosis, constricted pupil, unilateral anhidrosis, nasal congestion, and sometimes respiratory compromise.[37] These symptoms should be noted before surgery, to avoid any confusion in the neurologic examination later. This complication in a failed block indicates that the injection was placed too far anteriorly and too superficially.[21] Bilateral stellate ganglion block may result in profound bradycardia that is due to interruption of the cardioaccelerator fibers.[25]

Finally, occipital headaches have been described after some surgical procedures under cervical plexus blockade.[9] However, the cause appears to be hyperextension of the neck muscles and not the block itself. Headaches can also occur after carotid endarterectomy secondary to reperfusion of the cerebral circulation.

FUTURE TRENDS

Although cervical plexus blockade has been widely described in the literature, the use of this technique for surgical procedures has been limited. From the surgeon's standpoint, the potential for a delay in surgery because of the time required to perform the block and the potential for unsatisfactory anesthesia that would require further supplementation are deterrents to performing cervical plexus blockade. From the standpoint of the anesthesiologist, inexperience with performing the block and fear of complications reduce the use of this technique.[36]

The most common surgical procedure performed under cervical plexus blockade is the carotid endarterectomy. Since enormous progress in the past decade has validated the efficacy of this procedure, its use may increase.[47] In fact, a newer technique, percutaneous carotid angioplasty and stenting performed via direct common carotid access has been done successfully with cervical plexus blockade.[48] This technique may further broaden the indications for this type of nerve block. As the surgical population grows older and presents with more severe systemic illnesses, regional anesthesia may prove to be the safest form of anesthesia. Carotid endarterectomy performed under cervical plexus blockade has many benefits over general anesthesia, among them the opportunity to monitor the patient's neurologic status during the operation. Periodic examinations of the awake patient have proved to be more accurate than electroencephalography or any other form of monitoring in assessing neurologic status. Another advantage is that regional anesthesia allows for a trial of carotid clamping and carotid stump pressure measurements while neurologic status is monitored with the patient awake. Thus, routine shunting, which carries its own risks of morbidity and mortality, is avoided.[49]

Perioperative complications do occur during carotid endarterectomy under both cervical plexus blockade and general anesthesia. It appears that cervical plexus blockade is associated with greater activation of the sympathetic nervous system, which is manifested as hypertension and tachycardia, whereas general anesthesia is associated with a greater incidence of hypotension.[50, 51] On the other hand, postoperative blood pressure instability is less common in patients who have had cervical plexus blockade for the procedure.[13, 16, 17] A report from Karmody and colleagues[52] showed a statistically significant difference in neurologic complications between regional and general anesthesia during carotid endarterectomy, 0.6% and 4%, respectively.

In recent years, growing emphasis has been placed on cost containment by the government, third-party payors, and the public. A study by Godin and colleagues[49] recently confirmed that cervical plexus blockade is a safe, reliable, and less costly alternative to general anesthesia in patients undergoing carotid endarterectomy. As evidence accumulates to support the use of regional anesthetic techniques for carotid endarterectomy and other procedures and conditions, facility in performing cervical plexus blocks should be encouraged. Cervical plexus blockade should be considered an important regional technique in the armamentarium of any anesthesiologist.

REFERENCES

1. Wertheim HM, Rovenstine EA: Cervical plexus block. NY State J Med 39:1311–1315, 1939.
2. Winnie AP, Ramamurthy S, Durrani Z, Radonjic R: Interscalene cervical plexus block: A single-injection technique. Anesth Analg 54:370–375, 1975.
3. Collins VJ: Blocks of cervical spinal nerves. *In* Fundamentals of Nerve Blocks. Philadelphia, Lea & Febiger, 1960, pp 234–248.
4. Kappis H: Uber Leitunganasthesie am Bauch, Brust, Arm, und Hals durch Injection ans Foramen intervertebrale. Munchen Med Wschr 59:794–796, 1912.
5. Heidenhein L: Operations on the neck. *In* Braun H (ed): Local Anesthesia. Philadelphia, Lea & Febiger, 1914, pp 268–269.
6. Adriani J: Labat's Regional Anesthesia: Techniques and Clinical Applications, ed 3. Philadelphia, WB Saunders, 1967, pp 180–195.
7. Pai U, Raj P: Peripheral nerve blocks: Cervical plexus. *In* Raj P (ed): Handbook of Regional Anesthesia. New York, Churchill Livingstone, 1985, pp 163–167.
8. Katz J: Cervical plexus. *In* Katz J (ed): Atlas of Regional Anesthesia, ed 2. Norwalk, Conn, Appleton & Lange, 1994, pp 40–43.
9. Masters RD, Castresana EJ, Castresana MR: Superficial and deep cervical plexus block: Technical considerations. AANA J 63:235–243, 1995.
10. Rainer WG, McCrory CB, Feiler EM: Surgery on the carotid artery with cervical block anesthesia: Technical considerations. Am J Surg 112:703–705, 1966.
11. Stoneham MD, Doyle AR, Knighton JD, et al: Prospective, Randomized comparison of deep or superficial cervical plexus block for carotid endarterectomy surgery. Anesthesiology 89:907–912, 1998.
12. Stoneham MD: Correspondence—applied Anatomy of Cervical Plexus Blockade. Anesthesiology 90:1791, 1999.
13. Castresana MR, Balser JS, Newman WH, Stefansson S: Cervical block for carotid endarterectomy followed immediately by general anesthesia for coronary artery bypass and aortic valve replacement. Anesth Analg 77:186–187, 1993.
14. Davies MJ, Murrell GC, Cronin KD, et al: Carotid endarterectomy under cervical plexus block: A prospective clinical audit. Anaesth Intensive Care 18:219–223, 1990.
15. Jopling MW, deSanctis CA, McDowell DE, et al: Anesthesia for carotid endarterectomy: A comparison of regional and general techniques. Anesthesiology 59:A217, 1983.
16. Pick MJ, Taylor GW: Selective shunting on the basis of carotid clamping under regional anesthesia. Int Anesthesiol Clin 22:129–135, 1984.
17. Fried KS, Elias SM, Raggi R: Carotid endarterectomy under local anesthesia. NJ Med 87:795–797, 1990.
18. Muskett A, McGreevy J, Miller M: Detailed comparison of regional and general anesthesia for carotid endarterectomy. Am J Surg 152:691–694, 1986.
19. Andersen CA, Rich NM, Collins GJ, McDonald PT: Carotid endarterectomy: Regional versus general anesthesia. Am Surgeon 46:323–327, 1980.
20. Owitz S, Koppolu S: Nerve blocks: An anesthesiologist's approach to the relief of cancer pain. Mt Sinai J Med 53:550–553, 1986.
21. Cousins MJ, Bridenbaugh PO: Neural Blockade in Clinical Anesthesia and Management of Pain, 2nd ed. Philadelphia, JB Lippincott, 1988.
22. Brown DL: Cervcal plexus block. *In* Atlas of Regional Anesthesia, Philadelphia, WB Saunders, 1992, pp 165–170.
23. Moore DC: Regional block. *In* A Handbook for Use in the Clinical Practice of Medicine and Surgery, 2nd ed. Block of the Cervical Plexus Springfield, Ill, Charles C Thomas. 1957, pp 88–98.
24. Bonica JJ: General considerations of pain in the neck and upper limb. *In* The Management of Pain, ed 2. Philadelphia, Lea & Febiger, 1990, pp 823–825.

25. Carron H: Cervical plexus blocks. *In* Regional Anesthesia: Techniques and Clinical Applications. New York, Grune & Stratton, 1984, pp 10–15.
26. Mulroy MR: Peripheral nerve blockade. *In* Barash PG, Cullen BF, Stoelting RK (eds): Clinical Anesthesia, 2nd ed. Philadelphia, JB Lippincott, 1992, pp 847–849.
27. Stoneham MD, Bree SEP: Epileptic seizure during awake carotid endarterectomy. Anesth Analg 89:885–886, 1999.
28. Mehta Y, Juneja R: Regional analgesia for carotid artery endarterectomy by Winnie's single injection technique using a nerve detector. J Cardiothorac Vasc Anesth 6:772–773, 1992.
29. Merle JC, Mazoit JX, Desgranges P, et al: A comparison of two techniques for cervical plexus blockade: Evaluation of efficacy and systemic toxicity. Anesth Analg 89:1366–1370, 1999.
30. Allen BT, Anderson CB, Rubin BG, et al: The influence of anesthetic technique on perioperative complications after carotid endarterectomy. Vasc Surg 19:834–843, 1994.
31. Stoneham MD, Wakefield TW: Acute respiratory distress after deep cervical plexus block. J Cardiothorac Vasc Anesth 12:197–198, 1998.
32. Davies MJ, Murrell GC, Cronin KD, et al: Anaesthesia and intensive care: Carotid endarterectomy under cervical plexus block—a prospective clinical audit. Anaesth Intensive Care 18:219–223, 1990.
33. Tissot S, Frering B, Gagniew MC, et al: Plasma concentrations of lidocaine and bupivacaine after cervical plexus block for carotid surgery. Anesth Analg 84:1377–1379, 1997.
34. Davies MJ, Mooney PH, Scott DA, et al: Neurologic changes during carotid endarterectomy under cervical block predict a high risk of postoperative stroke. Anesthesiology 78:829–833, 1993.
35. Burke DL, Thomas P: Mandibular nerve block in addition to cervical plexus block for carotid endarterectomy. Anesth Analg 87:1034–1036, 1998.
36. Levelle JP, Martinez OA: Airway obstruction after bilateral carotid endarterectomy. Anesthesiology 63:220–222, 1985.
37. Satyanarayana T, Ali M, Ramanathan S, et al: Cervical plexus block for carotid endarterectomy. Anesthesiology 55:A170, 1981.
38. Dawson AR, Dysart RH, Amerena JV, et al: Arterial lignocaine concentrations following cervical plexus blockade for carotid endarterectomy. Anaesth Intens Care 19:197–200, 1991.
39. Neill RS, Watson R: Plasma bupivacaine concentrations during combined regional and general anaesthesia for resection and reconstruction of head and neck carcinomata. Br J Anaesth 56:485–491, 1984.
40. Goldberg MJ: Complications of cervical plexus block of fugue state. Anesth Analg 81:1108–1109, 1995.
41. Paul RS, Abadir AR, Spencer FC: Resection of an internal carotid artery aneurysm under regional anesthesia: Posterior cervical block. Ann Surg 168(1):147–153, 1968.
42. Kumar A, Battit GE, Froese AB, Long MC: Bilateral cervical and thoracic epidural blockade complicating interscalene brachial plexus block: Report of two cases. Anesthesiology 35:650–652, 1971.
43. Huang KC, Fitzgerald MR, Tsueda K: Bilateral block of cervical and brachial plexuses following interscalene block. Anaesth Intensive Care 14:87–88, 1986.
44. Winnie AP: Regional anesthesia. Surg Clin North Am 54 (4):880–881, 1975.
45. Emery G, Handley G, Davies MJ, Mooney PH: Incidence of phrenic nerve block and hypercapnia in patients undergoing carotid endarterectomy under cervical plexus block. Anaesth Intensive Care 26:377–381, 1998.
46. Castresana MR, Masters RD, Castresana EJ, et al: Incidence and clinical significance of hemidiaphragmatic paresis in patients undergoing carotid endarterectomy during cervical plexus block anesthesia. J Neurosurg Anesthesiol 6:21–23, 1994.
47. Gelb AW, Herrick IA: Anesthesia for carotid endarterectomy: IARS 1999. Review Course Lectures. New York, Elsevier, 1999, pp 45–48.
48. Alessandri C, Bergeron P: Local anesthesia in carotid angioplasty. J Endovasc Surg 3:31–34, 1996.
49. Godin MS, Bell WH, Schwedler M, Kerstein MD: Cost effectiveness of regional anesthesia in carotid endarterectomy. Am Surgeon 55:656–659, 1989.
50. Forssell C, Takolander R, Bergqust D, et al: Local versus general anaesthesia in carotid surgery. A prospective, randomised study. Eur J Vasc Surg 6:503–509, 1989.
51. Takolander R, Bergqust D, Hulthen UL, et al: Carotid artery surgery. Local versus general anaesthesia as related to sympathetic activity and cardiovascular effects. Eur J Vasc Surg 4:265–270, 1990.
52. Corson JD, Chang BB, Karmody AM: The influence of anesthetic choice on carotid endarterectomy outcome. Arch Surg 122:807–812, 1987.

CHAPTER • 30

Stellate Ganglion Block

P. Prithvi Raj, MD • Susan R. Anderson, MD

HISTORY

Selective block of the sympathetic trunk was first reported by Sellheim and, shortly thereafter, by Läwen, Kappis, and Finsterer, between 1905 and 1910. In 1924, reports were published by Brumm and Mandl and by Swertlow. After 1930, the technique and the indications were established by White in the United States and Leriche and Fontaine in Europe.

ANATOMY

Cell bodies for preganglionic nerves originate in the anterolateral horn of the spinal cord; fibers destined for the head and neck originate in the first and second thoracic spinal cord segments, whereas preganglionic nerves to the upper extremity originate at segments T2–T8, and occasionally T9. Preganglionic axons to the head and neck exit with the ventral roots of T1 and T2, then travel as white communicating rami before joining the sympathetic chain and passing cephalad to synapse at either the inferior (stellate), middle, or superior cervical ganglion. Postganglionic nerves either follow the carotid arteries (external or internal) to the head or integrate as the gray communicating rami before joining the cervical plexus or upper cervical nerves to innervate structures of the neck (Fig. 30–1).

To achieve successful sympathetic denervation of the head and neck, the stellate ganglion should be blocked, because all preganglionic nerves either synapse here or pass through on their way to more cephalad ganglia. Blockade of the middle or superior ganglion would miss the contribution of sympathetic fibers traveling from the stellate ganglion to the vertebral plexus and, ultimately, to the corresponding areas of the cranial vault supplied by the vertebral artery.[1]

Sympathetic nerves to the upper extremity exit T2–T8 through ventral spinal routes, travel as white communicating rami to the sympathetic chain, then pass cephalad to synapse at the second thoracic ganglion, first thoracic or inferior cervical (stellate) ganglion, and, occasionally, the middle cervical ganglion. Most postganglionic nerves leave the chain as gray communicating rami to join the anterior divisions at C5–T1, nerves that form the brachial plexus. Some postganglionic nerves pass directly from the chain to form the subclavian perivascular plexus and innervate the subclavian, axillary, and upper part of the brachial arteries.[2]

In most humans, the inferior cervical ganglion is fused to the first thoracic ganglion, forming the stellate ganglion. Although the ganglion itself is inconstant, it commonly measures 2.5 cm long, 1.0 cm wide, and 0.5 cm thick. It usually lies in front of the neck of the first rib and extends to the interspace between C7 and T1. When elongated, it may lie over the anterior tubercle of C7; in persons with unfused ganglia, the inferior cervical ganglion rests over C7, and the first thoracic ganglion over the neck of the first rib. From a three-dimensional perspective, the stellate ganglion is limited medially by the longus colli muscle, laterally by the scalene muscles, anteriorly by the subclavian artery, posteriorly by the transverse processes and prevertebral fascia, and inferiorly by the posterior aspect of the pleura (Fig. 30–2). At the level of the stellate ganglion, the vertebral artery lies anterior, having originated from the subclavian artery. After passing over the ganglion, the artery enters the vertebral foramen and is located posterior to the anterior tubercle of C6 (Fig. 30–3).

Because the classic approach to blockade of the stellate ganglion is at the level of C6 (Chassaignac's tubercle), the needle is positioned anterior to the artery. Other structures posterior to the stellate ganglion are the anterior divisions of the C8 and T1 nerves (inferior aspects of the brachial plexus). The stellate ganglion supplies sympathetic innervation to the upper extremity through gray communicating rami of C7, C8, T1, and, occasionally, C5 and C6. Other inconstant contributions to the upper extremity are from the T2 and T3 gray communicating rami, which do not pass through the stellate ganglion but join the brachial plexus and ultimately innervate distal structures of the upper extremity. These fibers have sometimes been implicated when relief of sympathetically mediated pain is inadequate despite evidence of a satisfactory stellate block.[3]

These anomalous pathways, termed *Kuntz's nerves*, can be reliably blocked only by a posterior approach.[3] Although the posterior approach is technically more difficult than the anterior approach taught traditionally, nerve imaging

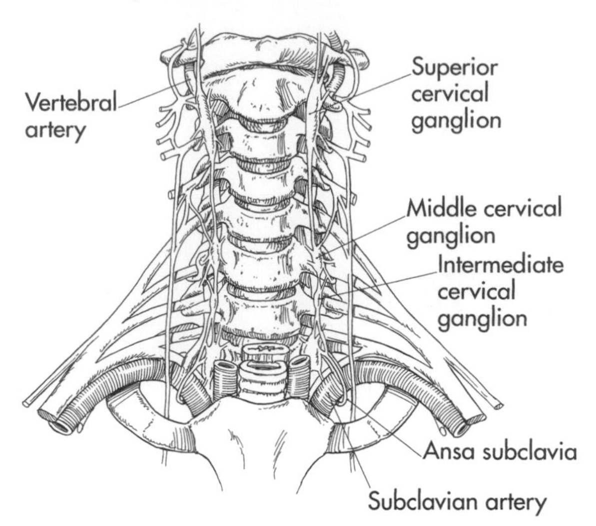

FIGURE 30–1 Cervical sympathetic ganglia and stellate ganglion. Note the relationship of structures to the respective ganglia. (From Raj PP [ed]: Practical Management of Pain, ed 2. St Louis: Mosby–Year Book, 1992.)

(e.g., computerized tomography or fluoroscopy) can help to prevent the major risk of pneumothorax. If a local anesthetic block via this approach is successful, neurolysis can be performed by radiofrequency thermocoagulation or using small amounts of either aqueous phenol or alcohol (2 to 3 mL). Because most, if not all, sympathetic fibers to the upper extremity pass through these upper thoracic ganglia, this neurolytic block can be quite successful.

Other efferent fibers from the stellate ganglion follow the major vascular structures, including the subclavian and common carotid arteries. The subclavian arterial plexus also receives contributions from the ansa cervicalis (originating from the stellate ganglion) and the intermediate cervical ganglion.

INDICATIONS

Stellate ganglion block is useful in the treatment of a variety of painful conditions, including Raynaud's disease, arterial embolism in the area of the arm, accidental intraarterial injection of drugs, and Meniere's syndrome. Although stellate ganglion block for treatment of Meniere's is controversial, several clinicians have had success with it. Stellate ganglion block is beneficial in the treatment of acute herpes zoster of the face and lower cervical and upper thoracic dermatomes. The technique may also be utilized for palliation of postherpetic neuralgia involving these anatomic areas.

The posttraumatic syndrome, which is often accompanied by swelling, cold sweat, and cyanosis, is an ideal indication for stellate ganglion block. Several clinical syndromes fall into this category, including complex regional pain syndromes type I (reflex sympathetic dystrophy) and type II (causalgia), and Sudeck's disease. Stellate ganglion block is also useful in the treatment of facial reflex sympathetic dystrophy.

For patients requiring vascular surgery on the upper extremities, stellate ganglion block has diagnostic, prognostic, and, in some cases, prophylactic value.

Stellate ganglion block can give rise to a number of complications, so simultaneous bilateral blocks are not advisable. Nevertheless, in cases of pulmonary embolism, bilateral stellate ganglion block is absolutely indicated as immediate therapy.

CONTRAINDICATIONS

Absolute contraindications of stellate ganglion block are as follows:

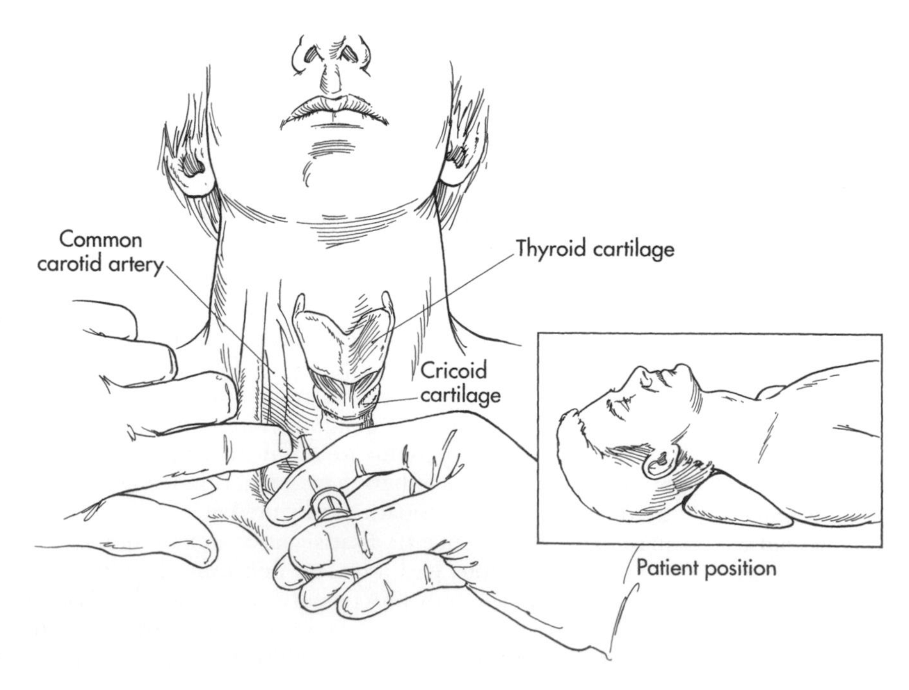

FIGURE 30–2 Stellate ganglion block. C6 anterior tubercle is directly beneath the operator's index finger. The carotid artery is retracted laterally when necessary. The needle is perpendicular to all skin planes and is inserted directly posterior from the point of entry. Inset, *Patient positioned for stellate ganglion block. A pillow or roll should be placed between the shoulders to extend the neck, bring the esophagus to the midline, and facilitate palpation of Chassaignac's tubercle. (From Raj PP [ed]: Practical Management of Pain, ed 2. St Louis: Mosby–Year Book, 1992.)*

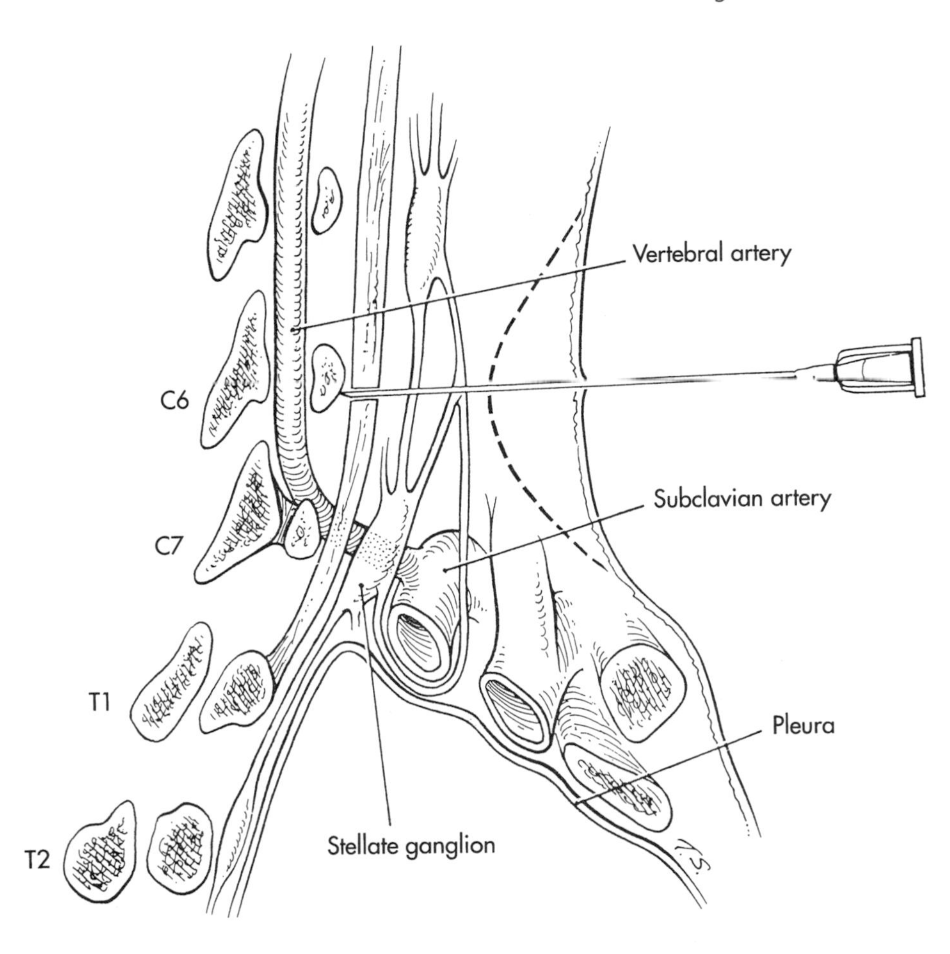

FIGURE 30–3 Sagittal view of the sympathetic chain. Note that the stellate ganglion is positioned directly posterior to the vertebral artery. The longus colli muscle separates the ganglia from the bone at the C6 level. The needle is superior to the stellate ganglion. (From Raj PP [ed]: Practical Management of Pain, ed 2. St Louis: Mosby–Year Book, 1992.)

- Anticoagulant therapy, because of the possibility of bleeding if there is vascular damage during insertion of the needle
- Pneumothorax and pneumonectomy on the contralateral side, because of the danger of additional pneumothorax
- Recent cardiac infarction, because stellate ganglion block cuts off the cardiac sympathetic fibers (accelerator nerves), with possible deleterious effects in this condition

Glaucoma can be considered a relative contraindication to stellate ganglion block, because provocation of glaucoma by repeated stellate ganglion blocks has been reported. Marked impairment of cardiac stimulus conduction (e.g., atrioventricular heart block) is also to be regarded as a relative contraindication, because blockade of the upper thoracic sympathetic ganglia aggravates bradycardia.

TECHNIQUE

Patient Preparation

Ideally, proper patient preparation for the initial block begins at the visit before the procedure. The patient is much more likely to remember discharge instructions and expected side effects if they are explained during a visit when the patient is not apprehensive about the imminent procedure. A patient booklet that explains in detail the procedure, what side effects may be expected, and potential complications allays the fears of most patients. Discussions of the realistic expectations of sympathetic blockade should be held before any procedure. The goals of blockade and the number of blocks in a given series differ with each pain syndrome, and these variables should be discussed, when possible, at visits before the actual blockade. Patients are much less likely to experience frustration or despair if they understand beforehand what can be expected. If the cause of pain is unclear and the intended block is considered diagnostic, a complete explanation allows the patient to record valuable information on the effectiveness of the procedure.

Informed consent must be obtained whenever sympathetic blockade is anticipated. Potential risks, complications, and possible side effects should be explained in detail. The patient should share responsibility for decision making and must understand the risks and the fact that complications do occur.

Placement of an intravenous (IV) line before the block is not mandatory at all pain clinics, but it facilitates use of IV sedation, when indicated, and provides access for administration of resuscitative drugs should a complication occur. In skilled hands, a stellate ganglion block can be performed quickly and relatively painlessly, so an IV may not be necessary. All standard resuscitative drugs, suction, oxygen, cardiac defibrillators, and instruments for endotracheal cannulation, however, need to be readily accessible. For anxious patients, and in teaching situations when the operator is inexperienced or when "hands-on" teaching is expected, preblock sedation through an IV line is beneficial.

Anterior Approach

The patient is asked to lie supine with the head resting flat on the table without a pillow. A folded sheet or thin pillow should be placed under the shoulders of most patients to facilitate extension of the neck and palpation of bony landmarks (see Fig. 30–2). The head should be kept midline with the mouth slightly open to relax the tension on the anterior cervical musculature. Hyperextension of the neck also causes the esophagus to move to midline, away from the transverse processes on the left.

The site of needle entry, Chassaignac's tubercle, at the C6 level, can be most readily identified by first locating the cricoid cartilage (see Fig. 24–3). In most persons, it is approximately 3.0 cm cephalad to the sternoclavicular joint. Palpation of the tubercle can be expected at the medial border of the sternocleidomastoid muscle, approximately 1.5 cm lateral to the midline. The location of the carotid artery should be noted; most often it lies lateral to the C6 tubercle. In some patients, it is necessary to retract the common carotid artery laterally, away from the site of entry.

To ensure proper needle positioning, the operator must correctly identify the C6 tubercle. Identification is most easily performed using firm pressure with the index finger. In either a left-handed or right-handed stellate ganglion block, the operator's nondominant hand should be used for palpating landmarks. Patients do not tolerate jabbing well; rather, gentle but firm probing can easily define the borders of the tubercle. A single finger, the index finger, relays the most specific tactile information. An alternative approach traps the tubercle between the index and middle fingers.[4]

The skin is antiseptically prepared, and the needle is inserted posteriorly, penetrating the skin at the tip of the operator's index finger. Making a skin wheal with local anesthetic is rarely necessary, except in some teaching situations or in patients with obese necks (in both situations, repeated punctures may be anticipated). A 23-gauge 4- to 5-cm needle (or a 22-gauge B-bevel needle) is used and should puncture the skin directly downward (posterior), perpendicular to the table in all planes. Although a smaller (e.g., 25-gauge) needle can be used, the added flexibility and smaller caliber make it more difficult to reliably ascertain when bone is encountered and then maintain the proper location for injection.

The needle passes through the underlying tissue until it contacts either the C6 tubercle or the junction between the C6 vertebral body and the tubercle. The depths of these structures differ, the tubercle itself being more anterior than the junction between body and tubercle. Regardless of the specific location encountered at C6, if the skin is being properly displaced posteriorly by the nondominant index finger, the depth is rarely more than 2.0 to 2.5 cm. The important difference between medial and lateral location of bone at C6 relates to the presence of the longus colli muscle, which is located over the lateral aspect of the vertebral body and the medial aspect of the transverse process. It does not cover the C6 tubercle; only the prevertebral fascia that invests the longus colli muscle also covers the C6 tubercle. Therefore, if the needle contacts the medial aspect of the transverse process at a depth somewhat greater than expected, the operator should be prepared to withdraw the needle 0.5 cm to avoid injecting into the longus colli muscle. Injection into the muscle belly can prevent caudad diffusion of local anesthetic to the stellate ganglion. Location of the needle on the superficial tip of the C6 anterior tubercle requires withdrawal of the needle from periosteum before injection.

The procedure is most easily performed if the syringe is attached before the needle is positioned. This prevents accidental dislodgement of the needle from the bone during syringe attachment after the needle is placed. Once bone is encountered, the palpating finger maintains its pressure, the needle is withdrawn 2 to 5 mm, and the medication is injected. Alternatively, once bone is met, the operator's palpating hand can release and fix the needle by grasping its hub, leaving the dominant hand free to aspirate and inject. Even though this technique can be performed blindly, more and more often fluoroscopy is used to confirm contrast spread (see Fig. 30–4). With fluoroscopy correct placement of the needle should be demonstrated by anteroposterior and lateral views with spread of the contrast solution. Once proper needle placement is confirmed, injection of medication must be performed in a routine and systematic fashion. A 50:50 mix of 2% lidocaine with 0.5% ropivacaine and 1 mL of 40 mg/mL of triamcinolone may be used. An initial test dose must be injected in all cases. Less than 1 mL of solution injected intravascularly has produced loss of consciousness and seizure activity. Before any injection, careful aspiration for blood and cerebrospinal fluid must be performed. If the aspiration is negative, 0.5 to 1.0 mL of solution is administered, and the patient is asked to raise the thumb to indicate the absence of adverse symptoms. The patient should be informed beforehand and reminded during the blockade procedure that talking might cause movement of the neck musculature that could dislodge the needle from its proper location. To communicate during the block, the patient can be asked to point a thumb or finger upward in response to questions. After the initial test dose, the operator can inject the remainder of the solution, carefully aspirating after each 3 to 4 mL.

During injection or needle placement, paresthesia of the arm or hand may be elicited. It should always be interpreted to mean that the needle has been placed deep to the anterior tubercle, adjacent to the C6 or C7 nerve root. Repositioning of the needle is necessary. Aspiration of blood or CSF also demands repositioning of the needle. Even though the needle may be in the correct position, sometimes it is necessary to confirm that the injected solution is not flowing where it is not desired. (Fig. 30–5 demonstrates brachial plexus spread and Fig. 30–6 demonstrates vascular spread.) The correct total volume of solution depends on what block is desired.[3] Properly placed, 5 mL of solution blocks the stellate ganglion, but this amount does not reliably block all fibers to the upper extremities because contributions from T2 and T3 may be present. Injection of 10 mL of solution more reliably blocks all sympathetic innervation to the upper extremity, even in patients with

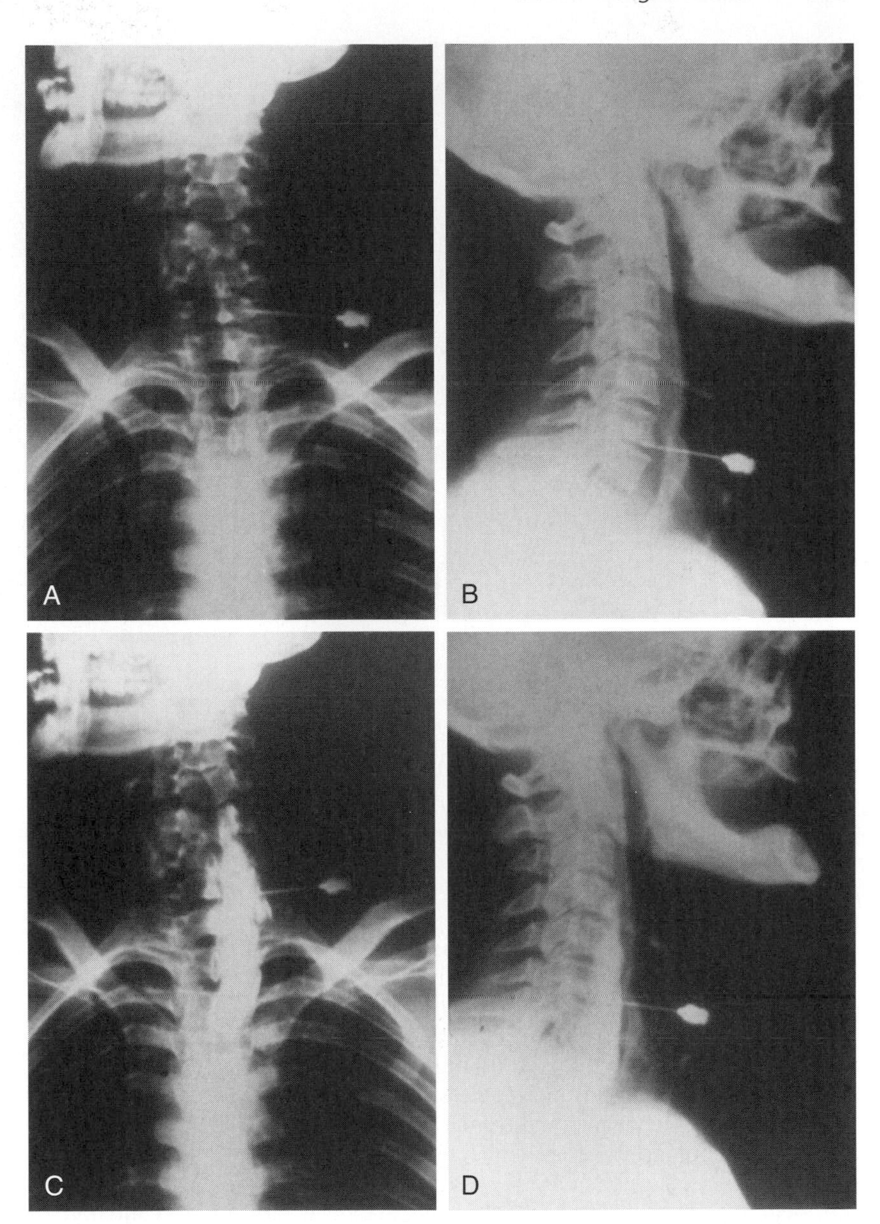

FIGURE 30-4 *Anteroposterior and lateral views of correct placement of the needle and the contrast spread after injection for stellate ganglion block.* A, *Anteroposterior and* B, *lateral views of needle placement.* C, *Anteroposterior and* D, *lateral views of contrast spread.*

the anomalous Kuntz's nerves. If blockade is being performed for sympathetic-mediated pain of the thoracic viscera, including the heart, 15 to 20 mL of solution should be administered.

EVIDENCE OF NERVE BLOCK

Sympathetic interruption to the head, supplied by the stellate ganglion, can easily be documented by evidence of Horner's syndrome: miosis (pinpoint pupil), ptosis (drooping of the upper eyelid), and enophthalmos (sinking of the eyeball). Associated findings include conjunctival injection, nasal congestion, and facial anhidrosis. These signs can be present without complete interruption of the sympathetic nerves to the upper extremity.

Evidence of sympathetic blockade to the upper extremity includes visible engorgement of the veins on the back of the hand and forearm, psychogalvanic reflex, plethysmographic and thermographic changes, and a positive sweat test. Skin temperature will also rise, provided that the preblock temperature did not exceed 33° to 34° C.

SIDE EFFECTS AND COMPLICATIONS

Side effects of a stellate ganglion block should be distinguished from complications. Most unpleasant side effects result from the Horner's syndrome—ptosis, miosis, and nasal congestion. Common complications of a stellate ganglion block result from diffusion of local anesthetic onto nearby nerve structures. These include the recurrent laryngeal nerve with complaints of hoarseness, feeling of a lump in the throat, and sometimes a subjective shortness of breath. Bilateral stellate blocks are rarely advised, because bilateral blocking of the recurrent laryngeal nerve can result in respiratory compromise and loss of laryngeal reflexes. Block of the phrenic nerve causes temporary pa-

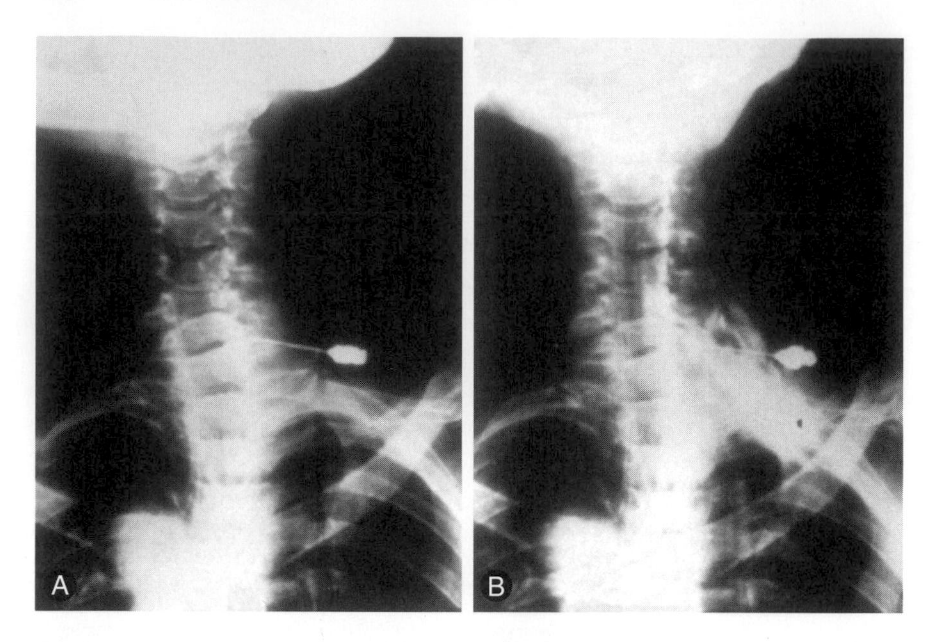

FIGURE 30–5 *Brachial plexus spread of contrast medium.*

ralysis of the diaphragm and can lead to respiratory embarrassment in patients whose respiratory reserve is already severely compromised. Partial brachial plexus block can also result secondary to spread along the prevertebral fascia[4] or positioning the needle too far posteriorly (Fig. 30–5). The patient should be discharged with the arm in a sling and given careful instructions on how to care for a partially blocked arm, should this complication occur.

The two most feared complications of stellate ganglion block are intraspinal injection and seizures induced by intravascular injection. Respiratory embarrassment and the need for mechanical ventilation can result from injection into either the epidural space (if high concentrations of local anesthetic are used) or the intrathecal space. Should either occur, patients need continual reassurance that everything is being appropriately managed and that they will recover without sequelae. Some sedation is required while the local anesthetic wears off. No drugs are necessary for endotracheal cannulation, because profound anesthesia of the larynx can be expected.

Intravascular injection most often involves the vertebral artery (Fig. 30–6). Small amounts of local anesthetic cause unconsciousness, respiratory paralysis, seizures, and sometimes severe arterial hypotension. Increased IV fluids, vasopressors if indicated, oxygen, and endotracheal intubation may be necessary. If the amount of drug injected into the artery is less than 2 mL, the sequelae just listed are short-lived and self-limiting, with oxygen and increased fluid administration often being the only therapy needed. Care must be taken during a stellate ganglion block to ensure that no air is injected from the syringe. Cerebral air embolisms have been reported from this procedure, and they are preventable.[2,5,6]

The risk of pneumothorax also attends the anterior approach. If the C7 tubercle is used and the needle is inserted caudally, the dome of the lung can be penetrated. This

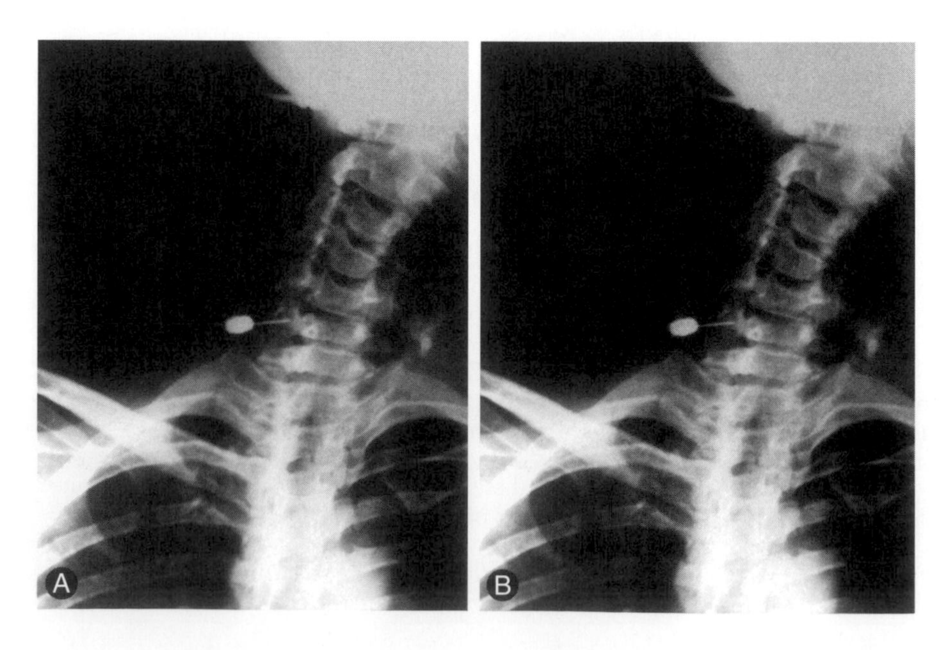

FIGURE 30–6 *Vascular spread of contrast medium.*

complication occurs more easily in thin, tall persons whose lung domes can extend farther cephalad.

ALTERNATIVE APPROACHES

C7 Anterior Approach

The anterior approach to the stellate ganglion at C7 is similar to the approach described at C6. Unlike C6, C7 has only a vestigial tubercle, which is very difficult to palpate. To identify C7, usually it is first necessary to find Chassaignac's tubercle (C6). Then the palpating finger moves one fingerbreadth caudad from the inferior tip. The patient must be positioned with a pillow under the shoulders to extend the cervical spine and to move the tubercle closer to the skin.

The advantage to blockade at C7 is manifested by the lower volume of local anesthetic needed to provide complete interruption of the upper extremity sympathetic innervation. Only 6 to 9 mL of solution suffices. The bothersome side effect of recurrent laryngeal nerve block is less common with this approach. The technique has two drawbacks: The less pronounced landmarks make needle positioning less reliable, and the risk of pneumothorax increases because the dome of the lung is close to the site of entry.

Posterior Approach

The ease of performing a stellate ganglion block by the anterior approach has rendered the posterior approach unnecessary, except for specific indications.[3,7] The posterior approach should be used for the patient who develops Horner's syndrome with an anterior approach but shows no other signs of sympathetic denervation to the upper extremity. Should this situation occur despite repeated, properly placed blocks, the patient may have a fascial tissue barrier that prevents caudad diffusion of the drug. The posterior approach at the T2 or T3 level provides sympathetic interruption to the upper extremity.

Patients chosen for chemical sympathectomy of the upper extremity should also be blocked with the posterior approach. Dilute solutions of phenol have been injected by the anterior approach at C6, but the smaller volume used may prevent reliable diffusion to the stellate ganglion.[8] Were the volume to be increased, the risk of spread to the recurrent laryngeal nerve, phrenic nerve, or brachial plexus would be unacceptably high. Horner's syndrome invariably develops when complete neurolytic destruction is achieved by the anterior approach. The posterior approach can often avert Horner's syndrome. The patient must understand and accept this potentially permanent complication before neurolysis.

A major disadvantage to sympathetic block by the posterior approach is the high risk of pneumothorax (Fig. 30–7). The apex of the lung lies close to the sympathetic chain at T2 and, for even the most experienced of operators, can be difficult to avoid. With the advent of computed tomography (CT), precise needle positioning can be more readily achieved.[7] Whenever neurolysis is anticipated, CT-guided needle placement should be employed.

Anatomy

The sympathetic chain lies close to the neck of the ribs in the thoracic space. In the cervical and lumbar regions the longus colli muscle and psoas muscle, respectively, separate the sympathetic chain from somatic nerves, but no muscle separates these structures in the thoracic region. The risk of intravertebral diffusion of drug during this block must be closely monitored. The pleura also abuts the sympathetic chain in the thoracic region, making precise needle location essential to avoiding pneumothorax. It has been reported that the risk of pneumothorax approaches 4% when this approach is employed.[4]

Technique

The posterior approach can be performed with the patient in either the prone or lateral position with the side to be blocked uppermost.[1,4] With new imaging techniques (e.g., fluoroscopy, CT), the prone position provides more useful information. This block was classically taught with needles inserted 6.0 cm from the midline. Entry at this point makes it extremely difficult, however, to position the needles properly along the vertebral body without passing through the pleura or parenchymal tissue (Fig. 30–8). Later, Bonica described a technique in which the needle was inserted 2.0 cm from the midline and advanced adjacent to the vertebral body. In many patients, however, 2.0 cm does not allow the needle to pass off the lamina without the operator directing it too far lateral, ultimately leading to pneumothorax. Rather, a distance of 3 to 4 cm from the midline facilitates proper needle alignment; the needle shaft should pass from the lamina and should be parallel with the sagittal plane. The needle should never be directed laterally, beyond the perpendicular plane. If the needle continues to contact lamina after being repositioned to the perpendicular plane, a new skin wheal should be raised, 1.0 cm lateral to the original wheal, and the process repeated.

The space lateral to the T1 spinous process can be used if local anesthetic is injected. If a neurolytic procedure is anticipated, either the T2 or T3 spinous process should be identified. After the area is prepared and draped, a skin wheal is raised 3 to 4 cm lateral to the spine. A 22-gauge, 8- to 10-cm needle is used to contact the ipsilateral lamina. The needle is then positioned laterally off the lamina until it passes through the anterior costotransverse ligament. This can be done by loss-of-resistance technique, one similar to that described for identification of the epidural space. Alternatively, a skin marker can be placed after contact with the lamina, requiring a depth of 2.0 cm once the needle passes from the lamina, at the junction of the anterior and the posterior halves of the vertebral body. At this point, 2 to 3 mL of radiographic contrast material should be injected. Characteristically, proper spread of the contrast is seen (Fig. 30–9). When contrast medium cannot be visualized, pleural or intravascular injection is likely. If neurolysis is anticipated, the intraspinal space must also be closely inspected for any back-diffusion of contrast medium before a neurolytic is injected. Once proper positioning is verified with contrast, 2 to 3 mL of local anesthetic or a neurolytic agent is injected slowly and with repeated aspirations.

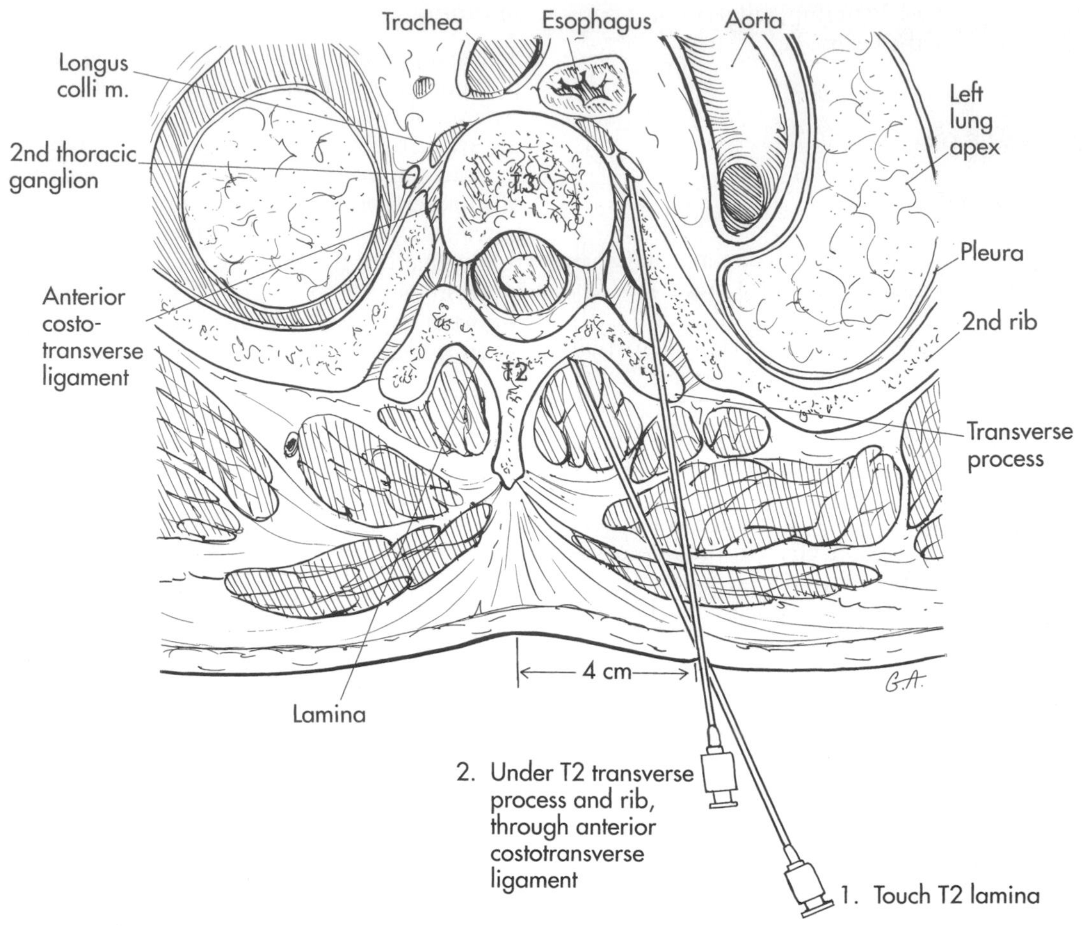

FIGURE 30–7 *Posterior approach to upper thoracic sympathetic chain block. The needle is introduced 4 cm from the midline, then "walked off" the T2 lamina. The needle should always be directed medially. 1, First insertion of the needle to touch the lamina. 2, Reinsertion of the withdrawn needle to lie under the T2 transverse process and the rib. (From Raj PP [ed]: Practical Management of Pain, ed 2. St Louis: Mosby–Year Book, 1992.)*

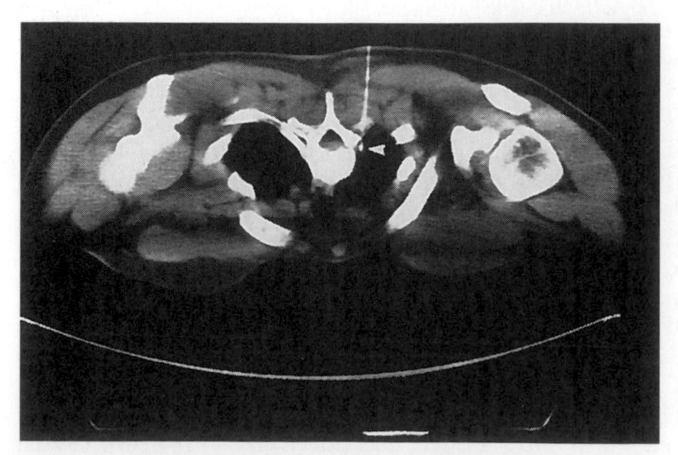

FIGURE 30–8 *Computed tomography view of upper thoracic sympathetic block. Contrast medium (arrow) is held close to the vertebral column by the endothoracic fascia and costotransverse ligament. (From Raj PP [ed]: Practical Management of Pain, ed 2. St Louis: Mosby–Year Book, 1992.)*

Neurolysis

Neurolysis of the stellate ganglion may be accomplished with phenol or with radiofrequency thermocoagulation. With either approach, imaging must be utilized.

PHENOL NEUROLYSIS

The approach for chemical neurolysis is similar to that for stellate ganglion block performed at C7. The patient must be positioned with a pillow under the shoulders to extend the cervical spine. Under direct anteroposterior fluoroscopy, the C7 vertebral body is identified. A skin wheal is raised over the ventrolateral aspect of the body of C7 with 1 mL of local anesthetic and a 25-gauge needle. A 22-gauge B-bevel needle is inserted through the skin wheal to contact the body of C7 in the ventrolateral aspect. This is at the junction of the transverse process with the vertebral body. Depth and direction should be confirmed with both anteroposterior and lateral views. The needle tip is positioned deep to the anterior longitudinal ligament. The longis colli lies lateral to the needle tip. The needle should be stabilized with a long-handled, heavy-duty Kelly clamp or hemostat. An IV extension should be attached to the needle and used for injection. Approximately 5 mL of water-soluble, nonirritating, nonionic, preservative-free,

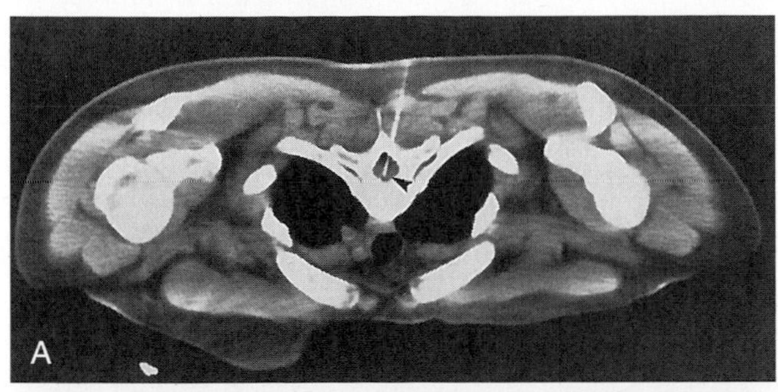

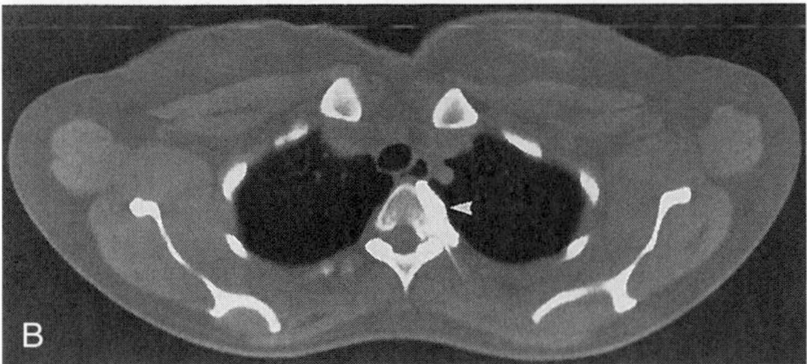

FIGURE 30–9 Potential complications of thoracic sympathetic block. A, Inadvertent placement of 22-gauge needle into the thoracic spine (arrow) *during upper thoracic sympathetic block. Leg and chest paresthesias were elicited, but no neurologic sequelae resulted.* B, *Placement of needle into the pleura* (arrow). *No pneumothorax was found on postblock chest radiographs. (From Raj PP [ed]: Practical Management of Pain, ed 2. St Louis: Mosby–Year Book, 1992.)*

hypoallergenic contrast is injected after negative aspiration. Dye should spread around the vertebra, avoiding intravascular, epidural, intrathecal, thyroidal, or myoneural (longus colli) uptake. If good spread of the contrast medium is visualized, a mix of local anesthetic, phenol, and steroid is injected. The total volume of 5 mL should consist of 2.5 mL of 6% phenol in saline, 1 mL of 40 mg triamcinolone, and 1.5 mL of 0.5% ropivacaine. (The total 5-mL dose contains a final mixture of 3% phenol.) The previously injected contrast material serves as a marker for the spread of the phenol. In the anteroposterior view, the contrast should spread caudad to the first thoracic sympathetic ganglion, cephalad to the inferior cervical ganglion, in the direction of the middle cervical sympathetic ganglion, and cephalad to the superior cervical ganglion. In the lateral view, spread should be observed in the retropharyngeal space and in front of the longis colli and anterior scalene muscles. After injection, the patient remains supine with the head elevated slightly for approximately 30 minutes, to prevent spread of the phenol to other structures.[8]

RADIOFREQUENCY NEUROLYSIS

Radiofrequency neurolysis of the stellate ganglion may be accomplished under fluoroscopic guidance. After the target area is identified for chemical neurolysis, a 16-gauge extracath is inserted through the skin wheal instead of the B-bevel needle. A 20-gauge, curved, blunt-tipped cannula with a 5-mm active tip is guided through the extracath at the superolateral aspect. The tip should rest at the junction of the transverse process and the vertebral body. The depth and direction should be confirmed with anteroposterior and lateral views. Correct placement may be confirmed conclusively with the injection of contrast medium. A sensory (50 Hz, 0.9 V) and a motor (2Hz, 2V) stimulation trial must be performed owing to the location of the phrenic nerve (lateral) and the recurrent laryngeal nerve (anterior and medial) relative to the proposed lesion. While motor stimulation is performed, the patient should say "*ee*," to ensure preservation of motor function. A small volume of local anesthetic (0.5 mL) should be injected before lesioning. The radiowave is applied for 60 seconds at 80°C. The cannula is then redirected to the most medial aspect of the transverse process in the same plane. Placement in the ventral aspect must be confirmed with a lateral view. Before lesioning, the patient must be retested for sensory and motor stimulation. A repeat dose of the local anesthetic should also be given through the cannula. A third (and final) lesion should be directed at the upper portion of the junction of the transverse process and the body of C7. Potential complications include injury to the phrenic or the recurrent laryngeal nerve, neuritis, and vertebral artery injury.[9, 10]

Neurolysis of the upper thoracic sympathetic chain via the posterior approach should be performed only when one of the image intensifiers is utilized, either CT or fluoroscopy. Needles can be misdirected (Fig. 30–10), with disastrous results if a neurolytic agent is injected.

For neurolysis, the T2 or T3 spinous process is utilized. Although Horner's syndrome may be avoided by this approach, the risk remains, and the patient must understand and accept the possibility. Once the needle is positioned, contrast material must be injected to check for interpleural spread, intraspinal diffusion, or intravascular injection. If good spread of contrast medium is demonstrated, 2 to 3 mL of 10% aqueous phenol is slowly injected.

Percutaneous radiofrequency sympathectomy is a more precise, controlled neurolysis. This is performed after diagnostic block produces a positive result. Before the procedure is undertaken, coagulopathy must be ruled out (i.e., prothrombin time, partial thromboplastin time, and bleeding time must be in the normal range). The patient is placed prone on the fluoroscopy table. The camera is placed in the oblique view (30 degrees) to place the shadow of the body lateral to the laminae. A cephalocaudad view is necessary to correct for the upper thoracic kyphosis (approximately 20 degrees). A 20-gauge, blunt, curved cannula with a 10-mm active tip is introduced through a 16-gauge extracath that has already pierced the skin approximately 3.5 cm from the midline. A tunnel view should demonstrate the cannula advancing toward the margin of the lamina. It is advanced along the lateral body until the tip is halfway between the anterior and the posterior border of the body. Proper needle placement must be assessed by the spread of the contrast medium, which should be spread paravertebrally under the pedicles in the anteroposterior view without intravascular, pleural, epidural, or intrathecal uptake. Sensory stimulation must be performed at 50 Hz and 0.9 V. More than 0.9 V produces a deep ache. Motor stimulation must be performed at 2 Hz and 2 V and found to be negative. Additionally, 1 mL of a local anesthetic-steroid mixture is injected after negative aspiration. A 30-sec delay should be observed before lesioning. Two lesions are performed at each level with the active tip turned cephalad for the first lesion and caudad for the second. The lesions should be made at 80 degrees for 90 seconds. A postoperative end-expiratory chest film is taken to rule

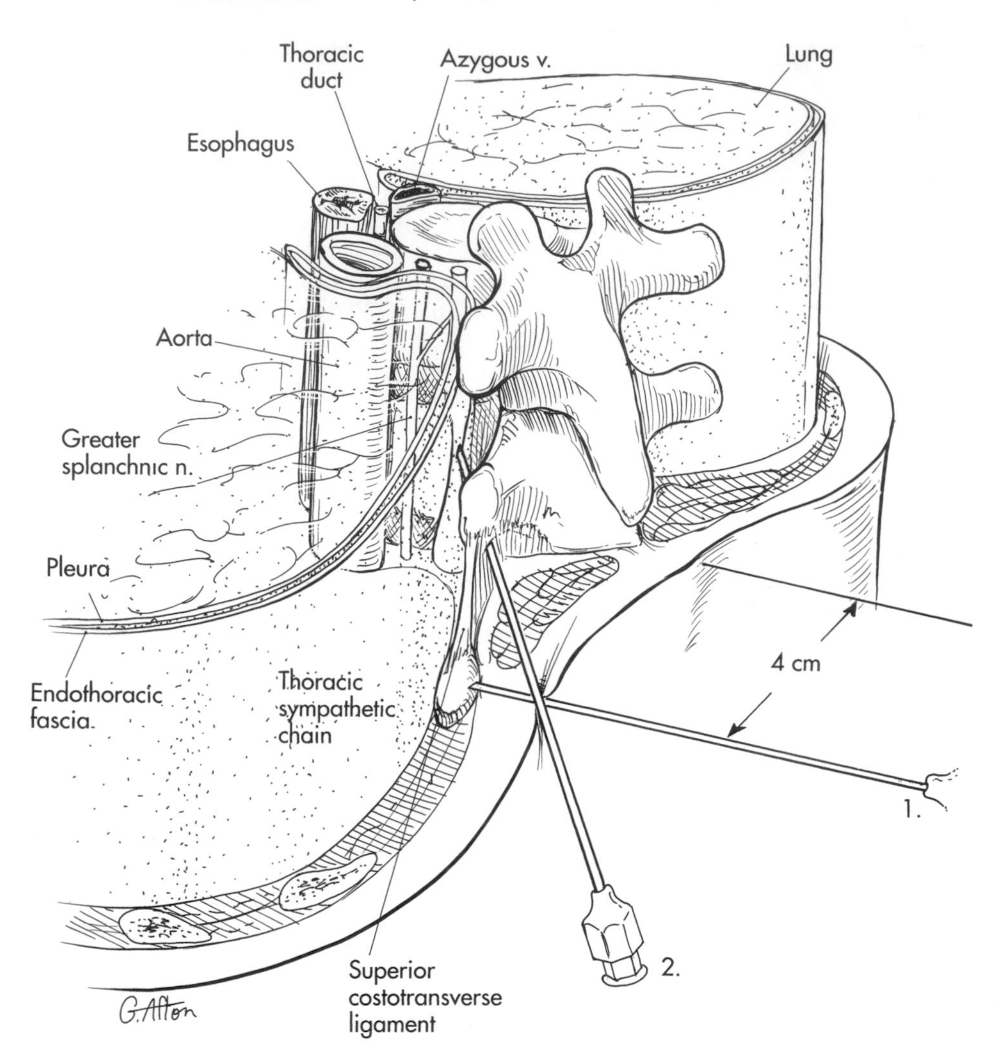

FIGURE 30–10 Midthoracic sympathetic block. (From Raj PP [ed]: Practical Management of Pain, ed 2. St Louis: Mosby–Year Book, 1992.)

out pneumothorax. Unfortunately, some 10% to 15% of patients suffer postprocedure neuritis. This can last 3 to 6 weeks.[8, 11]

COMPLICATIONS

The two principal complications of stellate ganglion block are pneumothorax and intraspinal injection (see Fig. 30–7). A third risk when neurolysis is performed is the possibility of persistent Horner's syndrome. Pneumothorax can be avoided with careful placement of the needle, and, if care is taken that the needle angulation is never lateral and that the needle is advanced through the costotransverse ligaments (posterior and anterior) slowly and cautiously utilizing the loss-of-resistance technique. Intraspinal injection most often occurs by diffusion through the intervertebral foramen and can be avoided by first injecting a water-soluble contrast dye and checking the needle position radiographically. The optimal method for checking needle position and solution spread is CT.[7]

To check for possible subsequent Horner's syndrome, the clinician can first inject local anesthetic into the region and inspect the patient after 15 to 30 minutes. This practice does not always obviate Horner's syndrome with neurolytic injection, however, and prior local anesthetic injection may not be considered optimal in all situations.

REFERENCES

1. Bonica JJ: The Management of Pain. Philadelphia, Lea & Febiger, 1953.
2. Moore DC: Stellate Ganglion Block. Springfield, Ill, Charles C Thomas, 1954.
3. Bonica JJ: Sympathetic Nerve Blocks for Pain Diagnosis and Therapy. New York, Breon Laboratories, 1984.
4. Bridenbaugh PO, Cousins MJ: Neural Blockade in Clinical Anesthesia and Management of Pain. Philadelphia, JB Lippincott, 1988.
5. Moore DC: Regional Block, ed 4. Springfield, Ill, Charles C Thomas, 1975.
6. Adelman MH: Cerebral air embolism complicating stellate ganglion block. J Mt Sinai Hosp 15:28–30, 1948.
7. Dondelinger RF, Kurdziel JC: Percutaneous phenol block of the upper thoracic sympathetic chain with computed tomography guidance. Acta Radiol 28:511–515, 1987.
8. Racz G: Techniques of Neurolysis. Boston, Kluwer Academic, 1989.
9. Wenger C, Christopher C: Radiofrequency lesions for the treatment of spinal pain. Pain Digest 8:1–16, 1998.
10. Sluijter ME: Radiofrequency Lesions in the Treatment of Cervical Pain Syndromes. Burlington, Mass, Radionics Inc, 1990, pp 1–19.
11. Skabelund C, Racz G: Indications and Technique of Thoracic$_3$ Neurolysis. Curr Rev Pain 3:400–405, 1999.

CHAPTER • 31

Cervical Epidural Nerve Block

Steven D. Waldman, MD, JD

Cervical epidural nerve block has a limited number of applications in surgical anesthesia. Consequently, this procedure has traditionally been identified as an exotic technique of only historical interest. Recognition of the clinical utility of cervical epidural nerve block in the management of head, face, neck, shoulder, and upper extremity pain has brought the technique into the mainstream of contemporary pain management. This chapter provides a practical overview of the indications for, technique of, and contraindications to cervical epidural nerve block.

HISTORICAL CONSIDERATIONS

Although Pagés's description[1] of the paramidline approach to the lumbar epidural space in 1921 is considered the first clinically relevant report of the technique of lumbar epidural nerve block, it appears that Dogliotti[2] was the first to describe the technique of epidural block in the cervical region.[3]

Owing to the problems inherent in complete sensory blockade of the cervical nerve roots when cervical epidural nerve block is performed for surgical anesthesia, many anesthesiologists believed that cervical epidural nerve block was too risky, given the general anesthetic techniques available at the time. This fact led to two persistent beliefs that, unfortunately, have colored contemporary thinking about the use of cervical epidural nerve block for pain management. The first belief is that cervical epidural nerve block is too risky for routine clinical use. The second belief is that it has a very limited number of applications. The documented clinical utility of cervical epidural administration of steroids to manage cervical radiculopathy, tension-type headache, and other painful conditions, along with cervical epidural opioids to manage cancer-related pain, combined with the clinical experience of most contemporary pain specialists simply refute both of these beliefs.

INDICATIONS AND CONTRAINDICATIONS

Indications for cervical epidural nerve block are summarized in Table 31–1. In addition to a limited number of applications for surgical anesthesia, cervical epidural nerve block with local anesthetics can be utilized as a diagnostic tool for differential neural blockade on an anatomic basis for the evaluation of head, neck, face, shoulder, and upper extremity pain.[4–8] If destruction of the cervical nerve roots is being considered, the technique is useful as a prognostic indicator of the extent of motor and sensory impairment that the patient may experience.

Cervical epidural nerve block with local anesthetics or opioids may be utilized to palliate acute pain emergencies during the wait for pharmacologic, surgical, or antiblastic methods to take effect.[9, 10] The technique is useful in the management of postoperative pain and pain secondary to trauma involving the head, face, neck, and lower extremities. The pain of acute herpes zoster and cancer-related pain are also amenable to epidural administration of local anesthetics, steroids, or opioids.[11] Additionally, this technique is of value for acute vascular insufficiency of the upper extremities secondary to vasospastic and vasoocclusive disease, including frostbite and ergotamine toxicity.[11] Evidence is increasing that the prophylactic or preemptive use of epidural nerve blocks in patients scheduled to undergo limb amputations for ischemia reduces the incidence of phantom limb pain.[12]

The administration of local anesthetics or steroids via the cervical approach to the epidural space is useful in the treatment of a variety of chronic benign pain syndromes, including cervical radiculopathy, cervicalgia, cervical spondylosis, cervical postlaminectomy syndrome, tension-type headache, phantom limb pain, vertebral compression fractures, diabetic polyneuropathy, chemotherapy-related peripheral neuropathy, postherpetic neuralgia, reflex sympathetic dystrophy, and neck and shoulder pain syndromes.[7, 13–15]

The cervical epidural administration of local anesthetics in combination with steroids or opioids is useful in the palliation of cancer-related pain of the head, face, neck, shoulder, upper extremity, and upper trunk.[16] This technique has been especially successful in relieving pain secondary to metastatic disease of the spine. The long-term epidural administration of opioids has become a mainstay in the palliation of cancer-related pain [17] The role of epidural opioids in the management of chronic benign pain syndromes is currently being evaluated.

TABLE 31–1 Indications for the Cervical Approach to The Epidural Space

Surgical, diagnostic, prognostic	Surgical anesthesia Differential neural blockade to evaluate head, neck, face, shoulder, and upper extremity pain Prognostic indicator before destruction of the cervical nerves
Acute pain	Palliation in acute pain emergencies Postoperative pain Head, face, neck, shoulder, and upper extremity pain secondary to trauma Pain of acute herpes zoster Acute vascular insufficiency of the upper extremities
Prophylactic and preemptive pain	Pain of tension-type headache Prior to amputation of ischemic limbs
Chronic benign pain	Cervical radiculopathy Cervical spondylosis Cervicalgia Vertebral compression fractures Diabetic polyneuropathy Postherpetic neuralgia Reflex sympathetic dystrophy Shoulder pain syndromes Upper extremity pain syndromes Phantom limb syndrome Peripheral neuropathy Postlaminectomy syndrome Pain of tension-type headache
Cancer-related pain	Pain secondary to head, face, neck, shoulder, and upper extremity malignancies Bony metastases to head, face, cervical spine, shoulder girdle, and upper extremity Chemotherapy-related peripheral neuropathy

Contraindictions to the cervical epidural nerve block are these:

- Local infection
- Sepsis
- Anticoagulant medication or coagulopathy
- Hypovolemia (relative contraindication)

Because of the potential for hematogenous spread via the epidural vasculature, local infection and sepsis represent absolute contraindications to using the cervical approach to the epidural space.[18] Unlike with the caudal approach to the epidural space, anticoagulation and coagulopathy are absolute contraindications to cervical epidural nerve block, owing to the risk of epidural hematoma.[19] Hypovolemia is a relative contraindication to cervical epidural nerve block with local anesthetics.[20]

CLINICALLY RELEVANT ANATOMY

Boundaries of the Cervical Epidural Space

The superior boundary of the cervical epidural space is the point at which the periosteal and spinal layers of dura fuse at the foramen magnum.[21] It should be recognized that these structures allow drugs injected into the cervical epidural space to travel beyond their confines if the volume of injectate is large enough. This fact probably explains many of the early problems associated with the use of cervical epidural nerve block for surgical anesthesia, when the large volumes of local anesthetics in vogue at the time were injected.

The epidural space continues inferiorly to the sacrococcygeal membrane.[22] The cervical epidural space is bounded anteriorly by the posterior longitudinal ligament and posteriorly by the vertebral laminae and the ligamentum flavum (Fig. 31–1). The ligamentum flavum is relatively thin in the cervical region and becomes thicker farther cauded, closer to the lumbar spine.[21] This fact has direct clinical implications, in that the loss of resistance felt during *cervical* epidural nerve block is more subtle than it is in the lumbar or lower thoracic region.

The vertebral pedicles and intervertebral foramina form the lateral limits of the epidural space (Fig. 31–2). The degenerative changes and narrowing of the intervertebral foramina associated with aging may be marked in the cervical region. Such changes reduce leakage of local anesthetic out of the foramina and account, in part, for the lower local anesthetic dose requirements of elderly patients undergoing cervical epidural nerve block. The distance between the ligamentum flavum and dura is greatest at the L2 interspace, measuring 5 to 6 mm in adults.[21] Because of the enlargement of the cervical spinal cord that corresponds to the neuromeres serving the upper extremities, this distance is only 1.5 to 2.0 mm at C7 (Fig. 31–3A).[21] It should be noted that flexion of the neck moves this cervical enlargement more cephalad, resulting in widening of the epidural space to 3.0 to 4.0 mm at the C7–T1 interspace (Fig. 31–3B).[22] This fact has important clinical implications if cervical epidural block is performed with the patient in the lateral or prone position (see Technique, later).

Contents of the Epidural Space

Fat

The epidural space is filled with fatty areolar tissue. The amount of epidural fat varies in direct proportion to the

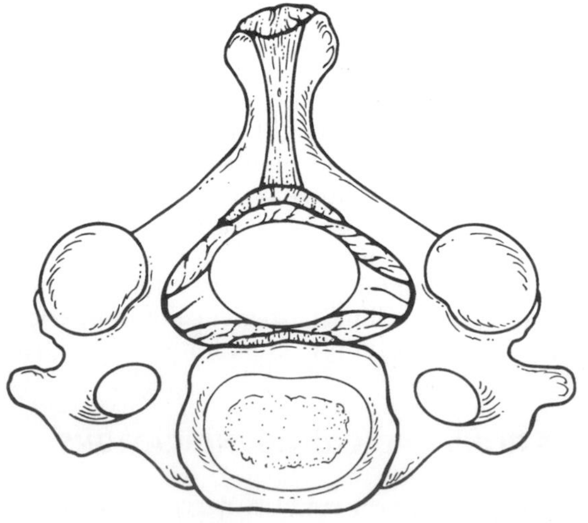

FIGURE 31–1 Cross-sectional anatomy of the cervical epidural space.

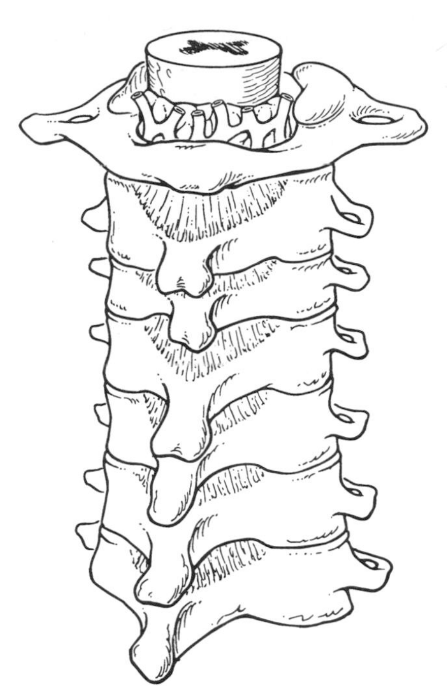

FIGURE 31–2 Posterolateral view of cervical epidural space.

amount of fat stored elsewhere in the body.[21] The epidural fat is relatively vascular and appears to change to a denser consistency with aging. This change in consistency may account for the significant variations in required drug doses in adults, especially with the caudal approach to the epidural space. The epidural fat appears to perform two functions: (1) It serves as a shock absorber for the other contents of the epidural space and for the dura and the contents of the dural sac. (2) It serves as a depot for drugs injected into the cervical epidural space. This second function has direct clinical implications for the choice of opioids for cervical epidural administration.

Epidural Veins

The epidural veins are concentrated principally in the anterolateral portion of the epidural space.[21] These veins are valveless and, so, transmit both intrathoracic and intraabdominal pressures. As pressure in either of these body cavities increases, owing to Valsalva's maneuver or compression of the inferior vena cava by a gravid uterus or a tumor mass, the epidural veins distend and reduce the volume of the epidural space. This decrease in volume can directly affect how much drug is needed to obtain a given level of neural blockade. Because this venous plexus serves the entire spinal column, it becomes a ready conduit for hematogenous infection.

Epidural Arteries

The arteries that supply the bony and ligamentous confines of the cervical epidural space as well as the cervical spinal cord enter the cervical epidural space via two routes, through the intervertebral foramina and via direct anastamoses from the intracranial portions of the vertebral arteries.[21,23] There are significant anastamoses between the epidural arteries, most of which lie in the lateral portions of the epidural space. Trauma to the epidural arteries can result in epidural hematoma formation and compromise the blood supply to the spinal cord itself.

Lymphatics

The lymphatics of the epidural space are concentrated in the region of the dural roots, where they remove foreign material from the subarachnoid and epidural spaces.

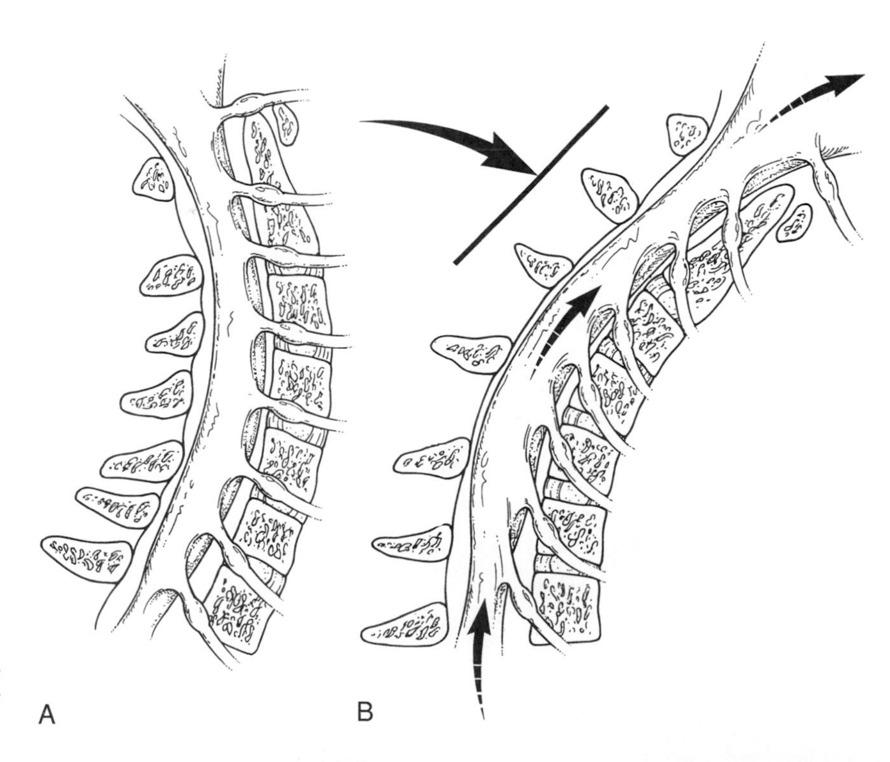

FIGURE 31–3 A, Lateral view of cervical spine in neutral position. B, Lateral view of cervical spine flexed and moving the neuromeres cephalad.

Structures Encountered During Midline Insertion of a Needle into the Cervical Epidural Space

In the cervical region, after traversing the skin and subcutaneous tissues, the styletted epidural needle impinges on the ligamentum nuchae, which runs vertically between the apices of the cervical spinous processes.[24] The ligamentum nuchae offers some resistance to the advancing needle (Fig. 31–4A). This ligament is dense enough to hold a needle in position even when the needle is released.

The interspinous ligament, which runs obliquely between the spinous processes, is encountered next and offers additional resistance to needle advancement (Fig. 31–4B). Because the interspinous ligament is contiguous with the ligamentum flavum, the operator may perceive a "false" loss of resistance when the needle tip enters the space between the interspinous ligament and the ligamentum flavum. This phenomenon is more pronounced in the cervical region than in the lumbar region because the ligaments are less well-defined.

A significant increase in resistance to needle advancement signals that the needle tip is impinging on the dense ligamentum flavum. Because the ligament is made up almost entirely of elastin fibers, resistance increases as the needle traverses the ligamentum flavum because of the drag of the ligament on the needle (Fig. 31–4C). A sudden loss of resistance occurs as the needle tip enters the epidural space (Fig. 31–4D). There should be essentially no resistance to injection of drug into the normal epidural space.

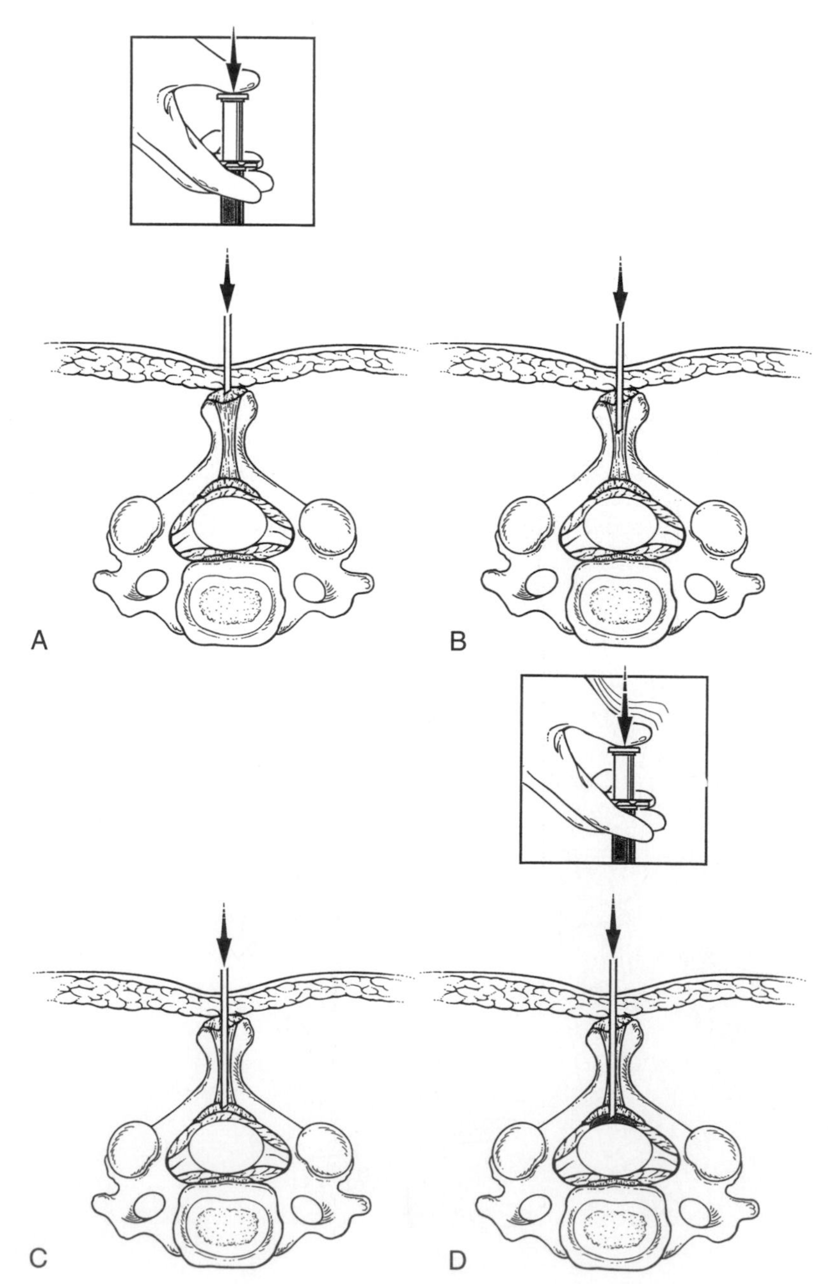

FIGURE 31–4 Midline ligaments of the cervical epidural space. A, Needle in supraspinous ligament. B, Needle in interspinous ligament. C, Needle in ligamentum flavum. D, Needle through ligamentum flavum with "animated" loss of resistance.

Pitfalls in Needle Placement

Although a comprehensive discussion of the pitfalls of needle placement for cervical epidural block is beyond the scope of this chapter, it suffices to say that close attention must be paid to the site of needle entry, the needle trajectory, and the final position of the needle tip; otherwise, the block may fail. Trauma to the nerves, arteries, veins, and to the dural sac and its contents may also occur, possibly with disastrous results.[25]

TECHNIQUE

All equipment—the needles and supplies for nerve block, the drugs, resuscitation equipment, oxygen supply, and suction—must be assembled and checked before the start of the cervical epidural nerve block, just as the patient's informed consent must be obtained.

Positioning of the Patient

Cervical epidural nerve block may be carried out with the patient in the sitting, lateral, or prone position. Each position has its advantages and disadvantages.

The Sitting Position

The sitting position is easiest for patient and pain management specialist alike. Not only does it enhance the operator's ability to identify the midline; it also ensures that the cervical spine is flexed, which widens the lower cervical epidural space. The sitting position avoids the rotation of the spine inherent in the lateral position, which makes identification of the epidural space difficult. The sitting position is not always an option, as with a patient with acute vertebral compression fractures. A history of vasovagal syncope with previous needle punctures precludes use of this position. In such situations, the lateral position is preferred unless the patient is first treated with intravenous ephedrine.

The Lateral Position

The lateral position is preferred for patients who cannot assume the sitting position or who are prone to vasovagal attacks. For the patient's comfort, the lateral position is more suitable for placement of tunneled epidural catheters or other implantable devices with an epidural terminus. If the lateral position is chosen, care must be taken to ensure that there is no rotation of the patient's spine, which would make epidural nerve block exceedingly difficult, if not impossible. Furthermore, flexion of the cervical spine is mandatory to maximize the width of the epidural space.

The Prone Position

The prone position is used principally for placement of tunneled epidural catheters and spinal stimulator electrodes. As with the other positions, care must be taken to flex the cervical spine to widen the epidural space. The prone position should be avoided if sedation is required because access to the airway is limited.

Preblock Preparation

After the patient is placed in optimal position, the skin is prepared with an antiseptic solution, such as povidone-iodine, so that all of the surface landmarks can be palpated aseptically. A fenestrated sterile drape is placed to avoid contamination by the palpating fingers. The interspace suitable for the intended epidural block is identified. At the level of this interspace, the operator's middle and index fingers are placed on either side of the spinous processes (Fig. 31–5A). The position of the interspace is confirmed again with palpation, using a rocking motion in the superior and inferior planes. The midline of the selected interspace is identified by palpating the spinous processes above and below the interspace with a lateral rocking motion, to ensure that the needle entry site is exactly in the midline (Fig. 31–5B). Failure to accurately identify the midline is the most common cause of difficulty in performing cervical epidural nerve block.

Choice of Needle

For the vast majority of adult patients the 18-gauge, 3.5-inch Hustead or Tuohy needle is suitable for cervical epidural block; however, with the sharper Tuohy needle the incidence of dural punctures may be higher.[26] Some centers are now using smaller epidural needles, with equally good results. These smaller needles decrease the amount of procedure-related and postprocedure pain.

Identification of the Epidural Space

The choice of technique for identifying the epidural space is usually based on the pain specialist's training and personal experience, rather than on scientific data. Most experts agree that the loss-of-resistance technique has significant advantages over the hanging-drop technique.[27] Because the hanging-drop method is associated with a 2.0% failure rate, as compared with less than 0.5% for the loss-of-resistance technique, the hanging-drop technique cannot be recommended.

The Loss-of-Resistance Technique

After careful identification of the midline at the chosen interspace using the technique described earlier, 1 mL of local anesthetic is utilized to infiltrate the skin, the subcutaneous tissues, and the supraspinous and interspinous ligaments. Large amounts of local anesthetic should be avoided, because they disrupt the ligamentous fibers and contribute to postprocedure pain.

The styletted needle is inserted exactly in the midline in the previously anesthetized area through the supraspinous ligament into the interspinous ligament.[27] The needle stylet is removed, and a well-lubricated 5-mL glass syringe filled with preservative-free sterile saline is attached. Because

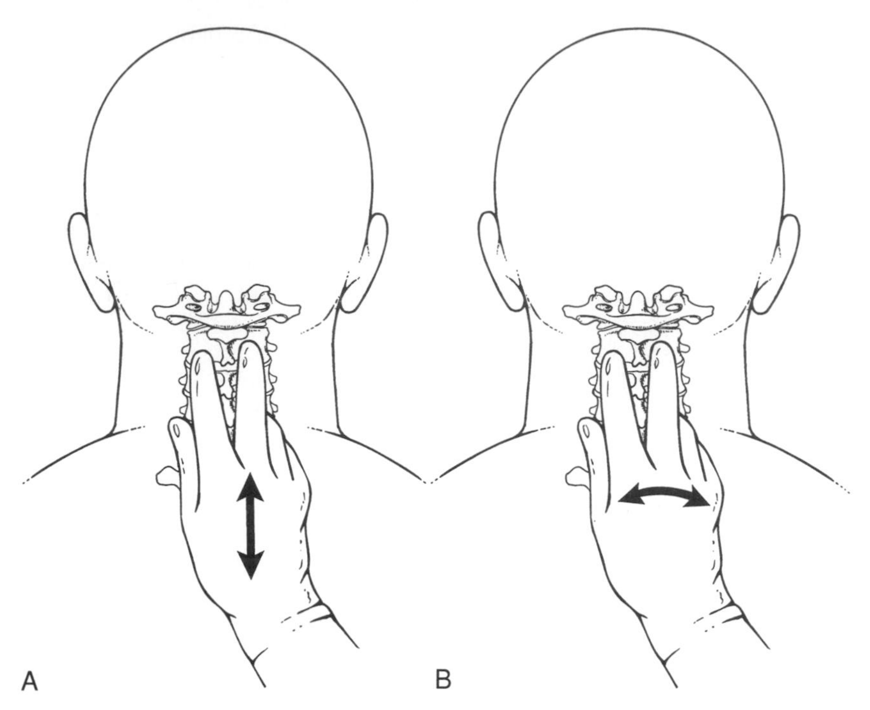

FIGURE 31–5 A, *Palpation of C6–7 intervertebral space with superoinferior rocking motion.* B, *Palpation of C6–7 midline with lateral rocking.*

saline is not compressible, it provides better tactile feedback than air. Additionally, saline avoids the risk of air embolism via the cervical epidural veins.[27]

The following instructions are written for right-handed physicians and should be reversed for left-handed physicians. The operator holds the epidural needle firmly at the hub with the left thumb and index finger. The left hand is placed firmly against the patient's neck to ensure against uncontrolled needle movements should the patient move unexpectedly (Fig. 31–6A). The right hand holds the syringe with the thumb exerting *continuous* firm pressure on the plunger.[28] Bromage[21] admonishes, "Never advance the needle without simultaneous pressure on the plunger to tell you where you are." Ballottement of the plunger, advocated by some clinicians, should not be used because it would increase the risk of inadvertent dural puncture.

As constant pressure is applied to the plunger of the syringe with the thumb of the physician's right hand, the needle and syringe are continuously advanced in a slow and deliberate manner with the left hand. As the needle bevel passes through the ligamentum flavum and enters the epidural space, there is a sudden loss of resistance and the plunger slides effortlessly forward (Fig. 31–6B). This loss of resistance provides the operator visual and tactile confirmation that the needle bevel has entered the epidural space. The syringe is gently removed from the needle.

An air or saline acceptance test is carried out by injecting 0.5 to 1.0 mL of air or sterile, preservative-free saline with a well-lubricated sterile glass syringe to help to confirm that the needle lies within the epidural space. The force required for injection should not exceed that necessary to overcome the resistance of the needle. Any significant pain or sudden increase in resistance during injection suggests incorrect needle placement. The injection should be stopped immediately and the position of the needle reassessed.

Injection of Drugs

When satisfactory needle position is confirmed, a syringe containing the drugs to be injected is carefully attached to the needle. Gentle aspiration is carried out to identify cerebrospinal fluid or blood.[28] Inadvertent dural puncture can occur in the best of hands, and careful observation for spinal fluid is mandatory.[29] If cerebrospinal fluid is aspirated, the epidural block may be attempted at a different interspace. In this situation, drug doses should be adjusted accordingly, because subarachnoid migration of drugs through the dural rent can occur. Aspiration of blood can be due either to damage to veins during insertion of the needle into the cervical epidural space or, less commonly, to intravenous placement of the needle.[28] If blood is aspirated, the needle should be rotated slightly and the aspiration test repeated. If no blood is present, incremental doses of local anesthetic and other drugs may be administered while the patient is monitored closely for signs of local anesthetic toxicity or untoward reactions to the other drugs.

Choice of Local Anesthetic

The spread of drugs injected into the cervical epidural space depends on the volume and speed of injection, the anatomic variations of the epidural space, the extent of dilatation of the epidural veins, and the position, age, and height of the patient.[30] Pregnant patients require signifi-

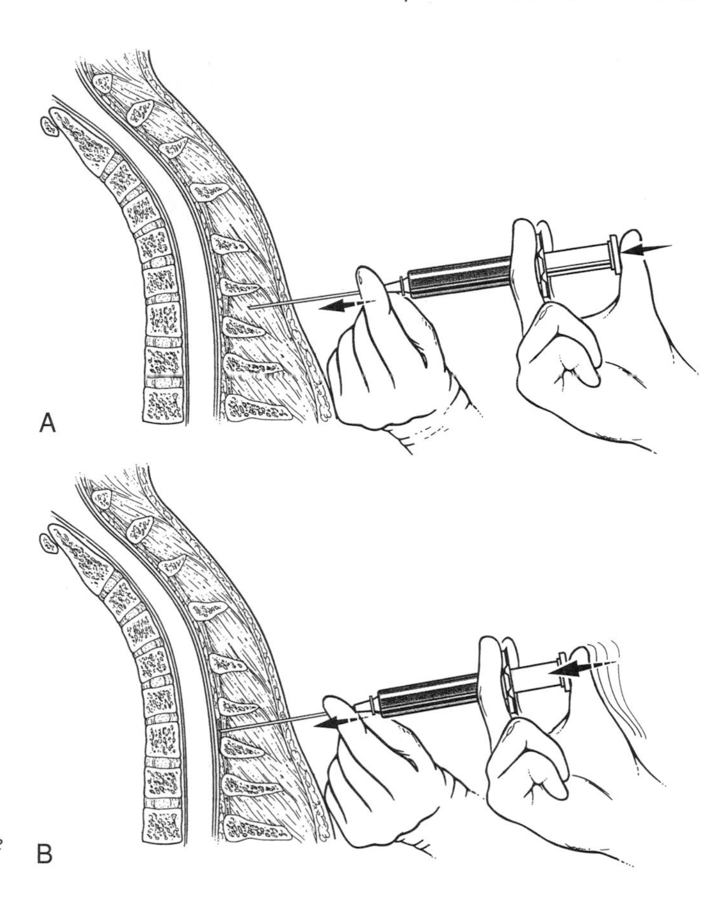

FIGURE 31 – 6 A, *Position of needle and hand for loss of resistance technique in cervical region.* B, *Sudden loss of resistance.*

cantly less drug to achieve a given level of blockade than do nongravid controls.[31]

Local anesthetics capable of producing adequate sensory block of the cervical nerve roots when administered via the cervical epidural route include 1.0% lidocaine, 0.25% bupivacaine, 2% 2-chloroprocaine, and 1.0% mepivacaine. Raising the concentration of drug increases the amount of motor block and speeds the onset of action. Adding epinephrine reduces systemic absorption and slightly prolongs the duration of action.[32] Generally, 5 to 7 mL of the previously listed agents is adequate for most pain management applications in the adult population.[7] Significant intrapatient variability exists, however, and additional incremental doses of local anesthetic may be needed to ensure adequate anesthesia in some adult patients. All local anesthetics administered via the cervical epidural route should be formulated for epidural use.[33]

For diagnostic and prognostic blocks, 1.0% preservative-free lidocaine is a suitable local anesthetic.[8] For therapeutic blocks, 0.25% preservative-free bupivacaine in combination with 80 mg of depot methylprednisolone (Depo-Medrol) is injected.[7, 8] Subsequent nerve blocks are carried out in a similar manner, with 40 mg of methylprednisolone instead of the initial 80-mg dose. Daily cervical epidural nerve blocks with local anesthetic or steroid may be required to treat the acute painful conditions described earlier.[3] Chronic conditions such as cervical radiculopathy, tension-type headache, and diabetic polyneuropathy are treated daily, every other day, or up to once a week, or as the clinical situation dictates.[3, 4, 7, 13]

If the cervical epidural route is chosen for administration of opioids, 0.5 mg of morphine sulfate formulated for epidural use is a reasonable initial dose for opioid-tolerant patients. More lipid-soluble opioids such as fentanyl must be delivered by continuous infusion via a cervical epidural catheter. All opioids administered via the cervical epidural route should be formulated for epidural use.[33]

Cervical Epidural Catheters

An epidural catheter may be placed into the cervical epidural space through a Hustead or Tuohy needle. The catheter is advanced approximately 2 to 3 cm beyond the needle tip. The needle is then carefully withdrawn over the catheter. Under no circumstance is the catheter withdrawn back through the needle, lest shearing of the catheter occur. After the injection hub is attached to the catheter, an aspiration test is carried out for blood or cerebrospinal fluid.[34] A test dose of 1 to 2 mL of local anesthetic is given via the catheter. The patient is observed for signs of local anesthetic toxicity and inadvertent subarachnoid injection. If no side effects are noted, a continuous infusion or intermittent boluses of local anesthetics or opioids may be administered through the catheter. Because the risk of infection limits the long-term use of percutaneous cervical epidural catheters, tunneling of the catheter is strongly recommended if it is anticipated that it will be in place for more than 48 hours.[35]

SIDE EFFECTS AND COMPLICATIONS OF THE CERVICAL APPROACH

Inadvertent Dural Puncture

In the hands of the experienced pain specialist, the prevalence of inadvertent dural puncture during cervical epidural nerve block is less than 0.5%.[25,29] Although postdural puncture headache is upsetting to patient and pain specialist alike, in and of itself, it should not result in permanent harm to the patient. Unfortunately, failure to recognize inadvertent dural puncture can. If an epidural needle or catheter is accidentally placed in the subarachnoid space and the problem goes unrecognized, injection of epidural doses of local anesthetics cause immediate total spinal anesthesia and associated loss of consciousness, hypotension, and apnea. If epidural doses of opioids are accidentally placed into the subarachnoid space, significant respiratory and central nervous system depression result. Should either of these problems occur, immediate supprotive measures must be taken to restore homeostasis.

Inadvertent Subdural Puncture

It is possible to inadvertently place a needle or catheter intended for the epidural space into the subdural space. If subdural placement goes unrecognized and epidural doses of local anesthetics are administered, the signs and symptoms are similar to those of massive subarachnoid injection, although the resulting motor and sensory block may be spotty.[36,37] The effect of inadvertent injection of large doses of opioids into the subdural space is probably similar to that of subarachnoid injection. Massive subdural injection of local anesthetics or opioids requires immediate supportive measures, as indicated, to restore homeostasis.

Inadvertent Intravenous Needle and Catheter Placement

The cervical epidural space is densely vascular. Intravenous placement of the epidural needle complicates approximately 0.5% to 1% of lumbar epidural anesthesia procedures.[21] The prevalence of inadvertent intravenous placement of the epidural needle in the cervical epidural space is assumed to be similar. This complication is more common in patients with distended epidural veins (e. g., parturients and patients with a large intraabdominal tumor mass). If the misplacement is unrecognized, injection of local anesthetic directly into an epidural vein results in significant local anesthetic toxicity.[38] Careful aspiration before injection of drugs into the epidural space is also mandatory to identify this potentially serious problem. Observation of the patient during and after the injection process is mandatory.

Hematoma and Ecchymosis

The epidural space is densely vascular. Needle trauma to the epidural veins may cause self-limited bleeding and, thus, postprocedure pain. Uncontrolled bleeding into the epidural space may result in compression of the spinal cord with the rapid development of neurologic deficit. Although the incidence of significant neurologic deficit secondary to epidural hematoma after cervical epidural block is exceedingly rare, this devastating complication should be considered whenever rapidly developing neurologic deficit follows cervical epidural nerve block.[39]

Infection

Although uncommon, infection in the epidural space is an ever present possibility, especially in immunocompromised patients or persons who have cancer.[40] Because of the nature of the epidural venous system, hematogenous spread throughout the central nervous system is a possibility when epidural infection occurs.[25] Because the offending organism in epidural infections is usually *Staphylococcus aureus*, initial antibiotic treatment should be directed at this organism until culture results are available.[41] If epidural abscess occurs, emergent surgical drainage to avoid spinal cord compression and irreversible neurologic deficit is usually necessary. Early detection and treatment of infection are crucial to avoiding potentially life-threatening sequelae.

Neurologic Complications

Neurologic complications of cervical nerve block are uncommon if proper technique is utilized. Direct trauma to the spinal cord or nerve roots is usually accompanied by pain. If significant pain occurs during placement of the epidural needle or catheter or during injection, the physician should immediately stop and ascertain the cause of the pain to avoid the possibility of additional neural trauma.[25] Intravenous sedation or general anesthesia before initiation of cervical epidural nerve block renders the patient unable to provide accurate verbal feedback if the needle is misplaced. Therefore, routine use of sedation or general anesthesia before cervical epidural nerve block is discouraged, because it takes away this important safeguard.[28]

Urinary Retention and Incontinence

The administration of local anesthetics and opioids into the cervical epidural space may be associated with a greater incidence of urinary retention as compared with cervical epidural block performed with local anesthetic and steroid.[34] This side effect is more common in elderly males and multiparous females whose bladders are ptotic. Overflow incontinence may occur when such patients are unable to void or bladder catheterization is not utilized. All patients undergoing cervical epidural nerve block should be able to empty their bladder before discharge from the pain center.

SUMMARY

Cervical epidural nerve block is quite useful in the management of a variety of acute, chronic, and cancer-related pain syndromes. Clinical experience has demonstrated that cervical epidural nerve block is safe as long as careful attention is paid to the technical aspects.

REFERENCES

1. Pagés E: Anestesia metamerica. Rev Sanid Mil Madr 11:351–385, 1921.
2. Dogliotti AM: Segmental peridural anesthesia. Am J Surg 20:107, 1933.
3. Waldman SD: Epidural nerve block. *In* Weiner RS (ed): Innovations in Pain Management. Orlando, Fla, PMD Press, 1990, pp 4–5.
4. Waldman SD: The role of neural blockade in the management of headaches and facial pain. Curr Rev Pain 1:346–352, 1997.
5. Waldman SD: Acute herpes zoster and postherpetic neuralgia. Intern Med 11:33–37, 1990.
6. Waldman SD: Reflex sympathetic dystrophy. Intern Med 11:62–68, 1990.
7. Cronen MC, Waldman SD: Cervical steroid epidural nerve blocks in the palliation of pain secondary to tension-type headaches. J Pain Symptom Manage 5:379–381, 1990.
8. Waldman SD: Acute and postoperative pain management. *In* Weiner RS (ed): Innovations in Pain Management. Orlando, Fla, PMD Press, 1993, pp 12–13.
9. Waldman SD: The role of spinal opioids in the management of cancer pain. J Pain Symptom Manage 5:163–168, 1990.
10. Waldman SD, Feldstein GS, Waldman HJ: Cervical implantable narcotic delivery systems in the management of upper body pain of malignant origin. Anesth Analg 66:780–782, 1987.
11. Waldman SD: Cervical Epidural Block. *In* Waldman SD: Atlas of Interventional Pain Management Techniques. Philadelphia, WB Saunders, 1998, pp 121–128.
12. Bonica JJ: Regional anesthesia with local anesthetics. *In* Bonica JJ (ed): The Management of Pain. Philadelphia, Lea & Febiger, 1990, p 1956.
13. Wilson WL, Waldman SD: Role of the epidural administration of steroids and local anesthetics in the palliation of pain secondary to vertebral compression fractures. Pain Digest 1:294–295, 1992.
14. Waldman SD, Waldman KA: Reflex sympathetic dystrophy of the face. Reg Anesth 12:15–17, 1987.
15. Cronen MC, Waldman SD: Cervical steroid epidural nerve block in the palliation of pain secondary to intractable muscle contraction headache. American Association for the Study of Headache 28:4;314–315, 1988.
16. Waldman SD, Portenoy RK: Recent advances in the management of cancer pain. Pain Manage 4:19, 1991.
17. Waldman SD, Coombs DW: Selection of implantable narcotic delivery systems. Anesth Analg 68:377–384, 1989.
18. Cousins MJ, Bromage PR: Epidural neural blockade. *In* Cousins MJ, Bridenbaugh DO (eds): Neural Blockade, ed 2. Philadelphia, JB Lippincott, 1988, pp 340–341.
19. Waldman SD, Feldstein GS, Waldman HJ: Caudal administration of morphine sulfate in anticoagulated and thrombocytopenic patients. Anesth Analg 66:267–268, 1987.
20. Bromage PR: Complications and contraindications. *In* Bromage PR (ed): Epidural Analgesia. Philadelphia, WB Saunders, 1978, pp 654–711.
21. Bromage PR: Anatomy. *In* Bromage PR (ed): Epidural Analgesia. Philadelphia, WB Saunders, 1978, pp 8–20.
22. Reynolds AF, Roberts PA, Pollay M, et al: Quantitative anatomy of the thoracolumbar epidural space. Neurosurgery 17:905, 1985.
23. Woollam DHM, Millen JW: An anatomical background to vascular disease of the spinal cord. Proc R Soc Med 51:540, 1958.
24. Katz J: Cervical approach—single injection technique. *In* Katz J (ed): Atlas of Regional Anesthesia. Norwalk, Conn, Appleton & Lange, 1994, pp 204–205.
25. Waldman SD: Cervical steroid epidural nerve blocks—a prospective study of complications occurring during 790 consecutive blocks. Reg Anesth 11:149–152, 1989.
26. Bromage PR: Epidural needles. Anesthesiology 22:1018, 1961.
27. Bromage PR: Identification of the epidural space. *In* Bromage PR (ed): Epidural Analgesia. Philadelphia, WB Saunders, 1978.
28. Cousins MJ, Bromage PR: Epidural neural blockade. *In* Cousins MJ, Bridenbaugh DO (eds): Neural Blockade. Philadelphia, JB Lippincott, 1988, pp 333–334.
29. Waldman SD, Feldstein GS, Allen ML: Cervical epidural blood patch for treatment of cervical dural puncture headache. Anesth Review 14:1;23–25, 1987.
30. Burn JM, Guyer PB, Langdon L: The spread of solutions injected into the epidural space: A study using epidurograms in patients with the lumbosciatic syndrome. Br J Anaesth 45:338, 1973.
31. Bromage PR: Mechanism of action. *In* Bromage PR (ed): Epidural Analgesia. Philadelphia, WB Saunders, 1978, pp 141–142.
32. Mather LE, Tucker GT, Murphy TM, et al: The effects of adding adrenaline to etidocaine and lignocaine in extradural anaesthesia. II: Pharmacokinetics. Br J Anaesth 48:989, 1976.
33. Waldman SD: Issues in selection of local anesthetics. Hosp Formulary 26:590–597, 1991.
34. Armitage EN: Lumbar and thoracic epidural. *In* Wildsmith JAW, Armitage EN (eds): Principles and Practice of Regional Anesthesia. New York, Churchill Livingstone, 1987, p 109.
35. Waldman SD: Placement of subcutaneous tunnelled epidural catheters. J Pain Symptom Manage 2:163–166, 1987.
36. Waldman SD: Horner's syndrome following epidural nerve block. Reg Anesth 17:55, 1992.
37. Waldman SD: Subdural injection as a cause of unexplained neurological symptoms. Reg Anest 17:55, 1992.
38. Braid DP, Scott DB: The systemic absorption of local analgesic drugs. Br J Anaesth 37:394, 1965.
39. Cousins MJ: Hematoma following epidural block. Anesthesiology 37:263, 1972.
40. Donohoe CD, Waldman SD: Headache in the AIDS patient. Intern Med 14:68–76, 1993.
41. Waldman SD: Cervical epidural abscess following cervical steroid epidural nerve block. Anesth Analg 72:717–718, 1991.

CHAPTER • 32

Brachial Plexus Block

Steven D. Waldman, MD, JD

HISTORICAL CONSIDERATIONS

Brachial plexus block was first performed by two famous surgeons—Halsted in 1884, and in 1887 Crile.[1] Both surgeons first surgically exposed the brachial plexus before applying cocaine to this neural structure under direct vision. The first percutaneous brachial plexus blocks were reported in 1911 by Hirschel and Hulenkampff.[2] Over the ensuing years, a variety of techniques, modifications, and advancements have made brachial plexus block one of the regional anesthetic techniques most frequently utilized in contemporary anesthesia practice. Recent work by Winnie has further elucidated the clinically relevant anatomy of the brachial plexus, which has led to further refinement of the technique and recognition of the role of brachial plexus block in the treatment of sympathetically maintained pain syndromes involving the upper extremity.[3]

CLINICALLY RELEVANT ANATOMY

A clear understanding of the clinically relevant anatomy of the brachial plexus is mandatory if the pain management specialist is to safely and successfully perform brachial plexus block, regardless of what technique is chosen. Failure to appreciate this fact will increase the incidence of failed blocks and complications. The brachial plexus is formed by the fusion of the anterior rami of the C5, C6, C7, C8, and T1 spinal nerves. There may also be a contribution of fibers from C4 and T2 spinal nerves. The nerves that make up the plexus exit the lateral aspect of the cervical spine and pass downward and laterally in conjunction with the subclavian artery. The nerves and artery run between the anterior scalene and the middle scalene muscle passing inferiorly behind the middle of the clavicle and above the top of the first rib to reach the axilla (Fig. 32–1). The scalene muscles are enclosed in an extension of prevertebral fascia that helps to contain drugs injected into this region.

Interscalene Block

Indications

The interscalence approach to the brachial plexus is the preferred technique for brachial plexus block when anesthesia or relaxation of the shoulder is desired.[4] In addition to applications for surgical anesthesia, interscalene brachial plexus nerve block with local anesthetics can be utilized as a diagnostic tool when performing differential neural blockade on an anatomic basis in the evaluation of shoulder and upper extremity pain. If destruction of the brachial plexus is being considered, this technique is useful as a prognostic indicator of the degree of motor and sensory impairment that the patient may experience. Interscalene brachial plexus nerve block with local anesthetic may be utilized to palliate acute pain emergencies including acute herpes zoster, brachial plexus neuritis, shoulder and upper extremity trauma, and cancer pain while waiting for pharmacologic, surgical, and antineoplastic methods to take effect.[5] Interscalene brachial plexus nerve block is also a useful alternative to stellate ganglion block when treating reflex sympathetic dystrophy of the shoulder and upper extremity.[4]

Destruction of the brachial plexus is indicated for the palliation of cancer pain, including invasive tumors of the brachial plexus and tumors of the soft tissue and bone of the shoulder and upper extremity.[6] Owing to the desperate nature of many patients' suffering from aggressively invasive tumors that have invaded the brachial plexus, blockade of the brachial plexus using the interscalene approach may be carried out in the presence of coagulopathy or anticoagulation by utilizing a 25-gauge needle, albeit with increased risk of ecchymosis and hematoma formation.

Technique

The patient is placed in a supine position with the head turned away from the side to be blocked. A total of 20 to 30 mL of local anesthetic is drawn up in a 30-mL sterile syringe. When treating painful or inflammatory conditions that are mediated via the brachial plexus, a total of 80 mg of depot steroid is added to the local anesthetic with the first block and 40 mg of depot steroid with subsequent blocks.

The patient is then asked to raise his or her head against the resistance of the pain specialist's hand to help to identify the posterior border of the sternocleidomastoid muscle. In most patients, a groove can be palpated between the posterior border of the sternocleidomastoid muscle and the

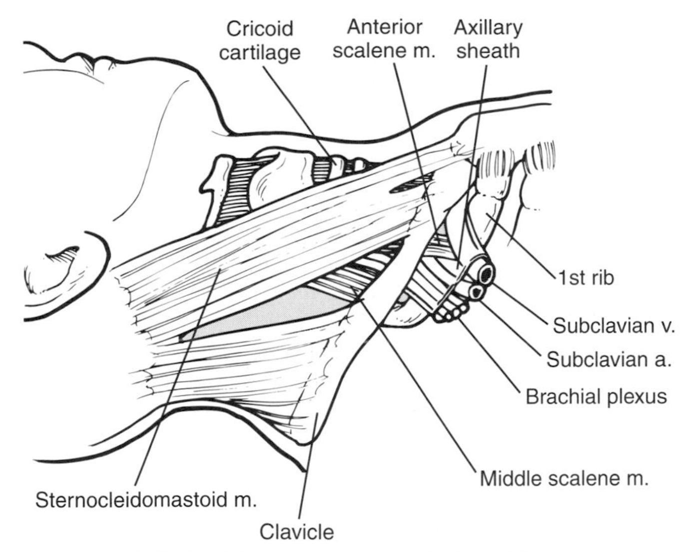

FIGURE 32–1 Anatomy of the brachial plexus.

anterior scalene muscle. Identification of the intrascalene groove can be facilitated by having the patient inhale strongly against a closed glottis. The skin overlying this area is then prepared with antiseptic solution. At the level of the cricothyroid notch (C6) at the interscalene groove, a 25-gauge 1 1/2-inch needle is inserted with a slightly caudad and inferior trajectory (Fig. 32–2). If the intrascalene groove cannot be identified, the needle is placed just slightly behind the posterior border of the sternocleidomastoid muscle. The needle should be advanced quite slowly as a paresthesia is almost always produced when the needle tip impinges on the brachial plexus as it traverses the interscalene space almost at a right angle to the needle tip. The patient should be warned that at some point a paresthesia will occur and to say, "There!" as soon as it is felt. Paresthesia should be encountered at a depth of approximately 3/4 to 1 inch. After paresthesia is elicited, gentle aspiration is carried out to identify blood or cerebrospinal fluid. If the aspiration test is negative and no paresthesia into the distribution of the brachial plexus persists, 20 to 30 mL of solution is slowly injected, as the patient is monitored closely for signs of local anesthetic toxicity or inadvertent subarachnoid injection. If surgical anesthesia is required for forearm or hand procedures, additional local anesthetic may have to be placed farther caudad along the brachial plexus to obtain adequate anesthesia of the lower portion of the plexus. Alternatively, specific nerves may be blocked farther distally if augmentation of the interscalene brachial plexus block is desired.[4]

Side Effects and Complications

The proximity of the brachial plexus to the subclavian artery and other large vessels suggests the potential for inadvertent intravascular injection or local anesthetic toxicity from intravascular absorption. Given the large doses of local anesthetic required for interscalene brachial plexus block, the pain specialist should carefully calculate the total milligram dose of local anesthetic that may safely be given. This vascularity also increases the incidence of postblock ecchymosis and hematoma formation. In spite of the vascularity of this anatomic region, this technique can safely be performed in the presence of anticoagulation by utilizing a 25- or 27-gauge needle, albeit at increased risk of hematoma, if the clinical situation dictates a favorable risk-benefit ratio. Risk for these complications can be decreased if manual pressure is applied to the area of the block immediately after injection. Application of cold packs for 20-minute periods after the block also decreases the amount of postprocedure pain and bleeding.

In addition to the potential for complications involving the vasculature, the proximity of the brachial plexus to the central neuroaxial structures and the phrenic nerve can result in side effects and complications. If the needle is placed too deep, inadvertent epidural, subdural, or subarachnoid injection is a possibility. If volume of local anesthetic utilized for this block is accidentally placed in any of these spaces, significant motor and sensory block will result. Unrecognized, these complications could be fatal. It should be assumed that the phrenic nerve will also be blocked during brachial plexus block utilizing the interscalene approach. In the absence of significant pulmonary disease, unilateral phrenic nerve block should rarely create respiratory embarrassment. However, blockade of the recurrent laryngeal nerve with its attendant vocal cord paralysis, combined with paralysis of the diaphragm, may make clearing pulmonary and upper airway secretions difficult. Although less likely than with the supraclavicular approach to brachial plexus block, pneumothorax is a possibility.

Clinical Pearls

The key to the safe and successful interscalene brachial plexus block is a clear understanding of the anatomy and careful identification of the necessary anatomic landmarks. Poking around for a paresthesia without first identifying the interscalene groove is a recipe for disaster. The pain specialist should remember that the brachial plexus is quite

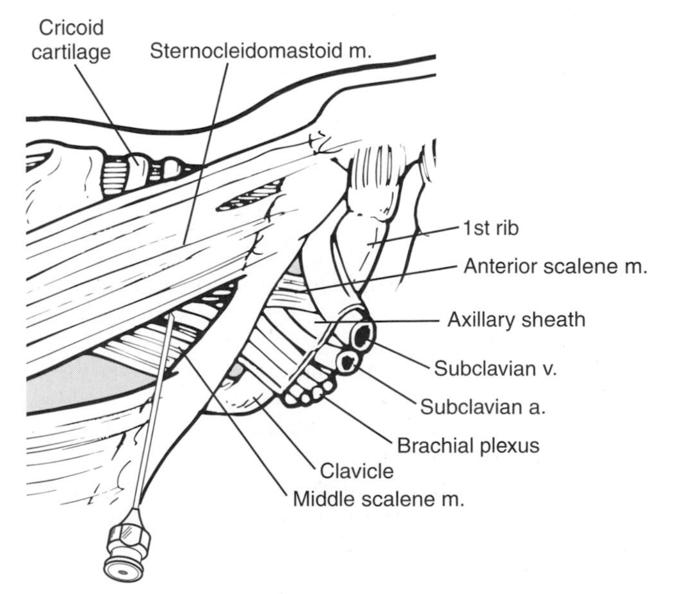

FIGURE 32–2 Needle placement for interscalene brachial plexus block.

close to the skin at the level where this block is performed. The needle should rarely be inserted deeper than 1 inch in all but the most obese patients. Supplementation of intrascalene brachial plexus block by more peripheral block of the ulnar nerve may be required, as the C8 fibers are not always adequately anesthetized when utilizing the interscalene approach. Careful neurologic examination for preexisting neurologic deficits that might later be attributed to the nerve block should be performed before beginning any brachial plexus block.

Supraclavicular Block

Indications

The supraclavicular approach to brachial plexus block is an excellent choice when dense surgical anesthesia of the distal upper extremity is required. This technique is less suitable for shoulder problems, as it almost always requires supplementation with cervical plexus block to provide adequate cutaneous anesthesia of the shoulder.[7] In addition to applications for surgical anesthesia, supraclavicular brachial plexus nerve block with local anesthetics can be utilized as a diagnostic tool when performing differential neural blockade on an anatomic basis to evaluate upper extremity pain. If destruction of the brachial plexus is being considered, this technique is useful as a prognostic indicator of the degree of motor and sensory impairment that the patient may experience. Supraclavicular brachial plexus nerve block with local anesthetic may be utilized to palliate acute pain emergencies, including that of acute herpes zoster, brachial plexus neuritis, upper extremity trauma, and cancer while waiting for pharmacologic, surgical, and antiplastic methods to take effect. Supraclavicular brachial plexus nerve block is also useful as an alternative to stellate ganglion block for treating reflex sympathetic dystrophy of the upper extremity.

Destruction of the supraclavicular brachial plexus is indicated for palliation of cancer pain, including invasive tumors of the brachial plexus, and tumors of the soft tissue and bone of the upper extremity.[6] Because of the potential for intrathoracic hemorrhage, the interscalene approach to brachial plexus block should be utilized in patients who are anticoagulated only if the clinical situation dictates a favorable risk-benefit ratio.

Technique

The patient is placed supine with the head turned away from the side to be blocked. A total of 10 mL of local anesthetic is drawn up in a 20-mL sterile syringe. When treating painful conditions that are mediated via the brachial plexus, a total of 80 mg of depot steroid is added to the local anesthetic with the first block and 40 mg of depot steroid is added with subsequent blocks.

The patient is then asked to raise his or her head against the resistance of the pain specialist's hand to aid in identifying the posterior border of the sternocleidomastoid muscle. The point at which the lateral border of the sternocleidomastoid attaches to the clavicle is then identified. At this point, just above the clavicle, after the skin is prepared with antiseptic solution, a 1.5-inch needle is inserted directly perpendicular to the table top (Fig. 32–3). The needle should be advanced quite slowly, as a paresthesia is almost always encountered at a depth of approximately 3/4 to 1 inch. The patient should be warned that a paresthesia will occur and to say, "There" as soon as it is felt. If a paresthesia is not elicited after the needle has been slowly advanced to a depth of 1 inch, the needle should be withdrawn and readvanced with a slightly more cephalad trajectory. This maneuver should be repeated until a paresthesia is elicited. Conversely, if the first rib is encountered before a paresthesia is induced, the needle should be walked laterally along the first rib until a paresthesia is elicited. The needle should never be directed in a more medial trajectory lest pneumothorax occur.

After paresthesia is elicited, gentle aspiration is carried out to identify blood or cerebrospinal fluid. If the aspiration is negative and no persistent paresthesia into the distribution of the brachial plexus remains, 20 to 30 mL of solution is slowly injected as the patient is monitored closely for signs of local anesthetic toxicity or inadvertent neuroaxial injection.

Side Effects and Complications

The proximity of the brachial plexus to the subclavian artery and other large vessels suggests the potential for inadvertent intravascular injection or local anesthetic toxicity from intravascular absorption. Given the large doses of local anesthetic required for supraclavicular brachial plexus block, the pain specialist should carefully calculate the total milligram dose of local anesthetic that may safely be given. This vascularity also increases the risk of postblock ecchymosis and hematoma formation. These complications can be minimized if manual pressure is applied to the area of the block immediately after injection. Applying cold packs for 20-minute periods after the block also reduces the amount of postprocedure pain and bleeding the patient may experience.

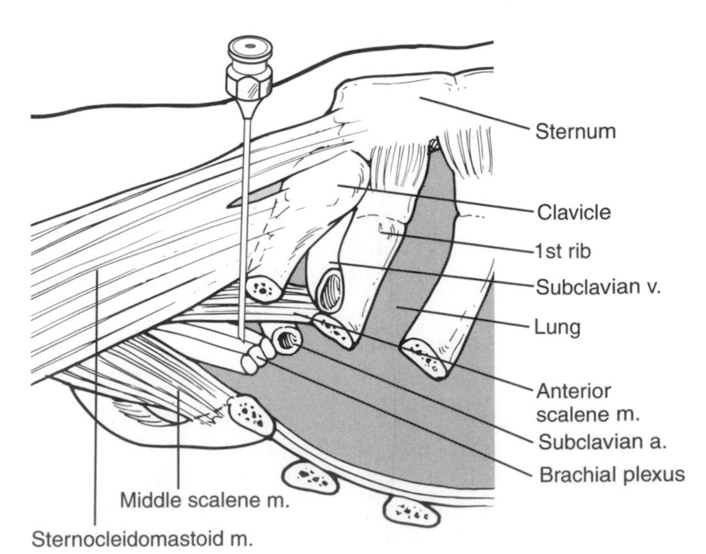

FIGURE 32–3 Needle placement for supraclavicular brachial plexus block.

In addition to the potential for complications involving the vasculature, the proximity of the brachial plexus to the central neuroaxial structures and the phrenic nerve can result in side effects and complications. Although these complications occur less frequently than with interscalene brachial plexus block, inadvertent epidural, subdural, or subarachnoid injection remains a possibility. If the volume of local anesthetic utilized for this block is accidentally placed in any of these spaces, significant motor and sensory block will result. Unrecognized, these complications could be fatal. It should be assumed that the phrenic nerve will also be blocked at least 30% of the time during brachial plexus block utilizing the supraclavicular approach. In the absence of significant pulmonary disease, unilateral phrenic nerve block should rarely create respiratory embarrassment.[7] Blockade of the recurrent laryngeal nerve with its attendant vocal cord paralysis, combined with paralysis of the diaphragm, may however make clearing pulmonary and upper airway secretions difficult. Owing to proximity of the apex of the lung, pneumothorax is a distinct possibility and the patient should be so informed.

Clinical Pearls

The key to performing safe and successful supraclavicular brachial plexus block is a clear understanding of the anatomy and careful identification of the necessary anatomic landmarks. Poking around for a paresthesia without first identifying the anatomic landmarks is a recipe for disaster. The pain specialist should remember that the brachial plexus is quite close to the surface at the level where this block is performed. The needle should rarely be inserted deeper than 1 inch in all but the most obese patients. If strict adherence to technique is observed and the needle is never advanced medially from the lateral border of the insertion of the sternocleidomastoid muscle on the clavicle, the incidence of pneumothorax should be less than 0.5%. Careful neurologic examination to identify preexisting neurologic deficits that might later be attributed to the nerve block should be performed before beginning any brachial plexus block.

Axillary Approach to the Brachial Plexus

Indications

The axillary approach to the brachial plexus is the preferred technique for brachial plexus block when dense anesthesia of the forearm and hand is required.[8] In addition to applications for surgical anesthesia, axillary brachial plexus block with local anesthetics can be utilized as a diagnostic tool when performing differential neural blockade on an anatomic basis to evaluate upper extremity pain. If destruction of the brachial plexus is being considered, this technique is useful as a prognostic indicator of the degree of motor and sensory impairment that the patient may experience. Axillary brachial plexus nerve block with local anesthetic may be utilized to palliate acute pain emergencies including that of acute herpes zoster, brachial plexus neuritis, shoulder and upper extremity trauma, and cancer pain while waiting for pharmacologic, surgical, and antiplastic methods to take effect. Axillary brachial plexus nerve block is also useful as an alternative to stellate ganglion block when treating reflex sympathetic dystrophy of the upper extremity.[8]

Destruction of the brachial plexus is indicated for the palliation of cancer pain, including invasive tumors of the distal brachial plexus and tumors of the soft tissue and bone of the upper extremity. Because of the desperation of many patients suffering from aggressively invasive tumors that have invaded the brachial plexus, blockade using the axillary approach may be carried out even in the presence of coagulopathy or anticoagulation by utilizing a 25-gauge needle, albeit with increased risk of ecchymosis and hematoma formation.

Clinically Relevant Anatomy

The brachial plexus is formed by the fusion of the anterior rami of the C5, C6, C7, C8, and T1 spinal nerves. There may also be a contribution of fibers from C4 and T2 spinal nerves. The nerves that make up the plexus exit the lateral aspect of the cervical spine and pass downward and laterally in conjunction with the subclavian artery. The nerves and artery run between the anterior scalene and the middle scalene muscle, passing inferiorly behind the middle of the clavicle and above the top of the first rib to reach the axilla. Because the sheath that encloses the axillary artery and nerves is less consistent than that which encloses the brachial plexus at the level where interscalene and supraclavicular brachial plexus blocks are performed, a single-injection technique is less satisfactory. The median, radial, ulnar, and musculocutaneous nerves surround the artery within this imperfect sheath. David Brown, M.D. has suggested that the position of these nerves relative to the axillary artery can best be visualized by placing them in the quadrants as represented on the face of a clock with the axillary artery at the center of the clock (Fig. 32–4).[9] The median nerve is found in the 12:00 to 3:00 o'clock quadrant, the ulnar nerve in the 3:00 to 6:00 o'clock quadrant, the radial nerve in the 6:00 to 9:00 o'clock quadrant, and the musculocutaneous nerve in the 9:00 to 12:00 o'clock quadrant.

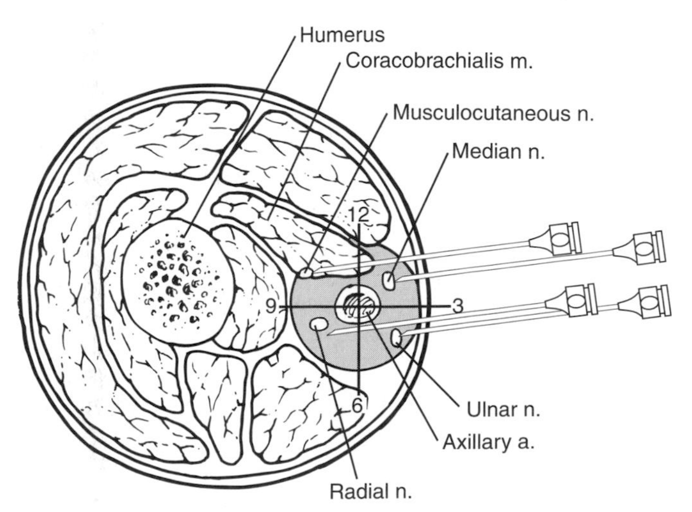

FIGURE 32–4 Relative locations of the median, radial, and ulnar nerves.

To ensure adequate block of these nerves, drugs must be injected into each quadrant to deposit it close in enough to each of these nerves.

Technique

The patient is placed in a supine position with the arm abducted 85 to 90 degrees and the fingertips resting just behind the ear. A total of 30 to 40 mL of local anesthetic is drawn up in a 50-mL sterile syringe. When treating painful or inflammatory conditions that are thought to be mediated via the brachial plexus, a total of 80 mg of depot steroid is added to the local anesthetic with the first block and 40 mg of depot steroid with subsequent blocks.

The pain specialist then identifies the pulsations of the axillary artery with the middle and index fingers of the nondominant hand and traces the course of the artery distally by following the pulsations. After the skin has been prepared with antiseptic solution, an 1-inch 25-gauge needle is inserted just below the arterial pulsations (Fig. 32–5). The needle should be advanced quite slowly, as a paresthesia is almost always induced as the needle tip impinges on the radial or ulnar nerve. The patient should be warned that a paresthesia will occur and asked to say "There" as soon as it is felt. Paresthesia should be encountered at a depth of approximately 1/2 to 3/4 inch. After paresthesia is elicited and its distribution identified, gentle aspiration is carried out to identify blood or cerebrospinal fluid. If the aspiration test is negative and no persistent paresthesia into the distribution of the brachial plexus remains, 8 to 10 mL of solution is slowly injected as the patient is monitored closely for signs of local anesthetic toxicity or inadvertent subarachnoid injection. If a radial paresthesia is elicited, the needle is withdrawn slightly into the 3:00 to 6:00 o'clock quadrant, which contains the ulnar nerve, and, after negative aspiration, an additional 8 to 10 mL of solution is injected. If an ulnar paresthesia is elicited, the needle is withdrawn and then slowly readvanced in a slightly more superior direction into the 6:00 to 9:00 o'clock quadrant, which contains the radial nerve, and the aspiration and injection technique is repeated. The needle is then withdrawn and redirected above the arterial pulsation to the 12:00 to 3:00 o'clock quadrant, which contains the median nerve. If aspiration is negative, 8 to 10 mL of solution is injected. The needle is then directed to the 9:00 to 12:00 o'clock quadrant, which contains the musculocutaneous nerve. If aspiration is negative, the remaining local anesthetic is injected. Alternatively, the musculocutaneous nerve can be blocked by infiltrating the solution into the mass of the coracobrachialis muscle.

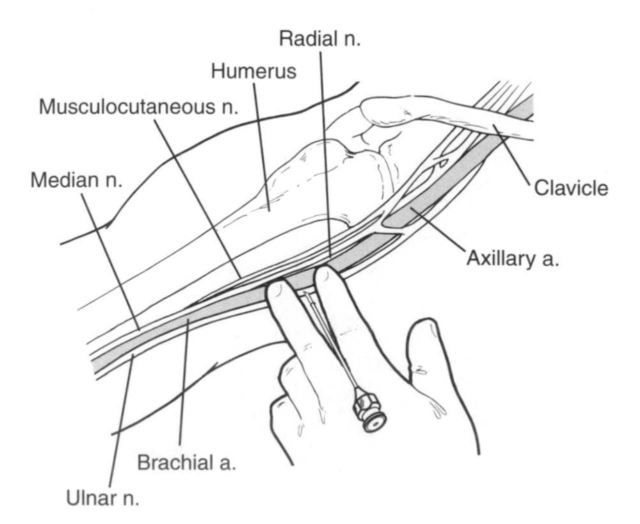

FIGURE 32–5 Needle placement for axillary approach to brachial plexus block.

Side Effects and Complications

The proximity of the nerves to the axillary artery and other large vessels carries the risk for inadvertent intravascular injection or local anesthetic toxicity from intravascular absorption.[10] Given the large doses of local anesthetic required for axillary brachial plexus block, the pain specialist should carefully calculate the total milligram dose of local anesthetic that may safely be given. The dense vascularity also increases the risk of postblock ecchymosis and hematoma formation. In spite of the vascularity of this anatomic region, this technique can safely be attempted in a patient taking anticoagulant by utilizing a 25- or 27-gauge needle, albeit at increased risk of hematoma, if the clinical situation dictates a favorable risk-benefit ratio. These complications can be reduced if manual pressure is applied to the area of the block immediately after injection. Applying cold packs for 20-min periods after the block also reduces the amount of postprocedure pain and bleeding.

The distance of the nerves to be blocked from the neuroaxis and phrenic nerve makes the complications associated with injection of drugs onto these structures highly unlikely, which is an advantage of the axial approach as compared with the intrascalene and supraclavicular approaches to brachial plexus block. Because paresthesias are elicited, the potential for post-block persistent paresthesia is a possibility and the patient should be so advised.

Clinical Pearls

The axillary approach to brachial plexus block is a safe and simple way to anesthetize the distal upper extremity. For pain above the elbow, the interscalene or supraclavicular approach is probably a better choice. Careful neurologic examination for preexisting neurologic deficits that might later be attributed to the nerve block should be performed before any brachial plexus block.

REFERENCES

1. Crile GW: Anesthesia of the nerve roots with cocaine. Cleve Med J 2:355, 1997.
2. Kulenkampff D: Anesthesia of the brachial plexus. Zentrabl Chir 38, 1337, 1911.
3. Winnie AP: Plexus Anesthesia: Perivascular Technique of Brachial Plexus Block, ed 2. Philadelphia, WB Saunders, 1990, pp 56–58.
4. Waldman SD: Brachial plexus block: Interscalene approach. *In* Waldman SD (ed): Atlas of Interventional Pain Management Techniques. Philadelphia, WB Saunders, 1998, pp 131–135.
5. Bonica JJ: Musculoskeletal disorders of the upper limb. *In* Bonica JJ (ed): The Management of Pain, ed 2. Philadelphia, Lea & Febiger, 1990, pp 891–893.

6. Bonica JJ: Neurolytic blockade. *In* Bonica JJ (ed): The Management of Pain, ed 2. Philadelphia, Lea & Febiger, 1990, pp 1996–1999.
7. Waldman SD: Brachial plexus block: Supraclavicular approach. *In* Waldman SD (ed): Atlas of Interventional Pain Management Techniques. Philadelphia, WB Saunders, 1998, pp 136–140.
8. Waldman SD: Brachial plexus block: Axiallary approach. *In* Waldman SD (ed): Atlas of Interventional Pain Management Techniques. Philadelphia, WB Saunders, 1998, pp 140–145.
9. Brown DL: Axillary block. *In* Brown DL (ed): Atlas of Regional Anesthesia. Philadelphia, WB Saunders, 1999, pp 49–56.
10. Katz J: Axillary block. *In* Katz J (ed): Atlas of Regional Anesthesia. Norwalk, Conn, Appleton-Century-Crofts, 1995, pp 70–72.

CHAPTER • 33

Suprascapular Nerve Block

Steven D. Waldman, MD, JD

HISTORICAL CONSIDERATIONS

Historically, suprascapular nerve block was utilized as a primary treatment for conditions that limited the range of motion of the shoulder, including adhesive capusulitis and calcific tendinitis and bursitis.[1] The advent of corticosteroids allowed earlier treatment of the maladies, and the use of suprascapular nerve block as a primary treatment modality for shoulder lesions declined. Recently, there has been renewed interest in suprascapular nerve block to allow early range of motion and rehabilitation after shoulder reconstruction or joint replacement.

INDICATIONS

Suprascapular nerve block with local anesthetics can be utilized as a diagnostic tool when performing differential neural blockade on an anatomic basis to evaluate shoulder girdle and shoulder joint pain.[2] If destruction of the suprascapular nerve is being considered, this technique is useful as a prognostic indicator of the degree of motor and sensory impairment that the patient might experience.[3] Suprascapular nerve block with local anesthetic may be utilized to palliate acute pain emergencies, including postoperative pain, pain secondary to trauma to the shoulder joint and girdle, and cancer pain while waiting for pharmacologic, surgical, or antiblastic treatment to become effective.[3] Suprascapular nerve block is also useful as adjunctive therapy for decreased range of motion of the shoulder secondary to reflex sympathetic dystrophy or adhesive capsulitis,[1, 3] and it can be utilized to allow the patient to tolerate more aggressive physical therapy after shoulder reconstructive surgery.[3]

Destruction of the suprascapular nerve is indicated for palliation of cancer pain, including that of invasive tumors of the shoulder girdle.[3] It can be performed in patients who are taking anticoagulants, if the clinical situation dictates a favorable risk-benefit ratio.

CLINICALLY RELEVANT ANATOMY

The suprascapular nerve is formed from fibers originating from the C5 and C6 nerve roots of the brachial plexus and, in most patients, some fibers from the C4 root. The nerve passes inferiorly and posteriorly from the brachial plexus to pass underneath the coracoclavicular ligament through the suprascapular notch.[4] The suprascapular artery and vein accompany the nerve through the notch. The suprascapular nerve provides much of the sensory innervation to the shoulder joint and innervation to two of the muscles of the rotator cuff, the supraspinatus and infraspinatus.

TECHNIQUE

The patient is placed in the sitting position with the arms hanging loosely at the side. A total of 10 mL of local anesthetic is drawn up in a 20-mL sterile syringe. When treating painful conditions that are mediated via the suprascapular nerve, a total of 80 mg of depot steroid is added to the local anesthetic with the first block and 40 mg of depot steroid with subsequent blocks.

The spine of the scapula is identified, and the pain specialist then palpates along the length of the scapular spine laterally to identify the acromion. At the point where the thicker acromion fuses with the thinner scapular spine, the skin is prepared with antiseptic solution. At this point, the skin and subcutaneous tissues are anesthetized utilizing a 1.5-inch needle. After adequate anesthesia is obtained, a 3 1/2-inch 25-gauge needle is inserted with an inferior trajectory toward the body of the scapula (Fig. 33–1). The needle should make contact with the body of the scapula at a depth of about 1 inch. The needle is then gently "walked" superiorly and medially until the tip walks off the scapular body into the suprascapular notch. If the notch is not identified, the same manuveur is repeated directing the needle superiorly and laterally until the needle tip is positioned in the suprascapular notch. A paresthesia is often encountered as the needle tip enters the notch, and the patient should be so warned. If a paresthesia is not elicited after the needle has entered the suprascapular notch, it is advance an additional 1/2 inch, to place the tip beyond the substance of the coracoclavicular ligament. The needle should never be advanced deeper, lest pneumothorax occur.

After paresthesia is elicited or the needle has been advanced into the notch as described above, gentle aspiration

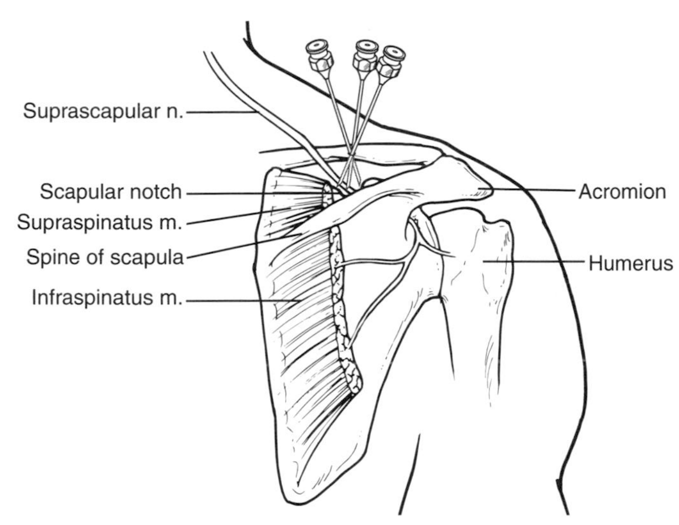

FIGURE 33–1 Needle placement for suprascapular nerve block.

is carried out to identify blood or air. If the aspiration test is negative, 10 mL of solution is slowly injected as the patient is monitored closely for signs of local anesthetic toxicity.

SIDE EFFECTS AND COMPLICATIONS

The proximity of the suprascapular nerve to the suprascapular artery and vein suggests the potential for inadvertent intravascular injection or local anesthetic toxicity from intravascular absorption. The pain specialist should carefully calculate the total (milligram) dose of local anesthetic that may safely be given for suprascapular nerve block. Owing to the proximity of the lung, should the needle be advanced too deep through the suprascapular notch, pneumothorax is a possibility.

CLINICAL PEARLS

Suprascapular nerve block is a safe and simple regional anesthesia technique that has many pain management applications. It is probably underutilized as an adjunct to rehabilitation after shoulder reconstruction and for the shoulder-hand variant of reflex sympathetic dystrophy. It is important that the pain specialist be sure that the physical and occupational therapists caring for the patient understand that suprascapular nerve block renders not only the shoulder girdle but also the shoulder joint insensate. This means that deep heat modalities and range of motion exercises must be carefully monitored to avoid burns and damage to the shoulder.

REFERENCES

1. Pitkin GP: Therapeutic nerve block. *In* Pitkin GP (ed): Conduction Anesthesia. Philadelphia, JB Lippincott, 1946, pp 884–886.
2. Katz J: Suprascapular nerve block. *In* Katz J (ed): Atlas of Regional Anesthesia. Norwalk, Conn, Appleton-Century-Crofts, 1995, pp 72–73.
3. Waldman SD: Suprascapular nerve block. *In* Waldman SD (ed): Atlas of Interventional Pain Management Techniques. Philadelphia, WB Saunders, 1998, pp 144–147.
4. Bonica JJ: Musculoskeletal disorders of the upper limb. *In* Bonica JJ (ed): The Management of Pain, ed 2. Philadelphia, Lea & Febiger, 1990, pp 891–893.
5. Pitkin GP: Anatomy of the crainial nerves. *In* Pitkin GP (ed): Conduction Anesthesia. Philadelphia, JB Lippincott, 1946, pp 56–57.

CHAPTER • 34

Thoracic Epidural Nerve Block

Somayaji Ramamurthy, MD

The technique of thoracic epidural nerve block is being utilized with increasing frequency in the practice of pain management. The presence of the spinal cord at the thoracic levels demands that the clinician have significant technical proficiency in performing epidural techniques without complications. A thorough knowledge of anatomic and physiologic changes associated with a thoracic epidural block is essential to avoiding complications. In this chapter I outline the anatomy, physiologic changes, indications, applications, and complications of thoracic epidural nerve block.

HISTORICAL CONSIDERATIONS

The development of thoracic epidural techniques followed the developments in lumbar epidural techniques. Modification of the Tuohy needle with the Huber tip to facilitate insertion of the catheter further increased their utility and safety as did the improvement in the catheter material and development of disposable, prepackaged sterile equipment. Advances in epidurally administered drugs such as the opioids, and the ability to implant catheters for the management of cancer pain further advanced the clinical applications of thoracic epidural block. The addition of implantable epidural electrodes to stimulate the spinal cord in the thoracic region has made this technique extremely useful.

INDICATIONS[1–6]

Surgical

Thoracic epidural catheters are increasingly utilized for providing intraoperative, and especially postoperative, analgesia for thoracic and upper abdominal surgical procedures. With the thoracic epidural, stress is significantly reduced.[6] It has been utilized for thoracotomy and cardiac surgery[7–12] in conjunction with light general anesthesia.[13] The benefits and safety of thoracic epidural analgesia for breast surgery are well-documented.[14–16]

Postoperative Analgesia

There has been much debate about whether thoracic epidural technique is indicated to provide postoperative analgesia. Many clinicians believe that a catheter placed in the lumbar epidural space, to deliver a narcotic, can provide significant analgesia in the thoracic area without risking the complications associated with the thoracic epidural technique.[17, 18] On the other hand, many studies show the superiority of the thoracic epidural technique.[19–24] With the thoracic epidural technique, the catheter can be placed very close to the nerve roots innervating the painful area. This becomes especially important when utilizing any local anesthetic. Small quantities of local anesthetics can be utilized to provide excellent analgesia with the thoracic approach.[20–22, 25] The lumbar epidural technique requires large volumes of local anesthetic to provide analgesia in the thoracic dermatomes.[17] This may result in significant hypotension and significant blood levels of the local anesthetic, thus limiting its usefulness.

Even with opioids such as morphine, which ascend in the cerebrospinal fluid, the thoracic epidural technique still has advantages because the onset of analgesia is faster.[20, 22] Morphine placed in the lumbar epidural space takes quite a while to ascend to the thoracic area and provide analgesia. With highly lipid-soluble drugs such as fentanyl and sufentanil, the doses required to maintain analgesia are such that either epidural technique may not offer any advantages over the intravenous route of administration.[18] Patient-controlled epidural analgesia has been used effectively and safely, even at thoracic levels.[26]

Thus, the thoracic epidural approach provides rapid onset of analgesia and minimizes the doses of both local anesthetics and opioids needed to provide excellent analgesia. Small doses of bupivacaine with morphine do not prevent ambulation.[27] This is very important, because small quantities of local anesthetic play a significant role in reducing pain related to motion and episodic pain.[20, 21, 25, 27] Thoracic epidural techniques have also been utilized in pediatric patients with good results. The analgesia obtained from the technique has been shown to be superior to that of interpleural or intravenous techniques.[28, 29]

Herpes Zoster and Postherpetic Neuralgia

Herpes zoster infection is most common in the thoracic area. Pain from the acute herpes zoster can be relieved by epidural administration of local anesthetic or steroids. For acute herpes zoster, the local anesthetic produces excellent pain relief and may prevent postherpetic neuralgia and limit eruption of more vesicles.[30] An epidural catheter placed very close to the involved nerve root can provide excellent analgesia, even with 2 to 3 mL of 0.25% bupivacaine. Usually, the catheter is left in only 2 or 3 days. The drug is injected once or twice a day.

Epidural Steroids

Herniated discs are not very common in the thoracic spine. The patient who has nerve root irritation secondary to a herniated intervertebral disc or inflammation of the nerve root secondary to cancer or radiation therapy responds extremely well to an epidural steroid injection. Methylprednisolone (Depo-Medrol), 80 mg, or triamcinolone (Aristocort), 25 to 50 mg, is given, alone or mixed with saline or local anesthetic.

Acute Pain Secondary to Trauma

Patients with multiple fractured ribs and fractured vertebra get excellent analgesia with a properly positioned epidural catheter. Local anesthetic, such as 0.125% to 0.25% bupivacaine and/or an opioid, can be utilized. Even with short-term administration of local anesthetic by the epidural route, the patient can have prolonged pain relief after the muscle spasm and other secondary phenomena are relieved.

Angina

Angina secondary to myocardial ischemia has been treated via the thoracic epidural technique.[1, 31, 32] It provides excellent analgesia and decreases myocardial oxygen consumption, anxiety associated with the pain, and catecholamine levels as well. It has also been used for long-term home self-treatment.[33] Spinal cord stimulation with the electrode placed in the epidural space has been used to control angina,[34, 35] and such stimulation does not mask the pain of acute myocardial infarction.[36]

Cancer Pain

Catheters placed in the thoracic epidural space can be utilized to provide long-term analgesia using opioids such as morphine or local anesthetic. Through a tunneled epidural catheter such as Du Pen or another catheter with external access, excellent long-term analgesia can be provided. Catheters can also be completely buried under the skin utilizing a reservoir which is accessed through the skin for injection. Epidural phenol[37] or alcohol[38] has also been used for analgesia in cancer patients. The catheter is placed in the area of the involved nerve roots. Alcohol is injected through the catheter in 0.5-mL increments to a maximum of 5 mL. Previous injection of local anesthetic and sedation help to reduce the pain associated with injection of the alcohol. The injection has to be repeated daily for at least 3 days. More than 79% of the patients report significant pain relief (50%). Phenol has also been used epidurally. The technique is similar to that of epidural alcohol: 5% phenol in dextrose or in 0.9% saline is injected slowly and repeated daily for 3 days. Both techniques have been reported to provide excellent analgesia without producing significant sensory or motor deficit.

Epidural clonidine can be a useful advancement for various types of cancer pain or benign neuropathic pain that has failed to respond to more traditional measures.

Spinal Cord Stimulation

Electrodes for spinal cord stimulation are commonly placed via the lumbar or thoracic area. The technique is similar to that of thoracic epidural catheter insertion, except that the needle is bevelled so that the catheter can be gently withdrawn and redirected. The procedure utilizes an image intensifier. Stimulation of the cervical spinal cord is usually approached through a thoracic epidurally placed electrode, which is advanced into the cervical area. The catheter is then tunneled subcutaneously and connected to a pulse generator.

Management of Acute Pancreatitis

Patients with severe pain secondary to acute pancreatitis benefit from an epidural catheter placed in the lower thoracic area to deliver local anesthetics such as bupivacaine and/or an opioid such as morphine.[6] The severe pain is thus controlled until the pancreatitis is under control.

CONTRAINDICATIONS

Contraindications are the same as those for any other epidural approach:

- Patient refusal.
- Infection in the area or septicemia.
- Bleeding or clotting disorders such as thrombocytopenia or current anticoagulant therapy.
- Uncorrected hypovolemia.

ANATOMY[1-5]

The thoracic epidural space extends from the lower margin of the C7 vertebra to the upper margin of L1. The vertebral column in the thoracic area normally has a kyphotic curvature with its apex at approximately T6. Slight scoliosis to the right can occur, even in normal persons. Significant scoliosis is associated with the rotation of the vertebral column, which can produce significant technical difficulty in performing this block. The inclination of the spinous processes is different at different levels of the thoracic vertebral column (Fig. 34–1). The spines from T1–T4 have very little inclination, whereas those of T5–T8 tilt significantly downward, making a midline approach to the epidural space practically impossible. The T9–T12 spines point dorsally without significant inclination, so the midline approach is possible. The ligamentum flavum is not as thick as it is in the lumbar spine, and, occasionally, the epidural space can be entered without encountering very much resistance. The attachment of the ligamentum flavum to the lower margin of the lamina on its inner aspect reduces the size of the epidural space, whereas the space is wider at the upper margin of the lamina, because the ligamentum flavum is attached to the outer aspect of the upper margin of the lower lamina. The epidural space is 3 to 4 mm wide in the thoracic area. The thoracic epidural space, just like the rest of the epidural space, contains loose areolar tissue, fat, and vertebral venous plexus.

Nerve Roots

The T1 nerve root is fairly large and participates in the formation of the brachial plexus. The nerve roots at T2 and below gradually increase in size but are still smaller than any of the lumbar or cervical roots. The epidural space communicates through the intervertebral foramina into the paravertebral space. The spinal cord has a lumbar enlargement at T9–T12. Even though the nerve roots in the subarachnoid space travel caudad for significantly increasing distances below T2 before they exit the intervertebral foramina, their course in the epidural space is horizontal. The dorsal and ventral roots unite just proximal to the intervertebral foramina.

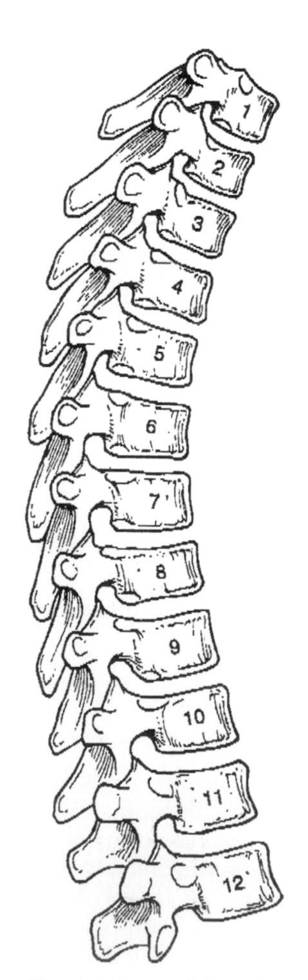

FIGURE 34–1 The inclination of the spinous processes from T1 to T12.

Epidural Pressure

The pressure in the thoracic epidural space is approximately −15 cm H_2O, being very close to that of the intrapleural pressure.[6] It is more pronounced in the sitting position. The negative pressure in the thoracic epidural space is also considered to be secondary to the tenting of the dura by a blunt epidural needle.[39] In 12% of patients, the pressure is not negative.

The insignificant amount of fat in the epidural space of children younger than 5 or 6 years makes it possible to thread a caudally introduced epidural catheter straight up into the thoracic epidural space.[40] Blanco and coworkers, however, report that lumbar epidural catheters were successfully advanced to T12 level only in 22% of the 199 patients.[41]

Physiologic Changes

Cardiovascular[4, 6]

The cardiovascular effects of a thoracic epidural nerve block depend on its level. The preganglionic sympathetic fibers are present in all of the thoracic anterior nerve roots. Levels of block up to T10 produce minimal cardiovascular changes. The degree of hypotension secondary to this level of block will depend on the blood volume and the position of the patient. The cardiovascular effects could be minimal because of the compensatory vasoconstriction in the upper extremities. If the local anesthetic block extends up to T6, the cardiovascular effects are mainly due to peripheral vasodilatation, venous pooling, decreased right heart filling, and hypotension. Blocking of the fibers to the abdominal viscera, including those to the adrenal medulla, can reduce the response to stress for lower abdominal and pelvic surgical procedures.

If the block extends up to T1, the sympathetic fibers innervating the heart are also affected. Thus, the block of the cardioaccelerator fibers can produce bradycardia and hypotension owing to the unopposed action of the parasympathetic fibers derived from the vagus nerve, sometimes resulting in cardiac standstill.[42] Studies have also shown decreased myocardial contractility.[43] The hypotension can be significant. It may respond to treatment with ephedrine initially but may require aggressive treatment with epinephrine and/or dopamine.

The myocardial oxygen consumption is reduced with a thoracic epidural. Blumberg and colleagues have shown that thoracic epidural analgesia can relieve the pain of angina, decrease stenosis, and also reduce the oxygen requirement, thus facilitating oxygenation of the myocardium.[31,32] Pulmonary hypertension[44] is decreased with thoracic epidural analgesia, and the ST-T segment changes can also be reversed.

Pulmonary

Weakening of the intercostal muscles can affect respiratory parameters. When a block affects all the intercostals, normal ventilation and Pa_{CO_2} can still be maintained by the activity of the diaphragm, since the phrenic nerve is not affected. Improved diaphragmatic shortening and tidal volume have been reported secondary to intercostal paralysis.[45] The inspiratory reserve volume and functional reserve capacity are significantly decreased, as is vital capacity. Thoracic or abdominal pain can produce shallow breathing and decreased oxygen saturation. Oxygenation can improve after pain relief because of the thoracic epidural block.[46]

Horner's Syndrome[47]

Thoracic epidural block of T1 nerve roots can result in unilateral or bilateral Horner's syndrome.

CLINICAL PEARLS

Placement of the thoracic epidural catheter can be done with the patient sitting or in the lateral decubitus position. The sitting position provides better alignment of the skin midline to the spine and facilitates identification of landmarks. But, a patient who is anxious may have a vasovagal reaction in the sitting position with hypotension and nausea. The procedure can also be done with the patient prone. Since there is no significant flexion and extension, flexion of the patient contributes very little to expanding the interlaminar space in the thoracic spine. Thousands of postoperative thoracic epidural procedures have been performed without complication and without radiographic guidance. Fluoroscopy or an image intensifier is required only for spinal cord stimulator placement. Verification of the position of the catheter using a nonionic contrast medium may be advisable before performing a neurolytic block.

Midline Approach

The midline approach (Fig. 34–2) is applicable in the upper part of the thoracic spine between C7 and T5 and in the lower part, including T9–L1, since the spinous processes project directly posteriorly and are horizontal. The level of the spinous process corresponds to the level of the vertebra. The epidural technique is similar to that used in the lumbar areas, with a 90-degree approach, but the author prefers starting at the lower part of the interspace, just above the lower spine, so that the needle is angled cephalad, which facilitates insertion and advancement of the catheter.

After infiltration of a local anesthetic such as lidocaine intradermally with a short, 25- or 27-gauge needle, injection of a local anesthetic with a slightly longer needle, such as a 1.5-inch, 22-gauge needle, into the paraspinal muscles on either side of the spine provides significant analgesia for the procedure by blocking the nerve fibers as they come from lateral areas toward the midline. I prefer to use a 16- to 18-gauge Tuohy needle 3.5 inches long. The Tuohy needle is advanced with the bevel cephalad so that the smooth part of the curvature will bounce off the lamina. The needle is advanced through the skin, subcutaneous tissue, supraspinous ligament, intraspinous ligament, and ligamentum flavum. If ligament resistance is encountered and the lamina is contacted after that, it is clear that the needle is at the upper margin of the lower lamina. Redirection farther cephalad facilitates entry into the epidural space, which entry is recognized by one of the many techniques described earlier.

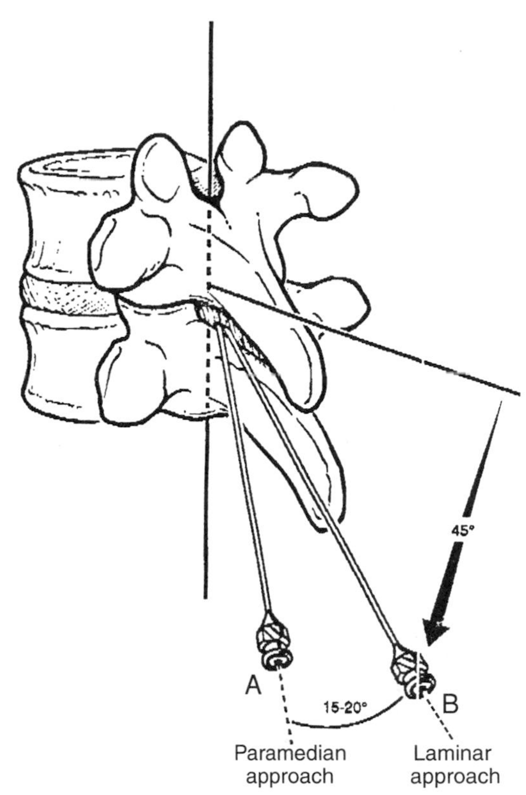

FIGURE 34–2 A, *Paramedian approach. Needle is inserted 1 cm lateral to the midline with a 45-degree cephalad angle and a 15- to 20-degree angle in the coronal plane to enter the ligamentum flavum in the midline.* B, *Laminar approach. Needle is inserted right next to the cephalad edge of the spine and is advanced straight forward without any deviation towards the midline.*

The most common one is the loss-of-resistance technique using air or a fluid-filled syringe containing a small bubble of air to allow compression (since a liquid is not compressible). If a liquid is used, the author prefers 0.9% saline without preservatives. Hanging-drop technique has been utilized, especially in the thoracic area, because of the significant negative pressure. Despite a low incidence of dural puncture, the drop is sucked in only 88% of the time. Since both hands are utilized to slowly advance the needle, entry into the epidural space is recognized even when the drop is not sucked in.

Some authors take the ability to advance the significant length of the catheters without difficulty as an indication of entry into the epidural space. If the needle is off course and enters the paraspinal muscles or a defect in the interspinous ligament, there could be misleading loss of resistance. This error can be identified by the paraspinal compression technique,[48] in which the index and middle fingers of the nondominant hand compress the paraspinal tissues on either side of the needle. If the resistance that was lost reappears, the tip of the needle is superficial to the ligamentum flavum. If the external pressure does not affect pressure in the syringe, the needle is deep to the ligamentum flavum.

A catheter is advanced 3 to 4 cm. As in any epidural technique, the catheter should not be withdrawn after it passes the tip of the needle as the catheter may be sheared off. Needles used for electrode placement in the epidural space are specially designed to allow for gentle withdrawal. Inserting the catheter too far may result in migration through the intervertebral foramen, epidural vein, or true knot formation. Tunneling the catheter for 5 cm utilizing another epidural needle reduces the risk of catheter migration.[49]

The author prefers to utilize the technique described by Raj[50] (Fig. 34–3) for taping the catheter, using the Steri-Strips Mystisol and Tegaderm. This technique reduces the possibility of catheter dislodgement and facilitates maintaining the catheter for a longer period of time. The catheter is connected to an adapter, a filter, and an injection site and then taped over the infraclavicular area to afford easy access for reinjection. An externalized catheter can be well-protected over the long term with a colostomy bag.[51]

Epidural Drugs

Choice of medication is similar to that used in the lumbar area, although smaller volumes of local anesthetics are needed. Positioning the catheter in the middle of the desired area of analgesia minimizes the necessary volume. The necessary doses depend on individual factors, such as age, height, weight, intercurrent disease (e.g., diabetes), and extent of desired analgesia. Short-acting and long-acting local anesthetics and opioids have been utilized for single administration or infusion. Concentrations are similar to those for lumbar epidural analgesia.

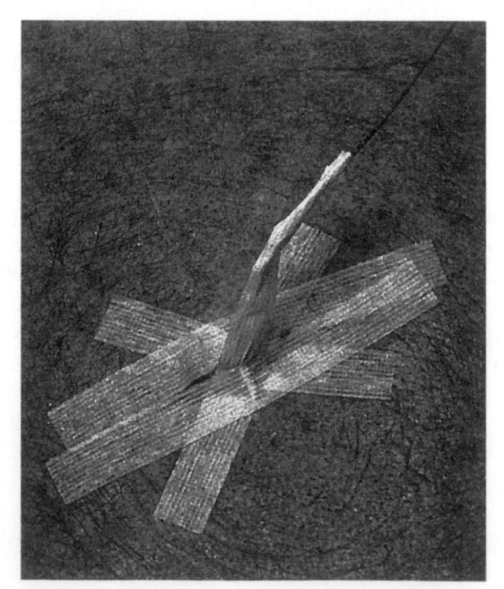

FIGURE 34–3 Technique of anchoring the epidural catheter for prolonged use.

Paramedian Lateral Approach

This technique can be utilized at any level of the thoracic spine. Usually, the starting point is 1 to 2 cm lateral to the superior margin of the spinous process. In the majority of patients, a 1.5-inch, 22-gauge needle can contact the lamina, and 1 mL of short-acting local anesthetic can be injected to decrease the pain related to "walking" on the lamina. The epidural needle is advanced at a 45- to 55-degree angle cephalad, and a 15- to 30-degree angle toward the midline. Extreme angles can result in nerve root contact on the opposite side of the spine, or the needle passing between the spinous processes into the paraspinal muscle without contacting the ligamentum flavum. The author prefers starting right next to the lateral margin of the cephalad edge of the spine, thus minimizing the angle required to make the puncture in the ligamentum flavum, close to the midline. Contacting the lamina with the epidural needle significantly increases the safety of the technique because the epidural space can be entered by walking off of the superior margin of the lamina. The steep angle required to enter the epidural space in the midthoracic area also facilitates the insertion of the catheter.

Laminar Approach

For a laminar approach the starting point is the same as that for the paramedian approach, but the needle is not angled toward the midline. Only the lateral portion of the epidural space is entered. The disadvantages of the technique are that the epidural space is narrower and veins are more numerous in the lateral portion of the epidural space. Also, if the starting point is too far lateral, or even with the slight lateral angle, the needle will contact the articular processes. Walking it more cephalad will not achieve entry into the epidural space. I prefer starting right next to the cephalad margin of the spinous process and minimizing the angle, which increases the chance of entering the epidural space. The laminar approach is more useful when attempting to get a predominantly unilateral block, especially while using epidural steroids. A small volume of injectate has a tendency to stay on one side for two to three segments.

PITFALLS

1. Since the spinal cord is present in the thoracic vertebral level, a thoracic epidural technique should be attempted only by an operator who has extensive experience doing lumbar epidurals. Bromage recommends that a person who performs a thoracic epidural should have done at least 50 consecutive lumbar epidurals without a dural puncture or a complication.
2. Because of the inclination of the spine in the midthoracic area, the technique could be technically difficult, although it can be mastered with some practice.

3. Because the nerve roots contain the sympathetics to the heart, a block of these fibers can produce significant bradycardia and hypotension.

Intercostal muscle weakness resulting from thoracic epidural block can produce significant difficulty, especially in obese patients and those with respiratory impairment. In a person with impaired function of the diaphragm, chronic obstructive lung disease, or obesity, intercostal paralysis can significantly contribute to the respiratory impairment.

COMPLICATIONS[52]

The complications of the thoracic epidural technique are similar to those of the lumbar epidural—infection, epidural hematoma, injury to the nerve roots, intravascular injection, respiratory depression, subdural and subarachnoid injection, among others. But, the presence of the spinal cord in the thoracic vertebral canal brings in the possibility of spinal cord damage. The incidence of spinal cord damage due to attempted thoracic epidural analgesia is not known. There are very few reports of this complication. In one series of 1071 postoperative patients, no long-term serious complications were reported. In a study of 4185 patients, absence of serious neurologic complications was documented.[53] Many studies document safety and absence of infection.[54, 55]

Infection

Epidural abscess[17, 56, 57] secondary to a thoracic epidural catheter left in place is a possibility, especially with the increasing use of long-term catheter placement for the management of cancer pain. There is some evidence that the incidence of infection is higher in the thoracic area than in other areas.[17]

Pleural Puncture[58]

Accidental pleural puncture and placement of the catheter was recognized during surgery. Although uncommon, this complication can be life-threatening if not recognized.

CONCLUSION

Thoracic epidural nerve block has become a mainstay of contemporary pain management. Careful attention to the functional anatomy of the thoracic spine will increase the clinician's success rate and decrease complications.

REFERENCES

1. Scott D: Central neural blockade. *In* (eds): Techniques of Regional Anaesthesia. Norwalk, Conn., McGraw-Hill, Appleton & Lange, 1989, pp 178–180.
2. Katz J, Renck H: Lumbar epidural block. *In* (eds): Handbook of Thoracoabdominal Nerve Block. Orlando, Fla., Grune & Stratton, 1987, pp 111–113.
3. Anderson JE: The back. *In* Grant's Atlas of Anatomy, 7th ed. Baltimore, Williams & Wilkins, 1978.
4. Bromage PR: Surgical applications. *In* Epidural Analgesia. Philadelphia, WB Saunders, 1978, pp 490–492.
5. Cousins MJ, Bridenbaugh PO: Epidural neural blockade. *In* Cousins MJ, Bridenbaugh PO (eds): Neural Blockade in Clinical Anesthesia and Management of Pain, ed 2. Philadelphia, JB Lippincott, 1988, pp 254, 261, 269, 273, 323, 331, 337, 341.
6. Lema MJ, Sinha I: Thoracic epidural anesthesia and analgesia. Pain Digest 4:3–11, 1994.
7. Liem TH, Booij LHDJ, Hasenbos MAWM: Coronary artery bypass grafting using two different anesthetic techniques: Part 1: Hemodynamic results. J Cardiothorac Vasc Anesth 6(2):148–155, 1992.
8. Liem TH, Hasenbos MAWM, Booij LHDJ: Coronary artery bypass grafting using two different anesthetic techniques: Part 2: Postoperative outcome. J Cardiothorac Vasc Anesth 6(2):156–161, 1992.
9. Mallick A, Bhaskaran NC: Thoracic epidural analgesia and coronary artery bypass graft surgery. Anaesthesia 53(5):511–512, 1998.
10. Turfrey DJ, Scott NB: Thoracic epidural analgesia started after cardiopulmonary bypass (Letter). Anaesthesia 52(9):914–916, 1997.
11. Turfrey DJ, Ray DA, Sutcliffe NP, et al: Thoracic epidural anaesthesia for coronary artery bypass graft surgery. Effects on postoperative complications. Anaesthesia 52(11):1090–1095, 1997.
12. Riedel BJ, Wright IG: Epidural anesthesia in coronary artery bypass grafting surgery. Curr Opin Cardiol 12(6):515–521, 1997.
13. Stenseth R, Berg EM, Bjella L, et al: The influence of thoracic epidural analgesia alone and in combination with general anesthesia on cardiovascular function and myocardial metabolism in patients receiving β-adrenergic blockers. Anesth Analg 77:463–468, 1993.
14. Lai CS, Yip WH, Lin SD, et al: Continuous thoracic epidural anesthesia for breast augmentation. Ann Plast Surg 36(2):113–116, 1996.
15. Lynch EP, Welch KJ, Carabuena JM, et al: Thoracic epidural anesthesia improves outcome after breast surgery. Ann Surg 222(5):663–669, 1995.
16. Nesmith RL, Herring SH, Marks MW, et al: Early experience with high thoracic epidural anesthesia in output submuscular breast augmentation. Ann Plast Surg 24(4):299–302, 1990.
17. Redekop GJ, Del Maestro RF: Diagnosis and management of spinal epidural abscess. Can J Neurol Sci 19:180–187, 1992.
18. Guinard JP, Mavrocordatos P, Chiolero R, et al: A randomized comparison of intravenous versus lumbar and thoracic epidural fentanyl for analgesia after thoracotomy. Anesthesiology 77:1108–1115, 1992.
19. Salomaki TE, Laitinen JO, Nuutiene LS: A randomized double-blind comparison of epidural versus intravenous fentanyl infusion for analgesia after thoracotomy. Anesthesiology 75:790–795, 1991.
20. Sawchuck WT, Ong B, Unruh HW, et al: Thoracic versus lumbar epidural fentanyl for postthoracotomy pain. Ann Thorac Surg 55:1472–1476, 1993.
21. George KA, Chisakuta AM, Gamble JAS, et al: Thoracic epidural infusion for postoperative pain relief following abdominal aortic surgery: Bupivacaine, fentanyl or a mixture of both? Anaesthesia 47:388–394, 1992.
22. George KA, Wright PMC, Chisakuta A: Continuous thoracic epidural fentanyl for post-thoracotomy pain relief: With or without bupivacaine? Anaesthesia 46:732–736, 1991.
23. Scott NB, James K, Murphy M, et al: Continuous thoracic epidural analgesia versus combined spinal/thoracic epidural analgesia on pain, pulmonary function and the metabolic response following colonic resection. Acta Anaesthesiol Scand 40(6):691–696, 1996.
24. Pelton JJ, Fish DJ, Keller SM: Epidural narcotic analgesia after thoracotomy. South Med J 86(10):1106–1109, 1993.
25. Mourisse J, Hasenbos M, Gielen MJM, et al: Epidural bupivacaine, sufentanil or the combination for post-thoracotomy pain. Acta Anaesthesiol Scand 36:70–74, 1992.
26. Liu SS, Allen HW, Olsson GL: Patient-controlled epidural analgesia with bupivacaine and fentanyl on hospital wards: Prospective experience with 1,030 surgical patients. Anesthesiology 88(3):688–695, 1998.
27. Moiniche S, Hjortso N-C, Blemmer T, et al: Blood pressure and heart rate during orthostatic stress and walking with continuous postoperative thoracic epidural bupivacaine/morphine. Acta Anaesthesiol Scand 37:65–69, 1993.
28. Tobias JD, Lowe S, O'Dell N, et al: Anaesthetic techniques: Thoracic epidural anaesthesia in infants and children. Can J Anaesth 40:879–882, 1993.

29. Tobias JD: Analgesia after thoracotomy in children: A comparison of interpleural, epidural, and intravenous analgesia. South Med J 84(12):158–161, 1991.
30. Winnie AP, Hartwell PW: Relationship between time of treatment of acute herpes zoster with sympathetic blockade and prevention of post-herpetic neuralgia: Clinical support for a new theory of the mechanism by which sympathetic blockade provides therapeutic benefit. Reg Anesth 18:277–282, 1993.
31. Blomberg S, Emanuelsson H, Kvist H, et al: Effects of thoracic epidural anesthesia on coronary arteries and arterioles in patients with coronary artery disease. Anesthesiology 73:840–847, 1990.
32. Blomberg S, Emanuelsson H, Ricksten SE: Thoracic epidural anesthesia and central hemodynamics in patients with unstable angina pectoris. Anesth Analg 69:558–562, 1989.
33. Blomberg SG: Long-term home self-treatment with high thoracic epidural anesthesia in patients with severe coronary artery disease. Anesth Analg 79(3):413–421, 1994.
34. Mannheimer C, Eliasson T, Augustinsson LE, et al: Electrical stimulation versus coronary artery bypass surgery in severe angina pectoris: The ESBY study. Circulation 97(12):1157–1163, 1998.
35. Hautvast RW, Blanksma PK, DeJongste MJ, et al: Effect of spinal cord stimulation on myocardial blood flow assessed by positron emission tomography in patients with refractory angina pectoris. Am J Cardiol 77(7):462–467, 1996.
36. Andersen C, Hole P, Oxhoj H: Does pain relief with spinal cord stimulation for angina conceal myocardial infarction? Br Heart J 71(5):419–421, 1994.
37. Racz GB, Heavner J, Haynsworth P: Repeat epidural phenol injections in chronic pain and spasticity. *In* Lipton S (ed): Persistent Pain: Modern Methods of Treatment. New York, Grune & Stratton, 1985, pp 157–179.
38. Korevaar WC: Transcatheter thoracic epidural neurolysis using ethyl alcohol. Anesthesiology 69:989–993, 1988.
39. Okutomi T, Watanabe S, Goto F: Time course in thoracic epidural pressure measurement. Can J Anaesth 40:1044–1048, 1993.
40. Gunter JB, Eng C: Thoracic epidural anesthesia via the caudal approach in children. Anesthesiology 76:935–938, 1992.
41. Blanco D, Llamazares J, Rincon R, et al: Thoracic epidural anesthesia via the lumbar approach in infants and children. Anesthesiology 84(6):1312–1316, 1996.
42. Ng KP: Complete heart block during laparotomy under combined thoracic epidural and general anaesthesia. Anaesth Intensive Care 24(2):257–260, 1996.
43. Goertz AW, Seeling W, Heinrich H, et al: Influence of high thoracic epidural anesthesia on left ventricular contractility assessed using the end-systolic pressure-length relationship. Acta Anaesthesiol Scand 37:38–44, 1993.
44. Armstrong P: Thoracic epidural anaesthesia and primary pulmonary hypertension. Anaesthesia 47:496–499, 1992.
45. Polaner DM, Kimball WR, Fratacci MD, et al: Thoracic epidural anesthesia increases diaphragmatic shortening after thoracotomy in the awake lamb. Anesthesiology 79:808–816, 1993.
46. Cicala RS, Voeller GR, Fox T, et al: Epidural analgesia in thoracic trauma: Effects of lumbar morphine and thoracic bupivacaine on pulmonary function. Crit Care Med 18(2):229–231, 1990.
47. Liu M, Kim PS, Chen CK, et al: Delayed Horner's syndrome as a complication of continuous thoracic epidural analgesia. J Cardiothorac Vasc Anesth 12(2):195–196, 1998.
48. Wilson MA, Swartzman S, Ramamurthy S: A simple test to confirm correct identification of the epidural space. Reg Anesth 8:158–162, 1983.
49. Bougher RJ, Corbett AR, Ramage DT: The effect of tunnelling on epidural catheter migration. Anaesthesia 51(2):191–194, 1996.
50. Raj P: Postoperative pain. *In:* Handbook of Regional Anesthesia. New York, Churchill Livingstone, 1985, p 106.
51. Kenworthy KL, Hoffman J, Rogers JN: A new dressing technique for temporary percutaneous catheters used for pain management (Letter to the editor). Anesthesiology 76:482–483, 1992.
52. Tanaka K, Watanabe R, Harada T, et al: Extensive application of epidural anesthesia and analgesia in a university hospital: Incidence of complications related to technique. Reg Anesth 18(1):34–38, 1993.
53. Giebler RM, Scherer RU, Peters J: Incidence of neurologic complications related to thoracic epidural catheterization. Anesthesiology 86(1):55–63, 1997.
54. Strafford MA, Wilder RT, Berde CB: The risk of infection from epidural analgesia in children: A review of 1620 cases. Anesth Analg 80(2):234–238, 1995.
55. Scherer R, Schmutzler M, Giebler R, et al: Complications related to thoracic epidural analgesia: A prospective study in 1071 surgical patients. Acta Anaesthesiol Scand 37(4):370–374, 1993.
56. Blomberg S, Curelaru I, Emanuelsson H, et al: Thoracic epidural anaesthesia in patients with unstable angina pectoris. Eur Heart J 10:437–444, 1989.
57. Yuste M, Canet J, Garcia M, et al: An epidural abscess due to resistant *Staphylococcus aureus* following epidural catheterization. Anaesthesia 52(2):163–165, 1997.
58. Zaugg M, Stoehr S, Weder W, et al: Accidental pleural puncture by a thoracic epidural catheter. Anaesthesia 53(1):69–71, 1998.

CHAPTER • 35

Thoracic Paravertebral Block

Steven D. Waldman, MD, JD

HISTORICAL CONSIDERATIONS

Historically, thoracic paravetebral nerve block was used principally to provide anesthesia for thoracic surgery.[1] The advent of endotracheal intubation and nondepolarizing muscle relaxants relegated thoracic paravertebral nerve block to a place in history. The technique has remained useful for certain applications.

INDICATIONS

Thoracic paravertebral nerve block is useful in the evaluation and management of pain involving the chest wall, upper abdominal wall, and thoracic spine.[2] Thoracic paravertebral nerve block with local anesthetics can be utilized as a diagnostic tool when performing differential neural blockade on an anatomic basis in the evaluation of chest, thoracic spine, and abdominal pain.[3] If destruction of the thoracic paravertebral nerve is being considered, this technique is useful as a prognostic indicator of the degree of motor and sensory impairment that the patient may experience.[3] With local anesthetic it can be utilized to palliate acute pain, including that of thoracic vertebral compression fracture, acute herpes zoster, and cancer until pharmacologic, surgical, and antiblastic methods take effect. Thoracic paravertebral nerve block with local anesthetic and steroid is also useful for treating postthoracotomy pain, posterior rib fractures, and postherpetic neuralgia.[3]

Destruction of the thoracic paravertebral nerve is indicated for palliation of cancer pain, including invasive tumors of the thoracic spine, posterior ribs, and chest and upper abdominal wall.[4] Owing to the desperation of many patients suffering from aggressively invasive malignancies, blockade of the thoracic paravertebral nerve using a 25-gauge needle may be carried out despite coagulopathy or anticoagulation, albeit with increased risk of ecchymosis and hematoma formation.[3]

CLINICALLY RELEVANT ANATOMY

The thoracic paravertebral nerves exit their respective intervertebral foramen just beneath the transverse process of the vertebra. Then it gives off a recurrent branch, which loops back through the foramen to provide innervation to the spinal ligaments, meninges, and its respective vertebra. The thoracic paravertebral nerve also interfaces with the thoracic sympathetic chain via the myelinated preganglionic fibers of the white rami communicantes and the unmyelinated postganglionic fibers of the gray rami communicantes. After providing these intercommunications with the thoracic sympathetic nervous system and with the recurrent branch, the thoracic paravertebral nerve divides into a posterior and an anterior primary division. The posterior division courses posteriorly, and, along with its branches, provides innervation to the facet joints and the muscles and skin of the back. The larger anterior division courses laterally to pass into the subcostal groove beneath the rib to become the respective intercostal nerves. The twelfth thoracic nerve courses beneath the twelfth rib and is called the *subcostal nerve.* The intercostal and subcostal nerves provide innervation to the skin, muscles, ribs, and parietal pleural and parietal peritoneum. Because blockade of the thoracic paravertebral nerve is performed at the point at which the nerve is beginning to give off its various branches, it is possible to block the anterior division, posterior division, and the recurrent and sympathetic components of each respective thoracic paravertebral nerve.

TECHNIQUE

The patient is placed prone with a pillow under the lower chest to slightly flex the thoracic spine. The spinous process of the vertebra just above the nerve to be blocked is palpated. At a point just below and 1.5 inches lateral to the spinous process, the skin is prepared with antiseptic solution. A 22-gauge, 3.5-inch needle is attached to a 12-mL syringe and is advanced perpendicular to the skin, being aimed at the middle of the transverse process. The needle should impinge on bone after being advanced approximately 1.5 inches. After contact is made with bone, the needle is withdrawn into the subcutaneous tissues and redirected inferiorly and "walked off" the inferior margin of the transverse process (Fig. 35–1). As soon as bony contact is lost, the needle is slowly advanced approximately

3/4 inch deeper until a paresthesia is elicited in the distribution of the thoracic paravertebral nerve to be blocked. Once the paresthesia has been elicited and careful aspiration reveals no blood or cerebrospinal fluid, 5 mL of 1.0% preservative-free lidocaine is injected. If there is an inflammatory component to the pain, the local anesthetic is combined with 80 mg of methylprednisolone and is injected in incremental doses. Subsequent daily nerve blocks are carried out in a similar manner substituting 40 mg of methylprednisolone for the initial 80-mg dose. Because of overlapping innervation of the posterior elements from the medial branch of the posterior division from adjacent vertebrae, the paravertebral nerves above and below the nerve suspected of subserving the painful condition will have to be blocked.

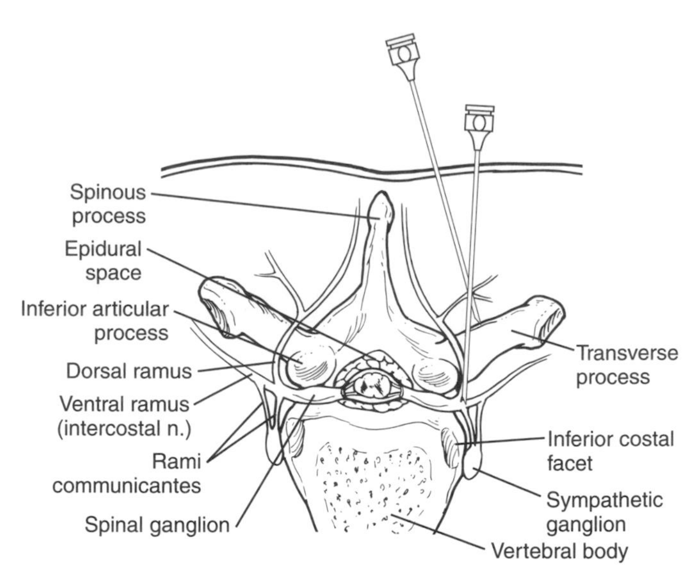

FIGURE 35–1 Needle placement for thoracic paravertebral block.

SIDE EFFECTS AND COMPLICATIONS

The proximity of the paravertebral nerve to the spinal cord and exiting nerve roots makes it imperative that this procedure be carried out only by an operator well-versed in the regional anatomy and experienced in performing interventional pain management techniques. Given the proximity of the pleural space, pneumothorax after thoracic paravertebral block is a distinct possibility. Needle placement too far medial may result in epidural, subdural, or subarachnoid injections or trauma to the spinal cord and exiting nerve roots. Placing the needle too deep between the transverse processes may injure the exiting thoracic nerve roots. Although uncommon, infection remains an ever present possibility, especially in immunocompromised patients. Early detection of infection is crucial to avoiding potentially life-threatening sequelae.

CLINICAL PEARLS

Thoracic paravertebral nerve block is a simple technique that can produce dramatic relief from certain types of pain. Neurolytic block with small quantities of phenol in glycerin or by cryoneurolysis or radiofrequency lesioning has been shown to provide long-term relief from postthoracotomy and cancer-related pain that is refractory to more conservative treatments. The proximity of the thoracic paravertebral nerve to the neuroaxis and pleural space makes careful attention to technique mandatory.

REFERENCES

1. Pitkin GP: Intercostal nerve block. *In* Pitkin GP (ed): Conduction Anesthesia. Philadelphia, JB Lippincott, 1946, pp 479–481.
2. Katz J: Thoracic paravertebral nerve block. *In* Katz J (ed): Atlas of Regional Anesthesia. Norwalk, Conn, Appleton-Century-Crofts, 1995, pp 94–95.
3. Waldman SD: Thoracic paravertebral nerve block. *In* Waldman SD (ed): Atlas of Interventional Pain Management Techniques. Philadelphia, WB Saunders, 1998, pp 212–215.
4. Bonica JJ: Cancer pain. *In* Bonica JJ (ed): The Management of Pain, ed 2. Philadelphia, Lea & Febiger, 1990, pp 240–242.

CHAPTER • 36

Thoracic Sympathetic Ganglion Block

Steven D. Waldman, MD, JD

HISTORICAL CONSIDERATIONS

Historically, blockade of the thoracic sympathetic ganglia was utilized in the palliation of pain secondary to malignancies of the thoracic contents, especially carcinoma of the esophagus.[1] It was also used to treat intractable cardiac arrhythmias.[2] The technique in the past has seen extensive use in the treatment of acute herpes zoster of the upper thoracic dermatomes. Treatment for this indication has largely been replaced by sympathetic block with local anesthetics via the epidural route. Recently interest has been renewed, since computed tomographic guidance makes the technique easier and safer.

INDICATIONS

Thoracic sympathetic ganglion block is useful in the evaluation and management of sympathetically mediated pain of the upper thorax, chest wall, and the thoracic and upper abdominal viscera.[3] Thoracic sympathetic ganglion block with local anesthetics can be utilized as a diagnostic tool when performing differential neural blockade on an anatomic basis for evaluation of chest, thoracic, and upper abdominal pain. If destruction of the thoracic sympathetic chain is being considered, the technique is a useful indicator of the degree of pain relief that the patient may experience. In the past, this block was used to treat intractable cardiac and abdominal angina. Thoracic sympathetic ganglion block with local anesthetic is also useful for treating post-thoracotomy pain, acute herpes zoster, postherpetic neuralgia, and phantom breast pain after mastectomy. Destruction of the thoracic sympathetic chain is indicated for palliation of pain syndromes that have responded to thoracic sympathetic blockade with local anesthetics.[4]

CLINICALLY RELEVANT ANATOMY

The preganglionic fibers of the thoracic sympathetics exit the intervertebral foramen along with the respective thoracic paravertebral nerves.[2] After exiting the intervertebral foramen, the thoracic paravertebral nerve gives off a recurrent branch that loops back through the foramen to provide innervation to the spinal ligaments, meninges, and its corresponding vertebra. The thoracic paravertebral nerve also interfaces with the thoracic sympathetic chain via the myelinated preganglionic fibers of the white rami communicantes and the unmyelinated postganglionic fibers of the gray rami communicantes. At the level of the thoracic sympathetic ganglia, preganglionic and postganglionic fibers synapse, and some of the postganglionic fibers return to their respective somatic nerves via the gray rami communicantes. These fibers provide sympathetic innervation to the vasculature, sweat glands, and pilomotor muscles of the skin. Other thoracic sympathetic postganglionic fibers travel to the cardiac plexus and course up and down the sympathetic trunk to terminate in distant ganglia.

The first thoracic ganglion is fused with the lower cervical ganglion to help make up the stellate ganglion. As the chain moves caudad, it changes its position, the upper thoracic ganglia lying just beneath the rib and the lower thoracic ganglia moving farther anterior to rest along the posterolateral surface of the vertebral body. The pleural space lies lateral and anterior to the thoracic sympathetic chain. Given the proximity of the thoracic somatic nerves to the thoracic sympathetic chain, the potential exists for both neural pathways to be blocked during blockade of the thoracic sympathetic ganglion.

TECHNIQUE

The patient is placed prone with a pillow under the lower chest to slightly flex the thoracic spine. The spinous process of the vertebra just above the nerve to be blocked is palpated. At a point just below and 1 1/2 inches lateral to the spinous process, the skin is prepared with antiseptic solution. A 22-gauge 3 1/2-inch needle is attached to a 12-mL syringe and is advanced perpendicular to the skin aiming for the middle of the transverse process. The needle should impinge on bone after being advanced approximately 1 1/2 inches. After contact is made with bone, the needle is withdrawn into the subcutaneous tissues and redirected inferiorly and "walked off" the inferior margin

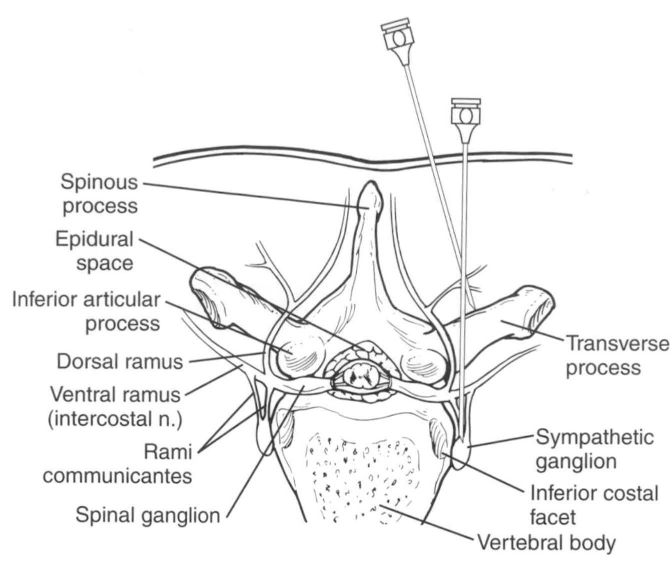

FIGURE 36–1 Needle placement for thoracic sympathetic ganglion block.

of the transverse process (Fig. 36–1). As soon as bony contact is lost, the needle is slowly advanced approximately 1 inch deeper. Given the proximity of the thoracic sympathetic chain to the somatic nerve, a paresthesia may be elicited in the distribution of the corresponding thoracic paravertebral nerve. If this occurs, the needle should be withdrawn and redirected slightly more cephalad, care being taken to keep the needle close to the vertebral body to avoid pneumothorax. Once the needle is in position and careful aspiration reveals no blood or cerebrospinal fluid, 5 mL of 1.0% preservative-free lidocaine is injected.

SIDE EFFECTS AND COMPLICATIONS

The proximity to the spinal cord and exiting nerve roots makes it imperative that this procedure be carried out only by someone well-versed in the regional anatomy and experienced in performing interventional pain management techniques. Given the proximity of the pleural space, pneumothorax after thoracic sympathetic ganglion block is a distinct possibility. The incidence of pneumothorax will be decreased if care is taken to keep the needle placed medially against the vertebral body. Placing it too far medial can result in epidural, subdural, or subarachnoid injection or trauma to the spinal cord and exiting nerve roots. Although infection is uncommon, it is an ever present possibility, especially in immunocompromised patients. Early detection of infection is crucial to avoid potentially life-threatening sequela.

CLINICAL PEARLS

Thoracic sympathetic ganglion block is a simple technique that can produce dramatic relief for patients suffering from certain types of pain. Neurolytic block with small quantities of phenol in glycerin or by cryoneurolysis or radiofrequency lesioning has been shown to provide long-term relief for sympathetically maintained pain that has been relieved with local anesthetics. The proximity of the thoracic sympathetic chain to the neuroaxis and pleural space makes careful attention to technique mandatory.

REFERENCES

1. Bonica JJ: Cancer pain. *In* Bonica JJ (ed): The Management of Pain, ed 2. Philadelphia, Lea & Febiger, 1990, pp 240–242.
2. Pitkin GP: Cervical and thoracic nerves. *In* Pitkin GP (ed): Conduction Anesthesia. Philadelphia, JB Lippincott, 1946, pp 891–893.
3. Katz J: Thoracic paravertebral nerve block. *In* Katz J (ed): Atlas of Regional Anesthesia. Norwalk, Conn, Appleton-Century-Crofts, 1995, pp 98–99.
4. Waldman SD: Thoracic sympathetic ganglion block. *In* Waldman SD (ed): Atlas of Interventional Pain Management Techniques. Philadelphia, WB Saunders, 1998, pp 224–225.
5. Bonica JJ: Neurolytic blockade and hypophysectomy. *In* Bonica JJ (ed): The Management of Pain, ed 2. Philadelphia, Lea & Febiger, 1990, pp 2012–2015.

CHAPTER • 37

Intercostal Nerve Block

Dan J. Kopacz, MD • Gale E. Thompson, MD

In the future, acute pain management will tend to emphasize the application of analgesic drugs directly to the surgical wound edges or to smaller peripheral nerve branches. In this way, we will avoid the many side effects (hypotension, itching, nausea, vomiting, urinary retention) that often accompany central neuraxis blockade. At some point, intercostal nerve block will finally and fully achieve a major role in pain management. Indeed, it will likely become the most often used peripheral nerve block. As we will show later, there must be one major development in local anesthetic drugs before this advance can be realized.

HISTORICAL CONSIDERATIONS

Upon reviewing the early writings of Schleich,[1] Braun,[2] Pauchet,[3] and Labat,[4] one is struck with the idea that the technique of intercostal nerve blockade developed through a series of evolutionary steps. At the turn of the 20th century, surgeons were fascinated by infiltration anesthesia. Elaborate descriptions and recipes defined how surgery of the chest and abdomen could be accomplished using large volumes (100 to 150 mL) of dilute solutions of local anesthetic drugs, procaine being the mainstay after it was synthesized in 1904. Over time, many of the descriptions and illustrations began to define the reality of blocking the intercostal nerve trunk, in preference to the more elaborate process of infiltration or "field block" of the more peripheral twigs and branches. In addition, paravertebral injections began to be utilized as an alternative to spinal injections.[5] These lumbar and thoracic blocks became popular because of increasing doubt and concern about possible neurotoxicity from the injection of cocaine and its synthetic allies directly into the spinal canal. Therefore, techniques were defined whereby major nerve trunks could be blocked after they exited the vertebral canal. Thus, proximal and more distal sites for blocking intercostal nerves were gradually defined. By 1922, Labat's textbook contained an elaborate description of intercostal nerve block that is quite similar to our present-day conceptions.

INDICATIONS

No method of pain relief is more specific and effective for fractured ribs than intercostal nerve block.[6] The pain from chest wall contusion, pleurisy, and flail chest is also quickly relieved.[7, 8] Often unappreciated is the fact that the pain from median sternotomy, pericardial window, or fractured sternum can be controlled successfully by blocks in the parasternal region (Fig. 37–1).[4] This point might well be applied to many cardiac and pulmonary surgery cases of today.[9, 10] Blockade of two or more nerves is a simple way to prepare for insertion of thoracostomy tubes and can also be used to provide analgesia for percutaneous biliary drainage or liver biopsy. Perhaps the most important but least exploited use of this block is for control of postoperative pain of the chest or abdomen.[11] A simple study by Bunting and McGeachie[12] vividly demonstrates this point. They simply performed lateral intercostal blocks of right T10, T11, and T12 at the conclusion of appendectomy. With this investment of a few milliliters of local anesthetic drug, the study patients required only a third as much postoperative narcotic as the patients who did not receive intercostal blocks.

Intercostal blocks (CPT Code 64420 [single], 64421 [multiple, regional block]) are also useful in several chronic pain scenarios. For instance, when combined or alternated with celiac plexus blockade, they can help resolve a not uncommon diagnostic dilemma and distinguish abdominal wall pain from visceral pain. A unilateral paravertebral T12 and L1 nerve block (CPT Code 64440 [single], 64441 [multiple, regional block]) can help unravel the question of nerve entrapment syndromes after inguinal hernia repair. Numerous references have been made to the diagnostic and therapeutic benefits of this block in patients with acute and chronic pain from herpes zoster.[13] There are also limited applications for a limited number of neurolytic intercostal blocks (CPT Code 64620) in some patients with terminal cancer.

ANATOMY

The intercostal nerves are composed of the ventral rami of the first through the twelfth thoracic nerves. The first,

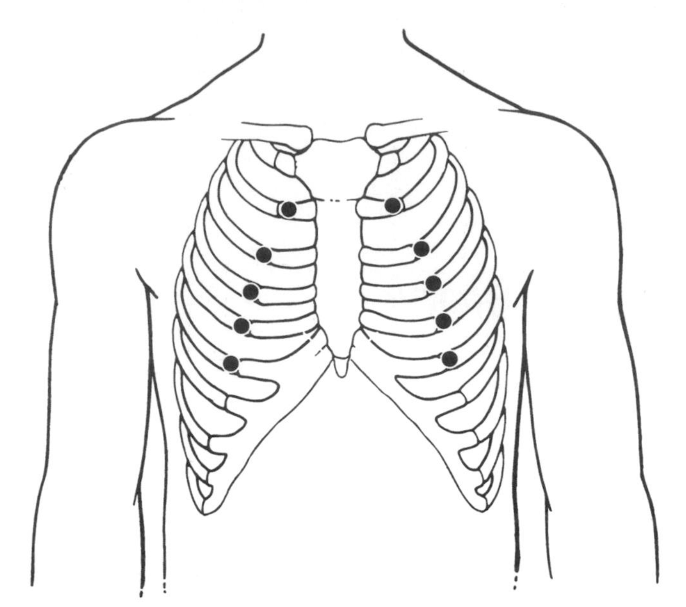

FIGURE 37–1 *Black dots indicate approximate sites for parasternal block of the upper anterior intercostal nerves. This is a very effective way to relieve pain from median sternotomy or a fractured sternum.*

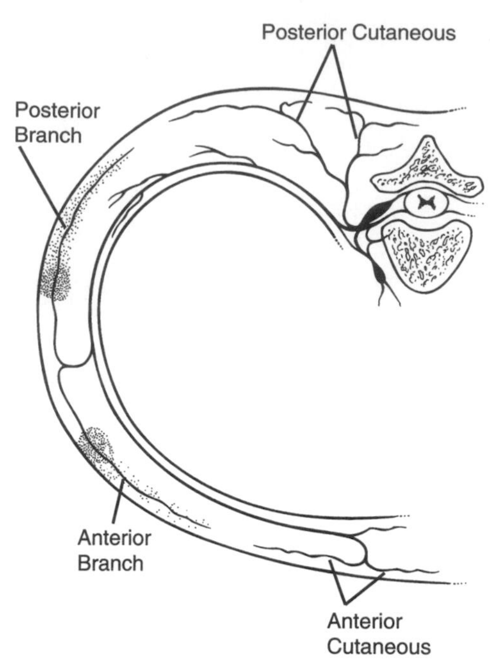

FIGURE 37–2 *The four branches of a typical intercostal nerve.*

second, and twelfth nerves differ from the other nine in several respects. T1 gives off a small contribution to the brachial plexus. T2–T3 sends cutaneous branches to the arm as the intercostobrachial nerve. T12 is not strictly an intercostal nerve but, rather, is more appropriately called a subcostal nerve. It runs its course in the abdominal wall below the twelfth rib and sends fibers to join L1.

Evidence from cadaver studies indicates that the classic medical school teaching that the intercostal vein, artery, and nerve are located in precise order and comfortably tucked into the subcostal groove is unrealistic. The nerve may actually vary from a subcostal to midcostal to supracostal location. In his cadaver study, Hardy[14] found the frequencies of these variations: classic subcostal, 17%; midzone, 73%; and supracostal, 10%.

Another anatomic subtlety for the anesthesiologist's appreciation is intercostal nerve branching, of which there are two types. First, the nerve may split into separate bundles that have no common enclosing fascial sheath. These may rejoin or subdivide further as the nerve continues its lateral course; thus, there is not necessarily a single, well-defined nerve at every site in the intercostal space. Second, each intercostal nerve gives off four well-defined branches as it proceeds on its circuitous route anteriorly (Fig. 37–2). The *first* is the gray rami communicantes, which goes to the appropriate sympathetic ganglion. The *second* branch arises as the posterior cutaneous branch and supplies skin and muscles in the paravertebral region and possibly as far lateral as the posterior axillary line. The *third* branch, the lateral cutaneous division, arises just anterior to the midaxillary line. The clinical importance of the takeoff of this branch historically has been emphasized, and perhaps exaggerated. This is a concern during blocking of intercostal nerves for pain relief, because the third branch sends subcutaneous fibers coursing both posteriorly and anteriorly, and a lateral injection could conceivably be directed too far anterior and miss the point of takeoff. The *terminal* or final branch is the anterior cutaneous branch, which provides cutaneous innervation to the midline of the chest and abdomen. Unlike the situation at the vertebral spines, there appears to be some slight overlap of sensory fibers across the anterior midline of the chest and abdomen.

The paravertebral space deserves separate discussion. The dura mater and the arachnoid membrane fuse with the epineurium as the nerve exits the vertebral foramen. This has two important implications (Fig. 37–3). Local anesthetics (or other drugs) injected directly intraneurally to the peripheral nerve may spread centrally, to the nerve roots or spinal cord. It is also possible to produce epidural or spinal anesthesia if a large volume of local anesthetic is injected into the paravertebral region and then flows centrally around the nerve in the vertebral foramen. Conacher[15] has nicely demonstrated that even quick-setting

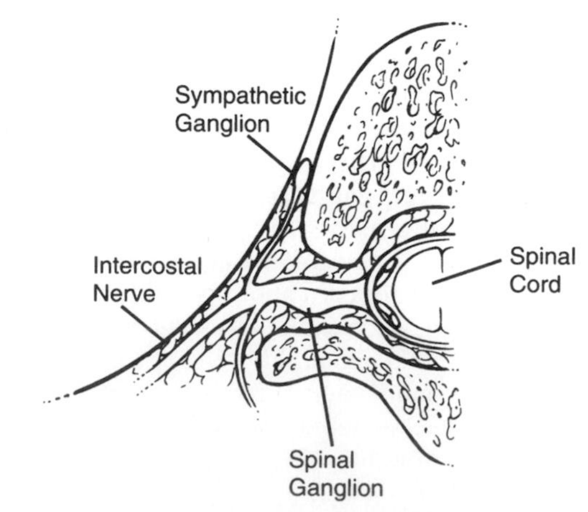

FIGURE 37–3 *Possible central neuraxial spread of solutions injected into the paravertebral space or intercostal nerve.*

resin can be thus propelled into the vertebral epidural space. He also showed that correctly placed paravertebral intercostal injections can spread over several intercostal spaces and can even dissect the pleura laterally from the vertebral bodies. In transverse section, the paravertebral space is wedge shaped. The posterior wall is the costotransverse ligament; anterolaterally is the parietal pleura; and medially lie the vertebral body and vertebral foramen. From the paravertebral space to the posterior angle of the rib, there is no structure between the intercostal nerve and the pleura. At the angle of the rib, the internal intercostal muscle arises and lies internal to the nerve, all the way around to the costosternal cartilages.

In the paravertebral region, the intercostal artery and vein are usually singular structures. Laterally, they show multiple branches. This has implications for intercostal block, because vessel puncture can lead to hematoma formation or rapid uptake of local anesthetic drug. Flank hematomas can become quite extensive in a patient taking anticoagulants.[16] Other high-risk scenarios involve patients with neurofibromatosis, Marfan's syndrome, and arterial dilatation or stretching, as for example, in coarctation of the aorta or severe scoliosis.[17]

TECHNIQUE: PEARLS AND PRINCIPLES

The Classic Approach

In the classic approach, intercostal nerve block is performed posteriorly at the angle of the ribs and just lateral to the sacrospinalis group of muscles (Fig. 37–4).[18] At this point, the thickness of the rib is about 8 mm. Thus, if the needle is advanced 3 mm into the triangular fat-filled space where the nerve runs, there is a 5-mm margin of safety before it penetrates the pleura. In most instances, the blocks are easiest to learn and perform with the patient in a prone position with a pillow under the midabdomen. This position is optimal for rib identification by posterior palpation of the intercostal spaces. The patient's arms are kept hanging over the sides of the cart or operating table to rotate the scapuli laterally and make it easier to block the nerves under the upper ribs. After the patient is positioned, it is helpful to use a skin-marking pen to identify the inferior edge of each rib. This constitutes a map to illustrate and review anatomic detail and ultimately makes the process of blocking smoother and quicker. First, a vertical line is drawn connecting the posterior thoracic vertebral spines. Then, by palpation, the lateral edge of the sacrospinalis group of muscles is identified and marked as another vertical line on each side. This lateral line is usually 7 to 8 cm from the posterior midline and should angle medially at the upper levels to avoid the scapulae. The inferior border of each rib is then marked along these two lateral vertical lines.

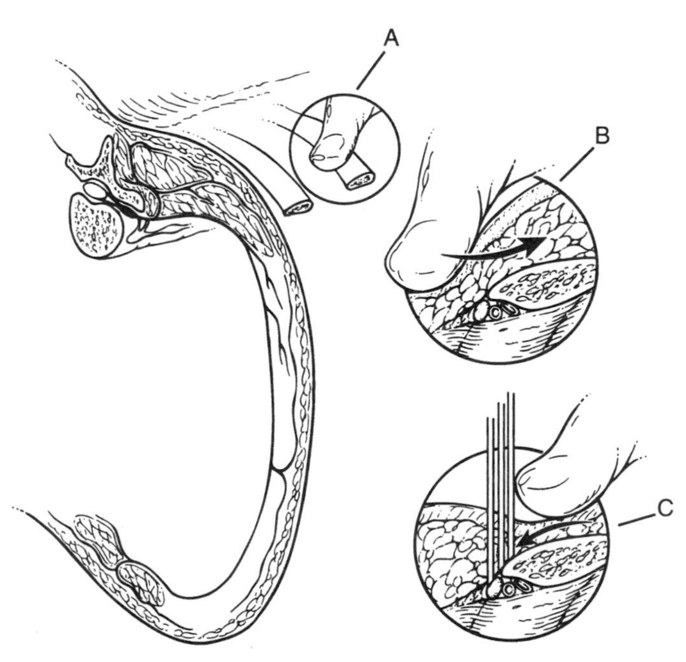

FIGURE 37–4 An overview of anatomy and technique for performing the classic posterior approach to intercostal block. A, The left index finger palpates to identify the rib. B, The skin and subcutaneous tissues are retracted cephalad. C, The needle is advanced until contact is made with the rib and then is withdrawn into the subcutaneous tissue. The needle is then "walked" off the inferior border of the rib.

Once these markings and local anesthetic mixing preparations have been completed, the initial step is to raise skin wheals (30-gauge needle) at each of the previously marked intersections of vertical and horizontal lines. A 2- to 3-cm, 22- or 23-gauge needle is then used to inject each intercostal nerve. If a disposable long-beveled needle is used, the operator must remember that the tip may easily be bent with the repeated bone contacts necessary to do this block. The needle can thus become barbed and possibly cause bleeding or nerve damage.

The practitioner's hand and finger position is of utmost importance to performing this block properly (Fig. 37–5). Beginning at the lowest rib, a right-handed operator uses the index finger of the left hand to pull the skin up and over at the lower edge of the rib. The needle is then introduced to the rib as the palpating left index finger defines it. Obviously, care should be taken to prevent the needle's penetrating beyond this palpated depth, because it could enter the interpleural or intraalveolar space. The practitioner should think of the palpating finger as having sonar capabilities. Once the needle reaches the rib, the right hand pushes to maintain firm contact between needle and rib. The left hand is then shifted to gain control of the needle by holding the hub and shaft with thumb and the index and middle fingers. In addition, firm placement of the left hand's hypothenar eminence against the patient's back is crucial. This allows precise and constant control of needle depth as the left hand now "walks" the needle off the lower edge of the rib. While the needle is being advanced, a slight loss of resistance is often felt as the tip enters the correct space. From 3 to 5 mL of local anesthetic solution is injected at each interspace. The left hand then walks the needle back onto the rib and finally releases control to the right hand and to the left index finger for palpation of the next higher rib. Keeping the needle in firm contact with the previously injected rib until the next space is identified serves to avoid missing a rib or doing a second block of the same rib.

This process is repeated for each of the nerves to be blocked. An experienced operator can safely and success-

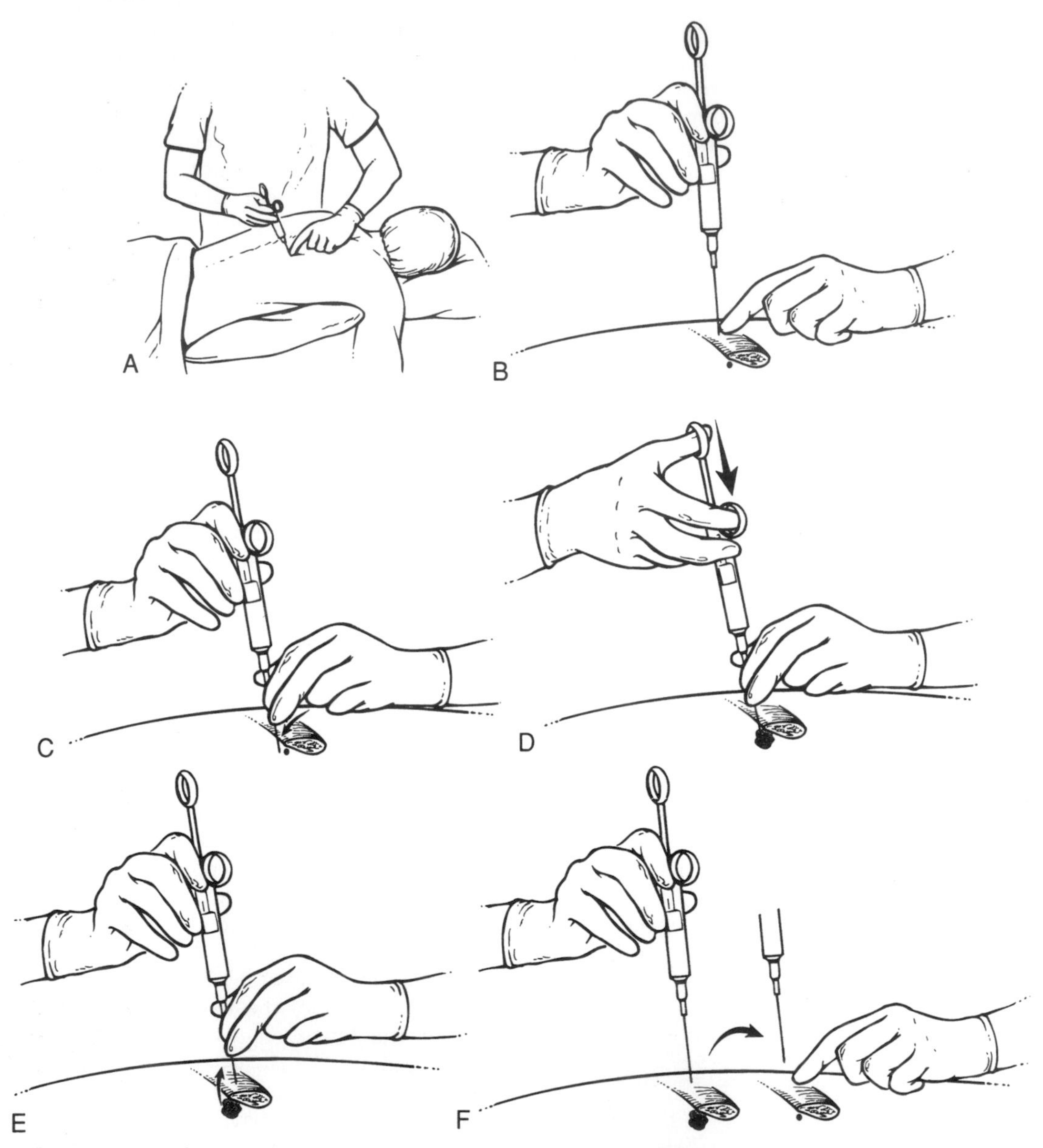

FIGURE 37–5 *A, Ideal overview of a posterior intercostal block. The right-handed physician stands on the left side of the prone patient, whose arms hang down to retract the scapulae laterally. In parts* B *to* F, *black dots indicate block sites.* B, *The palpating left index finger identifies the rib to determine depth and direction for the advancing needle.* C, *The depth of the needle is then firmly controlled by the anesthesiologist's left hand, which is constantly in contact (hypothenar eminence) with the patient's back.* D, *Now the right hand is shifted to inject 3 to 5 mL of solution. Note again that the depth of the needle is controlled by the* left *hand.* E, *The left hand again controls return of the needle to the "safety" of osseous contact.* F, *The previous steps are repeated at the next higher rib level.*

fully block 12 to 14 ribs in 3 to 5 minutes. Intercostal blocks may be repeated as needed.

Midaxillary Approach

It is quite reasonable to perform intercostal nerve blocks in the midaxillary line (Fig. 37–6). Some authors have advised against this approach, out of concern that it might be more likely to cause pneumothorax and to miss anesthetizing the lateral cutaneous branch of the nerve, which takes off near the midaxillary line and becomes superficial to innervate the skin of the anterolateral chest wall. Two realities make intercostal block effective, however, when done at a midaxillary site.[19] First, the solution always spreads longitudinally in the intercostal groove for a distance of several centimeters from the site of injection. Second, the final milliliter of solution can be injected as the needle is being moved away from the rib toward the skin, to anesthetize the lateral cutaneous branch in its subcutaneous site.

This midaxillary approach makes intercostal block much more feasible in patients who cannot be turned to a supine or lateral position, such as postoperative and trauma pa-

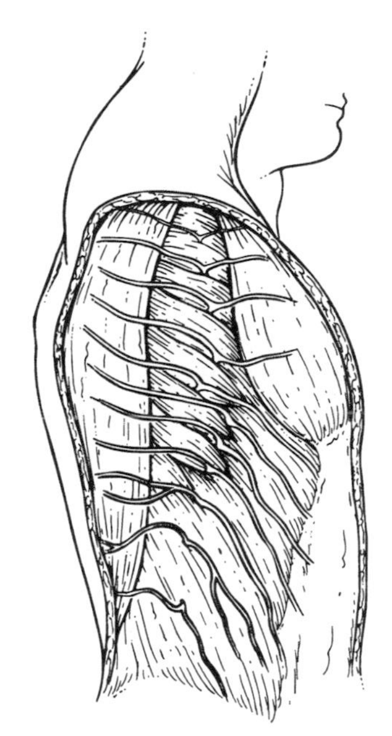

FIGURE 37–6 The lateral branches of the intercostal nerves near the midaxillary line. Blocks made at or near these sites are effective and can be easily done on the supine patient.

tients who experience severe pain with any motion. This block can also be used to complement a general anesthetic after induction and intubation of a supine patient. The anesthesiologist can reach down and quickly do a series of unilateral or bilateral midaxillary line blocks without even leaving the position at the head of the operating table. If the patient is being ventilated during this time, it is advisable to synchronize the block with the ventilator (i.e., to avoid walking the needle off the rib at the point of maximum inspiration) to help to avoid pneumothorax as a complication.

The upper intercostal nerves can be blocked by raising the patient's arm and palpating the ribs high in the axilla. Good analgesia can also be produced by blocking the intercostal nerve even farther anterior than the midaxillary line. For instance, parasternal blocks can provide good pain relief after median sternotomy. Rectus sheath block is yet another variation.[20]

Paravertebral Approach

Intercostal blocks can be performed posteriorly at any site medial to the posterior angle of the ribs. Obviously, there is some point medially at which every intercostal block is best characterized as a paravertebral block. In some sense, the distinction is moot, but there are two very interesting clinical concerns or observations. One is that central neuraxis spread of solution becomes ever more worrisome farther medially. The other is that subpleural spread of anesthetic from one intercostal space to another becomes more likely as injections are placed closer to the spine. Although some physicians believe that paravertebral somatic block is now of more interest to historians than to practicing anesthesiologists, there are still reasons to explore the technique. For instance, a catheter can be inserted here for a variation on the theme of interpleural anesthesia or "continuous" intercostal nerve block. Such a catheter would lie in the extrapleural space.[21, 22]

To perform a paravertebral block, a skin wheal is raised 2.5 to 3.0 cm from the posterior midline at the superior edge of the vertebral spinous process of the nerve to be blocked. It is not impossible to palpate the ribs at this point, because they are tilted steeply inward toward their attachments to the vertebral bodies and are covered by the thick paraspinous muscles. If palpation is commenced laterally at the angle of the rib, however, it is usually possible to project a mental image of its attachment to the spine. A 10-cm, 22-gauge needle is inserted perpendicular to the skin at the site of the skin wheal. Contact with the transverse process is usually made at a depth of 2 to 4 cm. With that depth now defined, the needle is withdrawn to a subcutaneous position and angled slightly inferior (caudal) to "walk off" the inferior edge of the transverse process. As it passes 1.0 to 1.5 cm deep to the transverse process, a loss of resistance may be felt as the needle pierces the costotransverse ligament. After negative aspiration, a total of 3 to 6 mL of local anesthetic solution is injected.

If a paravertebral catheter is to be used, the steps described earlier can be taken. An 18-gauge Tuohy needle is used to locate the loose areolar tissue of the paravertebral space. A catheter should be advanced only 1 to 2 cm beyond the tip of the needle: otherwise it could enter the epidural space. A 3-mL test dose of local anesthetic drug should be used to rule out intravascular and central neuraxis injection. Eason and Wyatt[23] report that one 15-mL injection can be expected to cover four intercostal spaces.

PITFALLS

Use of Sedative Drugs

Intercostal nerve block may cause significant skin and periosteal stimulation that can be easily relieved by giving light sedation before the procedure. This is not to say that these nerve blocks cannot be performed without sedation. In fact, it may be mandatory to use little or no sedation when the blocks are performed on seriously ill patients or when a block is being utilized to help solve a diagnostic pain dilemma. Drugs commonly used to supplement these blocks include midazolam, fentanyl, ketamine, thiopental, and propofol.[24] The clinical situation should dictate which agent(s) should be used. Is there need for hypnosis, analgesia, tranquilization, or some combination of these effects? It is important to titrate all sedative drugs in small intravenous doses while observing closely for the desired action.

Local Anesthetic Drugs

In preparing a solution of local anesthetic for bilateral intercostal nerve block, the following calculations are made:

- Total volume of solution.
- Effective concentration of drug.
- Total dose of drug.

- Volume of epinephrine to be added.
- Total dose of epinephrine.

There are safe or ideal limits for each of these interrelated variables. Volume multiplied by concentration determines total dose. Excessive volume or concentration may be tolerated by some patients, but toxic effects are more likely to occur. On the other hand, small volumes or low concentrations of drug produce ineffective anesthesia. Any block might be termed ineffective were it inadequate in area, duration, or extent of motor or sensory fiber blockade. The drug should be tailored to the block, and doing so requires more than just a vague knowledge of local anesthetic drug doses and effective concentrations (Table 37–1).

For each local anesthetic, recommendations for maximum total dose are approved. These recommendations may vary from country to country or region to region, according to the prevailing bias, custom, or regulatory agencies. Many regional techniques (e.g., subarachnoid block) require drug doses far smaller than the maximum recommended dose. To perform multiple bilateral intercostal blocks, however, the anesthesiologist often needs to approach the maximum recommended dose to achieve a successful result. Blood levels of local anesthetic drug are higher after multiple intercostal nerve blocks than after any other commonly used regional anesthetic procedure. Tucker and colleagues[25] measured arterial plasma levels after epidural, caudal, intercostal, brachial plexus, and sciatic-femoral nerve block with a single injection of 500 mg of mepivacaine. The blocks were performed using both 1% and 2% mepivacaine, with and without epinephrine. The highest plasma concentrations (5 to 10 μg/mL) were observed after intercostal nerve blocks without epinephrine. When a 1:200,000 concentration of epinephrine was added to the injected solution, plasma levels fell to the range of 2 to 5 μg/mL. These lower blood levels were similar to those found with the other regional block procedures.

Respiratory Effects

Intercostal blockade produces effective analgesia with little central respiratory depression and minimal interference with pulmonary function. With the exception of peak expiratory flow, indices of respiratory function are essentially unaltered in healthy volunteers.[26] After thoracotomy, lung function is better in patients with intercostal blocks than in nonblocked controls.[27] Good information or comparative studies of patients with underlying pulmonary disease not available.

TABLE 37–1 *Drugs for Intercostal Nerve Block for Pain Relief*

Drug	Duration (hr)	Concentration	Dose (mg/kg)
Bupivacaine	8–12	0.25–0.5	2–3
Ropivacaine	8–12	0.25–0.5	2–3
Mepivacaine	4–8	0.5–1.5	7.0
Lidocaine	4–7	0.5–1.5	7.0

COMPLICATIONS

Pneumothorax

The most feared complication of intercostal nerve block is pneumothorax. Many physicians avoid this block because they believe the risk of pneumothorax is too high. With proper attention to technique, however, the risk should be extremely low. Moore and Bridenbaugh[28] reported an incidence of pneumothorax of only 0.082% in an analysis of 17,000 patients. The majority of the blocks reported in their study were done by residents in training. Other authors have reported incidences of pneumothorax closer to 1% or 2%.[29] In these series, the lesions were generally silent, asymptomatic, and were discovered only on follow-up chest radiographs.

An asymptomatic pneumothorax is of little clinical consequence and usually requires no treatment beyond close observation. If further treatment is required, needle aspiration usually suffices. Reabsorption of a small pneumothorax can also be aided by administration of oxygen. A thoracostomy tube should be placed only if there is continued ventilatory embarrassment or a steady increase in the size of the pneumothorax.[30, 31]

To produce a pneumothorax from an intercostal injection, the needle must puncture not only the parietal pleura but also the visceral pleura, to allow air to leak from the lung into the pleural cavity. With coughing, over time, this condition can progress to tension pneumothorax. The most common technical error that results in pneumothorax is improper positioning of the hands during the performance of the block—thus, failure to control needle depth.

Systemic Toxicity

A second type of complication from intercostal block is the toxic effects of absorbed local anesthetic drugs. This problem is most likely to occur when large amounts of concentrated drug are injected. Systemic toxic reactions are less likely with blocks for diagnosis or postoperative pain relief, as ordinarily smaller volumes of more dilute local anesthetic solution are used.

Hypotension and Respiratory Failure

A third complication of intercostal block is hypotension.[32] Usually, it has occurred when intrathoracic intercostal blocks were performed under direct vision by the surgeon. It appears that, in each case a high epidural or total spinal block resulted from central spread of solution and subsequently to a rapid and profound drop in blood pressure. Hypotension develops on occasion, when intercostal blocks are performed to provide postoperative pain relief for patients in the intensive care unit. Although the cause is unclear, hypotension appears to occur in patients who are hypovolemic and vasoconstricted because of severe pain.

When analgesia is produced by the intercostal blocks, the compensatory vasoconstriction eases and the patient becomes hypotensive.

In a somewhat similar manner, intercostal nerve block can lead to respiratory failure when pain relief from the block unmasks the ventilatory depression of previously administered, but ineffective, parenteral narcotics.[33]

FUTURE CONSIDERATIONS

The success rate of intercostal nerve block should approach 100%. The problem is not in the doing but in the duration of this block. Currently available local anesthetic drugs give analgesia for only 8 to 12 hours. Cryoanalgesia has been advocated as a method of obtaining blocks of long duration by freezing the nerves. This technique, however, is unreliable, cumbersome, and declining in use.[34, 35]

Another future consideration is that techniques might be developed that do not require needle injections. For example, there are reports of using the jet injection system originally designed and used for mass inoculations, which has also been adapted to intercostal and other superficial peripheral nerve blocks. The injector jet is applied directly to the skin but does not penetrate it. The injectate is forced through the skin and is subsequently absorbed into the bloodstream. Advantages purportedly include little or no risk of pneumothorax and capability for performing multiple blocks easily and rapidly. The procedure is not totally painless; however, transdermal spread of local anesthetic drug is unpredictable, and the jet gun has some major deficits. One is that only 1 mL of solution can be ejected per "shot." Although this limitation could conceivably be overcome by design modifications, larger volume would likely be more painful when injected. Seddon[36] reported using 1 mL of 1.5% bupivacaine, which was specially prepared for his study, as this concentration is not available commercially.[36] This drug concentration did not appear to be neurotoxic, and the results compared favorably with postcholecystectomy pain relief from intramuscular narcotics. Katz and associates[37] compared two separate 1-mL injections of 0.75% bupivacaine with more traditional intercostal nerve blocks (3 mL) by needle injection. It is interesting to note that neither patient group appeared to receive effective analgesia in that study.

New drug formulations are currently being developed which may prolong the duration of intercostal blockade from hours to days, or even weeks. The incorporation of bupivacaine into liposomes and polymer microspheres has been shown to greatly extend its duration of action.[38, 39] The duration of sensory anesthesia after intercostal blockade in sheep is increased from 4 to 13 days after the injection of bupivacaine in microspheres (8 to 80 mg/kg). Despite this extremely large load of bupivacaine within the microspheres, plasma concentrations (<0.25 μg/mL) are only a fraction of what is detected after injection of aqueous bupivacaine.[40] When these new formulations become available, the slight pain and time involved in performing intercostal blockade will be more than offset by the benefits and duration of pain relief.

REFERENCES

1. Schleich DS: Schmerzlöse Operationen. Berlin, J Springer, 1894.
2. Braun H: Local Anesthesia: Its Scientific Basis and Practical Use. Philadelphia, Lea & Febiger, 1914.
3. Pauchet V, Sourdat P, Labat G: L'Anesthesie Regionale, ed 3. Paris, Librairie Octave Doin, 1921.
4. Labat G: Regional Anesthesia; Its Technic and Clinical Application. Philadelphia, WB Saunders, 1922.
5. Mandl F: Paravertebral Block. New York, Grune & Stratton, 1947.
6. Moore DC, Bridenbaugh LD: Intercostal nerve block in 4333 patients: Indications, technique, and complications. Anesth Analg 41:1, 1962.
7. Moore DC: Intercostal nerve block for postoperative somatic pain following surgery of thorax and upper abdomen. Br J Anaesth 47:284, 1975.
8. Mozell EJ, Sabanathan S, Mearns AJ, et al: Continuous extrapleural intercostal nerve block after pleurecotomy. Thorax 46:21, 1991.
9. Conacher I, Kokri M: Postoperative paravertebral blocks for thoracic surgery. Br J Anaesth 59:155, 1987.
10. Baxter AD, Jennings FO, Harris RS, et al: Continuous intercostal blockade after cardiac surgery. Br J Anaesth 59:162, 1987.
11. Nunn JF, Slavin C: Posterior intercostal nerve block for pain relief after cholecystectomy. Br J Anaesth 52:253, 1980.
12. Bunting P, McGeachie JF: Intercostal nerve blockade producing analgesia after appendicectomy. Br J Anaesth 61:169, 1988.
13. Sihota MK, Holmblad BR: Horner's syndrome after interpleural anesthesia with bupivacaine for post-herpetic neuralgia. Acta Anesth Scand 32:593, 1988.
14. Hardy PAJ: Anatomical variation in the position of the proximal intercostal nerve. Br J Anaesth 61:338, 1988.
15. Conacher ID: Resin injection of thoracic paravertebral spaces. Br J Anaesth 61:657, 1988.
16. Baxter AD, Flynn JF, Jennings FO: Continuous intercostal nerve blockade. Br J Anaesth 56:665, 1984.
17. Butchart EG, Grott GJ, Barnsley WC: Spontaneous rupture of an intercostal artery in a patient with neurofibromatosis and scoliosis. J Thorac Cardiovasc Surg 69:919, 1975.
18. Thompson GE, Brown DL: The common nerve blocks. *In* Nunn FF, Utting JE, Brown BR (eds): General Anaesthesia, ed 5. London, Butterworth, 1989, p 1070.
19. Moore D, Bush W, Scurlock J: Intercostal nerve block: A roentgenographic anatomic study of technique and absorption in humans. Anesth Analg 59:815, 1980.
20. Smith BE, Suchak M, Siggins D, Challands J: Rectus sheath block for diagnostic laparoscopy. Anaesthesia 43:947, 1988.
21. Kvalheim L, Reistad F: Interpleural catheter in the management of postoperative pain. Anesthesiology 61:A231, 1984.
22. Murphy DF: Continuous intercostal nerve blockade: An anatomical study to elucidate its mode of action. Br J Anaesth 56:627, 1984.
23. Eason MJ, Wyatt R: Paravertebral thoracic block—a reappraisal. Anaesthesia 34:638, 1979.
24. Thompson GE, Moore DC: Ketamine, diazepam and Innovar: A computerized comparative study. Anesth Analg (Cleve) 50:458, 1971.
25. Tucker GT, Moore DC, Bridenbaugh PO, et al: Systemic absorption of mepivacaine in commonly used regional block procedures. Anesthesiology 37:276, 1972.
26. Jakobson S, Fridiksson H, Hedenstrom H, Ivarsson I: Effects of intercostal nerve blocks on pulmonary mechanics in healthy men. Acta Anaesthesiol Scand 24:482, 1980.
27. Hecker BR, Fjurstrom R, Schoene RB: Effect of intercostal nerve blockade on respiratory mechanics and CO_2 chemosensitivity at rest and exercise. Anesthesiology 70:13, 1989.
28. Moore DC, Bridenbaugh LD: Pneumothorax: Its incidence following intercostal nerve block. JAMA 174:842, 1960.
29. Bridenbaugh PO, DuPen SL, Moore DC, et al: Postoperative intercostal nerve block analgesia versus narcotic analgesia. Anesth Analg (Cleve) 52:81, 1973.
30. Jones JS: A place for aspiration in the treatment of spontaneous pneumothorax. Thorax 40:66, 1985.
31. Vallee P: Sequential treatment of a simple pneumothorax. Ann Emerg Med 17:936, 1988.

32. Skretting P: Hypotension after intercostal nerve block during thoracotomy under general anesthesia. Br J Anaesth 53:527, 1981.
33. Cory PC, Mulroy MF: Postoperative respiratory failure following intercostal block. Anesthesiology 54:418, 1981.
34. Lloyd JW, Barnard JDW, Glynn, CJ: Cryoanalgesia, a new approach to pain relief. Lancet 2:932, 1976.
35. Maiwand O, Makey AR: Cryoanalgesia for relief of pain after thoracotomy. Br Med J 282:1749, 1981.
36. Seddon SJ: Intercostal nerve block by jet injection. Anaesthesia 39:484, 1984.
37. Katz J, Knarr D, Juneja M: Intercostal nerve block by jet injection. Anaesthesia 75:A726, 1991.
38. Curley J, Castillo J, Hotz J, et al: Prolonged regional nerve blockade. Anesthesiology 84:1401, 1996.
39. Mowat JJ, Mok MJ, MacLeod BA, Madden TD: Liposomal bupivacaine. Anesthesiology 85:635, 1996.
40. Drager C, Benziger D, Gao F, Berde CB: Prologed intercostal nerve blockade in sheep using controlled-release of bupivacaine and dexamethasone from polymer microspheres. Anesthesiology 89:969, 1998.

CHAPTER • 38

Interpleural Catheters: Indications and Techniques

Kathleen A. O'Leary, MD • Anthony T. Yarussi, MD • David P. Myers, MD

The concept of interpleural anesthesia (IPA) was originally described by Mandl[1] in 1947, who used 6% phenol injected into the interpleural space of experimental animals and produced no signs of pleural irritation or necrosis. IPA resurfaced in 1986, when it was used as an investigational tool for postoperative pain relief after breast surgery, kidney surgery, and cholecystectomy by Reiestad and Stromskag.[2] In their study, a single 20-mL dose of bupivacaine, 0.5%, with epinephrine was administered after surgery. Of the 81 enrolled patients, 78 required no additional analgesic measure during the first 24 hours postoperatively. Duration of analgesia ranged from 6 to 27 hours.

Most recently, interest in IPA for chronic pain management has increased. Durrani and colleagues[3] alleviated pancreatic carcinoma pain using interpleural bupivacaine. Fineman[4] used IPA for metastatic bronchogenic carcinoma pain in the pleura and chest wall.

MECHANISMS OF ACTION

Three theories of the mechanism of action of IPA have been advanced. First is diffusion of local anesthetic from the pleural space through the parietal pleural and the innermost intercostal muscles, producing multiple unilateral intercostal nerve blocks. Second, a unilateral block of the thoracic sympathetic chain and the splanchnic nerves is produced by drug traversing the parietal pleural paraspinally. Finally, diffusion of the anesthetic to the ipsilateral brachial plexus produces analgesia to the arm.

Riegler and Vadeboncouer[5] used evoked potential monitoring in dogs to demonstrate that IPA produces multiple sensory nerve blocks. Clinical studies by Durrani and colleagues,[3] Reiestad and Kvalheim,[6] and Alhburg and coworkers,[7] in which sympathetically mediated pain syndromes were treated with IPA, imply that autonomic blockade can also occur. Ramajoli and DeAmici[8] proposed that bilateral block of the sympathetic and splanchnic nerves occurs after unilateral IPA. In their patients with diffuse visceral pain, they noted marked reduction in pain scores bilaterally and bilateral increases in cutaneous temperatures as compared with controls after injection of 20 mL of 0.25% or 0.5% bupivacaine via an interpleural catheter. They hypothesized that the anesthetic agent diffused through the pleura at the costovertebral margin to the mediastinum to reach the ipsilateral and contralateral sympathetic chains. The force of aspiration is caused by the greater negative pressure in the mediastinum (−25 to −30 cm H_2O) as compared with the pleura (−5 to −10 cm H_2O).[9]

Diffusion of local anesthetic into the brachial plexus and stellate ganglion has produced relief for head and neck and upper extremity pain syndromes. Horner's syndrome is commonly seen if the drug is allowed to diffuse cephalad to block the stellate ganglion.

INDICATIONS

Interpleural analgesia is commonly used for unilateral subcostal postoperative pain relief. It also provides anesthesia for minor surgical procedures and chronic pain. Table 38–1 lists procedures in which IPA has been effective for either analgesia or anesthesia. It is important to remember that IPA is considered a unilateral block and is not currently recommended for pain extending across the midline. Moreover, bilateral interpleural analgesia should never be attempted, lest bilateral pneumothoraces occur, unless catheters can be placed under direct surgical vision.

Interpleural analgesia has been used effectively to treat chronic pain in terminally ill patients with pancreatic, renal cell, and breast cancers and lymphomas.[10] For those whom traditional methods of analgesic therapy have failed and whose expected survival is short, IPA can produce immediate pain relief. For patients with advanced cancer who may survive >3 months, interpleural phenol injections have been used with good results. Phenol injections into the pleural cavity of one cancer patient produced no microscopic or macroscopic changes in lung, pleura, or nerve tissue despite excellent analgesia over a 3-month period

TABLE 38–1 ***Indications for Use of Intrapleural Anesthesia***

Postoperative analgesia
- Cholecystectomy
- Breast surgery
- Renal surgery
- Other subcostal incisions
- Multiple rib fractures
- Thoracotomy
- Cardiac surgery

Surgical anesthesia
- Breast biopsy and lumpectomy
- Percutaneous hepatic and renal drainage procedures
- Lithotripsy

Chronic pain management
- Chronic pancreatitis
- Postherpetic neuralgia
- Reflex sympathetic dystrophies of the arm/face
- Frozen shoulder
- Upper abdominal cancer pain
- Chest wall and thoracic visceral pain
- Pain of pancreatic cancer and other abdominal cancer
- Upper limb ischemia
- Cystic fibrosis

until his death.[11] Tunneled interpleural catheters have also been useful in the palliation of chronic cancer-related pain. The interpleural catheter is tunneled in the same manner as an epidural catheter.

IPA has also been used for symptomatic management of acute herpes zoster,[12] postherpetic neuralgia,[13–15] reflex sympathetic dystrophy,[16] upper limb ischemia,[17] and cystic fibrosis.[18]

CONTRAINDICATIONS

Relative contraindications to the use of IPA include pleuritis, pulmonary fibrosis, pleural adhesions, emphysema, hemothorax, pleural effusions, empyema, bronchopleural fistula, and surgical or chemical pleurodesis. These processes either increase the risk of pneumothorax or cause erratic distribution and absorption of local anesthetic as well as difficulty in identifying the interpleural space. If a patient is being ventilated with positive end-expiratory pressure (PEEP) at the time of catheter insertion, the risk of pneumothorax is greatly increased.

Absolute contraindications to IPA include allergy to local anesthetic, extensive infection around the catheter insertion site, and bleeding diatheses.

PATIENT POSITIONING

Proper patient positioning is exceeded only by correct catheter placement and successful injection into the pleural space as critical determinants of the extent of the resulting block. Table 38–2 describes the three best positions for IPA. In all blocks except multiple intercostal rib blocks sparing the thoracic sympathetic chain, the patient must be positioned with the *affected side up*. Because the block sets up by mass action, delivery of local anesthetic agent along the paravertebral gutter by gravitational flow is essential to have the bulk of solution bathe the affected nerves (Fig. 38–1). The position of the patient after injection of local anesthetic into the pleural space also determines, in large part, the nature, intensity, and extent of the resulting blockade. The preferred approach for unilateral blockade of cervical or superior thoracic segments is to place the patient in a lateral decubitus position with the head down 20 degrees for 20 to 30 min after the injection.

Patients who are suffering from somatic or visceral pain, such as that from pancreatic carcinoma, may also benefit from interpleural analgesia.[3] For those who are unable to lie prone or in lateral decubitus position owing to pain, celiac plexus blockade is not an option. IPA can be provided by putting the patient in either the sitting or reverse Trendelenburg position, depending on the patient's tolerance.

INSERTION OF CATHETERS

In a 70-kg man, the pleural space is 10 to 20 μm wide and occupies a surface area of 2000 cm^2. This cavity is created between the visceral pleura lining the heart and lungs and the parietal pleura covering the thoracic cage and diaphragm. Pleural pressure varies from −12 cm H_2O in the apical portion of the lungs to less negative values (−5 cm H_2O) at the bases. This negative interpleural pressure is

TABLE 38–2 ***Patient Positioning for Intrapleural Anesthesia***

Purpose of Block	Recommended Position and Comments
Unilateral blockade of cervical and superior thoracic segments of sympathetic chain	Lateral decubitus position with affected side up and head down about 20 degrees for 20–30 min after injection of local anesthetic Partial blockade of ipsilateral brachial plexus is also achieved by this position, as demonstrated by hypesthesia in C3–T1 dermatomes and motor weakness of shoulder, arm, and forearm
Surgical anesthesia for unilateral breast tumor resection	Lateral decubitus position with affected side down and head down about 20 degrees for 20–30 min after injection of local anesthesia Produces unilateral blockade of intercostal nerves from T1–T9 with complete skin anesthesia
Postoperative pain management, including chest trauma	Side-lying position at angle of about 20 degrees with the affected side up during injection and injection time of 5–6 min for 30 mL of local anesthetic: after injection, patient is turned supine. Produces blockade of both sympathetic chain and intercostal nerves of affected side

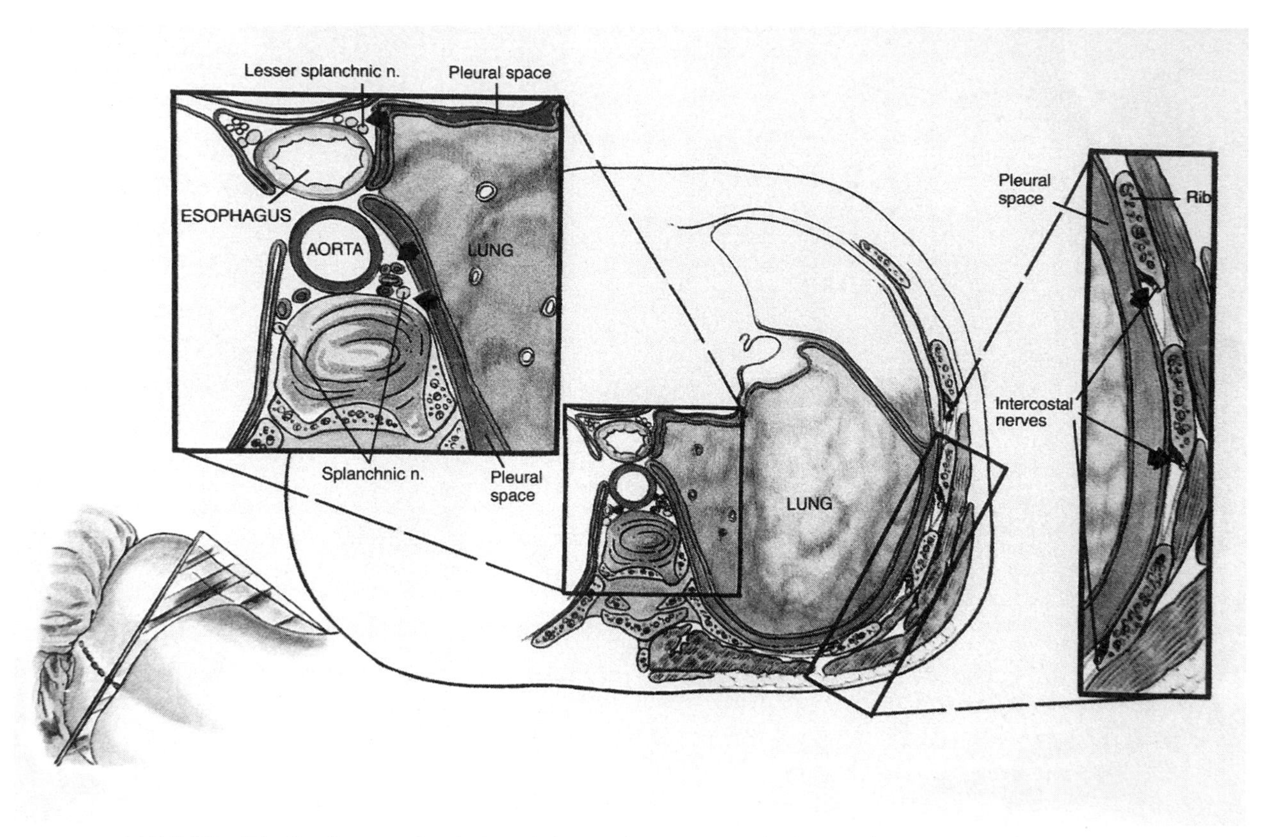

FIGURE 38–1 *Cross-sectional view of thorax shows paravertebral gutter between visceral and parietal pleura. (From Brown DL: Atlas of Regional Anesthesia, Philadelphia, WB Saunders, 1992.)*

the key to proper identification of the pleural space and is a function of the elastic recoil of the chest outward and the tendency of the lungs to collapse.

Blood pressure, heart rate, and respiration should be monitored during and immediately after placement of the interpleural catheter. The patient lies in the lateral decubitus position with the affected side up. An interpleural kit (Arrow) is ideal, but a continuous epidural tray will suffice. The major advantages of the interpleural kit are its blunter needle and softer-tipped catheter (Flexitip), which reduce the chance of pneumothorax.

With sterile technique, an area is identified for insertion, most commonly the T7–T8 intercostal space. The site of puncture is 8 to 10 cm from the posterior midline (Fig. 38–2A). After local anesthetic injection (Fig. 38–2B), the blunt-tipped needle is introduced in a medial direction with the cutting edge uppermost until it reaches the lower rib of the selected interspace (Fig. 38–2C). When the parietal pleura is penetrated, which is perceived as a clicking sensation (Fig. 38–2D), the negative pleural pressure and the plunger weight itself cause the air to escape into the thorax (Fig. 38–2E). The syringe is then removed, and the catheter is introduced 6 to 8 cm into the pleural space (Fig. 38–2F). The needle is removed next and the catheter left in place (Fig. 38–2G). After aspiration for blood and air, the catheter is taped in place.

A test dose of local anesthetic with epinephrine can then be administered. If there are no adverse reactions, a bolus dose can be given. Upon return of pain, additional bolus doses may be given, again with the patient in the lateral decubitus position and the affected side up.

Although this has been the standard technique for interpleural catheter placement, the introduction of air into the interpleural space is difficult to avoid as the Tuohy needle is open to air to allow passage of the catheter. As much as 20 ml of air can be entrained into the pleural space during insertion, and the resulting air pockets can be responsible for patchy blocks which may sometimes be encountered with interpleural anesthesia. Modified techniques have been developed to create a closed system and reduce the chance of air entering the interpleural space.[19, 20]

Gomar and associates used an electronic device (Episensor [Palex, Spain]) that detects negative pressure under -1.8 cm H_2O to identify the interpleural space.[21] This technique was used in 25 patients postoperatively and catheter positions confirmed radiographically. None of the patients developed pneumothorax. Electronic devices may prove to be useful adjuncts to interpleural catheter placement, especially in obese patients or those with pleural disease.

DOSAGE

Various dosing regimens have been advocated for IPA, but controversy about the optimal dosage, volume, and concentration of local anesthetic persists. The need for adequate analgesia must be balanced with the risk of possible toxicity, because the margin of safety with IPA is small.

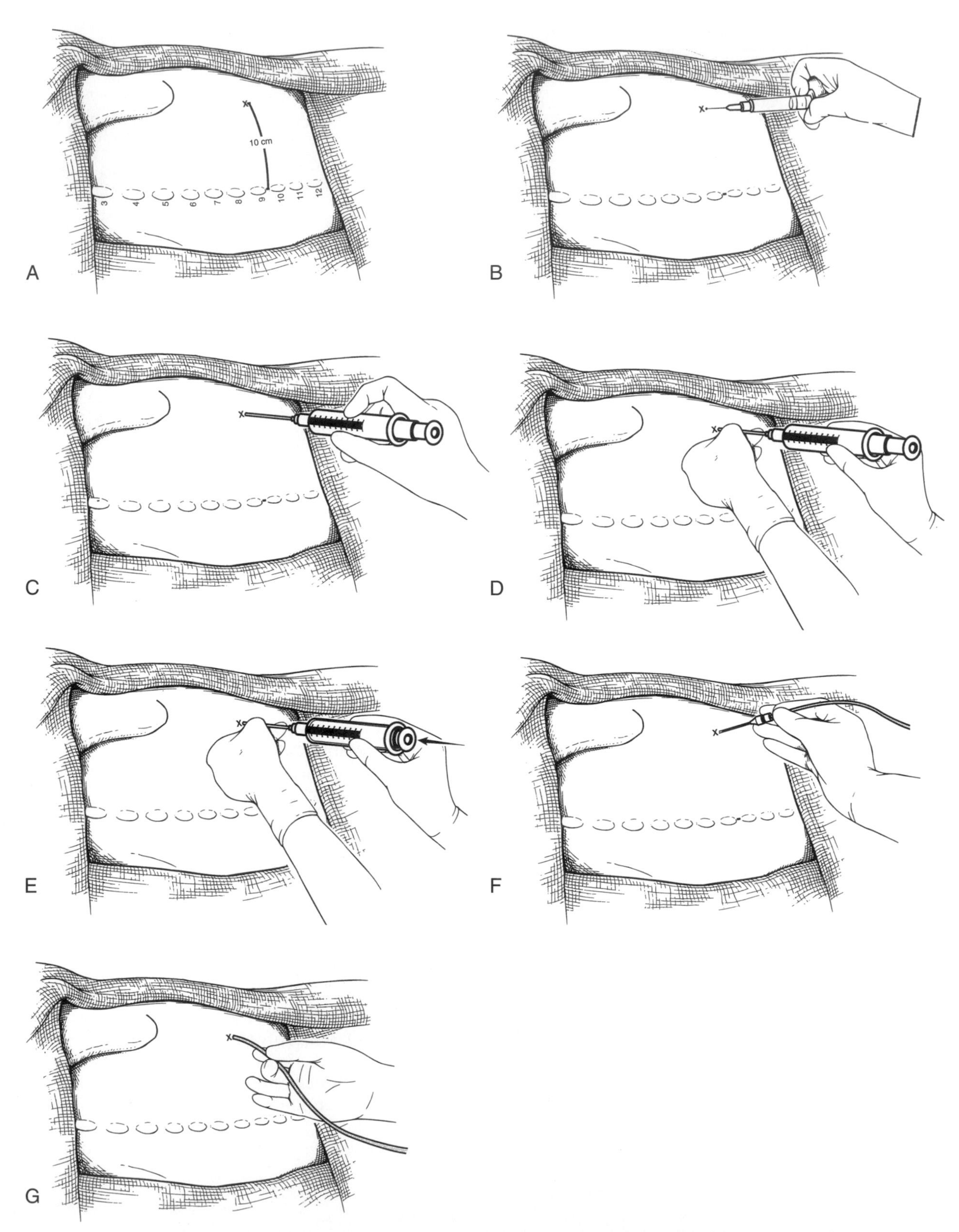

FIGURE 38–2 *A, Mark skin 10 cm from posterior line between T7–T10. B, Mark skin wheal with a local anesthetic (1% lidocaine). C, After making a small skin incision, insert an epidural needle with the bevel up and 4 cc of air in the syringe. D, Using passive loss of resistance and a two-handed technique, advance the needle slowly until a pop of the parietal pleura is felt. E, Air will be drawn in by the negative pressure of the thoracic space. F, Quickly insert and advance the catheter through the needle lumen to avoid entrainment of additional air. G, Remove the needle and secure the catheter with Steri-Strips and a clear plastic dressing.*

Perhaps the most common method of delivering IPA is the intermittent bolus method. Typically, a bolus dose is given at the end of the surgical procedure, prior to the conclusion of the general anesthetic. This initial dose is followed up with doses given either at established intervals (usually every 6 hours) or as needed when the patient experiences pain.

Bolus doses using 20 mL of both 0.25% and 0.5% bupivacaine with epinephrine 1:200,000 have proved efficacious for postoperative analgesia.[2, 22] Stromskag and colleagues[23] compared the analgesic effects of 40 mL of 0.25% bupivacaine with epinephrine and 20 mL of 0.5% bupivacaine with epinephrine in postcholecystectomy patients. They found no difference between the two groups, concluding that, as long as the amount of drug administered is adequate, the volume of bupivacaine with epinephrine has little effect within the range of 20 to 40 mL.

Continuous infusion of bupivacaine has also been utilized. Laurito and associates[24] compared continuous infusions of 0.25% bupivacaine (plain) at a rate of 0.125 mL/kg/hr with bolus doses of 0.5% bupivacaine with epinephrine 1:200,000 at 0.4 mL/kg every 6 hours in postcholecystectomy patients. They found that the continuous infusion produces better analgesia and lower plasma bupivacaine levels than bolus dosing. Van Kleef and co-workers[25] compared continuous infusions of 0.25% and 0.5% bupivacaine with epinephrine 1:200,000 at 5 mL/hr in postoperative patients who had either flank or subcostal incisions. They found comparable clinical effects but lower plasma concentrations in the group who received 0.25% bupivacaine.

Thus, continuous infusions of 0.25% bupivacaine with epinephrine are safe, effective, and less labor intensive than intermittent bolus doses. When continuous infusions are not possible, intermittent bolus doses of 20 to 30 mL of 0.25% bupivacaine with epinephrine can safely be utilized. In either situation, the patients should be monitored for evidence of systemic toxicity during the course of treatment.

Clinical studies have also been done to evaluate the effect of interpleural opioids on postoperative pain control.[26, 27] Welte and colleagues found that interpleural morphine had no beneficial effect in reducing postoperative pain scores or improving pulmonary function after thoracotomy, as compared with the intravenous route.[27] Morphine via the interpleural route does not appear to activate peripheral opioid receptors at primary afferent neurons, thus giving it no greater effect than if administered intravenously.

COMPLICATIONS

Although the IPA technique has been very safe in clinical use, there has been some disagreement about its safety. Gomez and colleagues[28] demonstrated a high malposition rate with intraoperative placement of 18 catheters. They concluded that the procedure was unsafe, but several factors contributed to the high failure rate. They inserted catheters to 30 cm and used sharp-tipped needles and stiffer epidural catheters. The patients also received positive-pressure ventilation during insertion of the interpleural catheter.

The risks of inserting an interpleural catheter (see Table 38–3) are low if one takes the time to slowly advance a catheter with a soft, flexible tip to a distance of 6 to 8 cm. The use of a blunt epidural-style needle and a heavier-barreled 10-mL glass syringe allow for easier confirmation of positioning in the interpleural space. Despite meticulous care, however, complications can occur.

Clinically significant pneumothorax is the most common complication (reported incidence <5%). Thus, a chest radiograph is mandatory after placement of an interpleural catheter. In such cases, a small pocket of air may be seen over the apex of the lung. This finding represents injected air that entered the pleural space during positioning of the interpleural catheter, not air leaking from a perforated lung. This air is rapidly absorbed and presents no clinical problem. One tension pneumothorax[29] has been reported. It resulted from use of the loss-of-resistance technique to identify the interpleural space.

The reported prevalence of systemic toxicity from local anesthetics is 1.3%.[29] The clinical manifestations are neurologic, ranging from somnolence and disorientation to seizure activity. It is likely that absorption of local anesthetic is increased in patients with inflamed pleura, and they are the ones most at risk for systemic toxicity.

Pleural effusion after IPA is rare (incidence 0.4%).[30] Causes include damage to intercostal vessels, minor trauma from needle insertion, failure of local anesthetic absorption, and diaphragmatic tracking of inflammatory fluid after abdominal surgery. Other reported complications include catheter displacement, Horner's syndrome, empyema, and formation of a bronchopleural fistula.[30]

SUMMARY

The correct technique for placement of interpleural catheters is relatively easy as compared with other anesthetic procedures such as thoracic epidural catheter insertion. Another advantage of IPA is the development of a unilateral sympathetic block, versus the bilateral sympathetic and somatic block produced by thoracic epidural analgesia. Unilateral sympathetic blockade avoids bradycardia and hypotension, because the contralateral sympathetic chain is intact.

In spite of the advantages of this technique, IPA has not gained momentum in anesthesiology. To many, the risk of inserting a needle into the thoracic cavity for routine postoperative analgesia far outweighs the benefits. Its suc-

TABLE 38–3 **Complications of Interpleural Anesthesia**

Pneumothorax
Pleural effusion
Horner's syndrome
Catheter displacement
Catheter loss
Systemic reaction
Empyema
Bronchopleural fistula
Laceration of intercostal neurovascular bundle

cess in relieving subdiaphragmatic chronic organ pain, however, makes it an intriguing alternative to the more complex plexus blocks for pain management.

At present, IPA appears to be most clinically useful for analgesia for subdiaphragmatic incisions, chronic benign pain, and neurolytic cancer pain in terminally ill persons. Further clinical studies will continue to elucidate the place of IPA in the armamentarium of the regional anesthesiologist.

REFERENCES

1. Mandl F: Paravertebral Block. New York, Grune & Stratton, 1947, pp 34–37.
2. Reiestad F, Stromskag K: Interpleural catheter in the management of postoperative pain. Reg Anesth 11:89–91, 1986.
3. Durrani Z, Winnie A, Ikuta P: Interpleural catheter analgesia for pancreatic pain. Anesth Analg 67:479–481, 1988.
4. Fineman S: Long-term postthoracotomy cancer pain management with interpleural bupivacaine. Anesth Analg 68:694–697, 1989.
5. Riegler F, Vadeboncouer T: Interpleural anesthetics in the dog: Differential somatic neural blockade. Anesthesiology 71:744–750, 1989.
6. Reiestad F, Kvalheim L: Continuous intercostal blocks for post operative pain relief. Norweg Med Assoc J 104:485–487, 1984.
7. Ahlburg P, Noreng M, Molgaard J, Egebo K: Treatment of pancreatic pain with interpleural bupivacaine: An open trial. Acta Anesthesiol Scand 34:156–157, 1990.
8. Ramajoli F, DeAmici D: Is there a bilateral block of the thoracic sympathetic chain after unilateral intrapleural analgesia? Anesth Analg 87:360–367, 1998.
9. Miserocchi GM, Pistoleis M, Miriati M, et al: Pleural liquid pressure gradients and intrapleural distribution of injected bolus. J Appl Physiol 56:526–532, 1984.
10. Myers DP, Lema MJ, deLeon-Casasola OA, Bacon DR: Interpleural analgesia for the treatment of severe cancer pain in terminally ill patients. J Pain Symptom Manage 8:505–510, 1993.
11. Lema MJ, Myers DP, deLeon-Casasola OA, Penetrante R: Pleural phenol therapy for treatment of chronic esophageal pain. Reg Anesth 17:166–170, 1992.
12. Johnson LR, Racco AG, Fellonte FM: Continuous subpleural-paravertebral block in acute thoracic herpes zoster. Anesth Analg 67:1105–1108, 1988.
13. Reiestad F, McIlvaine WB, Barnes M, et al: Interpleural analgesia in the treatment of severe thoracic post herpetic neuralgia. Reg Anesth 15:113–117, 1990.
14. Reiestad F, Stokke T, Barnes M: Interpleural analgesia in chronic pain. Acta Anaesth Scand 33:A101, 1989.
15. Sihuta MK, Holmblad BR: Horner's syndrome after intrapleural anesthesia with bupivacaine for postherpetic neuralgia. Acta Anaesth Scand 32:593–597, 1988.
16. Reiestad F, McIlvaine WB, Kvalheim L, Stokke T, Pettersen B: Interpleural analgesia in the treatment of upper extremity reflex sympathetic dystrophy. Anesth Analg 69:671–673, 1989.
17. Perkins G: Interpleural anesthesia in the management of upper limb ischemia. A report of three cases. Anaesth Intensive Care 19:575–578, 1991.
18. Bruce DL, Gerken MV, Lyon GD: Post cholecystectomy pain relief by intrapleural bupivacaine in patients with cystic fibrosis. Anesth Analg 66:1187–1189, 1987.
19. Marsh B, McDonald P: A modified technique for the insertion of an interpleural catheter. Anaesthesia 46(10):889, 1991.
20. Ho A, Cortardi L: A simple technique to facilitate interpleural catheter placement. Anesth Analg 79:614–615, 1994.
21. Gomar C, Cabres L, DeAndres T, Nalda MA, Caltrava P: An electronic device (Episensor) for detection of the interpleural space. Reg Anesth 16:112–115, 1991.
22. Stromskag KE, Reiestad F, Holmquist ELO: Intrapleural administration of 0.25%, 0.37%, and 0.5% bupivacaine with epinephrine after cholecystectomy. Anesth Analg 67:430, 1988.
23. Stromskag KE, Minor BG, Lindeberg A: Comparison of 40 milliliters of 0.25% intrapleural bupivacaine with epinephrine with 20 milliliters of 0.5% intrapleural bupivacaine with epinephrine after cholecystectomy. Anesth Analg 73:397, 1991.
24. Laurito CE, Kirz LI, Vadeboncouer TR, et al: Continuous infusion of interpleural bupivacaine maintains effective analgesia after cholecystectomy. Anesth Analg 72:516, 1991.
25. Van Kleef JW, Logeman A, Burns AGL, et al: Continuous interpleural infusion of bupivacaine for postoperative analgesia after surgery with flank incisions: A double-blind comparison of 0.25% and 0.5% solutions. Anesth Analg 75:268, 1992.
26. Schulte-Steinberg H, Weringer G, Jokisch O, et al: Intraperitoneal versus interpleural morphine or bupivacaine for pain after laparoscopic cholecystectomy. Anesthesiology 82:634–640, 1995.
27. Welte M, Haimerl E, Groh J, et al: Effect of interpleural morphine on postoperative pain and pulmonary function after thoracotomy. Br J Anaesth 69:637–639, 1992.
28. Gomez MN, Symreng T, Rossi NP, Chiang CK: Interpleural bupivacaine for intraoperative analgesia: A dangerous technique? Anesth Analg 67:578, 1988.
29. Stromskag KE, Minor B, Steen PA: Side effects and complications related to interpleural analgesia: An update. Acta Anaesth Scand 34:473–477, 1990.
30. Harrison P, Kent E, Lema M: Interpleural analgesia: Its use and complication in a quadriplegic patient with chronic pain. J Pain Sympt Manage 8:238–241, 1993.

CHAPTER • 39

Lumbar Epidural Nerve Block

Steven D. Waldman, MD, JD

Probably no other regional anesthesia technique has been studied and used as extensively as lumbar epidural nerve block. The applications for this technique in the areas of surgical and obstetric anesthesia and pain management continue to expand. This chapter offers the pain specialist a practical overview of the role of lumbar epidural nerve block in contemporary pain management.

HISTORICAL CONSIDERATIONS

The description of the paramidline approach to the lumbar epidural space proposed by Pagés[1] in 1921 is considered the first clinically relevant report of the technique of lumbar epidural nerve block. Pagés's technique used the tactile feedback from the needle's impinging on and passing through the ligamentum flavum as the means of identifying the epidural space. Confirmation of needle placement in the epidural space was based on obstruction of free flow of spinal fluid from the needle and the lack of resistance to injection of local anesthetic. This approach was obviously technically demanding and was associated with a significant failure rate.

The problems inherent in this technique led to further refinements in the lack-of-resistance technique. Forestier and Sicard advocated attaching a fluid-filled syringe to a needle and injecting continuously while advancing the needle through the ligaments of the spine.[2] Sicard envisioned that the injectate served as a "fluid trocar" that atraumatically pushed the dura away from the advancing needle.

In 1933, drawing from the work of Sicard and Forestier, Dogliotti[3] introduced the loss-of-resistance technique into clinical practice. Dogliotti's technique relied on the sudden loss of resistance to injection when the needle bevel passed from the dense ligamentum flavum into the epidural space.

Independently and in the same year, Gutierrez[4] suggested that the negative pressure of the epidural space might be used to identify the epidural space and devised the hanging-drop technique. This technique involves placing a drop of local anesthetic into the open hub of the needle, which is then advanced toward the epidural space. Gutierrez postulated that, as the needle bevel passes through the ligamentum flavum into the negative pressure of the epidural space, the drop of local anesthetic is sucked through the needle into the epidural space. Later measurements of epidural pressures have caused this mechanism to be called into question.[5]

In spite of these technical advances, many anesthesiologists in the first half of the 20th century considered epidural anesthesia an unreliable anesthetic technique as compared with spinal anesthesia. For this reason, epidural anesthesia remained popular with a limited number of enthusiasts. The introduction of neuromuscular blocking agents in 1946 led to a decline in the use of all regional anesthetic techniques, including epidural anesthesia.

Interestingly, it was a needle rather than new drugs that renewed interest in epidural anesthesia. The Tuohy needle not only reduced the incidence of inadvertent dural punctures but allowed the anesthesiologist to maintain analgesia for prolonged periods through the use of indwelling catheters placed through the needle.[6] The introduction of lidocaine into clinical practice in the early 1950s added a greater margin of safety for epidural anesthesia and led to increased use of epidural anesthesia in obstetrics. Bupivacaine, introduced in the early 1960s, enabled anesthesiologists to provide long-lasting neural blockade from a single injection and made epidural nerve block an option in a variety of new clinical situations. The discovery of the clinical utility of the epidural administration of steroids in the management of radiculopathy and other painful conditions and of opioids in the management of cancer-related pain brought epidural nerve block into the mainstream of pain management.[7]

INDICATIONS AND CONTRAINDICATIONS

Indications for lumbar epidural nerve block are summarized in Table 39–1. In addition to surgical and obstetric anesthesia, lumbar epidural nerve block using local anesthetic can be used as a diagnostic tool when one is performing differential neural blockade on an anatomic basis in the evaluation of lower abdominal, back, groin, pelvic, bladder, perineal, genital, rectal, anal, and lower extremity pain.[8] When destruction of the lumbar nerve roots is being considered, lumbar epidural nerve block is useful as an indica-

TABLE 39–1 **Indications for the Lumbar Approach to the Epidural Space**

Surgical, obstetric, diagnostic, prognostic
Surgical anesthesia
Obstetric anesthesia
Differential neural blockade to evaluate lower abdominal, back, groin, pelvic, bladder, perineal, genital, rectal, anal, and lower extremity pain
Prognostic indicator before destruction of the lumbar nerves
Acute pain
Palliation of acute pain emergencies
Postoperative pain
Back, lower abdominal, pelvic, and lower extremity pain secondary to trauma
Pain of acute herpes zoster
Acute vascular insufficiency of the lower extremities
Pain of ureteral calculi
Prophylactic and preemptive pain
Before amputation of ischemic limbs
Chronic benign pain
Lumbar radiculopathy
Spinal stenosis
Low back syndrome
Vertebral compression fractures
Diabetic polyneuropathy
Postherpetic neuralgia
Reflex sympathetic dystrophy
Orchalgia
Proctalgia
Pelvic pain syndromes
Phantom limb syndrome
Chemotherapy-related peripheral neuropathy
Postlaminectomy syndrome
Cancer-related pain
Pain secondary to pelvic, perineal, genital, and rectal malignancy
Bone metastases to pelvis
Chemotherapy-related peripheral neuropathy

tor of the extent of motor and sensory impairment that the patient may experience.

Lumbar epidural nerve block with local anesthetics or opioids may be utilized to palliate acute pain until pharmacologic, surgical, or antiblastic treatment becomes effective.[9, 10] This technique is useful in the management of postoperative pain and pain secondary to trauma involving the lower abdomen, back, retroperitoneum, pelvis, and lower extremity. The pain of acute herpes zoster, ureteral calculi, and cancer is also amenable to treatment with epidurally administered local anesthetics and opioids.[11] Additionally, this technique is useful in patients suffering from acute vascular insufficiency of the lower extremities secondary to vasospastic and vasoocclusive disease, including frostbite and ergotamine toxicity.[12] There is growing evidence that prophylactic or preemptive use of lumbar epidural nerve blocks in patients scheduled to undergo lower extremity amputation for ischemia results in a decreased incidence of phantom limb pain.[13]

The administration of local anesthetics or steroids via the lumbar approach to the epidural space is useful in a variety of chronic benign pain syndromes, including lumbar radiculopathy, low back syndrome, spinal stenosis, postlaminectomy syndrome, phantom limb pain, vertebral compression fractures, diabetic polyneuropathy, chemotherapy-related peripheral neuropathy, postherpetic neuralgia, reflex sympathetic dystrophy, orchalgia, proctalgia, and pelvic pain syndromes.[13–15] There is an increasing body of evidence that the caudal epidural route of administration may prove more efficacious than the lumbar approach for some pain management applications.[14]

Lumbar epidural administration of local anesthetics in combination with steroids and/or opioids is useful in the palliation of cancer-related lower abdominal, groin, back, pelvic, perineal, and rectal pain.[16] This technique has been especially successful in the relief of pain secondary to metastatic disease of the spine from breast and prostate cancer and other malignancies. The long-term epidural administration of opioids has become a mainstay in the palliation of cancer pain. The role of epidural opioids in the management of chronic benign pain syndromes is currently being evaluated.

Contraindications to the lumbar epidural nerve block are these:

- Local infection
- Sepsis
- Anticoagulant therapy or coagulopathy
- Hypovolemia (relative contraindication)

Because of the potential for hematogenous spread via Batson's plexus, local infection and sepsis are absolute contraindications to the lumbar approach to the epidural space.[17] Owing to the risk of epidural hematoma, anticoagulation and coagulopathy are absolute contraindications to lumbar epidural nerve block, as they are not to the caudal approach. Hypovolemia represents a relative complication to lumbar epidural nerve block with local anesthetics.[17]

CLINICALLY RELEVANT ANATOMY

The Boundaries of the Epidural Space

The superior boundary of the epidural space is the fusion of the periosteal and spinal layers of dura at the foramen magnum.[19] The epidural space is bounded inferiorly by the sacrococcygeal membrane, anteriorly by the posterior longitudinal ligament, and posteriorly by the vertebral laminae and the ligamenta flava (Fig. 39–1). The vertebral pedicles and intervertebral foramina form the lateral limits

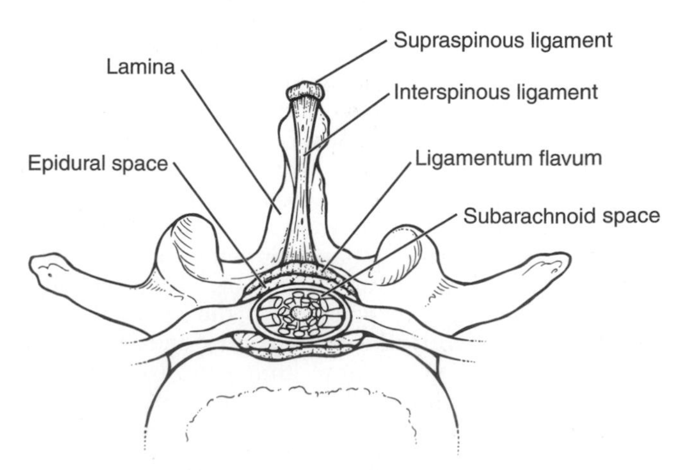

FIGURE 39–1 *Cross-sectional anatomy of the epidural space.*

of the epidural space (Fig. 39–2). The distance between the ligamentum flavum and the dura is greatest at the L2 interspace, where it measures 5 to 6 mm in adults.[20]

The Contents of the Epidural Space

Fat

The epidural space is filled with fatty areolar tissue. The amount of epidural fat varies in direct proportion to the amount of fat stored elsewhere in the body.[21] The epidural fat is relatively vascular and appears to become denser in consistency with age. This change in consistency may account for the significant variations in required drug doses in adults, especially for the caudal approach to the epidural space. The epidural fat appears to perform two functions: (1) as a shock absorber for the other contents of the epidural space and the dura and contents of the dural sac and (2) as a depot for drugs injected into the epidural space. This second function has direct clinical implications for the choice of the proper opioids for epidural administration.

Epidural Veins

The epidural veins are concentrated primarily in the anterolateral portion of the epidural space.[21] These veins are valveless and thus transmit both intrathoracic and intraabdominal pressures. When pressure in either of these body cavities increases—due to Valsalva's maneuver or compression of the inferior vena cava by the gravid uterus or tumor mass—the epidural veins distend and reduce the volume of the epidural space. This decrease in volume can directly affect the volume of drug needed to produce a given degree of neural blockade. This venous plexus serves the entire spinal column, so it is a ready conduit for the spread of hematogenous infection.

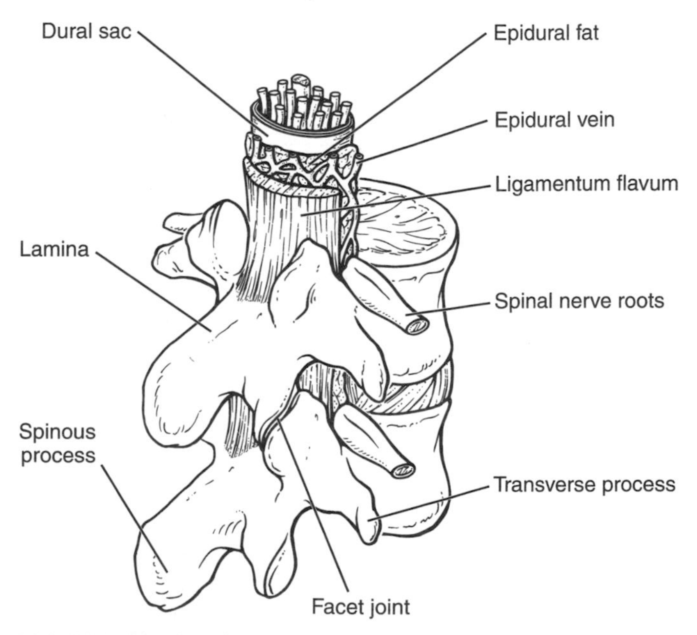

FIGURE 39–2 Three-quarters view. Anatomy of the epidural space.

Epidural Arteries

The arteries that supply the bony and ligamentous confines of the epidural space and the spinal cord enter the epidural space via the intervertebral foramina.[22] There are significant anastamoses between the epidural arteries. The epidural arteries lie primarily in the lateral portions of the epidural space. Trauma to the epidural arteries can result in epidural hematoma formation or compromise of the blood supply to the spinal cord itself.

Lymphatics

The lymphatics of the epidural space are concentrated in the region of the dural roots, where they help to remove foreign material from the subarachnoid and epidural spaces.[21]

Structures Encountered During Midline Insertion of a Needle into the Lumbar Epidural Space

After traversing the skin and subcutaneous tissues, the styleted epidural needle impinges on the supraspinous ligament, which runs vertically between the apices of the spinous processes (Fig. 39–3).[23] The supraspinous ligament offers some resistance to the advancing needle (Fig. 39–3B). This ligament is dense enough to hold a needle in position, even when it is released by the operator.

The interspinous ligament, which runs obliquely between the spinous processes, is next encountered and offers additional resistance to needle advancement. Because the interspinous ligament is contiguous with the ligamentum flavum, the clinician may perceive a "false" loss of resistance when the needle tip enters the space between the interspinous ligament and the ligamentum flavum.

A significant increase in resistance to needle advancement signals that the needle tip is impinging on the dense ligamentum flavum. Because the ligament is made up almost entirely of elastin fibers, resistance increases as the needle traverses the ligamentum flavum, owing to the drag of the ligament on the needle (Fig. 39–3C). A sudden loss of resistance occurs as the needle tip enters the epidural space (Fig. 39–3D). There should be essentially no resistance to injection of the drugs into the normal epidural space.

Pitfalls in Needle Placement

Although a comprehensive discussion of the pitfalls of needle placement is beyond the scope of this chapter, it is sufficient to say that, if careful attention is not paid to the site of needle entry, the needle trajectory, and the final position of the needle tip, a failed block may result. Trauma to nerves, arteries, veins, or the dural sac and its contents may also occur, with the potential for disastrous results.[24]

TECHNIQUE OF LUMBAR EPIDURAL NERVE BLOCK

All equipment, including the needles and supplies for nerve block, drugs, resuscitation equipment, oxygen supply, and

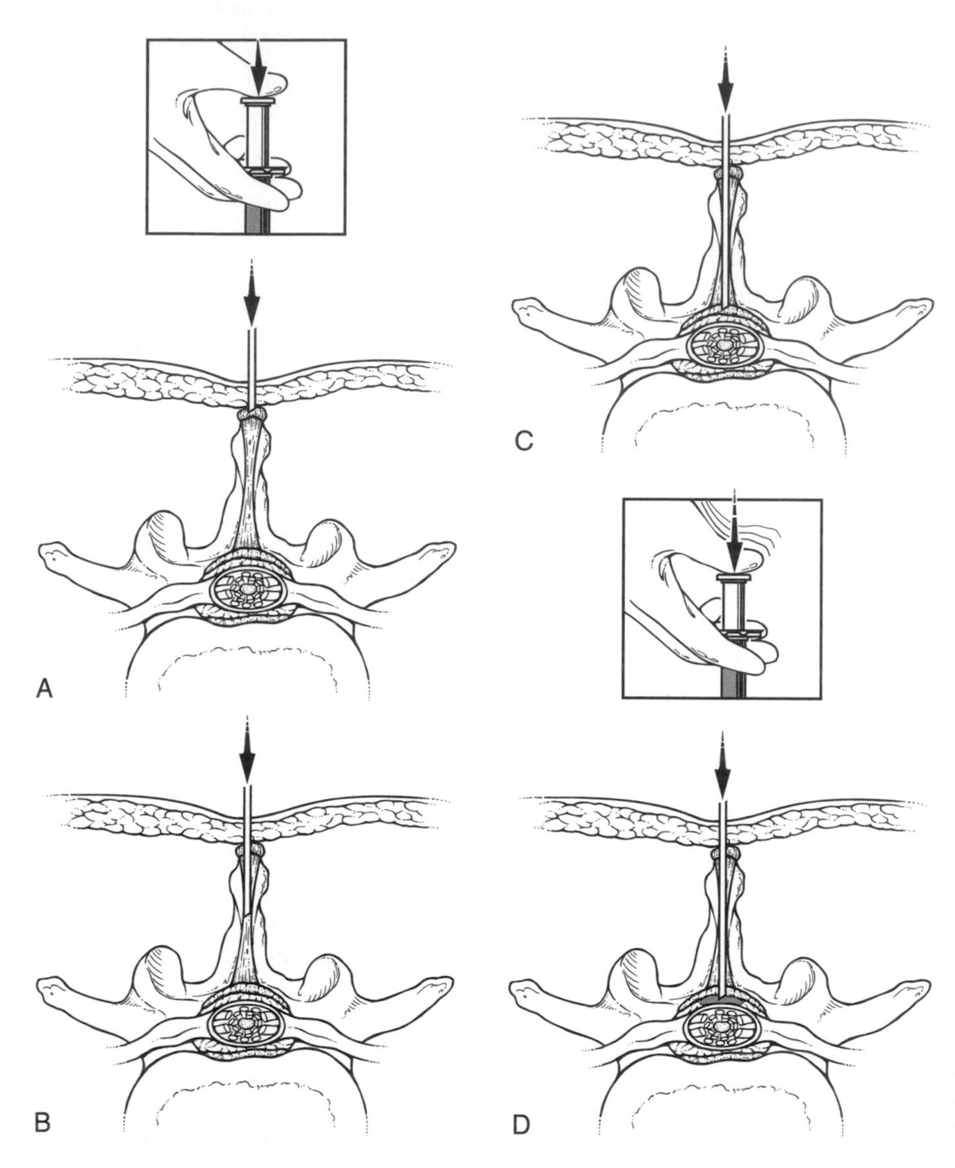

FIGURE 39–3 A, B, *Needle in supraspinous ligament.* C, *Needle in ligamentum flavum.* D, *Needle in epidural space.*

suction must be assembled and checked before lumbar epidural nerve block is undertaken. Informed patient consent is also obtained before lumbar epidural nerve block.

Positioning of the Patient

Lumbar epidural nerve block is carried out with the patient in the sitting, lateral, or prone position, each position having its advantages and disadvantages.

Sitting Position

The sitting position is easiest for patient and clinician alike. This position enhances the ability to identify the midline and avoids the problem of rotation of the spine inherent to the lateral position, which may make identification of the epidural space difficult. Some investigators believe that the effects of gravity on local anesthetics are enhanced in the sitting position, thereby improving the ability to block the S1 nerve roots, the size of which can make the nerve difficult to block.[25]

The use of the sitting position may be limited by a patient's inability to assume this position, such as a patient with acute vertebral compression fractures. A history of vasovagal syncope with previous needle punctures precludes the use of the sitting position. For such patients, the lateral position is preferred.

Lateral Position

The lateral position is preferred for patients who cannot assume the sitting position or who are prone to vasovagal attacks. The lateral position causes the patient less discomfort during placement of tunneled epidural catheters or other implantable devices with an epidural terminus. If the lateral position is chosen, care must be taken to prevent any rotation of the patient's spine, which would make epidural nerve block exceedingly difficult, if not impossible.

Prone Position

The prone position is used principally for placement of tunneled epidural catheters and spinal stimulator electrodes. If sedation is required, this position should be avoided, because it limits access to the airway.

Preblock Preparation

After the patient is placed in the optimal position, the skin is prepared with an antiseptic solution such as povidone-iodine so that all of the surface landmarks can be palpated aseptically. A fenestrated sterile drape is placed to avoid contamination of the palpating fingers.

The interspace suitable for the intended epidural block is identified. At the level of this interspace, the pain management specialist's middle and index fingers are placed on each side of the spinous processes (Fig. 39–4A). The position of the interspace is reconfirmed with palpation using a rocking motion in the superior and inferior planes. The midline of the selected interspace is then identified by palpating the spinous processes above and below the interspace, using a lateral rocking motion, to ensure that the needle entry site is exactly in the midline (Fig. 39–4B). Failure to accurately identify the midline is the most common reason for difficulty in performing epidural nerve block.

Choice of Needle

A 3.5-inch, 18-gauge Hustead or Tuohy needle is suitable for lumbar epidural block in the vast majority of adult patients. The sharper Tuohy needle may be more likely to cause dural puncture.[26] Some centers are now using smaller epidural needles with equally good results. Smaller needles decrease the amount of procedure-related and postprocedure pain.

Identification of the Epidural Space

The choice of technique to identify the epidural space is usually based on the operator's previous training and personal experience rather than on scientific data. It is the consensus of most experts that the loss-of-resistance technique has significant advantages over the hanging-drop technique.[23] This is especially true in the lower thoracic and lumbar epidural space, where the absence of negative pressure (notably in the sitting position) seriously compromises the reliability of the hanging-drop technique.[27] Bromage[2] has remarked, "It is illogical to use the hanging drop test in the lumbar region at all."

The Loss-of-Resistance Technique

After careful identification of the midline at the proper interspace (using the technique described earlier), 1 mL of local anesthetic is used to infiltrate the skin, subcutaneous tissues, and supraspinous and interspinous ligaments. Large amounts of local anesthetic should be avoided because they disrupt the ligamentous fibers and contribute to postprocedure pain.

The styleted needle is inserted exactly in the midline in the previously anesthetized area through the supraspinous ligament into the interspinous ligament.[2] The needle stylet is removed, and a well-lubricated, 5-mL glass syringe filled with preservative-free sterile saline is attached. Because saline is not compressible, it provides better tactile feedback

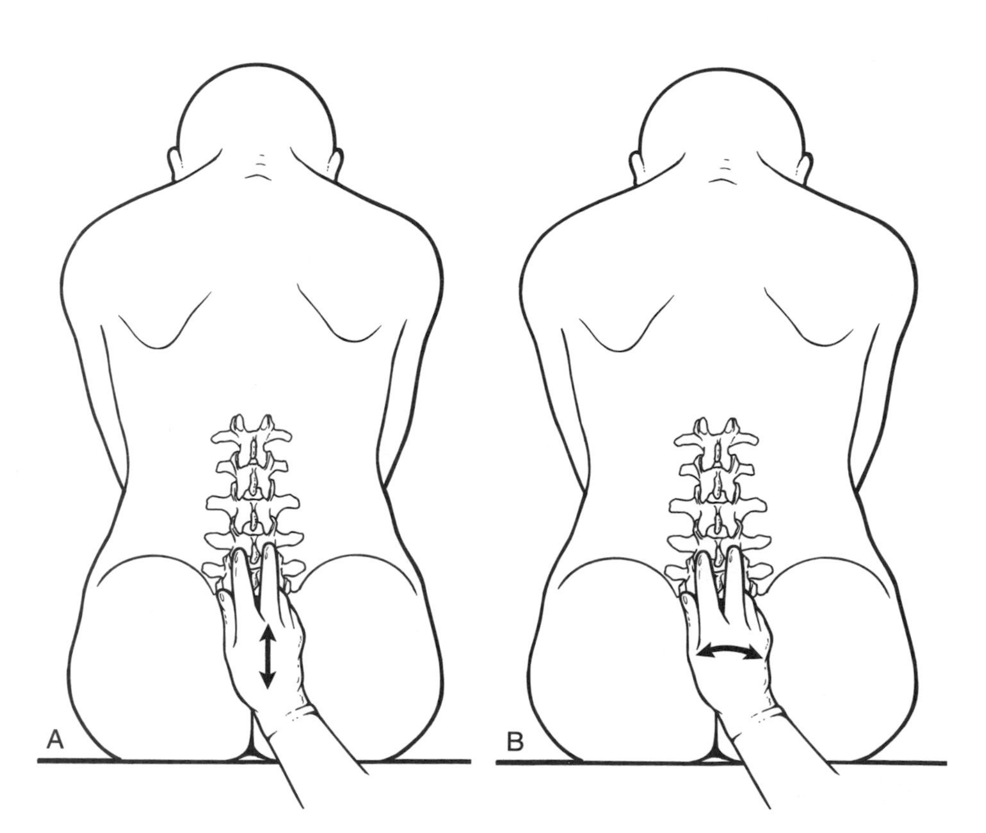

FIGURE 39–4 *A, Palpating the spinous process superoinferior plane. B, Palpating spinous process lateral plane.*

than air. Additionally, use of saline avoids the risk of air embolism via the epidural veins. A right-handed operator holds the epidural needle firmly at the hub with the left thumb and index finger. The left hand is placed firmly against the patient's back to ensure against uncontrolled needle movements if the patient moves unexpectedly (Fig. 39–5A). The right hand holds the syringe with the thumb exerting continuous firm pressure on the plunger.[28] Bromage[2] admonishes, "Never advance the needle without simultaneous pressure on the plunger to tell you where you are." Ballottement of the plunger as advocated by some clinicians, should not be used because it increases the incidence of inadvertent dural puncture.

While constant pressure is applied to the plunger of the syringe with the thumb of the right hand, the needle and syringe are continuously advanced in a slow and deliberate manner with the left hand. As soon as the needle bevel passes through the ligamentum flavum and enters the epidural space, there is a sudden loss of resistance to injection, and the plunger effortlessly surges forward (Fig. 39–5B). This loss of resistance provides the clinician visual and tactile evidence that the needle bevel has entered the epidural space. The syringe is gently removed from the needle.

An air or saline acceptance test is carried out by injecting 0.5 to 1.0 mL of air or preservative-free sterile saline with a well-lubricated sterile glass syringe to confirm that the needle is within the epidural space. The force required for injection should not exceed that necessary to overcome the resistance of the needle. Any significant pain or sudden increase in resistance during injection suggests incorrect needle placement, and the operator should *stop injecting immediately* and reassess the position of the needle.

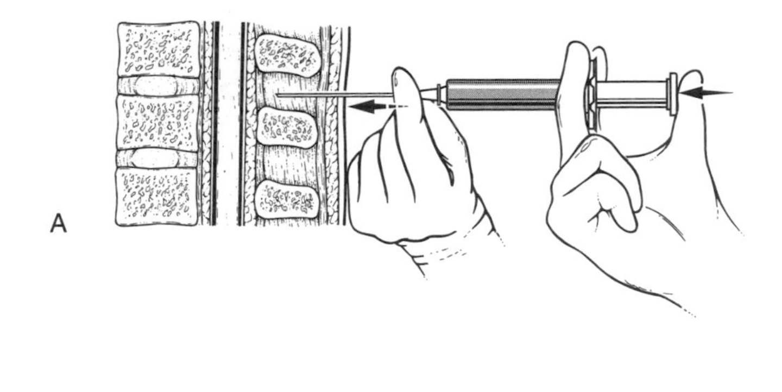

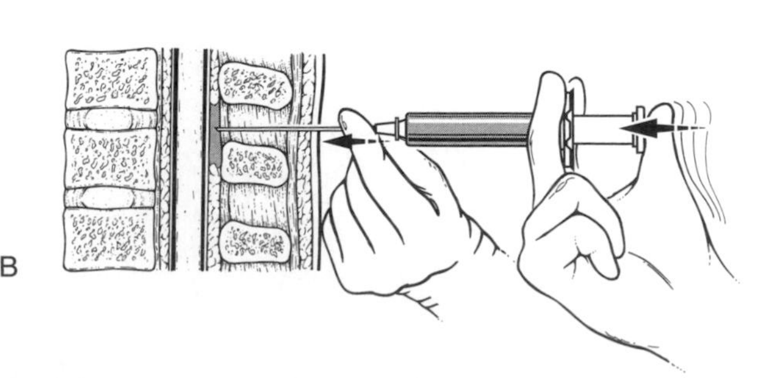

FIGURE 39–5 *A, Loss-of-resistance technique. B, Needle in epidural space.*

Injection of Drugs

When satisfactory needle position is confirmed, a syringe containing the drugs to be injected is carefully attached to the needle. Gentle aspiration is carried out to identify cerebrospinal fluid or blood.[2] Inadvertent dural puncture can occur in the best of hands; therefore, careful observation for spinal fluid is mandatory. If cerebrospinal fluid is aspirated, the epidural block can be converted to a spinal (subarachnoid) block, with a corresponding change in drug dose if clinically appropriate.[17] When a spinal block would be unsuitable, the epidural block may be repeated at a different interspace. In such a situation, drug dosages should be adjusted accordingly, because subarachnoid migration of drugs can occur through the dural rent.

Aspiration of blood can be due either to damage to veins during insertion of the needle into the lumbar epidural space or, less commonly, to intravenous placement of the needle.[17] If aspiration of blood occurs, the needle should be rotated slightly and the aspiration test repeated. If no blood is aspirated, incremental doses of local anesthetic and other drugs may be administered while the patient is monitored carefully for signs of local anesthetic toxicity and untoward reactions to the other drugs injected.

Choice of Local Anesthetic

The spread of drugs injected into the lumbar epidural space depends on the volume and speed of injection, the anatomic variations of the epidural space, the degree of dilatation of the epidural veins, and the position, age, and height of the patient.[29] The pregnant patient requires a significantly lower volume to achieve the same level of blockade as a nongravid control.[30]

Local anesthetics capable of producing adequate sensory block of the lower lumbar and sacral nerve roots when administered via the lumbar epidural route include 1.0% lidocaine, 0.25% bupivacaine, 2% 2-chloroprocaine, 0.5% ropivacaine, and 1.0% mepivacaine. Raising the concentration of drug increases the amount of motor block and speeds onset of action. The addition of epinephrine decreases the amount of systemic absorption and slightly prolongs the duration of action.[31] Generally, 12 to 15 mL of any of the listed drugs is adequate in adult patients for most pain management applications.[8] Significant intrapatient variability exists, however, and additional incremental doses of local anesthetic may have to be administered to ensure adequate anesthesia in some adult patients. All local anesthetics administered via the lumbar epidural route should be formulated for epidural use.[32]

For diagnostic and prognostic blocks, 1.0% preservative-free lidocaine is a suitable local anesthetic.[8] For therapeutic blocks, 0.25% preservative-free bupivacaine or ropivacaine in combination with 80 mg of depot methylprednisolone (Depo-Medrol) is injected.[8, 10] Subsequent nerve blocks are carried out in a similar manner using 40 mg of methylprednisolone. Daily lumbar epidural nerve blocks with local anesthetic or steroid may be required to treat the acute painful conditions described as indications for the procedure.[10] Chronic conditions such as lumbar radiculopathy and diabetic polyneuropathy are treated every other day, once a week, or as the clinical situation dictates.[8]

If the lumbar epidural route is chosen for administration of opioids, 4 to 5 mg of morphine sulfate formulated for epidural use is a reasonable initial dose. More lipid-soluble opioids, such as fentanyl, must be delivered by continuous infusion via a lumbar catheter. All opioids administered via the lumbar epidural route should be formulated for epidural use.[32]

Lumbar Epidural Catheters

An epidural catheter may be placed into the lumbar epidural space through a Hustead or Tuohy needle. The catheter is advanced approximately 2 to 3 cm beyond the needle tip. The needle is then carefully withdrawn over the catheter. Under no circumstances is the catheter withdrawn back through the needle, to avoid shearing of the catheter. After the injection hub is attached to the catheter, an aspiration test is carried out to identify the presence of blood or cerebrospinal fluid.[33] A test dose of local anesthetic is given via the catheter. The patient is observed for signs of local anesthetic toxicity and inadvertent subarachnoid injection. If no side effects are noted, a continuous infusion or intermittent boluses of local anesthetics or opioids are administered through the catheter. Because the risk of infection limits long-term use of percutaneous lumbar epidural catheters, tunneling is strongly recommended if it is anticipated that the catheter will be left in place for more than 48 hours.[34]

SIDE EFFECTS AND COMPLICATIONS OF THE LUMBAR APPROACH TO THE EPIDURAL SPACE

Inadvertent Dural Puncture

In the hands of an experienced pain specialist, inadvertent dural puncture during lumbar epidural nerve block should occur in fewer than 0.5% of cases.[24] Although post–dural puncture headache is upsetting to patient and pain specialist alike, this side effect in and of itself should not cause permanent harm to the patient, but, unfortunately, failure to recognize inadvertent dural puncture can. If an epidural needle or catheter is accidentally placed in the subarachnoid space and the problem goes unrecognized, injection of epidural doses of local anesthetics causes immediate total spinal anesthesia with associated loss of consciousness, hypotension, and apnea. If epidural doses of opioids are accidentally placed in the subarachnoid space, significant respiratory and central nervous system depression result. Should either of these problems occur, immediate supportive measures are indicated to restore homeostasis.

Inadvertent Subdural Puncture

It is possible to inadvertently place a needle or catheter intended for the epidural space into the subdural space. If subdural placement goes unrecognized and epidural doses of local anesthetics are administered, the signs and symptoms are similar to those of massive subarachnoid injection, although the resulting motor and sensory block may be spotty.[35] The effect of inadvertent injection of large doses of opioids into the subdural space is probably similar to that of subarachnoid injection. Massive subdural injection of local anesthetics or opioids requires immediate supportive measures, as indicated, to restore homeostasis.

Inadvertent Intravenous Needle and Catheter Placement

The lumbar epidural space is highly vascular. Intravenous placement of the needle occurs in approximately 0.5% to 1% of patients undergoing lumbar epidural anesthesia.[24] This complication is more likely in patients with distended epidural veins (i.e., parturients) or a large intraabdominal tumor mass. If the misplacement is not recognized, injection of local anesthetic directly into an epidural vein results in significant local anesthetic toxicity.[36] Careful aspiration before injection of drugs into the epidural space is mandatory to identify this potentially serious problem. Observation of the patient during and after the injection process is mandatory.

Hematoma and Ecchymosis

The epidural space is densely vascular. Needle trauma to the epidural veins may result in self-limited bleeding, which may cause postprocedural pain. Uncontrolled bleeding into the epidural space may result in compression of the spinal cord with the rapid development of neurologic deficit. Although significant neurologic deficit secondary to epidural hematoma after lumbar epidural block is exceedingly rare, this devastating complication should be considered whenever there is rapidly developing lower extremity weakness or symptoms of cauda equina syndrome after epidural nerve block.[37]

Infection

Although uncommon, infection in the epidural space remains an ever present possibility, especially in immunocompromised patients with AIDS or cancer.[38] Because of the nature of the epidural venous system, hematogenous spread throughout the central nervous system is a possibility when epidural infection occurs.[24] Because the offending organism in epidural infections is usually *Staphylococcus aureus*, initial antibiotic treatment should be directed at this organism until culture results are available.[39] If epidural abscess develops, emergency surgical drainage is usually required to avoid spinal cord compression and irreversible neurologic deficit. Early detection and treatment of infection are crucial to avoid potentially life-threatening sequelae.

Neurologic Complications

Neurologic complications of lumbar nerve block are uncommon if proper technique is utilized. Usually, such complications are associated with a preexisting neurologic lesion or with surgical or obstetric trauma rather than with the lumbar block itself.[33] Direct trauma to the spinal cord or nerve roots is usually accompanied by pain. Any significant pain that occurs during placement of the epidural needle or catheter or during injection should warn the clinician to stop the procedure immediately and ascertain the cause of the pain, to avoid the possibility of additional neural trauma.[24] Intravenous sedation or general anesthesia before epidural nerve block would render the patient unable to provide accurate verbal feedback if the needle were misplaced, and should therefore be avoided.[17]

Urinary Retention and Incontinence

Application of local anesthetics and opioids to the lumbar and sacral nerve roots results in a higher incidence of urinary retention.[33] This side effect of lumbar epidural block is more common in elderly men, in multiparous women, and in patients who have undergone inguinal or perineal surgery. Overflow incontinence may occur if such a patient is unable to void or bladder catheterization is not done. All patients undergoing lumbar epidural block should demonstrate the ability to void the bladder before being discharged from the pain center.

CONCLUSION

Lumbar epidural nerve block has great utility in the management of a variety of acute, chronic, and cancer-related pain syndromes. Careful attention to the technical aspects of lumbar epidural nerve block enables the pain specialist to perform the procedure simply and safely.

REFERENCES

1. Pagés E: Anestesia metamerica. Rev Sanid Mil Madr 11:351–385, 1921.
2. Bromage PR: Identification of the epidural space. *In* Bromage PR (ed): Epidural Analgesia. Philadelphia, WB Saunders, 1978, p 178.
3. Dogliotti AM: Segmental peridural anesthesia. Am J Surg 20:107, 1933.
4. Gutierrez A: Valor de la aspiracion liquada en al espacio peridural en la anestesia peridural. Rev Circ 12:225, 1933.
5. Usubiaga JE, Wikinski JA, Usubiaga LE: Epidural pressure and its relation to spread of anesthetic solutions in epidural space. Anaesthesia 46:440, 1967.
6. Bromage PR: Introduction. *In* Bromage PR (ed): Epidural Analgesia. Philadelphia, WB Saunders, 1978, p 3.
7. Lievre JA, Block-Michel H, Attali P: L'hydrocortisone transsacrée, étude clinique et radiologique. Bull Soc Med Hôp Paris 73:1110–1117, 1957.
8. Waldman SD: Epidural nerve block. *In* RS Weiner (ed): Innovations in Pain Management. Orlando, Fla, PMD Press, 1990, pp 4–5.
9. Waldman SD: Management of acute pain. Postgrad Med 87:15–17, 1992.
10. Waldman SD: Acute and postoperative pain management. *In* Weiner RS (ed): Innovations in Pain Management. Orlando, Fla, PMD Press, 1993, pp 12–13.
11. Waldman SD: Acute herpes zoster and postherpetic neuralgia. Intern Med 11:33–38, 1990.
12. Raj PP: Chronic pain. *In* Raj PP (ed): Handbook of Regional Anesthesia. New York, Churchill Livingstone, 1985, pp 103–107.
13. Waldman SD: Lumbar epidural block. *In* Waldman SD: Atlas of Interventional Pain Management Techniques. Philadelphia, WB Saunders, 1998, pp 308–317.
14. Waldman SD, Greek CR, Greenfield, MA: The caudal administration of steroids in combination with local anesthetics in the palliation of pain secondary to radiographically documented lumbar herniated disc—a prospective outcome study with six-month follow-up. Pain Clinic 11:43, 1998.
15. Wilson WL, Waldman SD: Role of the epidural administration of steroids and local anesthetics in the palliation of pain secondary to vertebral compression fractures. Pain Digest 1:294–295, 1992.
16. Portenoy RK, Waldman SD: Managing cancer pain non-pharmacologically. Contemp Ob/Gyn 39:82–87, 1994.
17. Cousins MJ, Bromage PR: Epidural neural blockade. *In* Cousins MJ, Bridenbaugh DO (eds): Neural Blockade. Philadelphia, JB Lippincott, 1988, pp 340–341.
18. Waldman SD, Feldstein GS, Waldman HJ: Caudal administration of morphine sulfate in anticoagulated and thrombocytopenic patients. Anesth Analg 66:267–268, 1987.
19. Katz J: Lumbar approach—single injection technique. *In* Katz J (ed): Atlas of Regional Anesthesia. Norwalk, Conn, Appleton & Lange, 1994, pp 178–179.
20. Reynolds AF, Roberts PA, Pollay M, et al: Quantitative anatomy of the thoracolumbar epidural space. Neurosurgery 17:905, 1985.
21. Bromage PR: Anatomy. *In* Bromage PR (ed): Epidural Analgesia. Philadelphia, WB Saunders, 1978, p 14.
22. Woollam DHM, Millen JW: An anatomical background to vascular disease of the spinal cord. Proc R Soc Med 51:540, 1958.
23. Brown DL: Lumbar epidural block. *In* Brown DL (ed): Atlas of Regional Anesthesia. Philadelphia, WB Saunders, 1999, pp 329–346.
24. Bromage PR: Complications and contraindications. *In* Bromage PR (ed): Epidural Analgesia. Philadelphia, WB Saunders, 1978, pp 654–711.
25. Galindo A, Hernandez J, Benavides O, et al: Quality of spinal extradural anaesthesia: The influence of spinal nerve root diameter. Br J Anaesth 47:41, 1975.
26. Bromage PR: Epidural needles. Anesthesiology 22:1018, 1961.
27. Bryce-Smith R: Pressures in the extradural apace. Anaesthesia 5:213, 1950.
28. Moore DC: Single-dose lumbar anesthesia. *In* Moore DC (ed): Regional Block, ed 4. Springfield, Ill, Charles C Thomas, 1965, p 417.
29. Burn JM, Guyer PB, Langdon L: The spread of solutions injected into the epidural space: A study using epidurograms in patients with the lumbosciatic syndrome. Br J Anaesth 45:338, 1973.
30. Bromage PR: Mechanism of action. *In* Bromage PR (ed): Epidural Analgesia. Philadelphia, WB Saunders, 1978, pp 141–142.
31. Mather LE, Tucker GT, Murphy TM, et al: The effects of adding adrenaline to etidocaine and lignocaine in extradural anaesthesia. Part II: Pharmacokinetics. Br J Anaesth 48:989, 1976.
32. Waldman SD: Issues in selection of local anesthetics. Hosp Formulary 26:590–597, 1991.
33. Armitage EN: Lumbar and thoracic epidural. *In* Wildsmith JAW, Armitage EN (eds): Principles and Practice of Regional Anesthesia. New York, Churchill Livingstone, 1987, p 109.
34. Waldman SD, Coombs DW: Selection of implantable narcotic delivery systems. Anesth Analg 68:377–384, 1989.
35. Waldman SD: Subdural injection as a cause of unexplained neurological symptoms. Reg Anesth 17:55, 1992.
36. Braid DP, Scott DB: The systemic absorption of local analgesic drugs. Br J Anaesth 37:394, 1965.
37. Cousins MJ: Hematoma following epidural block. Anesthesiology 37:263, 1972.
38. Portenoy RK, Waldman SD: Managing cancer pain. Contemp Oncol 3:33–41, 1993.
39. Hancock DO: A study of 49 patients with acute spinal extradural abscess. Paraplegia 10:285, 1973.

CHAPTER • 40

Continuous Regional Analgesia

P. Prithvi Raj, MD • Susan R. Anderson, MD

Infusion techniques in the epidural space and on the peripheral nerves are now commonly utilized for acute and chronic pain. It has been found to be beneficial for the acute pain of trauma, after surgery, and of acute medical conditions. Similarly, it is useful for chronic pain—rehabilitation of patients with chronic back pain, reflex sympathetic dystrophy, peripheral neuropathy, or cancer pain.

Continuous epidural analgesia is not new.[1–3] The first use of this technique in 1949 described intermittent bolus doses of a local anesthetic administered for 1 to 5 days postoperatively.[4] Although effective analgesia was obtained, significant sympathetic blockade accompanied the pain relief, with fluctuating levels of analgesia. Continuous epidural analgesia with intermittent bolus injections is labor intensive and requires skilled personnel to reassess and reinject the patient every few hours. Because of these shortcomings, *continuous infusion* of epidural local anesthetics has now become commonplace (Fig. 40–1).

CONTINUOUS INFUSION VERSUS INTERMITTENT BOLUS INJECTION

Continuous epidural infusion offers many therapeutic advantages over intermittent bolus injection. The primary advantage is the continuity of analgesia as compared with intermittent doses. Although single boluses of opioids such as epidural morphine may provide 12 hours of pain relief, wide variability has been reported in the duration of effective analgesia, ranging from 4 to 24 hours.[5, 6] Thus, it becomes difficult to titrate dosing to provide a consistent level of analgesia. Continuous infusions are easy to titrate, particularly when shorter-acting opioids such as fentanyl and sufentanil are employed. Epidural fentanyl has an onset of action within 4 to 5 min and peak effect within 20 min.[7–9] This rapid onset facilitates adjustment of dosage, because the patient can quickly gauge the relief.

Another disadvantage of the intermittent bolus technique is the need for action when pain relief subsides, 4 to 6 hours after epidural administration of morphine. The clinician must decide whether to inject a second dose of epidural opioid or to supplement the bolus with a systemic analgesic. Supplementation with parenteral narcotic or sedative drugs increases the risk of respiratory depression in a patient who earlier received epidural narcotic. For the intermittent bolus technique to be successful, a longer-acting agent such as morphine or hydromorphone is required to provide analgesia of reasonable duration. These opioids are associated with a higher risk of delayed-onset respiratory depression.[6]

The third disadvantage of the intermittent bolus technique is the tachyphylaxis that develops with repeat boluses.[10, 11] In contrast, continuous infusion of the analgesia with the same dose actually increases the intensity of the block, and the rate of infusion has to be reduced to maintain the desired level of analgesia over time.

Continuous epidural infusion of analgesic agents, especially opioids, has the advantage of fewer fluctuations in cerebrospinal fluid drug concentrations. The fact that it takes several hours to infuse enough of a long-acting opioid such as morphine to provide adequate analgesia is, however, a major drawback. It can be overcome by administering a 5- to 10-mL "loading" bolus of epidural local anesthetic at the beginning of the infusion or a bolus of short-acting opioid such as fentanyl or sufentanil. It usually takes 5 half-lives for the infused drug to reach a steady state (which for morphine or bupivacaine is about 15 to 18 hours).

CATHETER LOCATION

Segmental limitation of epidural analgesia mandates placement of an epidural catheter at a site adjacent to the dermatome that is the site of the pain. This practice reduces dose requirements and increases the specificity of spinal analgesia.[12, 13] Interspaces where catheters are usually located for epidural analgesia are shown in Table 40–1.

ANALGESIC AGENTS

Epidural analgesia is commonly provided with one of the following choices:

- A local anesthetic.
- An opioid.
- An opioid combined with a local anesthetic.

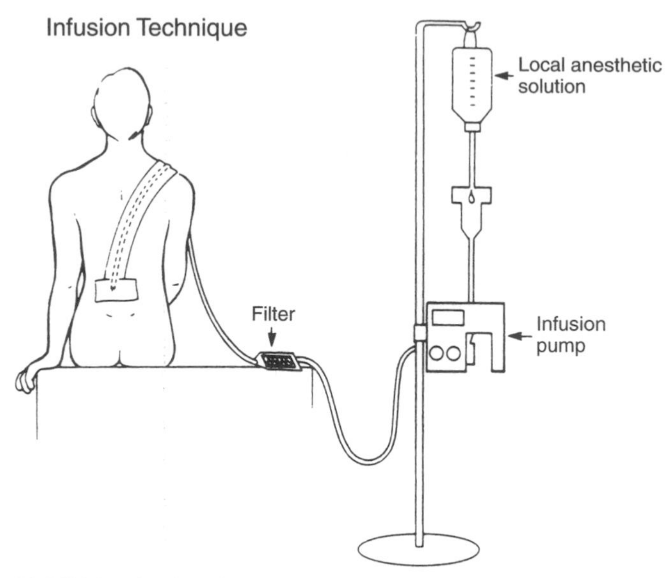

FIGURE 40–1 The assembly of analgesic solution, infusion pump, and catheter connection with a filter for epidural infusion technique.

Local Anesthetics

Local anesthetic agents are best used to provide analgesia and anesthesia for postoperative pain relief. Lidocaine, bupivacaine, and more recently, ropivacaine effectively produce and sustain analgesia.[10, 11] In general, lidocaine is limited to use in a bolus form to establish or "rescue" a block, whereas bupivacaine is used as an infusion. Ropivacaine is becoming more widely used for infusions owing to its shorter time to onset, shorter duration of motor block, greater selectivity for A-delta and C fibers, and decreased cardiotoxicity as compared with bupivacaine.[14–20] A problem inherent in bolus dosing of a local anesthetic through the epidural catheter is tachyphylaxis, which, however, has not developed when bupivacaine is administered as an infusion.

Continuous infusion of dilute local anesthetic solutions has simplified maintenance and improved analgesic consistency; however, concentrations sufficient to produce pain relief usually have produced progressive sensorimotor blockade. Such deficits are undesirable, because the patient's ability to walk is compromised. Used alone, local anesthetic agents can accumulate in the systemic circulation.[10, 21] This effect is more pronounced with the short-acting amides such as lidocaine than with the longer-acting ones, a phenomenon that, in turn, has been attributed to greater nonspecific binding of the longer-acting agents in the fat of the epidural space. Even when bupivacaine was infused for 72 hours after abdominal surgery, the serum bupivacaine level increased, peaking at 48 to 60 hours.[22] A local anesthetic is less toxic when the agent accumulates slowly, but there is the ever present risk of central nervous system depression, convulsions, or cardiac arrest.

The concentration of local anesthetic affects the analgesia and the profile of side effects. A constant-rate infusion of bupivacaine (at least 0.25%) is associated with hypotension, muscle weakness, sensory block, and, sometimes, accumulation of toxic systemic levels of drug.[10] Plasma levels may be higher in elderly or frail patients. Side effects may be attenuated by using lower concentrations of bupivacaine. Low-dose, constant-rate epidural infusion of bupivacaine (0.03% to 0.06%) close to the dermatomal level desired for pain relief reduces the incidence of side effects. Although the low dose of bupivacaine is effective, it provides less profound analgesia than does either a combination of bupivacaine and epidural morphine in low concentration or opioids alone.[10, 23, 24]

Opioids

The ideal intraspinal opiate would be hydrophilic, have high affinity for the opiate receptor, have to contact a small percentage of receptors to provide analgesia, demonstrate prolonged duration of analgesia, and be free of side effects. The drugs commonly used spinally are morphine, meperidine, fentanyl, and sufentanil. Morphine remains the only opiate that is approved by the U.S. Food and Drug Administration for epidural dosing. In the postoperative period, morphine sulfate has been given by intermittent injection and by continuous infusion. Meperidine has also been injected epidurally and possesses local anesthetic properties. The accumulation of its metabolite normeperidine is a concern. Fentanyl has achieved widespread popularity during the past 7 to 10 years. Its advantage over morphine sulfate is that rostrad spread is less than that of morphine. Whether the effect after intraspinal injection is spinal or systemic, the rapid onset of analgesia after epidural fentanyl makes it the drug of choice for acute, unacceptable pain. Sufentanil has been used epidurally. The characteristics of the lipid-soluble fentanyl are magnified with sufentanil. Its theoretical advantage relates to its strong affinity for mu receptors, a feature relevant to cancer management.

Combination of Opioid with Local Anesthetic

In an effort to combine the desirable analgesic properties of local anesthetics with those of epidural opioids, several investigators studied epidural infusion of the combination of morphine and bupivacaine.[25–28] Studies demonstrated either additive or synergistic analgesic activity between a variety of opioids and dilute concentrations of bupivacaine.[27–29] Such combinations appear to provide pain relief of greater magnitude than does either agent alone, and the incidence and severity of side effects are minimized. This

TABLE 40–1 ***Suggested Interspace(s) for Catheter Insertion for Continuous Infusion of Analgesic Solutions After Surgery***

Location of Surgery	Interspace(s) for Catheter
Thorax	T2–T8
Upper abdomen	T4–L1
Lower abdomen	T10–L3
Upper extremity	C2–C8
Lower extremity	T12–L3

advantage may be explained by the different analgesic properties of each class of agents and their ability to block pain at two different sites in the spinal cord. Opioids produce analgesia by specific binding and activation of opiate receptors in the substantia gelatinosa, whereas local anesthetics act by blocking impulse transmission at the nerve roots and dorsal root ganglia.

Bupivacaine has been used most often in concentrations of 0.03% to 0.125% with morphine, fentanyl, or meperidine. The combination of morphine and bupivacaine has produced effective analgesia after thoracic, abdominal, and general surgery.[10, 24, 30, 31] Fentanyl combined with bupivacaine, however, produced fewer side effects than the morphine-bupivacaine combination. Bupivacaine (0.03% to 0.125%) mixed with fentanyl (2 to 3 g/mL) infused at the rate of 8 to 10 mL/hr in a 70-kg adult usually produces excellent analgesia with minimal respiratory depression and sensorimotor blockade. Bupivacaine (0.03%) with 0.005% morphine or 2 to 3 g/mL fentanyl infused at 8 to 10 mL/hr produces similar results for patients with chronic pain. Ropivacaine may be used in place of bupivacaine in concentrations ranging from 0.1% to 0.2% with either morphine or fentanyl.

Concentrations of drugs and rates of infusion should be tailored to the individual patient. For example, it is possible to treat or prevent significant hypotension by (1) decreasing the local anesthetic concentration, (2) eliminating the local anesthetic, (3) decreasing the rate of a combined local anesthetic–opioid infusion, or (4) infusing intravenous fluids. Sedation or carbon dioxide retention can be treated by (1) changing the specific epidural opioid, (2) decreasing the concentration of the opioid, (3) decreasing the overall infusion rate, or (4) eliminating the opioid from the infusion.

MANAGEMENT OF INADEQUATE ANALGESIA

Although continuous epidural infusion techniques provide excellent results in most patients, pain relief is occasionally inadequate. In these cases, the reason for inadequate analgesia must be determined. Most often, catheter placement is tested in two stages. First, 5 mL of the epidural infusion solution is administered, and the patient's analgesia is reassessed after 30 min. Second, if the analgesia remains inadequate, a total of 5 to 10 mL of 2% lidocaine is administered in two fractionated doses.

This test dose generally yields one of three results. If bilateral sensory block occurs in a few segmental dermatomes, correct catheter placement is confirmed. In this case, insufficient volume of the infusion mixture was the likely cause of inadequate analgesia, which can be rectified by increasing the rate of infusion. A unilateral sensory block most likely indicates that the catheter tip was placed too far laterally into the epidural space (i.e., at the foramen). The catheter can be withdrawn 1 to 2 cm and the test dose repeated. Finally, failure to produce any sensory block indicates that the epidural catheter is no longer in the epidural space. The catheter is then removed, and the operator has the option of placing another epidural catheter or administering alternative therapy.

COMPLICATIONS OF CONTINUOUS INFUSION EPIDURAL ANESTHESIA

Complications of continuous epidural anesthesia include accidental intrathecal administration of the analgesic drug, infection, epidural hematoma, and respiratory depression. To decrease the incidence of these complications, the following guidelines are offered:

1. The use of appropriate concentrations of local anesthetics (e.g., 0.03% to 0.125% bupivacaine) allows one to prevent serious hypotension and to diagnose subarachnoid catheter migration more readily by providing progressive levels of sensory blockade where none would have been expected. Another safety feature is the combination of dilute local anesthetic solution with half the usual dose of an opioid, such as 0.5 to 1 mg of morphine or 1 μg of fentanyl.
2. Daily examination of catheter insertion sites, monitoring of temperature, and periodic evaluation for neurologic signs of meningism is essential. If findings are consistent with infection, the catheter should be removed and the infection treated. We have experience of one case of epidural abscess in 2000 epidural infusion cases, which resolved in 6 weeks with aggressive antibiotic therapy. Infections limited to the cutaneous superficial and subcutaneous tissues resolve with local conservative therapy.
3. If epidural catheters are placed at least 1 hour before heparin is given, the incidence of epidural hematoma is not significant. Epidural catheters may be inserted safely in patients who receive warfarin postoperatively, as long as their coagulation status is normal at the time of catheter insertion.

LIMITATIONS OF CONTINUOUS EPIDURAL ANALGESIA

There are limitations to epidural infusion analgesia. First, alone it cannot control pain from multiple sites. Epidural analgesia normally can provide analgesia for five to seven dermatomes in continuity, such as L4–S5 or T2–T8. Patients with multiple injuries may require another form of pain management.

The site of the epidural catheter influences the adequacy of pain relief and the maintenance of normal vital functions. In general, placing the catheter within the dermatomal distribution of the pain achieves the best result with the smallest amount of drug. For example, pain from a thoracotomy is best treated with a thoracic epidural infusion, and pain in the lower extremity with a lumbar infusion.

PATIENT-CONTROLLED EPIDURAL ANALGESIA

Patient-controlled epidural analgesia (PCEA) has been offered to patients with acute postoperative pain after abdominal, major orthopedic, or thoracic surgery or for chronic pain such as that of cancer. The technique has several potential advantages. The patient can titrate analgesic doses in proportion to the pain. Given the range of individual variations in pain relief,[32] this is important in optimizing spinal opioid analgesia. Most of the published work on PCEA comes from Europe.[32] Chrubasik and colleagues[33,34] compared three different epidural opioids for PCEA. The findings were remarkable in that the morphine dosage required to provide effective analgesia with PCEA was much smaller than the amount utilized with continuous epidural infusion or intravenous patient-controlled analgesia (PCA).[35–37] Serum morphine levels used in these studies were very low. Table 40–2 lists various studies and the opioids used, along with appropriate hourly dosing.

Sjöström and colleagues[32] demonstrated the efficacy of morphine PCEA. They employed 1-mg intermittent boluses with a 30-min lockout period. The average consumption was about 0.5 mg/hr, and serum morphine levels were well below the minimum effective plasma concentrations usually associated with parenteral delivery. Marlowe and coworkers[38] compared constant infusion of epidural opioid with PCEA and found the self-administration technique to be superior in that less opiate was required to provide similar levels of analgesia. Walmsley and associates[39] reported high efficacy of PCEA in their evaluation of more than 4000 surgical cases.

The following advantages are cited for PCEA as compared with conventional epidural infusion analgesia:

- increased efficiency
- Higher satisfaction
- Decreased sedation
- Reduced opioid use

The following advantages are cited for PCEA as compared with intravenous PCA:

- Self-adjustment by patient
- Self-satisfaction and resulting decrease in anxiety
- Reduced opioid requirement

PCEA TECHNIQUE USING MORPHINE[31]

Loading Dose

Lower thoracic or upper lumbar catheters are placed preoperatively or intraoperatively using standard techniques. Patients are "loaded" with 2 to 3 mg of preservative-free morphine and a basal infusion of 0.4 mg/hr started as a 0.02% solution. Patients are allowed to self-administer 0.2 mg morphine every 10 to 15 min with a maximum dose of 1 to 2 mg/hr. The loading dose is administered only after a local anesthetic test dose (2 to 3 mL of 2% lidocaine) has demonstrated that the catheter is not in the subarachnoid space. The optimal loading dose and timing of administration have yet to be determined; however, given morphine's latency to peak effect, the loading dose must be given as early as possible. Breakthrough pain is common in these patients during the first 6 to 8 hours postoperatively.

Breakthrough pain is treated with epidural morphine boluses at 0.5 to 1.0 mg/hour. If two doses are inadequate to provide analgesia, the catheter needs to be retested with local anesthetic to confirm epidural placement and to rule out dislodgement. The loading dose can be augmented with epidurally administered fentanyl, 50 to 100 μg. This drug speeds onset of the analgesia, possibly because of dual action (i.e., rapid vascular uptake) and rapid spinal cord neural uptake. Residual levels of intraoperative local anesthetics augment initial epidural morphine analgesia and contribute to subsequent postoperative pain relief.

TABLE 40–2 ***Consumption of Opioids used with Patient-Controlled Analgesia***

Investigators*	Epidural Opiates	Average Consumption (mg/hr)
Sjöström et al[25]	Morphine sulfate	0.52
Marlowe et al[31]	Demerol	18.0
Walmsley et al[32]*	Hydromorphone	0.1
Chrubasik and	Morphine sulfate	0.47
Wiener[26]*	Morphine sulfate	0.25

* Infusion and PCEA were both used.

Lockout

The short lockout period usually set with PCEA is somewhat controversial in view of the longer latency of morphine's epidural effect. Sjöström and coworkers[32] thus chose 30 min as the lockout period. There are few problems with morphine's longer latency to peak epidural effect, however, provided that a suitable loading dose has been administered 90 to 120 min before PCEA is begun. It is possible that patients perceive early analgesic benefits from the small increase in the serum morphine levels that occurs soon after a PCA bolus. The shorter latency of response to a single PCA bolus may be related to the "primed" or "loaded" state of spinal cord tissues during infusion and an optimal interval between the load and the initiation of PCEA opioid. Alternatively, patients may be satisfied by the placebo effect associated with all self-administration techniques.

The size of the intermittent PCEA dose should be limited to avoid excessive accumulations of morphine. Small boluses with short lockouts are safe and do not lead to excessive accumulation of drug before the initial dose takes effect.

Continuous Infusion

A continuous infusion provides the major portion of morphine administered epidurally. The typical postoperative patient does not develop tolerance to morphine when continuous infusions are added to PCEA. Several authors believe that continuous infusions, by avoiding peaks and valleys in cerebrospinal fluid levels, provide a more stable level of analgesia while reducing the incidence of side effects.[35,36] Serum levels at 24 hours are low: 90% of 20 samples studied contained less than 6.5 ng/mL.[39] This finding indicates that the systemic absorption of morphine contributes very little to the overall level of analgesia. Breakthrough pain is treated with small morphine boluses. Changing the rate of infusion alone has little effect over the short term, because it takes 5 half-lives to reach the new equilibrium.

ALTERNATIVE ANALGESIC AGENTS FOR PCEA

Lipophilic Opioids

Fentanyl, sufentanil, and hydromorphone may be used with a PCEA infusion technique; however, the amount of drug necessary to provide effective analgesia appears to be much greater than equivalent doses of morphine. Giving lipophilic opioids by continuous infusion or PCEA, or both, has been questioned by several authors.[40, 41] Estok and coworkers[41] showed that fentanyl administered by intravenous PCA or PCEA provided equivalent analgesia.

Epidurally administered lipophilic opioids are most appropriately administered via thoracic epidural catheters. They may be of special use in the following applications:

- To speed the onset of epidural opioid analgesia.
- In large volumes of dilute solution or combined with local anesthetics. Cohen and associates[42, 43] compared combinations of fentanyl, bupivacaine, and buprenorphine-bupivacaine for PCEA. The average hourly doses of opioid were minimized, presumably because of the effective analgesia provided by bupivacaine administered concurrently, so that 24-hour serum concentrations were low.
- For breakthrough pain, especially in the first few hours after surgery.

Local Anesthetics

The use of PCEA with local anesthetics during labor has been reported to be safe and effective. The technique (Table 40–3) was first described in 1988 by Gambling and colleagues,[44] who compared bupivacaine (0.125%) PCEA with continuous infusion alone. They found PCEA better than continuous epidural infusion of bupivacaine. Patients in the PCEA group required significantly smaller doses of bupivacaine to provide comparable analgesia. The technique was believed to be safe and reliable and not to be associated with excess sensory blockade.

Lysak and associates[45] evaluated 0.125% bupivacaine in combination with fentanyl in three different concentrations to find the optimum regimen for PCEA. The control group received continuous infusion of plain bupivacaine. Their results suggested greater safety of PCEA when monitoring hemodynamics, sensory level, and duration of labor and concluded that the optimal concentration of fentanyl for PCEA hourly dosing was 1 μg/mL.[46, 47]

Bupivacaine-fentanyl administered by PCEA with infusion also demonstrated greater safety and efficacy (i.e., fewer top-ups and lower infusion rates) than when administered by continuous infusion. Naulty and coworkers,[48] used bupivacaine-sufentanil combinations during labor, demonstrating no particular benefits for PCEA with this combination of drugs; in fact, total drug requirements were greater in the PCEA group. Whether this finding was attributable to the drugs or to the PCEA regimen (small volume of self-administered dose) remains to be seen.

Dilute local anesthetic (0.03% to 0.06% bupivacaine) solutions can be used in certain postoperative patients. The use of local anesthetics should, however, be limited to the first 12 to 24 hours after surgery to avoid interfering with ambulation. They are probably best employed with segmentally placed catheters in patients recovering from major upper abdominal or thoracic surgery. Though the incidence is small, hypotension and lower extremity weakness are associated with the PCEA technique.

Conclusion

PCEA is a relatively new technique that may offer adequate analgesia with lower opioid doses than intravenous PCA while providing greater control and greater patient satisfaction than continuous infusion. There is also the potential for fewer dose-dependent side effects with PCEA. Its clinical advantages may outweigh its greater cost and the inva-

TABLE 40–3 ***Studies Comparing Patient-Controlled Epidural Analgesia (PCEA) with Continuous Infusion (CI) Analgesia***

Investigators*	Analgesic Drug	Additional Drug	Continuous Infusion (mL/hr)	PCEA Dose (mL)	Duration of Lockout* (min)	Comment
Gambling et al[37]	Bupivacaine, 0.125%	Epinephrine, 1:400,000	–	4	20	Greater satisfaction with PCEA than with CI
Gambling et al[39]	Bupivacaine, 0.125%	–	4	4	20	PCEA group used less local anesthetic than CI group
Lysak et al[38]	Bupivacaine, 0.125%	Fentanyl, 1 (μg/mL)	6	4	10	Fewer top-ups needed with PCEA than with CI
Viscomi and Eisenach[40]	Bupivacaine, 0.125%	Fentanyl, 1 (μg/mL)	4	4	10	Fewer top-ups needed with PCEA than with CI
Naulty et al[41]	Bupivacaine, 0.063%	Sufentanil, 0.3 (g/mL)	5	2	6	No advantage of PCEA over CI

* Inactivation of the PCEA pump during the period.

siveness of the technique. More data need to be analyzed, however, when choosing IVPCA, continuous infusion, or PCEA for analgesia of acute or chronic pain.

CONTINUOUS PERIPHERAL REGIONAL ANALGESIA

A prolonged peripheral nerve block may be placed as a continuous peripheral technique to provide perioperative pain relief for trauma or postoperative pain.[49] This continuous technique is performed very much like a single-injection technique.[50] After the needle is placed in the correct position, a catheter may be threaded into the perivascular compartment and secured for up to 7 to 10 days. In addition to perioperative pain relief, these catheters may be placed for a sympathetic block in patients with vascular compromise,[51] or intractable pain from complex regional pain syndromes I and II, or phantom limb pain.[52]

Continuous Brachial Plexus Infusion[53]

Indications for continuous brachial plexus infusion include perioperative pain and postoperative pain, vascular compromise, intractable pain from complex regional pain syndromes I and II, and phantom limb pain.

Anatomy

The brachial plexus is an ideal site for a continuous regional technique because of its well-defined perivascular compartment and its proximity to the many nerves that supply the upper extremity. All techniques of brachial plexus blockade have been described as continuous techniques but some are easier to achieve than others.[53] The infraclavicular approach has been preferred because the catheter can remain long in the same position, sometimes as long as 3 weeks.[53]

Technique

The patient lies supine with the head turned away from the arm to be blocked. The arm is abducted to 90 degrees and allowed to rest comfortably. The physician stands on the side opposite the arm to be blocked. The whole length of the clavicle is identified after palpation or fluoroscopic imaging. The midpoint of the clavicle is marked. The brachial artery is palpated in the arm and marked. The C6 tubercle on the same side is palpated in the neck and marked. A line is drawn from the C6 tubercle to the brachial artery in the arm. This line goes through the midpoint of the clavicle (Fig. 40–2). This is the surface marking of the brachial plexus. The ground electrode of a peripheral nerve stimulator is attached to the opposite shoulder. A skin wheal is raised 2 cm below the inferior border of the clavicle at its midpoint. An 18-gauge needle is used to pierce the skin. A 19-gauge Becton, Dickinson Longwell needle/catheter (or 16-gauge Racz epidural needle with appropriate epidural catheter to follow) is introduced through the skin wheal. The needle point is directed laterally towards the brachial artery. The exploring needle is then attached to either the stem or the hub of the needle with a sterile alligator clip. The current of the peripheral nerve stimulator is set to deliver 3 mA, and the needle is advanced at an angle of 45 degrees to the skin. As the needle approaches the fibers of the brachial plexus, the muscles supplied by those fibers will move. The forearm and hand are carefully observed for these movements. Flexion or extension of the elbow, wrist, or digits confirms that the needle point is close to nerve fibers of the brachial plexus. The current of

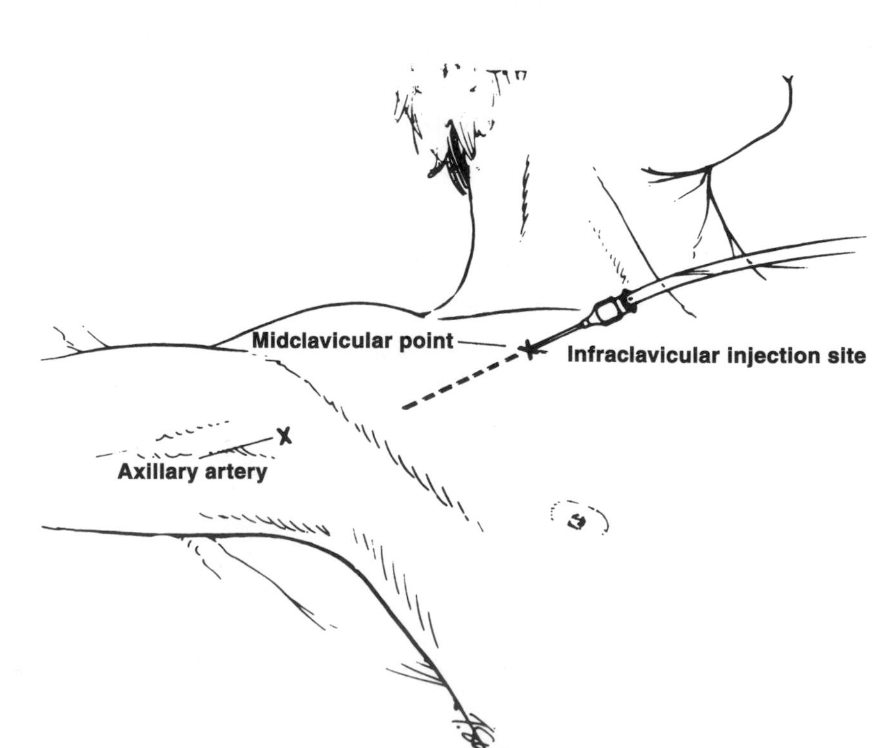

FIGURE 40–2 Raj's technique of the infraclavicular approach. The drawing illustrates the surface markings of the brachial plexus. The needle is directed laterally at 45 degrees to the skin at the point of entry. The point of entry is 1 inch inferior to the midpoint of the clavicle. The artery is identified in the upper arm and the needle is directed toward it. (From Raj PP, Pai U, Rawal N: Techniques of regional anesthesia in adults. In Raj PP [ed]: Clinical Practice of Regional Anesthesia. New York, Churchill-Livingstone, 1991. Reprinted with permission.)

the impulse is decreased to 0.5 mA. The needle is then advanced. The muscle movements previously seen increase as the needle tip moves closer to the brachial plexus. The needle is advanced until the muscle movements start to decrease. When this happens, the needle tip has passed the nerve, and it must be slowly withdrawn until muscle movements are maximal and then held in that position. Water-soluble contrast medium may be injected (approximately 3 mL) to observe spread in the nerve sheath (Figs. 40–3, 40–4). Two milliliters of 2% lidocaine is then injected through the needle, with the 1-impulse/second button on the peripheral nerve stimulator activated. If the needle is placed correctly on the nerve fibers, the muscle movements seen previously cease within 30 sec. If they do not, the needle should be withdrawn slightly and the process repeated.[54] The catheter is then threaded through the needle and approximately 3 to 5 cm beyond the needle tip. Further confirmation of proper catheter placement can be made with contrast dye. Twenty to 30 mL of 0.2% ropivacaine is then injected in divided doses through a bacteriostatic filter for immediate pain relief. The needle is withdrawn under direct fluoroscopic guidance. The catheter is sutured into place. The site is covered with antibiotic ointment and biocclusive dressing. The brachial plexus catheter is then connected to a constant infusion of 0.1% ropivacaine fentanyl (5 μg/mL) at 6 to 10 mL/hr. Occasional bolus doses may be required and may be administered by the patient (patient controlled with 3-mL doses, 15-min lockout, and a maximum of 6 mL/hr). The continuous infusion is reliably efficacious for up to 48 hours. After that period, the efficacy for A-delta fiber blocking drops precipitously. Sympathetic block can still be maintained as long as 2 to 3 weeks with 0.1% to 0.2% ropivacaine in a securely anchored catheter.[53]

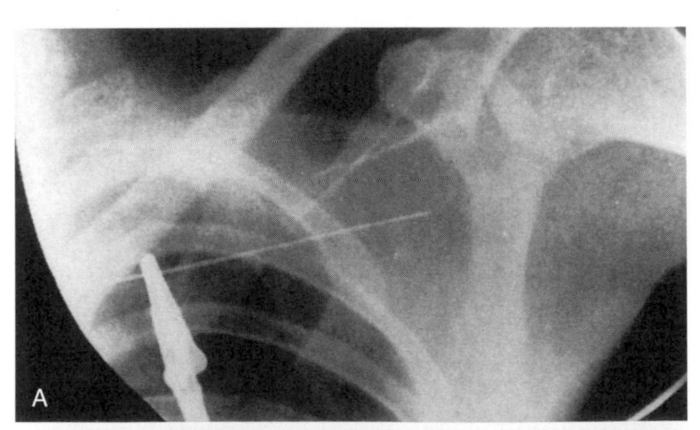

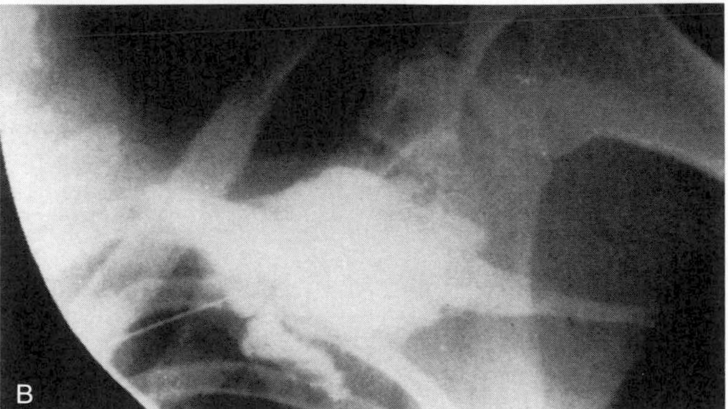

FIGURE 40–3 A, *Radiograph shows needle in final position after infraclavicular block. Note that the needle tip approaches the scapula as it goes deeper.* B, *The spread of the contrast material (20 ml) when the needle is on the brachial plexus in the infraclavicular region. (From Raj PP, Montgomery SJ, Nettles D, et al: Infraclavicular brachial plexus block: A new approach. Anesth Analg 52:897–904, 1973. Reprinted with permission.)*

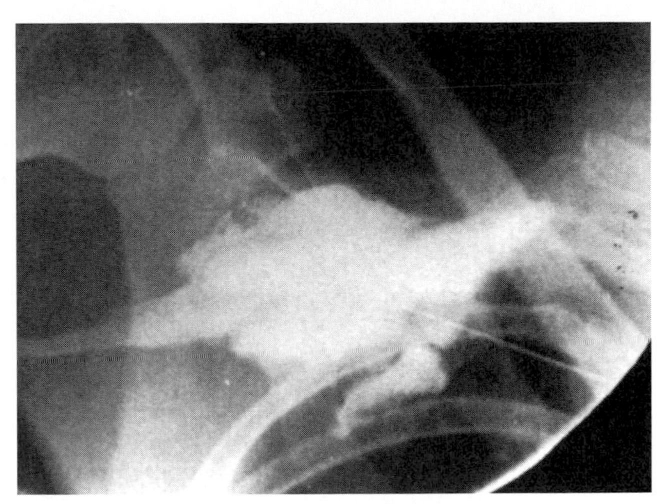

FIGURE 40–4 Details of 20 ml of contrast solution injected in the infraclavicular region. Note the cephalad spread under the midclavicular region and the filling of the axillary sheath in the upper arm (caudad spread). The spilling of the solution in the midportion suggests a sievelike brachial plexus sheath in the infraclavicular region. The spilling of contrast solution outside the sheath at this level usually blocks the intercostobrachial nerve, an obvious advantage of this block. (From Raj PP, Montgomery SJ, Nettles D, et al: Infraclavicular brachial plexus block: A new approach. Anesth Analg 52:897–904, 1973. Reprinted with permission.)

Complications

The complications of continuous brachial plexus infusion are similar to those of a brachial plexus block: bleeding, infection, intravascular or intrathecal injection, pneumothorax, and phrenic nerve paralysis. The severity and length of phrenic nerve paralysis is related to the site of catheter placement (e.g., interscalene, supraclavicular) and what local anesthetic is used.[55–61] The plasma concentration and pharmacokinetics of the constant infusion in steady state are similar to those observed in epidural infusion. Once steady state is reached, the drugs do not accumulate if infused at the same rate. The metabolites also remain at insignificant levels without causing any deleterious effects.[54]

Continuous Sciatic Nerve Infusion

Indications

Patients with complex regional pain syndrome I or II, vascular insufficiency, or unilateral leg edema (of many causes) are frequently managed with lumbar epidural catheters. There are, however, inherent risks with long-term placement of an epidural catheter. The sciatic catheter can be an alternative for such patients. It can eliminate the risk of epidural abscess, hematoma formation, and catheter erosion of the dura. The affected limb can be specifically treated without numbing or weakening the contralateral limb. Thus, ambulation is maintained. Contraindications include (1) anticoagulant therapy, (2) septicemia, (3) local infection, (4) recent injury at the site of injection to the nerve, and (5) inability of the patient to lie prone.

Anatomy

The sciatic nerve is formed from the nerve roots of L4–L5 and S1–S3 at the sciatic notch, and passes through the gluteal region between the greater trochanter and the ischial tuberosity. In the buttocks, it runs posterior to the gemelli and the obturator internus. It lies anterior to the piriformis muscle as it descends to the thigh first described by Labat in 1923.[62] Our approach is based on the identification of the piriformis muscle and placement of the catheter on the sciatic nerve in the gluteal region.

Technique

The patient is placed in the prone position. The gluteal region ipsilateral to the affected side is sterilized and draped. Landmarks are located by fluoroscopy—(1) the posterior superior iliac spine, (2) the greater trochanter, and (3) the ischial tuberosity. A line is drawn connecting the posterior iliac spine and the greater trochanter. The midpoint is identified and a perpendicular line drawn in a caudal direction. A second line is drawn from the greater trochanter to the ischial tuberosity. This line is divided into 3 parts. A third line is drawn vertically from the medial third mark upward to intersect the other line. The point of entry is where the two lines meet (Figs. 40–5, 40–6). A skin wheal is raised at the site with a 25-gauge needle. A larger needle (16- or 18-gauge) can pierce the skin. A blunt 16-gauge, 7-in needle is introduced perpendicularly,

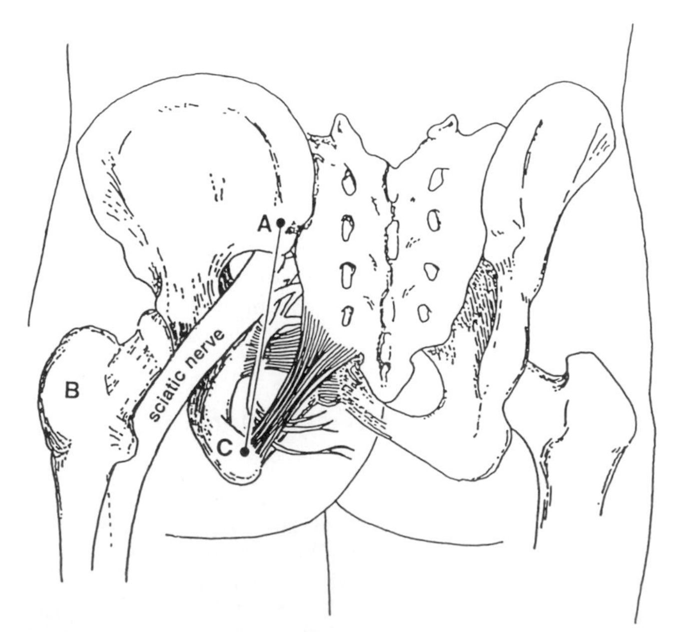

FIGURE 40–5 Drawing depicting the landmarks to be identified by fluoroscopy: (A), posterior superior iliac spine, (B), greater trochanter, and (C), ischial tuberosity.[63, 64]

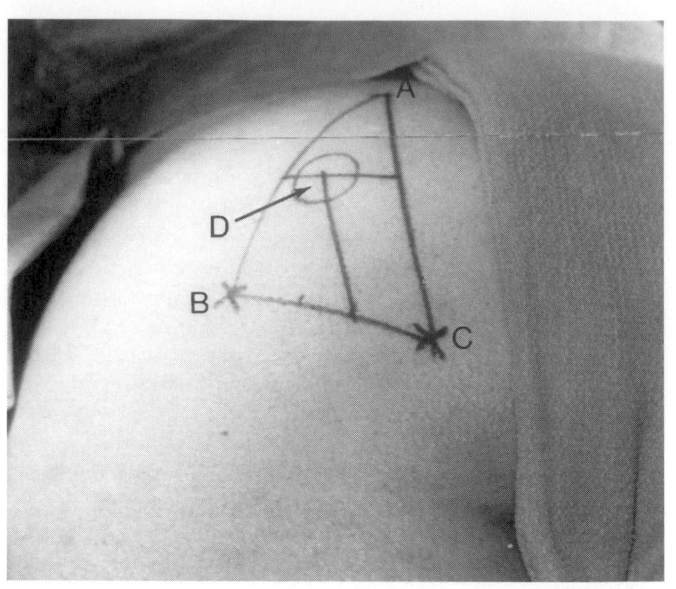

FIGURE 40–6 Surface landmarks and entry point of needle: (A) posterior superior iliac spine, (B) greater trochanter, (C) ischial tuberosity, and (D) insertion site.[63, 64]

approximately 1 cm through the skin to reach the piriformis muscle. A 22-gauge needle is inserted subcutaneously and attached to a positive lead from the Medtronic test stimulator (or a comparable peripheral nerve stimulator). The Medtronic test stimulator should be set to deliver 6 to 8 V at 1 impulse/sec. (If a peripheral nerve stimulator is used, the current should be adjusted from 3 to 0.5 mA at 1 impulse/sec.) The needle is slowly advanced anteriorly until the piriformis muscle, which is identified by contrast solution, is twitching. The needle is further advanced until the piriformis muscle stimulation stops and foot twitching (dorsiflexion) is observed in the affected limb. A stimulating catheter is then inserted through the needle (Fig. 40–7). The negative lead of the stimulator is attached to the distal connect wire of the catheter. The catheter is passed to the level of the lesser trochanter for foot movement. The needle is then removed and the catheter is attached to the hub connector. Placement can be confirmed with 3 mL of contrast dye introduced via the catheter (Figs. 40–8, 40–9). Another 3 mL of 0.2% ropivacaine may be injected, and stimulation of the sciatic nerve should cease.[63] Through an attached bacteriostatic filter 15 to 30 mL of 2% lidocaine or 0.2% ropivacaine is injected in divided doses for immediate pain relief and nerve blockade. The constant infusion of 0.1% ropivacaine with fentanyl (5 μg/mL) may range from 4 to 10 mL/hr. Occasional bolus doses may be required and may be delivered by the patient through the pump with a bolus of 5 mL and a 30-min lockout.[64] The catheter may be connected to a drug infusion balloon for outpatient care through home health services. This balloon delivers 4 mL/hr of the drug to the patient for 24 hours. (The volume of the balloon reservoir is 100 mL.)

Complications

Potential complications with the continuous sciatic catheter include bleeding, infection, hematoma, intravascular injection, or residual dysesthesia.

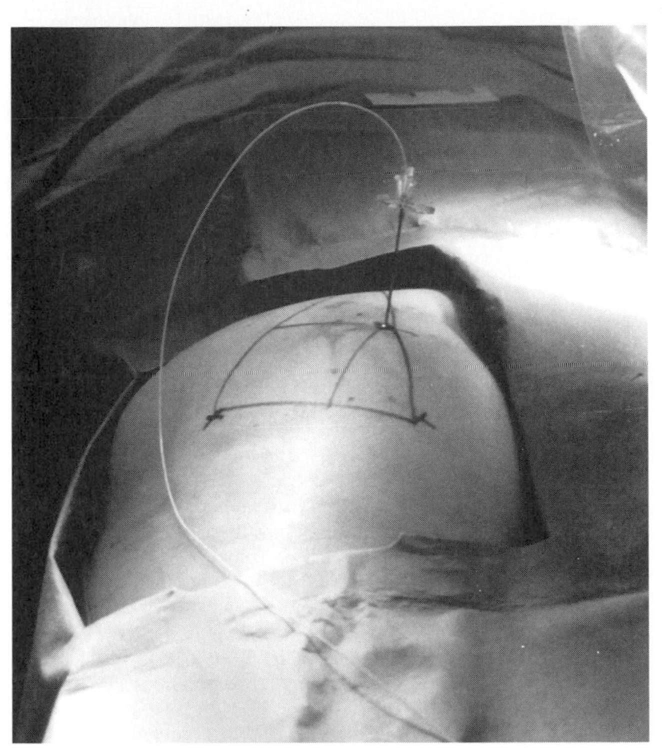

FIGURE 40 – 7 Surface view of the catheter after placement.[63, 64]

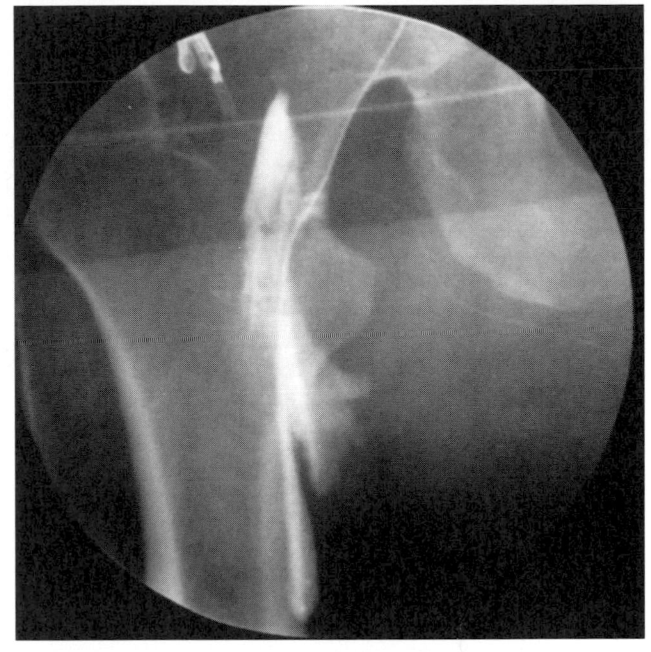

FIGURE 40 – 9 Fluoroscopic image of the catheter with contrast solution following the sciatic nerve sheath.[63, 64]

CONCLUSION

Continuous regional analgesia, whether central or peripheral, is safe and efficacious. The infusions may utilize local anesthetics, opioids, or a combination of the two. These infusions are performed when prolonged analgesia is required for moderate to severe acute, chronic, or cancer pain.[53]

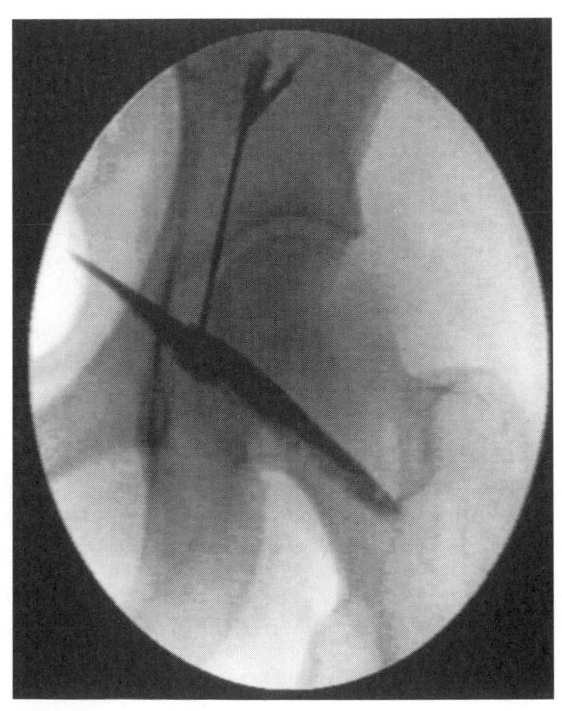

FIGURE 40 – 8 Fluoroscopic image of catheter with the piriformis muscle superficially and with contrast solution over the sciatic nerve.[63, 64]

REFERENCES

1. Green R, Dawkins CJM: Postoperative analgesia: The use of continuous drip epidural block. Anaesthesia 21:372, 1966.
2. Spoerel WE, Thomas A, Gerula GR: Continuous drip analgesia: Experience with mechanical devices. Can Anaesth Soc J 17:37, 1970.
3. Rosenblatt RM, Raj PP: Experience with volumetric infusion pumps for continuous epidural analgesia. Reg Anaesth 4:3–5, 1979.
4. Cleland JG: Continuous peridural caudal analgesia in surgery and early ambulation. Northwest Med 48:266, 1949.
5. Akerman B, Arwenström E, Post C: Local anesthetics potentiate spinal morphine antinociception. Anesth Analg 67:943–948, 1988.
6. Bromage PR, Camporesi E. Chestnut D: Epidural narcotics for postoperative analgesia. Anesth Analg 59:473–480, 1980.
7. Cousins MJ, Mather LE: Intrathecal and epidural administration of opioids. Anesthesiology 61:276–310, 1984.
8. Rutler DV, Skewes DG, Morgan M: Extradural opioids for postoperative analgesia. Br J Anaesth 53:915–920, 1981.
9. Van der Auwera D, Verborgh C, Camu F: Analgesic and cardiorespiratory effects of spidural sufentanil and morphine in humans. Anesth Analg 66:999–1003, 1987.
10. Scott NB, Mogensen T, Bigler D, et al: Continuous thoracic extradural 0.05% bupivacaine with or without morphine: Effect on quality of blockade, lung function and the surgical stress response. Br J Anaesth 62:253–257, 1989.
11. Raj PP, Denson D, Finnason R: Prolonged epidural analgesia: Intermittent or continuous? *In* Meyer J, Nolte H (eds): Die kontinuerliche peridural Anesthesia: 7th International Symposium uber die Regional Anesthesia AM, January 7, 1982, Minden. Stuttgart, George Thieme, 1983, pp 26–38.
12. Lubenow TR, Durrani Z, Ivankovish AD: Evaluation of continuous epidural fentanyl/butorphanol infusion for postoperative pain. Anesthesia 69:381, 1988.
13. Rosseel PMJ. Van Der Broeck J, Boer EC, Prakash O: Epidural sufentanil for intraoperative and postoperative analgesia in thoracic

surgery: A comparative study with intravenous sufentanil. Acta Anaesthesiol Scand 32:193–198, 1988.
14. Scott DB, Lee A, Fagan D, Bowler GMR, Bloomfield P, Lundh R: Acute toxicity of ropivacaine compared with that of bupivacaine. Anesth Analg 69:563–569, 1989.
15. Markham A, Faulds D: Ropivacaine: A review of its pharmacology and therapeutic use in regional anaesthesia. Drugs 52(3):429–449, 1996.
16. Akerman B, Hellberg IB, Trossvik C: Primary evaluation of the local anaesthetic properties of the amino amide agent ropivacaine. Acta Anaesthesiol Scand 32:571–578, 1988.
17. Feldman HS, Covino BG: Comparative motor-blocking effects of bupivacaine and ropivacaine, a new amino amide local anesthetic, in the rat and dog. Anesth Analg 67:1047–1052, 1988.
18. Reiz S, Haggmark S, Johansson G, Nath S: Cardiotoxicity of ropivacaine—a new amide local anesthetic agent. Acta Anaesthesiol Scand 33:93–98, 1989.
19. Finucane BT: Ropivacaine—a worthy replacement for bupivacaine? Can J Anaesth 37(7):722–725, 1990.
20. Arthur GR, Feldman HS, Covino BG: Comparative pharmacokinetics of bupivacaine and ropivacaine, a new amide local anesthetic. Anesth Analg 67:1053–1058, 1988.
21. Tucker GT, Cooper S, Littlewood D, Buckley SP: Observed and predicted accumulation of local anesthetics during continuous extradural analgesia. Br J Anaesth 49:237, 1977.
22. Schweitzer SA, Morgan DJ: Plasma bupivacaine concentrations during postoperative continuous epidural analgesia. Anaesth Intensive Care 15:425–430, 1987.
23. Gregory MA, Brock-Utne JC, Bux S, Downing JW: Morphine concentration in brain and spinal cord after subarachnoid morphine injection in baboons. Anesth Analg 64:929–932, 1985.
24. Rawal N, Sjöstrand U, Dahlström B: Postoperative pain relief by epidural morphine. Anesth Analg 60:726–731, 1981.
25. Chestnut DH, Owen CL, Bates JN, et al: Continuous infusion epidural analgesia during labor: A randomized double-blind comparison of 0.0625% bupivacaine/0.0002% fentanyl versus 0.125% bupivacaine. Anesthesiology 68:754–759, 1988.
26. Cullen M, Staren E, Ganzouri A, et al: Continuous thoracic epidural analgesia after major abdominal operations: A randomized prospective double-blind study. Surgery 98:718–728, 1985.
27. Fisher R, Lubenow TR, Liceaga A, et al: Comparison of continuous epidural infusion of fentanyl-bupivacaine and morphine-bupivacaine in the management of postoperative pain. Anesth Analg 67:559–563, 1988.
28. Logas WG, El-Baz NM, El-Ganzouri A, et al: Continuous thoracic epidural analgesia for postoperative pain relief following thoracotomy: A randomized prospective study. Anesthesiology 67:787–791, 1987.
29. Hjortso NC, Lund C, Mogensen T, et al: Epidural morphine improves pain relief and maintains sensory analgesia during continuous epidural bupivacaine after abdominal surgery. Anesth Analg 65:1033–1036, 1986.
30. Magora F, Olshwand DL, Eimei D, et al: Observation on extradural morphine analgesia in various pain conditions. Br J Anaesth 52:247–252, 1980.
31. Rutberg H, Hakannson E, Anderberg B, et al: Effects of extradural administration of morphine or bupivacaine on the endocrine response to upper abdominal surgery. Br J Anaesth 56:233–238, 1984.
32. Sjöström S, Hartvig D, Tamsen A: Patient controlled analgesia with extradural morphine or pethidine. Br J Anaesth 60:358, 1988.
33. Chrubasik J, Wieners K: Continuous–plus–on demand epidural infusion of morphine for postoperative pain relief by means of a small, externally worn infusion device. Anesthesiology 62:263, 1985.
34. Chrubasik J, Wust H, Schulte-Monting J, et al: Relative analgesic potency of epidural fentanyl, alfentanil and morphine in treatment of postoperative pain. Anesthesiology 68:929, 1988.
35. Downing JE, Stedman PM, Busch EH: Continuous low volume infusion of epidural morphine for postoperative pain. Reg Anesth 13(Suppl):84, 1988.
36. Planner RS, Cowie RW, Babarczy AS, et al: Continuous epidural morphine analgesia after radical operations upon the pelvis. Surg Gynecol Obstet 166:229, 1988.
37. Rauck R, Knarr D, Denson D, Raj P: Comparison of the efficacy of epidural morphine given by intermittent injection or continuous infusion for the management of postoperative pain. Anesthesiology 65:A201, 1986.
38. Marlowe S, Engstrom R, White PF: Epidural patient-controlled analgesia (PCA): An alternative to continuous epidural infusions. Pain 37:97, 1989.
39. Walmsley PNH, McDonnell FJ, Colclough GW, et al: A comparison of epidural and intravenous PCA after gynecological surgery. Anesthesiology 73:A684, 1989.
40. Loper KA, Ready LB, Sandler AN: Epidural and IV fentanyl infusions are clinically equivalent following knee surgery. Anesthesiology 71:A1149, 1989.
41. Estok PM, Glass PSA, Goldberg JS, et al: Use of PCA to compare IV to epidural administration of fentanyl in the postoperative patient. Anesthesiology 67:A230, 1987.
42. Cohen S, Amar D, Pantuck CB: Continuous epidural-PCA post-cesarean section: Buprenorphine-bupivacaine 0.03% vs. fentanyl-bupivacaine 0.03%. Anesthesiology 73:A975, 1990.
43. Cohen S, Amar D, Pantuck CB: Continuous epidural-PCA for cesarean section: Buprenorphine-bupivacaine 0.015 with epinephrine vs. fentanyl-bupivacaine 0.015 with and without epinephrine. Anesthesiology 73:A918, 1990.
44. Gambling DR, Yu P, Cole C, et al: A comparative study of patient controlled epidural analgesia (PCEA) and continuous infusion epidural analgesia (CIEA) during labour. Can J Anaesth 35:249–254, 1988.
45. Lysak SZ, Eisenach JC, Dobson CE: Patient-controlled epidural analgesia during labor: A comparison of three solutions with a continuous infusion control. Anesthesiology 72:44–49, 1990.
46. Gambling DR, McMorland GH, Yu P, et al: Comparison of patient controlled epidural analgesia and conventional intermittent "top-up" injections during labor. Anesth Analg 70:256–261, 1990.
47. Viscomi C, Eisenach JC: Patient-controlled epidural analgesia during labor. Obstet Gynecol 77:A685, 1989.
48. Naulty JS, Barnes D, Becker R, et al: Epidural PCA vs. continuous infusion of sufentanil-bupivacaine for analgesia during labor and delivery. Anesthesiology 73:A963, 1990.
49. Fisher A, Meller Y: Continuous postoperative regional analgesia by nerve sheath block for amputation surgery: A pilot study. Anesth Analg 72:300–303, 1991.
50. Raj P: Continuous brachial plexus analgesia. 21st Annual Meeting. American Society of Regional Anesthesia, San Diego. Abstract Book. 1996, pp 501–502.
51. Matsuda M, Kato N, Hosoi M: Continuous brachial plexus block for replantation in the upper extremity. Hand 14:129–134, 1982.
52. Hartrick C: Pain due to trauma including sports injuries. *In* Raj PP (ed): Practical Management of Pain, ed 2. St. Louis, Mosby–Year Book, 1992, pp 409–433.
53. Raj PP: Continuous regional analgesia. *In* Raj PP (ed): Practical Management of Pain, ed 3. St. Louis, Mosby–Year Book, 2000.
54. Raj PP, Montgomery SJ, Nettles D, et al: Infraclavicular brachial plexus block—a new approach. Anesth Analg 52(6):897–904, 1973.
55. Pere P, Pitkanen M, Rosenberg PH, et al: Effect of continuous interscalene brachial plexus block on diaphragm motion and on ventilatory function. Acta Anaesthesiol Scand 36:53–57, 1992.
56. Urmey WF, Talts KH, Sharrock NE: One hundred percent incidence of hemidiaphragmatic paresis associated with interscalene brachial plexus anesthesia as diagnosed by ultrasonography. Anesth Analg 72:498–503, 1991.
57. Urmey WF, McDonald M: Hemidiaphragmatic paresis during interscalene brachial plexus block: Effects on pulmonary function and chest wall mechanics. Anesth Analg 74:352–357, 1992.
58. Knoblanche GE: The incidence and etiology of phrenic nerve blockade associated with supraclavicular brachial plexus block. Anaesth Intensive Care 7:346–349, 1979.
59. Dhuner K-G, Moberg E, Onne L: Paresis of the phrenic nerve during brachial plexus block analgesia and its importance. Acta Chir Scand 109:53–57, 1955.
60. Farrar MD, Scheybani M, Nolte H: Upper extremity block: Effectiveness and complications. Reg Anesth 6:133–134, 1981.
61. Kulenkampff D: Die Anasthesia des plexus brachialis. Zentralbl Chir 38:1337–1340, 1911.

62. Adriani J: Labat's Regional Anesthesia: Techniques and Clinical Applications. Philadelphia, WB Saunders, 1967.
63. Racz G, Raj P, Lou L, Lewandowski E, Heavner JE: Posterior sacral approach to the sciatic nerve for continuous lidocaine infusion: A new technique. Presented at 1997 ASA, San Diego, Calif. and the 1997 PGA, New York, NY; and 1998 IARS, Orlando, Fla.
64. Racz G, Raj P, Lou L, Day M, Harris C, Anderson S, Heavner JE: Posterior sacral approach to the sciatic nerve for continuous ropivacaine infusion: A new technique. Presented at 1998 PGA, New York, NY.

BIBLIOGRAPHY

Lubenow TR: Epidural analgesia: Considerations and delivery methods. *In* Sinatra RS, Hord AH, Ginsberg B, Preble LM (eds): Acute Pain: Mechanisms and Management. St Louis, Mosby–Year Book, 1992, pp 233–242.

Walmsley PNH: Patient controlled epidural analgesia. *In* Sinatra RS, Hord AH, Ginsberg B, Preble LM (eds): Acute Pain: Mechanisms and Management. St Louis, Mosby–Year Book, 1992, pp 312–320.

CHAPTER • 41

Percutaneous Epidural Neuroplasty

Leland Lou, MD MPH • Gabor Racz, MD
James Heavner, DVM

HISTORY

Epidural fibrosis and adhesions can have many causes. Leakage of the substance of the nucleus pulposus into the epidural space has been documented to cause an inflammatory response and a resultant increase in fibrocystic deposition. Postsurgical bleeding and the associated healing process frequently produce scarring. Epidural adhesions alone do not cause pain. The associated irritation or inducement of epidural venous engorgement may contribute to pain production. Whether by the direct mechanical encasement of nerve roots within scar tissue or the secondary process of epidural venous congestion with increasing nerve root edema, pain is produced by movement of the swollen inflamed nerve root.[1]

DIAGNOSIS OF EPIDURAL ADHESIONS

Magnetic resonance imaging (MRI) can be used to detect epidural fibrosis, but it is not a perfect test. It has been documented that myelography, computed tomography (CT), and MRI have been unsuccessful.[2] A method used with great success is epidurography, a technique initially reported in 1921 by Sicard and Forestier.[3] Bogduk and colleagues stated that a volume of 10 mL was sufficient to reach the L5 segmental level.[4, 5] The experience at Texas Tech University and a study performed by Manchikanti and colleagues found that the caudal epidurogram was effective in correlating a filling defect with the patient's reported level of pain.[6, 7]

RADIOLOGIC LANDMARKS OF THE CAUDAL CANAL

On the lateral view (Fig. 41–1A), the caudal canal appears as a translucent layer posterior to the sacral segments. The median sacral crest is seen as an opaque line posterior to the caudal canal. The sacral hiatus is usually visible as a translucent opening at the base of the caudal canal. The coccyx can be seen articulating with the inferior surface of the sacrum. On the anteroposterior view (Fig. 41–1B), the intermediate sacral crests are opaque vertical lines on either side of the midline. The sacral foramina are seen as translucent nearly circular areas lateral to the intermediate sacral crests. Bowel gas can make recognition of these structures difficult.

TECHNIQUE

Consent must be obtained from the patient before beginning this procedure. The consent form should include all possible complications related to the procedure. These include bruising, transient hypotension, transient breathing difficulty, numbness of the extremities, bowel or bladder dysfunction, paralysis, infection, sexual dysfunction, and the possibility that the catheter might shear. Laboratory studies to be ordered are complete blood cell count, urinalysis, prothrombin time, partial prothrombin time, and bleeding time.

Intravenous access is recommended in anticipation of accidental injection of local anesthetic into the subarachnoid space, subdural space, or vascular structure. It may be necessary to sedate the patient with 1 to 2 mg midazolam and 25 to 50 μg fentanyl. Injection of solutions into the epidural space of a patient with adhesions is usually quite painful because of distention of affected nerve roots. The patient typically experiences pain in the dermatomal distribution of the nerve roots being stretched. Although sedation is given, it is important that the patient be awake and responsive during the procedure to ensure that the spinal cord is not compressed during the injection. During the injection of local anesthetic and steroids, the patient is asked to report any motor weakness or numbness after each bolus dose given to monitor for a "nonepidural" injection.

Fluoroscopy is essential for adhesion lysis. It is preferable to use a unit with memory capabilities to decrease radiation exposure. For documentation, videotaping the fluoroscopy screen during the procedure or making printouts for subsequent review is recommended. To minimize radiation exposure, the physician should use appropriate protective measures, such as leaded gloves, apron, thyroid shield, and

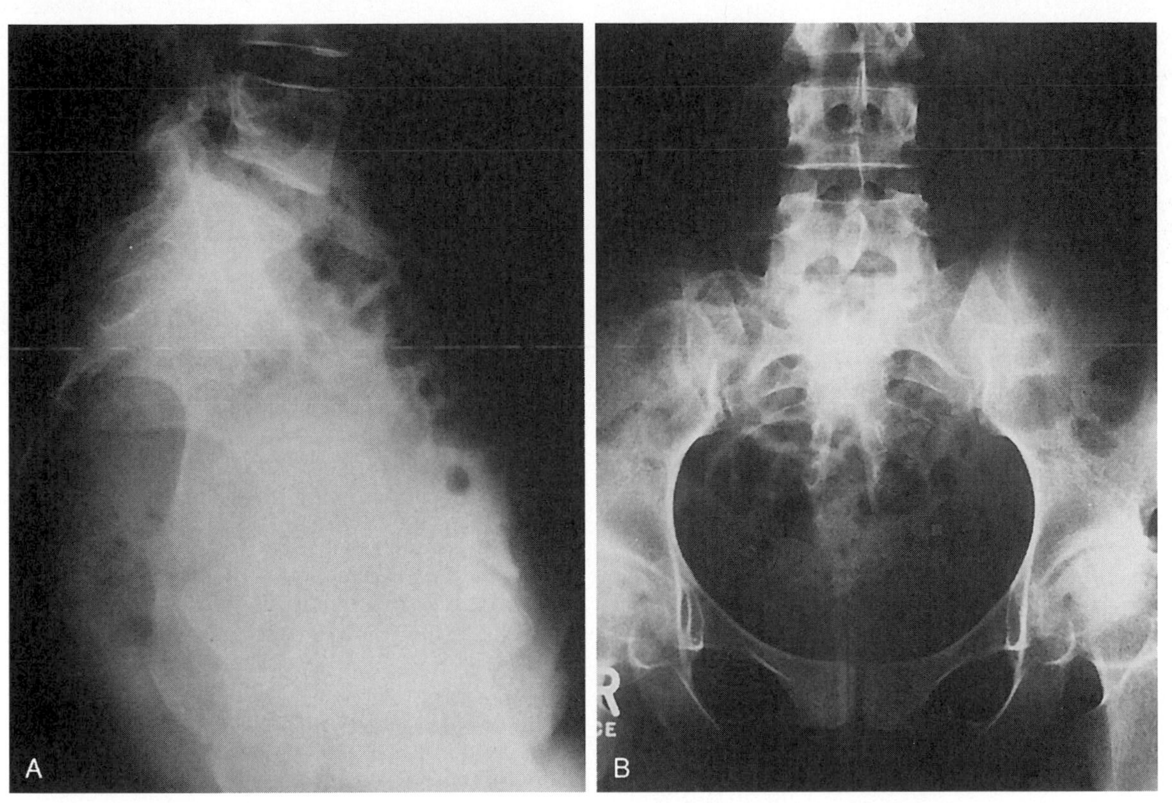

FIGURE 41–1 *A, Lateral radiograph of the sacrum. B, Anteroposterior radiograph of the sacrum.*

leaded glasses. Although epidural catheters are frequently placed without radiographic guidance, fluoroscopy is important to optimize the success of this procedure (i.e., for verification of needle placement, visualization of dye spread, and proper catheter placement).

A water-soluble, nonionic contrast medium is used because of the possibility of unintended subarachnoid injection. Even in the most careful hands, scar tissue may dissect during injection of contrast and enter the subarachnoid space. Non–water-soluble ionic contrast medium in the subarachnoid space can cause spinal cord irritation, spinal cord seizures or clonus, arachnoiditis, and paralysis.[8]

The steroid that we currently use for this procedure is triamcinolone acetate. Methylprednisolone, which we have used in the past, clumps when mixed with local anesthetics or normal saline. A particulate steroid can occlude the catheter or possibly cause infarction of spinal tissue via vascular injection. Because the particle size of triamcinolone acetate is about 20 microns, it cannot be injected through a bacteriostatic filter.

Hypertonic saline is used to prolong pain relief because of its local anesthetic effect.[9] The mechanism of action of hypertonic saline is not fully understood. A direct effect may be lysis of scar tissue. The indirect effect is attributed to the osmotic outflow of "free water" in the edematous neural tissue to the area of the hypertonic saline.

THE CAUDAL AREA

On the fluoroscopy table the patient is placed prone with a pillow under the abdomen to straighten the lumbar spine. Monitors are applied, including electrocardiography sensors, pulse oximeter, and a blood pressure cuff (preferably an automated one). The sacral area is then prepared with sterile technique and draped from the top of the iliac crest to the bottom of the buttocks. Abduction of the legs and inversion of the feet ("pigeon toe") facilitates entry into the sacral hiatus. The sacral cornua and the sacral hiatus are palpated with the index finger of the operator's nondominant hand. The entry point through the skin, approximately 1 to 2 cm lateral and 2 cm inferior to the sacral hiatus, is in the gluteal fold opposite the affected side. This allows the needle and the catheter to be directed toward the affected side. Lateral needle placement also tends to avoid penetration of the dural sac or subdural area with either the needle or the catheter. The entry point is infiltrated with a local anesthetic such as lidocaine. A 16-gauge epidural needle (preferably an R-K needle) is passed through the described entry point and into the sacral hiatus, using the sacral cornua as landmarks to locate the hiatus (Fig. 41–2). The needle is advanced to a point below the S3 foramen to prevent S3 nerve root damage. Placement is confirmed by a lateral fluoroscopic view before any injections, to verify that the needle is within the bony canal (Fig. 41–3A). This is important, because anatomic variations of the sacrum could lead to incorrect needle placement that nevertheless "feels" correct (Fig. 41–3B). Next, an anteroposterior view should verify that the needle tip points toward the affected side (Fig. 41–4).

After aspiration is negative for blood and cerebrospinal fluid (CSF), 10 mL of iohexol (Omnipaque-240) or metrizamide (Amipaque) is injected under fluoroscopy. If venous runoff is noted, the needle tip is moved during injec-

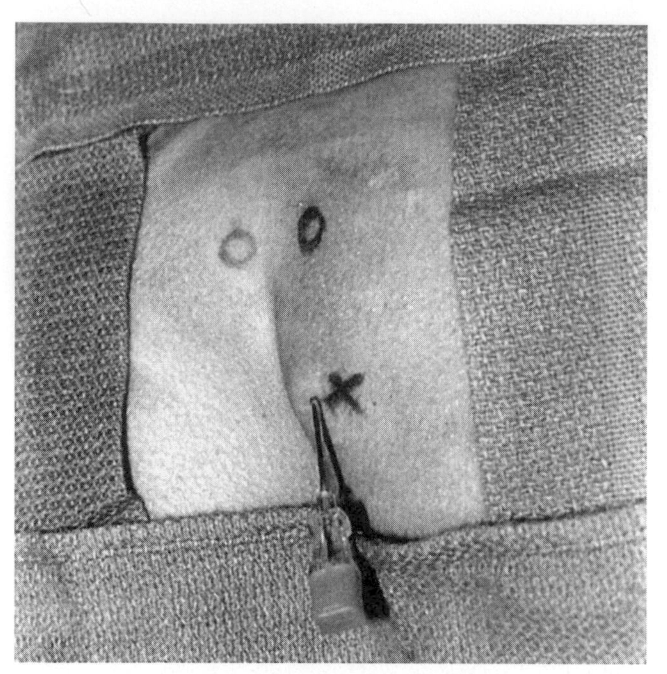

FIGURE 41–2 Entry point into the caudal canal. Note lateral placement of the needle, as described in the text, as compared with the classic midline approach. The circles *indicate the sacral cornua.*

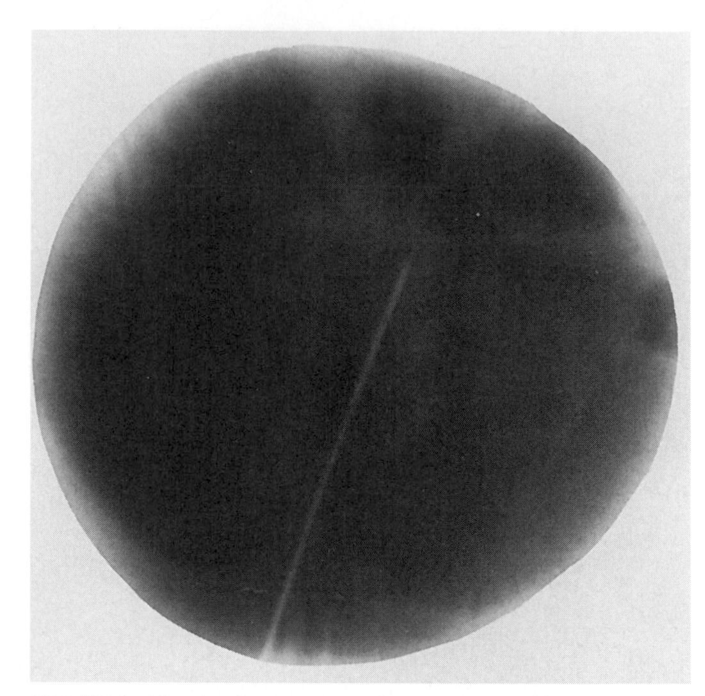

FIGURE 41–4 On anteroposterior view, the needle is seen pointing to the affected side.

tion until contrast medium is seen spreading within the epidural space. As the medium is injected into the epidural space, a Christmas-tree shape develops as the dye spreads into the perineural structures inside the bony canal and along the nerves as they exit the vertebral column. Epidural adhesions prevent dye spread, so dye does not outline the involved nerve roots (Fig. 41–5A). A lateral view likewise shows no dye outlining the scarred nerve roots.

When the needle tip is in the subarachnoid space, dye spreads centrally and cephalad (Fig. 41–6), as it does when the needle tip is subdural (but not as extensively as with subarachnoid injection). The contrast medium enhances

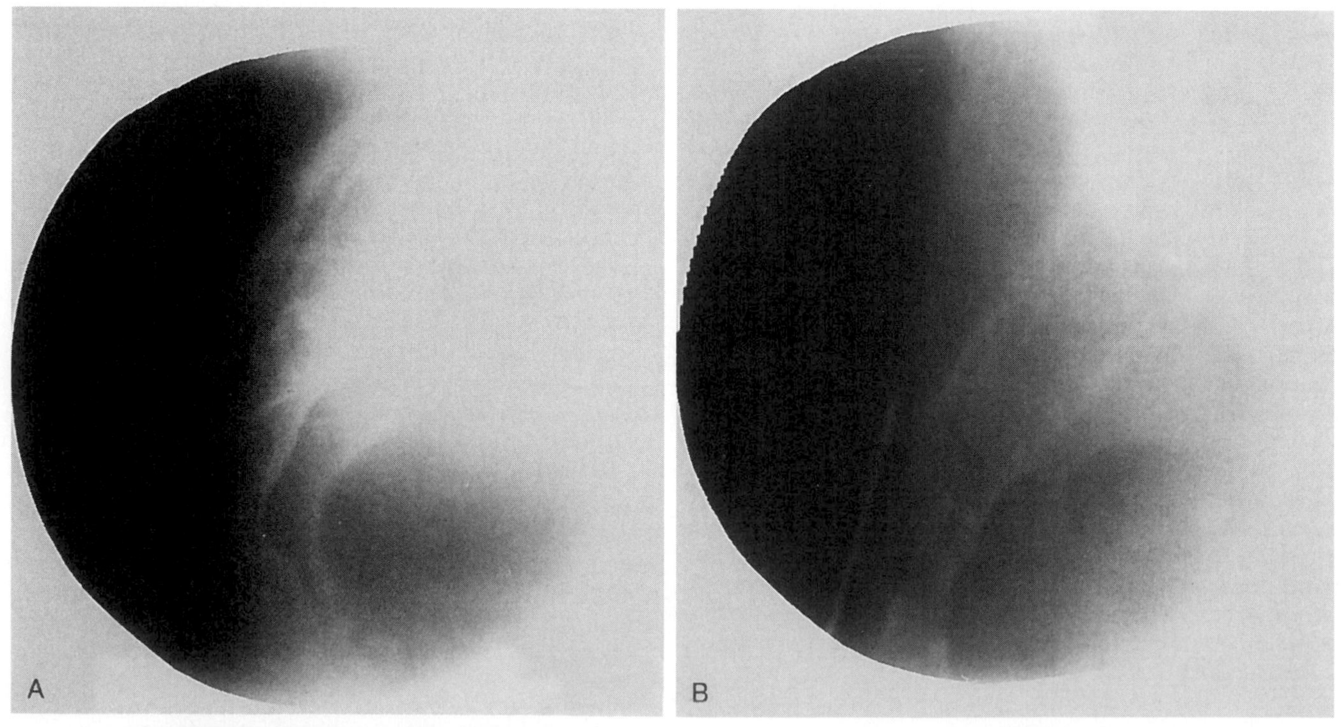

FIGURE 41–3 A, Correct needle placement into the caudal canal. B, Incorrect needle placement into the subcutaneous tissue.

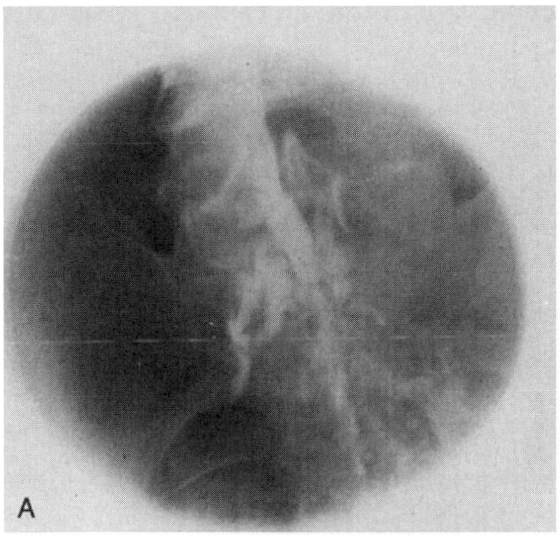

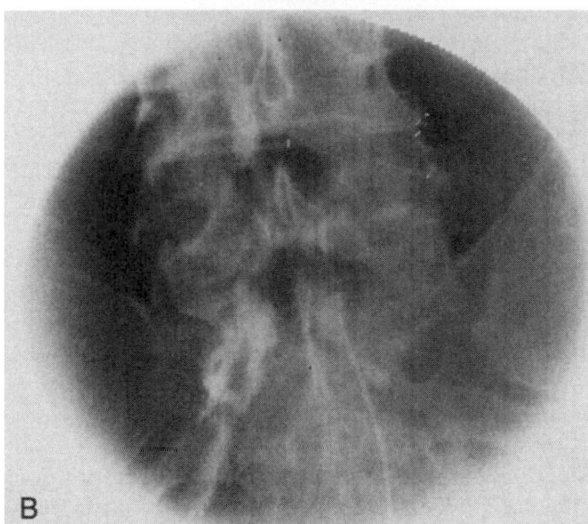

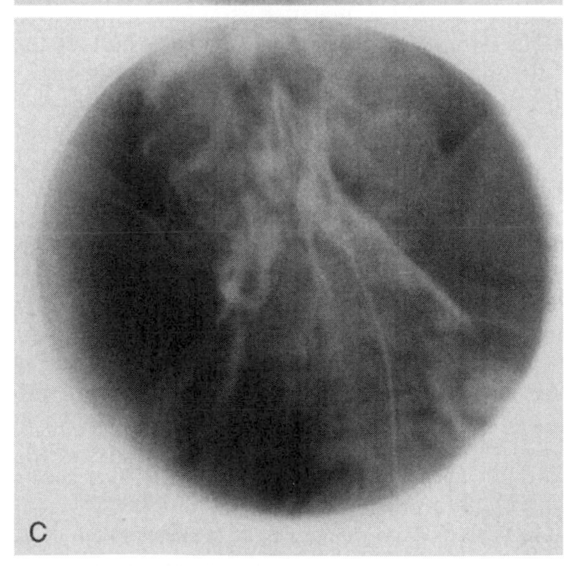

FIGURE 41–5 *A, After injection of 10 mL of contrast medium, the medium spreads to the left side of the epidural space, avoiding the right side, from whence the symptoms are originating. B, The Racz Tun-L-Kath epidural catheter is threaded to the right side of the epidural space into the area scarred. C, Injection of 5 mL of contrast medium shows spread into the area scarred previously. This was followed by injection of 9 mL of 0.2% ropivacaine with 40 mg (1 mL) triamcinolone and, 30 min later, by 10 mL 10% saline. The patient had complete pain relief after the procedure.*

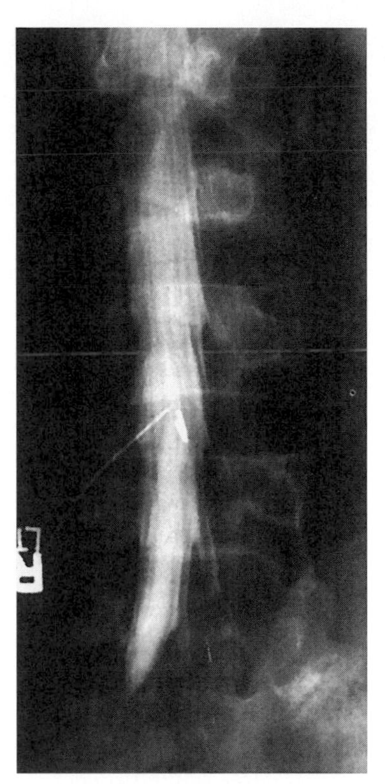

FIGURE 41–6 *Subarachnoid spread of contrast medium.*

the outline of the nerve roots and the dura from the circumferential spread within the less resistant subdural space (Fig. 41–7). Injection of local anesthetic into the subarachnoid or subdural space will result in a motor block that is notably more profound and of more rapid onset than that subsequent to injection into the epidural space. A subdural block is often typified by a segmental motor block with a diffuse sensory block to the level expected from a subarachnoid injection of local anesthetic.

If CSF is aspirated, it is best to abort the procedure and repeat it another day. If blood is aspirated, the needle is

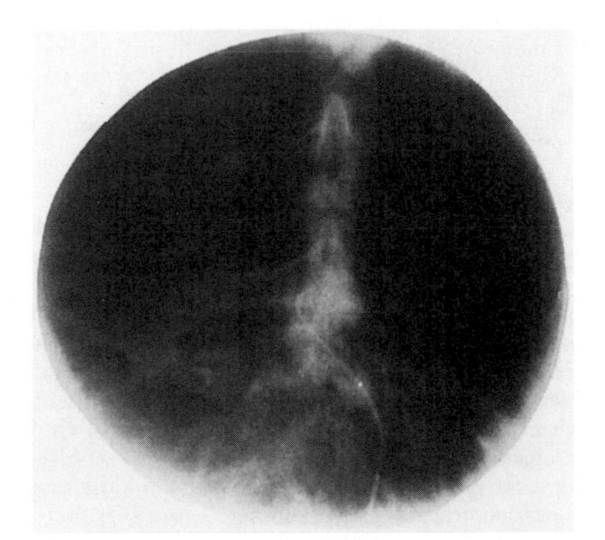

FIGURE 41–7 *Subdural spread of contrast medium. Observe the contrast medium spreading centrally, without a "Christmas tree" configuration. The catheter is in the central part of the canal.*

first retracted caudad in the sacral canal until no blood can be aspirated. If this is unsuccessful, an attempt can be made to proceed with catheter placement into the proper site. Aspiration through this catheter should be negative for blood, and lack of venous runoff should be confirmed with injection of contrast medium.

The ideal epidural catheter is a stainless steel, fluoropolymer-coated, spiral-tipped Racz Tun-L-Kath-XL.[10, 11] A Racz catheter is passed through the needle into the scar tissue (see Fig. 41–5B). The bevel of the needle should face the ventrolateral aspect of the caudal canal on the affected side. This facilitates passage of the catheter to the desired side and decreases the chance of shearing the catheter. Because scar formation is usually uneven, multiple passes may be necessary to place the catheter into the scarred area. For this reason, it is best to use a 16-gauge R-K epidural needle, which has been specially designed to allow multiple passes of the catheter.[12] To facilitate steering of the catheter into the desired location, a 15-degree bend is placed at its distal end. After final placement of the catheter and negative aspiration, another 5 to 10 mL of contrast medium is injected through the catheter. This additional dye should spread into the area of the previous filling defect and outline the targeted nerve root (see Fig. 41–5C). Then, 1500 units of Wydase (hyaluronidase) in 10 mL of preservative-free saline is injected rapidly. Afterward and after negative aspiration, 10 mL of 0.2% ropivacaine and 40 mg of triamcinolone are injected through the catheter in divided doses. This additional volume promotes further lysis of adhesions, because the catheter tip is in the scar tissue. The area of scarring and subsequent scar dissection should be noted and recorded. Because steroids cannot be injected through the 0.2 micron bacteriostatic filter, the steroid must be injected before the in-line filter is installed.

If contrast medium is not used because of an allergic history, the procedure is the same except for the absence of dye. Aspiration should be negative for CSF and blood before any injection. Additionally, a test dose of local anesthetic should be given to verify that the needle, and, subsequently, the catheter are not subarachnoid or subdural. When the needle is properly placed, the patient will often report pain with injection in the dermatomal distribution of the scarred area.

When the procedure is completed, the catheter should be secured to the skin with 2-0 nylon on a cutting needle. Caution must be exercised to avoid puncturing the catheter with the needle or cutting the catheter coating while wrapping it. The puncture site where the catheter exits is covered by a large clump of a triple-antibiotic ointment such as polymyxin, and two 2 × 2-inch split venous gauze dressings are used to cover the antibiotic ointment and prevent its spread outside the area of the gauze. The surrounding skin is sprayed or covered with tincture of benzoin, and, with a single curve of the catheter toward the midline, all of the above is covered with a 4 × 6-inch Opsite (Tegaderm) dressing. On top of the transparent dressing, we place two 4 × 4-inch gauzes over the course of the catheter from the puncture site and the subcutaneous portion of it toward the sacral hiatus, and apply over the area four 6-inch pieces of Hypafix tape. Hypafix has the unique properties of being elastic yet porous, so the patient will not "sweat it off" during the 3 days while the catheter remains in place. Before the sterile field is undraped, the catheter is connected to an adapter and to a bacteriostatic filter that is not removed until the three daily injections have been completed. The filter is capped, and the catheter is taped to the flank of the patient. During the hospitalization, the patient is given intravenous antibiotics in the form of cephalosporin (Rocephin), 1 g/day, to prevent bacterial colonization that is especially hazardous because of the epidurally administered steroid. It is also our practice to send a patient home with 5 more days' dosing of oral antibiotic for epidural abscess prophylaxis.

Once the patient is taken to the recovery room and vital signs are checked, 9 mL of 10% hypertonic saline is infused over 20 to 30 min. Occasionally, the patient may complain of severe burning pain during the infusion. The cause is usually the introduction of hypertonic saline into unanesthesized epidural tissue. Should this occur, the infusion must be stopped and another 3- to 5-mL bolus of local anesthetic is given. After 5 min, the hypertonic saline infusion can be restarted without incident. After completion of the hypertonic saline infusion, 1.5 mL of preservative-free normal saline is used to flush the catheter. Once this task is completed the cap is replaced on the filter.

The hypertonic saline has a mild, reversible local anesthetic effect and reduces edema in previously scarred or inflamed nerve roots.[13, 14] Injection of a hypertonic solution into the normal epidural space is quite painful unless local anesthetic is given first. If the hypertonic saline spreads farther than the area covered by the local anesthetic, the patient may have severe pain. The pain caused by the hypertonic saline in the epidural space rarely persists longer than 5 min.

The catheter is left in place for 3 days. On the second and third days, it is injected once a day with 10 mL of 0.2% ropivacaine after negative aspiration from the catheter. Fifteen minutes later, 10 mL of 10% saline is infused over 20 min for patient comfort. As in any hypertonic saline infusion series, the catheter must be flushed with 1.5 mL of preservative-free normal saline. On the third day, the catheter is removed 10 min after the last injection. A triple antibiotic ointment is placed on the wound and is covered with a bandage or another appropriate dressing.

While the catheter is indwelling, the patient should keep the insertion site dry. We also recommend that it be kept dry for the first 48 hours after removal to reduce the chance of infection. Showering is permitted thereafter. Immersing the wound, as in a bathtub or therapy pool, should be avoided for at least 7 to 10 days.

This procedure is usually followed by significant improvement in pain and motor function. As pain is relieved, it is important to initiate aggressive physical therapy to improve muscle strength and tone, which are usually reduced by disease secondary to pain. Often, it is not possible to lyse existing epidural adhesions completely because of the extensive scar tissue. If necessary, we repeat the procedure. Because of the steroids, a 3-month delay between procedures is necessary, during which time the patient should be encouraged to continue intensive physical therapy. This therapy should begin immediately, when possible. Neural flossing, especially while the local anesthetic is still active, provides a prime opportunity to maximize adhesiolysis with the least discomfort to the patient. One month of aquatic therapy followed by aggressive, graded physical therapy and work hardening is also recommended.

CERVICAL, THORACIC, AND LUMBAR AREAS

The technique for lysis of epidural adhesions in these areas of the spinal cord must be modified to ensure that initially the needle is positioned in the epidural space and to avoid spinal cord compression by subsequent injections.

The patient is placed in the left lateral position on the fluoroscopy table. When placing the catheter in the cervical region, it is necessary to tilt the patient's right shoulder forward slightly, to move the shoulder out of the way. With the fluoroscopy C arm in the vertical position, which actually provides a lateral view of the spine, the bases of the spinous processes are visualized. This allows a view of the spinous processes, which would otherwise be obscured by the ribs. After preparation and draping using sterile technique, a 16-gauge epidural needle (preferably an R-K needle) is advanced with the stylet in place to the ligamentum flavum. In the cervical and thoracic regions, a paramedian approach is usually easier than a midline approach because of the angle of the spinous processes. When placing a catheter in the cervical area, the C7–T1 or T1–T2 interspaces are usually the easiest points of entry. Skin entry should be 1.5 to 2 levels below the desired epidural entry point to facilitate catheter placement. After local anesthetic is used on the skin, an 18-gauge needle is inserted through the same puncture site to form an entry wound. Through the puncture site, a 16-gauge epidural needle is first advanced under fluoroscopic guidance (anteroposterior view) to determine the *direction* of the needle. Next, in the lateral view, the needle is advanced to the point just before the "straight line" formed by the fluoroscopic image of the anterior border of the spinous process in the lateral view (the insertion site of the ligamentum flavum). The lateral view under fluoroscopy demonstrates the *depth* of needle placement. Last, an anteroposterior view is checked again to confirm the *direction* of the needle. When the direction is satisfactory, the loss-of-resistance technique with a Pulsator (Concord Labs) syringe filled halfway with normal (0.9%) saline and halfway with air is used to advance the needle into the epidural space.

A Racz Tun-L-Kath or Racz Tun-L-Kath-XL epidural catheter is passed in an anterocephalad direction toward the filling defect outlined by the dye, until the catheter tip enters the scarred area. The catheter adapter is attached to the external end of the catheter for injection. After negative aspiration, 1 to 3 mL of nonionic dye is injected while observing the fluoroscope screen for spread within the adhesions (Fig. 41–8). Once an outflow or runoff tract is seen (i.e., either opening of the neuroforamina or caudal spread), 3 to 5 mL of 0.9% preservative-free saline with 1500 units hyaluronidase is injected. Last, 0.2% ropivacaine (4 mL) and 40 mg (1 mL) triamcinolone diacetate are injected after negative aspiration, watching for displacement of the dye. For safety purposes, the local anesthetic is given in divided doses to first rule out intrathecal subdural (1–2 mL), or intravascular injection. Five minutes later

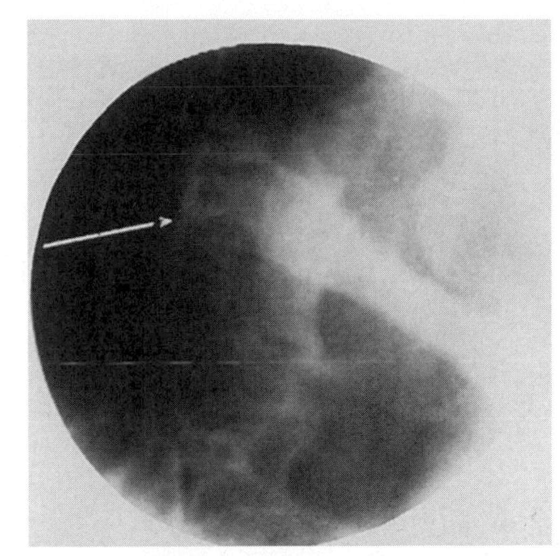

FIGURE 41–8 Epidurogram of the cervical area shows contrast medium spreading proximally and caudally, as indicated by the arrows.

the rest of the volume of the local anesthetic and steroid is injected.

The volume of ropivacaine injected depends on the level where the tip of the catheter lies. If the tip is in the cervical region (Fig. 41–9), we use 4 mL of 0.2% ropivacaine and triamcinolone diacetate. If it is in the thoracic region, we use 8 mL; and if the tip is in the lumbar region, 10 mL. The catheter is then secured, as described for the caudal approach. Thirty minutes later, 10% saline is injected after negative aspiration, as described before, in small increments on slow infusion over 20 min. Again, the volume used is dependent on the location of the tip of the catheter. We use 4 mL of hypertonic saline in the cervical area, 7 mL in the thoracic area, and 9 mL in the lumbar area.

After noting negative aspiration, all solutions should be injected slowly. Initially, the fluoroscopic images often reveal massive epidural scar formation (Fig. 41–10). In Figure 41–10A, after 10 mL of Omnipaque-240, the dye can be seen to preferentially spread toward the right-hand side, opening up the right L4–L5 S1–S2 nerve roots, whereas on the left there is a complete filling defect of L4–S1 and partial filling of the L5 nerve root. In Figure 41–10B, a Racz Tun-L-Kath-XL catheter is threaded into the L5 neural foramen area, and through this, an injection of an additional 10 mL of Omnipaque is seen to open up the L5–S1 nerve root (see Fig. 41–10C) and to spread cephalad as evidenced by the disappearance of the L4–L5 disc space as the space is masked by the spreading contrast medium (see Fig. 41–10D). This is followed by the injection of 10 mL of preservative-free saline, 1500 units of hyaluronidase spreading to L4 and L5, and finally the 10 mL of 0.2% ropivacaine and 40 mL of triamcinolone (see Fig. 41–10E). In Figure 41–10F, the contrast is spreading up to L4, L5, and then to S1, evenly, almost in the shape of a Christmas tree. The foot drop dramatically improved the following day as a result of the decompression of the L4–S1 nerve roots by dissection of the perineural space with the injected material.

We inject only one dose of steroid and do it in the operating room under strictly sterile conditions. After the

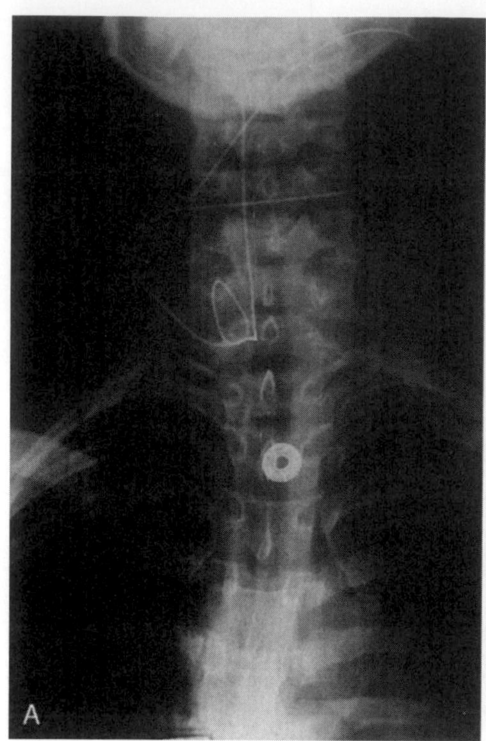
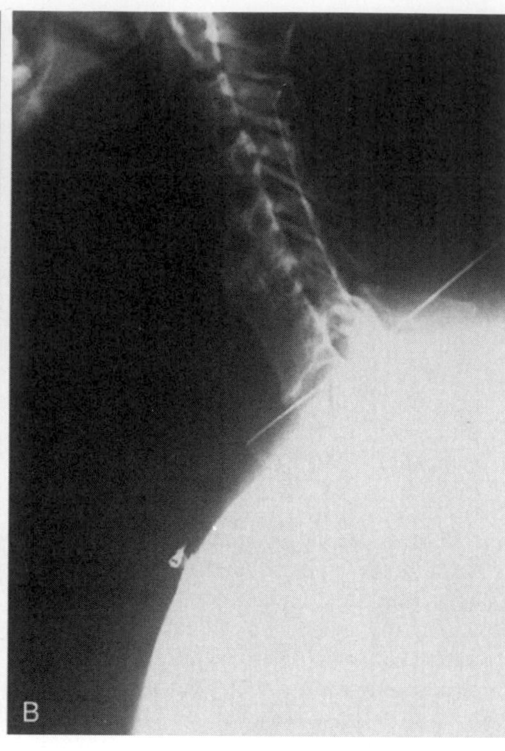

FIGURE 41–9 A, Anteroposterior view of a cervical catheter shows placement on the right side of the epidural space in a patient with right arm pain. B, Lateral view of cervical catheter.

bacteriostatic filter is placed, it is not removed during the subsequent series of injections. We have demonstrated in our laboratory that, when methylprednisolone (Depo-Medrol plus local anesthetic or triamcinolone (Aristocort) and local anesthetic are injected through a bacteriostatic filter, the filter screens out virtually all of the steroid.[15]

When scarring is severe, a transforaminal approach is used in the lumbar region. Using fluoroscopy in an oblique view (approximately 18 degrees to the ipsilateral side and 18 degrees caudocephalad), the designated foraminal level is targeted for skin entry with a Kelly's clamp. Lidocaine, 1%, is injected at the selected entry site with a 25-gauge needle. Through the same puncture site, an 18-gauge needle is used to enlarge the wound for easier entry of the epidural needle. Before insertion of the R-K epidural needle, a 15-degree bend is made 1.0 cm from the tip. While inserting the epidural needle, the top of the ear of the "Scottie dog," or the superior pars articularis, should first be hit with the tip of the needle. After bone is hit, the needle is turned laterally to slide past the pars articularis. Just as the needle slides into the foramen, a "pop" is felt. The advance of the needle should be stopped before the nerve root is contacted. Insertion is stopped and the needle bevel turned medially. A Racz Tun-L-Kath is passed through the needle, slid by the anterior nerve root, and placed in the anterior spinal canal, just medial to the pedicle in the anteroposterior view. To confirm proper placement, 1 to 3 mL of nonionic contrast can be used. The catheter is secured in place as for the caudal catheter (see earlier). If both this catheter and a catheter placed caudally are being used, 5 to 6 mL of local anesthetic and steroids are injected in divided doses. The volume of the caudally placed catheter is reduced to 7 to 8 mL of local anesthetic and steroids. Hypertonic saline infusion volume is likewise decreased to match the volume of local anesthetic and steroids injected.

PATIENT DATA

We have reviewed data from 4500 patients treated by the lysis-of-adhesions technique between the beginning of 1989 through 2000. We randomly selected 100 patients. Fifty had one dose of triamcinolone plus local anesthetic followed by hypertonic saline on the first day, and on the second and third days only the local anesthetic injection. The other 50 patients had, in addition, 1500 units of hyaluronidase injected in the operating room before the injection of local anesthetic and steroid, followed by 10% sodium chloride. The patient data were reviewed for demographics and duration of pain relief. Telephone follow-up was carried out by a disinterested third party, who strictly tabulated the patient responses, which, in some instances, were collected as long as 3 years after treatment. The results are tabulated in Figures 41–11 and 41–12, where the patients are separated according to hyaluronidase therapy and by gender, and their experience categorized as having had no relief, being completely pain free at the time of review, and having had partial relief, measured in months. In the "non-hyaluronidase" group, the failure rate was 18%; 14% of the patients were pain-free at the time of the review; and 68% of the patients reported pain relief measured in months. In the hyaluronidase group, the complete failure rate was 6.1%; persistent relief, 12.3%; and pain relief of some duration, 81.6%.

A prospective study involving 83 patients evaluated the efficacy of isotonic saline, hypertonic saline, hypertonic saline with hyaluronidase, and isotonic saline with hyal-

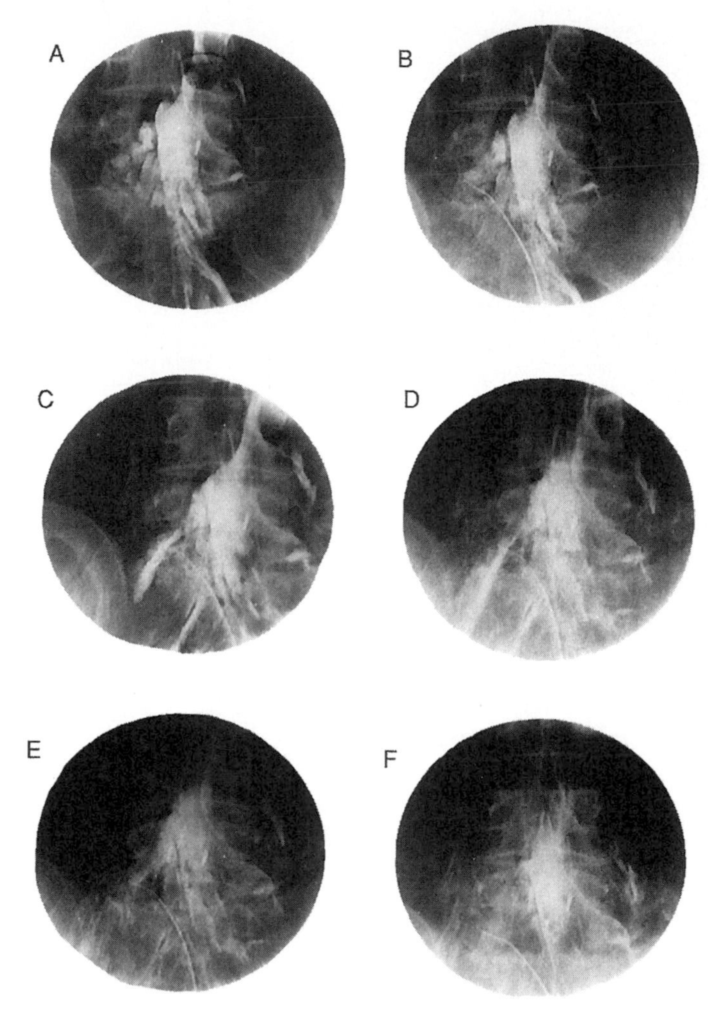

FIGURE 41–10 *Radiographs from patient with left lower extremity pain and footdrop.* A, *After 10 mL of Omnipaque 240. Note complete filling defect on left at L4 and S1 and partial filling of the L5 spinal nerve.* B, *Racz Tun-L-Kath XL threaded into L5 neural foramen.* C, *After injection of another 10 mL of Omnipaque, note opening of L5–S1 nerve root and cephalad spread of contrast medium.* D–F, *Further opening of filling defect and cephalad spread of contrast medium.*

uronidase. Of the 83 patients recruited, 59 completed the study. From this group the reported relief was greatest immediately after treatment, and 25% of the 59 patients reported residual benefit after 1, 3, 6, 9, and 12 months).[16] The 1-year follow-up of these patients did reveal 49% persistent pain relief in the area of the targeted lesion.[17]

COMPLICATIONS

Potential hazards of this neuroplasty include unintentional subarachnoid or subdural injection of local anesthetic or hypertonic saline, paralysis, bowel or bladder dysfunction, and infection. Careful attention to sterile technique is necessary, because steroids suppress the immune system, so the risk of infection is increased. Hypertonic saline injected into the subarachnoid space has been reported to cause cardiac arrhythmias, paresis, and loss of sphincter control.[9]

All injections should be made slowly. Rapid injections into the epidural space may cause large increases in CSF pressure, which could, in turn, produce cerebral hemorrhage, visual disturbances, headache, or compromised spinal cord blood flow.

At our institution, we have performed the technique described above for lysis of epidural adhesions in more than 4500 patients, with very few complications. We have rarely had a subarachnoid or subdural injection of local anesthetic. The two patients who developed meningitis responded to antibiotic therapy. We have had no patients with paralysis from this procedure, although one did have transient motor weakness after a caudal procedure where solid proximal adhesions prevented runoff of injected solution. We have seen no significant bowel or bladder problems using this technique, although a few patients have noted mild difficulty voiding for as long as 2 weeks after the procedure. Occasionally, transient perineal numbness has been reported, which is usually self-limiting and resolves in 1 to 2 months.

In one patient who had extremely severe failed back surgery syndrome with partial paralysis and inversion of a foot, the gradual development of arachnoiditis was not recognized because of the hardware in her back. The patient had not had interventional radiologic studies. The patient underwent lysis of adhesions, but the proce-

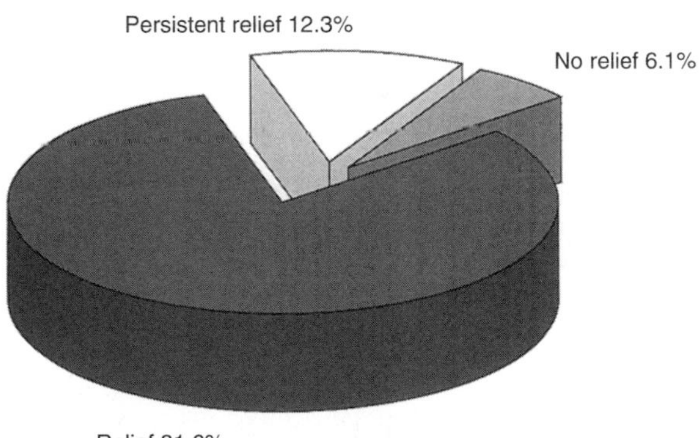

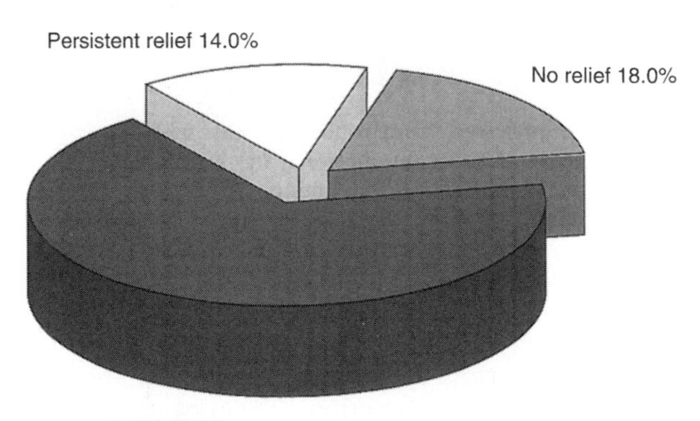

FIGURE 41–11 *Pain relief in patients treated,* A, *with and,* B, *without hyaluronidase. Percentages of the 50 patients treated are shown.*

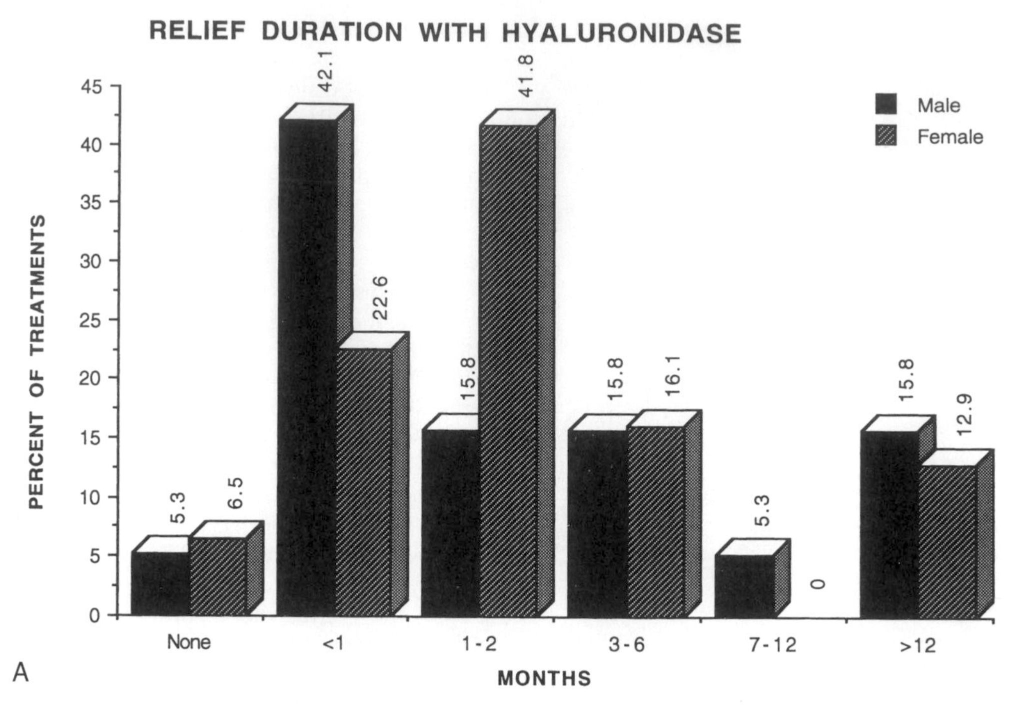

FIGURE 41–12 *Duration of pain relief in patients treated,* A, *with and,* B, *without hyaluronidase.*

dure was aborted because of the development of a motor block after injection of local anesthetic without any injection of hypertonic saline. The patient had preexisting bowel and bladder dysfunction; however, the full extent of her neurologic deficit was not appreciated because of the overwhelming concern for her partial paralysis, spasm, and pain. After she recovered motor function, the patient was left with bowel and bladder deficits. She was not able to void without catheterization and developed fecal incontinence. Subsequent diagnostic studies (myelography) showed massive constrictive arachnoiditis. Her pain was subsequently managed by the placement of a subarachnoid morphine pump. The fecal incontinence slowly resolved, but, because of the arachnoiditis and preexisting neurogenic bladder, the patient must do self-catheterization.

The concern regarding preexisting neurogenic bladders in multisurgical failed back or spinal cord injury patients has resulted in increased awareness and cooperation with our urologist for the purpose of carrying out urodynamic studies and documenting the preexistence of neurogenic bladders. The typical experience is improvement in bladder function and in male sexual function after lysis of adhesions. Advanced documentation of neurogenic bladder has resulted in our getting better informed consent from our patient population, who certainly are at highest risk for ongoing constrictive arachnoiditis and, in turn, the development of clinically recognized bowel, bladder, and sexual dysfunction. In certain cases, patients are shown a videotape of the procedure which lists all of the possible complications and the expectations from the intractable progressive failed back syndrome dilemma. The surprising finding has been improvement in bladder function rather than the feared development of neurogenic bladder and related problems. Additionally, patients are warned that epidural infection is a distinct possibility because of both the instrumentation and the steroid injection, especially during the first 2 to 6 weeks after the procedure. Until it is proved otherwise, nausea, vomiting, neck stiffness, new pain, different pain, bigger pain, weakness, numbness, and/or paralysis that develop are considered to be signs and symptoms of procedurally related epidural infection. The patient needs to understand and report, either to the physician who performed the procedure or to the patient's own physician, any of these signs or symptoms, so that prompt intravenous antibiotic therapy can be given and the patient hospitalized until the condition clears up. As indicated earlier, this has not been a problem in our patient population, but that does not mean that watchfulness and caution can be relaxed. An unrecognized and untreated epidural abscess has potentially devastating consequences.

In our practice, catheter shearing does seem to occur every time we have a new group of pain fellows, until they develop the sensation of absence of free, smooth-flowing catheter within the needle, as we often have to withdraw through the specially designed RK needle to secure optimal positioning. The sheared catheter usually becomes hung up in the subcutaneous tissues or at the sacral hiatus. Of late, we have made it part of our consent form that, if a catheter is sheared, we will request surgical intervention to retrieve it. To date, we have had five such incidents. This technical "pearl" is worth remembering: To retrieve the sheared catheter, under fluoroscopic guidance, place two needles from different angles that will pinpoint the end of the sheared catheter. This makes removal through a half-inch incision a very simple affair. The view that sheared catheters are best left behind is simply not shared by those in our institution.

DISCUSSION

Clearly, lysis of adhesions in the epidural space is a procedure that must be used *after* simpler procedures, such as rest, nonsteroidal antiinflammatory medications, muscle relaxants, physical therapy, activity programs, two or three single shots of epidural steroid, and transcutaneous electrical nerve stimulation. Better-informed patients will opt for procedures such as lysis of adhesions rather than surgery. The results clearly show a dramatic decline in the need for further surgical interventions in our patient population and complete avoidance of surgical intervention in appropriately selected patients with clearly documented herniated discs and nerve root compression. This awareness is gaining support by having the United States regulatory agencies, as well as courts, recognize the effectiveness of lysis of adhesions.[6]

Scarring in the epidural space frequently occurs after surgery and causes no problems. Scarring can follow leakage of nucleus pulposus material into the epidural space.[1] The pain associated with the scar formation originates from the nerve itself, which is irritated, swollen, and angry looking and has no room to move freely. Normally, epidural scarring involves the nerves as they enter the neural foramina and the epidural veins when surrounding scar obstructs venous runoff. The obstruction raises intravenous pressure, which promotes additional edema formation in the epidural space.

The technique described above overcomes the obstacle of being able to get the medication to a lesion specific site by placing the tip of a soft spring catheter within the scar and letting the injected fluid under pressure find the path of least resistance within the scar and open up the perineural space. Thus, steroid can reach the inflamed, angry nerve root and produce its antiinflammatory effect. The hyperosmolar sodium chloride solution will reach and block the nerve roots (together with the local anesthetic) and give additional pain relief. Our previous studies demonstrate that the chloride ion does not readily move across the dura, which very likely is the explanation for the absence of feared complications that previously were reported after subarachnoid infusion of hypertonic saline.[18–27] Hitchcock's early work with iced saline irrigation of the subarachnoid space in cancer pain was followed by complications, which included bowel or bladder dysfunction, hypertension, paralysis, raised intracranial pressure, seizures as a consequence of the chloride ion, and hyperosmolar solution expanding and putting pressure on the spinal cord and the central nervous system.[28] Injection of hypertonic saline into the epidural space causes extremely severe pain. Therefore, the operator must inject local anesthetic before injecting hypertonic saline. If there is a significant sensory and motor block after 0.2% ropivacaine, that in itself should be enough reason to abort the procedure without injecting the hypertonic saline. This is very likely the explanation for why we have done such a large series of procedures without many or serious complications.

The addition of hyaluronidase has resulted in threefold reduction of outright failures in our patient population, and this needs to be investigated further to determine whether we are looking at a volume effect or if the addition of hyaluronidase really makes the difference. We are sufficiently convinced that the hyaluronidase is helpful that we are continuing to inject it. Hyaluronidase has been studied from the first report of this enzyme in 1929 by Duran-Reynals, when he labeled it *spreading factor*.[29] In 1520 epidural administrations of hyaluronidase Moore reported a 3% rate of sensitivity reactions.[29] We believe that we have not seen this rate in our series because we place the steroid exactly at the site where the hyaluronidase is deposited and the steroid leaves the space more slowly than does hyaluronidase. We are looking very carefully for evidence of sensitivity reaction in our patients who receive hyaluronidase. The threefold reduction of outright therapeutic failure, we believe, is sufficient justification to continue the administration of hyaluronidase in our patients.

Patients who benefit from lysis of adhesions include those with failed back surgery, disc disruption, vertebral body compression fracture, spinal stenosis, metastatic carcinoma, multilevel degenerative arthritis, facet pain, epidural scarring after infection, meningitis or severe pain that spinal cord stimulator or spinal opioids fail to control, compression fracture secondary to cancer metastases, and osteoporotic compression fractures—generally speaking, conditions that lead to radiculopathy.

The overall principle is always to start the injection from below the problem area. Especially in the cervical thoracic area, the rate of injection has to be very slow. Continuous cooperation and discussion with the patient must be maintained, and fluoroscopic evidence for fluid runoff is to be observed continuously. We use the lateral approach in dissecting the adhesions, especially in the cervical area, where placement of the catheter near the neural foramina is less likely to lead to spinal cord compression in the anteroposterior direction. It is not unusual to succeed in freeing up cervical nerve roots all the way up to the C2 area after three or four attempts and, subsequently, gratifying pain relief or the ability to place a spinal cord stimulator if the pain relief is judged to be less than satisfactory by the patient. A lesion that responds very well to the three daily injections of local anesthetic and hypertonic saline frequently indicates a good outcome. Not infrequently, we can do only one side and come back 3 months later to repeat the injection series on the other side.

Measuring pain is always difficult, but the effectiveness of lysis is evidenced, for example, in patients who have ongoing morphine subarachnoid infusion but do not have adequate pain relief. For example, one patient was receiving 120 mg/day of morphine through a Synchromed pump. Within 4 days after the lysis-of-adhesions procedure, we were able to reduce the morphine dose to 60 mg. This effect lasted 9 months, and the patient described the experience as "the best 9 months I have had in years." By the time the procedure had to be repeated, 1 year after the original one, the morphine dose was up to 80 mg/day. The repeat lysis of adhesions for the intractable back and leg pain in this failed back surgery patient again allowed us to reduce the daily dose of morphine. We have had numerous similar experiences with patients in whom spinal cord stimulation failed to give satisfactory relief. After lysis of adhesions on the most extensively involved nerve root area, a dramatic improvement resulted; this finding suggests synergism between neuroaugmentation by cord stimulation and lysis of adhesions.

For a very important subgroup of patients who suffer from cancer pain, oral or spinal opioids do not control movement-related pain. Inevitably, this is due to painful, swollen, angry nerve roots that are involved in compression fracture a condition no different from other similar mechanical irritants of the nerve roots. Based on our experience, the enhancement of the spinal or oral opioid will last some 3 to 4 months in this patient population, which makes a big difference in their movement-related pain and, therefore, their activities of daily living.

In summary, epidurography is a valuable diagnostic tool for locating filling defects that prevent the application of pain medications to angry, swollen, spinal epidural nerves. When patient selection criteria and the treatment method described here are used, the therapeutic success rate is high.

REFERENCES

1. McCarron RF, Wimpee MW, Hudkins PG, Laros GS: The inflammatory effect of the nucleus pulposus: A possible element in the pathogenesis of low back pain. Spine 12:760–764, 1987.
2. Barsa JE, Charlton JE: Diagnosis of epidural scarring and its possible contribution to chronic low back pain syndrome. Pain S4:S376, 1984.
3. Sicard JA, Forestier J: Methode radiographique d'exploration de la cavite epidurale par le Lipiodol. Rev Neurol 2; 8:1264, 1921.
4. Bogduk N, Brazenor G, Christiophidis N, et al: Epidural use of steroids in the management of back pain and sciatica of spinal origin. Commonwealth of Australia, National Health and Medical Research Council, 1994, pp 7–76.
5. Bogduk N, Aprill C, Derby R: Epidural steroid injections. *In* White AH, Schofferman JA (eds): Spinecare: Diagnosis and Conservative Treatment, vol 1. St Louis, CV Mosby, 1995, pp 302–343.
6. Racz GB, Holubec JT: Lysis of adhesions in the epidural space. *In* Racz GB (ed): Techniques of Neurolysis. Boston, Kluwer Academic, 1989, pp 57–72.
7. Manchikanti L, Bakhit CE, Pampati V: Role of epidurography in caudal neuroplasty. Pain Digest 8:277–281, 1998.
8. Gupta RC, Gupta SC, Dubey RK: An experimental study of different contrast media in the epidural space. Spine 9:778–781, 1984.
9. Racz GB, Heavner JE, Singleton W, Carline M: Hypertonic saline and corticosteroid injected epidurally for pain control. *In* Racz GB (ed): Techniques of Neurolysis. Boston, Kluwer Academic, 1988, pp 73–86.
10. Racz GB, Sabonghy M, Gintautas J, Kline WM: Intractable pain therapy using a new epidural catheter. JAMA 248:579–581, 1982.
11. Racz GB, Haynsworth RF, Lipton S: Experiences with an improved epidural catheter. Pain Clinic 1:21–27, 1986.
12. Racz GB, Kline WN: New epidural adapter and epidural needle. *In* Racz GB (ed): Techniques of Neurolysis. Boston, Kluwer Academic, 1988.
13. Katz J (ed): Atlas of Regional Anesthesia. Norwalk, Conn., Appleton-Century-Crofts, 1985, p 124.
14. MacNab I: The mechanism of spondylogenic pain. *In* Hirsch C, Zotterman Y (eds): Cervical Pain. Oxford, Pergamon, 1972, pp 89–94.
15. Racz GB, Heavner JE: Aristocort and Depo-Medrol passage through a 0.2-micron filter (Abstract). Reg Anesth 15(1S):25, 1991.
16. Heavner JE, Racz GB, Raj P: Percutaneous epidural neuroplasty: Prospective evaluation of 0.9% NaCl versus 10% NaCl with or without hyaluronidase. Reg Anesth Pain Med 24:202–207, 1999.
17. Racz GB, Heavner JE, Raj PP: Percutaneous epidural neuroplasty: Prospective one-year follow-up. Pain Digest 9:97–102, 1999.
18. Hitchcock E: Osmolytic neurolysis for intractable facial pain. Lancet 1:434–436, 1969.
19. Myers RR, Katz J: Neuropathology of neurolytic and semidestructive agents. *In* Cousins MJ, Bridenbaugh PO (eds): Neural Blockade, ed 2. Philadelphia, JB Lippincott, 1990, pp 567–568.
20. Lake DA, Barnes CD: Effects of changes in osmolality on spinal cord activity. Exp Neurol 68:555–567, 1980.
21. Ventafridda V, Spreavice R: Subarachnoid saline perfusion. Adv Neurol 4:477–484, 1974.
22. Squire AW, Calvillo O, Bromage PR: Painless intrathecal hypertonic saline. Can Anesth Soc J 21:308–314, 1974.
23. Jewett DL, King JS: Conduction block of monkey dorsal rootlets by water and hypertonic saline solutions. Exp Neurol 33:225–237, 1971.
24. King JS, Jewett DL, Sundberg HR: Differential blockade of cat dorsal root C-fibers by various chloride solutions. J Neurosurg 36:569–583, 1972.
25. Kukita F, Yamagishi KF: Excitation of squid giant axons in hypotonic and hypertonic solutions. Jpn J Physiol 20:669–681, 1979.

26. Swerdlow M: Complications of neurolytic neural blockade. In Cousins MJ, Bridenbaugh PO (eds): Neural Blockade. Philadelphia, JB Lippincott, 1980, pp 543–553.
27. Hitchcock ER: Hypothermic subarachnoid irrigation. Lancet 1:330, 1967.
28. Payne JN, Ruff NY: The use of hyaluronidase in caudal block anesthesia. Anesthesiology 12:162–172, 1951.
29. Moore DC: The use of hyaluronidase in local and nerve block analgesia other than spinal block: 1520 cases. Anesthesiology 12:611–626, 1951.

CHAPTER • 42

Facet Block and Neurolysis

Dan P. Gray, MD • Zahid H. Bajwa, MD
Carol A. Warfield, MD

HISTORY

Spinal pain, especially lumbar and cervical, is very prevalent in our society. Chronic low back pain is second only to the common cold as the most common affliction of mankind and is perhaps the most common chronic pain syndrome.[1] In most industrialized countries the lifetime prevalence of back pain is greater than 60%, and the annual incidence is at least 5%.[1–4] Some recent studies have suggested that the chronicity or recurrence of low back pain is actually 35% to 79% of patients.[5] Back pain incapacitates up to 20% of workers for long periods (>4 weeks), and absorbs approximately 40% of the cost of workers' compensation. The estimated total annual cost in the United States was $15 billion in 1984, then $24 billion in 1990, and now is most certainly even higher.[5–7] In 1998 in the United Kingdom, the direct healthcare cost was estimated to be £1632 million and the cost of informal care and production losses was estimated to be an additional £10,668 million.[8]

The lumber facet (zygapophyseal) joint has long been considered by some to be a significant source of low back pain. The prevalence of cervical pain approaches that of lumbar spine pain,[9] and recently the cervical facet joint has been shown to be a significant source of chronic neck pain.[10–12] The thoracic facet joints are a less firmly established cause of back pain.

Goldthwait, in 1911, first stated that the peculiarities of the facet joints were responsible for low back pain and instability.[12a, 13, 14] Like many clinicians of that time, he was struck by the asymmetry of the facet joints seen on x-ray studies. He believed that the joint asymmetry could cause pain from nerve root pressure.[15, 16] The Italian surgeon Putti published an article in 1927 that supported Goldthwait's earlier findings and focused specifically on articular facet degeneration as a cause of pain.[14, 17] In 1933, Ghormley[16] was the first to describe *facet syndrome*, which he defined as lumbosacral pain with or without sciatic pain, particularly occurring suddenly after a twisting or rotatory strain of the lumbosacral region. In addition, his initial discussion focused on the role of the facet joints, not the intervertebral discs, in creating nerve pressure and sciatica. In 1934, however, Mixter and Barr[18] described protrusion of lumbar discs as the most likely cause of low back pain. This description then overshadowed the role of facet joint disorders as a source of low back pain and sciatica.[19, 20]

In 1941, Badgley[21] made a plea to focus attention on the facets to explain the large numbers of patients with low back pain whose symptoms were not due to a ruptured disc. He showed that facet joint pathology could cause symptoms, including radiation of pain into the lower extremity. Badgley was the first clinician to associate facet arthritis with nerve root irritation as a cause of low back pain and sciatica. Hirsch and colleagues,[22] in 1963, were the first to demonstrate that low back pain distributed along the sacroiliac and gluteal areas with radiation to the greater trochanter could be induced by injecting hypertonic saline in the region of the facet joints. These findings were confirmed by Mooney and Robertson,[23] who in 1976 performed intraarticular facet injections with hypertonic saline and noted that the pain produced could be relieved by intraarticular injection of local anesthetics. In addition, Pawl[24] reported the reproduction of pain in patients after injecting hypertonic saline into their cervical facet joints.[25]

No specific therapeutic approach to facet syndrome emerged until the 1970s. Credit for advancing the concept of facet joint denervation as a therapy rests with the Australian physician W. E. S. Rees,[26] who proposed a surgical approach to severing the posterior sensory nerve.[27, 28] Subsequent dissections established the anatomy of dorsal facet innervation more precisely and thus paved the way for the more accurate and simpler percutaneous denervation techniques described by Shealy.[29] In fact, Shealy was the first to report the use of fluoroscopic localization of the facet joint in an attempt to specifically treat facet syndrome.[15, 29] Since then, much work has been done, particularly by N. Bogduk and his collaborators, to delineate the anatomy, incidence, and techniques for blocking spinal facet pain.

ANATOMY OF THE FACET JOINTS

The spine is usually made up of seven cervical, twelve thoracic, and five lumbar vertebrae. The vertebrae articu-

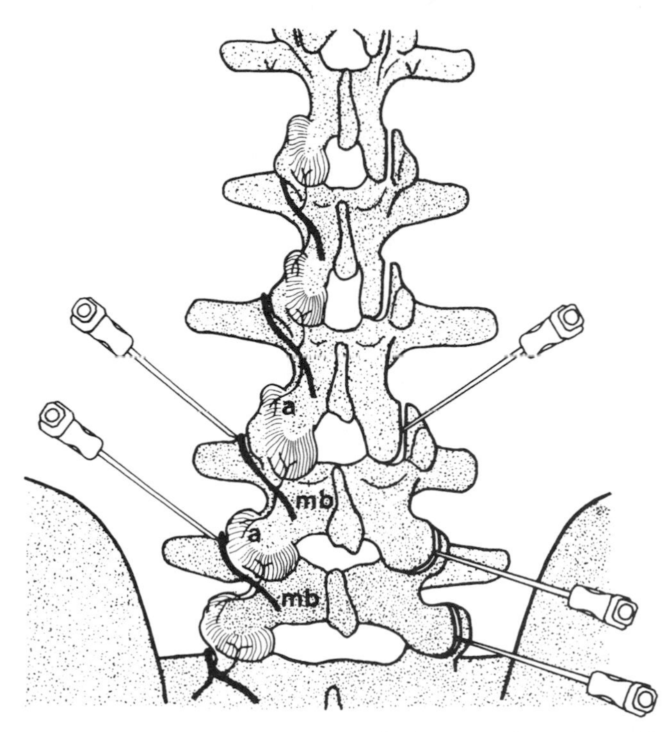

FIGURE 42–1 Sketch of the needle placements for lumbar medial branch blocks and lumbar intraarticular zygapophyseal blocks. On the left, the courses of the medial branches of the lumbar dorsal rami (mb) and their articular branches (a) are shown. Needles have been introduced onto the L3 and L4 medial branches, which would be anesthetized to block the L4–L5 joint. On the right, the needle placement for intraarticular blocks of the L3–L4, L4–L5, and L5–S1 zygapophyseal joints is depicted. (Bogduk N: Back pain: Zygapophyseal blocks and epidural steroids. In Cousins MJ, Bridenbaugh PO (eds): Neural Blockade in Clinical Anesthesia and Management of Pain, ed 2. Philadelphia, JB Lippincott, 1988, pp 935–946.)

late anteriorly through the discs and posteriorly through two facet joints (one right and one left). The facet joints are paired diarthrodial synovial joints formed by the inferior articular process of one vertebra and the superior articular process of the subjacent vertebra (Fig. 42–1).[2, 30–32] Biomechanically, this produces a complex, tripod structure that has evolved into distinctive patterns at each spinal level.

The facet joints share the same general characteristics of synovial joints. The articular surfaces are covered by cartilage, and a synovial membrane bridges the margins of the cartilages of the two facets in each joint. Covering the synovial membrane superiorly, posteriorly, and inferiorly is a thick fibrous joint capsule; however, anteriorly the synovial membrane lacks a true fibrous capsule and instead is in direct contact with the ligamentum flavum. Immediately anterior to the ligamentum flavum covering the facet joint is some adipose tissue in the epidural space. This adipose tissue is in direct contact with the nerve root dural sleeve (Fig. 42–2). The dural sleeve is so close to the anterior aspect of the facet joint that it is possible to pass a needle completely through the facet joint into cerebrospinal fluid.[33] Enlarged and osteophytic joints can contribute to significant narrowing of the neuroforaminal opening and compression of the nerve root.[34]

Superiorly and inferiorly, the fibrous joint capsule balloons out to form a pocket connected to the lumbar facet joint. Between the capsule pocket and the synovium are two structures. The first has been referred to as *meniscoid.* There are several descriptions of these menisci, but probably they are best understood as a fold of synovium that contains adipose tissue, collagen, and some blood vessels. The normal function of these meniscoids is not clear.[9, 34, 35] In diseased facet joints they have been implicated as a source of damage to the articular cartilage, causing

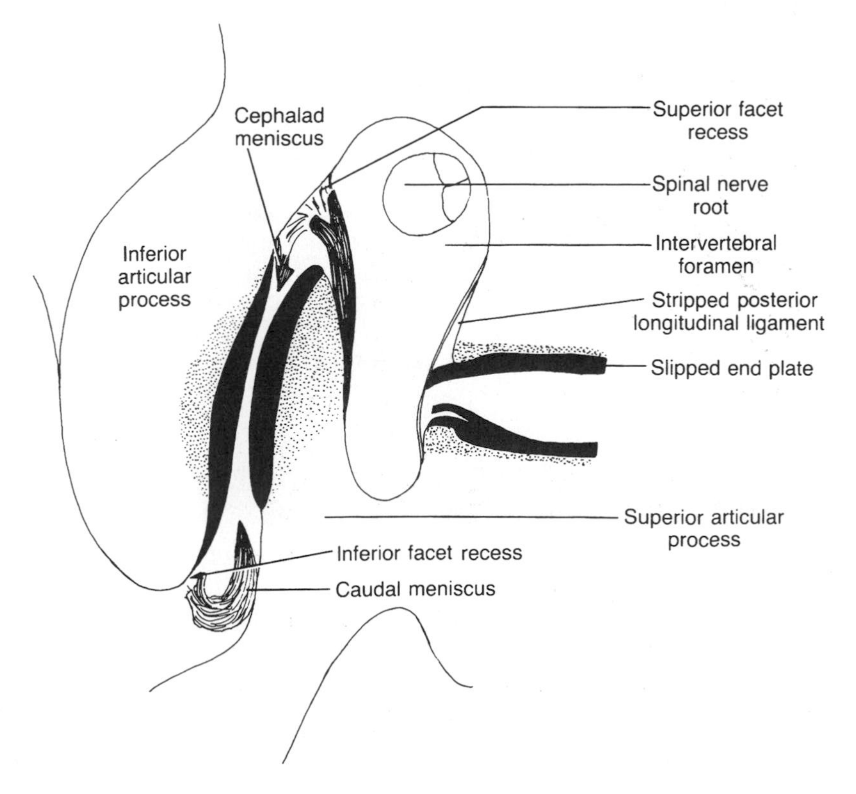

FIGURE 42–2 A segmental cross section through the facet joint and intervertebral foramen shows the mixed nerve root high up in the foramen close to the weakened upper portion of the facet capsule and superior articular recess. (Paris SV: Anatomy as related to function and pain. Orthop Clin North Am 14(3):475–489, 1983.)

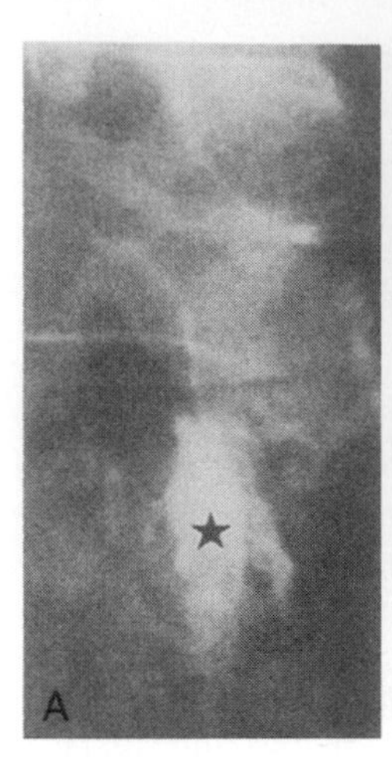

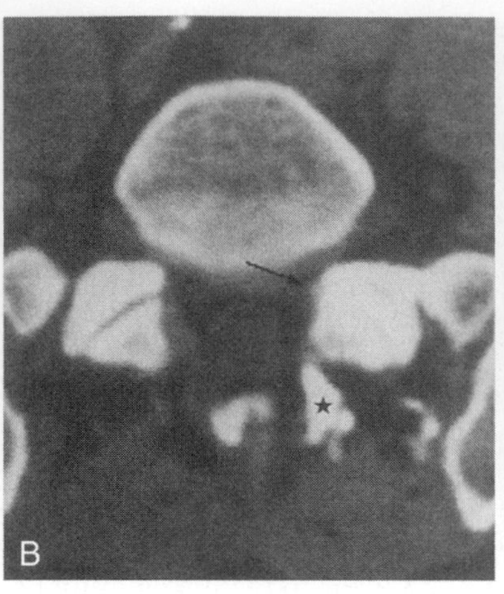

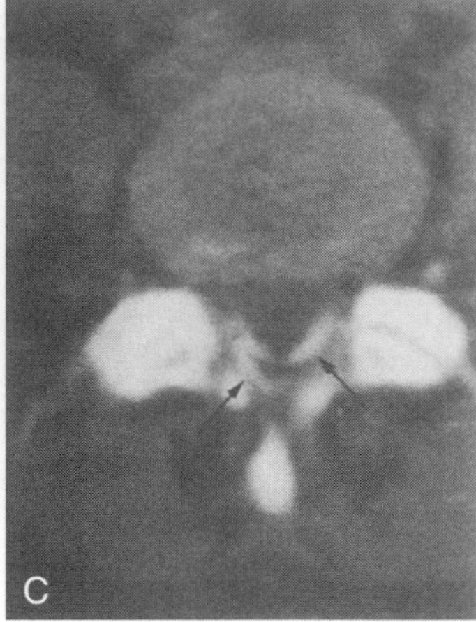

FIGURE 42–3 A, *L5–S1 left joint. Contrast medium leakage* (star) *at the inferior aspect of the capsule is seen after opacification.* B, *CT scan of the same patient demonstrates localization of the contrast medium leakage* (star). *Note the medial side of the capsule bulging slightly* (arrow) *near the intervertebral foramen.* C, *CT scan at L4–L5 disc level. The epidural space is opacified* (arrows) *after arthrography of both joints. (Dory MA: Arthrography of the lumbar facet joints. Radiology 140:23–27, 1981.)*

the facet joints to lock. The second structure is simply adipose tissue, which fills up any leftover space beneath the capsule. The superior and inferior parts of the capsule each have a hole. The superior hole connects the intracapsular fat to the epidural space.

The space enclosed by the articular cartilage and synovium contains synovial fluid. Computed tomography (CT), magnetic resonance imaging (MRI), or intraarticular contrast medium may demonstrate the extensions of the joint space along both the dorsal and medial aspects of the lumbar facet joint (Figs. 42–3, 42–4, 42–5).[36, 37] The lumbar joint space can distend to accommodate an additional 1 mL of fluid, and perhaps as much as 2 mL. Somewhere between 1 and 2 mL, the joint capsule will likely rupture and the excess fluid be extravasated into adjacent tissues.[38] Joint rupture may be manifested by spread of contrast dye injected to confirm intraarticular needle placement. The joint capsule may rupture at the inferior joint recess (Fig. 42–6)[39] or anteriorly through the ligamentum flavum into the epidural space overlying the dural sleeve (Fig. 42–7).[38] Joint rupture might also be suspected with a significant increase, and then a decrease, in resistance to intraarticular injection. In the thoracic spine the facet joint volume is the least of the three levels', and capsule rupture may occur after injection of 0.4 to perhaps 0.6 mL.[40, 41] The volume of injectate that will rupture a cervical facet joint is between 0.5 and 1 mL.[12, 42–44] In addition, abnormal communications between ipsilateral and contralateral lumbar facet joints are opened by spondylitic pars interarticularis defects, increasing the spread of injected agent (Figs. 42–8, 42–9).[37] This occurs because the pars defect is actually enclosed by the joint capsule; however, the spread between ipsilateral and contralateral facets is frequently seen with injection into cervical facet joints, although this may be more a function of volume injected with anterior extravasation.[42, 45]

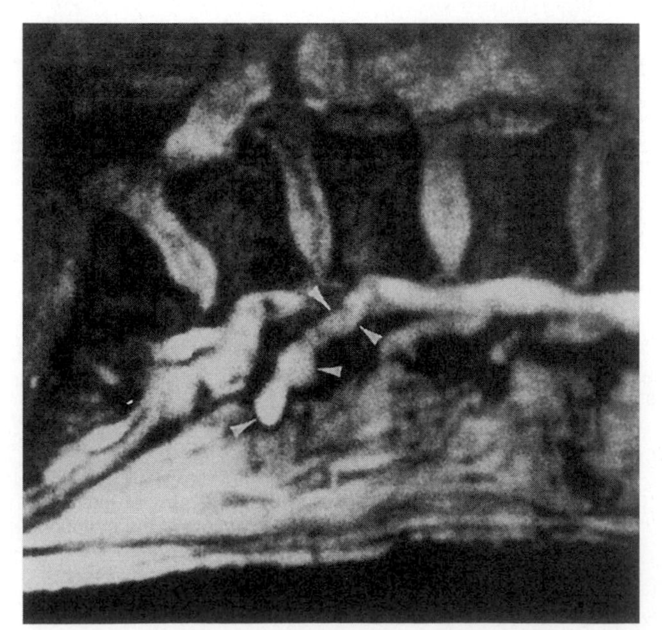

FIGURE 42–4 Fluid in facet joints. Distended superior synovial recess compressed thecal sac in a 66-year-old man who had progressively more severe lower back pain for 10 days. Sagittal T_2-weighted MR image (multiplanar, gradient-recalled fast scan; 500/15, flip angle 15) through medial aspect of facet joints on right side shows fluid-distended superior and inferior recesses at L4–L5 facet joint (arrowheads). *Patient reported relief from pain after fluid was drained. (El-Khoury GY, Reinfrew DL: Percutaneous procedures for the diagnosis and treatment of low back pain: Diskography, facet-joint injection, and epidural injection. AJR Am J Roentgenol 157:685–691, 1991.)*

In the upper lumbar spine, approximately 80% of the facet joints are curved and 20% are flat. In the lower lumbar spine the situation is reversed and approximately 80% of the facet joints are flat.[46] The upper lumbar facets are more oriented in the sagittal plane, and by the L5–S1 level they have rotated to a more oblique angle. The facet joints are oriented lateral to the sagittal plane from the midline posteriorly as follows: the L1–L2 joint 30 degrees or less, the L2–L3 joint 15 to 45 degrees, the L3–L4 joint 30 to 60 degrees, and the L4–L5 and L5–S1 joints 30 to 75 degrees.[46–51] The lumbar facets are all almost vertically oriented, being tipped approximately 10 degrees with the cephalad end of the joint farther anterior than the caudad end of the joint (Figs. 42–10, 42–11).[51] Because of the curvature of the upper lumbar facet joints, the posterior opening is usually more in the sagittal plane than the overall angle of the joint. This usually means that the accessible posterior joint space opening is usually 5 to 10 degrees less oblique than the best fluoroscopic image, which shows the angle of the joint overall.

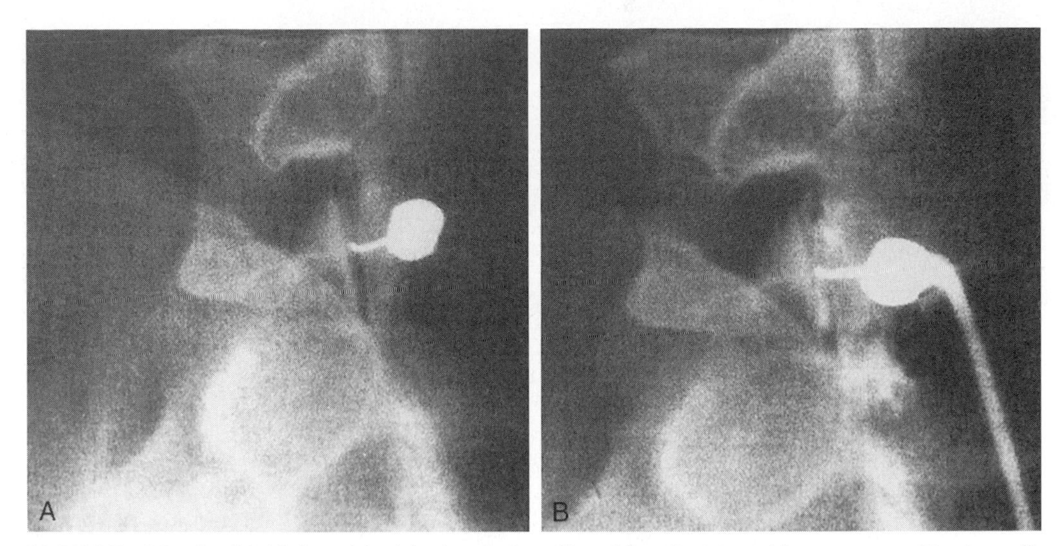

FIGURE 42–5 L4–L5 facet joint injection. A, Spot film with patient turned from prone position to profile facet joint being injected (L5–S1). Needle is advanced perpendicular to the joint until its tip is within the joint. B, During injection, contrast material flows away from the needle; typically, contrast material collects in superior and inferior recesses and to a lesser extent between articulating facets. (El-Khoury GY, Reinfrew DL: Percutaneous procedures for the diagnosis and treatment of low back pain: Diskography, facet-joint injection, and epidural injection. AJR Am J Roentgenol 157:685–691, 1991.)

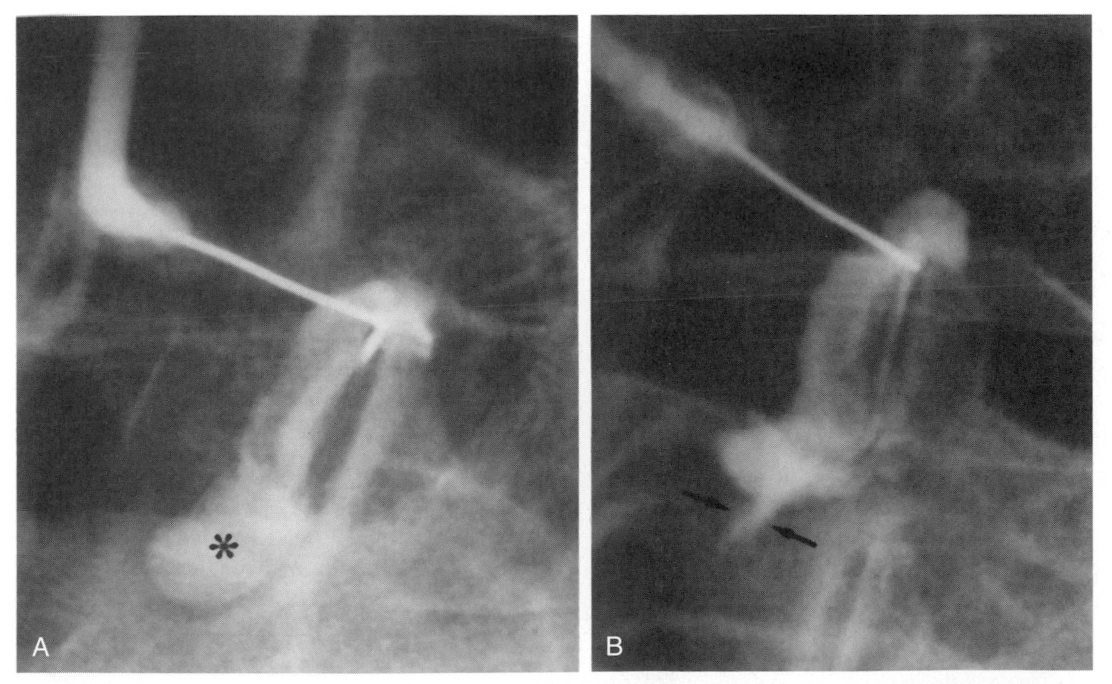

FIGURE 42–6 A, L5–S1 right facet joint (patient prone) during opacification. Note the large inferior recess (star). B, L4–L5 right facet joint (patient prone) at the end of opacification. The capsule has ruptured at the inferior recess (arrows). (Dory MA: Arthrography of the lumbar facet joints. Radiology 140:23–27, 1981.)

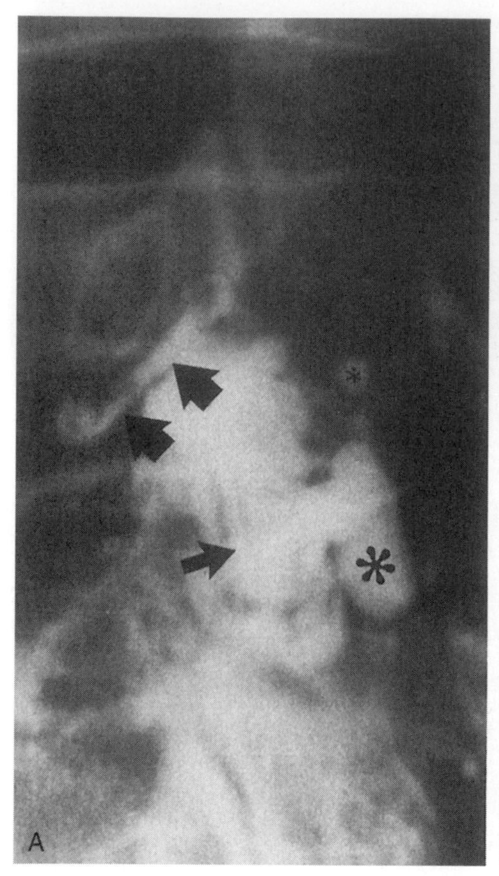

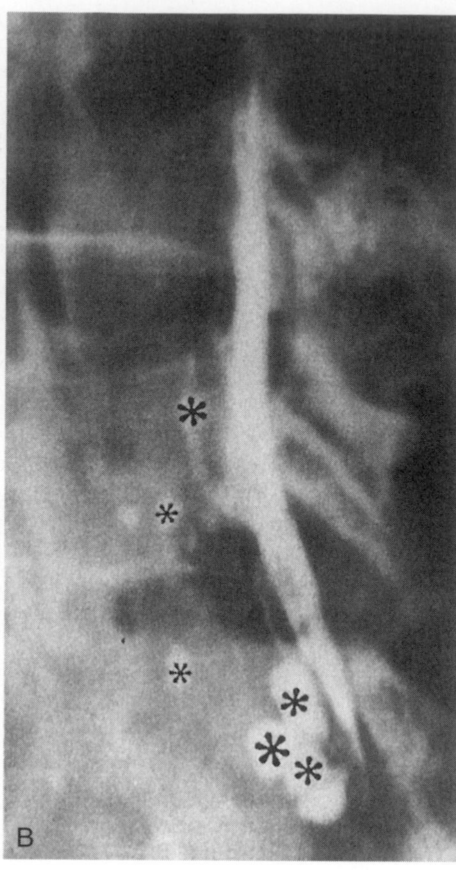

FIGURE 42–7 A, Arthrography after injection of 1.5 mL metrizamide. The contrast material is present in the joint space (small arrow). Extravasation into the intervertebral foramen is documented by opacification of the epidural space below the segmental nerve (large arrows). B, Injection of a total volume of 3 mL (same patient, opposite oblique projection) resulted in epidurography. Note persisting oily contrast material in the subarachnoid space from a previous myelogram. (Raymond J, Dumas J: Intraarticular facet block: Diagnostic test or therapeutic procedure? Radiology 151:333–336, 1984.)

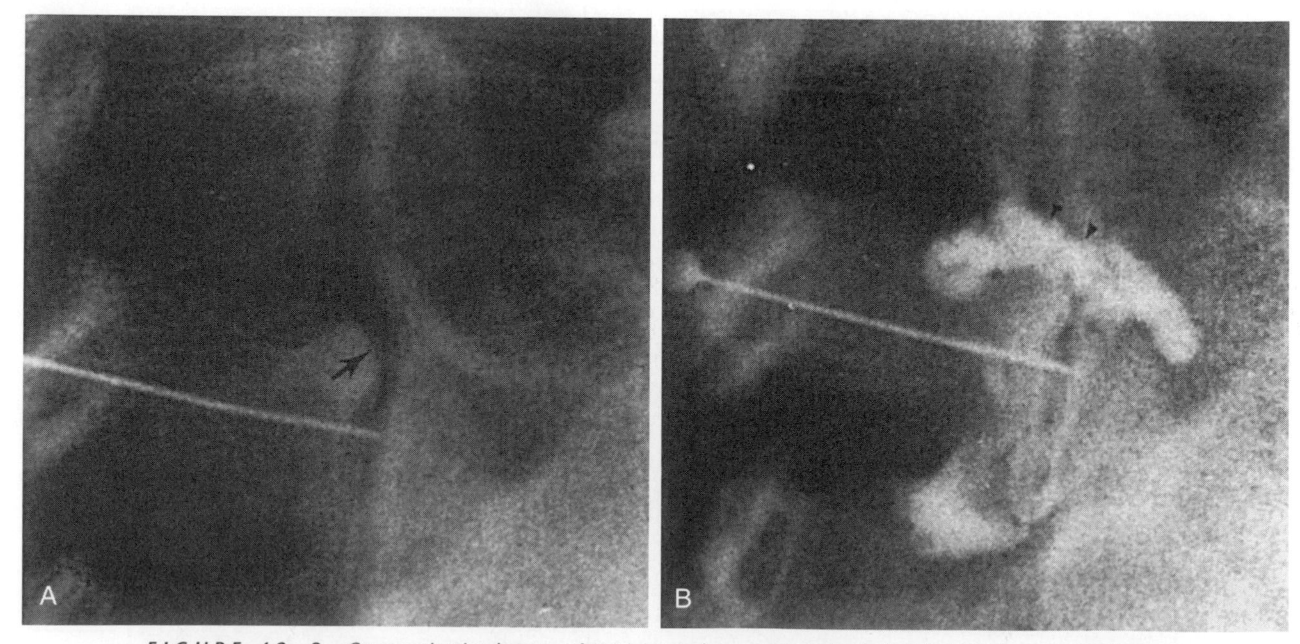

FIGURE 42–8 Communication between facet joint and a pars interarticularis defect. Such a communication is important if pars defect is believed to be a source of lower back pain. Injecting local anesthetic into facet joint could also block pain originating in pars defect. A, Radiograph shows needle in L5–S1 facet joint and pars defect (arrow) superior to joint. B, After injection of contrast material, both facet joint and pars defect (arrowheads) fill simultaneously. (El-Khoury GY, Reinfrew DL: Percutaneous procedures for the diagnosis and treatment of low back pain: Diskography, facet-joint injection, and epidural injection. AJR Am J Roentgenol 157:685–691, 1991.)

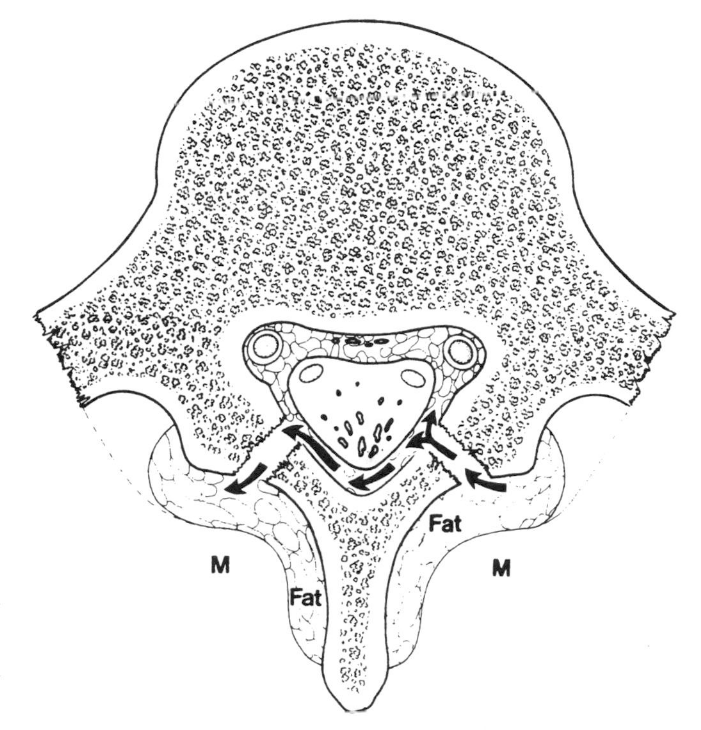

FIGURE 42–9 Diagram of a horizontal section of L5, based on Figure 42–8. The fat behind each lamina is part of the extracapsular inferior recess of L4–L5, which is enclosed by the attachments of the multifidus muscle (M); on each side, the recess communicates with the L4–L5 joint space above through a gap in the inferior joint capsule. Bilateral pars interarticularis defects establish communication between the inferior recesses of the two facet joints through the epidural space. Arrows indicate the route of spread of contrast medium. (McCormick CC, Taylor JR, Twang LT: Facet joint arthrography in lumbar spondylolysis: Anatomic basis for spread of contrast medium. Radiology 171:193–196, 1989.)

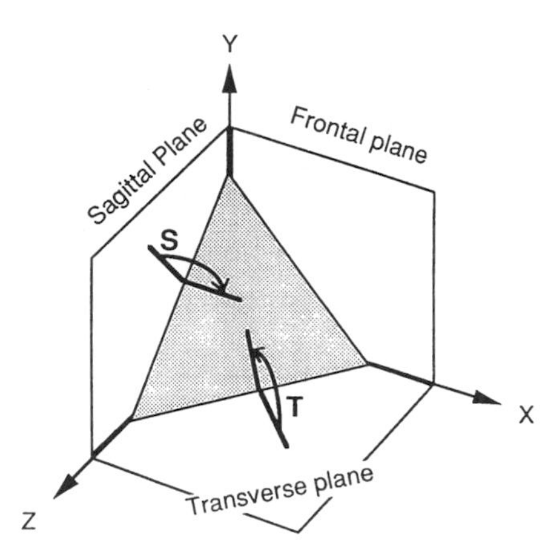

FIGURE 42–10 Facet surface was approximated by a plane. The orientation of the plane was defined by two angles made by the facet plane with the anatomic planes, sagittal (S) and transverse (T). (Panjabi MM, Oxland T, Takata K, et al: Articular facets of the human spine: Quantitative three-dimensional anatomy. Spine 18(10):1298–1310, 1993.)

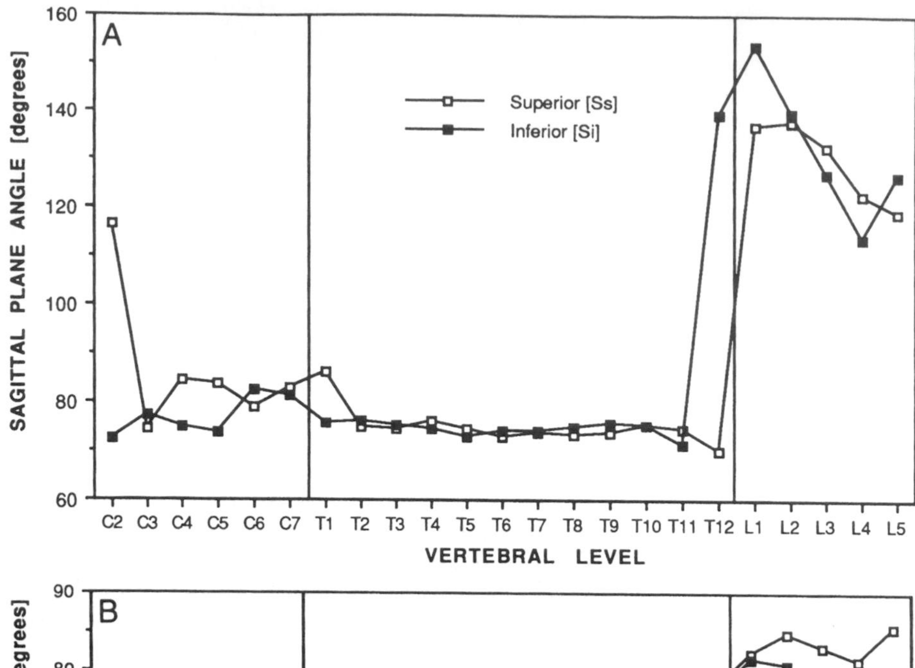

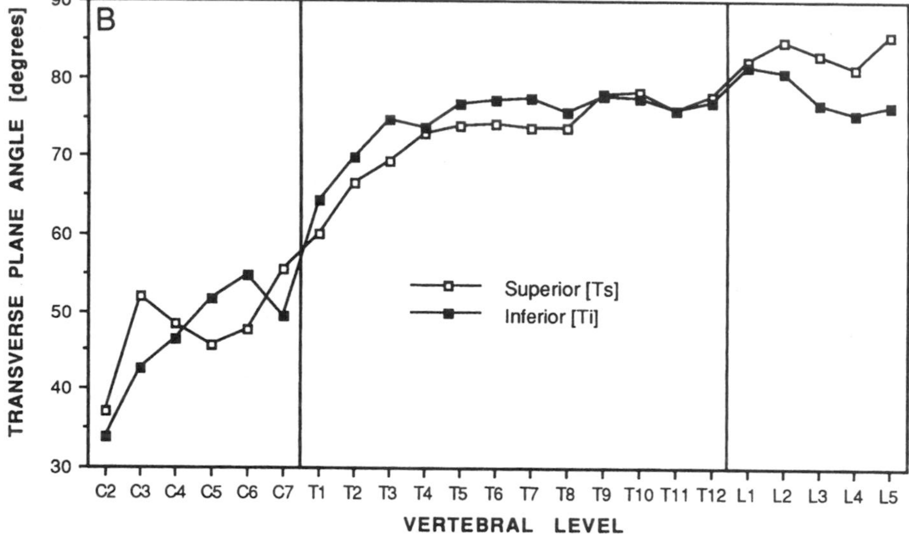

FIGURE 42–11 Angles made by the facet plane with the two anatomic planes as functions of vertebral level. A, sagittal plane, B, transverse plane. (Panjabi MM, Oxland T, Takata K, et al: Articular facets of the human spine: Quantitative three-dimensional anatomy. Spine 18(10):1298–1310, 1993.)

The T1–T2 facet joint is angled 66 degrees from a transverse plane, with the cephalad end more anterior than the caudad end.[51, 52] The angle steepens to 75 degrees by the T3–T4 facet joint and then remains constant to the T11–T12 facet joint. The T1–T2 to the T11–T12 facet joints are uniformly angled 110 degrees from the midline posterior sagittal plane. The thoracic facet joints are thus mostly vertically oriented and almost parallel to the coronal plane (Figs. 42–12, 42–13). The transition from the thoracic to the lumbar facet joints occurs primarily at the T11–T12, and T12–L1 joints.[49] There is some variability at the T11–T12 facet joint, but it is essentially oriented vertically (perpendicular to the sagittal plane) and faces directly anterior (parallel to the coronal plane). The T12–L1 facet joint assumes the more lumbar orientation and is approximately 25 degrees obligue to the sagittal plane from the midline posteriorly (Fig. 42–14).

The anatomy of the cervical facets is quite different from that of the lumbar facets (Fig. 42–15).[9, 53] The atlantooccipital and atlantoaxial joints are, technically, the C0–C1 and C1–C2 facet joints. Their structure, function, and innerva-

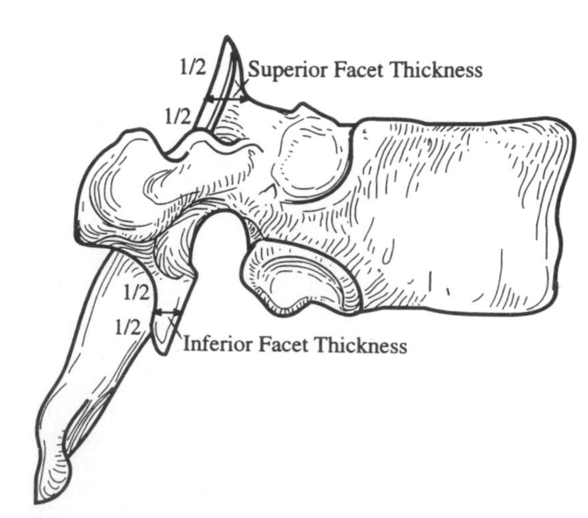

FIGURE 42–12 Typical thoracic facet showing orientation of facet joints and spinous processes, and facet thickness. (Ebraheim NA, Xu R, Ahmad M, et al: The quantitative anatomy of the thoracic facet and the posterior projection of its inferior facet. Spine 22(16):1811–1818, 1997.)

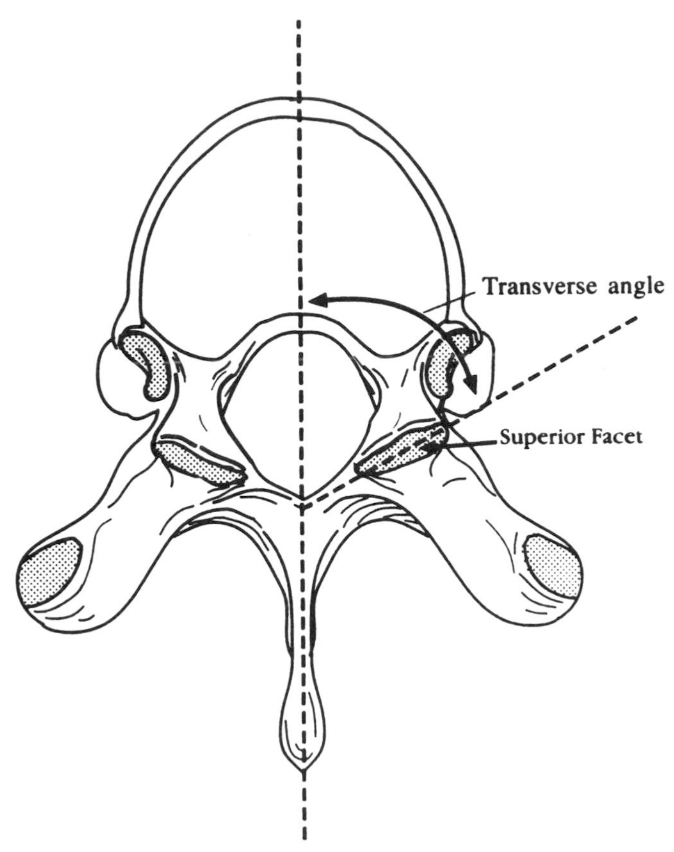

FIGURE 42–13 *Typical thoracic facet showing the transverse angle of a superior facet. (Ebraheim NA, Xu R, Ahmad M, et al: The quantitative anatomy of the thoracic facet and the posterior projection of its inferior facet. Spine 22(16):1811–1818, 1997.)*

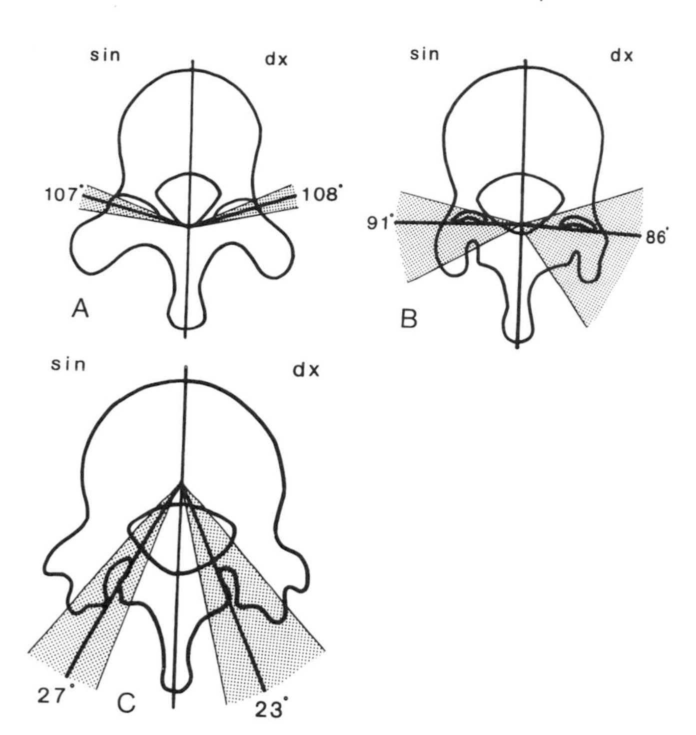

FIGURE 42–14 *Median and 10th and 90th percentiles of facet joint angles of 24 cadaver spines. A, T10–T11. Facet orientation was nearly always frontal. B, T11–T12. Facet angles showed widest variation. C, T12–L1. Facet orientation was usually of lumbar type, and nearly sagittal. (Malmivaara A, Videman T, Kuosma E, et al: Facet joint orientation, facet and costovertebral joint osteoarthrosis, disc degeneration, vertebral body osteophytosis, and Schmorl's nodes in the thoracolumbar junctional region of cadaveric spines. Spine 12(5):458–463, 1987.)*

tion are unique and their disorders will be discussed only minimally. The C2–C3 through C5–C6 facet joints are angled 35 degrees from the coronal plane. The C6–C7 joint is in transition between the orientation of the C5–C6 facet joint and that of C7–T1, which is tipped 22 degrees from the coronal plane.[51, 54] All of the cervical facet joints from C2–C3 caudad to C7–T1 are angled 110 degrees from the midline posterior sagittal plane. This makes their orientation very much like that of the thoracic facet joints, only not quite as close to the vertical plane. The cervical facet joints play a physically larger role in the spinal articular tripod structure, and are actually best described as the superior and inferior ends of articular pillars. Also unique to the cervical spine is the vertebral artery, which passes through the transverse foramen of the transverse processes of C6–C1 vertebra.[55]

Given this description, the facet joints appear anatomically designed to restrain excessive mobility and distribute axial loading over a broad area. They help to resist the shearing motion produced by forward bending and the compression produced by rotation.[31] The orientation and shape of the facet joints appear to be specifically suited to the stresses and movements at each spinal level.

Neuroanatomy

The poor localization of facet joint pain is explained in part by the pattern of profuse overlapping of sensory

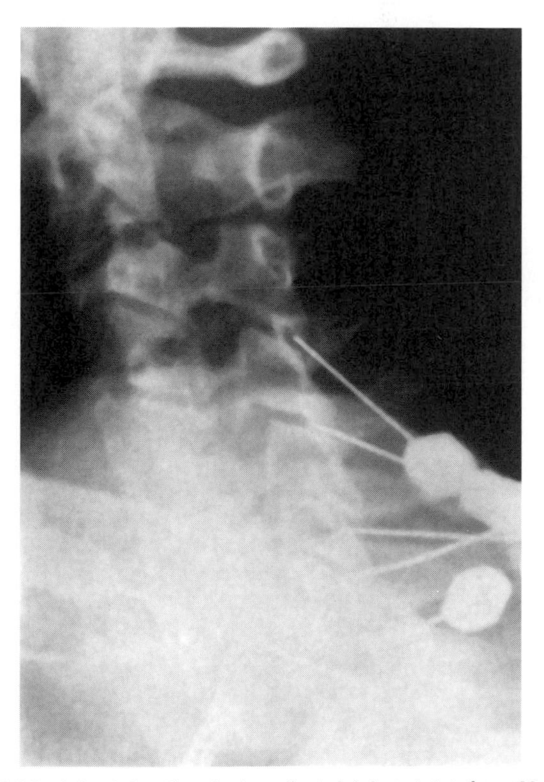

FIGURE 42–15 *Six spinal needles in left facet joints from C3–C4 to T1–T2. (Hove B, Gyldensted C: Cervical analgesic facet joint arthrography. Neuroradiology 32:456–459, 1990.)*

innervation of these joints (Fig. 42–16). Initially, the posterior and anterior primary rami of a nerve root diverge at the intervertebral foramen. The posterior ramus passes dorsally and caudally through a foramen in the intertransverse ligament.[56] At a point 5 mm from its origin, it divides into medial, lateral, and intermediate branches. The medial branch supplies the lower pole of the facet joint at its own level and the upper pole of the facet joint below.[15, 57] Therefore, each of the facet joints receives its innervation from a medial branch nerve of two posterior primary rami. One branch arises from the nerve at the same level as the joint, and the other from the segmental level above.[58] For example, the facet joint between the L4 and L5 vertebral bodies is innervated by the medial branch nerves from the L3 and L4 nerve roots (Fig. 42–17).

In the lumbar region, the medial branch of the posterior ramus lies in a groove on the base of the superior articular facet, where it lies in direct contact with the base of the superior surface of the transverse process, passing between the mammillary and accessory processes. The nerve actually passes under the mammilloaccessory ligament, and this is the most reliable site for locating the nerve in the lumbar spine. This ligament can become calcified, especially at the L3, L4, and L5 levels (20% at the L5 level).[59, 59a] It is suspected that this could even lead to entrapment of the medial branch nerve at this location. The medial branch nerve then progresses posteriorly and inferiorly, first sending fibers cephalad to innervate the caudad capsular margin of the adjacent superior joint capsule before sending fibers to the next lower level at its cephalad capsular margin.[60] The course of the L5 medial branch is somewhat modified, because the transverse process is replaced by the ala of the sacrum (Figs. 42–18, 42–19).[56, 61] An additional abnormality at the lumbosacral junction is the proposal that a branch from the posterior opening of the S1 nerve root in the sacrum runs cephalad to supply the L5–S1 facet

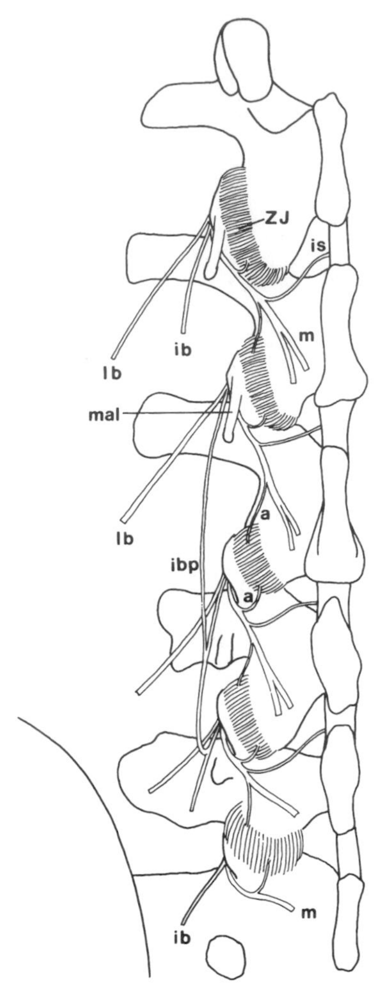

FIGURE 42–17 A sketch of a dorsal view of the branches of the left lumbar dorsal rami. Mammilloaccessory ligaments (mal) have been left in situ covering the L1 and L2 medial branches. ZJ, *zygapophyseal (facet) joint;* m, *medial branch;* lb, *lateral branch;* ib, *intermediate branch;* ibp, *intermediate branch plexus;* is, *interspinous branch,* a, *articular branches. (Bogduk N. The innervation of the lumbar spine. Spine 8(3):286–293, 1983.)*

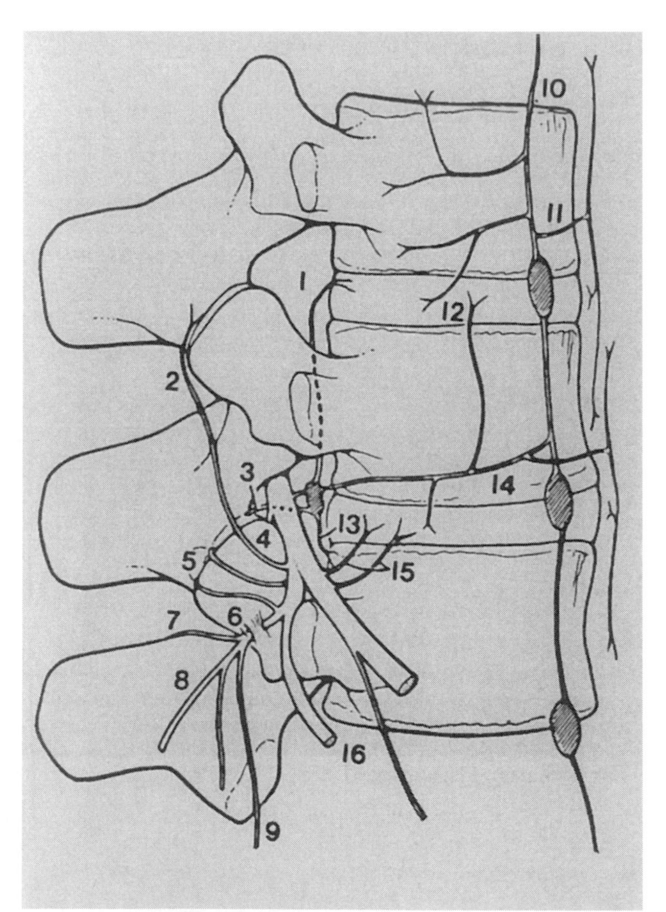

FIGURE 42–16 Neuroanatomic definition of the lumbar motion segment: 1, ascending branch of sinuvertebral nerve; 2, ascending facet branch; 3, sinuvertebral nerve to facet; 4, direct branch to facet; 5, branches to multifidus; 6, medial branch of posterior primary ramus; 7, local facet branch; 8, descending facet branch; 9, branch to sacroiliac; 10, sympathetic chain; 11, branch under anterior longitudinal ligament; 12, branches from gray ramus to disc; 13, sinuvertebral to disc; 14, gray ramus communicans; 15, branches from anterior primary ramus to disc; 16, lateral branch of posterior primary ramus. (Mooney V: Facet syndrome: Clinical entities. In Weinstein JN, Wiesel SW (eds): The Lumbar Spine. Philadelphia, WB Saunders, 1990, pp 422–441.)

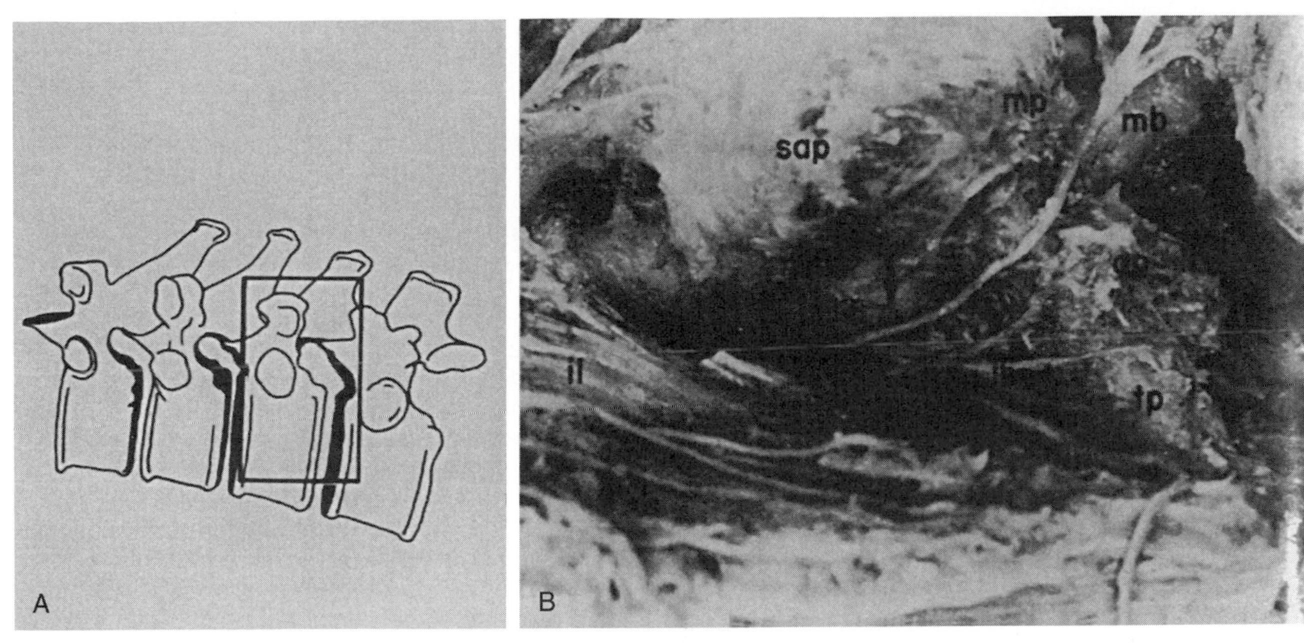

FIGURE 42–18 *The proximal part of the course of the L2 medial branch (*mb*). The medial branch rises dorsally and caudally across the root of the L3 superior articular process (*sap*).* mp, *Mammillary process;* tp, *transverse process;* ap, *accessory process;* il, *intertransversarii laterales;* lb, *lateral branches. Arrow indicates the target point for medial branch neurotomy. This is the junction of the lateral surface of the superior articular process with the most medial end of the superior border of the transverse process. (Bogduk N, Long D: The anatomy of the so-called "articular nerves" and their relationship to facet denervation in the treatment of low back pain. J Neurosurg 51:172–177, 1979.)*

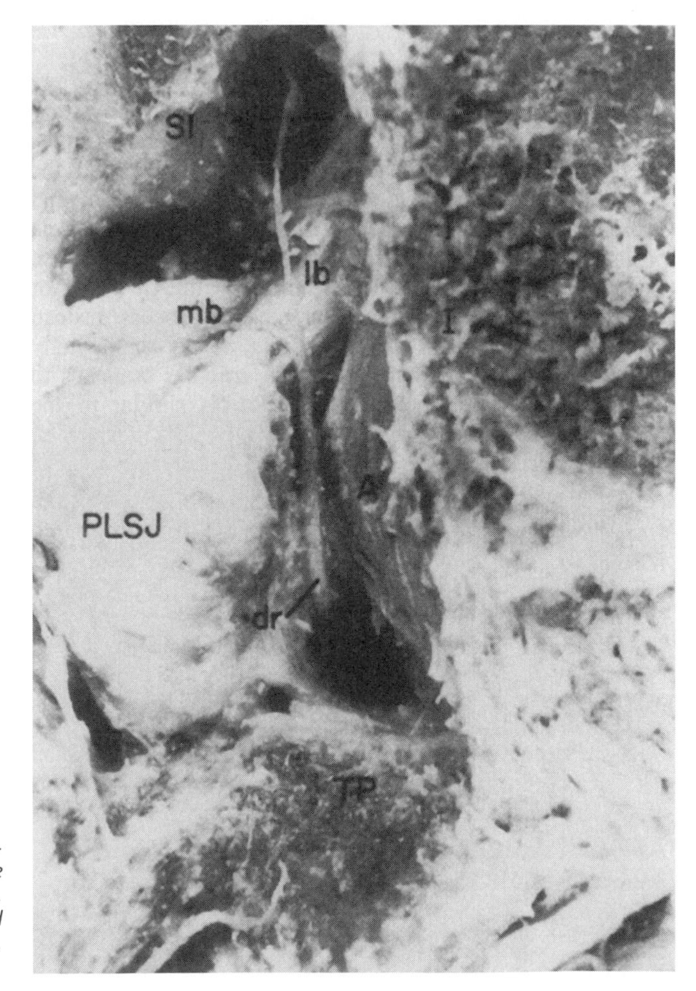

FIGURE 42–19 *The course of the L5 dorsal ramus (*dr*).* PLSJ, *posterior lumbosacral joint;* I, *ilium (resected);* A, *ala of sacrum;* TP, *L5 transverse process;* mb, *medial branch;* lb, *lateral branch;* S1, *S1 dorsal foramen. (Bogduk N, Long D: The anatomy of the so-called "articular nerves" and their relationship to facet denervation in the treatment of low back pain. J Neurosurg 51:172–177, 1979.)*

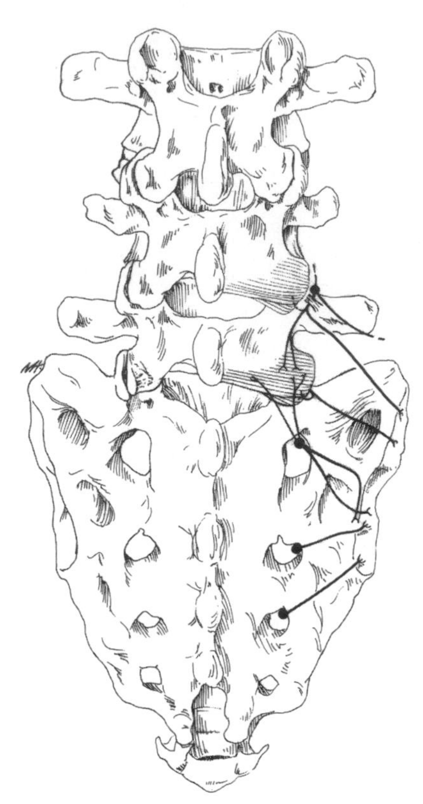

FIGURE 42–20 *Illustration of the medial branch of L4 innervating the L4–L5 and L5–S1 facet joints, and possibly the posterior sacroiliac joint. The L5 medial branch innervates the L5–S1 facet joint and the posterior sacroiliac joint. Additionally, the S1 nerve sends one or two ascending branches to the L5–S1 facet joint, as well as a branch to the sacroiliac joint. (Paris SV: Anatomy as related to function and pain. Orthop Clin North Am 14(3):475–489, 1983.)*

joint (Fig. 42–20).[62,66] This would result in the L5–S1 facet joint's being innervated by three nerves, and this third nerve would also need to be blocked to completely anesthetize this joint.

Each medial branch of the posterior primary ramus also supplies the multifidus, interspinales, and intertransversarii mediales muscles and the ligaments and periosteum of the neural arch.[22,61,63] However, there is considerable segmental overlap of this sensory innervation. Therefore, blockade of the two medial branch nerves, which have been shown to be the main source of nociceptive signals from an individual facet joint, can reasonably be expected to be specific for the facet joint.[64]

In summary, each joint has dual segmental innervation, and each segmental nerve supplies two facet joints plus the soft tissues overlying them. Because of the duality of segmental innervation, each joint must be denervated at two segmental levels (and perhaps three for the L5–S1 joint), both at and above the level of the involved joint.

Controversy once surrounded the question of whether there is innervation from a third ascending branch that arises from the mixed spinal nerve just anterior to the intertransverse fascia (ligament). The proposed nerve branch apparently ascends, well clear of the transverse process, through the soft tissue into the posterior aspect of the facet above (see Fig. 42–16).[31,60,65,66] Although this has been proposed, more recent anatomic studies have failed to find such an ascending nerve. It likely does not exist, and even if it actually does exist it appears to be very small and inconsistent and likely clinically insignificant. Additional articular branches to the ventral aspect of the facet joints from the dorsal ramus have also been described, but subsequent studies also failed to locate them.[61] If these branches actually exist, they seem likewise to be very small and inconsistent, and likely not clinically significant.

There is evidence in rats and humans of multilevel innervation of the lumbar facet joints which includes not only the posterior primary ramus but also the sympathetic and parasympathetic ganglia.[61,67] The sympathetic fibers innervating the lumbar facet joints have been found to pass through the dorsal root ganglion and to go directly into rami communicantes, on their way to the paravertebral sympathetic trunk. The origins of these nerves have been found to be several segmental levels away from the innervated facet joint. The sympathetic fibers have been reported to regulate the activity of sensory neurons, and this is compatible with some reports that the sympathetic trunk contributes to low back pain.

Medial branch nerves from two segmental levels innervate each thoracic facet. As in the lumbar spine, the nerves innervate the joint at the same level plus the joint below. Below the T3 level this pattern is consistent, but it seems that the C7 and C8 nerves may travel caudad as far as the T2 and T3 levels.[40]

Because of the precise, consistent anatomic descriptions of the location of the medial branch nerves in the lumbar and cervical spine, it has been assumed that the position would be essentially identical in the thoracic spine.[68] Because of the limited clinical interest to date in the thoracic facets as a significant source of pain, this assumption was only recently assessed by an anatomic study.[69] Although only a small study, it shows a significantly different path for the medial branch nerve than had been thought (Figs. 42–21, 42–22). The medial branch arises from the dorsal ramus within 5 mm of the lateral margin of the intervertebral foramen. It then passes dorsally, inferiorly, but primarily laterally within the intertransverse space, posterior to the superior costotransverse ligament. Opposite the tip of the transverse process the medial branch curves dorsally through the intertransverse space, aiming for the superolateral corner of the transverse process. It then makes its first bony contact by crossing this corner and entering the posterior compartment of the back. It then runs caudad along the posterior surface of the tip of the transverse process, lying in the cleavage plane between the origins of the multifidus medially and the semispinalis laterally. Ascending articular branches arise from the medial branch as it passes caudad to the facet joint and enters the inferior aspect of the joint capsule. A descending articular branch arises from the medial branch as it crosses the superolateral corner of the transverse process. It then follows a path between the fascicles of the multifidus to reach the superior aspect of the joint capsule below.

Exceptions to this configuration occur at the midthoracic level, where the nerve does not even reliably make bony contact with the superolateral corner of the transverse process. Also, the T11 branch runs across the lateral surface of the root of the relatively smaller T12 transverse process.

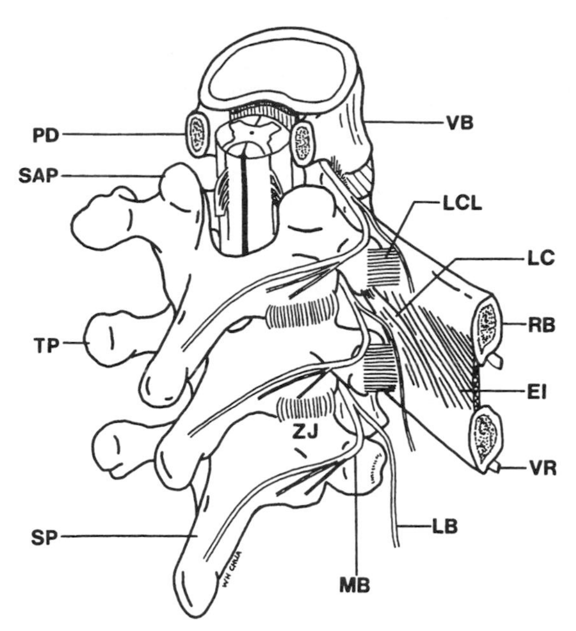

FIGURE 42–21 *A sketch of the archetypical course and relations of the thoracic dorsal rami viewed from a right superior aspect.* Sp, *spinous process;* TP, *transverse process;* SAP, *superior articular process;* PD, *pedicle;* ZJ, *zygapophyseal (facet) joint;* MB, *medial branch;* LB, lateral branch; VR, *ventral ramus,* EI, *external intercostals;* RB, *rib;* LC, *levator costae;* LCL, *lateral costotransverse ligament;* VB, *vertebral body. (Chua WH, Bogduk N: The surgical anatomy of thoracic facet denervation. Acta Neurochir 136:140–144, 1995.)*

At the T12 level the medial branch assumes a course analogous to those of the lumbar medial branches.

The medial branch nerves in the thoracic region swing laterally to circumvent the multifidus, which arises from the distal end of the transverse process. At no point are nerves encountered crossing the superomedial corner of the transverse process. The only consistent point of contact of the medial branch nerve with the transverse process is at least 12 mm lateral to the root of the transverse process. This is important because the maximum radius of the coagulated tissue from the thermocouple electrodes used for denervation is 1.1 mm. This apparent anatomic abnormality is actually in keeping with the homologous anatomy of the transverse processes between the thoracic and lumbar spine, which is explained in more detail in the referenced article.[69]

Therefore, more work needs to be done before a reliable technique for thoracic facet denervation can be proposed. First, the anatomic dissection needs to be repeated, and with a larger sample. Second, once the bony location of the medial branch nerve in the thoracic region is reliably identified, a double-blind controlled trial must confirm the effectiveness of the modified technique.

The medial branches of the cervical posterior rami are somewhat different in that they supply mainly the facet joints and have limited innervations of the posterior neck muscles—the multifidus, interspinalis, semispinalis cervicis, and semispinalis capitis (Fig. 42–23).[55] The C3 dorsal ramus is the only cervical dorsal ramus below C2 that has a cutaneous distribution. Therefore, if neck pain or headache is due to cervical facet disease, it is likely to be relieved by cervical facet joint or medial branch blocks, without significantly affecting neck muscle strength or skin sensation.

The upper cervical synovial joints—the atlantooccipital (C0–C1) and lateral atlantoaxial (C1–C2)—are not innervated by cervical dorsal rami. They receive branches from the C1 and C2 ventral rami. Therefore the only interventional procedure for these joints is direct intraarticular injection. Because of the high risk associated with such injections, few physicians routinely perform them. The anatomic description of these injections is probably best learned *by* those already very experienced at interventional procedures and *from* others already skilled at the injections.

The C2–C3 facet joint is innervated mainly by the large third occipital nerve, which is one of the two medial branches of the C3 dorsal ramus, and to some degree also by the C2 dorsal rami (see Fig. 42–22).[53,70,71] The C2 dorsal ramus has five branches. The medial branch is commonly known as the *greater occipital nerve.* There are several communicating branches between the dorsal branches of C1, C2, and C3, which may play a role in the anatomic basis for cervicogenic headache. Unfortunately, there are no reliable radiologic coordinates for the C2 dorsal ramus, since it runs in the soft tissue dorsal to the C2 lamina. Because there are eight cervical nerves but only seven cervical vertebrae, the first seven cervical nerve roots exit the spine *above* the vertebral body whose "number" they share. Therefore,

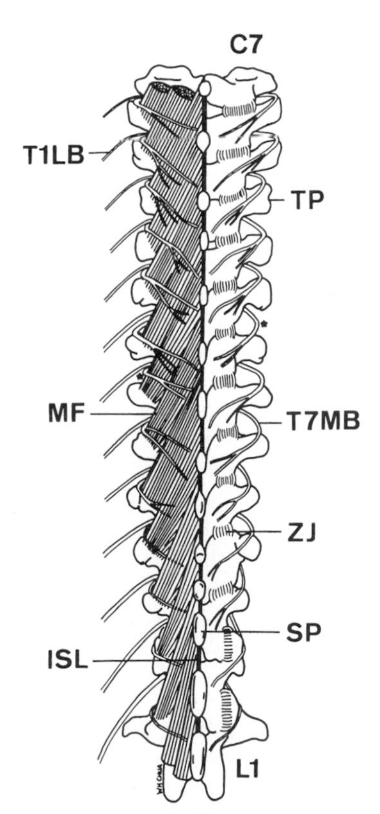

FIGURE 42–22 *A sketch of the medial branches of the thoracic dorsal rami viewed from behind. On the right side, the multifidus and lateral branches are not shown.* TP, *transverse process;* MB, *medial branch;* ZJ, *zygapophyseal (facet) joint;* SP, *spinous process;* LB, *lateral branch;* MF, *multifidus;* ISL, *interspinous ligament;* C, *cervical vertebra;* L, *lumbar vertebra;* (star) *atypical medial branch. (Chua WH, Bogduk N: The surgical anatomy of thoracic facet denervation. Acta Neurochir 136:140–144, 1995.)*

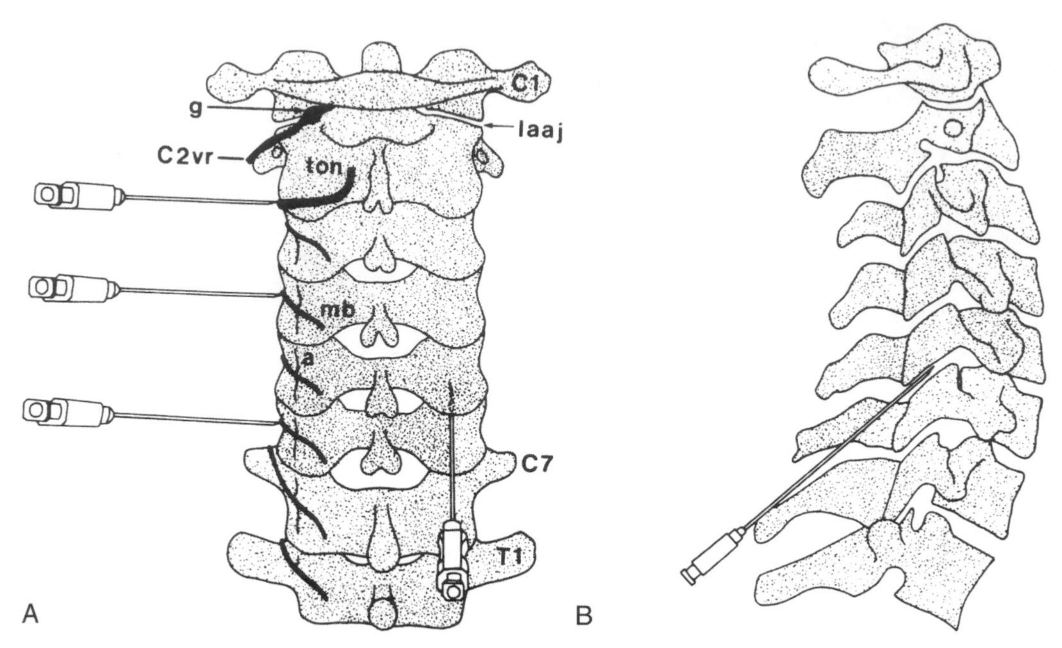

FIGURE 42–23 Illustrations of the needle placement for cervical medial branch blocks and intraarticular zygapophyseal blocks. A, *Posterior view of the cervical spine showing the location of the C2 ganglion* (g) *behind the lateral atlantoaxial joint* (laaj), *the C2 ventral ramus* (C2vr), *the courses of the medial branches of the cervical dorsal rami* (mb), *their articular branches* (a), *and the third occipital nerve* (ton). *Needles are shown in position as they would be used for blocks of the C4 and C6 medial branches and the third occipital nerve. The articular pillar of C7 may be obscured by the shadow of the large C7 transverse process, in which case the C7 medial branch can be located midway between the lateral convexities of the C6–C7 and C7–T1 zygapophyseal joints.* B, *Lateral view of the cervical spine showing the course of a needle into the cavity of the right C5–C6 zygapophyseal joint. (Bogduk N: Back pain: Zygapophyseal blocks and epidural steroids.* In *Cousins M, Bridenbaugh PO (eds): Neural Blockade in Clinical Anesthesia and Management of Pain, ed 2. Philadelphia, JB Lippincott, 1988, pp 935–946.)*

the C3 nerve root exits via the intervertebral foramen between the C2 and C3 vertebral bodies. The C3 dorsal ramus curves dorsally through the intertransverse space.

Two medial branches usually arise separately from the C3 dorsal ramus. The superior and larger branch is the third occipital nerve (also known as the superficial medial branch), and the inferior branch is the deep medial branch. The third occipital nerve curves dorsally and medially around the superior articular process of the C3 vertebra. It crosses the C2–C3 facet joint either just below or across the joint margin. The innervation of the C2–C3 facet joint may come from the third occipital nerve and an articular nerve that branches off the dorsal ramus itself. Because the C2–C3 facet innervation is complex, the practical implication is that blocking the third occipital nerve on the C3 articular process will denervate this joint (Fig. 42–24).[72] The deep medial branch of the C3 dorsal ramus is parallel but caudad to the third occipital nerve in the C3 articular pillar. The location of this nerve on the articular pillar is essentially the same as those of nerves C4–C8.

The C3–C4 to C7–T1 facet joints are supplied by the medial branches of the cervical posterior rami at the same level and from the segmental level above.[55, 70] Therefore, the C3–C4 facet is innervated by the C3 and C4 medial branch nerves. These nerves arise from the posterior primary rami in the cervical intertransverse spaces and then curve dorsally and medially to wrap around the waists of their respective articular pillars.[24] As they start to wrap around the articular pillars, the nerves are 2.2 mm (C3) to 1.2 mm (C7) in vertical extent.[73] They are also 7.3 mm (C3) to 5.5 mm (C7) caudad to the tip of the superior at this location. The medial branches are bound to the periosteum by an investing fascia and are held against the articular pillars by tendons of the semispinalis capitis.[53, 70, 72] The medial branches are seen on a lateral view of the cervical spine to pass through the "centroid" of the articular pillar (Fig. 42–25). Rostral and caudal branches from each nerve then pass into the joints immediately above and below. The C7 medial branch crosses the root of the C7 transverse process and therefore lies higher on the lateral projection of the C7 articular pillar (Figs. 42–23, 42–26, 42–27).[74]

PATHOPHYSIOLOGY OF THE FACET SYNDROME

A growing body of research shows clearly that the medial branch nerves transmit nociceptive signals, in addition to proprioceptive ones, from the facet joints.[67, 75–85] These nociceptive signals may result from a combination of inflammatory and mechanical joint stress, possibly in the presence of additional central sensitization. Neurophysiologic studies have identified substance P, calcitonin gene–related peptide, vasoactive intestinal peptide, and C-flanking peptide of neuropeptide Y, all neuromodulators of nociception, within the facet joint capsule, and synovium.[56, 77, 82, 83, 85] These are found on the type 1 articular receptors. In addition, there are mechanosensitive somatosensory units found within the facet joint classifed as the type 2, 3, and

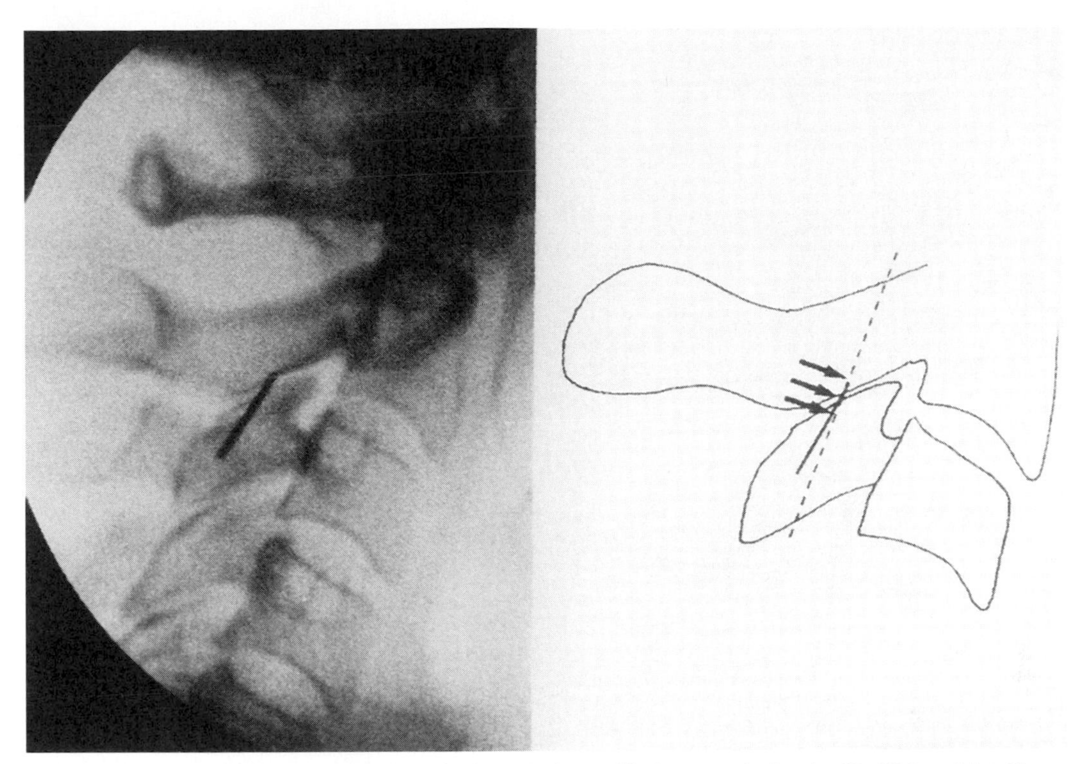

FIGURE 42–24 *Target points for a third occipital nerve block to anesthetize the C2–C3 facet joint. Three injections are placed vertically along a midline through the C2–C3 articular pillar (*dotted line*). The injections are placed over the joint line (*middle arrow*), immediately above the subchondral plate of the inferior articular facet of C2 (*upper arrow*) and immediately below the subchondral plate of the superior articular facet of C3 (*lower arrow*). (Barnsley L, Bogduk N: Medial branch blocks are specific for the diagnosis of cervical zygapophyseal joint pain. Reg Anesth 18:343–350, 1993.)*

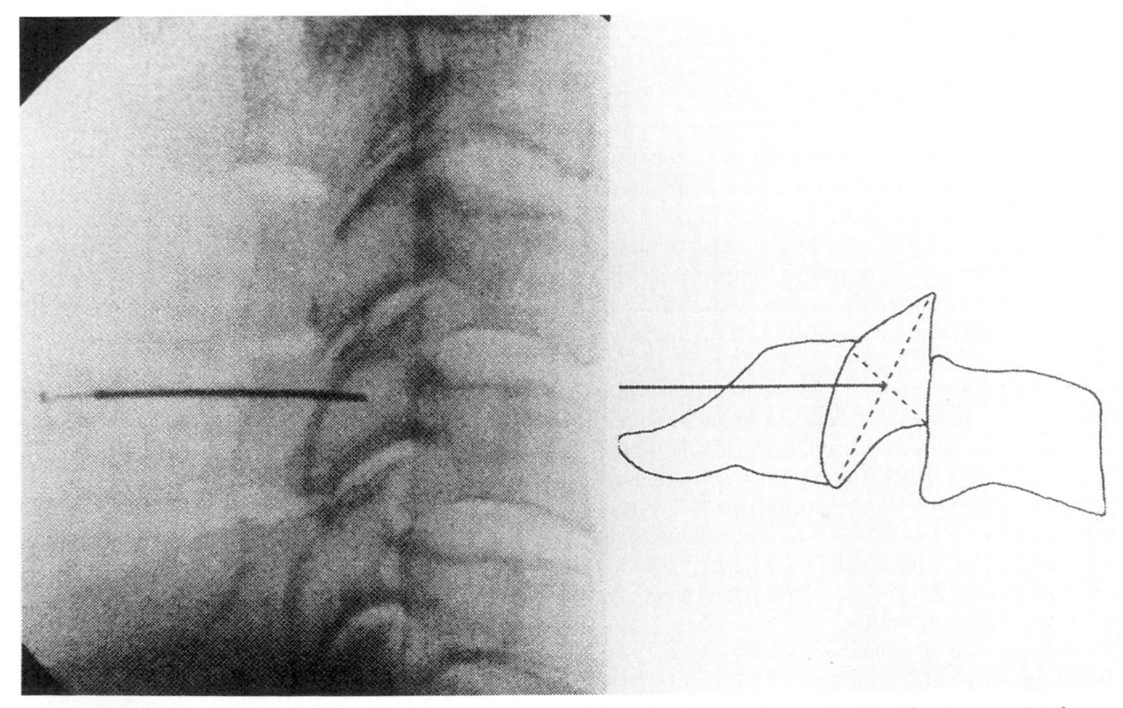

FIGURE 42–25 *Target points for cervical medial branch blocks at levels C3–C7. The target point for injection is the centroid of the articular pillar as seen in a true lateral view of the cervical spine. The dotted lines intersect at the centroid. (Barnsley L, Bogduk N: Medial branch blocks are specific for the diagnosis of cervical zygapophyseal joint pain. Reg Anesth 18:343–350, 1993.)*

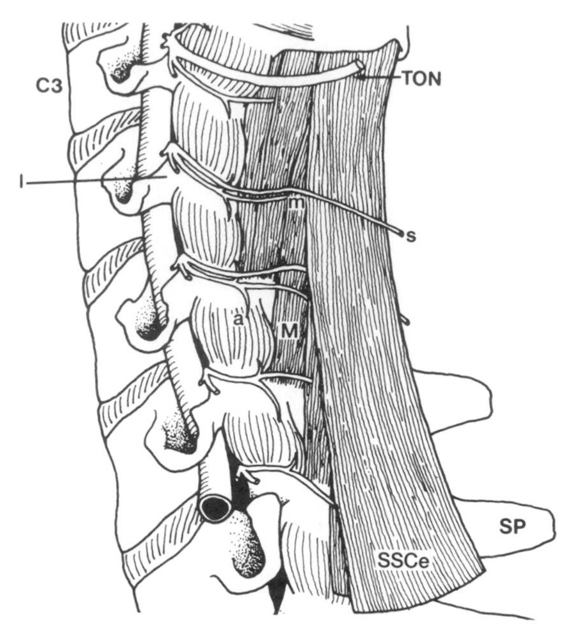

FIGURE 42–26 *Lateral view of the anatomy of the left cervical dorsal rami in the plane of the multifidus. The lateral branches of the cervical dorsal rami (*I*) have been cut at their origin. The C2–C3 facet joint is supplied by the third occipital nerve (*TON*) as it crosses the dorsolateral aspect of the joint or by the communicating branch (c) between the C2 and C3 dorsal rami. Below C2–C3, the deep medial branches (*m*) send articular (*a*) branches to the facet joints before ramifying in multifidus (*M*). The superficial (*s*) branches pass deep or dorsal to the semispinalis cervicis (*SSCe*) to become cutaneous.* C3, *Vertebral body of C3;* SP, *spinous process of C7. (Lord SM, Barnsley L, Bogduk N: Percutaneous radiofrequency neurotomy in the treatment of cervical zygapophyseal joint pain: A caution. Neurosurgery 36(4):732–739, 1995.)*

4 articular receptors. These are all thought to modulate nociception.[38–40]

With chronic inflammation, these synovial joints can fill with fluid and distend. Their distension could cause pain due to stimulation of the capsule. The distension of the articular recesses could compress the nerve root in the spinal canal and neural foramina, especially if the size of the foramen is reduced by osteophytes. This hypothesis may explain some of the radiating pain found in the facet syndrome.[39] It is also possible that some of this radiating pain is referred pain from the facet joints themselves. The referred pain can be quite difficult to assess because the referral can be to the limb dermatome, myotome, or sclerotomes (Fig. 42–28).[86]

Other osteochondral and capsular abnormalities could also cause facet pain by mechanisms similar to those in any other arthritic joint.[87] In fact, an anomalous ossicle of the inferior facet has been described that predisposes the facet joint to trauma, degenerative changes, and pain.[88, 89] There are also numerous reports of synovial cysts causing pain because of distension and mass effect on nearby structures,[90–93] calcification of the cysts,[94, 95] unilateral facet hypertrophy,[96] and facet osteomyelitis.[97]

Finally, intervertebral disc space narrowing can cause the facet joints to undergo subluxation, which can impose abnormal stresses on the joint and cause nerve root impingement (Fig. 42–29).[98, 99] Capsular irritation and local inflammation follow and sometimes cause reflex spasm of the posterior erector spinae muscles. Chronic irritation may lead to new bone formation and osteophyte production, which can further limit the range of pain-free movement.[96, 100] In the absence of specific facet joint disease noted earlier, degenerative changes in the lumbar facets are in fact unlikely to occur without lumbar disc degeneration.[101, 102] Some 75% of lumbar disc degeneration occurs without evidence of facet arthritis. However, almost universally, where there is facet arthritis, there is disc degeneration at that same level.[102a]

Overall, depending upon the clinical group of chronic low back pain patients that is being assessed, the lumbar facets seem to be the major pain generator in fewer than 5% to as many as 40% of the patients studied.[103, 104] In reviews of primary care patient populations, the lumbar facets seem to be responsible for about 6% of patients with chronic low back pain.[105] In a general referral pain practice, the incidence seems to be at least 10% to 15%, and in some referral populations it has been found to be as high as 40%.[106–108]

The pathophysiology of thoracic facet joint pain can likely be attributed to processes similar to those in the lumbar and cervical spine, although the specific details of the frequency, causes, and differences from the adjacent spinal levels have not been determined at this time.[68, 69]

Patients with cervical pain may have progressive facet joint arthritis and may develop vertical, lateral, and rotatory subluxation of the odontoid process with lateral mass collapse (Fig. 42–30). This often causes neurologic deterioration as well as pain.[70, 109] Whiplash injuries of the cervical spine causing musculoligamentous sprains of the cervical

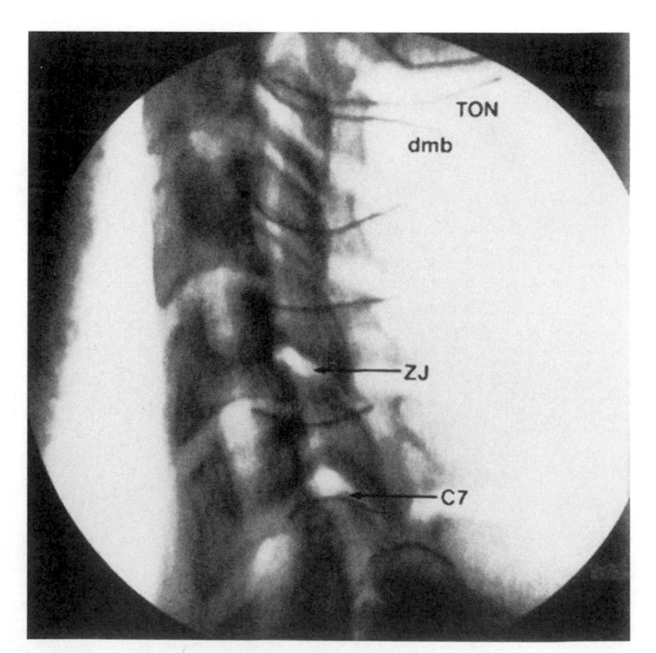

FIGURE 42–27 *Lateral x-ray of a cadaver with wires fixed to the medial branches of the cervical dorsal rami. In this specimen, the third occipital nerve (*TON*) crosses the inferior pole of the C2–C3 facet joint, running close to the C3 deep medial branch (*dmb*). The C4–C6 medial branches course around the waists of the articular pillars. The C7 medial branch (*C7*) crosses the root of the C7 transverse process, and thus lies higher on the lateral projection of the C7 articular pillar.* ZJ, *C5–C6 zygapophyseal (facet) joint. (Lord SM, Barnsley L, Bogduk N: Percutaneous radiofrequency neurotomy in the treatment of cervical zygapophyseal joint pain: A caution. Neurosurgery 36(4):732–739, 1995.)*

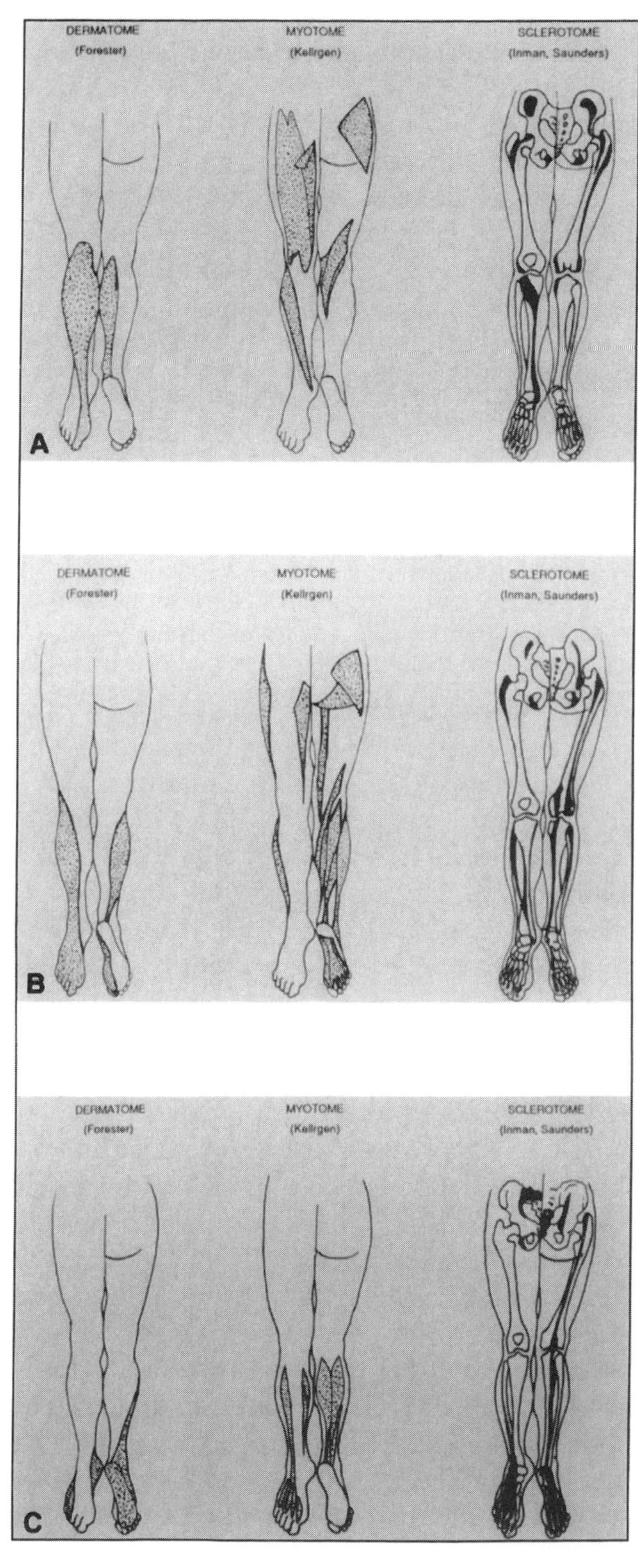

FIGURE 42–28 Dermatome, myotome, and sclerotome patterns of: A, L4; B, L5; C, S1. (Simmons JW, Ricketson R, McMillin JN: Painful lumbosacral sensory distribution patterns: Embryogenesis to adulthood. Orthop Rev 10:1110–1118, 1993.)

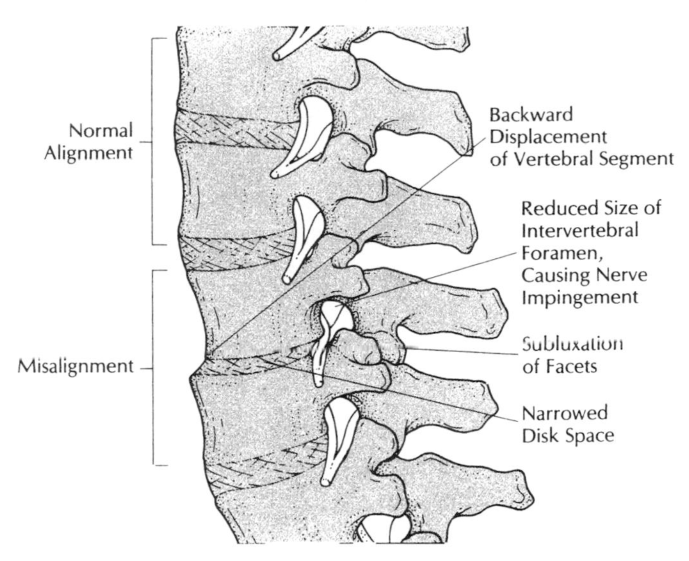

FIGURE 42–29 Disc space narrowing produces derangement of the mechanics of the spine, with consequent subluxation of the facet joints. Sequelae include nerve impingement, backward displacement of vertebral segment, and restriction of vertebral rotation. (Warfield CA: Facet syndrome and the relief of low back pain. Hosp Pract 23(10A):41–48, 1988.)

facet joints with periosteal tearing have also been suggested as the most common cause of neck pain and nerve root irritation.[110] In fact, recent research strongly suggests that for 50% to 60% of postwhiplash neck pain patients the cervical facet joints are the primary source of pain.[10, 111, 112] There is also growing evidence that the upper cervical spine (C1–C3), including the facet joints, contribute significantly to neck and head pain of cervicogenic headaches.

FACET BLOCK

Indications

The clinical picture of the facet joint syndrome is difficult to describe. Typically, it has been discussed in relation to

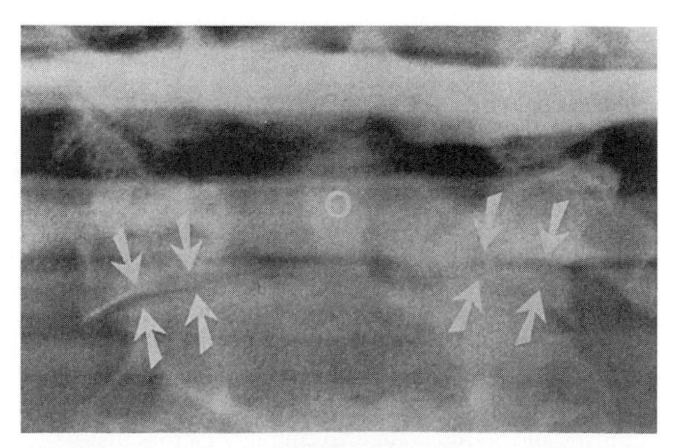

FIGURE 42–30 Panographic zonography examination demonstrates erosion of the odontoid process (O) and destruction of the atlantoaxial facet joints (arrows). (Santavirta S, Hopfner-Hallikainen D, Paukku P, et al: Atlantoaxial facet joint arthritis in the rheumatoid cervical spine: A panoramic zonography study. J Rheumatol 15:217–223, 1988.)

low back pain, although it can be applied to any spinal facet joint. As yet, there is no known anatomic, imaging, or histopathologic standard for identifying a painful facet joint. The greatest difficulty in evaluating patients with suspected facet syndrome lies in selecting those with symptomatic facets and deciding at which levels to make the injections.[113] Facet-induced pain is currently a diagnosis of exclusion supported by reproduction of the pain during arthrography (in the lumbar spine)—although the reliability of this sign has been challenged—and abolition of pain after injection of local anesthetic into the joint or onto the two medial branch nerves supplying the joint.

To help clarify the lumbar spine facet syndrome, referral patterns of pain from the lumbar spine have been identified during operations under local anesthesia,[114, 115] and via percutaneous injections. These have clearly shown the lumbar facet joints, particularly the capsule more than the synovium, to be sources of pain and the articular cartilage to be pain-free. Further study to identify the referral patterns for pain from the lumbar facet joints, has been disappointing. Nonetheless, some conclusions are worth noting.[116–118] There is considerable overlap in the pain patterns of the lumbar facets, the low back region being the common site of pain. All of the joints from L2–L3 to L5–S1 could refer pain into the groin. Only the L3–L4 to L5–S1 joints refer pain into the buttock or greater trochanter region. Coccygeal pain is very unlikely to be referred from facet joints. Although some studies have shown radiation of pain into the legs, the primary site of pain is the low back. Pain in the posterior thigh occurs inconsistently, and pain distal to the knee is very uncommon. Keeping in mind the close relation of the facet joint to the spinal nerve root, however, and the existence of dermatomes, myotomes, and sclerotomes, it would not be unreasonable for a painful facet joint also to cause radicular symptoms.

In 1933, Ghormley first described the facet syndrome. Since then, many attempts have been made to redefine which clinical features are most sensitive and specific for the diagnosis.[6, 13, 19, 20, 27, 119–125] The results have been generally disappointing. Part of the problem has been that the gold standard for making the diagnosis is the abolition of facet joint pain by injection. Unfortunately, the varying specificity of the several injection techniques, different criteria for pain relief (50%, 75%, 100%), and single and double blocks for diagnosis, have made most of these findings unreliable or difficult to interpret—and comparisons among studies invalid. It seems that even apparently specific blocks may have a 38% false-positive rate; that is, a second block fails to relieve pain when the first one did.[126] Also, placebo injections can produce pain relief 32% of the time. In one study using double diagnostic blocks, no clinical criteria were found to be predictive of pain relief after the first and repeat facet injection.[127] The only significant finding in this study was a negative one: none of the patients with central (as opposed to unilateral or bilateral) back pain, had pain relief with both injections. A second study using double diagnostic blocks also failed to find any factors that would predict which patients would have pain relief.[108] Some progress has been made in identifying possible predictive criteria based on a single diagnostic block.[128] Seven criteria were found to be predictive of pain relief after a facet block:

- No exacerbation of pain on rising from forward flexion
- Good pain relief with recumbency
- No exacerbation of pain with coughing
- No exacerbation with combined extension and rotation
- No exacerbation with hyperextension
- No exacerbation with forward flexion
- Age older than 65 years

Even when five of these seven variables are present, however, the odds are only one in three that the patient will derive pain relief from a facet injection. More work needs to be done to identify variables that will better predict who will respond to facet blocks. It does not seem likely that a reliable clinical picture of the lumbar facet syndrome will emerge anytime soon.

The classically unreliable features of the lumbar facet syndrome on history and physical examination that need further clarification are as follows: The patient's primary symptom is low back pain, either unilateral or bilateral, with tenderness over the facet joints. The pain is generally a deep, dull ache that is difficult to localize. Facet syndrome low back pain can be referred to the buttock, groin, hip, or posterior and lateral thigh. It occasionally radiates below the knee, but not into the foot (Fig. 42–31). Some patients

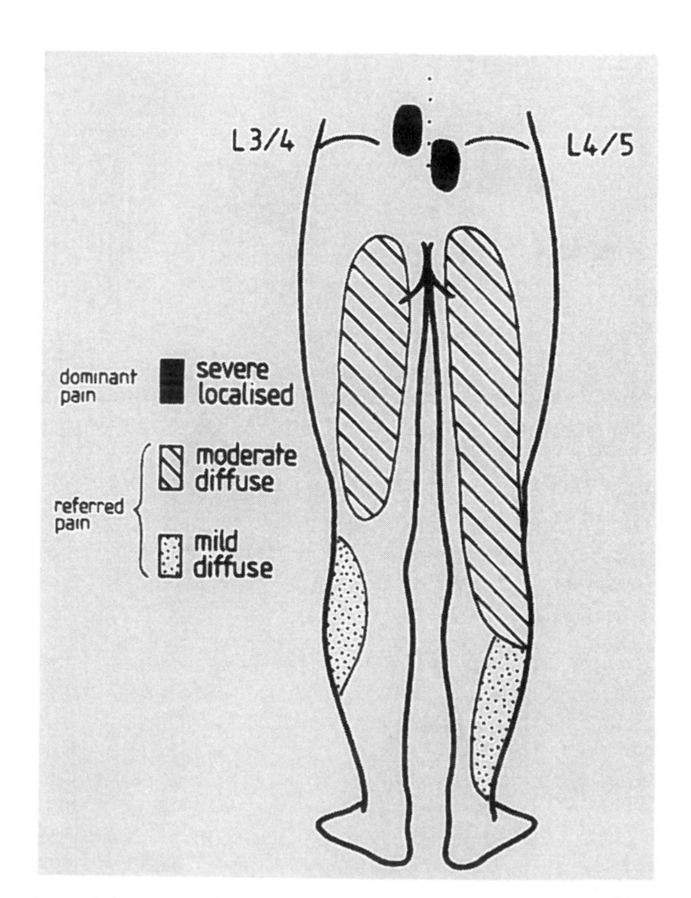

FIGURE 42–31 Pain distribution in the facet syndrome. Referred pain patterns from facet joints reflect the distribution of the segmental nerve supply at each level involved. Distal reference to the buttocks relates to the caudad migration of posterior branches, whereas limb distribution mimicking root pain results from pain reference in the anterior division of each segmental nerve. (Bous RA: Facet joint injections. In Stanton-Hicks M, Bous RA (eds): Chronic Low Back Pain. New York, Raven, 1982, pp 199–211.)

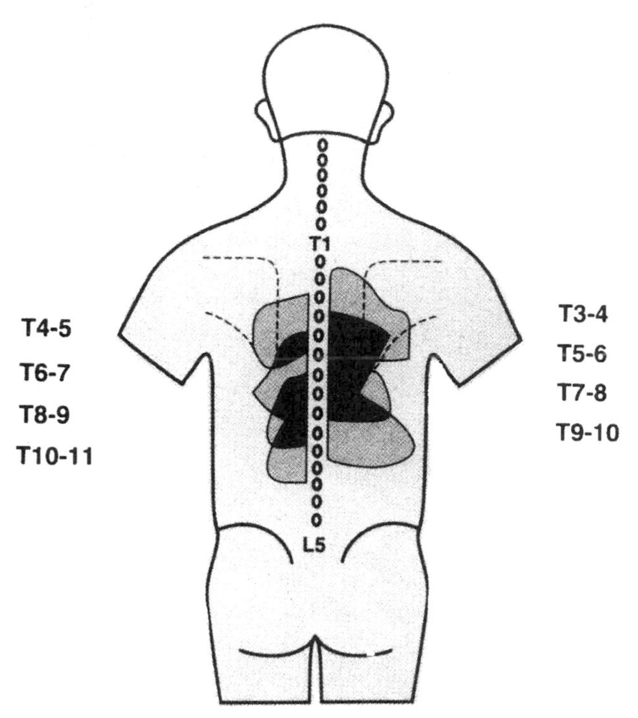

FIGURE 42–32 *A composite map showing referral patterns from the T3–T4 to T10–T11 thoracic facet joints. (Dreyfuss P, Tibiletti C, Dreyer S: Thoracic zygapophyseal joint pain patterns. Spine 19(7):807–811, 1994.)*

Nonetheless, pain referral patterns from injection into normal joints have been described (Figs. 42–32 through 42–34).[40, 41] Distension of normal joints was not painful in 27.5% of volunteers, but, when it was painful, the referral patterns were always unilateral and reproducible for most of the thoracic spine. In all subjects for the T2–T3 to T11–T12 levels, the area of most intense pain was one segment inferior and slightly lateral to the involved joint and never crossed the midline. Although significant overlap occurred, pain was not referred more than 2 1/2 segments inferior to the joint injected. At the C7–T1 joint, pain was felt in the paravertebral area over the injected joint, which extended superiorly toward the superior angle of the scapula and inferiorly toward the inferior angle of the scapula. The pain was sometimes also referred toward the shoulder joint and suprascapular region. At the T1–T2 joint, pain was felt in the paravertebral region over the joint, below the inferior angle of the scapula, and sometimes into the suprascapular region. Because of the considerable overlap, the pain maps for the C7–T1 through T2–T3 joints were not felt to be reliable enough to identify the joint of origin.

Patients who have chronic undiagnosed neck pain without objective neurologic signs or distinguishing radiographic features, can be divided into those who have a history of neck trauma and those who do not. The first group are considered to have whiplash syndrome. When there are associated headaches they may be cervicogenic

describe sudden onset of pain, usually in association with twisting, bending, or rotatory movements. Patients may report that they have more pain on extension or lateral bending than on flexion, although the reliability of this clinical feature has been challenged.[19] Pain may be more prominent in the morning and with inactivity. Pain may be aggravated by sitting, not increased by standing, and relieved by walking. It may also be aggravated on extension after forward flexion in the standing position. Typically, there is no exacerbation with Valsalva's maneuver.

On examination, patients may have paralumbar tenderness localized over the facet joints and some associated muscle spasm. They usually have no neurologic findings except perhaps some subjective hypalgesia or hyperalgesia in the skin over the painful region, subjective nondermatomal extremity sensory loss with other sensory complaints as far distal as the foot, and pain-inhibited weakness.[27, 127, 129] Flexion is generally normal or only slightly restricted in some descriptions of lumbar facet syndrome. Others, however, have reported decreased range of motion in all planes, especially on extension and rotation. Straight-leg raising is essentially negative for nerve root irritation or tension, but patients may complain of hip, buttock, or back pain.[6, 13–15, 58, 100, 117, 119, 120, 124]

The clinical picture of painful thoracic facet joints is thought to be analogous to that in the lumbar region, although there are very little data at this time. No clearly delineated thoracic facet syndrome exists, and the research to date has been based on vague clinical features: continuous or nearly continuous unilateral or bilateral paravertebral pain and tenderness in a clearly identified thoracic area of the back, without objective neurologic signs.[68]

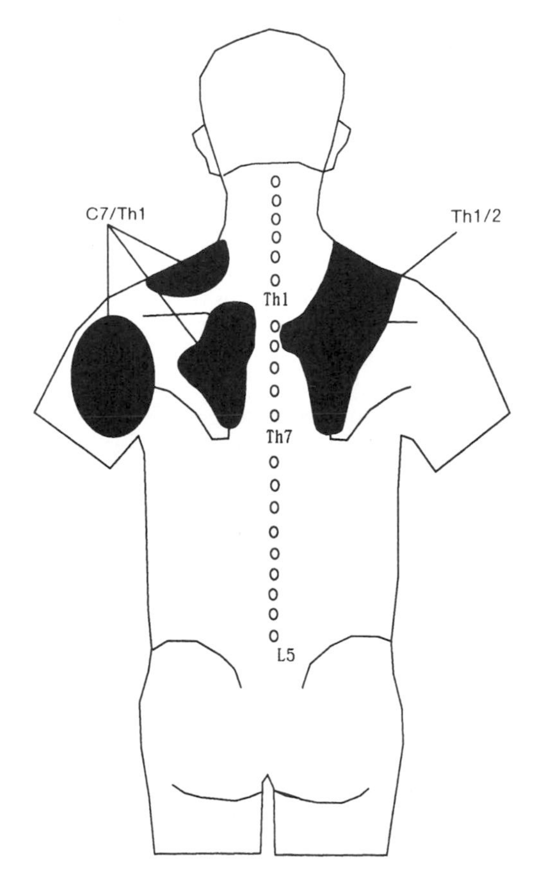

FIGURE 42–33 *A composite map shows referral patterns from the C7–T1 and T1–T2 thoracic facet joints. (Fukui S, Ohseto K, Shiotani M: Patterns of pain induced by distending the thoracic zygapophyseal joints. Reg Anesth 22(4):332–336, 1997.)*

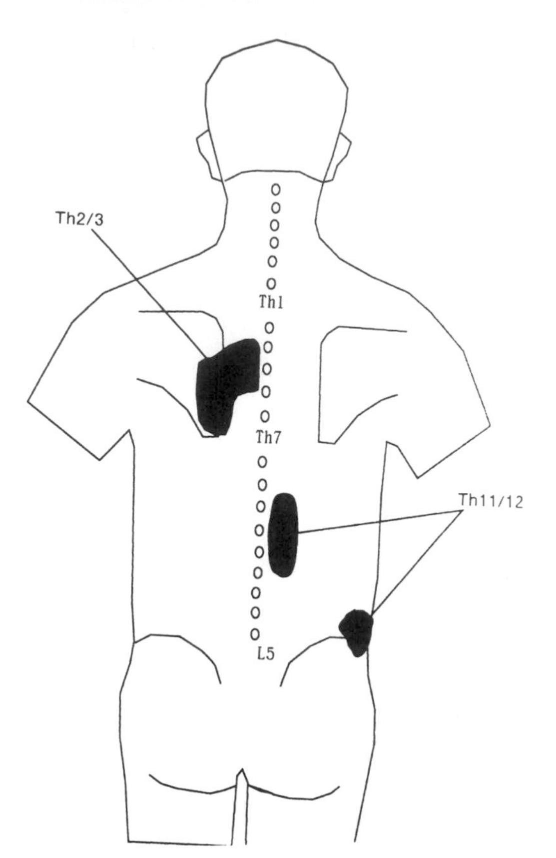

FIGURE 42–34 *A composite map shows referral patterns from the T2–T3 and T11–T12 thoracic facet joints. (Fukui S, Ohseto K, Shiotani M: Patterns of pain induced by distending the thoracic zygapophyseal joints. Reg Anesth 22(4):332–336, 1997.)*

in origin. Patients with no history of trauma may have degenerative facet disease as a significant pain generator.

The Quebec Task Force on Whiplash in 1993 did not focus on the pathology, pathophysiology, and diagnosis of whiplash[130]; however, it now seems that the likely pathology includes injuries to the facet joints.[10, 12, 55, 111, 131] A conservative estimate is that 25% of these patients have cervical facet joint pain, and the real figure may be as high as 60%.[10, 12, 111] The most common levels for symptomatic joints were C2–C3 and C5–C6. With cervicogenic headaches, the C2–C3 facet joint may be a significant pain generator.[71, 132–135] Performing a third occipital nerve block should relieve pain from the C2–C3 facet. Among patients with headache after whiplash, blockade of the third occipital nerve relieved it in 27% to 53%.[132]

In patients with degenerative disease of the cervical spine but no trauma, the facet joints may be a significant pain generator. When these patients present with the vague clinical picture of undiagnosed neck pain without objective neurologic signs or distinguishing radiographic features, the facet joints should be considered in the differential diagnosis.[6] Neck tenderness overlying a suspected involved facet joint does not appear to be a reliable sign. An Australian study of 20 such patients, however, showed 100% specificity and 100% sensitivity of a manipulative therapist in identifying those patients who did not have facet pain (12) and those who did (8).[136] The manual testing of the mechanical properties of the cervical joints was even able to identify the specific involved joint that was identified on diagnostic injection. These promising findings need to be independently confirmed with a larger group of patients.

For cervical facet joints, distinctive upper, lower, and pancervical neck pain syndromes have been described.[55] The pain is described as deep and aching.[42] It extends beyond the immediate vicinity of the joint and, therefore, is to some degree referred pain. Pain from the atlantooccipital joint (C0–C1) is referred unilaterally to the suboccipital area (Fig. 42–35).[137] Pain from the atlantoaxial joint (C1–C2) is described as unilateral, focused at the occipitocervical junction, and radiating to the postauricular region (Fig. 42–36). There may be associated physical signs, such as limited head rotation, tender trigger points confined to the occipital area, palpable cervical crepitus, and abnormal head position.[138] Pain from the C2–C3 facet joint pattern is located in the upper cervical region and extends at least to the occiput and sometimes into the head, toward the ear, vertex, forehead, or eye.[42, 43, 139] The C3–C4 facet joint produces pain over the posterolateral cervical region, following the course of the levator scapulae muscle. It extends craniad as far as the suboccipital region and then caudad over the posterolateral aspect of the neck without entering the region of the shoulder girdle. The C4–C5 facet joint pain involves a triangular area, its two sides consisting of the posterior midline and posterolateral border of the neck and its base running parallel to the spine of the scapula in the same horizontal plane as the lateral third of the clavicle. The C5–C6 facet joint produces pain in a triangular distribution with the apex directed toward the midcervical region posteriorly, the main area draped over the top of the shoulder girdle, both front and back, and the base coinciding

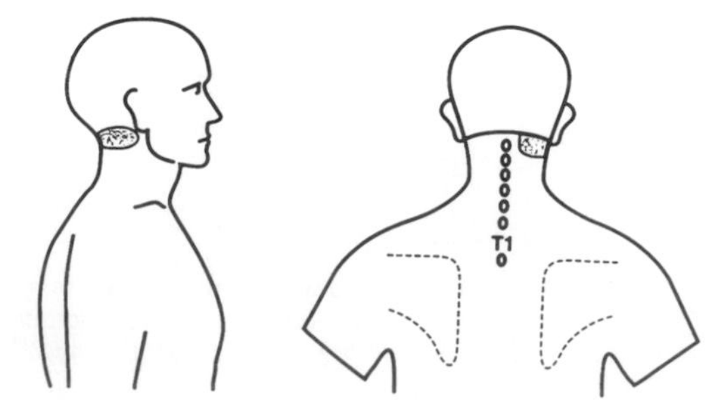

FIGURE 42–35 *A composite map shows referral pattern for the right atlantoaxial (C1–C2) joint. (Dreyfuss P, Michaelsen M, Fletcher D: Atlanto-occipital and lateral atlanto-axial joint pain patterns. Spine 19(10):1125–1131, 1994.)*

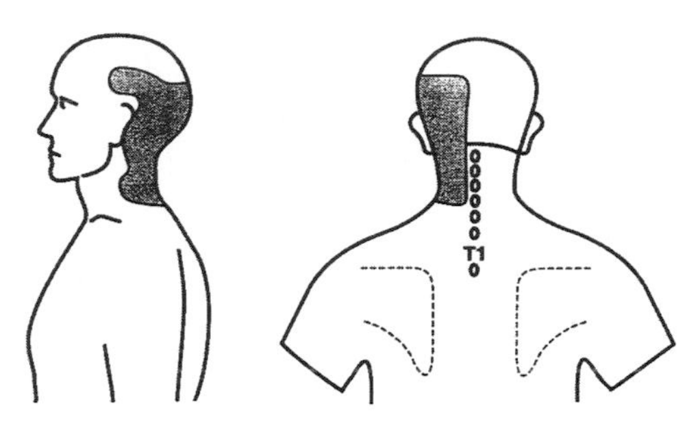

FIGURE 42–36 *A composite map shows the referral pattern for the left atlantooccipital (C0–C1) joint. (Dreyfuss P, Michaelsen M, Fletcher D: Atlanto-occipital and lateral atlanto-axial joint pain patterns. Spine 19(10):1125–1131, 1994.)*

with the spine of the scapula. The C6–C7 facet joint produces pain described as covering the supraspinous and infraspinous fossae (Figs. 42–37 through 42–39).[43, 140]

Radiographic facet joint changes are very common in adults; thus, they are a nonspecific finding. Routine lumbar radiographs can be normal or can reveal facet joint arthrosis, such as subchondral cysts or joint line irregularities, and this almost always occurs in conjunction with degenerative changes in the discs. It is also worth noting that a transitional vertebra between the lumbar and sacral spine seems to produce abnormal loading onto the adjacent superior facet joints. Such transitional vertebrae occur in only 4% to 7% of the population, and, when present, do not seem to increase the incidence of low back pain as compared with that in the normal population. However, when degenerative disease of the lumbar spine does occur, it is not spread incrementally across the spine, with 35% of the degenerative changes at the L5–S1 level, 30% at the L4–L5 level.[141] Instead, 90% of the degenerative changes, when they occur, affect the junction immediately superior to the transitional vertebra.[142]

Arthrography can show the spread of dye into a lumbar pars interarticularis defect followed by spread into the contralateral joint space (although this contralateral joint

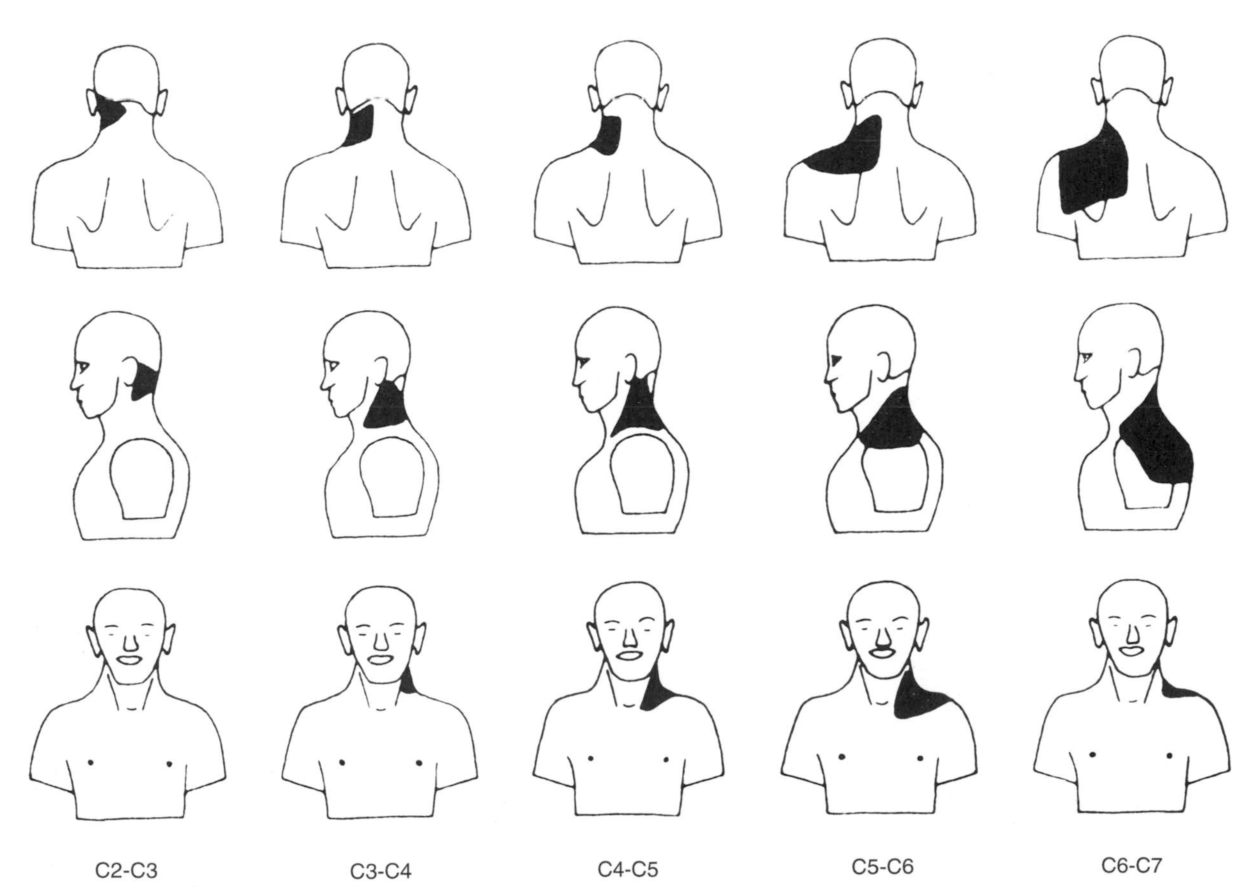

FIGURE 42–37 *Patterns of pain evoked in the first volunteer by stimulating the zygapophyseal joints at segments C2–C3 to C6–C7. (Dwyer A, Aprill C, Bogduk N: Cervical zygapophyseal joint pain patterns. I: A study in normal volunteers. Spine 15:453–457, 1990.)*

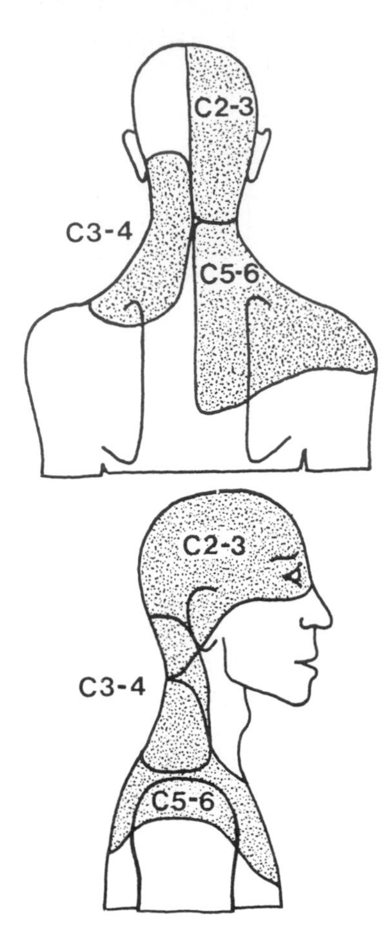

FIGURE 42–38 *A sketch of the distributions of pain reported by patients (*stippled areas*) and the segmental levels of the zygapophyseal joints found to be responsible for the pain in the majority of cases. (Bogduk N, Marsland A: The cervical zygapophyseal joints as a source of neck pain. Spine 13:610–617, 1988.)*

spread is common in the cervical spine).[39, 45, 143] The pars interarticularis communicates with the facet joint, being covered by the joint capsule. The pars interarticularis defect occurs with spondylolisthesis of the vertebral column. Before or after a therapeutic joint injection, arthrography can also demonstrate a ruptured disc capsule.

CT and MRI examinations can also be nonspecific. Some studies, however, have suggested that CT may be very helpful in diagnosing significant abnormalities of facet joints, such as joint narrowing, subchondral irregularities, and erosions.[47,107,143–147] These abnormalities may correlate well clinically with the facet joint syndrome.[113] Recently, single photon emission CT (SPECT) has been proposed as a tool to assess clinically significant facet joint disease. Although not difficult to do, SPECT has not yet been shown to be of value for that application.[148, 149] Although degenerative changes of the facet joints are common but nonspecific, clinically, it seems that a completely radiographically normal joint is unlikely to be a significant source of pain.

The clinical criteria for facet syndrome are nonspecific and still unreliable. Intraarticular facet injections or medial branch blocks should be reserved for patients with no neurologic deficit, when no other cause for their chronic pain can be identified. Also, the pain should be unresponsive to simpler therapies such as rest during acute exacerbations and oral medications, including nonsteroidal antiinflammatory drugs. The facets to be blocked can be identified by physical examination and analysis of the patient's symptoms. If the patient has marked tenderness to palpation over a particular facet joint or if pain increases with motion or loading of the joint, trial blockade of the joint should be considered.

Which joint or joints are to be blocked depends on the overall assessment. In the lumbar spine, the joint most often involved is L5–S1, and, next, L4–L5. Together, these two levels likely account for two thirds of painful joints in the lumbar spine. If there is tenderness or pain and radiographic changes suggestive of involvement at a more

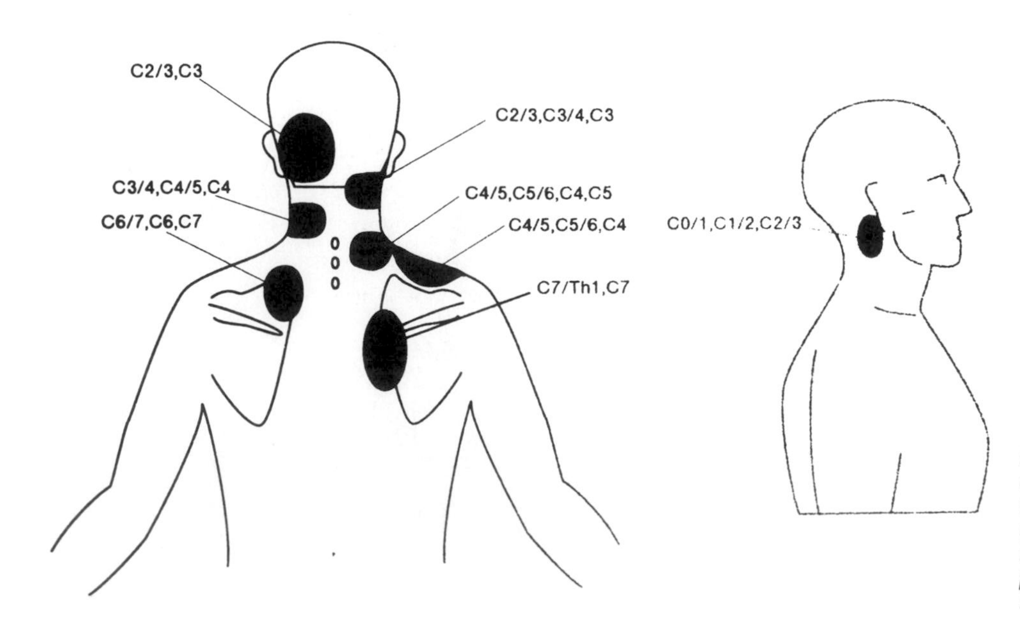

FIGURE 42–39 *Main referral pain distributions for the facet joints from C0–C1 to C7–T1, and the dorsal rami of C3–C7. (Fukui S, Ohseto K, Shiotani M, et al: Referred pain distribution of the cervical zygapophyseal joints and cervical dorsal rami. Pain 68:79–83, 1996.)*

cephalad level, then the injections should be made into a more cephalad lumbar joint. If the pain is primarily unilateral, the lowest one to three facet joints are usually implicated. With bilateral low back pain, bilateral injections at L5–S1, and perhaps also at L4–L5, may be in order.

When there is a transitional vertebra, the diseased joints are usually the pair of facet joints at the level between the transitional vertebra and the next most cephalad vertebra.[142]

In the thoracic spine, the joint(s) to be injected should be chosen according to the clinical picture, as in the lumbar spine. In the cervical spine, the choice of joint(s) should be based on the clinical picture, and usually no more than two joints are injected at one time (one bilaterally or two on one side). In patients with a history of neck trauma, the joint most often involved is C2–C3 or C5–C6 level. Using the location of maximum pain and tenderness, in conjunction with radiographic abnormalities, the diseased joint can be fairly reliably identified.

Contraindications

There are no absolute contraindications to facet blockade other than those for any regional block. Facet blocks should not be performed in patients with coagulopathy, systemic infection, or infection at the site of injection, nor in patients who are allergic to the medication to be injected or who refuse the procedure.

Techniques

Lumbar Facet Blocks

The patient is placed prone with the hips supported by pillows. This position flexes the back slightly and allows optimal visualization of the lumbar facet joints. Using fluoroscopy, the joint(s) to be blocked are identified and marked before making the injection(s) (Fig. 42–40). It may be necessary to count the vertebral bodies from T12 to the sacrum to properly identify the joint to be blocked. At each joint to be blocked, the caudal edge of the spinous process corresponding to the level of the facet joint is identified (e.g., the L4 process corresponding to the L4–L5 facet). This helps to identify the facet joint if it is hard to see.

After sterile preparation and draping, local anesthetic is used to infiltrate the skin and deeper layers overlying the facet joint. Either a 20- or a 22-gauge, 10-cm spinal needle or a thin probe designed for cryoneurolysis or radiofrequency facet denervation is then advanced to the desired position before injection or neurolysis is performed (Fig. 42–41). For intraarticular injection, the spinal needle is inserted into the joint. To do this it is best to visualize the joint by rotating the fluoroscope beam obliquely 10 to 40 degrees lateral from the midline posteriorly. Once this is done, the needle can be directed down the path of the beam into the joint. The posterior joint space may be difficult to see and to enter if there is significant arthritis. Also, the best fluoroscopic image of the joint may be obtained at an angle 5 to 10 degrees more oblique than the best angle for the needle to enter the joint. Radiocontrast dye, 0.25 to 0.5 mL, may be injected to visualize the

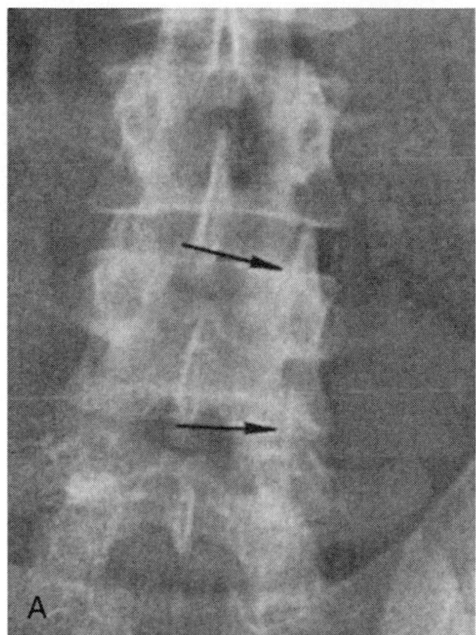

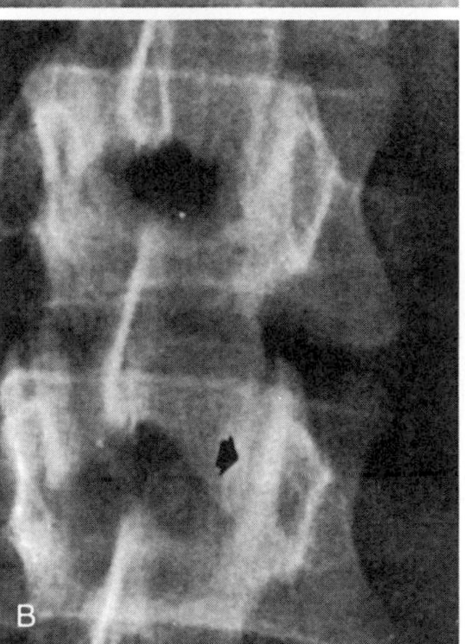

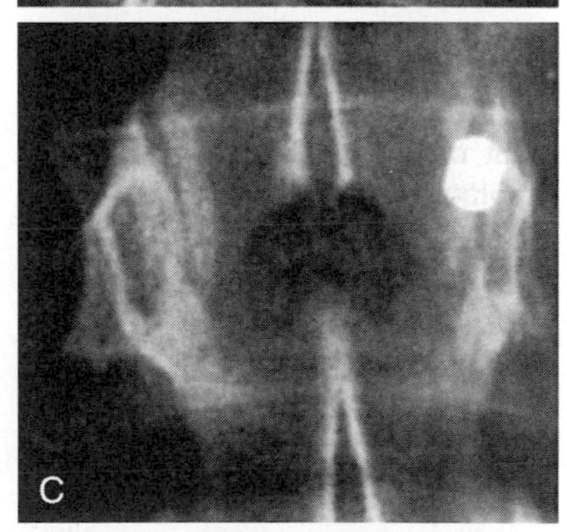

FIGURE 42–40 *A, Facet joint spaces are seen at L3–L4 and at L4–L5* (arrows) *with the patient prone (sagittal beam). In each case, the joint space is the portion of the joint farthest posterior and most accessible to puncture from the back.* B, *Fluoroscopic spot radiograph with the patient rotated slightly into a minimally oblique position (affected side up). The posterior portion of the facet joint is clearly identified* (arrowhead) *and readily accessible to puncture.* C, *Fluoroscopic spot radiograph taken during insertion of a 20-gauge spinal needle vertically into the L3–L4 facet joint. The needle is advanced until the posterior joint opening is contacted. A direct vertical puncture ensures that the tip enters the joint space. (Carrera GF: Lumbar facet joint injection in low back pain and sciatica. Radiology 137:661–664, 1980.)*

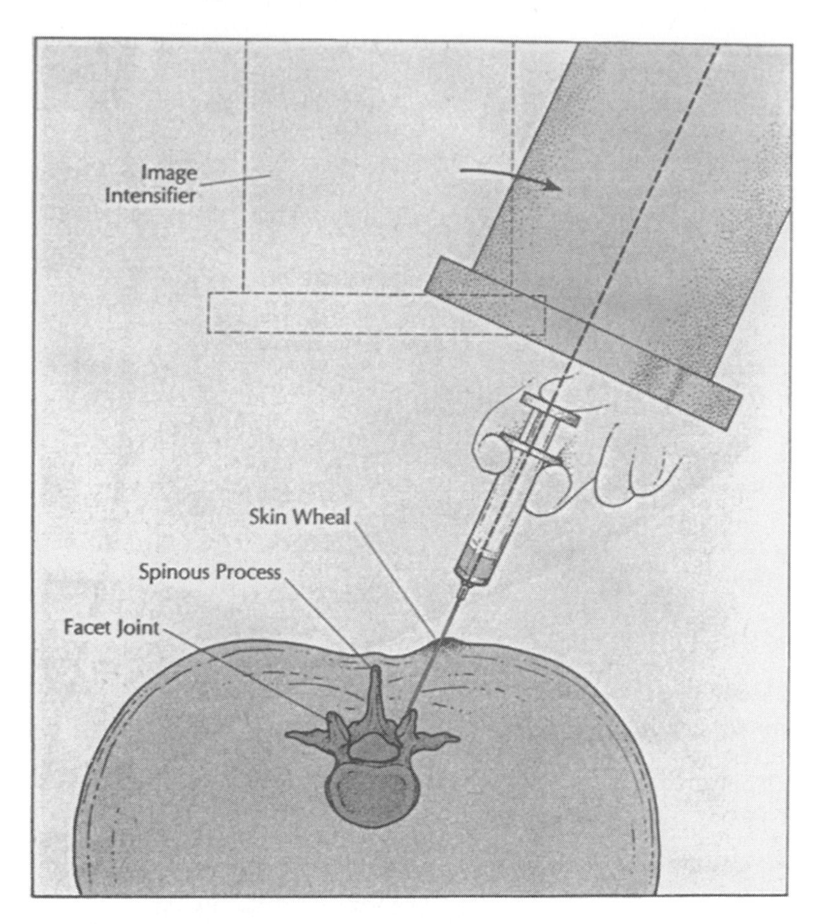

FIGURE 42–41 The only way to make a definitive diagnosis of facet syndrome is to inject local anesthetic into the facet joint or its nerve supply. Relief of pain confirms the diagnosis. The procedure may also be therapeutic when conservative treatment has failed. Needle can be accurately positioned within the facet joint under fluoroscopic guidance. (Warfield CA: Facet syndrome and the relief of low back pain. Hosp Pract 30(10A):41–48, 1988.)

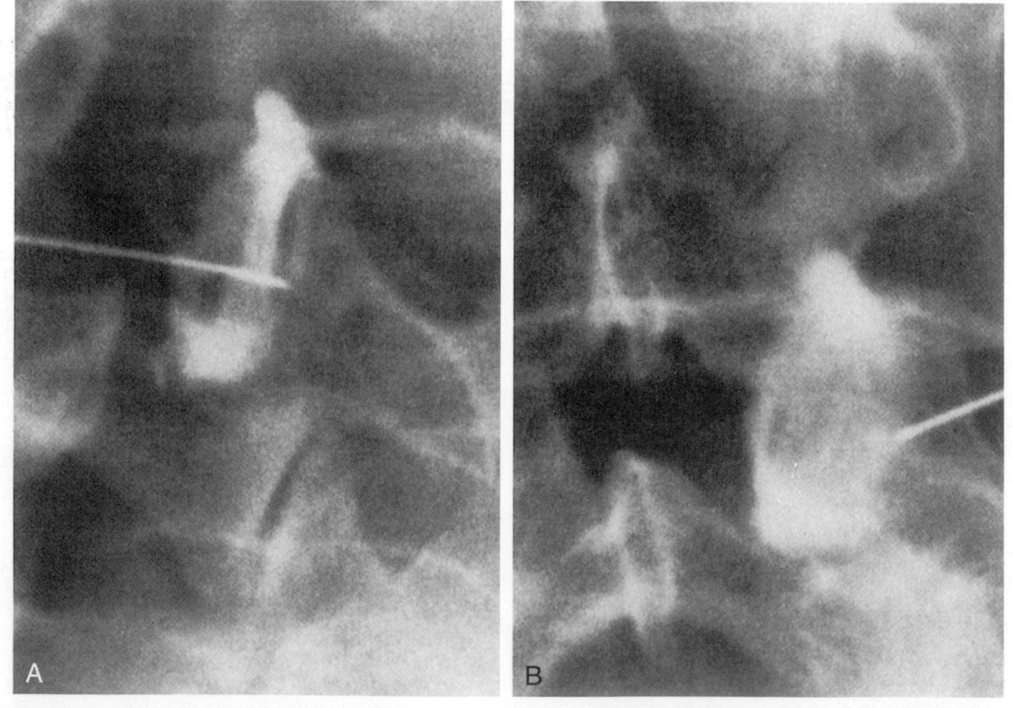

FIGURE 42–42 Normal facet arthrogram. A, Oblique view of an L4–L5 facet joint after injection of 1 mL of Conray-60. The normal joint capsule has a smooth, sigmoid configuration. B, Posterior view of the same facet joint shows a smooth, oval joint capsule. (Destouet JM, Gilula LA, Murphy WA, Mousees B: Lumbar facet joint injection: Indication, technique, clinical correlation, and preliminary results. Radiology 145:321–325, 1982.)

S-shaped joint space and confirm proper needle placement before injection of 1 to 1.5 mL of medication (i.e., 2% lidocaine with 10 to 20 mg triamcinolone or methylprednisolone; Fig. 42–42). Before the radiocontrast dye is injected, the physician must confirm that the patient has no allergy. The use of radiocontrast dye helps to insure that the articular injection is accurately placed and that there is no capsule rupture and extravasation of dye. The needle's position can also be confirmed clinically by the feel of the needle walking off the bone and then into the joint. The patient can then be rolled 10 to 20 degrees under fluoroscopic guidance with one of the operator's hands cephalad and the other caudad to the inserted needle and outside the fluoroscopic beam. The needle can be seen to be inside the joint, and typically bends 1 to 2 cm proximal from the needle tip, confirming that it is fixed in the joint.

In medial branch blocks, using a spinal needle, the needle is introduced approximately 5 cm lateral from the midline and directed obliquely, to avoid the overhang of the articular processes. From L1–L4, the medial branch is blocked where it lies in a gutter on the dorsal surface of the transverse process, just caudal to the most medial end of the superior edge of the transverse process. At the lumbosacral level, the posterior primary ramus of L5 is blocked as it runs in the groove between the ala of the sacrum and the superior articular process of the sacrum (Figs. 42–1 through 42–45).[56, 150] For the injection to be reliably diagnostic, the needle location needs to be precisely placed and preferably with the bevel opening facing medially and inferiorly. The ideal target point is midway between the upper border of the transverse process and the mamilloaccessory ligament. For the L1–L4 medial branch nerves, this is at position 1 on Figures 42–44 and 42–45. The analogous location for the L5 nerve is a point midway between position 1 and 2 on Figures 42–44 and 42–45. This is midway between the junction of the superior border of the ala of the sacrum with the superior articular process of the sacrum, and the mamilloaccessory ligament. Blocking a single joint requires that two medial branch nerves be injected, and, for completeness, at the L5–S1 level the S1 nerve should also be blocked. It is usually located just cephalad to the S1 posterior opening in a line between the S1 opening and the L5–S1 facet joint. Finding it may require walking the needle tip in a medial to lateral direction, crossing the path of the nerve as it travels caudad to cephalad along the periosteum. To minimize unwanted spread of injectate, the injection is precisely targeted, and only a small volume of local anesthetic is used (0.5–1.0 mL). The rate of injection is important.

If the injection is to be done for diagnostic purposes, either a low-volume intraarticular or medial branch block should be performed. Both are equally reliable, and the choice depends on the ease of visualization and insertion of the needle into the joint, or simply on the operator's preference. For therapeutic purposes, with perhaps less specificity, a periarticular injection using up to 4 mL of injectate per joint can be performed.

Thoracic Facet Block

Only three studies of thoracic facet denervation have been conducted, and, unfortunately, the results are unreliable because the anatomic location of the medial branch nerves in the thoracic spine has since been shown to be 12 mm away from the site of denervation.[68, 69] Therefore, until a reliable technique is developed, the only injection for thoracic facets is either intraarticular or periarticular. These may be useful therapeutically, and perhaps also diagnostically.

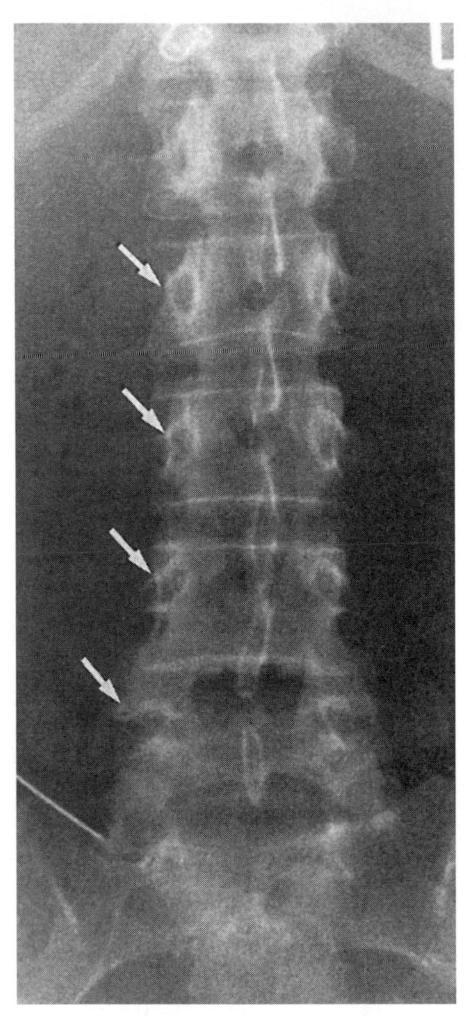

FIGURE 42–43 Posteroanterior radiograph of the lumbar spine shows a needle in position for L5 medial branch block. Target points for the other lumbar medial branches are indicated by arrows. (Bogduk N: Back Pain: Zygapophyseal blocks and epidural steroids. In Cousins MJ, Bridenbaugh PO (eds): Neural Blockade in Clinical Anesthesia and Management of Pain, ed 2. Philadelphia, JB Lippincott, 1988, pp 935–946.)

For the articular injection technique the patient is positioned prone. The joint to be blocked is identified by counting the ribs from T1 caudad and from T12 cephalad. Once the joint is identified, a radiopaque marker on the skin over the joint may help in needle localization. Because of the steep angle of the thoracic facet joints, the skin entry point may need to overlie the pedicle one or two segments caudad. After sterile preparation and draping, local anesthetic is injected into the skin and tissues along the needle path. A 20- or 22-gauge, 10-cm spinal needle is then directed steeply cephalad toward the joint. Using the skin marker and a combination of anteroposterior and lateral fluoroscopic images, the needle is then advanced into the joint. As in the lumbar spine, a combination of dye injection

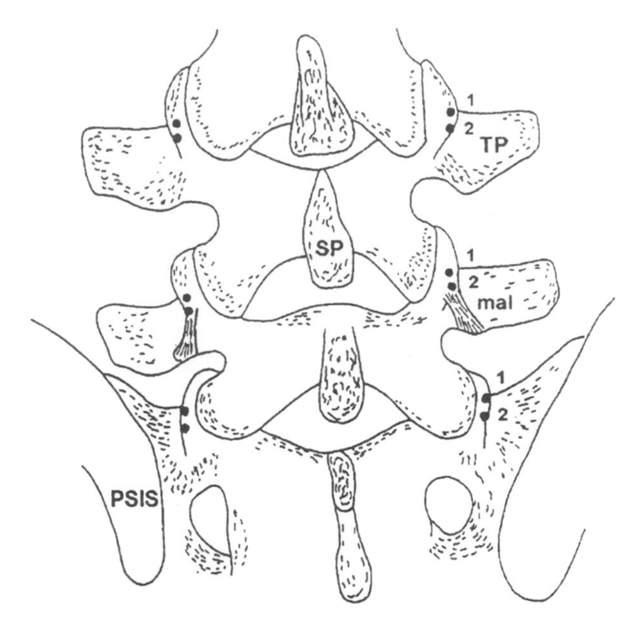

*FIGURE 42–44 Posterior view of the lower lumbar spine shows the location of the upper (1) and lower (2) target points for the L3 and L4 medial branch blocks and L5 dorsal rami blocks. The mammilloaccessory ligament (*mal*) is shown. TP, transverse process; SP, spinous process; PSIS, posterior superior iliac spine. (Dreyfuss P, Schwarzer AC, Lau P, et al: Specificity of lumbar medial branch and L5 dorsal ramus blocks. Spine 22(8):895–902, 1997.)*

and needle "feel" confirms proper needle placement. The thoracic facet joints are very small and can hold only 0.4 to 0.6 mL of injectate. Therefore, the mixture of dye, local anesthetic, and steroid should not exceed this total joint volume. Additional solution may be injected periarticularly for therapeutic purposes.

Cervical Facet Block

For medial branch nerve blocks of C3 through C7, the patients are positioned laterally with the side to be blocked uppermost. A 22-gauge spinal needle or a shorter 22- or 25-gauge block needle is inserted with sterile technique using a posterolateral approach with fluoroscopic guidance. The target point for the third through the seventh medial branches is the periosteum at the "centroid" of the projection of the articular pillar as seen on the lateral fluoroscopic image (Fig. 42–25).[72] To establish that the contralateral articular process is not being mistaken for the ipsilateral process, the x-ray beam is rotated slightly to and fro around a longitudinal axis. This causes the two images of the ipsilateral and contralateral articular processes to separate, and the ipsilateral articular process is identified as the one that rotates in the same direction as the needle. After aspiration to check for blood or cerebrospinal fluid, 0.5 mL of local anesthetic is injected (Figs. 42–23, 42–46). The medial

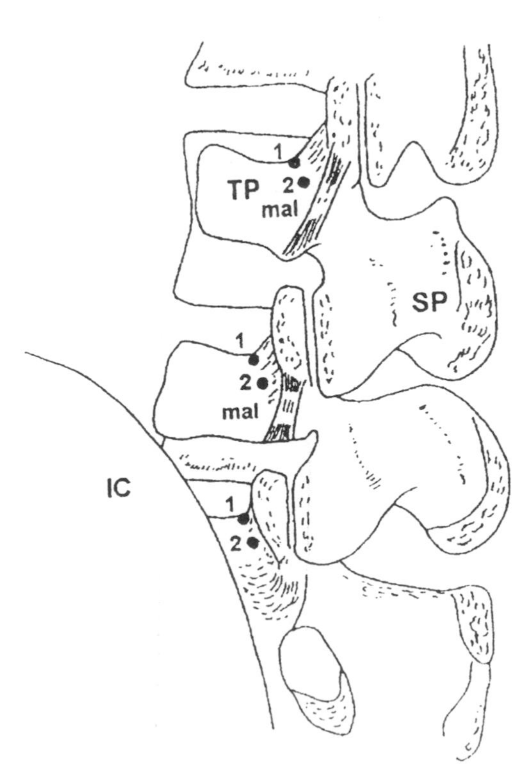

*FIGURE 42–45 Oblique lateral view of the lower lumbar spine shows the upper (1) and lower (2) target points for L3 and L4 medial branch blocks and L5 dorsal rami blocks. The mammilloaccessory ligament (*mal*) is shown. TP, transverse process; SP, spinous process; IC, iliac crest. (Dreyfuss P, Schwarzer AC, Lau P, et al: Specificity of lumbar medial branch and L5 dorsal ramus blocks. Spine 22(8):895–902, 1997.)*

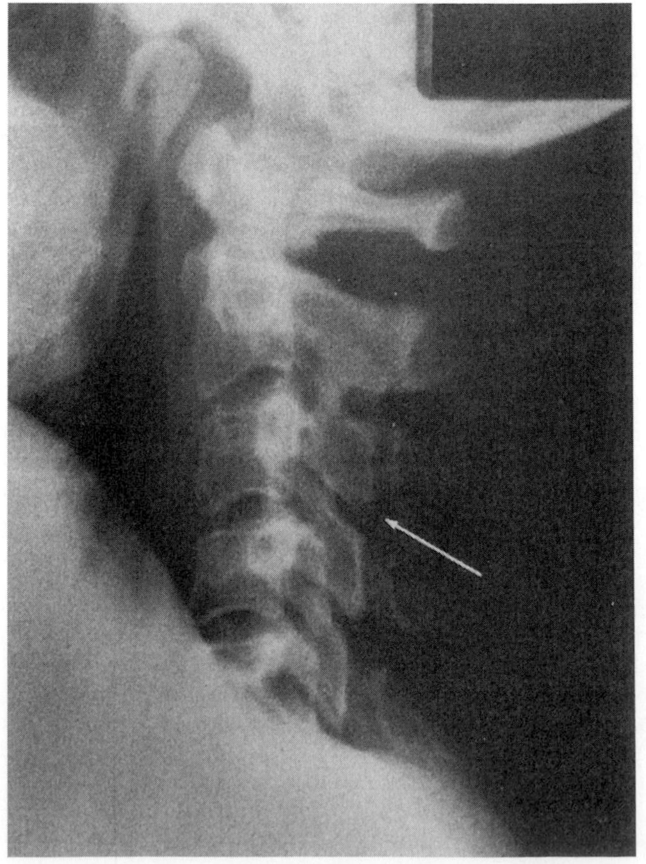

FIGURE 42–46 Needle in position for facet desensitization. (Selby DK, Paris SV: Anatomy of facet joints and its clinical correlation with low back pain. Contemp Orthopaed 3:1097–1103, 1981.)

branch of the C8 posterior ramus crosses the root of the T1 transverse process. Instead of wrapping around an articular pillar, it hooks medially onto the lamina of T1, whence it sends articular branches to the C7–T1 facet joint. This orientation is similar to the innervation of the lumbar facet joints. Therefore, using 0.5 mL of local anesthetic, the target point is modified to block the medial branch nerve as it crosses the lamina of T7.

Intraarticular blockade of cervical facets C3–C7 can also be performed (Figs. 42–23, 42–47). A 22-gauge, 10-cm spinal needle should be inserted one to two levels below the joint to be blocked. The needle is then advanced upward and forward into the middle of the joint under fluoroscopic guidance. Radiocontrast dye, 0.25 to 0.5 mL, can be used to confirm proper intraarticular placement. No more than 1 mL of medication, including the dye, can be injected before the facet joint ruptures.

To block the innervation of the C2–C3 facet joint requires locating the third occipital nerve. The patient is positioned in the lateral position with the side to be blocked uppermost. The needle is advanced using a posterolateral approach until it contacts the C2–C3 facet joint and then is redirected laterally until it reaches the lower half of the lateral margin of the facet (see Fig. 42–24).[72] The target points are located along a vertical line bisecting the articular pillar of C3 and injections are made immediately above the subchondral plate of the C2 inferior articular process, immediately below the subchondral plate of the C3 superior articular process, and at a point midway between these two. At each of these three sites, 0.5 mL of local anesthetic is injected. The patient should be assessed for suboccipital numbness, which indicates adequate blockade of the third occipital nerve and innervation of the C2–C3 facet joint.

The atlantoaxial joint can be blocked using a 25-gauge spinal needle to enter the joint posterolaterally and then directing the needle onto the lateral half of the posterior capsule under fluoroscopic guidance.[137] To do this, the patient is placed in the lateral decubitus position with the side to be injected uppermost. The head is rotated toward the table approximately 45 degrees and the neck slightly flexed. The mastoid process and occipital prominences are located through palpation, and skin marks are placed. Between these two marks is a palpable cleft. A third mark is placed over this cleft, below the occipital brim. With oblique imaging, the C arm and skull/neck are moved slowly until the third skin mark is located over the superior, posterior, and lateral aspect of the joint (the target point). A skin wheal of local anesthetic is injected at this point, and the needle is advanced along this path to the target point. The needle is advanced slowly, using confirmation with posteroanterior open-mouth, lateral, and oblique views to ensure that the needle is in the middle of the joint before injecting medication (Figs. 42–48, 42–49). Up to 0.5 mL of radiocontrast dye can also be used to document proper needle placement. The practitioner should be aware that the epidural space lies immediately medial to the joint capsule and that the vertebral artery passes just lateral to it. Aspiration for blood or cerebrospinal fluid should be performed before each injection. Using more than 1.0 mL total volume of injectate may result in leakage outside the joint capsule with subsequent blockade of the cervical spinal nerve roots.

Bogduk and associates[24, 55] recommend medial branch nerve blocks rather than intraarticular injections in the cervical area, for the following reasons:

- Medial branch nerve blocks are easier to perform, and possibly less traumatic, than intraarticular injections.
- The medial branch nerves lie fairly superficial and are easily accessible after penetration of the neck muscles by the needle.
- Intraarticular blocks require skillful insertion of the needle into a narrow joint space, often after several adjustments.
- Medial branch nerve blocks can be successfully performed in patients with facet joint disease that has obliterated the joint space.

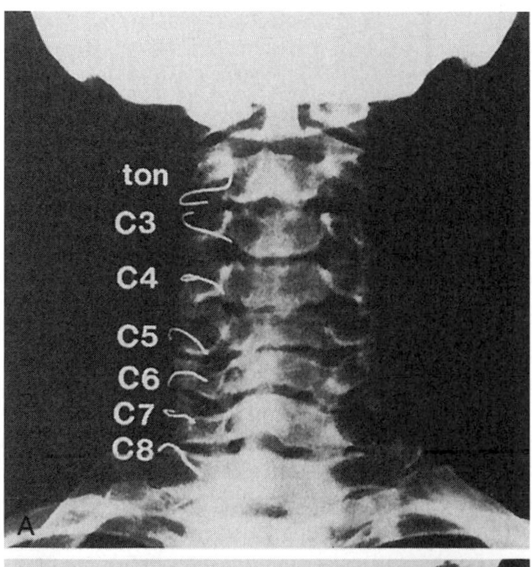

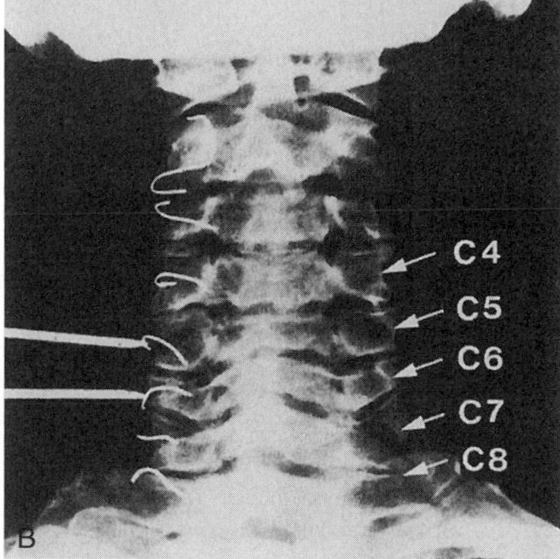

FIGURE 42–47 Radiographic anatomy of the cervical medial branches. A, *Posteroanterior radiograph of a specimen in which wires were placed along the proximal portions of the third occipital nerve (*ton*) and the C3–C8 medial branches to indicate their course in relation to bone.* B, *Suggested needle placements and target points* (arrows) *for medial branches suitable for selective local anesthetic blocks or percutaneous coagulation. Note how the tips of the needles rest directly on the dissected medial branches, whose positions are indicated by the wires. (Bogduk N: The clinical anatomy of the cervical dorsal rami. Spine 7:319–330, 1982.)*

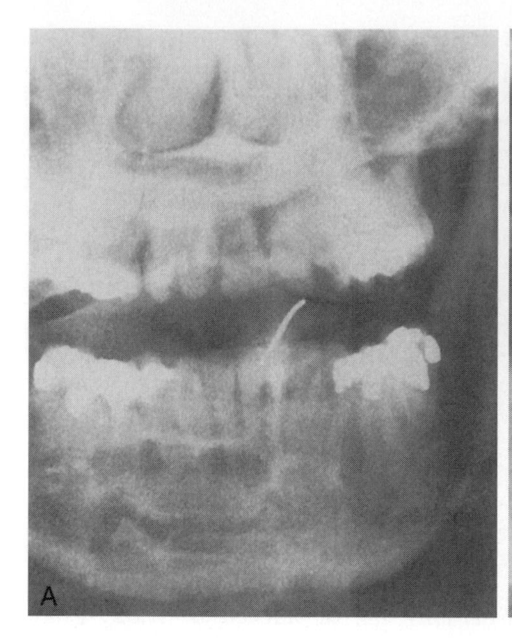

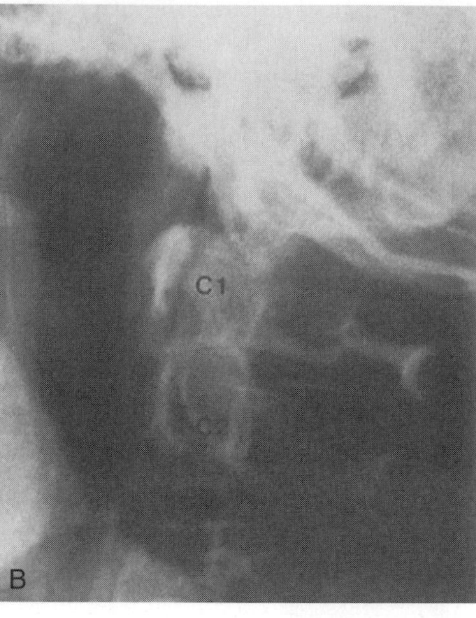

FIGURE 42–48 Radiographs showing the appearance of a needle introduced into the right lateral atlantoaxial joint. A, *Posteroanterior view;* B, *lateral view. (Bogduk N: Back pain: Zygapophyseal blocks and epidural steroids.* In *Cousins M, Bridenbaugh PO (eds): Neural Blockade in Clinical Anesthesia and Management of Pain, ed 2. Philadelphia, JB Lippincott, 1988, pp 935–946.)*

- The approach to medial branch nerve block allows the needle to remain on the dorsolateral aspect of the cervical spine; therefore, theoretically there is less risk of penetration of a vertebral artery, the epidural space, or the dural sac than with intraarticular injections.
- No studies indicate greater therapeutic success or diagnostic specificity with the intraarticular approach as compared with blockade of the medial branches innervating the facet joints.

Although needle placement has traditionally been done with fluoroscopic guidance, techniques have also been developed that use ultrasound, CT, and MRI.[64, 151–153]

What those trying to set the standard have not been able to agree on is the definition of a *successful block*. Generally, in the past, pain during the injection of a single diagnostic block that was relieved by a local anesthetic was considered diagnostic. Pain with intraarticular injection has since been shown to be much less reliable diagnostically.[154, 155] Single diagnostic blocks have been shown to produce false-positive results in the lumbar spine in 38%, and in the cervical spine in 27% of patients (these results being determined with double diagnostic blocks). Patients do not necessarily require double diagnostic blocks before medial branch denervation, as this procedure seems to be fairly safe. The research on outcomes needs to be based on this new standard of double diagnostic blocks, however.

Even when the block relieves pain, there is no consistent standard for what is considered significant pain relief. The standard for defining pain relief has been set at 50% by some, 75% by others, and even 100% by a few. The difficulty with accepting 50% pain relief, even with double diagnostic blocks, is the lack of specificity this may lead to. It has been proposed that 10% to 15% of chronic low back pain can be attributed to the facet joints, and degenerative disc disease accounts for another 40%. How-

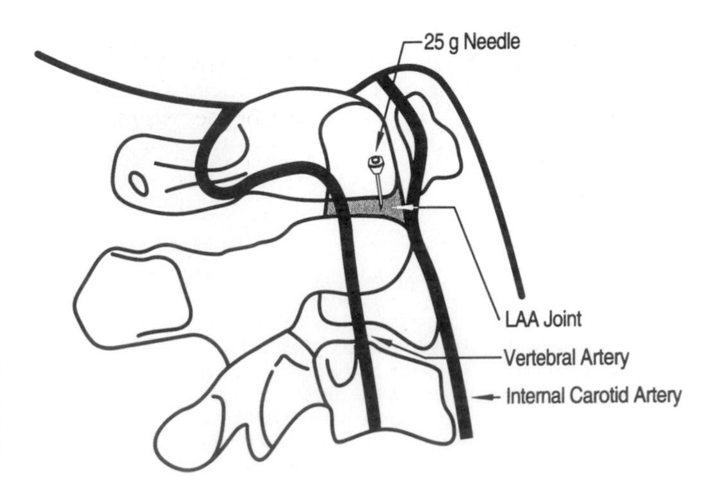

FIGURE 42–49 Diagram depicting placement of a 25-gauge spinal needle into the lateral atlantoaxial (LAA) joint using a lateral approach. The relationship of the needle to the vertebral and internal carotid arteries is shown. (Dreyfuss P, Michaelsen M, Fletcher D: Atlanto-occipital and lateral atlanto-axial joint pain patterns. Spine 19(10):1125–1131, 1994.)

ever, back pain is usually multifactorial. To focus on the facet joints to the exclusion of other possible factors, based on 50% pain relief, may lead to an excessive number of facet or medial branch injections.

Facet Denervation

Facet denervation is performed on the medial branch nerves with the same technique used to locate the nerves for medial branch blocks. This means that a single lumbar facet denervation requires that two nerves be treated, and three in the case of the L5–S1 facet joint. Two nerves are also denervated for each of the cervical facets from C3–C4 to C7–T1. The technique of denervation of these cervical facets is slightly different from block technique and is described below. The C2–C3 facet joint requires three denervation target points as described earlier. The results of previous diagnostic blocks will determine which facet joints will be denervated. Because denervation is obviously destructive to the nerves, there must be clear indications for proceeding. One potential concern is the development of deafferentation pain, although this risk seems to be very small. Ideally, to avoid doing the procedure when it could produce no benefit, the selection criteria should be strict. Currently the best proposal is to use "clear pain relief" after two diagnostic blocks as the indication. *Clear pain relief* is defined as at least 50%—and preferably 75% to 100%—pain relief. This avoids unnecessarily "denervating" 38% of lumbar pain patients, and 27% of the cervical pain patients when the first diagnostic block is false-positive.[126, 156] Too strict criteria, on the other hand, would deny the denervating procedure to those 8% of patients whose first result is false-negative.

In theory, the denervation can be performed with radiofrequency lesioning, cryotherapy, or chemical ablation. In practice, chemical denervation is not done because of the potential for inadvertent spread and morbidity. Cryotherapy is a viable technique, although in practice radiofrequency denervation is the most popular technique. There is a large body of literature on the techniques for lumbar[65, 157–173] and cervical spine denervation.[74, 112, 163, 174–176] Because of the lack of a reliable technique for thoracic medial branch block, no technique for thoracic medial branch denervation is recommended at this time.

Medial branch denervation uses a radiofrequency lesioning probe and fluoroscopic guidance (see Fig. 42–48). Several sizes of probes are available for various locations to be denervated (22-gauge, 54-mm; 22-gauge, 105-mm; and 20-gauge, 145-mm). These standard probes require that, after proper needle positioning, the probe be removed from the needle so that local anesthetic can be injected before the denervation. This could potentially result in movement of the needle tip and failure of denervation. To avoid this, some operators have simply performed the denervation without local anesthetic, although this can be quite painful for the patient. It is, however, usually possible to gradually increase the probe tip temperature to 80°C over one minute, typically with a 15-second pause at 50°C for patient comfort.

Radionics has made radiofrequency lesioning probes that allow local anesthetic to be injected via connecting tubing without having to remove the probe after the nerve has been located. These probes are available in 23-gauge, 60-mm, and 22-gauge, 100-mm sizes. Once the probe has been positioned, an electrical stimulator provides confirmation that the tip of the probe is not too close to the anterior primary ramus. If the probe is properly positioned, the patient may complain of greater than usual pain at 50 Hz and less than 1 V, and ideally at less than 0.5 V. If the probe is not in good position, muscle twitching or leg movements may be seen at 2 Hz and at less than 2 V. Between 1 and 2 mL of local anesthetic should be injected before a radiofrequency lesion is made using the coagulation current. The current is sustained for 60 to 90 sec, when the temperature of the probe tip reaches 80° C (Radionics Lesiongenerator RFG-3B). At this temperature, the tissue surrounding the tip of a 22-gauge probe produces a consistent lesion that extends 1.1 mm distal to the tip and radially 1.9 mm from the shaft of the probe. The resulting lesion is sausage-shaped, approximately 7 mm long, and 4 mm wide. Because the medial branch nerves are generally 1 to 1.5 mm across, the most reliable probe position is with the shaft of the probe parallel to the path of the nerve. Coagulating the nerve off the tip of the probe is more likely to fail.[177] Because it is relatively easy to coagulate the nerve incompletely, two to three lesions are recommended parallel to the path of the nerve in the lumbar spine, moving the probe 1 mm cephalad and caudad from the ideal target point with the skin entry point posterior to the nerve and the probe directed straight anterior.

Because of the need to have the probe parallel to the nerve and because the success of cervical medial branch denervation has been mediocre, the cervical denervation technique is slightly different from that of medial branch block.[74, 112, 176] For cervical spine denervation, the patient is placed in a prone position and two skin entry points are used, one directly anteroposterior and the second angled 30 degrees and slightly cephalad in orientation (Figs. 42–50 through 42–54). These are done with fluoroscopic guidance using anteroposterior and lateral views. The first probe is inserted from a posterior approach along a parasagittal plane, tangential to the articular pillar and directed to the medial branch target point. The probe tip is advanced just medial to the lateral margin of the articular pillar until bony resistance is felt on the back of the pillar. This prevents over insertion of the probe. The probe is then walked laterally off the pillar in very small increments until a loss of bony resistance is felt, and the electrode gently slips forward tangential to the pillar. The second probe is directed 30 degrees obliquely from a slightly more caudad skin entry point and, therefore, directed slightly cephalad. It is advanced as for the parasagittal approach. The remainder of the technique is the same as that for the lumbar spine, each probe being repositioned 1 mm cephalad and 1 mm caudad from the target point, for a total of six lesions. This process is more reliable but also more time-consuming. For the C2–C3 facet denervation, the probe passes are at the level of maximum convexity of the C2–C3 joint, at a point just above the waist of the C3 articular pillar and at one point between the two.

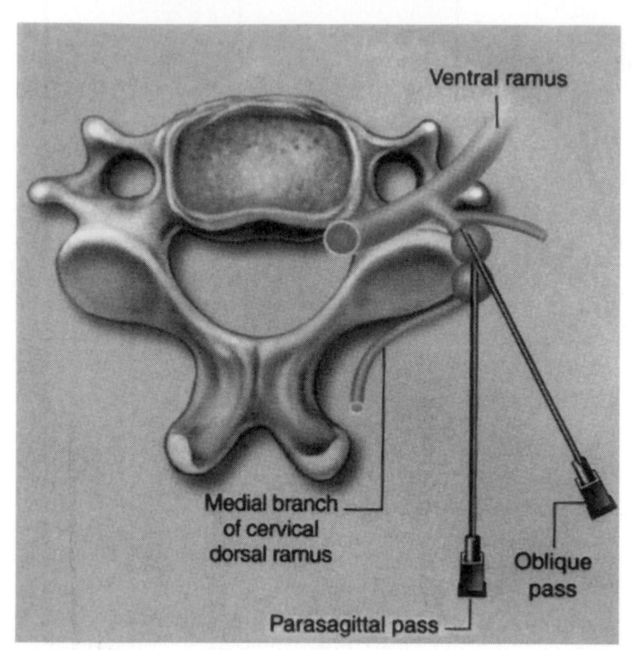

FIGURE 42–50 *The use of electrodes to coagulate a medial branch of a cervical dorsal ramus is shown on a cross section through the C5 vertebra. An oblique pass is used to reach the nerve over the anterolateral aspect of the articular pillar. A parasagittal pass is used to reach the nerve over the lateral aspect of the pillar. (Lord SM, Barnsley L, Wallis BJ, et al: Percutaneous radio-frequency neurotomy for chronic cervical zygapophyseal joint pain. N Engl J Med 335(23):1721–1726, 1996. Copyright © 1996, Massachusetts Medical Society. All rights reserved.)*

Unfortunately, the success rate of the C2–C3 facet denervation technique is poor, and further modifications need to be made so that a reliable technique can be recommended.[74]

More recently, pulse radiofrequency denervation has been proposed as an improvement on the standard technique.[178] With pulse radiofrequency denervation, the tip temperature is increased to 42° C or the delivered voltage reaches 60 V. The generator then delivers 20-msec bursts every 0.5 sec for 120 sec. The therapeutic effect of this is not clear at this time. However, because the denervation takes place at a lower temperature, the pulse radiofrequency denervation is thought to be more selective for the C fibers, less likely to damage motor fibers, and less likely to produce neuritic changes. More studies need to be done to assess the potential benefit and role of pulse radiofrequency for denervating procedures.

Complications

Complications secondary to lumbar facet block have usually been temporary and infrequent. The problem most often cited is a transient exacerbation in pain (about 2% incidence) lasting (in rare cases) as long as 6 weeks to 8 months.[58] Spinal anesthesia has occurred after facet joint injection.[179, 180] Several reports of chemical meningitis after lumbar facet block have also been published.[181, 182] Both of these complications are thought to have occurred after inadvertent dural puncture. Paraspinal infections have also been reported after facet injections.[183, 184] Facet capsule rupture also occurs, especially when more than 2.0 mL of injectate is used for intraarticular injections in the lumbar spine, more than 0.6 mL in the thoracic spine, and more than 1.0 mL in the cervical spine. It is not clear at this time whether capsular rupture exacerbates chronic back or neck pain.

Cervical facet blockade carries the risks of entry into the intervertebral foramen and puncture of the vertebral artery, two structures that lie directly anterior to the cervical facet joints. This complication occurs more frequently with the intraarticular technique than with blockade of the medial branches innervating the cervical facets, because intraarticular blocks require deeper penetration by the needle. The epidural space lies immediately medial to the joint, and the cervical nerve roots exit via the intervertebral foramen very close to the joint capsule. Local anesthetic could leak out of the joint into these areas, causing motor and sensory deficits.[24, 42, 55]

Third occipital nerve blocks can cause transient ataxia and unsteadiness secondary to partial blockade of the upper cervical proprioceptive afferents.[24, 55] After radiofrequency

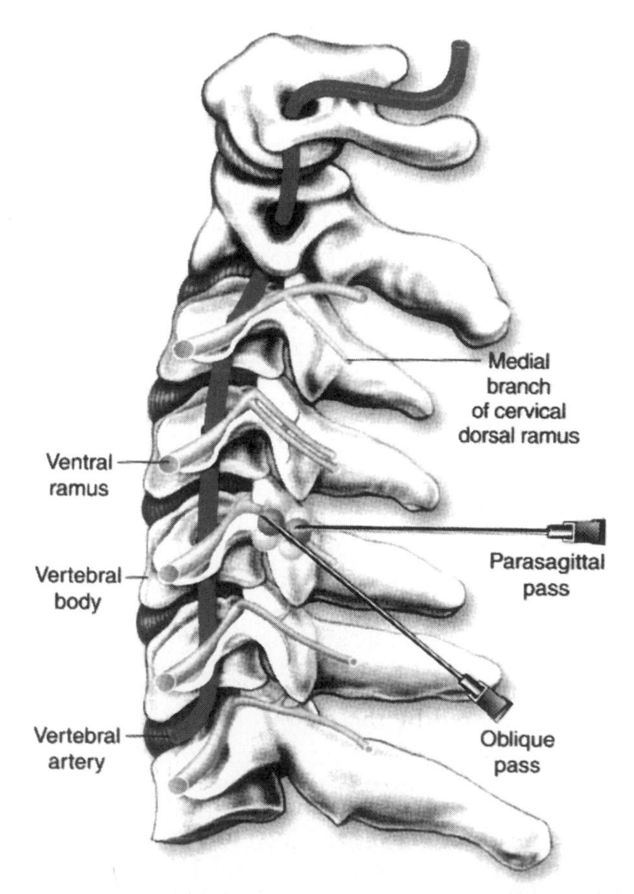

FIGURE 42–51 *The use of electrodes to coagulate a medial branch of a cervical dorsal ramus, shown for the left C5 vertebra. With the oblique and parasagittal passes, lesions are placed at, above, and below the cephalocaudad center of the pillar. Ideally, a total of six lesions are made for each nerve. (Lord SM, Barnsley L, Wallis BJ, et al: Percutaneous radio-frequency neurotomy for chronic cervical zygapophyseal joint pain. N Engl J Med 335(23):1721–1726, 1996. Copyright © 1996, Massachusetts Medical Society. All rights reserved.)*

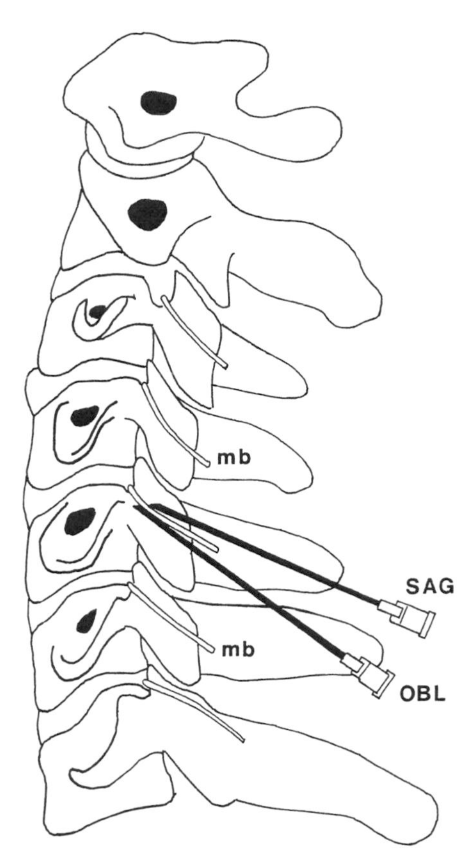

FIGURE 42–52 *Sketch of a lateral view of the cervical spine showing the course of the medial branches of the cervical dorsal rami (*mb*), placement of electrodes along a sagittal path (*SAG*), and an oblique path (*OBL*), to coagulate the nerve. (McDonald GJ, Lord SM, Bogduk N: Long-term follow-up of patients treated with cervical radiofrequency neurotomy for chronic neck pain. Neurosurgery 45(1):61–68, 1999.)*

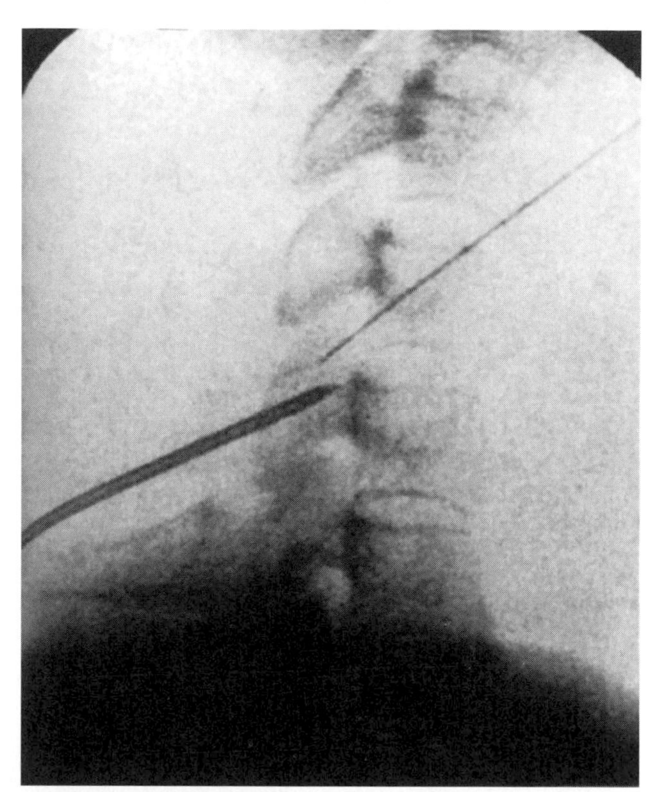

FIGURE 42–54 *Lateral x-ray showing an electrode in position for the performance of radiofrequency neurotomy of the medial branch of a C5 dorsal ramus. Lesions would be made at the site illustrated and at one electrode width above and below. (McDonald GJ, Lord SM, Bogduk N: Long-term follow-up of patients treated with cervical radiofrequency neurotomy for chronic neck pain. Neurosurgery 45(1):61–68, 1999.)*

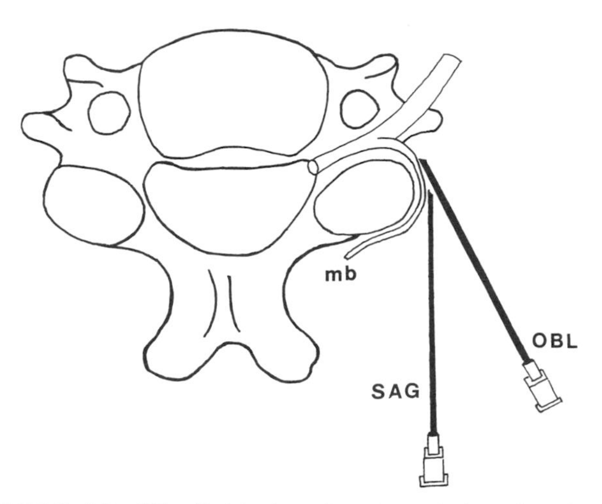

FIGURE 42–53 *Sketch of top view of a cervical vertebra, showing the course of the medial branch (*mb*) and the orientation of electrodes placed along the sagittal path (*SAG*), and an oblique path (*OBL*), to coagulate the nerve. (McDonald GJ, Lord SM, Bogduk N: Long-term follow-up of patients treated with cervical radiofrequency neurotomy for chronic neck pain. Neurosurgery 45(1):61–68, 1999.)*

denervation of the cervical facets, 13% of the patients in one study complained of postprocedure pain that resolved in 2 to 6 weeks and 4% complained of occipital hypesthesia, probably secondary to a lesion of the third occipital nerve, which resolved in 3 months. No persistent motor or sensory deficits developed.[185]

One final concern is the development of a Charcot joint as a result of facet denervation. In theory, a facet joint could be damaged because it lacks protective surrounding muscles. This appears to be mainly a theoretical concern for procedures in the lumbar and cervical spine, as the denervation is not permanent and only a small portion (20% across a segment?) of the paraspinal muscles are denervated when the neurotomy is restricted to one or two segments.[185a]

Pearls and Pitfalls

When the fluoroscope's C arm is properly positioned for lumbar facet blockade, a "Scottie dog" configuration can be clearly seen (Figs. 42–42, 42–43, 42–55, 42–56). The back of the head and the ears of the "Scottie dog" are formed by the inferior articular process, and the front feet by the superior articular process of the vertebra below. Rotation of the fluoroscope's C arm to maximize visualization of the joint space facilitates needle insertion into the

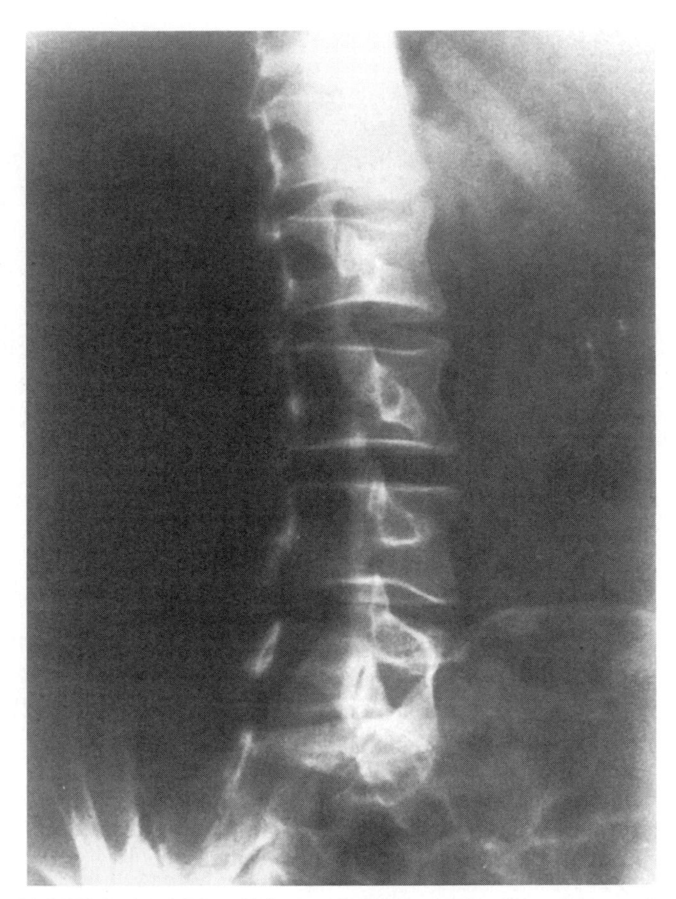

FIGURE 42–55 *Oblique radiograph of spine shows degenerative changes at L5–S1 facet. Radiographic finding is, however, not specifically diagnostic of facet syndrome. (Warfield CA: Facet syndrome and the relief of low back pain. Hosp Pract 23(10A):41–48, 1988.)*

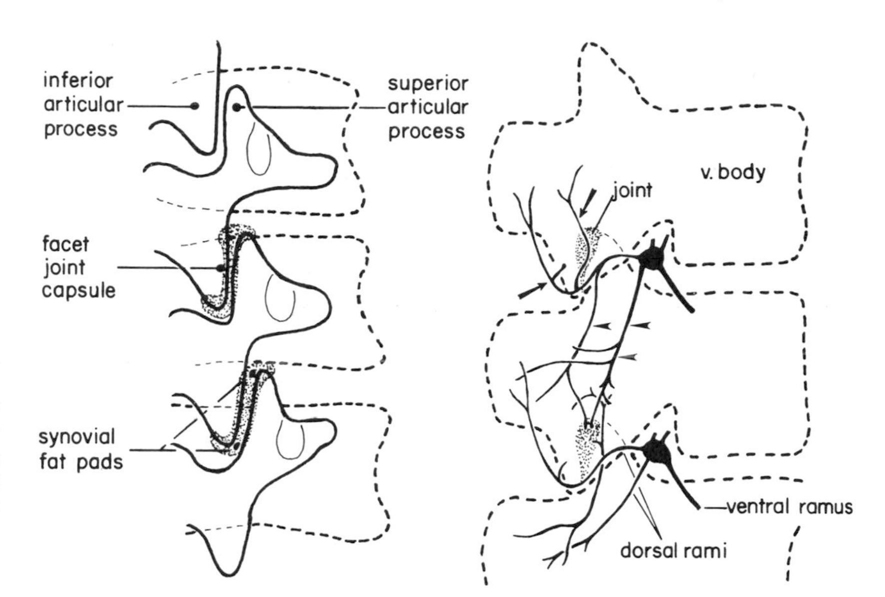

FIGURE 42–56 Sketch of the "Scottie-dog" image seen on an oblique x-ray view of the lumbar spine. The ear is formed by the tip of the superior articular process; the front leg by the tip of the inferior articular process; and the nose by the transverse process. The eye of the Scottie-dog is formed by the pedicle. (Destouet JM, Gilula LA, Murphy WA, Mousees B: Lumbar facet joint injection: Indication, technique, clinical correlation, and preliminary results. Radiology 145:321–325, 1982.)

joint capsule, which is defined by the ears and back of the head of one "Scottie dog" and by the front feet of the "Scottie dog" above. From 0.25 to 0.5 mL of radiocontrast dye injected into the joint space should reveal an S-shaped facet joint.

Sometimes injection can be difficult because of anatomic abnormalities. In the lumbar spine area, the distance to the target point can be surprisingly long when the needle is directed along the fluoroscopic beam. It is prudent to have available long needles for these situations. Sometimes the ideal fluoroscopic image is difficult to find because of significant joint disease. In such cases it may be possible to approximate the joint space by averaging the location from the joint above and below the intended joint. This is reasonable if the injection is intended to be periarticular, for therapeutic but not diagnostic benefit. Ideally the injection should be changed to block the medial branch nerves with the intent that the block be diagnostic for possible future radiofrequency ablation. Sometimes the posterior superior iliac crest obstructs ideal fluoroscopic imaging of the L5–S1 joint. In this situation, while maintaining joint space visualization, the operator angles the C arm more cephalad to allow the needle to pass by the iliac crest. In the cervical spine, similar difficulty can be encountered when the patient has a short neck and the shoulder gets in the way, especially for the lower medial branch nerves. In this case the patient may have to reach down to a knee with the uppermost hand or perhaps even to have the shoulder gently pulled caudad and held out of the way with tape.

When the patient has significant degenerative disease of the spine or has had spine surgery (particularly fusion), the difficulty increases and the success rate decreases. In the case of previous surgery, it is possible that pain may result from scar or bony entrapment of the nerves.[186] Sometimes it simply takes longer to do the procedure—and sometimes it is simply wiser to abandon the procedure.

Some practitioners advocate use of larger volumes (2–5 mL) for pericapsular, rather than intraarticular, injection. This type of injection bathes the ligaments, paraspinal muscles, and supporting structures with local anesthetic and steroid in a nonspecific manner and has been beneficial to some patients with chronic low back pain, probably because the pain has multiple causes and the volume used provides analgesic and antiinflammatory effects over a larger area of affected tissue.

In the thoracic spine, because there is no precise technique for medial branch blocks, the only reliable injection technique is intraarticular or periarticular injection. Because of the steep angle of the thoracic joints, the intraarticular injection may be technically difficult. Unfortunately no data comparing thoracic intraarticular to periarticular injections have been published. Also, because of the unfavorable anatomy of the thoracic medial branch nerves, there is no reliable technique to denervate the thoracic facet joints at this time.

Because of the anatomy of the cervical facets, medial branch block is the superior procedure. Although the medial branches of the dorsal rami innervate both joints and neck muscles, pain that is relieved by medial branch block is most likely coming from the facet joint and not from the overlying muscles and ligaments.[150, 187] The small-volume diagnostic injections for medial branch nerves, although fairly specific for assessing facet pain, produce false-negative results 8% of the time in the lumbar spine. This complication occurs when the injectate is inadvertently delivered to the vessels accompanying the medial branch nerves (an event confirmed with radiocontrast dye). The result is that the injectate is either carried away or diluted by a small hematoma, and the pain is not relieved. It is then often falsely assumed that facet joint pain is not the problem. A similar problem may happen in the cervical spine, but this is not proven at this time.

There are several conflicting reports on the success of treating low back pain with facet denervation. Some studies have shown intraarticular saline to be as effective as local anesthetic or steroid. Advocates of the procedure argue that there is little to lose, and something to gain, by offering facet denervation to patients who have exhausted other therapies and continue to have disabling pain. No one can deny that some patients do experience benefit.

Until the role of the facet as a cause of low back and neck pain is better defined, it is likely that, in clinical practice, facet joint denervation will continue to be considered for patients with intractable back and neck pain not responsive to conservative therapies and epidural steroid injections.

Efficacy

The success associated with facet joint injections has varied widely. Rate of effectiveness of lumbar intraarticular facet joint injection of local anesthetic and steroid is between 16% and 69%. Cervical intraarticular facet joint injection or medial branch nerve block have afforded slightly higher success rates, between 69% and 86%.[24] There appears to be no significant difference in outcome between intraarticular facet joint injections and medial branch nerve blocks.[75, 188] The success rate of lumbar radiofrequency facet denervation has also varied over a wide range, from 17% to 83%.* These different results occur for a variety of reasons, including the technical adequacy of facet joint entry or medial branch denervation, the selection of the correct facet joint or the number of joints to be denervated, the total volume of medication used, and, most important, the patient population selected. For proper selection of patients for facet joint therapy, other causes of low back pain, such as muscle strain, displaced discs, disc space infection, tumor, and ankylosing spondylitis, must first be ruled out.[189]

Early studies of facet joint injections with steroids and local anesthetics for diagnosis and therapy were encouraging. Carrera[87] reported immediate relief in 13 of 20 patients, and six had relief for more than 6 months after injection. Mooney and Robertson[23] found that 62% of chronic low back pain patients received initial pain relief when their facet joints were injected with local anesthetics and that 20% had complete relief at 6-month follow-up. Destouet and coworkers[30] reported 59% initial improvement and 27% long-term relief rates. Lewinnek and Warfield[119] found that 75% of patients had an initial response, and 33% had a lasting response. Forty-three percent of Lippitt's[120] patients reported good to excellent relief of symptoms after facet joint injection. In one study by Silvers,[27] 69% of patients had pain relief after injection of 0.5 to 1 mL of 0.4% phenol in glycerine. However, he concurrently injected 1 mL of 0.5% bupivacaine and 20 mg of methylprednisolone. This result is comparable to those obtained from using local anesthetic and steroid alone. Therefore, there is no obvious advantage to using phenol and glycerine at this time. Results of many of these earlier studies have been questioned because the trials were not randomized and controlled. Some used large volumes of medication which had the potential to produce capsular rupture with extravasation.[23]

Studies that have prevented extravasation by restricting the total volume of medication injected to 1 mL have shown conflicting results. Raymond and Dumas,[28] in a study of 25 patients, reported only 16% temporary relief and no long-term relief. Moran and colleagues[38] achieved only a 13% success rate. The study by Lynch and Taylor,[57] however, contradicts these results; they administered two injections of 1 mL each of fluid containing corticosteroids in 50 patients and demonstrated that intraarticular injections were more effective than extraarticular injections for long-term pain relief.

In two prospective, randomized, controlled studies of facet joint injections, Lilius and colleagues[122] and Carette and associates[190] concluded that facet joint injections were of little value in treating low back pain. Both studies showed that intraarticular injections of steroid or steroid with local anesthetic did not differ clinically or statistically in effectiveness from injections of placebo. A major criticism of both of these studies, however, involves patient selection. In the Lilius study, 109 patients who had unilateral low back pain for over 3 months were studied, and some patients had "minor, mainly subjective neurological deficiencies."[122] In the Carette study, the initial group consisted of patients with low back pain, buttock pain, or both lasting for at least 6 months.[190] Clearly, both of these studies had broad patient inclusion criteria, and therefore, many of the patients in the studies likely did not really have the facet syndrome. This fact may well explain their discouraging results.

Even the second phase of the Carette study, in which facet joints were injected with 2 mL of 1% lidocaine and patients with relief of 50% or more were identified as having facet syndrome, has flaws. In lumbar pain syndromes, single diagnostic local anesthetic blocks are potentially nonspecific. Also, these blocks commonly have poorly predicted the results of permanent procedures for chronic benign pain syndromes such as spinal fusion.[191] It would be desirable to identify those patients who have back pain on the basis of facet joint disease and to conduct randomized, prospective, clinical trials using only these patients to evaluate the efficacy of facet joint therapy.[192]

Helbig and Lee[20] have advocated stricter diagnostic criteria for the lumbar facet syndrome in order to select a population of patients with a high likelihood of successful response to facet joint treatments. They reviewed 22 consecutive patients with a clinical diagnosis of lumbar facet syndrome, made by conventional diagnostic criteria previously mentioned, who were then treated with facet joint injections. The treatment responses were reviewed, and new diagnostic criteria were formulated on the basis of a scoring system derived from the values observed in the review. The scoring system has a total of 100 points, allocated as follows: back pain associated with groin or thigh pain, 30 points; well-localized paraspinal tenderness, 20; reproduction of pain with extension or rotation, 30; corresponding radiographic changes, 20; and pain below the knee, −10 points. In this study, a score of 60 points or more selected a population of patients who had 100% prolonged response. A score of 40 points or more

*See references 14, 23, 24, 28, 30, 38, 39, 57, 75, 119, 122, 190, 191.

predicted 78% prolonged response. Helbig and Lee[20] concluded that the scorecard may allow clinicians to bring together the constellation of clinical symptoms and more reliably select patients for successful facet joint treatment.

More recently, double diagnostic blocks with (1) local anesthetic as compared with saline or (2) lidocaine as compared with bupivacaine—have attempted to identify predictors of pain relief from facet blocks and to improve the accuracy of patients selected for radiofrequency denervation.[106, 108, 127, 128] No clear factors have emerged to suggest what a facet syndrome is. However, Schwarzer, Bogduk, and coworkers have shown that, for the lumbar spine, single diagnostic blocks have a false-positive rate of 38%. Unfortunately, this implies that the data and conclusions from most of the earlier work are much less compelling.

Similar work was done by Lord, Barnsley, and Bogduk on pain after whiplash.[10, 12, 55, 111, 132, 193] Using double diagnostic blocks again, they found that third occipital nerve headaches occur in at least 27% of individuals complaining of pain after whiplash. They also showed that the prevalence of cervical facet joint pain after whiplash is likely 60%. Psychological assessment of whiplash patients by Wallis and associates showed that those who had pain relief after cervical radiofrequency denervation also had their psychological distress relieved, and those who had ongoing pain were still distressed.[194] The implication of this is profound, because, in spite of the generally held belief that whiplash is a psychological problem, this shows that a large percentage of whiplash patients can have their pain relieved, and that their psychological distress is secondary to the pain, not the source of it.

Work on evaluating radiofrequency denervation of the medial branch nerves is now one step behind the improved assessment of patients for facet pain; however, a recent randomized trial of lumbar radiofrequency denervation by Van Kleef found significant alleviation of pain and functional disability that lasted 12 months. The main criticism of this study is that patients were selected for denervation based on a single diagnostic block, but, even so, their results were significant. For the cervical spine, recent work on assessing radiofrequency denervation was done by Van Kleef, Lord, Barnsley, and Bogduk.[74, 112, 176, 195] The rate of relief for patients chosen for denervation based on a positive response to double diagnostic blocks was 71%. The median duration of relief was 422 days for those who had a successful outcome on the first procedure. Unfortunately, the subgroup of patients denervated at the C2–C3 facet had a poor response, and this needs further work.

FUTURE CONSIDERATIONS

Spinal fusion has been used extensively to stabilize vertebrae that cause severe pain with abnormal movement. It has been suggested that stabilization of facets by bone graft and the fusion that subsequently occurs may alleviate such pain. Stein and coworkers[2] performed percutaneous facet joint fusion in dogs. They determined that such a procedure is feasible and that, with further development, it may be beneficial to humans suffering from painful facet joints.

Most importantly, extensive studies of patients with low back pain, thoracic back pain, and cervicogenic pain must be conducted to confirm the role that facet joints seem to play in these pain syndromes. In addition, outcome studies need to be done to determine which therapies are most successful for facet syndrome. Selecting patients for surgery has not been reliably linked to the diagnosis and treatment of facet pain, and this connection needs to be explored further.[196–198]

REFERENCES

1. Frymoyer JW: Back pain and sciatica. N Engl J Med 318:291–300, 1998.
2. Stein M, Elliott D, Glen J, Morara-Protzner I: Percutaneous facet joint fusion: Preliminary experiences. Vasc Interv Radiol 4:69–74, 1993.
3. Borenstein DG: Epidemiology, etiology, diagnostic evaluation, and treatment of low back pain. Curr Opin Rheumatol 9(2):144–150, 1997.
4. Frymoyer JW: An overview of the incidences and costs of low back pain. Orthop Clin North Am 22(2):263–271, 1991.
5. Manchikanti L: Facet joint pain and the role of neural blockade in its management. Curr Rev Pain 3:348–358, 1999.
6. El-Khoury GY, Reinfrew DL: Percutaneous procedures for the diagnosis and treatment of low back pain: Diskography, facet-joint injection, and epidural injection. AJR 157:685–691, 1991.
7. Haldeman S: Failure of pathology to predict back pain. Spine 15:718–724, 1990.
8. Maniadakis N, Gray A: The economic burden of back pain in the UK. Pain 84:95–103, 2000.
9. Bland JH, Boushey DR: Anatomy and physiology of the cervical spine. Semin Arthritis Rheum 20(1):1–20, 1990.
10. Lord SM, Barnsley L, Wallis BJ, et al: Chronic cervical zygapophysial joint pain after whiplash. Spine 21(15):1737–1745, 1996.
11. Bogduk N, Aprill C: On the nature of neck pain, discography, and cervical zygapophysial joint blocks. Pain 54:213–217, 1993.
12. Aprill C, Bogduk N: The prevalence of cervical zygapophyseal joint pain. Spine 17(7):744–747, 1992.

12a. Goldthwait JE: The lumbosacral articulation: An explanation of many cases of lumbago, sciatica, and paraplegia. Boston Med Surg J 164:365, 1911.

13. Jackson RP: The facet syndrome: Myth or reality? Clin Orthop 279:110–121, 1992.
14. Jackson RP, Jacobs RR, Montesano PX: Facet joint injection in low back pain: A prospective statistical study. Spine 13:966–971, 1988.
15. Mooney V: Facet syndrome: Clinical entities. *In* Weinstein JN, Wiesel SW (eds): The Lumbar Spine. (The International Society for the Study of the Lumbar Spine.) Philadelphia, WB Saunders, 1990, pp 422–441.
16. Ghormley RK: Low back pain with special reference to the articular facet, with presentation of an operative procedure. JAMA 101:1773–1777, 1993.
17. Putti V: Lady Jones' lecture on new concepts in pathogenesis of sciatic pain. Lancet 2:53–60, 1927.
18. Mixter WJ, Barr JS: Rupture of the intervertebral disk with involvement of the spinal canal. N Engl J Med 211:210–215, 1934.
19. Revel ME, Listrat VM, Chevalier XJ, et al: Facet joint block for low back pain: Identifying predictors of a good response. Arch Phys Med Rehabil 73:824–828, 1992.
20. Helbig T, Lee C: The lumbar facet syndrome. Spine 13:61–64, 1988.
21. Badgley CE: The articular facets in relation to low back pain and sciatic radiation. J Bone Joint Surg Am 23:481–496, 1941.
22. Hirsch C, Ingelmark B, Miller M: The anatomical basis for low back pain. Acta Orthop Scand 33:1, 1963.
23. Mooney V, Robertson J: The facet syndrome. Clin Orthop 115:149–156, 1976.
24. Pawl RP: Headache, cervical spondylosis, and anterior cervical fusion. Surg Ann 9:391, 1971.

25. Bogduk N: Back pain: Zygapophysial blocks and epidural steroids. *In* Cousins MJ, Bridenbaugh PO (eds): Neural Blockade in Clinical Anesthesia and Management of Pain, ed 2. Philadelphia, JB Lippincott, 1988, pp 935–946.
26. Rees WES: Multiple bilateral subcutaneous rhizolysis of segmental nerves in the treatment of the intervertebral disk syndrome. Ann Gen Pract 16:126, 1971.
27. Silvers RH: Lumbar percutaneous facet rhizotomy. Spine 15:36–40, 1990.
28. Raymond J, Dumas J: Intraarticular facet block: Diagnostic test or therapeutic procedure? Radiology 151:333–336, 1984.
29. Shealy CN: Percutaneous radiofrequency denervation of spinal facets: Treatment for chronic back pain and sciatica. J Neurosurg 43:448–451, 1975.
30. Destouet JM, Gilula LA, Murphy WA, Mousees B: Lumbar facet joint injection: Indication, technique, clinical correlation, and preliminary results. Radiology 145:321–325, 1982.
31. Selby DK, Paris SV: Anatomy of facet joints and its clinical correlation with low back pain. Contemp Orthop 3:1097–1103, 1981.
32. Maldague B, Mathurien P, Malghern J: Facet joint arthrography in lumbar spondylolysis. Radiology 140:29–36, 1981.
33. Marks R, Semple AJ: Spinal anaesthesia after facet injection. Anaesthesia 43:65–66, 1988.
34. Bogduk N, Anat D, Engel R: The menisci of the lumbar zygapophyseal joints. Spine 9(5):454–460, 1984.
35. Bogduk N: Clinical Anatomy of the Lumbar Spine and Sacrum, ed 3. Edinburgh, Churchill Livingstone, 1997.
36. Xu GL, Hayerton VM, Carrera GF: Lumbar facet joint capsule: Appearance at MR imaging and CT. Radiology 177:415–420, 1990.
37. McCormick CC, Taylor JR, Twang LT: Facet joint arthrography in lumbar spondylolysis: Anatomic basis for spread of contrast medium. Radiology 171:193–196, 1989.
38. Moran R, O'Connell D, Walsh M: The diagnostic value of facet joint injections. Spine 13:1407–1410, 1988.
39. Dory MA: Arthrography of the lumbar facet joints. Radiology 140:23–27, 1981.
40. Fukui S, Ohseto K, Shiotani M: Patterns of pain induced by distending the thoracic zygapophyseal joints. Reg Anesth 22(4):332–336, 1997.
41. Dreyfuss P, Tibiletti C, Dreyer S: Thoracic zygapophyseal joint pain patterns. Spine 19(7):807–811, 1994.
42. Dwyer A, Aprill C, Bogduk N: Cervical zygapophyseal joint pain patterns I: A study in normal volunteers. Spine 15:453–457, 1990.
43. Aprill C, Dwyer A, Bogduk N: Cervical zygapophyseal joint pain patterns II: A clinical evaluation. Spine 15:458–461, 1990.
44. Hove B, Gyldensted C: Cervical analgesic facet joint arthrography. Neuroradiology 32:456–459, 1990.
45. Okada K: Studies on the cervical facet joints using arthrography of the cervical facet joint. Jpn J Orthop 55:563–580, 1981.
46. Horvitz T, Smith RM: An anatomical, pathological, and roentgenological study of the intervertebral joints of the lumbar spine and of the sacroiliac joints. Am J Roentgenol 43:173–186, 1940.
47. Tournade A, Patay Z, Krupa P, et al: A comparative study of the anatomical, radiological, and therapeutic features of the lumbar facet joints. Radiology 34:257–261, 1992.
48. Maldjian C, Mesgarzadeh M, Tehranzadeh J: Diagnostic and therapeutic features of facet and sacroiliac joint injection. Radiol Clin North Am 36(3):497–508, 1998.
49. Malmivaara A, Videman T, Kuosma E, et al: Facet joint orientation, facet and costovertebral joint osteoarthrosis, disc degeneration, vertebral body osteophytosis, and Schmorl's nodes in the thoracolumbar junctional region of cadaveric spines. Spine 12(5):458–463, 1987.
50. Tulsi RS, Hermanis GM: A study of the angle of inclination and facet curvature of superior lumbar zygapophyseal facets. Spine 18(10):1311–1317, 1993.
51. Panjabi MM, Oxland T, Takata K, et al: Articular facets of the human spine: Quantitative three-dimensional anatomy. Spine 18(10):1298–1310, 1993.
52. Ebraheim NA, Xu R, Ahmad M, et al: The quantitative anatomy of the thoracic facet and the posterior projection of its inferior facet. Spine 22(16):1811–1818, 1997.
53. Bogduk N, Anat D: The clinical anatomy of the cervical dorsal rami. Spine 7(4):319–330, 1982.
54. Milne N: The role of zygapophyseal joint orientation and uncinate processes in controlling motion in the cervical spine. J Anat 178:189–201, 1991.
55. Bogduk N, Marsland A: The cervical zygapophyseal joints as a source of neck pain. Spine 13:610–617, 1988.
56. Bogduk N, Long D: The anatomy of the so-called "articular nerves" and their relationship to facet denervation in the treatment of low back pain. J Neurosurg 51:172–177, 1979.
57. Lynch MC, Taylor JF: Facet joint injection for low back pain: A clinical study. J Bone Joint Surg 68B:138–141, 1986.
58. Bous RA: Facet joint injections. *In* Stanton-Hicks M, Bous R (eds): Chronic Low Back Pain. New York, Raven, 1982, pp 199–211.
59. Maigne J-Y, Maigne R, Guerin-Surville H: The lumbar mamillo-accessory foramen: A study of 203 lumbosacral spines. Surg Radiol Anat 13:29–32, 1991.
59a. Giles LGF: The relationship between the medial branch of the lumbar posterior ramus and the mamillo-accessory ligament. J Manip Physiol Therap 14:189–192, 1991.
60. Rashbaum RF: Radiofrequency facet denervation: A treatment alternative in refractory low back pain with or without leg pain. Orthop Clin North Am 14:569–575, 1983.
61. Bogduk N: The innervation of the lumbar spine. Spine 8(3):286–293, 1983.
62. Jerosch J, Castro WHM, Liljenqvist U: Percutaneous facet coagulation: Indication, technique, results, and complications. Neurosurg Clin North Am 7(1):119–134, 1996.
63. Bogduk N, Wilson AS, Tynan W: The human lumbar dorsal rami. J Anat 134(2):383–397, 1982.
64. Murtagh FR: Computed tomography and fluoroscopy guided anesthesia and steroid injection in facet syndrome. Spine 13:686–689, 1988.
65. Schuster GD: The use of cryoanalgesia in the painful facet syndrome. J Neurol Orthop Surg 3:271–274, 1982.
66. Paris SV: Anatomy as related to function and pain. Orthop Clin North Am 14(3):475–489, 1983.
67. Suseki K, Takahashi Y, Takahashi K, et al: Innervation of the lumbar facet joints. Spine 22(5):477–485, 1997.
68. Stolkre RJ, Vervest ACM, Groen GJ: Percutaneous facet denervation in chronic thoracic spinal pain. Acta Neurochir 122:82–90, 1993.
69. Chua WH, Bogduk N: The surgical anatomy of thoracic facet denervation. Acta Neurochir 136:140–144, 1995.
70. Santavirta S, Hopfner-Hallikainen D, Paukku P, et al: Atlantoaxial facet joint arthritis in the rheumatoid cervical spine: A panoramic zonography study. J Rheumatol 15:217–223, 1988.
71. Bovim G, Berg R, Gunnar Dale L: Cervicogenic headache: Anesthetic blockades of cervical nerves and facet joint (C2/C3). Pain 49:315–320, 1992.
72. Barnsley L, Bogduk N: Medial branch blocks are specific for the diagnosis of cervical zygapophyseal joint pain. Reg Anesth 18:343–350, 1993.
73. Ebraheim NA, Haman ST, Xu R, et al: The anatomical location of the dorsal ramus of the cervical nerve and its relation to the superior articular process of the lateral mass. Spine 23(18):1968–1971, 1998.
74. Lord SM, Barnsley L, Bogduk N: Percutaneous radiofrequency neurotomy in the treatment of cervical zygapophyseal joint pain: A caution. Neurosurgery 36(4):732–739, 1995.
75. Marks RC, Houston T, Thulbourne T: Facet joint injection and facet nerve block: A randomised comparison in 86 patients with chronic low back pain. Pain 49:325–328, 1992.
76. Yamashita T, Cavanaugh JM, El-Boly AA, et al: Mechanosensitive afferent units in the lumbar facet joint. J Bone Joint Surg 72A:865–870, 1990.
77. Ashton IK, Aston BA, Gibson SJ, et al: Morphological basis for back pain: The demonstration of nerve fibers and neuropeptides in the lumbar facet joint capsule but not in ligamentum flavum. J Orthop Res 10:72–78, 1992.
78. Cavanaugh JM, Ozaktay AC, Yamashita T, et al: Mechanisms of low back pain: A neurophysiologic and neuroanatomic study. Clin Orthop 335:166–180, 1997.
79. Beaman DN, Graziano GP, Glover RA, et al: Substance P innervation of lumbar spine facet joints. Spine 18(8):1044–1049, 1993.
80. Gronblad M, Weintein JN, Santavira S: Immunohistochemical observations on spinal tissue innervation. Acta Orthop Scand 62(6):614–622, 1991.

81. Gronblad M, Korkala O, Konttinen YT, et al: Silver impregnation and immunohistochemical study of nerves in lumbar facet joint plical tissue. Spine 16(1):34–38, 1991.
82. Gilees LGF, Taylor JR: Human zygapophyseal joint capsule and synovial fold innervation. Br J Rheumatol 26:93–98, 1987.
83. Wyke B: The neurology of joints: A review of general principles. Clin Rheum Dis 7(1):223–239, 1981.
84. Cavanaugh JM: Neural mechanisms of lumbar pain. Spine 20(16):1804–1809, 1995.
85. Yamashita T, Cavanaugh JM, Ozaktay AC, et al: Effect of substance P on mechanosensitive units of tissues around and in the facet joint. J Orthop Res 11:205–214, 1993.
86. Simmons JW, Ricketson R, McMillin JN: Painful lumbosacral sensory distribution patterns: Embryogenesis to adulthood. Orthop Rev 10:1110–1118, 1993.
87. Carrera GF: Lumbar facet joint injection in low back pain and sciatica. Radiology 137:661–664, 1980.
88. Raymond J, Dumas J: Anomalous ossicle of the articular process: Arthrography and facet block. Am J Radiol 141:1233–1234, 1983.
89. Kofod S, Boll K: Anomalous ossicle in a lumbar facet joint. Arch Orthop Trauma Surg 106:333–334, 1987.
90. Howington JU, Edward MD, Connolly ES, et al: Intraspinal synovial cysts: A ten year experience at the Ochsner Clinic. J Neurosurg (Spine) 91:193–199, 1999.
91. Shirado O, Kaneda K: Large osteoarthritic bone cyst of the facet joint causing low back pain and sciatica. Orthopedics 20(5):472–475, 1997.
92. Sabo RA, Tracy PT, Weinger JM: A series of 60 juxtafacet cysts: Clinical presentation, the role of spinal instability, and treatment. J Neurosurg 85:560–565, 1996.
93. Hsu KY, Zucherman JF, Shea WJ, et al: Lumbar intraspinal synovial and ganglion cysts (facet cysts). Spine 20(1):80–89, 1995.
94. Rapin PA, Gerster JC: Calcified synovial cyst of a zygapophyseal joint. J Rheumatol 20(4):767–768, 1993.
95. Wendling D, Ferraud D: Calcified synovial cysts of zygapophyseal joints. J Rheumatol 21(1):373–374, 1994.
96. Wilde GP, Szypryt EP, Mulholland RC: Unilateral lumbar facet joint hypertrophy causing nerve root irritation. Ann R Coll Surg Engl 70:307–310, 1988.
97. Louic T, Morgan B, Standiford HC: Facet and facet-joint infections: Case report and review. Clin Infect Dis 26:510–512, 1998.
98. Yang KH, King AI: Mechanism of facet load transmission as a hypothesis for low back pain. Spine 9(6):557–565, 1984.
99. Cavanaugh JM: Lumbar facet pain: Biomechanics, neuroanatomy and neurophysiology. J Biomech 29(9):1117–1129, 1996.
100. Warfield CA: Facet syndrome and the relief of low back pain. Hosp Pract 23:41–48, 1988.
101. Butler D, Trafimow JH, Andersson GBJ, et al: Discs degenerate before facets. Spine 15(2):111–113, 1990.
102. Revel M, Poiraudeau S, Auleley GR, et al: Capacity of the clinical picture to characterize low back pain relieved by facet joint anesthesia. Spine 23(18):1972–1977, 1998.
102a. Lord SM, Bogduk N: Treatment of chronic cervical zygapophyseal joint pain. N Engl J Med 336(21):1530–1531, 1997.
103. Dreyer S, Dreyfuss PH: Low back pain and the zygapophyseal (facet) joints. Arch Phys Med Rehabil 77:290–300, 1996.
104. Pang WW: Application of spinal pain mapping in the diagnosis of low back pain—analysis of 104 cases. Acta Anaesthesiol Sin 36(2):71–74, 1998.
105. Newton W, Curtis P, Witt P, et al: Prevalence of subtypes of low back pain in defined population. J Fam Pract 45(4):331–335, 1997.
106. Schwarzer AC, Aprill CN, Derby R, et al: The relative contributions of the disc and zygapophyseal joint in chronic low back pain. Spine 19(7):801–806, 1994.
107. Schwarzer AC, Wang S, O'Driscoll D, et al: The ability of computed tomography to identify a painful zygapophyseal joint in patients with chronic low back pain. Spine 20(8):907–912, 1995.
108. Schwarzer AC, Wang S, Bogduk N, et al: Prevalence and clinical features of lumbar zygapophyseal joint pain: A study in an Australian population with chronic low back pain. Ann Rheumatic Dis 54:100–106, 1995.
109. Halla JT, Hardin JG: The spectrum of atlantoaxial facet joint involvement in rheumatoid arthritis. Arthritis Rheum 33:325–329, 1990.
110. Kirby NG, Maimaris C: Unilateral facet joint hypertrophy causing nerve root irritation. Ann R Coll Surg Engl 71:267–268, 1989.
111. Barnsley L, Lord SM, Wallis BJ, et al: The prevalence of chronic cervical zygapophyseal joint pain after whiplash. Spine 20(1):20–26, 1995.
112. Lord SM, Barnsley L, Wallis BJ, et al: Percutaneous radio-frequency neurotomy for chronic cervical zygapophyseal joint pain. N Engl J Med 335(23):1721–1726, 1996.
113. Carrera GF: Lumbar facet joint injection in low back pain and sciatica. Radiology 137:665–667, 1980.
114. Smyth MJ, Wright V: Sciatica and the intervertebral disc. J Bone Joint Surg 40A(6):1401–1418, 1958.
115. Kuslich SD, Ulstrom CL, Michael CJ: The tissue of origin of low back pain and sciatica. Orthop Clin North Am 22(2):181–187, 1991.
116. McCall IW, Park WM, O'Brein JP: Induced pain referral from posterior lumbar elements in normal subjects. Spine 4(5):441–446, 1979.
117. Marks R: Distribution of pain provoked from lumbar facet joints and related structures during diagnostic spinal infiltration. Pain 39:37–40, 1989.
118. Fukui S, Ohseto K, Shiotani M, et al: Distribution of referred pain from the lumbar zygapophyseal joints and dorsal rami. Clin J Pain 13:303–307, 1997.
119. Lewinnek GE, Warfield CA: Facet joint degeneration as a cause of low back pain. Clin Orthop 213:216–222, 1986.
120. Lippit AB: The facet joint and its role in spine pain. Spine 9(7):746–750, 1984.
121. Destouet JM, Murphy WA: Lumbar facet block: Indications and technique. Orthop Rev 14(5):280–288, 1985.
122. Lilius G, Laasonen EM, Myllynen P, et al: Lumbar facet syndrome: A randomized clinical trial. J Bone Joint Surg 71B(4):681–684, 1989.
123. Hourigan CL, Bassett JM: Facet syndrome: Clinical signs, symptoms, diagnosis, and treatment. J Manipulative Physiol Ther 12(4):293–297, 1989.
124. Lilius G, Harilainen A, Laasonen EM, Myllynen P: Chronic unilateral low back pain: Predictors of outcome of facet joint injections. Spine 15:780–782, 1990.
125. Mehta M, Parry CBW: Mechanical back pain and the facet joint. Disability Rehabil 16(1):2–12, 1994.
126. Schwarzer AC, Aprill CN, Derby R, et al: The false positive rate of uncontrolled diagnostic blocks of the lumbar zygapophyseal joints. Pain 58:195–200, 1994.
127. Schwarzer AC, Aprill CN, Derby R, et al: Clinical features of patients with pain stemming from the lumbar zygapophyseal joints. Spine 19(10):1132–1137, 1994.
128. Revel M, Poiraudeau S, Auleley GR, et al: Capacity of the clinical picture to characterize low back pain relieved by facet joint anesthesia. Spine 23(18):1972–1977, 1998.
129. Fairbank JCT, Park WM, McCall IW, et al: Apophyseal injection of local anesthetic as a diagnostic aid in primary low-back pain syndromes. Spine 6(6):598–605, 1981.
130. Cassidy JD (ed): Scientific monograph of the Quebec task force on whiplash-associated disorders: Redefining "whiplash" and its management. Spine 20(8S):1S–47S, 1995.
131. Taylor JR, Twomey LY: Acute injuries to cervical joints: An autopsy study of neck sprain. Spine 18(9):1115–1122, 1993.
132. Lord SM, Barnsley L, Wallis BJ, et al: Third occipital nerve headache: A prevalence study. J Neurol Neurosurg Psychiatry 57:1187–1190, 1994.
133. Nilsson N: The prevalence of cervicogenic headache in a random population sample of 20–59 year olds. Spine 20(17):1884–1888, 1995.
134. Wilson PR: Cervicogenic headache. Am Pain Soc J 1(4):259–264, 1992.
135. Sjaastad O, Fredriksen TA, Plaffenrath V: Cervicogenic headache, diagnostic criteria. Headache 30:725–726, 1990.
136. Jull G, Bogduk N, Marsland A: The accuracy of manual diagnosis for cervical zygapophysial joint pain syndromes. Med J Austral 148:233–236, 1988.
137. Dreyfuss P, Michaelsen M, Fletcher D: Atlanto-occipital and lateral atlanto-axial joint pain patterns. Spine 19(10):1125–1131, 1994.
138. Halla JT, Hardin JG: Atlantoaxial (C1-C2) facet joint osteoarthritis: A distinctive clinical syndrome. Arthritis Rheum 30:577–582, 1987.

139. Santavirta S, Konttinen Y, Lindqvist C, Sandelin J: Occipital headache in rheumatoid cervical facet joint arthritis. Lancet 2:695, 1986.
140. Fukui S, Ohseto K, Shiotani M, et al: Referred pain distribution of the cervical zygapophyseal joints and cervical dorsal rami. Pain 68:79–83, 1996.
141. Elster AD: Bertolotti's syndrome revisited: Transitional vertebrae of the lumbar spine. Spine 14(12):1373–1377, 1989.
142. Vergauwen S: Distribution and incidence of degenerative spine changes in patients with a lumbo-sacral transitional vertebra. Eur Spine J 6(3):168–172, 1997.
143. Rosa M, Capellini C, Canaveri MA, et al: CT in low back and sciatic pain due to lumbar canal osseous changes. Neuroradiology 28:237–240, 1986.
144. Demaerel P, Wilms G, Goffin J, et al: Osteoarthritis of the facet joints and its role in low back pain: Evaluation with conventional tomography. J Belge Radiol 75:81–86, 1992.
145. Jensen MC, Brant-Zawadzki MN, Obuchowski N, et al: Magnetic resonance imaging of the lumbar spine in people without back pain. N Engl J Med 331(2):69–73, 1994.
146. Savage RA: The relationship between the magnetic resonance imaging appearance of the lumbar spine and low back pain, age and occupation in males. Eur Spine J 6(2):106–114, 1997.
147. Weishaupt D: MR imaging and CT in osteoarthritis of the lumbar facet joints. Skeletal Radiol 28(4):215–219, 1999.
148. Holder LE, Machin JL, Asdourian PL, et al: Planar and high-resolution SPECT bone imaging in the diagnosis of facet syndrome. J Nucl Med 36:37–44, 1995.
149. Dolan AL, Ryan PJ, Arden NK, et al: The value of SPECT scans in identifying back pain likely to benefit from facet joint injection. Br J Rheumatol 35:1269–1273, 1996.
150. Dreyfuss P, Schwarzer AC, Lau P, et al: Specificity of lumbar medial branch and L5 dorsal ramus blocks. Spine 22(8):895–902, 1997.
151. Jerosch J, Tappiser R, Assheuer J: MRI controlled facet block—technique and initial results. Biomed Tech (Berlin) 43(9):249–252, 1998.
152. Kullmer K, Rompe JD, Lowe A, et al: Ultrasound image of the lumbar spine and the lumbosacral transition. Ultrasound anatomy and the possibilities for ultrasonically controlled facet joint infiltration. Z Orthop Ihre Grenzgeb 135(4):310–314, 1997.
153. Schleifer J, Fenzl G, Wolf A, et al: Treatment of lumbar facet joint syndrome by CT-guided infiltration of the intervertebral joints. Radiologe 34(11):666–670, 1994.
154. Schwarzer AC, Derby R, Aprill CN, et al: The value of the provocation response in lumbar zygapophyseal joint injections. Clin J Pain 10(4):309–313, 1994.
155. Bough B, Thakore J, Davies M, et al: Degeneration of the lumbar facet joints. Arthrography and pathology. J Bone Joint Surg Br 72(2):275–276, 1990.
156. Barnsley L, Lord S, Wallis B, et al: False-positive rates of cervical zygapophyseal joint blocks. Clin J Pain 9(2):124–130, 1993.
157. Lora J, Long D: So-called facet denervation in the management of intractable back pain. Spine 1(2):121–126, 1976.
158. Burton CV: Percutaneous radiofrequency facet denervation. Appl Neurophysiol 39:80–86, 1976.
159. Shealy CN: Facet denervation in the management of back and sciatic pain. Clin Orthop 115:157–164, 1976.
160. Florez G, Eiras J, Ucar S: Percutaneous rhizotomy of the articular nerve of Luschka for low back and sciatic pain. Acta Neurochir Suppl 24:67–71, 1997.
161. Hickey RFJ, Tregonning GD: Denervation of spinal facet joints for treatment of chronic low back pain. NZ Med J 85:96–99, 1977.
162. Ogsbury JS, Simon RH, Lehman RAW: Facet "denervation" in the treatment of low back syndrome. Pain 3:257–263, 1977.
163. Schaerer JP: Radiofrequency facet rhizotomy in the treatment of chronic neck and low back pain. Int Surg 63:53–59, 1978.
164. Ignelzi RJ, Cummings TW: A statistical analysis of percutaneous radiofrequency lesions in the treatment of chronic low back pain and sciatica. Pain 8:181–187, 1980.
165. Bogduk N, Long DM: Percutaneous lumbar medial branch neurotomy: A modification of facet denervation. Spine 5(2):193–200, 1980.
166. Andersen KH, Mosdal C, Vaernet K: Percutaneous radiofrequency facet denervation in low back and extremity pain. Acta Neurochir (Wein) 87:48–51, 1987.
167. Savitz MH: Percutaneous radiofrequency rhizotomy of the lumbar facets: Ten years' experience. Mount Sinai J Med 58(2):177–178, 1991.
168. North RB, Han M, Zahurak M, Kidd DH: Radiofrequency lumbar facet denervation: Analysis of prognostic factors. Pain 57:77–83, 1994.
169. Jerosch J, Castro WH, Halm H, et al: Long-term results following percutaneous facet coagulation. Z Orthop Ihre Grenzgeb 131(3): 241–247, 1993.
170. Goupille P, Cotty P, Fouquet B, et al: Denervation of the posterior lumbar vertebral apophyses by thermocoagulation in chronic low back pain. Result of the treatment of 103 patients. Rev Rheum Ed Fr 60(11):791–796, 1993.
171. Gocer AI, Cetinalp E, Tuna M, et al: Percutaneous radiofrequency rhizotomy of lumbar spine facets: The results of 46 cases. Neurosurg Rev 20:114–116, 1997.
172. Cho J, Park YG, Chung SS: Percutaneous radiofrequency lumbar facet rhizotomy in mechanical low back pain syndrome. Stereotact Funct Neurosurg 68:212–217, 1997.
173. Van Kleef M, Barendse GAM, Kessels A, et al: Randomized trial of radiofrequency lumbar facet denervation for chronic low back pain. Spine 24(18):1937–1942, 1999.
174. Sluijter ME, Koestveld-Baart CC: Interruption of pain pathways in the treatment of the cervical syndrome. Anesthesia 35:302–307, 1980.
175. Suijlekom HA, Van Kleef M, Barendse GAM, et al: Radiofrequency cervical zygapophyseal joint neurotomy for cervicogenic headache: A prospective study of 15 patients. Funct Neurol 13:297–303, 1998.
176. McDonald GJ, Lord SM, Bogduk N: Long-term follow-up of patients treated with cervical radiofrequency neurotomy for chronic neck pain. Neurosurgery 45(1):61–68, 1999.
177. Bogduk N, Macintosh J, Marsland A: Technical limitations to the efficacy of radiofrequency neurotomy for spinal pain. Neurosurgery 20(4):529–535, 1987.
178. Vaisman J: Pulse radiofrequency: A new and ingenious modality for pain management. N Engl Pain Assoc Newslett 4(2):4, 7, 1999.
179. Goldstone JC, Pennant JH: Spinal anaesthesia following facet joint injection: A report of two cases. Anaesthesia 42:754–756, 1987.
181. Thomson SJ, Lomax DM, Collett BJ: Chemical meningism after lumbar facet joint block with local anaesthetic and steroids. Anaesthesia 46:563–564, 1991.
182. Berrigan T: Chemical meningism after lumbar facet joint block. Anaesthesia 47:905–906, 1992.
183. Magee M, Kannangara S, Dennien B: Paraspinal abscess complicating facet joint injection. Clin Nucl Med 25:71–73, 2000.
184. Cook NJ, Hanrahan P, Song S: Paraspinal abscess following facet joint injection. Clin Rheumatol 8(1):52–53, 1999.
185. Vervest AM, Stolker RJ: The treatment of cervical pain syndromes with radiofrequency procedures. Pain Clinic 4:103–112, 1991.
185a. Fujiwara A, Tamai K, Yamamoto M, et al: The relationship between facet joint osteoarthritis and disc degeneration of the lumbar spine: An MRI study. Eur Spine J 8(5):396–401, 1999.
186. Busch EH, Lamer TJ: Injection of the facetectomy remnant in the evaluation and treatment of postsurgical back pain: Case reports. Clin J Pain 6:125–127, 1990.
187. Kaplan M, Dreyfuss P, Halbrook B, et al: The ability of lumbar medial branch blocks to anesthetize the zygapophyseal joint: A physiologic challenge. Spine 23(17):1847–1852, 1998.
188. Barnsley L, Lord S, Wallis B, Bogduk N: Lack of effect of intraarticular corticosteroids for chronic pain in the cervical zygapophyseal joints. N Engl J Med 330:1047–1050, 1994.
189. Bogduk N: Neck pain. Aust Fam Physician 13:26–30, 1984.
190. Carette S, Marcoux S, Truchon R, et al: A controlled trial of corticosteroid injections into facet joints for chronic low back pain. N Engl J Med 325:1002–1007, 1991.
191. Essess SI, Moro JK: The value of facet joint blocks in patient selection for lumbar fusion. Spine 18:185–190, 1993.
192. Murphy WA: The facet syndrome. Radiology 151:533, 1984.
193. Lord SM, Barnsley L, Bogduk N: The utility of comparative local anesthetic blocks versus placebo-controlled blocks for the diagnosis of cervical zygapophyseal joint pain. Clin J Pain 11:208–213, 1995.

194. Wallis BJ, Lord SM, Bogduk N: Resolution of psychological distress of whiplash patients following treatment by radiofrequency neurotomy: A randomized, double-blind, placebo-controlled trial. Pain 73:15–22, 1997.
195. Van Suijlekom HA, Weber WEJ, Van Kleef M, et al: Radiofrequency cervical zygapophyseal joint neurotomy for cervicogenic headache: A short term follow-up study. Funct Neurol 13(1):82–83, 1998.
196. Lovely TY, Rastogi P: The value of provocative facet blocking as a predictor of success in lumbar spinal fusion. J Spinal Disorders 10(6):512–517, 1997.
197. Grob D: Surgery in the degenerative cervical spine. Spine 23(24):2674–2683, 1998.
198. North RB, Kidd DH, Zahurak M, et al: Specificity of diagnostic nerve blocks: A prospective randomized study of sciatica due to lumbosacral spine disease. Pain 65:77–85, 1996.

CHAPTER • 43

Lumbar Sympathetic Nerve Block and Neurolysis

Michael Stanton-Hicks, MB, MD

Conduction block of the lumbar sympathetic trunk is particularly useful as an aid to the diagnosis, prognosis, and therapy of certain pain states in the pelvis and lower extremity.

HISTORICAL CONSIDERATIONS

The first report of lumbar sympathetic block is that by Brunn and Mandl,[1] who in a 1924 article described Selheim's technique of injecting the lumbar sympathetic nerves as a component of his paravertebral approach to blocking the mixed spinal outflow in the lumbar region. Eighteen years after Novocain was released in 1905, Kappis[2] described both the technique of lumbar sympathetic block and surgical resection of the lumbar sympathetic nerves. Other names associated with the technique of lumbar sympathetic block are von Gaza,[3] Mandl,[4] and Läwen[5] in Germany; Jonnesco[6] and Lériche and Fountain[7] in France; and White[8] in the United States. During the 1950s, Bonica,[9] Moore,[10] and Arnulf[11] described in detail the importance of lumbar sympathetic blockade, particularly its relationship to the treatment of causalgia and post-traumatic reflex dystrophies in servicemen after World War II. Although the technique described by Mandl[4] in 1926 remains one of the most popular approaches to the lumbar sympathetic trunk, Reid and colleagues,[12] in a large series published in 1970, described a more lateral approach that avoids contact with the transverse process. Two techniques are described in this chapter: the "classic" technique first described by Kappis[2] and Mandl[4] and the lateral technique first described by Mandl[4] and redefined by Reid and colleagues.[12]

INDICATIONS

The indications for lumbar sympathetic block may be divided into three broad categories: (1) circulatory insufficiency in the leg, including arteriosclerotic vascular disease, diabetic gangrene, Buerger's disease, Raynaud's phenomenon and disease, and reconstructive vascular surgery after arterial embolic occlusion; (2) pain from renal colic, reflex sympathetic dystrophy, or causalgia (chronic regional pain syndrome [CRPS] types I and II), intractable urogenital pain, amputation stump pain, phantom pain, and frostbite; and (3) other conditions, such as hyperhidrosis, phlegmasia alba dolens, erythromelalgia, acrocyanosis, and trench foot.

The rationale for sympathetic blocks, particularly in the treatment of pain, is based on the observation that pain under certain conditions is potentiated or mediated by sympathetic activity. Laboratory evidence has demonstrated that the sympathetic postganglionic neuron may act not only at its effector terminal but also on the primary afferent (PA) neuron in certain pathologic conditions; it may communicate with the PA neuron at other sites (direct and indirect coupling).[13] Although the mechanism remains unclear, blocks of the sympathetic nervous system may have two actions: (1) interruption of preganglionic and postganglionic sympathetic efferents may influence function of the PA neuron[14, 15] or (2) visceral afferents from deep visceral structures in the leg that travel with the sympathetic nerves may be blocked.[16] As a diagnostic and prognostic tool, sympathetic blocks are helpful in determining the nature of the pain (i.e., whether it is sympathetically maintained [SMP] or whether it is independent of sympathetic function [SIP]). Such procedures are always used to test the effects of destructive (neurolytic, chemical) sympatholysis or surgical sympathectomy.

CONTRAINDICATIONS

Contraindications to sympathetic blocks are a bleeding diathesis, local infection, and certain anatomic anomalies, which may be considered relative contraindications if they are likely to render the procedure difficult or hazardous.

FUNCTIONAL ANATOMY

The general anatomy of the sympathetic nervous system consists of central and peripheral components. The central components are the hypothalamus, midbrain, pons, medulla, and lateral columns of the spinal cord extending from T1 to L2. Peripherally, the sympathetic nervous system consists of preganglionic and postganglionic efferent fibers that innervate deep somatic structures, skin, and viscera. The two paravertebral sympathetic trunks are connected segmentally by preganglionic neurons, whose cell bodies are situated in the lateral horn, intermediate nucleus, and paracentral nuclei of the thoracolumbar cord. The cell bodies responsible for vasoconstriction in the lower limbs are in the lower three thoracic and first three lumbar segments. The preganglionic fibers pass by way of their corresponding nerves as white rami communicantes, which communicate with considerable convergence in the paravertebral ganglia with postganglionic efferents and in the prevertebral ganglia by postganglionic efferents to the pelvic viscera. A small percentage of postganglionic fibers pass directly to ganglia in the aortic plexus and the superior and inferior hypogastric plexuses. The postganglionic fibers leave the sympathetic trunk as gray rami communicantes, some passing to the L1 nerve to contribute to the iliohypogastric and genitofemoral nerve territories, some to the L2–L5 nerves, and some to the upper three sacral nerves, where they pass on to their respective destinations in the lumbosacral plexus.

Intermediate ganglia found in the psoas and iliacus muscles also communicate with postganglionic fibers that pass through the segmental lumbar and sacral nerves. The S1 and S2 nerves contain the largest numbers of postganglionic fibers. Most of these represent gray rami communicantes that subserve vasomotor, pilomotor, and sudomotor functions. It has been determined that, although each root of the lumbosacral plexus receives one group of gray rami communicantes, the S1–S3 nerves contain several (i.e., a large convergence),[17] because they innervate the blood vessels in the lower extremity. Each lumbar sympathetic chain enters the retroperitoneal space under the right and left crura, continuing inferiorly in the interval between the anterolateral aspect of the vertebral bodies and the origin of the psoas muscle to enter the pelvis at the L5–S1 disc. Posteriorly, the periosteum overlies the vertebral bodies and the fibroaponeurotic origin of the psoas muscles and their fascial coverings. Anterior is the parietal reflection of the peritoneum, the aorta lying anteromedial to the left trunk and the vena cava anterior to the right trunk. It should be noted that the white and gray rami communicantes pass to their respective ganglia beneath the fibrous arcades of psoas attachments to each vertebral body. Also, they tend to pass alongside the middle of the vertebral body, an observation that is important to positioning of the blocking needle.

The sympathetic ganglia of the lumbar sympathetic chains are variable in both numbers and position. Rarely are five ganglia found on each side in the same individual.[18] In most cases, only four are found. There tends to be fusion of L1 and L2 ganglia in most patients, and ganglia are aggregated at the L2–L3 and L4–L5 discs. Also, there is considerable variability in the size of the ganglia, some being fusiform and as long as 10 to 15 mm, others being round and approximately 5 mm long.[19] Because of this aggregation and the fact that the right crus extends to L3 and the left to L2, sympathetic blockade is more efficacious when performed at the L3, L4, or L5 level rather than at the L2 vertebral body, as is most common. It should be noted that, although most postganglionic sympathetic efferents join spinal nerves that form the lumbar plexus and pass distally as components of the femoral, sciatic, and obturator nerves, their branches distribute segmentally to their respective vessels in the lower limb. Block of L2–L3 ganglia should therefore interrupt most of the efferent sympathetic supply to the lower limb. It should also be noted that, in patients whose sympathetic pathways bypass the sympathetic chain and make synapses with their respective postganglionic efferents in somatic spinal nerves, complete sympathetic interruption is not achieved after surgical sympathectomy.[20] Important branches of the lumbar sympathetic trunk contain postganglionic efferents, visceral afferents, and lumbar somatic afferents that supply the axial skeleton, musculoskeletal structures in the hip and the lower limbs. Clearly with this understanding, there can be no "pure" sympathetic block. Some component of somatosensory block, if only a small one, will always be present with every sympathetic-blocking procedure.

TECHNIQUE

Although the "classic" or paramedian technique describes the insertion of three needles from L2 to L4, this method has been modified to one using only two needles at L2 and L4[21] and, more recently, a single-needle technique[22] at either L2 or L3. It should be noted that, when a neurolytic procedure is to be undertaken, it is important to use at least two needles, if not three, to prevent too much local pressure developing at the injection sites. For neurolytic blockade, an image intensifier (fluoroscopy) or computed tomography (CT) should be mandatory. Because of the expense and, not infrequently, the inconvenience of scheduling CT, they are used in only a small percentage of cases.

The prone position is most convenient for lumbar sympathetic blockade, but pain or anatomic deformity may make it necessary to place the patient in the left or right lateral decubitus position.

Classic or Traditional Technique[23]

After sterile preparation of the skin and draping of the area, wheals are made 5 to 6 cm lateral to the spinous processes and on lines that are drawn through the upper margins of the second, third, and/or fourth lumbar spinous processes. This placement can be verified by anteroposterior (AP) fluoroscopy (Fig. 43–1). With a 22-gauge, 8-cm needle, a local anesthetic solution is infiltrated down to the respective transverse processes, forming tracts through which the 20-gauge, 15-cm sympathectomy needle and stylet can be introduced. Each sympathectomy needle in turn is introduced at an angle of 5 to 10 degrees from the parasagittal plane and is advanced so as to contact the transverse process (Fig. 43–2). At this point, a lateral view with the image intensifier is taken to observe the alignment, and any small adjustments necessary are made to set up the proper angle so that the needle will reach the anterolateral

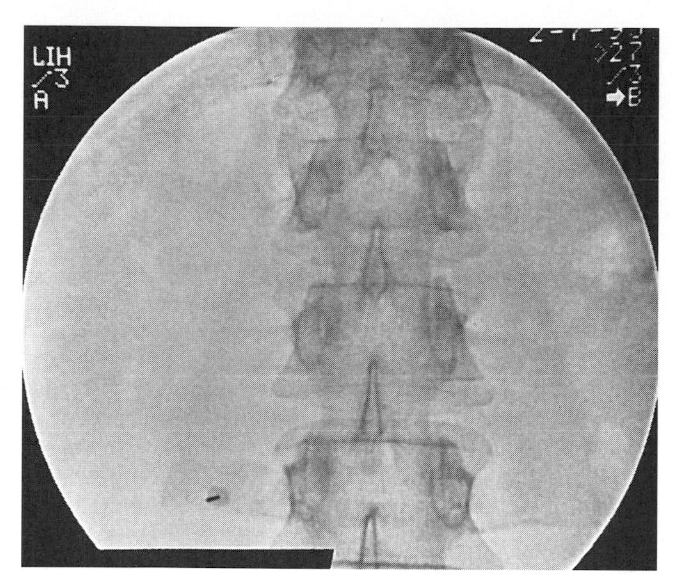

FIGURE 43–1 *Anteroposterior view of the needle seen end-on after being introduced to the transverse process of L3.*

aspect of the vertebral body (Fig. 43–3). The latter view is obtained by "looking down the needle" with the image intensifier. The needle is then introduced by following the axis of the image intensifier camera, and an imaginary line is subtended to reach the anterolateral aspect of the vertebral body of interest. The needle depth can be determined by taking a lateral view (Fig. 43–4). Care should be taken when the needle is passed below the transverse process, because it may contact the posterior or anterior primary rami at that level. Should the needle contact the vertebral body, medial pressure on the paraspinous muscle usually induces sufficient bend in the needle to deflect it from the side of the vertebral body and allow it to pass forward through the psoas muscle and its investing fascia to reach the retroperitoneal space (Fig. 43–5).[24]

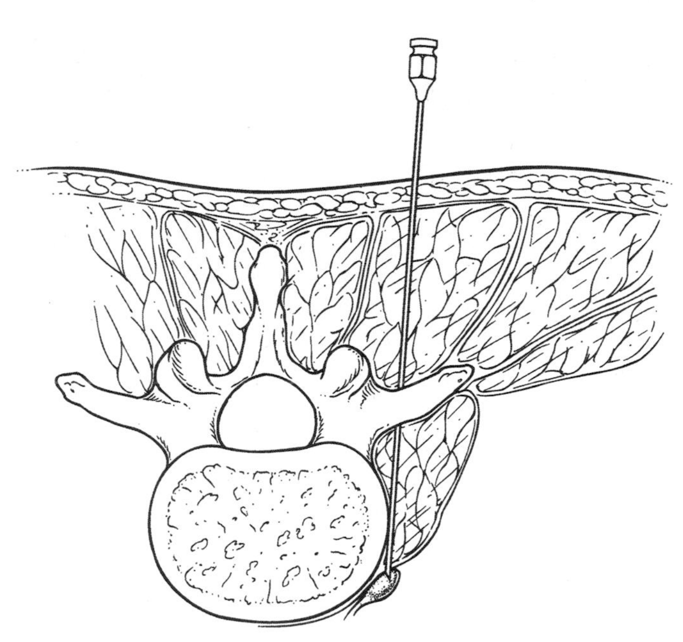

FIGURE 43–3 *Needle tip in correct portion for lumbar sympathetic block.*

With a loss-of-resistance syringe and light percussion with the tip of a finger, the retroperitoneal space may be

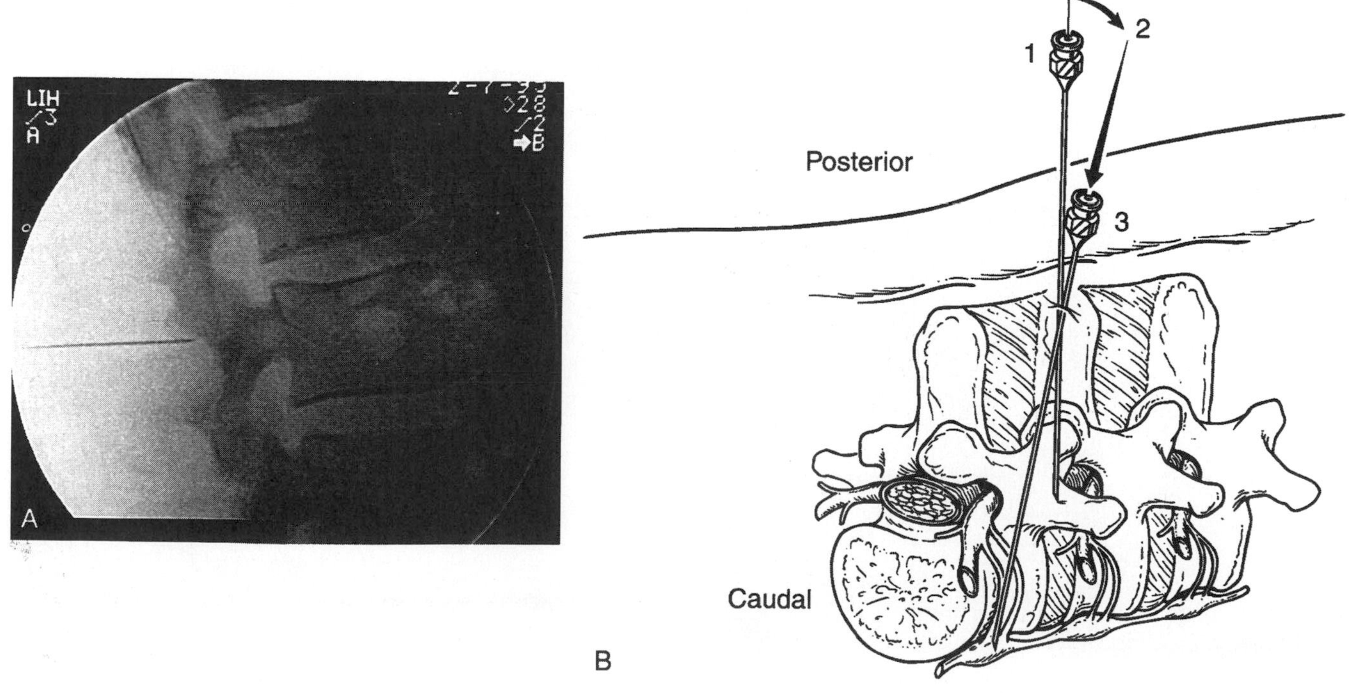

FIGURE 43–2 A, *Lateral radiograph shows proper needle position.* B, *Lateral view shows the needle tip and alignment on the inferior aspect of the transverse process of L3.*

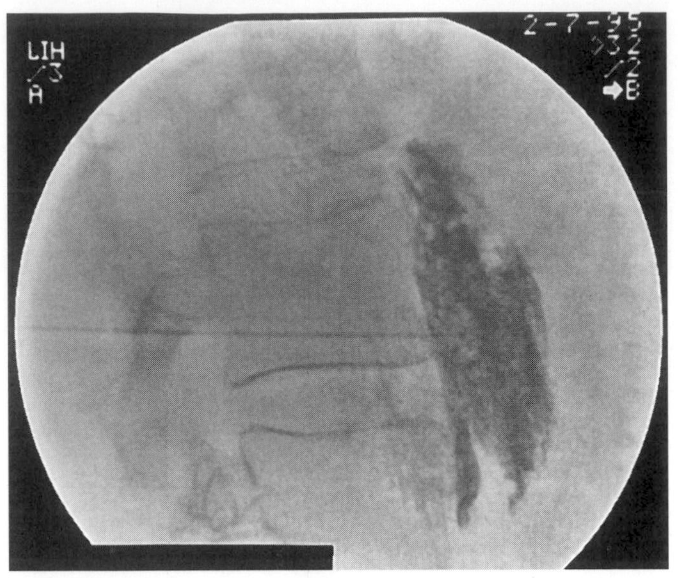

FIGURE 43–4 Lateral image shows the needle at the anterolateral aspect of the vertebral body with the retroperitoneal space identified by longitudinal spread of contrast material.

identified (Fig. 43–6).[25] The position of the needle tip can be verified by injection of either a small amount of air to produce an "airogram" or nonionizable, water-soluble contrast material.[26, 27]

The technique just described is repeated at each additional level. If the needles have been placed in the correct space (retroperitoneal), the injected contrast material should be confluent at each vertebral level (Figs. 43–4, 43–7B). If the contrast material has been placed within the substance of the psoas or just beneath its fascia, the appearance will be as shown in Figure 43–7A. This position produces only incomplete sympatholysis.

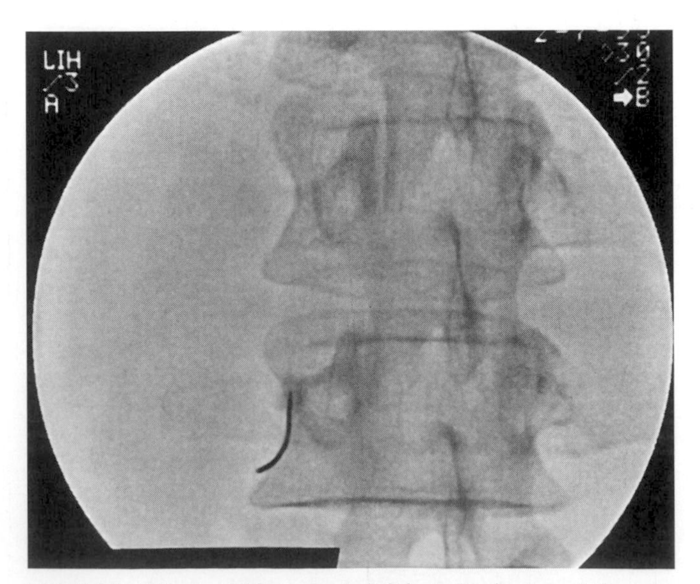

FIGURE 43–5 Oblique (and slightly inclined) view of the spine shows deflection of the needle produced by lateral pressure on the trunk and slight curving of the needle to allow it to pass alongside the vertebral body.

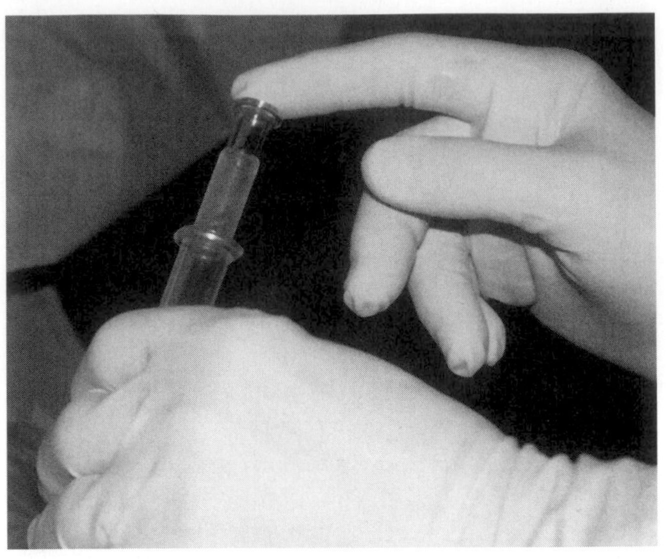

FIGURE 43–6 The retroperitoneal space is identified using a loss-of-resistance syringe and light percussion with the tip of the finger.

Lateral Technique[12]

The lateral technique is favored over the paramedian technique, because it causes less discomfort for the patient, because it does not require contact with the transverse process, is unlikely to encounter a segmental nerve, and provides a direct path and optimal position to contact the lumbar sympathetic trunk and its ganglia. This technique requires only two needles, and, with experience, a single-needle technique can be used successfully in almost 80% of cases.[28]

It is not necessary to measure the point of needle insertion; rather, this point is determined by using the fluoroscope's C arm as a sighting device (Figs. 43–8, 43–9). Distance from the midline, depending on the girth of the

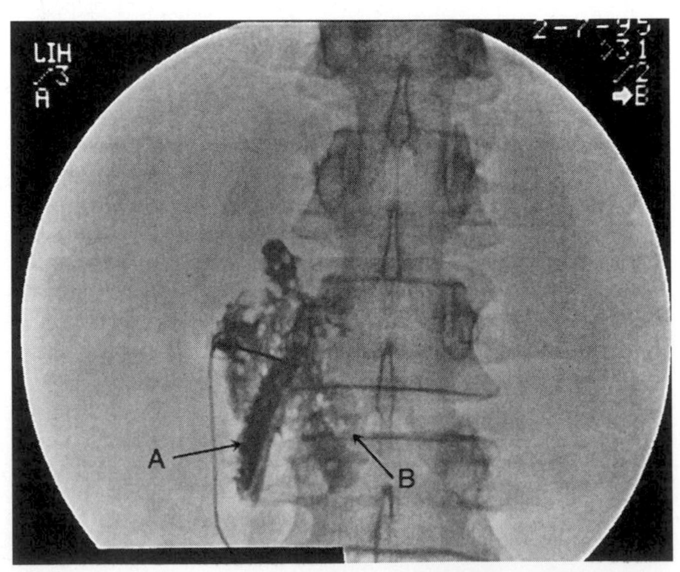

FIGURE 43–7 Compound figure shows the correct position of the needle, and contrast is depicted in two tissue planes: A, The striated linear spread is within the psoas fascia and is incorrect. *B, The "vacuolated" appearance is retroperitoneal and the spread of contrast material is in the* correct *plane.*

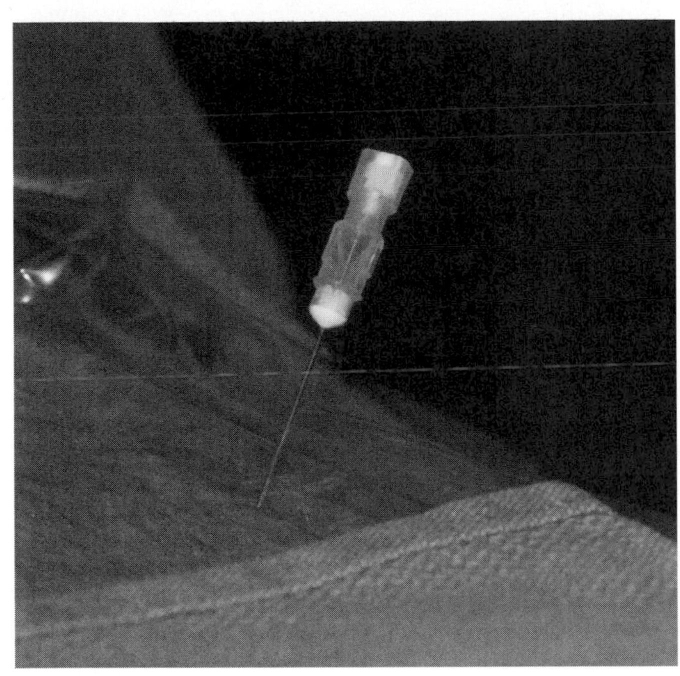

FIGURE 43–8 View of the needle entry site for the Reid or lateral approach.

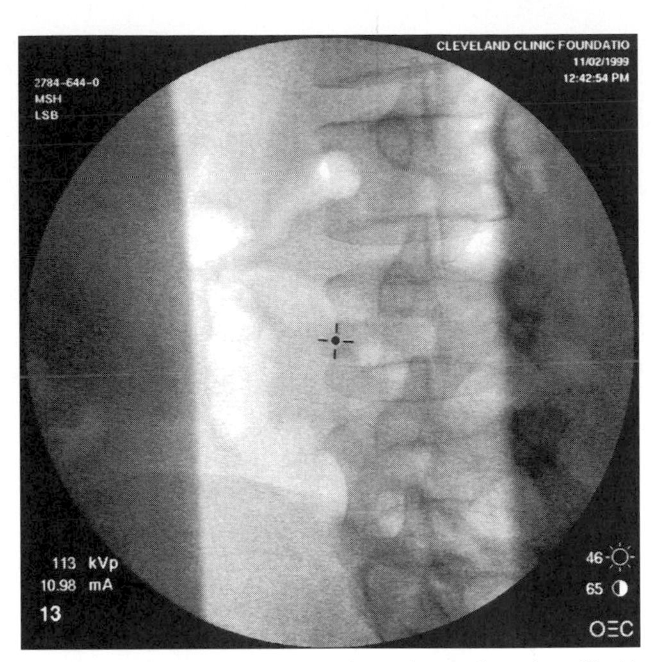

FIGURE 43–10 Oblique view shows the needle end-on ("looking down the needle") as it is introduced into the retroperitoneal space. Note that the image intensifier has also been rotated caudad to allow a clear path for the needle to reach the lower third of the vertebral body without contacting the transverse process.

patient, is between 8 and 12 cm. After a skin wheal is raised, a track of local anesthetic can be infiltrated using a 22-gauge spinal needle. The 20-gauge, 15-cm sympathetic block needle is then introduced at an angle that allows it to arrive at the anterolateral aspect of the vertebral body margin. The axis of the C-arm camera, when positioned to "look down the needle," (Fig. 43–10) should facilitate insertion of the needle into the retroperitoneal space (Fig. 43–11). Using a lateral view to check its depth (Fig. 43–12), the final few millimeters of the needle's travel can be undertaken by the loss-of-resistance syringe until the retroperitoneal space is reached. If the needle should contact the side of the vertebral body, the needle may be deflected from this position by first being withdrawn 2 to 3 cm and then being passed alongside the vertebral body by medial pressure on the paraspinous musculature (see Fig. 43–5). Correct alignment of the needle and its position in the retroper-

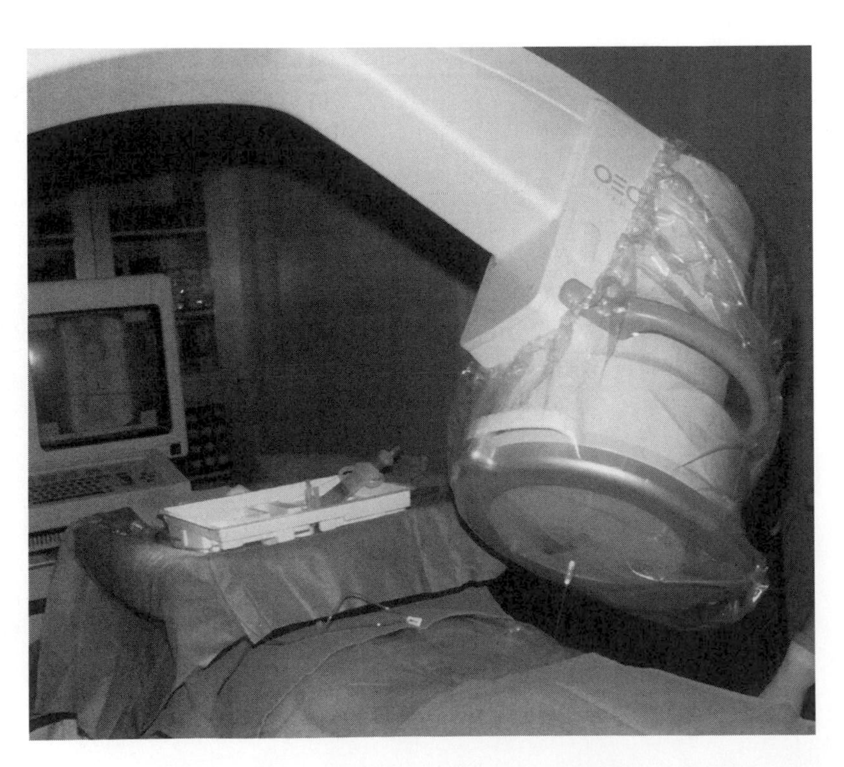

FIGURE 43–9 View of the image intensifier positioned to "look down" the needle during the Reid or lateral approach.

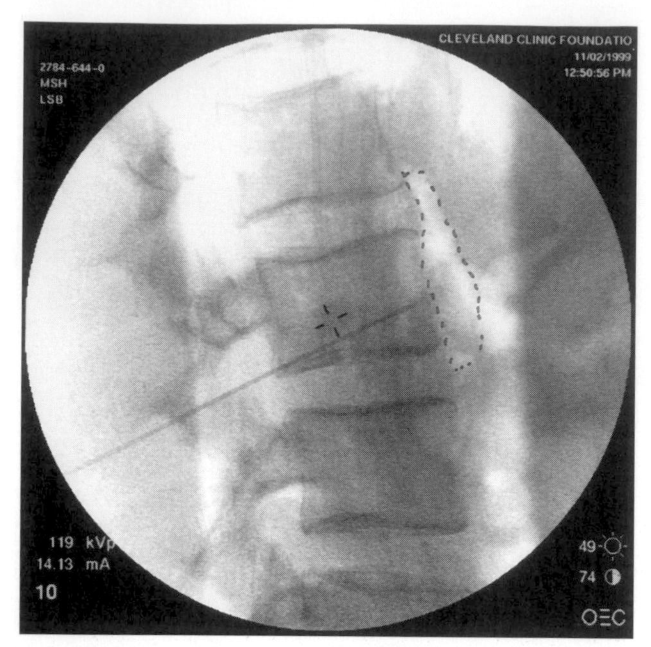

FIGURE 43–11 *Transverse view shows position of the needle tip at the sympathetic trunk using the Reid or lateral approach.*

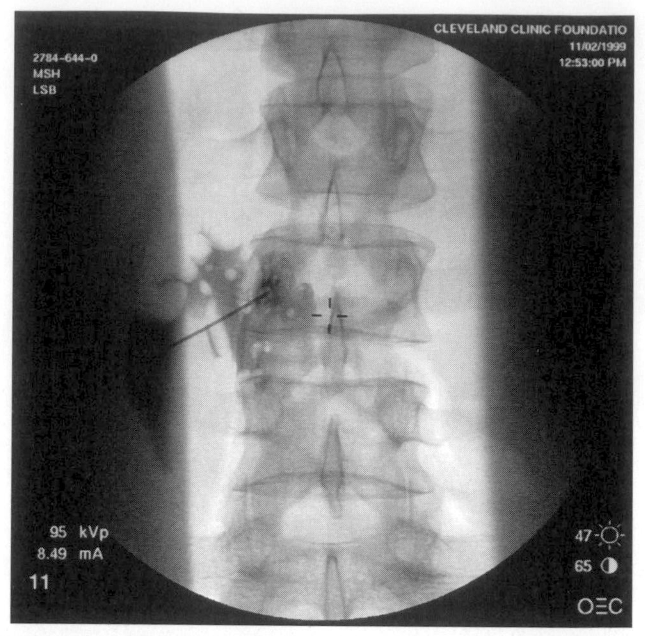

FIGURE 43–13 *Anteroposterior projection of contrast spread in patient shown in Figure 43–12.*

itoneal space can be determined by injecting either a small amount of air to produce an "airogram" (Fig. 43–12A) or nonionizable, water-soluble contrast (Fig. 43–12B). Use of CT as an aid to needle placement is shown in Figure 43–14.

Comment

When determining loss of resistance, it is necessary to ballotte the plunger of the syringe gently with a finger, because the thumb is too insensitive in most cases to feel the small change in pressure as the needle tip enters the retroperitoneal space. Sometimes, as a result of previous (1) retroperitoneal surgery, (2) peritoneal inflammatory disease, or (3) neurolytic sympatholysis, the retroperitoneal space is obliterated and no loss of resistance is recognizable. Under such circumstances, it may be necessary to place the needle tip anatomically in relation to the vertebral body, taking advantage of biplanar views, and to dissect the space by injection of saline and contrast material. I have used this technique successfully in most instances.

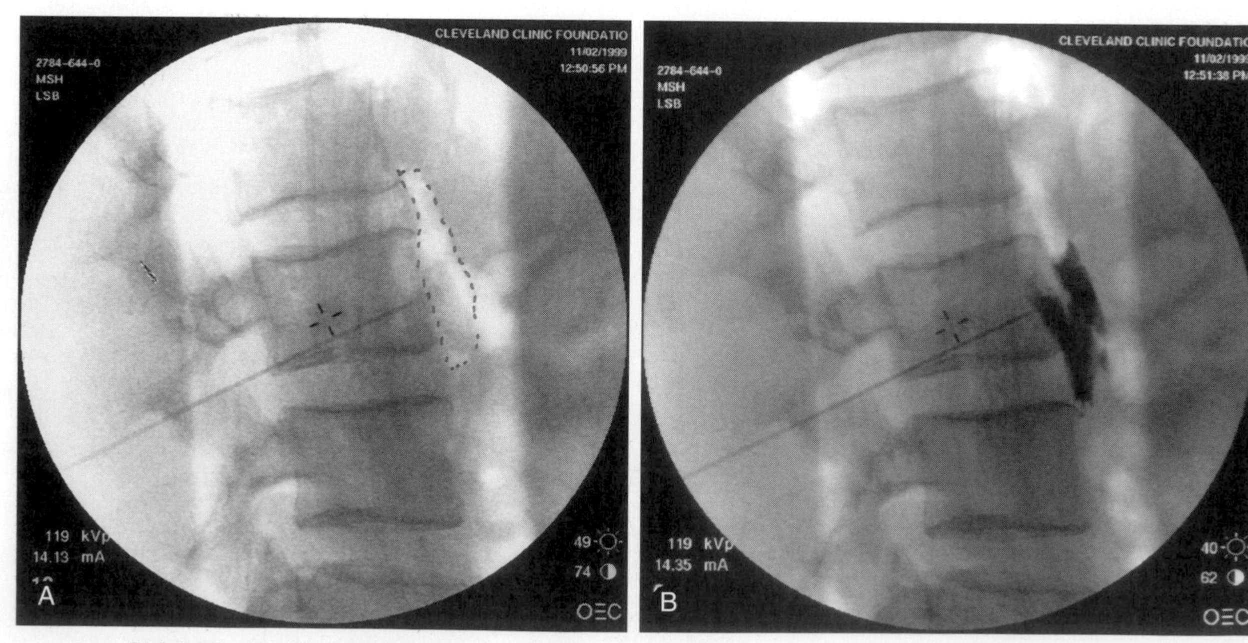

FIGURE 43–12 *A, Lateral image of needle in position with "airogram" obtained after injection of 2 mL air. B, Lateral image of needle in same patient after the injection of 2 mL of radiopaque contrast.*

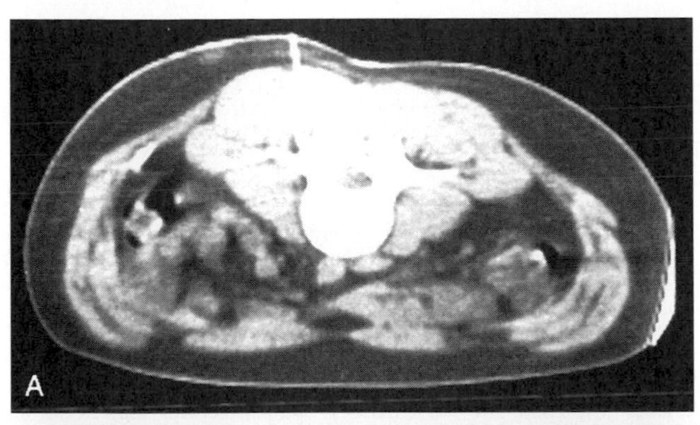

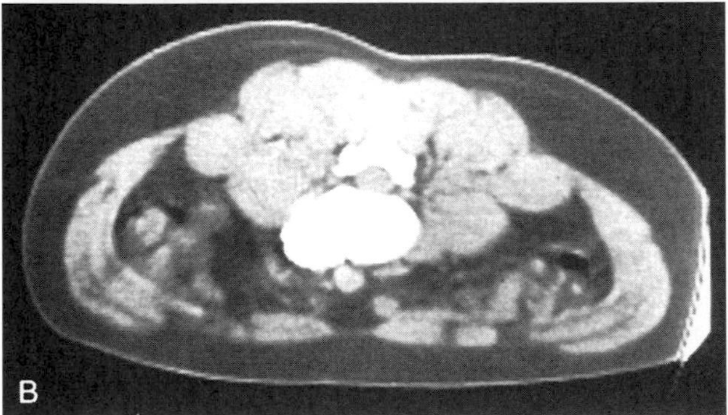

FIGURE 43–14 *A, CT-guided needle placement for lumbar sympathetic block. B, Proper spread of contrast medium outlining the sympathetic chain.*

Injection of any therapeutic or diagnostic solutions should be monitored by continuous imaging. Movement of the contrast tracer confirms its correct dispersion and alerts the observer to any anomalous spread. Injected solutions may enter a lymphatic, vein, or artery and may spread in an unwanted tissue plane, such as alongside the rami communicantes to the lateral foramen. Obviously, imaging time should be kept to a minimum, but the progress of injection should always be monitored throughout. Bonica[9] has suggested that, in the presence of an unexpectedly poor sympatholysis, it may be necessary to undertake prognostic blocks of the lower thoracic sympathetic ganglia in addition to the lumbar ganglia, in case postganglionic fibers have taken other routes than the lumbar trunk to reach the lower extremities.

MEDICATIONS EMPLOYED FOR SYMPATHOLYSIS

Although short-acting local anesthetics are commonly used for prognostic and therapeutic sympathetic blocks, I believe that a long-acting agent such as bupivacaine is advantageous for both therapy and prognosis, because it provides the patient a longer time to evaluate the effects of sympatholysis and any effect this might have on the pain, quite apart from any greater duration that may accrue with physiologic adaptation. A concentration of 0.375% bupivacaine gives optimal duration without the need for an added vasoconstrictor. The disadvantage of bupivacaine is its relatively long latency, from 5 to 8 minutes. It may be shortened by mixing 2% 2-chloroprocaine and 0.75% bupivacaine in equal proportions, or using a small 5- to 6-mL injection of 2% 2-chloroprocaine as a test solution.

A solution of 10% to 16% phenol in diatrizoate sodium (Renografin) is very suitable for neurolysis. Although an "older" ionized contrast material, it is the only solution that has undergone stability testing, and it has a long shelf life.[29] This combination has not been associated with any hypersensitivity response in my experience.

COMPLICATIONS

Like all regional anesthetic blocks, sympatholysis may result in intravascular injection; however, the chance of intravenous injection should be negligible if fluoroscopic guidance is used throughout the injection.[30, 31] The most common complication associated with lumbar sympatholysis is neuralgia of the genitofemoral nerve, particularly for the lateral approach.[32] The incidence of genitofemoral neuralgia has been reported to be as high as 15%, but it may be as low as 4% with a single-needle technique. Most cases are transient and resolve with nonprescription analgesics, but the condition may last as long as 6 weeks. A repeat local anesthetic sympathetic block commonly produces immediate remission. Similarly, intravenous lidocaine may be used in a dose of 1 to 2 mL/kg, or transcutaneous nerve stimulation may be employed over the thigh for genitofemoral neuralgia.

Other complications are necrosis of the psoas muscle and sloughing of the ureter (D. Reed, personal communication, 1985). Bleeding may occur in a person with a clotting deficiency, which, in any case, would be a contraindication to sympathetic block. Otherwise, any bleeding from needle puncture should be self-limiting. Patients should be warned that they may have some hypotension immediately after sympatholysis, and male patients should be apprised that they may experience impotence or failure of ejaculation, particularly if a neurolytic procedure is undertaken. No incidence has been established for this latter complication.

INTERPRETATION OF AND RESPONSES TO LUMBAR SYMPATHETIC BLOCK

It is important to understand the patient's personality when interpreting the subsequent effects of sympatholysis. Although evidence of sympatholysis—vasodilatation, increased temperature, and reduction of edema—is important, it is the qualitative effect on the preexisting symptoms, which may be manifested as continuous pain, hyperalgesia, or touch-evoked pain such as allodynia, that requires careful assessment after sympatholysis. It should be remembered that technical failure may be the cause of therapeutic failure, even on repeated occasions. A placebo response is normal and may merely be the response of a grateful patient to the fact that something fundamental has been done to unravel a particular medical condition. It should also be noted that the amount of local anesthetic used for sympatholysis may, as the result of its own uptake, have an effect on multisynaptic pathways in the central nervous system, producing central inhibition of nociception, an effect that may erroneously be attributed to sympatholysis.[33] Lumbar sympatholysis is associated with surprisingly few complications and is normally a very reproducible technique when carried out with proper imaging guidance. Appropriate knowledge of anatomy and good technique are required to minimize the risk of harm to the patient, and the procedure is valuable in the management of a comparatively small but treatment-refractory group of painful conditions.

Finally, Treede and coworkers have questioned the efficacy and reproducibility of sympathetic block (as did Bonica[9]), particularly in relation to pain relief, as a response. Nevertheless, carefully performed, sympathetic block is a useful and important therapeutic diagnostic procedure.[35]

REFERENCES

1. Brunn F, Mandl F: Die paravertebrale Injektion zur Bekämpfung visceraler Schmerzen. Wien Klin Wochenschr 37:511, 1924.
2. Kappis M: Weitere Erfahrungen mit der Sympathektomie. Klin Wochenschr 2:1441, 1923.
3. von Gaza W: Die Resektion der paravertebralen Nerven und die isolierte Durchschneidung des Ramus communicans. Arch Klin Chir 133:479, 1924.
4. Mandl F: Die Paravertebrale Injektion. Vienna, J Springer, 1926.
5. Läwen A: Über segmentare Schmerzaufhegungen durch paravertebrale Novokaininjektion zur differential Diagnose intraabdominaler Erkrankungen. München Med Wochenschr 69:1423, 1922.
6. Jonnesco R: Angine de poitrien guérié par le résection du sympathique cervico-thoracique. Bull Acad Med 84:93, 1920.
7. Lériche R, Fountain R: L'Anesthésie isolée du ganglion étoile: Sa technique, ses indications, ses résultats. Presse Med 42:849, 1934.
8. White JC: Diagnostic novocaine block of the sensory and sympathetic nerves. Am J Surg 9:264, 1930.
9. Bonica JJ: The Management of Pain. Philadelphia, Lea & Febiger, 1953.
10. Moore DC: Stellate Ganglion Block. Springfield, Ill., Charles C Thomas, 1954.
11. Arnulf G: Practique des Infiltrations Sympathetiques. Lyon, Camugli, 1954.
12. Reid W, Watt JK, Gray RG: Phenol injection of the sympathetic chain. Br J Surg 57:45, 1970.
13. Devor M, Wall PD, Jänig W: Cross-excitation of dorsal root ganglion neurons in nerve injured rats by neighboring afferents and by postganglionic sympathetic efferents. Soc Neurosci 17:439, 1991.
14. Procacci P, Francini F, Zoppi M, Maresca M: Cutaneous pain threshold changes after sympathetic block in reflex dystrophies. Pain 1:167, 1975.
15. Price D, Bennett GJ, Raffi A: Psychophysical observations on patients with neuropathic pain relieved by sympathetic block. Pain 36:273–288, 1989.
16. Mense G: Slowly conducting afferent fibers from deep tissues: Neurological properties and central nervous actions. Prog Sensory Physiol 6:139–219, 1986.
17. Gabella G: Structure of the Autonomic Nervous System. London, Chapman and Hall, 1976.
18. Hovelacque A: Anatomie des Nerfs Craniens et Rachidens et du Systeme Grand Sympathique chez 1 'Homme. Paris, G Doin, 1927.
19. Rocco AG, Palomgi D, Raeke D: Anatomy of the lumbar sympathetic chain. Reg Anesth 20:13–19, 1995.
20. Bonica JJ, Buckley FP. Regional analgesia with local anesthetics. *In* Bonica JJ (ed): The Management of Pain, ed 2. Philadelphia, Lea & Febiger, 1990, pp 883–966.
21. Boas RA, Hatangdi VS: Chemical sympathectomy techniques and responses. *In* Yokua T, Dubner R (eds): Current Topics in Pain Research and Therapy—Proceedings of the International Symposium on Pain, Kyoto, December 19, 1982. Amsterdam, Excerpta Medica, 1983.
22. Hatangdi VS, Boas RA: Lumbar sympathectomy: A single needle technique. Br J Anaesth 57:285, 1985.
23. Bergan JJ, Conn JJR: Sympathectomy for pain relief. Med Clin North Am 52:147–159, 1968.
24. Eriksson E: Illustrated Handbook of Local Anaesthesia. Copenhagen, Munksgaard, 1980.
25. Stanton-Hicks MDA: Blocks of the sympathetic nervous system. *In* Stanton-Hicks MDA (ed): Pain and the Sympathetic Nervous System. Boston, Kluwer Academic, 1990, p 155.
26. Boas RA, Hatangdi VS, Richards EG: Lumbar sympathectomy—a percutaneous technique. Adv Pain Res Ther 1:685, 1976.
27. Eaton AC, Wright M, Cullum KG: The use of the image intensifier in phenol lumbar sympathetic block. Radiography 46:298, 1980.
28. Loh L, Nathan PW: Painful peripheral states and sympathetic blocks. J Neurol Neurosurg Psychiatry 41:664–671, 1978.
29. Gregg RV, Constantini TH, Ford DJ, Raj PP: Electrophysiologic investigation of phenol in diatrizoate sodium as a neurolytic agent. Reg Anesth 10:46–47, 1985.
30. Walsh JA, Glynn CJ, Cousins MJ, Basedow RW: Blood flow, sympathetic activity and pain relief following lumbar sympathetic blockade or surgical sympathectomy. Anaesth Intensive Care 13:18–24, 1984.
31. Cousins MJ, Reeve TS, Glynn CJ, et al: Neurolytic lumbar sympathetic blockade: Duration of denervation and relief of rest pain. Anaesth Intensive Care 7(2):121, 1979.
32. Dam WH: Therapeutic blockade. Acta Chir Scand Suppl 343:89, 1965.
33. Woolf CJ, Wiesenfeld-Hallin Z: The systemic administration of local anaesthetics produces a selective depression of C-afferent fibre evoked activity in the spinal cord. Pain 23:361–374, 1985.
34. Rowbotham MC, Fields HL: Topical lidocaine reduces pain in postherpetic neuralgia. Pain 38:297–301, 1989.
35. Treede RD, David KD, Campbell JN, Rajc SN: The plasticity of cutaneous hyperalgesia during sympathetic ganglionic blockade in patients with neuropathic pain. Brain 115:607–621, 1992.

CHAPTER • 44

Celiac Plexus and Splanchnic Nerve Block

Steven D. Waldman, MD, JD • Richard B. Patt, MD

HISTORICAL CONSIDERATIONS

In 1914, Kappis[1] introduced a percutaneous technique for blockade of the splanchnic nerves and celiac plexus with local anesthetic.* He described a posterior approach intended to be used primarily for surgical anesthesia, that utilized two needles, the tips of which were placed into the retroperitoneum via a retrocrural approach. He rapidly gained experience with this technique and reported on it in a series of 200 patients in 1918.[2]

The same year, Wendling[3] described a method of blocking the celiac plexus and splanchnic nerves utilizing a single needle placed anteriorly through the liver. Judged to be riskier than Kappis's posterior approach, it rapidly fell into disfavor.

Labat, Farr, and others introduced further modifications of Kappis's technique over the ensuing 30 years.[4–6] Because of the technical demands and variable results of celiac plexus and splanchnic nerve block as a surgical anesthetic, over time, this technique was supplanted by spinal anesthesia and segmental blockade of the somatic paravertebral nerves.[7]

In the classic textbook *Conduction Anesthesia*, published in 1946, Pitkin,[8] surveying the status of the use of splanchnic nerve block for surgical anesthesia, wrote, "Posterior splanchnic block gained some popularity with a limited number of anesthetists, but because of unsatisfactory results it was never continued beyond the experimental stage." There is no doubt that, as with many other regional anesthesia techniques, the introduction of neuromuscular blocking agents into the clinical practice of anesthesia led to the final demise of celiac plexus and splanchnic nerve block for surgical anesthesia, except at a limited number of institutions.

As celiac plexus and splanchnic nerve blocks were falling into disuse for surgical anesthesia, the clinical utility of these techniques was becoming apparent in the new specialty of pain management. In 1947, Gage and Floyd[9] described the use of celiac plexus and splanchnic nerve block in the management of pain secondary to pancreatitis. Esnaurrizar[10] and others recommended it to palliate abdominal pain secondary to a variety of causes. Recognizing the difficulty in distinguishing the somatic and visceral components of abdominal pain, Popper[11] recommended the use of splanchnic nerve block with local anesthetic as a diagnostic tool.

Alcohol neurolysis of the splanchnic nerves and celiac plexus for long-lasting relief of abdominal pain was first described by Jones,[12] in 1957. Bridenbaugh and colleagues[13] reported on the role of neurolytic celiac plexus block to treat the pain of upper abdominal malignancy. In 1965, Moore[14] further modified Kappis's original technique and brought celiac plexus block into the mainstream of pain management practice.

In spite of these modifications over the last 80 years, Kappis's classic posterior approach to blockade of the celiac plexus and splanchnic nerves continues to serve as the basis for contemporary techniques. Interestingly, there is renewed interest in the anterior approach to celiac plexus block, utilizing computed tomography or ultrasound to allow more accurate needle placement.[15, 16]

INDICATIONS

Indications for celiac plexus block are several. Celiac plexus block with local anesthetic is indicated as a diagnostic tool to determine whether flank, retroperitoneal, or upper abdominal pain is sympathetically mediated via the celiac plexus.[17] Daily celiac plexus blocks with local anesthetic are also useful in the palliation of pain secondary to acute pancreatitis.[18, 19] Clinical reports suggest that early implementation of celiac plexus block with local anesthetic and/

* Note: There is significant confusion about the nomenclature for the neural structures that innervate the abdominal viscera. Different investigators have used a variety of terms, including *splanchnic plexus*, *splanchnic nerve*, *solar plexus*, and *abdominal brain of Bichat*, to describe all or some of the same structures. In this chapter, we have tried to utilize all neuroanatomic nomenclature in an "anatomically correct" manner whenever possible.

or steroid markedly reduces the morbidity and mortality associated with acute pancreatitis.[20, 21] Celiac plexus block is also used successfully to palliate the acute pain of arterial embolization of the liver for cancer therapy and to reduce the pain of abdominal "angina" associated with visceral arterial insufficiency.[22] Celiac plexus block with local anesthetic may be utilized for prognosis before performing celiac plexus neurolysis.[23]

Neurolysis of the celiac plexus with alcohol or phenol is indicated to treat pain secondary to malignancies of the retroperitoneum and upper abdomen.[24,25] Neurolytic celiac plexus block may also be useful in some chronic benign abdominal pain syndromes, including chronic pancreatitis, in carefully selected patients.[26, 27] Most investigators report a lower success rate when utilizing celiac plexus and splanchnic nerve block to treat patients suffering from chronic nonmalignant abdominal pain as compared with the rate for abdominal pain of neoplastic origin.[23]

CONTRAINDICATIONS

Owing to the proximity to vascular structures, celiac plexus block is contraindicated in patients who are on anticoagulant therapy or suffer from coagulopathy secondary to congenital abnormality, antiblastic cancer therapies, or liver abnormalities associated with ethanol abuse.[23, 25] Local or intraabdominal infection and sepsis represent absolute contraindications to celiac plexus block.

Because blockade of the celiac plexus results in greater bowel motility, the technique should be avoided in patients with bowel obstruction.[20] Neurolytic celiac plexus block should probably be deferred in patients who suffer from chronic abdominal pain, who are chemically dependent, or who exhibit drug-seeking behavior until these relative contraindications have been adequately addressed.[18] The use of alcohol as a neurolytic agent should be avoided in patients on disulfiram therapy for alcohol abuse.

CLINICALLY RELEVANT ANATOMY

To perform celiac plexus and splanchnic nerve block safely and effectively, it is necessary to understand the anatomy of the autonomic nervous system and the relationships of the anatomic structures surrounding the celiac plexus. Computed tomography (CT) has enhanced the understanding of the region's functional anatomy and better documents where injected drugs are ultimately deposited. This information has been used to improve the efficacy and safety of celiac plexus and splanchnic nerve block.

The Autonomic Nervous System

The sympathetic innervation of the abdominal viscera originates in the anterolateral horn of the spinal cord (Fig. 44–1).[28] Preganglionic fibers from T5 through T12 exit the spinal cord in conjunction with the ventral roots, to join the white communicating rami on their way to the sympathetic chain. Rather than synapsing with the sympathetic chain, these preganglionic fibers pass through it, ultimately to synapse on the celiac ganglia.[29]

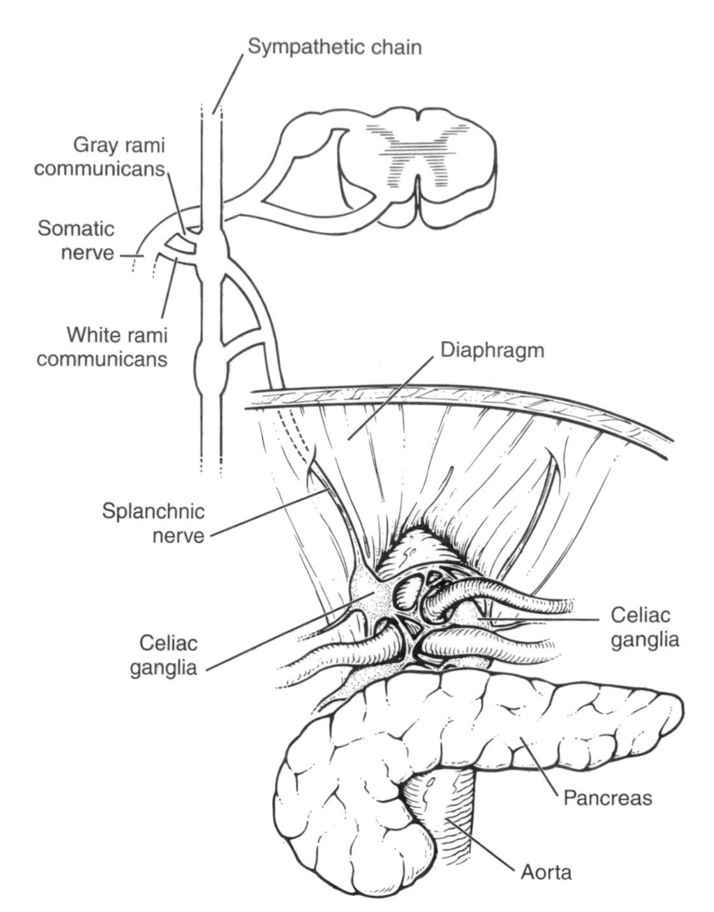

FIGURE 44–1 The sympathetic innervation of the abdominal viscera.

The Splanchnic Nerves

The greater, lesser, and least splanchnic nerves provide the major preganglionic contribution to the celiac plexus (Fig. 44–2).[30] The greater splanchnic nerve has its origin from the T5–T10 spinal roots. The nerve travels along the thoracic paravertebral border, through the crus of the diaphragm, and into the abdominal cavity, ending on the ipsilateral celiac ganglion. The lesser splanchnic nerve arises from the T10–T11 roots and passes with the greater nerve to end at the celiac ganglion. The least splanchnic nerve arises from the T11–T12 spinal roots and passes through the diaphragm to the celiac ganglion. It is important to note that the greater, lesser, and least splanchnic nerves are *preganglionic* structures that synapse at the celiac ganglia.[20] Blockade limited solely to these nerves is properly termed *splanchnic nerve block* (see later).

The Celiac Ganglia

The three splanchnic nerves synapse at the celiac ganglia (see Fig. 44–1). Despite significant variability from patient

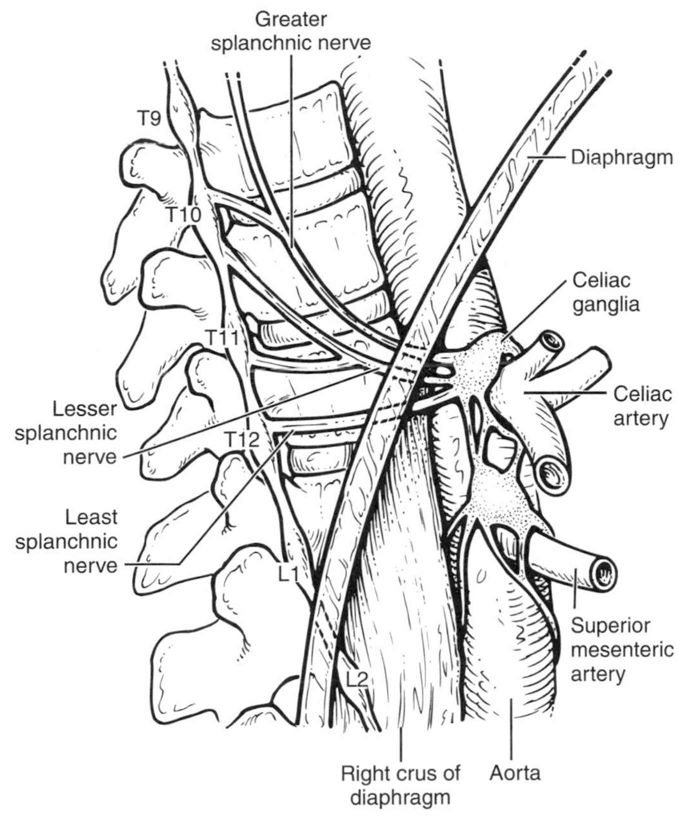

FIGURE 44–2 *The splanchnic nerves.*

to patient of the anatomy of the celiac ganglia, the following generalizations can be drawn from anatomic studies.[31] The number of ganglia ranges from one to five and their diameters from 0.5 to 4.5 cm. The ganglia lie anterior and anterolateral to the aorta. The ganglia located on the left are uniformly farther inferior than their right-sided counterparts by as much as a vertebral level, but both groups of ganglia lie below the level of the celiac artery. In most instances, the ganglia lie approximately at the level of L1.

Postganglionic fibers radiate from the celiac ganglia along the course of the blood vessels that innervate the abdominal viscera, which are derived from the embryonic foregut[25]: much of the distal esophagus, stomach, duodenum, small intestine, ascending and proximal transverse colon, adrenal glands, pancreas, spleen, liver, and biliary system.

The Celiac Plexus

Ganglia and *plexus* are often used interchangeably, but, in point of fact, it is the ganglia and their respective dense network of preganglionic and postganglionic fibers that constitute the celiac plexus. Anatomically, the celiac plexus arises from the preganglionic splanchnic nerves, vagal preganglionic parasympathetic fibers, sensory fibers from the phrenic nerve, and postganglionic sympathetic fibers.[28]

The celiac plexus is anterior to the diaphragmatic crura.[32] It extends in front of and around the aorta, the greatest concentration of fibers being anterior to the aorta (see Fig. 44–1). Blockade of these neural structures, which include the afferent fibers carrying nociceptive information, is properly termed *celiac plexus block*. It should be noted that the phrenic nerve also transmits nociceptive information from the upper abdominal viscera,[28] which may be perceived as poorly localized pain referred to the supraclavicular region.

Structures Surrounding the Celiac Plexus

The relationship of the celiac plexus to the surrounding structures is depicted in Figure 44–3. The normal configuration of these structures may be dramatically distorted owing to organomegaly or tumor. The aorta lies anterior and slightly to the left of the anterior margin of the vertebral body. The inferior vena cava lies to the right of the midline, and the kidneys are posterolateral to the great vessels. The pancreas lies anterior to the celiac plexus. All of these structures lie within the retroperitoneal space.

TECHNIQUE OF CELIAC PLEXUS AND SPLANCHNIC NERVE BLOCK

The Classic Retrocrural Technique

The technique of celiac plexus block that is traditionally taught and, thus, most commonly utilized by anesthesiologists for blocking the celiac plexus, is the retrocrural technique first described by Kappis[2] and subsequently refined and popularized by Moore.[14]

As with other techniques for celiac plexus and splanchnic nerve block, preparation includes administration of intravenous fluids to attenuate the hypotension associated with neural blockade of these structures. Evaluation for coagulopathy is especially indicated in those patients who have undergone antiblastic therapy or have a history of significant alcohol abuse.[23] If radiographic contrast is to be utilized, evaluation of the patient's renal function is indicated as well.

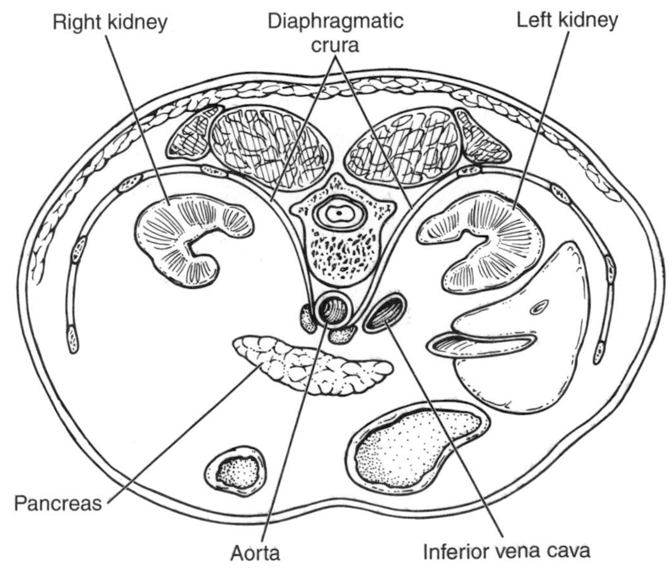

FIGURE 44–3 *The structures surrounding the celiac plexus.*

The patient is placed in the prone position with a pillow beneath the abdomen to reverse the thoracolumbar lordosis. This position increases the distance between the costal margins and the iliac crests and between the transverse processes of adjacent vertebral bodies. For comfort, the patient's head is turned to the side, and the arms are permitted to hang freely off either side of the table. The operative field is prepared and draped in standard aseptic manner.

Some clinicians find it beneficial to delineate the pertinent landmarks on the skin with a sterile marker. The landmarks include the iliac crests, 12th ribs, dorsal midline, vertebral bodies (T12–L2), and lateral borders of the paraspinal (sacrospinalis) muscles (Fig. 44–4). Moore[14] recommends that the intersection of the 12th rib and the lateral border of the paraspinal muscles on each side (which corresponds to L2) be marked and connected with lines to each other and to the cephalic portion of the L1 spine, forming an isosceles triangle, the sides of which serve as an additional guide to needle positioning.

The skin and underlying subcutaneous tissues and musculature are infiltrated with 1.0% lidocaine at the points of needle entry, which is about four fingerbreadths (7.5 cm) lateral to the midline, just beneath the 12th ribs. Either 20- or 22-gauge, 13-cm styleted needles are inserted bilaterally through the previously anesthetized areas. The needles are initially oriented 45 degrees toward the midline and about 15 degrees cephalad, to ensure contact with the L1 vertebral body (Fig. 44–5). Once contact with the vertebral body has been verified, the depth at which bone contact occurred is noted. (Some clinicians find it useful to actually mark this measurement on the shaft of the needle with a sterile gentian violet marker after the needle is withdrawn.)

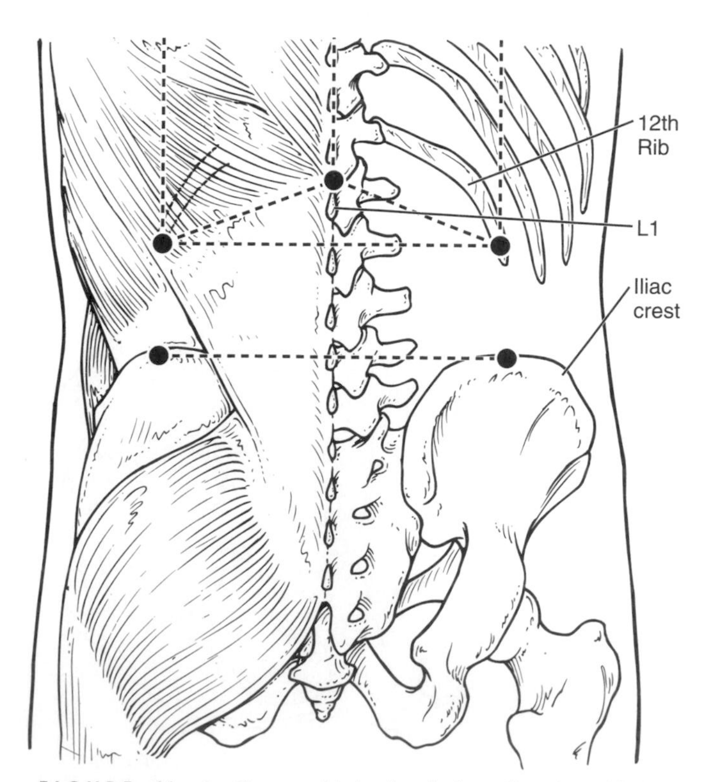

FIGURE 44–4 Topographic landmarks for celiac plexus block.

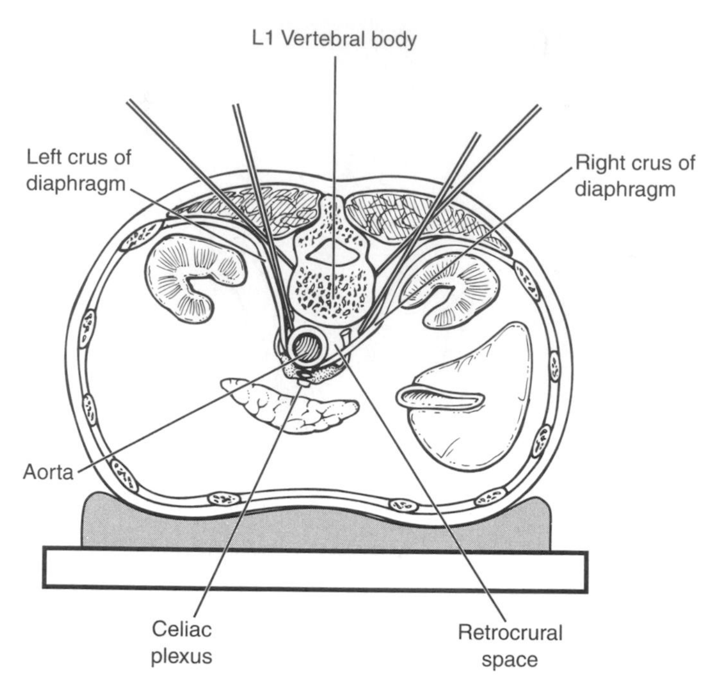

FIGURE 44–5 Needle placement for "classic" celiac plexus block.

After bone contact is made and the depth is noted, the needles are withdrawn to the level of the subcutaneous tissue and redirected slightly less mesiad (about 60 degrees from the midline) so as to "walk off" the lateral surface of the L1 vertebral body. The needles are reinserted to the depth at which contact with the vertebral body was first noted. At this point, if no contact with bone is made, the left-sided needle is gradually advanced 1.5 to 2 cm or until the pulsations emanating from the aorta and transmitted to the advancing needle are felt.[33, 34] The right-sided needle is then advanced slightly farther (i.e., 3–4 cm past contact with the vertebral body). Ultimately, the tips of the needles should be just posterior to the aorta on the left and to the anterolateral aspect of the aorta on the right (see Fig. 44–5).

The stylets are removed, and the needle hubs are inspected for blood, cerebrospinal fluid, and urine. If radiographic guidance is being utilized, a small volume of contrast material is injected bilaterally and its spread is observed radiographically.

Ideally, on the fluoroscopic anteroposterior view, contrast material is confined to the midline and concentrated near the L1 vertebral body (Fig. 44–6). A smooth posterior contour can be observed that corresponds to the psoas fascia on the lateral view (Fig. 44–7).

Alternatively, if CT guidance is used, contrast material should appear lateral to and behind the aorta. If contrast material is confined entirely to the retrocrural space, the needles should be advanced to the precrural space to minimize the risk of posterior spread of local anesthetic or neurolytic agent to the somatic nerve roots (see later).[35]

If radiographic guidance is not utilized, a local anesthetic with rapid onset and in sufficient concentration to produce motor block (such as 1.5% lidocaine or 3.0% 2-chloroprocaine) is given before administration of neurolytic agents. If the patient experiences no motor or sensory

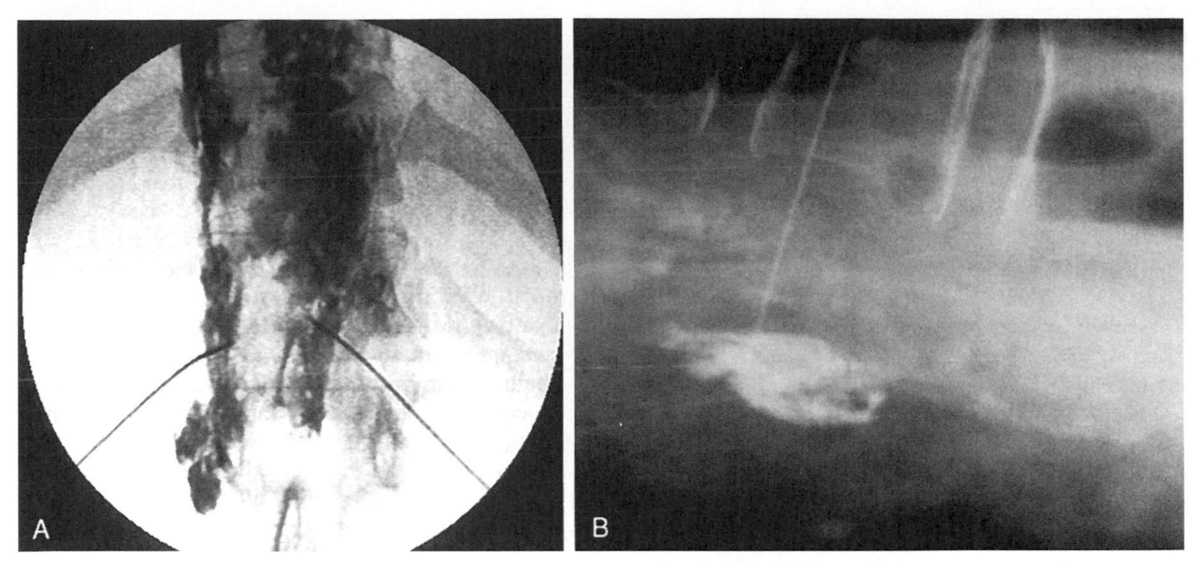

FIGURE 44–6 Anteroposterior fluoroscopic view of the midline placement of contrast agent at L1.

block after an adequate waiting time, it is likely that additional drugs injected through the needles will not reach the somatic nerve roots if given in similar volumes.

For diagnostic and prognostic block utilizing the retrocrural technique, 12 to 15 mL of 1.0% lidocaine or 3.0% 2-chloroprocaine is administered through each needle.[18] For therapeutic local anesthetic block, 10 to 12 mL of 0.5% bupivacaine is administered through each needle. Owing to the potential for local anesthetic toxicity, all local anesthetics should be administered in incremental doses.[24] For treatment of the pain of acute pancreatitis, an 80-mg dose of depot methylprednisolone is advocated for the initial celiac plexus block, and 40 mg for subsequent blocks.[36]

Most investigators suggest that 10 to 12 mL of 50% ethyl alcohol or 6.0% aqueous phenol be injected through each needle for retrocrural neurolytic block. Thomson and colleagues,[34] however, strongly recommend that 25 mL of 50% ethyl alcohol be injected via each needle.

After the neurolytic solution has been injected, each needle should be flushed with sterile saline solution. (There have been anecdotal reports of neurolytic solution being tracked posteriorly along with the needles as they are withdrawn.) Radiographic guidance, in particular CT guidance, offers the pain specialist an added margin of safety when performing neurolytic celiac plexus block and thus should be utilized whenever possible.

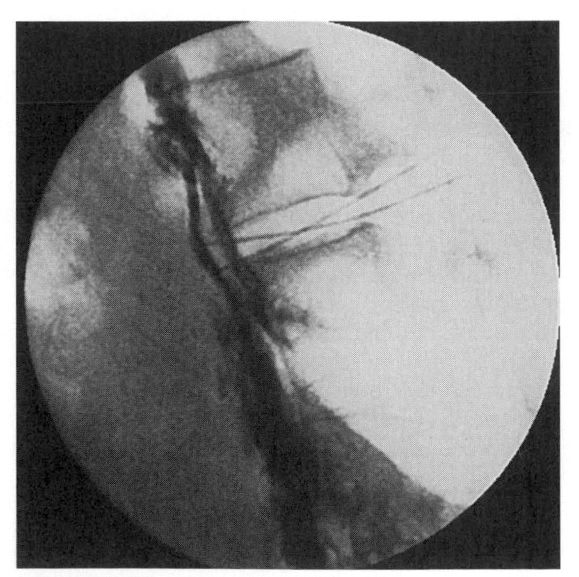

FIGURE 44–7 Lateral fluoroscopic view of contrast agent bounded by psoas fascia.

Transcrural Techniques

The diaphragm separates the thoracic and abdominal cavities but permits the passage of the thoracoabdominal structures, including the aorta, vena cava, and splanchnic nerves. The diaphragmatic crura are bilateral structures that arise from the anterolateral surfaces of the upper two or three lumbar vertebrae and discs. The crura of the diaphragm serve as a barrier to effectively separate the splanchnic nerves from the celiac ganglia and plexus below.[28]

In the modified Kappis approach to celiac plexus block described previously, the needles are behind the crura in almost all instances. That is to say, the needles and injected solution are placed posterior and cephalad to the crura of the diaphragm. On the basis of CT and cadaver studies, it has been suggested that the classic method of retrocrural block is more likely to produce splanchnic nerve block rather than blockade of the celiac plexus. Instead of depositing injected material around and anterior to the aorta and directly onto the celiac plexus at the level of the L1 vertebral body, as was previously thought, the injectate appears to (1) concentrate posterior to the aorta and in front of and along the side of the L1 vertebral body, where it may anesthetize retroaortic celiac fibers; (2) diffuse cephalad to anesthetize the splanchnic nerve at a site rostrad to the origin of the plexus, and (3) only finally encircle the aorta at the site of the celiac plexus when a sufficient volume of drug is injected to transgress the diaphragm by diffusing caudad through the aortic hiatus.[33, 37]

Although the retrocrural approach has been shown to be generally effective and safe, advocates of the transcrural approaches believe that simple modifications maximize the spread of injected solutions anterior to the aorta, where the celiac plexus is most concentrated, and minimize the risk of somatic nerve root blocks. The term *transcrural* reflects placement of needle tips and drug anterior and caudal to the diaphragmatic crura.

Singler[37] and Boas[62] recommend a transcrural approach using, respectively, CT and fluoroscopic guidance as important modifications of the traditional retrocrural technique. Transcrural block is carried out in a manner essentially the same as that for retrocrural block, except that needles are advanced farther anteriorly. Slightly smaller volumes of local anesthetic and neurolytic agents are utilized for the bilateral transcrural approach. Efficacy equal to or slightly greater than that of the classic retrocrural approach is reported by most investigators.[38]

Transaortic Techniques

In 1983, Ischia and colleagues[39] introduced a new approach to transcrural celiac plexus block that involved placing a single needle on the left side and posteriorly through the aorta, to ensure that the injected drugs are placed in the precrural space directly onto the celiac plexus. This method is, in some respects, analogous to the transaxillary approach to brachial plexus block. The safety of the transaortic approach is suggested by previous experience with both axillary block and translumbar aortograms.[40]

Despite concerns about the potential for aortic trauma and subsequent occult retroperitoneal hemorrhage with the transaortic approach to celiac plexus block, it may, in fact, be safer than the classic two-needle posterior approach.[41, 42] The lower incidence of complications is thought to be due in part to the use of a single fine needle rather than two larger ones. The fact that the aorta is relatively well-supported in this region by the diaphragmatic crura and prevertebral fascia also contributes to the technique's apparent relative safety.[41]

The transaortic approach to celiac plexus block has three additional advantages over the classic two-needle approach. First, it avoids the risks of neurologic complications related to posterior retrocrural spread of drugs. Second, the aorta provides a definitive landmark for needle placement when radiographic guidance is not available. Third, much smaller volumes of local anesthetic and neurolytic solutions are required to achieve efficacy equal to or greater than that of the classic retrocrural approach.[42]

Fluoroscopically Guided Transaortic Celiac Plexus Block

The fluoroscopically guided transaortic approach utilizes the usual landmarks for the posterior placement of a left-sided, 22-gauge, 13-cm styleted needle. Some investigators use a needle entry point 1.0 to 1.5 cm closer to the midline than that for the classic retrocrural approach, combined with a needle trajectory closer to the perpendicular, to reduce the incidence of renal trauma.

The needle is advanced with the goal of passing just lateral to the anterolateral aspect of the L1 vertebral body. If that vertebral body is encountered, the needle is withdrawn into the subcutaneous tissues and redirected in a manner analogous to that for the classic retrocrural approach. The styleted needle is gradually advanced until its tip rests in the posterior periaortic space. As the needle impinges on the posterior aortic wall, the operator feels transmitted aortic pulsations via the needle and greater resistance to its passage.

Passing the needle through the wall of the aorta has been likened to passing a needle through a large rubber band. Presence of the needle within the aortic lumen is evidenced by free flow of arterial blood when the stylet is removed. The stylet is replaced, and the needle is advanced until it impinges on the intraluminal anterior wall of the aorta. At this point, the operator again feels increased resistance to needle advancement. A pop is felt as the needle tip passes through the anterior aortic wall, indicating that it probably lies within the preaortic fatty connective tissue and the substance of the celiac plexus. A saline loss-of-resistance technique, as described earlier, may help in identification of the preaortic space.

Because the needle is sometimes inadvertently advanced beyond the retroperitoneal space into the peritoneal cavity, confirmatory fluoroscopic views of injected contrast medium are advised, especially when neurolytic blockade is to be done. On anteroposterior views, the contrast medium should be confined to the midline, with a tendency toward greater concentration around the lateral margins of the aorta. Lateral views should demonstrate a predominantly preaortic orientation extending from around T12 through L2, sometimes accompanied by pulsations.[25] Incomplete penetration of the anterior wall is indicated by a narrow longitudinal "line image."

Failure of the contrast medium to completely surround the anterior aorta may occur in the presence of extensive infiltration of the preaortic region by tumor or in patients who have undergone previous pancreatic surgery or radiation therapy. It is our experience that the chance of success is smaller when poor or irregular preaortic spread of contrast is observed. In this setting, selective alcohol neurolysis of the splanchnic nerves may provide better pain relief.

For diagnostic and prognostic block using the fluoroscopically guided transaortic technique, 10 to 12 mL of 1.5% lidocaine or 3.0% 2-chloroprocaine is administered through the needle. For therapeutic block, 10 to 12 mL of 0.5% bupivacaine is administered. Owing to the potential for local anesthetic toxicity, all local anesthetics should be administered in incremental doses. For treatment of the pain of acute pancreatitis, the same dosages of depot methylprednisolone mentioned previously for the retrocrural and transcrural techniques are indicated. Absolute alcohol or 6.0% aqueous phenol, 12 to 15 mL, is utilized for neurolytic block.

CT-Guided Transaortic Celiac Plexus Block

The CT-guided transaortic celiac plexus block is probably the safest way to achieve neurolysis of the celiac plexus.

CT allows the pain management physician to clearly identify the clinically relevant anatomy, including the crura of the diaphragm, aorta, vena cava, and kidneys, to ensure accurate precrural needle placement. Observation of the spread of contrast medium, as described here, enables the physician to know exactly where the injectate is deposited, and provides an added margin of patient safety in comparison with fluoroscopic or blind techniques.

The patient is prepared for CT-guided transaortic celiac plexus block just as for the techniques described earlier. After proper positioning on the CT scanning table, a scout film is obtained to identify the T12–L1 interspace (Fig. 44–8). A CT image is then taken through the interspace. The scan is reviewed for the position of the aorta relative to the vertebral body, the position of intraabdominal and retroperitoneal organs, and any distortions of normal anatomy by tumor, previous surgery, or adenopathy (Fig. 44–9). The aorta at this level is evaluated for significant aortic aneurysm, mural thrombus, or calcifications; any of these would recommend against use of a transaortic approach.[23]

The level at which the scan was taken is identified on the patient's skin and marked with a gentian violet marker. The skin is prepared with antiseptic solution. The skin, subcutaneous tissues, and muscle at a point approximately 2.5 in from the left of the midline is anesthetized with 1.0% lidocaine. A 13-cm, 22-gauge styleted needle is placed through the anesthetized area and is advanced until the posterior wall of the aorta is encountered, as evidenced by transmission of arterial pulsations and greater resistance to needle advancement. The needle is advanced into the lumen of the aorta. The stylet is removed, and the needle hub is observed for free flow of arterial blood (Fig. 44–10).

A well-lubricated 5-mL glass syringe filled with preservative-free saline is attached to the needle hub. The needle and syringe are then advanced through the anterior wall of the aorta using a loss-of-resistance technique in the same way that it is used to identify the epidural space.[43] The glass syringe is removed, and 3.0 mL of 1.5% lidocaine in solution with an equal amount of water-soluble contrast medium is injected through the needle.

A CT scan at the level of the needle's tip is taken. The scan is reviewed for the placement of the needle and, most importantly, for the spread of contrast medium,[23] which should be seen in the preaortic area and surrounding the aorta (Fig. 44–11). No contrast medium should be observed in the retrocrural space (Fig. 44–12). After proper needle placement and spread of contrast medium is confirmed, 12 to 15 mL of absolute alcohol or 6% aqueous phenol is injected through the needle.[42] The needle is flushed with a small amount of sterile saline and then removed. The patient is observed carefully for hemodynamic changes, including hypotension and tachycardia secondary to the resulting profound sympathetic blockade.

Lieberman and Waldman[43] reported on the success and efficacy of transaortic celiac plexus block utilizing the loss-of-resistance technique in a large series of patients suffering

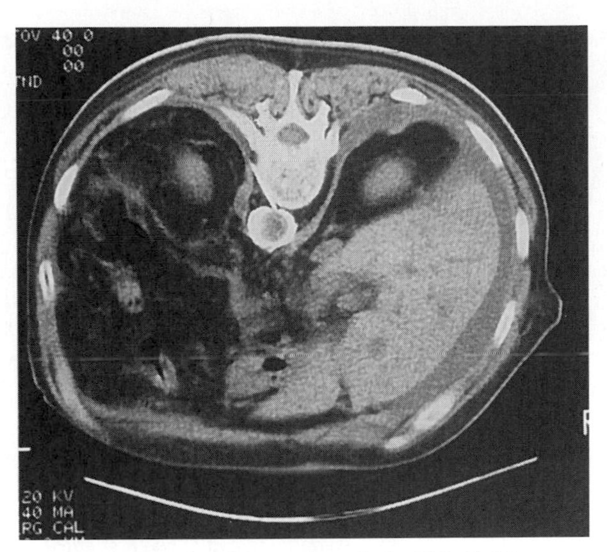

FIGURE 44–9 CT scan through the T12–L1 interspace.

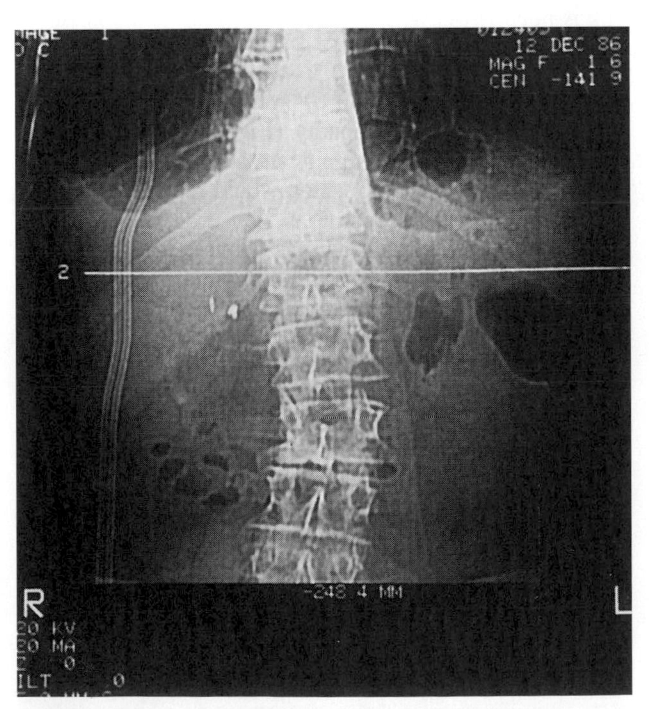

FIGURE 44–8 Identification of the T12–L1 interspace for CT-guided transaortic celiac plexus block.

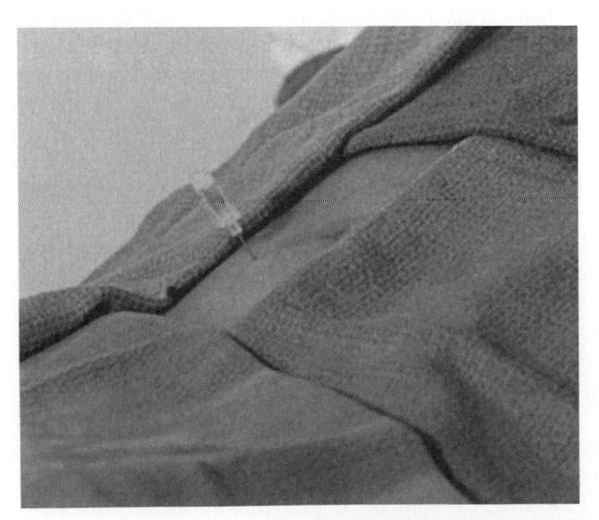

FIGURE 44–10 Needle in position with tip in lumen of aorta.

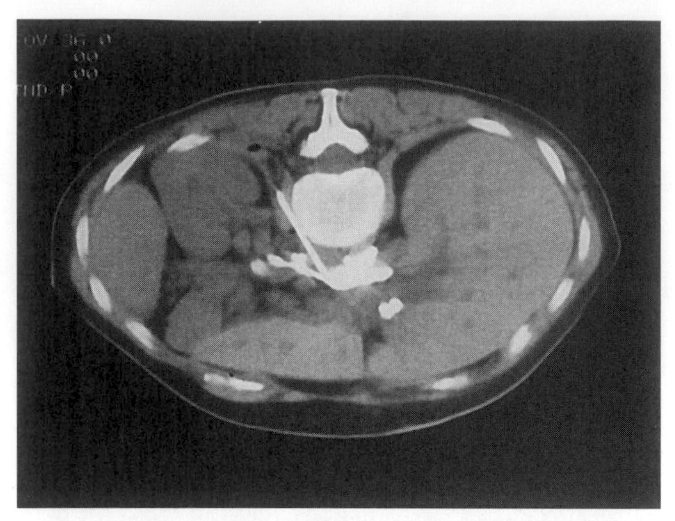

FIGURE 44–11 Preaortic spread of contrast agent.

from cancer pain.[43] In this study, 91% of patients reported marked immediate pain relief after CT-guided transaortic celiac plexus block utilizing the loss-of-resistance technique. At 6 weeks, 39% of surviving patients were pain-free and did not require opioid analgesics. An additional 50% of patients reported great improvement but required adjunctive treatment with opioids. No unusual complications or side effects were encountered in this large series of patients.

Anterior Approaches to Celiac Plexus Block

Percutaneous Gangliolysis

A percutaneous anterior approach to the celiac plexus was advocated early in this century, only to be abandoned because of the high incidence of complications.[3, 44] The advent of fine needles, improvements in radiologic guidance technology, and the maturation of the specialty of interventional radiology have since led to renewed interest in the anterior approach to blockade of the celiac plexus.

Extensive experience with transabdominal fine-needle aspiration biopsy has confirmed the relative safety of this approach and provides the rationale and method for the modification of this radiologic technique for anterior celiac plexus block. The anterior approach to the celiac plexus necessarily involves the passage of a fine needle through the liver, stomach, intestine, vessels, and pancreas. Surprisingly, it is associated with very low rates of complications.[45–48]

Advantages of the anterior approach to blocking the celiac plexus include its relative ease, speed, and reduced periprocedural discomfort as compared with posterior techniques.[16, 25] Perhaps the greatest advantage of the anterior approach is the fact that patients are spared having to remain prone for long, which can be a significant problem for patients suffering from intraabdominal pain. The supine position is also advantageous for patients with iliostomies and colostomies.

The anterior approach is probably associated with less discomfort because only one needle is used. Furthermore, the needle does not impinge on either periosteum or nerve roots or pass through the bulky paraspinous musculature. Because needle placement is precrural, there is less risk of accidental neurologic injury related to retrocrural spread of drug to somatic nerve roots or epidural and subarachnoid spaces.

Potential disadvantages of the anterior approach to celiac plexus block include the risks of infection, abscess, hemorrhage, and fistula formation.[46] Although preliminary findings indicate that these complications are exceedingly rare, further experience is needed to draw a definitive conclusion. By the same token, although preliminary data suggest the efficacy of the anterior approach, further experience is needed to permit adequate comparisons with better-established techniques.

The anterior technique can be carried out under CT or ultrasound guidance. Patient preparation is similar to that for posterior approaches to celiac block. The patient is placed in the supine position on the CT or ultrasound table. The skin of the upper abdomen is prepared with antiseptic solution. The needle entry site is identified 1.5 cm below and 1.5 cm to the left of the xyphoid process (Fig. 44–13).[45] At that point, the skin, subcutaneous tissues and musculature are anesthetized with 1.0% lidocaine. A 22-gauge, 15-cm needle is introduced through the anesthetized area perpendicular to the skin and advanced to the depth of the anterior wall of the aorta, as calculated using CT or ultrasound guidance (Figs. 44–14, 44–15).

If CT guidance is being utilized, 4 mL of water-soluble contrast in solution with an equal volume of 1.0% lidocaine is injected to confirm needle placement (Fig. 44–16). If ultrasound guidance is being used, 10 to 12 mL of sterile saline can be injected to help confirm needle position (Fig. 44–17).[16] After satisfactory needle placement is confirmed, diagnostic and prognostic block is carried out using 15 mL of 1.5% lidocaine or 3.0% 2-chloroprocaine. Therapeutic block is performed with an equal volume of 0.5% bupivacaine. Owing to the potential for local anesthetic toxicity, all local anesthetics should be administered in incremental doses.

Matamala and associates[16] recommend 35 to 40 mL of 50% ethyl alcohol for neurolytic blocks of the celiac plexus via the anterior approach. Other investigators have had

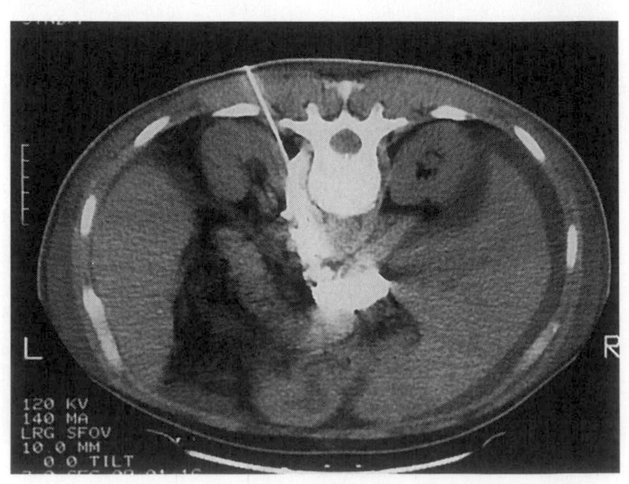

FIGURE 44–12 Retrocrural spread of contrast agent.

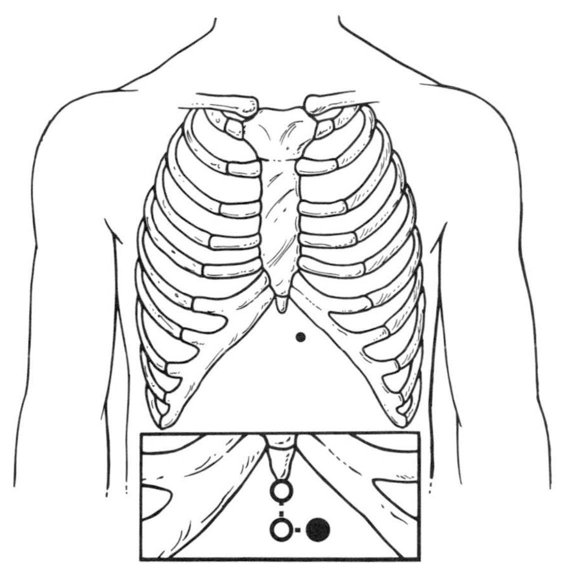

FIGURE 44 – 13 Needle entry site for anterior celiac plexus block. Inset, The site is located 1.5 cm below and 1.5 cm to the left of the xyphoid process.

equally good results utilizing 15 to 20 mL of absolute alcohol.

An alternative technique uses fluoroscopy to guide the passage of a single needle just to the right of the center of the L1 vertebral body, after which it is withdrawn 1 to 3 cm.[45] Important precautions for the anterior approach to celiac plexus block include the administration of prophylactic antibiotics and the use of needles no larger than 22 gauge to minimize the risks of infection and trauma to the vasculature and viscera.

Intraoperative Gangliolysis

The intraoperative anterior approach to the blockade of the celiac plexus and splanchnic nerves was first advocated by Braun[4] in 1921 as a means to provide intraoperative

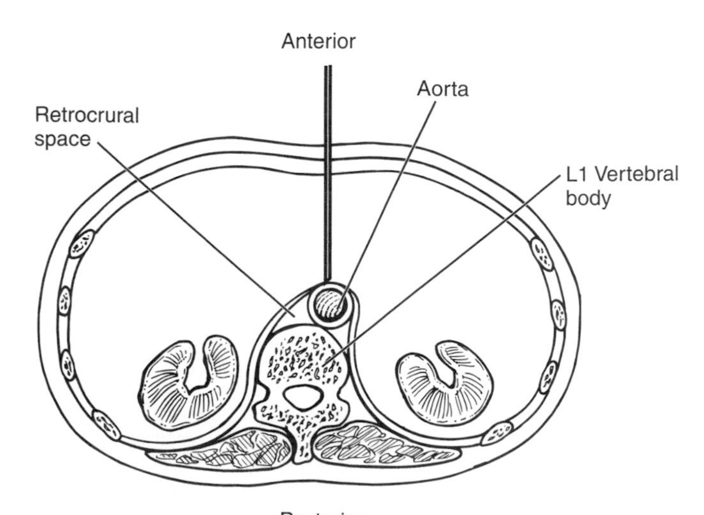

FIGURE 44 – 14 Needle placement for anterior celiac plexus block.

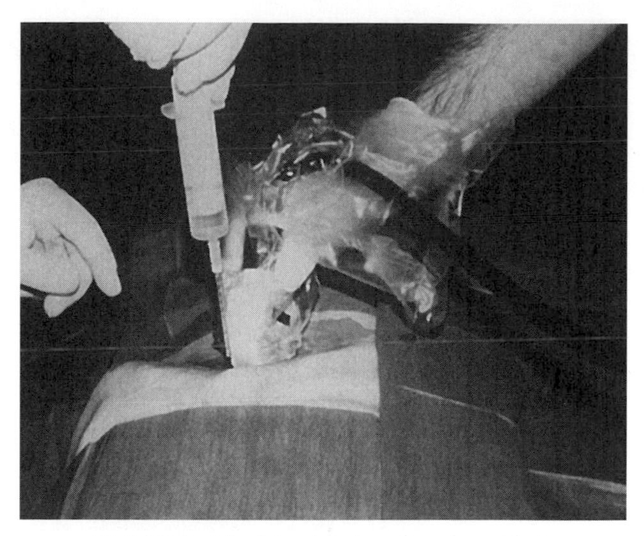

FIGURE 44 – 15 Anterior celiac plexus block.

visceral anesthesia. This technique was used in combination with field block of the abdominal wall. Braun's approach involved gentle retraction of the stomach and placement of a digit between the aorta and vena cava to serve as a guide to the injection of an anesthetic over the ventral surface of the L1 vertebral body. This technique enjoyed only limited acceptance for surgical anesthesia for abdominal operations.

In 1978, Kraft and associates described a similar approach to block the splanchnic nerves and celiac plexus for pain management.[49, 50] They identified the origin of the celiac artery and advanced a 20-gauge spinal needle over the exploring finger. Then, 15 to 20 mL of 6% aqueous phenol was injected intraoperatively.

The main advantage of intraoperative celiac block is the elimination of a separate procedure for pain control. In addition, intraoperative celiac block provides an opportunity to prophylactically treat the patient with only mild or no pain who is known to have an intraabdominal malignancy that in all likelihood will produce pain as it progresses.

Disadvantages of intraoperative anterior celiac plexus neurolysis include the unfamiliarity of most surgeons with (1) the functional regional anatomy, (2) injection techniques, and (3) the use of neurolytic agents required for the block.[25] Furthermore, safe access to the specified injec-

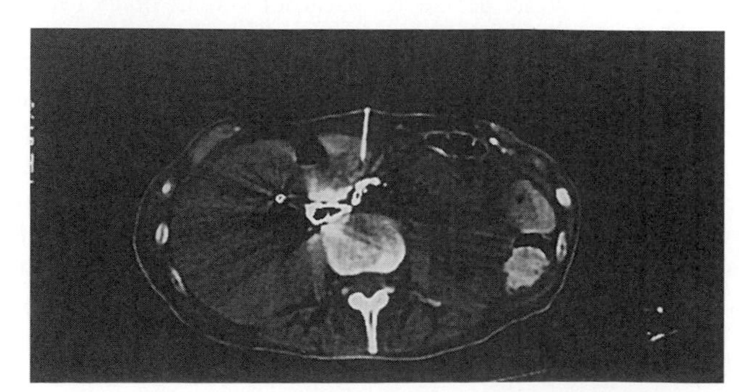

FIGURE 44 – 16 CT confirms proper needle placement for anterior celiac plexus block.

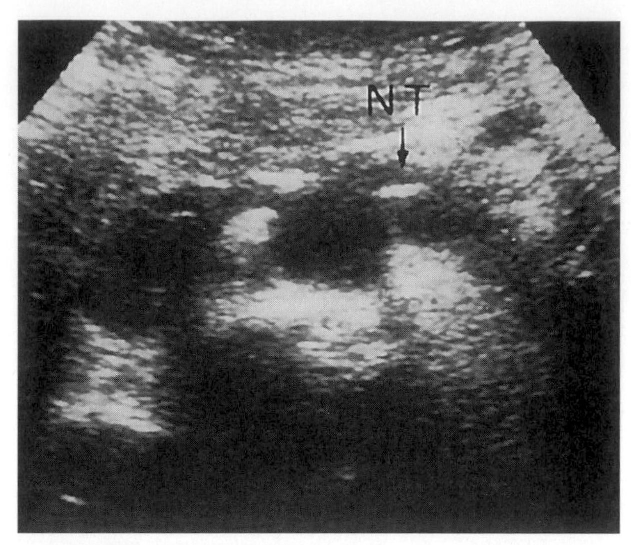

FIGURE 44–17 *Ultrasonogram confirms proper needle placement for anterior celiac plexus block.*

tion site may be prohibited by bulky intraabdominal disease and phlegmon. Because intraoperative dissection may result in leakage of the injected solution out of the intended injection site, the risk of neurologic injury is increased and the overall efficacy decreased.[25] Concurrent general anesthesia renders a test dosing with local anesthetic invalid and further raises the patient's risk, because of the patient's inability to report untoward reactions to the local anesthetic.

Given the current availability of effective percutaneous methods of achieving celiac block, intraoperative celiac plexus block cannot be recommended except when laparotomy is already planned for exploration or bypass of the gastrointestinal or biliary tract.[49] Even in these cases, the efficacy and relative safety of the technique are controversial. A valuable alternative in such cases is placement of surgical clips in the vicinity of the celiac axis to facilitate postoperative neural blockade.[51]

Catheter Techniques

Anecdotal reports documenting the efficacy and safety of temporary periaortic catheters to facilitate daily celiac nerve blocks have been presented.[52, 53] A percutaneous polytetrafluoroethylene periaortic catheter was in place for 14 days in a patient with pancreatitis, during which time serial injections of local anesthetic were administered before a definitive neurolytic block was performed.[54] Fluoroscopy and CT performed 13 days after placement revealed no catheter migration and no perivascular erosion or pleural reaction. A second report, documenting a single case of intraoperative placement of a percutaneously tunneled epidural catheter that was used after surgery to produce neurolysis suggests another potential treatment option.[55] In a third report, after a temporary periaortic catheter was placed percutaneously, the patient had persistent hematuria, and evidence of transrenal catheter placement was obtained. That case suggests that CT guidance may be advisable during placement of percutaneous catheters for celiac plexus block.[28]

At present, indications for periaortic catheterization are ill-defined. If shown to be safe and efficacious, this approach may ultimately prove beneficial in patients with chronic nonmalignant conditions.

Splanchnic Nerve Block

The recognition that splanchnic nerve block may provide relief of pain in a subset of patients who fail to obtain relief from celiac plexus block has renewed interest in this technique.[25, 56] The splanchnic nerves transmit the majority of nociceptive information from the viscera.[28] These nerves are contained in a narrow compartment made up by the vertebral body and the pleura laterally, the posterior mediastinum ventrally, and the pleural attachment to the vertebra dorsally. This compartment is bounded caudally by the crura of the diaphragm. Abram and Boas[56] have determined that the volume of this compartment is approximately 10 mL on each side.

The technique for splanchnic nerve block differs little from the classic retrocrural approach to the celiac plexus, except that the needles are aimed more cephalad so as to rest ultimately at the anterolateral margin of the T12 vertebral body (Fig. 44–18). It is imperative that both needles be placed medially against the vertebral body to reduce the incidence of pneumothorax.

An alternative approach to splanchnic nerve block utilizes 22-gauge, 3.5-inch spinal needles.[57] The needles are placed 3 to 4 cm lateral to the midline, just below the 12th ribs. Their trajectory is slightly mesiad, so that the tips come to rest at the anterolateral margin of the T12 body.

Abram and Boas[56] have described a simplified technique for splanchnic nerve block that uses a paravertebral transthoracic approach. Standard 22-gauge, 3.5-in spinal needles are introduced bilaterally 6 cm from the midline through the 11th intercostal space (see Fig. 44–18). The needle is advanced to rest against the anterolateral aspect of the T11 vertebral body. Precautions include attendance to a medial entry point and observation of the lower limit of the lung, which during quiet breathing is generally observed to lie one segment higher in the costophrenic angle. These precautions allow the needles to safely traverse the transpleural spaces. If experience eventually demonstrates that this simplified technique is comparable in safety and efficacy to the more difficult classic technique, it will clearly become the procedure of choice for splanchnic nerve block.

For diagnostic and prognostic splanchnic nerve block, 7 to 10 mL of 1.5% lidocaine or 3.0% 2-chloroprocaine is administered through the needle; for therapeutic block, 7 to 10 mL of 0.5% bupivacaine. Owing to the potential for local anesthetic toxicity, all local anesthetics should be administered in divided doses. A 10-mL volume of absolute alcohol or 6.0% aqueous phenol is utilized for neurolytic block.

The risks of splanchnic nerve block are similar to those of celiac plexus block. Additionally, the rates of pneumothorax, thoracic duct injury, and inadvertent spread of injected drugs to the somatic nerve roots are higher than those for transcrural approaches to celiac plexus block.[56]

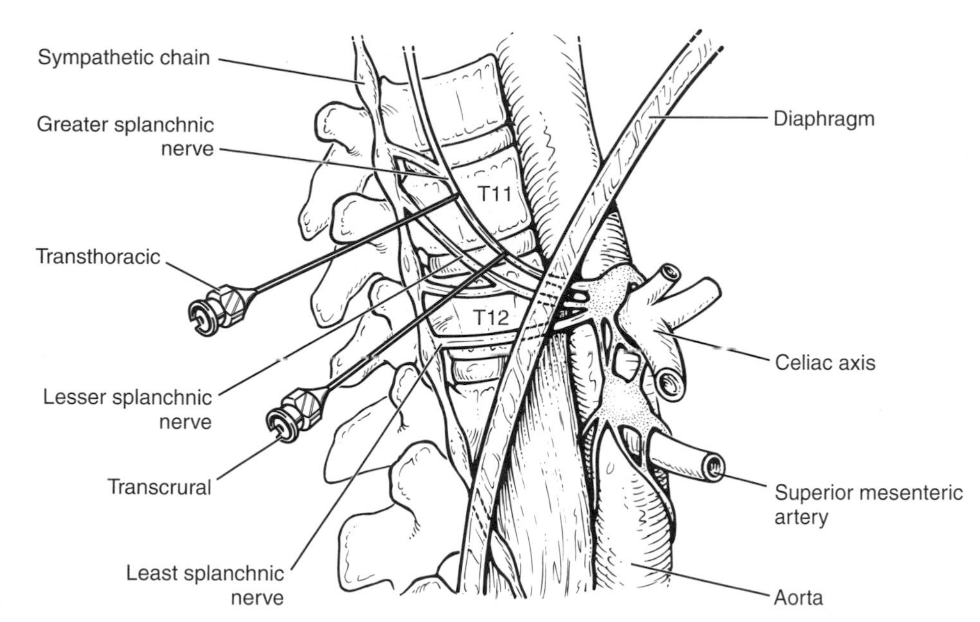

FIGURE 44–18 *Splanchnic nerve block.*

Because of the need for accurate needle placement, it is advisable to perform splanchnic nerve block under fluoroscopic or CT guidance.

CHOICE OF AGENT, VOLUME, NEEDLE, RADIOGRAPHIC GUIDANCE, AND TECHNIQUE

Choice of Agent

Investigators tend to disagree about the ideal volume, concentration, or drug for celiac plexus and splanchnic nerve blocks. Diagnostic and prognostic celiac plexus and splanchnic nerve blocks should be performed with a local anesthetic that has rapid onset and is sufficiently concentrated to produce sensory and motor block. For the classic two-needle retrocrural approach, a total volume of 20 to 25 mL of 1.0% lidocaine or 3.0% 2-chloroprocaine is appropriate. A volume of 12 to 15 mL is adequate for a single-needle transcrural approach to the celiac plexus block. Splanchnic nerve block is performed with 7 to 10 mL of 1.5% lidocaine or 3.0% 2-chloroprocaine. Similar volumes (as specified for each technique) of longer-acting local anesthetics such as 0.5% bupivacaine are utilized for therapeutic nerve block. Owing to the potential for local anesthetic toxicity, all local anesthetics should be administered in incremental doses. For the pain of inflammatory conditions such as pancreatitis, depot preparations of methylprednisolone may be administered in an initial dose of 80 mg and subsequent doses of 40 mg.

Neurolytic blockade of the celiac plexus and splanchnic nerves may be carried out with either ethyl alcohol or aqueous phenol. Because of limitations associated with the classic retrocrural technique, some authors have advocated 50-mL of 50% ethyl alcohol. Others have used concentrations of alcohol (25%–100%) in volumes ranging from 20 to 80 mL without apparent differences in efficacy or side effects.[27, 58, 59] Smaller volumes (12–15 mL) of absolute alcohol are recommended for single-needle transcrural techniques.

Many investigators believe that as a neurolytic agent alcohol is superior to phenol in duration of neural blockade; however, alcohol has the disadvantage of producing transient severe pain on injection. Furthermore, alcohol is not miscible with contrast medium. Unless alcohol is accidentally injected into a vessel, actual alcohol intoxication should not occur. Susceptible patients undergoing alcohol neurolysis may be subject to acetaldehyde syndrome, a relatively innocuous side effect (see discussion of complications).[34, 60, 61] Alcohol should be avoided in patients on disulfiram therapy for alcohol abuse.

Several workers have recommended 6% to 10% phenol for celiac plexus and splanchnic nerve block.[25, 49, 50] An advantage of phenol over alcohol is that it can be combined with contrast medium. The combination allows radiographic documentation of the distribution of neurolytic solution during and after injection, instead of relying on verification of needle placement before injection of neurolytic solution, as is necessary for alcohol injection. Mixtures of 10% phenol and iodinated contrast medium (Conray 420 or Renografin 76) remain stable up to 3 months.[62] The fact that phenol is not commercially available and must be prepared for each patient by a pharmacist is a practical disadvantage of this agent. The apparently greater affinity of phenol for vascular, rather than neurologic, tissue also represents a theoretical disadvantage, in view of the vascularity of the region surrounding the celiac plexus and splanchnic nerves.[63] Some investigators believe that phenol produces a block of shorter duration than that produced by alcohol, making it a less desirable agent for the intractable and progressive pain of cancer. It is important to note that controlled comparisons between alcohol and phenol for this application have not been conducted but they appear to be equally safe and efficacious.

Choice of Needles

Both 20- and 22-gauge needles have been advocated for celiac plexus and splanchnic nerve block. Thompson and

Moore[58] note that the resistance to injection provided by a long 22-gauge needle interferes with the appreciation of differences in tissue compliance, which can provide much useful information about needle position.[58] In addition, owing to the greater flexibility of 22-gauge needles, it is more difficult to maintain a straight trajectory during placement.[28] If 22-gauge needles are used, it is advisable to rely on radiologic guidance to confirm needle placement. A 22-gauge needle is preferred for anterior and transaortic approaches.[64]

Choice of Radiographic Guidance

The use of radiologic guidance for celiac plexus and splanchnic nerve block was once very controversial. Today, it is in favor. Provided that proper precautions are observed, celiac plexus and splanchnic nerve block with local anesthetic can safely be accomplished by experienced practitioners relying on topographic guidance alone.[34] In our opinion and that of others, radiologic guidance is virtually mandatory for neurolytic celiac plexus and splanchnic nerve block.[23, 35] Interestingly, when large series of cases are compared, it is not clear that the use of fluoroscopy actually reduces the incidence of complications.[64] It does appear, however, that CT guidance may add a margin of safety as compared with fluoroscopy, although a small number of serious complications have been reported when CT has been used for celiac plexus block.[43, 64] It is our strong belief that the use of radiographic guidance must still be encouraged on practical, empirical, and medicolegal grounds.

It is clear that even sophisticated radiologic guidance by itself does not ensure against complications. Routine application of simple precautionary measures, including careful serial aspiration and incremental injections of local anesthetic, is essential to minimize the likelihood of an adverse outcome. CT permits visualization of, not only bony structures, but also vascular and soft tissue elements (including diaphragmatic crura and tumor spread). It is particularly useful when anterior and transcrural approaches are planned. The disadvantages of CT include limited availability in some areas, the need for specialized support personnel, and the slightly higher cost relative to fluoroscopy.[28]

Choice of Technique

Numerous techniques have been advocated to achieve celiac plexus and splanchnic nerve block. Most of the experience is with the classic retrocrural technique, which, as a result, is regarded as the standard against which other techniques are compared. It is anticipated that the newer techniques for celiac plexus and splanchnic nerve block will gain greater acceptance as experience accrues, because they appear safe and efficacious and offer certain practical and theoretical advantages. The transaortic approach is particularly attractive, because it requires only a single needle whose position is easily verifiable, ensuring anterior deposition of the drug.[43] The anterior approach, although it requires CT or ultrasound guidance, is quick and relatively painless. It is an excellent option for patients who cannot assume the prone position.[16] The transcrural approach, with or without CT, is theoretically more desirable than retrocrural techniques, because injectate spreads reliably around the aorta, thus avoiding the somatic nerves.[28] Ultimately, the choice of technique should be individualized to the facility, the patient's physical status, the extent of tumor spread, and the clinician's experience and preparation.

COMPLICATIONS

In the hands of the skilled clinician, serious complications should rarely occur from celiac plexus and splanchnic nerve block. Because of the proximity of other vital structures, however, coupled with the use of large volumes of neurolytic drugs, the following side effects and complications may be seen:

- Hypotension
- Paresthesia of lumbar somatic nerve
- Intravascular injection (venous or arterial)
- Deficit of lumbar somatic nerve
- Subarachnoid or epidural injection
- Diarrhea
- Renal injury
- Paraplegia
- Pneumothorax
- Chylothorax
- Vascular thrombosis or embolism
- Vascular trauma
- Perforation of cysts or tumors
- Injection of the psoas muscle
- Intradiscal injection
- Abscess
- Peritonitis
- Retroperitoneal hematoma
- Urinary tract abnormalities
- Failure of ejaculation
- Pain during and after procedure
- Failure to relieve pain

Hypotension, Altered Gastrointestinal Motility, and Pain

Hypotension[65] and increased gastrointestinal motility occur to some extent in most patients following celiac plexus and splanchnic nerve block. The high frequency of these side effects dictates that they should be anticipated with either prophylactic treatment or a well-conceived management plan. Hypotension occurs as a result of regional vasodilation and pooling of blood within the splanchnic vessels. This side effect is more likely to occur in patients who are elderly, debilitated, and chronically or acutely dehydrated. Without prophylaxis, clinically significant hypotension can be expected in 30% to 60% of patients but may be prevented by administration of 500 to 1000 mL of balanced salt solution intravenously before the procedure.[58] Small increments of intravenous ephedrine are occasionally required, in addition to intravenous fluids, to maintain an adequate blood pressure. Careful monitoring of blood pressure during the procedure and the recovery period is mandatory. A gradual return to a sitting position is indicated to allow early identification and treatment of unrecognized orthostatic hypotension.

Gastrointestinal hypermotility may occur as a result of unopposed parasympathetic activity. It occasionally manifests as diarrhea, except in cancer patients, who tend to be chronically constipated from high doses of opioids. For them, the hypermotility improves bowel habits. Self-limited diarrhea lasting 36 to 48 hours has been reported in as many as 60% of patients after alcohol celiac block.[39] Unrecognized, this side effect can be life-threatening.[66]

Although not a complication per se, pain can occur during and after celiac plexus and splanchnic nerve block. The interval to maximal pain relief after the procedure is variable. In the majority of patients, relief is immediate and complete; in others, it develops over a few days.[59] It is not uncommon for a patient to experience transient self-limited back or pleuritic pain after the procedure.[55]

Neurologic and Vascular Complications

Among 3000 cases of celiac plexus and splanchnic nerve block, Moore[58] reported 18 episodes of dural puncture (0.006%). In all but one case, it was manifested as the appearance of clear fluid in the needle hub.[58] In the majority of these cases, radiographic guidance was not used. The results of a more contemporary series suggest that this complication can be avoided by consistent use of radiographic guidance, as can epidural puncture. One case of unilateral paraplegia was reported in a patient who, because of obesity and ascites, was positioned laterally.[34] No form of radiologic guidance was used in that case. It is probable that paraplegia was the result of unrecognized injection of the psoas muscle that accidentally produced neurolysis of lumbar somatic nerve roots.

With the classic retrocrural technique, the anesthetic may track posteriorly (even when "correct" needle placement has been confirmed) and be deposited near somatic nerve roots. The consequent neurologic injury may manifest as numbness over the anterior thigh and lower abdominal wall and quadriceps weakness.[26] This complication is less likely when transcrural techniques are used.[37, 43]

Another potential mechanism of neurologic injury is disruption of or accidental injection into the small nutrient vessels of the spinal cord (i.e., the artery of Adamkiewicz).[28] This mechanism was postulated to be responsible for the rapid development of persistent paraplegia after celiac plexus block with 6 mL of 6% aqueous phenol in a patient with carcinoma of the pancreas.[67] Neither test doses of local anesthetic nor radiologic guidance was used in this case. To avoid this serious complication, preneurolysis test doses of local anesthetic and either fluoroscopy to detect "vascular run off" or CT guidance should be used to confirm exact needle placement.[68] It is not uncommon for larger vessels to be entered, either by accident or by intention.[43, 64] Intermittent aspiration, an obvious and essential precaution, is not entirely reliable for detecting intravascular placement. Giving test doses of local anesthetics and using radiographic guidance decrease the incidence of this potentially lethal complication. Clinically significant bleeding and hematoma formation have not been reported in the literature, even after transaortic blocks. It is essential that each patient's coagulation status be investigated, and if necessary optimized, before the procedure.

Visceral Injury

The advent of CT guidance for celiac plexus and splanchnic nerve block revealed that perforation of adjacent viscera, including the kidney, occurred more often than we had appreciated. Renal puncture is characteristically a self-limited complication suggested by the appearance of transient hematuria. Accidental injection of an appreciable volume of neurolytic drug into the renal parenchyma, however, may produce serious injury and renal infarction. Moore[58] believes that renal puncture is more likely when (1) needles are inserted farther than 7.5 cm from the midline, (2) the needle tip comes to rest too far lateral to the vertebral body, and (3) a relatively higher vertebral body (T11) is targeted.

Careful attention to technique reduces the incidence of perforation of the viscera. The risk can be further reduced by using CT guidance. An obvious advantage of CT is the ability to visualize the anatomic relationships of visceral structures before and during needle placement.[36] This practice is particularly useful in patients whose normal anatomy is distorted because of a bulky tumor or a previous surgical insult.

Pneumothorax and Pleural Effusion

Pneumothorax may occur as a result of celiac plexus and splanchnic nerve block, even when the operator has radiologic guidance. This complication may or may not require tube thoracostomy. Pleural effusion after celiac plexus neurolysis has also been reported.[69] The proposed mechanism of pleural effusion is diaphragmatic irritation resulting from overflow of alcohol into the subdiaphragmatic space. Other suggested mechanisms include acute pancreatitis and hemorrhage. Chylothorax, an occasional complication of translumbar aortography, has been reported to have occurred on one occasion after phenol celiac plexus block.[70, 71] Ejaculatory failure has also been reported after celiac plexus neurolysis.[72]

Metabolic Complications

Although accidental intravascular injection of alcohol could conceivably produce intoxication, several investigators have measured serum ethanol levels after celiac block and have determined that circulating levels are insufficient to produce systemic effects.[61, 68, 73] After 50 mL of 50% alcohol administered via the classic retrocrural approach, peak serum ethanol levels ranged from 21 to 39 mg/dL. These levels are well below the legally defined levels for intoxication.

Accumulation of high levels of acetaldehyde has been observed in persons with an atypical phenotype for the enzyme aldehyde dehydrogenase. This genetic defect, which is more common in Asians, has been implicated in facial flushing, palpitations, and hypotension in susceptible persons.[60] Such patients report a history of facial flushing after ingesting small amounts of alcoholic beverages, which represents potentially useful data. The use of alcohol as a neurolytic agent should also be avoided in patients undergoing disulfiram therapy for alcoholism.

The finding that amylase levels measured before and after celiac plexus block remained normal in a series of 20 patients suggests that pancreatic injury does not typically occur with this procedure.[73] Alterations in creatine phosphokinase (CPK) levels were minimal in most of the patients studied, suggesting absence of significant skeletal muscle injury. Interestingly, the only two patients with significantly elevated CPK levels (4242 and 1640 IU/L) also experienced side effects consistent with damage to nearby muscle tissue (bilateral L1 neuritis and back pain). A single case of a generalized seizure and transient loss of consciousness has been reported after apparent accidental intravascular injection of phenol.[74]

FUTURE DIRECTIONS

Further technologic advances in radiology should produce continued improvements in the efficacy and safety of celiac plexus and splanchnic nerve blocks. Faster image acquisition and higher resolution will continue to make CT guidance a more attractive option for celiac plexus and splanchnic nerve block. Three-dimensional image reconstruction may also provide the pain specialist a better understanding of the functional clinical anatomy and allow further refinement of these neurolysis techniques. As more experience is gained with ultrasound, it will play a role in the evolution of the anterior approach. The development of safer and longer-acting local anesthetics and neurolytic agents would be a welcome advance for the pain management specialist who performs celiac plexus and splanchnic nerve block.

REFERENCES

1. Kappis M: Erfahrungen mit Lokalansthesie bei Bauchoperationen. Verh Dtsch Ges Circ 43:87, 1914.
2. Kappis M: Die Ansthesierung des Nervus splanchnicus. Zentralbl 45:709, 1918.
3. Wendling H: Ausschaltung der Nervi splanchnici durch Leitungsanesthesie bei Magenoperationen und anderen Eingriffen in der oberen Bauchule. Beitr Klin Chir 110:517, 1918.
4. Braun H: Ein Hilfsinstrument zur Ausfuhrung der Splanchnicusanesthesie. Zentralbl Chir 48:1544, 1921.
5. Labat G: L'anesthésie splanchnique dans les interventions chirurgicales et dans les affections douloureuses de la cavité abdominale. Gaz d'Hôp 93:662, 1920.
6. Roussiel M: Anesthésie des nerfs splanchniques et des plexus mésenteriques supérieur et inferieurs en chirurgie abdominale. Presse Med 31:4, 1923.
7. De Takats G: Splanchnic anesthesia: A critical review of the theory and practice of this method. Surg Gynecol Obstet 44:501, 1927.
8. Pitkin GP: Segmental block for visceral surgery. *In* Southworth JL, Hingson RA (eds): Conduction Anesthesia. Philadelphia, JB Lippincott, 1946, pp 517–518.
9. Gage M, Floyd JB: The treatment of acute pancreatitis: With discussion of mechanism of production, clinical manifestations and diagnosis and report of four cases. Treatment Symp South Aust 59:415, 1947.
10. Esnaurrizar M: The surgical relief of abdominal pain by splanchnic block. Ann R Coll Surg Engl 4:192, 1949.
11. Popper HL: Acute pancreatitis: An evaluation of the classification, symptomatology, diagnosis and therapy. Am J Digest Dis 15:1, 1948.
12. Jones RR: A technique of injection of the splanchnic nerves with alcohol. Anesth Analg 36:75, 1957.
13. Bridenbaugh LD, Moore DC, Campbell DD: Management of upper abdominal cancer pain: Treatment with celiac plexus block with alcohol. JAMA 190:877, 1964.
14. Moore DC: Regional Block, ed 4. Springfield, Ill. Charles C Thomas, 1965, pp 137–143.
15. Matamala AM, Lopez FV, Martinez LI: Percutaneous approach to the celiac plexus using CT guidance. Pain 34:285, 1988.
16. Matamala AM, Sanchez JL, Lopez FV: Percutaneous anterior and posterior approach to the celiac plexus: A comparative study using four different techniques. Pain Clinic 5:21–28, 1992.
17. Portenoy RK, Waldman SD: Managing cancer pain. Contemp Oncol 13:33–41, 1993.
18. Waldman SD: Management of acute pain. Postgrad Med 87:15–17, 1992.
19. Waldman SD: Celiac plexus block. *In* Waldman SD: Atlas of Interventional Pain Management Techniques. Philadelphia, WB Saunders, 1998, pp 269–277.
20. Raj PP: Chronic pain. *In* Raj PP (ed): Handbook of Regional Anesthesia. New York, Churchill Livingstone, 1985, pp 113–115.
21. Kune GA, Cole R, Bell S: Observations on the relief of pancreatic pain. Med J Aust 2:789, 1975.
22. Loper KA, Coldwell DM, Leck J, et al: Celiac plexus block for hepatic arterial embolization: A comparison with intravenous morphine. Anesth Analg 69:398, 1989.
23. Waldman SD: Celiac plexus block. *In* RS Weiner (ed): Innovations in Pain Management. Orlando, Fla., PMD Press, 1990, pp 10–15.
24. Waldman SD, Portenoy RK: Recent advances in the management of cancer pain. Part II. Pain Manage 4:19, 1991.
25. Patt RB: Neurolytic blocks of the sympathetic axis. *In* Patt RB (ed): Cancer Pain. Philadelphia, JB Lippincott, 1993, pp 393–411.
26. Bell SN, Cole R, Roberts-Thomson IC: Coeliac plexus block for control of pain in chronic pancreatitis. Br Med J 281:1604, 1980.
27. Hegedus V: Relief of pancreatic pain by radiography-guided block. AJR 133:1101, 1979.
28. Bonica JJ: Autonomic innervation of the viscera in relation to nerve block. Anesthesiology 29:793, 1968.
29. Lobstrom JB, Cousins MJ: Sympathetic neural blockade. *In* Cousins MJ, Bridenbaugh PO (eds): Neural Blockade, 2nd ed. Philadelphia, JB Lippincott, 1988, pp 479–491.
30. Brown DL: Celiac plexus nerve block. *In* Brown DL (ed): Atlas of Regional Anesthesia. Philadelphia, WB Saunders, 1999, pp 281–292.
31. Ward EM, Rorie DK, Nauss LA, et al: The celiac ganglion in man: Normal and anatomic variations. Anesth Analg 58:461, 1979.
32. Woodburne RT, Burkel WE: Essentials of Human Anatomy. New York, Oxford University Press, 1988, p 552.
33. Moore DC, Bush WH, Burnett LL: Celiac plexus block: A roentgenographic, anatomic study of technique and spread of solution in patients and corpses. Anesth Analg 60:369, 1981.
34. Thomson GE, Moore DC, Bridenbaugh PO, et al: Abdominal pain and celiac plexus nerve block. Anesth Analg 56:1, 1987.
35. Jain S: The role of celiac plexus block in intractable upper abdominal pain. *In* Racz GB (ed): Techniques of Neurolysis. Boston, Kluwer Academic, 1989, p 161.
36. Waldman SD: Acute and postoperative pain management. *In* RS Weiner (ed): Innovations in Pain Management. Orlando, Fla., PMD Press, 1993, pp 28–29.
37. Singler RC: An improved technique for alcohol neurolysis of the celiac plexus. Anesthesiology 56:137, 1982.
38. Brown D, Moore DC: The use of neurolytic celiac plexus block for pancreatic cancer: Anatomy and technique. Pain Sympt Manage 3:206, 1988.
39. Ischia S, Luzzani A, Ischia A, et al: A new approach to the neurolytic block of the celiac plexus: The transaortic technique. Pain 16:333, 1983.
40. Hessel SJ, Adams DF, Abrams HL: Complications of angiography. Radiology 138:273, 1981.
41. Ostheimer GW: Pain and its treatment. *In* Miller RD, Kirby RR, Ostheimer GW, et al (eds): Year Book of Anesthesia. Chicago, Year Book, 1984, p 364.
42. Feldstein GS, Waldman SD: Loss of resistance technique for transaortic celiac plexus block. Anesth Analg 65:1089, 1986.

43. Lieberman RP, Waldman SD: Celiac plexus neurolysis with the modified transaortic approach. Radiology 175:274, 1990.
44. Labat G: Splanchnic analgesia. *In* Labat G (ed): Regional Anesthesia: Its Technique and Clinical Application, ed 2. Philadelphia, WB Saunders, 1928, p 398.
45. Lieberman RP, Nance PN, Cuka DJ: Anterior approach to the celiac plexus during interventional biliary procedures. Radiology 167:562, 1988.
46. Mueller PR, van Sonnenberg E, Casola G: Radiographically guided alcohol block of the celiac ganglion. Semin Intervent Radiol 4:195, 1987.
47. Lieberman RP, Crummy AB, Matallana RH: Invasive procedures in pancreatic disease. Semin Ultrasound CT MR 1:192, 1980.
48. Wajsman Z, Gamarra M, Park JJ, et al: Transabdominal fine needle aspiration of retroperitoneal lymph nodes in staging of genitourinary tract cancer. J Urol 128:1238, 1982.
49. Flanigan DP, Kraft RO: Continuing experience with palliative chemical splanchnicectomy. Arch Surg 113:5089, 1978.
50. Copping J, Willix R, Kraft RO: Palliative chemical splanchnicectomy. Arch Surg 98:418, 1969.
51. Charlton JE: Relief of the pain of unresectable carcinoma of the pancreas by chemical splanchnicectomy during laparotomy. Ann R Coll Surg Engl 67:136, 1985.
52. Corbitz C, Leavens M: Alcohol block of the celiac plexus for control of upper abdominal pain caused by cancer and pancreatitis. J Neurosurg 34:575, 1971.
53. Balamoutsos NG: Infiltration block of the celiac plexus using plastic catheter. Reg Anesth 5:64, 1982.
54. Humbles FH, Mahaffey JE: Teflon epidural catheter placement for intermittent celiac plexus blockade and celiac plexus neurolytic blockade. Reg Anesth 15:103, 1990.
55. Illuminati M, Kizelshteyn G, Ackert M et al: Neurolytic celiac plexus block: Intraoperative catheter technique. Reg Anesth 14(Suppl):90, 1989.
56. Abram SE, Boas RA: Sympathetic and visceral nerve blocks. *In* Benumof JL (ed): Clinical Procedures in Anesthesia and Intensive Care. Philadelphia, JB Lippincott, 1992, p 787.
57. Parkinson SK, Mueller JB, Little WL: A new and simple technique for splanchnic nerve block using a paramedian approach and 3-1/2 inch needles. Reg Anesth 14(Suppl):41, 1989.
58. Moore DC: Celiac (splanchnic) plexus block with alcohol for cancer pain of the upper intra-abdominal viscera. *In* Bonica JJ, Ventafridda V (eds): Advances in Pain Research and Therapy, vol 2. New York, Raven, 1979, p 357.
59. Jones J, Gough D: Coeliac plexus block with alcohol for relief of upper abdominal pain due to cancer. Ann R Coll Surg Engl 59:46, 1977.
60. Noda J, Umeda S, Mori K, et al: Acetaldehyde syndrome after celiac plexus block. Anesth Analg 65:1300, 1986.
61. Jain S, Hirsh R, Shah N, et al: Blood ethanol levels following celiac plexus block with 50% ethanol. Anesth Analg 68(Suppl):S135, 1989.
62. Boas RA, Hatangdi VS, Richards EG: Lumbar sympathectomy: A percutaneous chemical technique. *In* Bonica JJ, Albe-Fessard D (eds): Advances in Pain Research and Therapy, vol 1. New York, Raven, 1976, p 685.
63. Nour-Eldin F: Preliminary report: Uptake of phenol by vascular and brain tissue. Microvasc Res 2:224, 1970.
64. Lieberman RP, Lieberman SL, Cuka DJ, et al: Celiac plexus block and splanchnic nerve block: A review. Semin Intervent Radiol 5:213, 1988.
65. Myhre J, Hilsted J, Tronier B, et al: Monitoring of celiac plexus block in chronic pancreatitis. Pain 38:269, 1989.
66. Matson JA, Ghia JN, Levy JH: A case report of a potentially fatal complication associated with Ischia's transaortic method of celiac plexus block. Reg Anesth 10:193, 1985.
67. Galizia EJ, Lahiri SK: Paraplegia following coeliac plexus block with phenol. Br J Anaesth 46:539, 1974.
68. Waldman SD: Avoiding complications when performing celiac plexus block. Pain Clinic 6:62–63, 1993.
69. Fujita Y, Takori M: Pleural effusion after CT-guided alcohol celiac plexus block. Anesth Analg 66:911, 1987.
70. Cook FE Jr, Flaherty RA, Willmarth CL, et al: Chylothorax: A complication of translumbar aortography. Radiology 75:251–253, 1960.
71. Fine PG, Bubela C: Chylothorax following celiac plexus block. Anesthesiology 63:454, 1985.
72. Black A, Dwyer B: Coeliac plexus block. Anaesth Intensive Care 1:315, 1973.
73. Lebenow TR, Ivankovich AD: Serum alcohol, CPK and amylase levels following celiac plexus block with alcohol. Reg Anesth 13(Suppl):64, 1988.
74. Benzon HT: Convulsions secondary to intravascular phenol: A hazard of celiac plexus block. Anesth Analg 58:150, 1979.

CHAPTER • 45

Ilioinguinal-Iliohypogastric and Genitofemoral Nerve Blocks

Lowell Reynolds, MD • Divakara Kedlaya, MD

HISTORICAL CONSIDERATIONS

Ilioinguinal-iliohypogastric neuropathy was first described in the literature by Magee in 1942 along with genitofemoral neuralgia.[1] Ilioinguinal entrapment neuropathy was distinctly described by Kopell and coworkers[2] in 1962 and Mumenthaler and coworkers[3] in 1966. In 1982, Stulz and Pfeiffer described ilioinguinal-iliohypogastric neuropathy as peripheral nerve injuries resulting from common surgical procedures in the lower portion of the abdomen.[4] They also described the diagnostic triad of ilioinguinal-iliohypogastric neuropathy: (1) typical burning or lancinating pain near the incision that radiates to the area supplied by the nerve, (2) clear evidence of impaired sensory perception of the nerve, and (3) pain relieved by infiltration with local anesthetic at the site where the two nerves leave the internal oblique muscle. The first elaborate description in the literature of ilioinguinal-iliohypogastric-genitofemoral nerve blocks for inguinal hernia repair was published by Braun in 1908.[5]

CLINICALLY RELEVANT ANATOMY

The first lumbar ventral ramus, joined by a branch from the 12th thoracic ramus splits into two divisions (Figs. 45–1, 45–2). The upper larger part divides again into iliohypogastric and ilioinguinal nerves. The lower smaller division unites with a second lumbar branch to form the genitofemoral nerve.[6]

The iliohypogastric nerve emerges from the upper lateral border of the psoas major. It perforates the transversus abdominis muscle and runs obliquely adjacent to the posterior aspect of the internal oblique muscle and supplies both muscles. It also divides into terminal anterior and lateral cutaneous branches. The lateral cutaneous branch pierces the internal and external oblique muscles above the iliac crest and supplies posterolateral gluteal skin. The anterior cutaneous branch pierces the internal oblique about 2 cm medial to the anterior superior iliac spine and the external oblique aponeurosis about 3 cm above the superficial inguinal ring. It supplies skin over the suprapubic region.

The ilioinguinal nerve is smaller than the iliohypogastric nerve, and it emerges from the lateral border of the psoas major, with or just caudal to the iliohypogastric nerve. It perforates the transversus abdominis and internal oblique muscles and traverses the inguinal canal below the spermatic cord. It emerges through the superficial inguinal ring to supply upper medial skin of the thigh and either skin over the penile root and upper part of the scrotum (males) or skin covering the mons pubis and adjoining labium majus (females).

The genitofemoral nerve descends obliquely forward through the psoas major, emerging on the abdominal surface near its medial border opposite L3 or L4. The nerve descends subperitoneally on the psoas major behind the ureter and divides into genital and femoral branches at a variable distance above the inguinal ligament. The genital branch enters the inguinal canal through the deep inguinal ring and supplies the cremaster and the scrotal skin. In females it accompanies the round ligament and supplies the skin of the mons pubis and labium majus. The femoral branch descends lateral to the external iliac artery, passes behind the inguinal ligament, and enters the femoral sheath lateral to the femoral artery. It innervates the skin anterior to the upper part of the femoral triangle.

ETIOLOGY AND PATHOGENESIS

Ilioinguinal-iliohypogastric neuralgias are frequently iatrogenic and appear after lower abdominal surgery, but they sometimes occur spontaneously.[7] Injury to these nerves may be due to suture or staple placement, fibrous adhesions, or neuroma formation. Iliohypogastric-ilioinguinal neuropathy has been reported after various gynecologic procedures, including laparoscopy, needle bladder suspension, open and laparoscopic hernia repairs, cesarean section, ne-

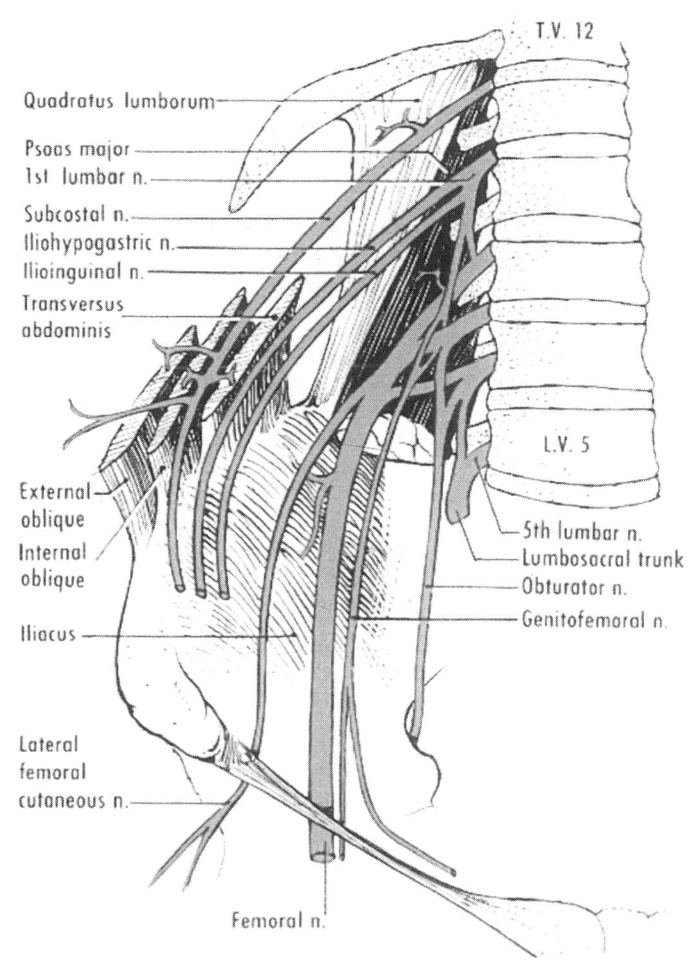

FIGURE 45–1 Schematic drawing shows origin, course, and relations of ilioinguinal–iliohypogastric—genitofemoral nerves. (Gardner E, Gray DJ, O'Rahilly R [eds]: Anatomy: A Regional Study of Human Structure, 5th ed. WB Saunders, 1986.) (Also in color; see Color Plates.)

phrectomy, appendectomy, abdominoplasty, and anterior superior iliac crest bone grafts.[4,8–10] It has also been reported to develop spontaneously during pregnancy or post partum.[11]

The majority of genitofemoral neuralgias occur after inguinal herniorrhaphy, but they can also be associated with appendectomy or cesarean section.[12–14] Rarely psoas abscess, mass, or blunt trauma to the groin is the cause.[15] Sometimes genitofemoral neuralgia occurs along with ilioinguinal-iliohypogastric neuralgia. Comparative features of ilioinguinal, iliohypogastric, and genitofemoral neuralgias are set forth in Table 45–1.

INDICATIONS

Blockade of the ilioinguinal and iliohypogastric nerves has long been used to provide anesthesia and postoperative analgesia in surgical procedures.[16, 17] Some of the procedures are inguinal herniorrhaphy, orchiopexy, and cesarean section. These blocks have also been used to diagnose and treat chronic pain associated with nerve entrapments, neuromas, and neuralgias.[11]

Genitofemoral nerve block is done in conjunction with ilioinguinal and iliohypogastric nerve blocks for inguinal herniorrhaphy, orchiopexy, or hydrocelectomy. It is also done with femoral nerve block for long saphenous vein stripping.[18] It is also used to diagnose and treat genitofemoral neuralgia[12] and to investigate chronic testicular pain.[19]

CONTRAINDICATIONS

Absolute contraindications are sepsis, local infection, and allergic history to the injectate. Relative contraindications include coagulopathy. In affected patients if there is strong clinical indication, the procedure should be done with extreme caution and using a 25-gauge needle.

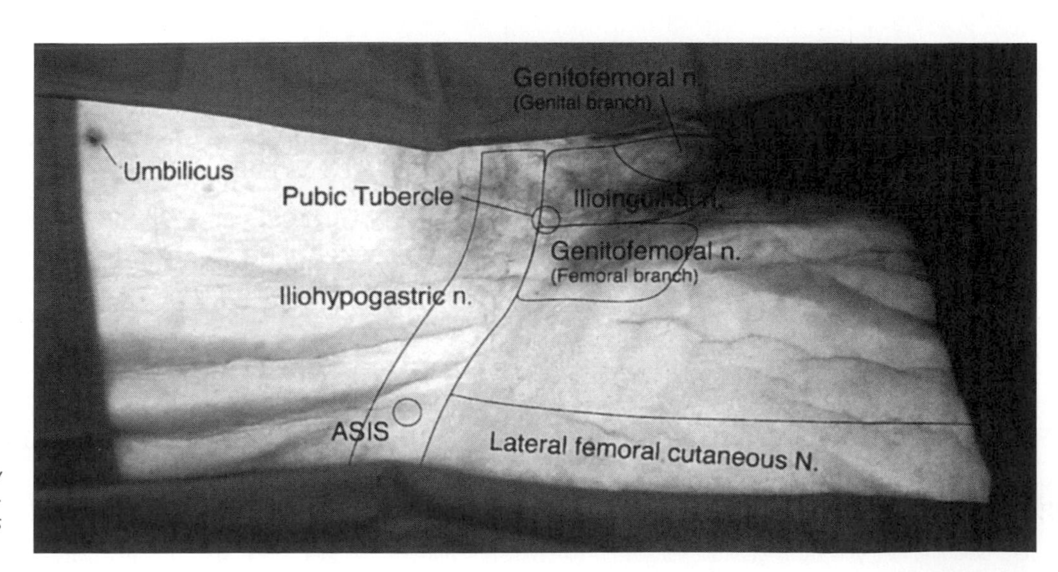

FIGURE 45–2 Anterior view of right lower trunk, groin, perineum, and thigh shows cutaneous nerve distributions.

TABLE 45–1 ***Features of Ilioinguinal, Iliohypogastric, and Genitofemoral Neuralgias***

Variable	Ilioinguinal	Iliohypogastric	Genitofemoral
Pain location	Inguinal region, radiating to upper medial thigh and scrotum or labium majus	Mainly localized to hypogastric region, occasionally in inguinal region	Inguinal region with radiation to the genitalia and upper anteromedial thigh
Altered sensation	Inguinal region	Hypogastric and suprapubic region	Upper anterior thigh and genitalia
Lesion site	Near anterior superior iliac spine	Near anterior superior iliac spine	Posterior abdominal wall or inguinal region
Point tenderness	Medial to anterior superior iliac spine	Medial to anterior superior iliac spine	Internal inguinal ring
Exacerbating positions	Hip extension and internal rotation	Hip extension and internal rotation	Hip extension
Treatment	Nerve block, analgesics, membrane-stabilizing agents, neurectomy	Nerve block, analgesics, membrane-stabilizing agents, neurectomy	Nerve block, analgesics, membrane-stabilizing agents, neurectomy

TECHNIQUE

Ilioinguinal-Iliohypogastric Block

The anterior superior iliac spine is identified when the patient is lying supine. A point is marked on the skin 2 cm medial and 2 cm cephalad to the anterior superior iliac spine, and this should be on the imaginary line drawn from the anterior superior iliac spine to the umbilicus. The skin is prepared with povidone-iodine or alcohol, and a skin wheal is raised at the marked point with lidocaine 1% using a 25- or 27-gauge needle. A 22- to 25-gauge, 3.75-cm needle connected to the syringe containing 5 to 10 mL of 0.25% bupivacaine, with or without 40 to 80 mg methylprednisolone is introduced through the wheal perpendicularly until it reaches the fascia of the external oblique muscle. Half the volume is injected at that site and remaining content is injected around that area using fan-like needle movements.[17, 20] This technique is illustrated in Figures 45–3 and 45–4.

Genitofemoral Nerve Block

With the patient in supine position, the pubic tubercle, anterior superior iliac spine, inguinal ligament, inguinal crease, and femoral artery are identified. The skin is prepared in usual aseptic fashion. The femoral branch of the genitofemoral nerve is blocked by inserting a 22- to 25-gauge, 3.75-cm needle at the lateral border of the femoral artery at the inguinal crease and "fanlike" infiltration is done with 5 to 10 mL of 0.25% bupivacaine. Caution should be exercised to avoid injecting into the blood vessel by repeatedly aspirating. The genital branch of the genitofemoral nerve is blocked by infiltrating 5 to 10 mL of 0.25% bupivacaine just lateral to the pubic tubercle below the inguinal ligament.[18, 21] This technique is illustrated in Figure 45–5.

Transpsoas technique of genitofemoral nerve block was described by Hartrick.[22] With the patient in the prone position, a 15-cm, 21-gauge needle is introduced paravertebrally, approximately 5 cm from the midline at the level of the L3–L4 interspace. The needle is advanced toward the transverse process of either L3 or L4. After the depth

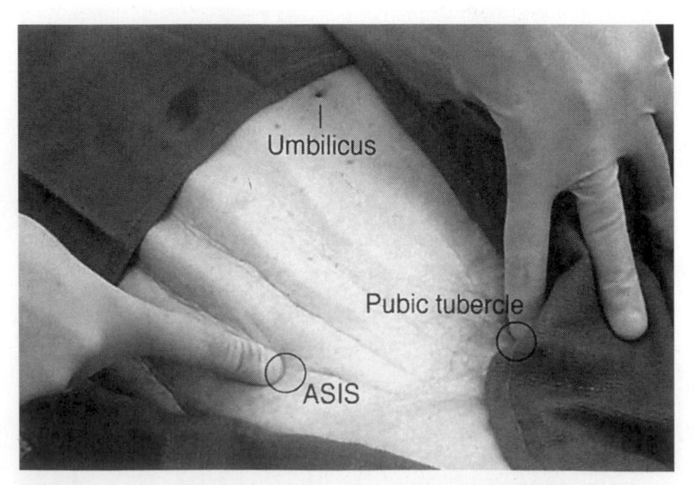

FIGURE 45–3 Anterior view shows important anatomic landmarks for ilioinguinal-iliohypogastric-genitofemoral nerve blocks. ASIS = anterior superior iliac spine.

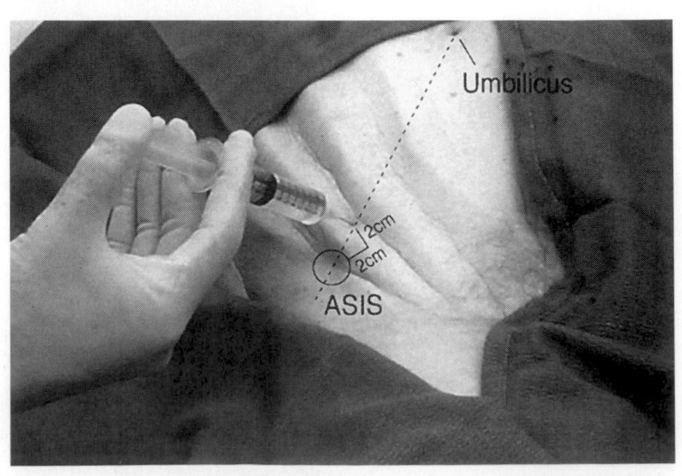

FIGURE 45–4 Technique of ilioinguinal-iliohypogastric nerve block. ASIS = anterior superior iliac spine.

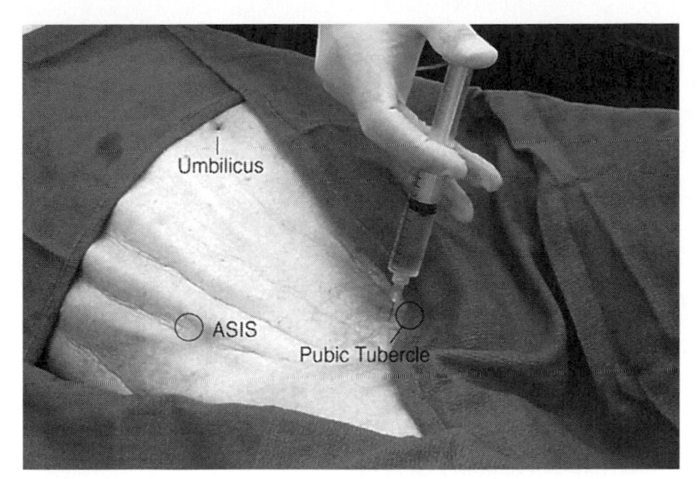

FIGURE 45–5 Technique of genitofemoral nerve block (genital branch). ASIS = anterior superior iliac spine.

of the processes is noted, the needle is redirected to pass between the transverse processes in perpendicular fashion. The loss of resistance is used to identify the psoas muscle compartment first, and further advancement locates the space anterior to the psoas major muscle. At this point, 2 to 3 mL of 0.25% bupivacaine is injected to block the genitofemoral nerve.

Cryoneurolysis

Cryoneurolysis of ilioinguinal nerve for herniorrhaphy pain was first described by Wood and coworkers, in 1979.[23] Although initial studies suggested benefit from cryoanalgesia of the iliohypogastric-ilioinguinal nerves after hernia repair,[24] two recent prospective, randomized, controlled trials did not show any significant pain relief.[25, 26] No study has been done, however, to evaluate the effect of cryoneurolysis in the treatment of ilioinguinal-iliohypogastric and genitofemoral neuralgias. When treating these neuralgias it is very important to localize the nerve precisely using a sensory nerve stimulator.

Complications

Complications from these procedures are extremely rare. Hemorrhage, peritoneal puncture, local hematoma formation, and unwanted motor blockade of the femoral nerve are possible.[27, 28] Performing these procedures without proper attention to technique and local anatomy would increase the risk of complications. There is a report of colonic puncture during ilioinguinal nerve block in a child.[29]

SUMMARY

While diagnosing and treating atypical lower abdomen, groin, and genital region pain, the possibility of ilioinguinal-iliohypogastric-genitofemoral neuropathy should be kept in mind, although other common causes should be excluded before making one of these diagnoses. Ilioinguinal-iliohypogastric-genitofemoral nerve blocks help to diagnose and treat these uncommon but painful and functionally incapacitating conditions.

REFERENCES

1. Magee RK: Genitofemoral causalgia (a new syndrome). Can Med Assoc J 46:326–329, 1942.
2. Kopell HP, Thompson WAL: Peripheral entrapment neuropathy of ilioinguinal nerve. N Engl J Med 266:16–19, 1962.
3. Mumenthaler A, Mumenthaler M, Luciani G, Kramer J: The ilioinguinal syndrome. German Med Monthly 11:91–95, 1966.
4. Stulz P, Pfeiffer KM: Peripheral nerve injuries resulting from common surgical procedures in the lower portion of the abdomen. Arch Surg 117(3):324–327, 1982.
5. Hirschel G: Textbook of Local Anesthesia for Students and Practitioners. English, New York, William Wood & Company, 1914, pp 106–107.
6. William PL (ed): Gray's Anatomy, The Anatomical Basis of Medicine and Surgery, ed 38. New York, Churchill Livingstone, 1995, pp 1277–1279.
7. Knockaert DC, D'Heygere FG, Bobbaers HJ: Ilioinguinal nerve entrapment: A little known cause of iliac fossa pain. Postgrad Med J 65:632–635, 1989.
8. Melville K, Schultz EA, Dougherty JM: Ilioinguinal-iliohypogastric nerve entrapment. Ann Emerg Med 19:925–929, 1990.
9. Smith SC, DeLee JC, Ramamurthy S: Ilioinguinal neuralgia following iliac bone grafting. J Bone Joint Surg 66A:1306–1308, 1984.
10. Liszka TG, Dellon AL, Manson PN: Iliohypogastric nerve entrapment following abdominoplasty. Plast Reconstr Surg 93(1):181–184, 1994.
11. Racz GB, Hagstrom D: Iliohypogastric and ilioinguinal nerve entrapment: Diagnosis and treatment. Pain Digest 2:43–48, 1992.
12. Harms BA, DeHass DR, Starling JR: Diagnosis and management of genitofemoral neuralgia. Arch Surg 119:339–341, 1984.
13. Starling JR, Harms BA: Diagnosis and treatment of genitofemoral and ilioinguinal neuralgia. World J Surg 13:586–591, 1989.
14. Lyon EK: Genitofemoral causalgia. Can Med Assoc J 53:213–216, 1945.
15. O'Brien MD: Genitofemoral neuropathy. Br Med J 1:1052, 1979.
16. Bunting P, McConachie I: Ilioinguinal nerve blockade for analgesia after cesarean section. Br J Anaesth 61(6):773–775, 1988.
17. Amid PK, Shulman AG, Lichtenstein IL: Local anesthesia for inguinal hernia repair: Step-by-step procedure. Ann Surg 220(6):735–737, 1994.
18. Vloka JD, Hadzíc A, Mulcare R, et al: Femoral and genitofemoral nerve blocks versus spinal anesthesia for outpatients undergoing long saphenous vein stripping surgery. Anesth Analg 84(4):749–752, 1997.
19. Reynolds LW, Schultz DE, Waldman SD: Testicular pain (orchialgia). Pain Digest 8:177–185, 1998.
20. Mutroy MF: Peripheral nerve block. *In* Barash PG, Cullen BF, Stoelting RK (eds): Clinical Anesthesia, ed 2. Philadelphia, JB Lippincott, 1992, p 864.
21. Carron H, Korbon GA, Rowlingson JC: Abdominal blocks. *In* Korbon GA, Rowlingson JC (eds): Regional Anesthesia. Techniques and Clinical Applications. Orlando, Fla., Grune & Stratton, 1984, pp 82–95.
22. Hartrick CT: Genitofemoral nerve block: A transpsoas technique. Reg Anesth 19(6):432–433, 1994.
23. Wood GJ, Lloyd JW, Evans PJ, et al: Cryoanalgesia and day-case herniorrhaphy. Lancet 2:479, 1979.
24. Wood GJ, Lloyd JW, Bullingham RE, et al: Postoperative analgesia for day case herniorrhaphy patients: A comparison of cryoanalgesia, paraveretebral blockade and oral analgesia. Anaesthesia 36:603–610, 1981.
25. Callesen T, Bech K, Thorup J, et al: Cryoanalgesia: Effect on postherniorrhaphy pain. Anesth Analg 87(4):896–899, 1998.
26. Khiroya RC, Davenport HT, Jones JG: Cryoanalgesia for pain after herniorrhaphy. Anaesthesia 41(1):73–76, 1986.
27. Ang BL: Transient quadriceps paresis after ilioinguinal nerve block. Singapore Med J 38(2):83–84, 1997.
28. Leng SA: Transient femoral nerve palsy after ilioinguinal nerve block. Anesth Intensive Care 25(1):92, 1997.
29. Johr M, Sossai R: Colonic puncture during ilioinguinal nerve block in a child. Anesth Analg 88(5):1051–1052, 1999.

CHAPTER • 46

Lateral Femoral Cutaneous Nerve Block

Lowell Reynolds MD • Divakara Kedlaya MD

HISTORICAL ASPECTS

Lateral femoral cutaneous neuralgia was first described in 1878 by Bernhardt[1] and again in 1885 by Hegar.[2] In 1895, a Russian physician, Roth, described five patients with lateral femoral cutaneous neuralgia.[3] Thus, this condition is also called *Bernhardt-Roth syndrome*. Roth used a Greek term to name the condition *meralgia paresthetica* (*meros*, thigh; *algos*, pain). In 1895, Sigmund Freud published his own personal impression of the symptoms of meralgia paresthetica.[4] The first reported publication on lateral femoral cutaneous nerve block was by Nystrom in 1909.[5] The classic fan-wise technique of lateral cutaneous nerve block was first described by Labat in 1922 as *external cutaneous nerve block*.[6]

CLINICALLY RELEVANT ANATOMY

The lateral femoral cutaneous nerve is a pure sensory nerve that originates from the dorsal branches of the second and third lumbar ventral rami. It emerges from the lateral border of the psoas major muscle, crossing the iliacus muscle obliquely toward the anterior superior iliac spine.[7] (According to one recent anatomic study, the average medial distance from anterior superior iliac spine to lateral femoral cutaneous nerve was 20.4 mm.[8]) Then it passes through or behind the inguinal ligament, in five different variable relations to the anterior superior iliac spine[9]:

1. Posterior to the anterior superior iliac spine, across the iliac crest (prevalence 4%).
2. Anterior to the anterior superior iliac spine and superficial to the origin of the sartorius muscle but within the substance of the inguinal ligament (27%).
3. Medial to the anterior superior iliac spine, ensheathed in the tendinous origin of the sartorius muscle (23%).
4. Medial to the origin of the sartorius muscle, in an interval between the tendon of the sartorius muscle and thick fascia of the iliopsoas muscle, deep to the inguinal ligament (26%).
5. Farthest (of the five) medial and embedded in loose connective tissue, deep to the inguinal ligament (20%).

The first three courses of the nerve are considered most susceptible to mechanical trauma and compression. Distal to the inguinal ligament, the nerve divides into anterior and posterior branches in the thigh. The anterior branch becomes superficial about 10 cm distal to the anterior superior iliac spine, supplying the skin of the anterior and lateral thigh as far as the knee. The posterior branch pierces the fascia lata higher than the anterior branch, dividing to supply the skin on the lateral surface from the greater trochanter to about mid-thigh (Figs. 46–1, 46–2).

ETIOLOGY AND PATHOGENESIS OF MERALGIA PARESTHETICA

Different causes have been described in the literature, although in some cases the cause cannot be identified conclusively (Table 46–1).

Meralgia paresthetica is considered to be due to either compression or injury to the lateral femoral cutaneous nerve near the anterior superior iliac spine as it passes through or under the inguinal ligament. It has been proposed that erect human posture, combined with the particular course of the lateral femoral cutaneous nerve, cause tension, mechanical friction, and irritation of the nerve. All of these contribute to the development of pseudoganglion and play a role in the pathogenesis of meralgia paresthetica.[28]

INDICATIONS AND CONTRAINDICATIONS

Lateral femoral cutaneous nerve block is commonly used for diagnosing and treating lateral thigh pain and paresthesia of meralgia paresthetica.[29, 30] It is important to keep in mind, however, that it can have several causes, especially occult tumors, and that each patient should be properly investigated. A combination of local anesthetic with depot

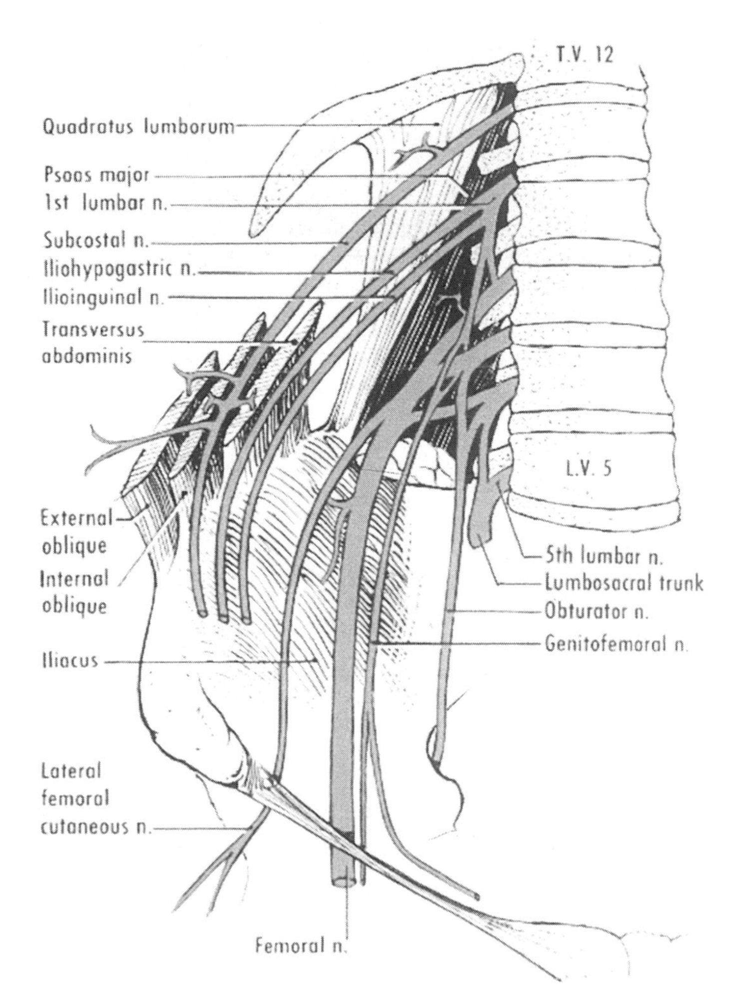

FIGURE 46-1 *Schematic drawing shows origin, course, and relations of lateral femoral cutaneous nerve. (Gardner E, Gray DJ, O'Rahilly R (eds): Anatomy: A Regional Study of Human Structure, 5th ed. Philadelphia, WB Saunders, 1986.) (Also in color; see Color Plates.)*

TABLE 46-1 ***Causative Factors in Meralgia Paresthetica***[10-27]

Causative Factors
Orthopedic
Fracture of anterior superior iliac spine
Iliac crest bone graft
Pelvic osteotomy
Shelf operation
Total hip arthroplasty
Leg length discrepancy
Spinal stenosis
General Surgery
Laparoscopic herniorrhaphy
Laparoscopic myomectomy
Laparoscopic cholecystectomy
Appendectomy
Coronary artery bypass graft
Transfemoral angiography
Abdominal aortic aneurysm
Metabolic and Endocrine
Diabetes mellitus
Hypothyroidism
Tumors
Pelvic
Psoas
Lumbar metastasis
Iliac metastasis
External causes
Tight trousers
Seat belt
Heavy wallet
Waist belts and girdles
Sports trauma
Obesity or recent weight gain
Ascites
Chronic urinary retention
Other
Pelvic inflammatory disease
Leprosy
Systemic lupus erythematosus, scleroderma
Hemophilia

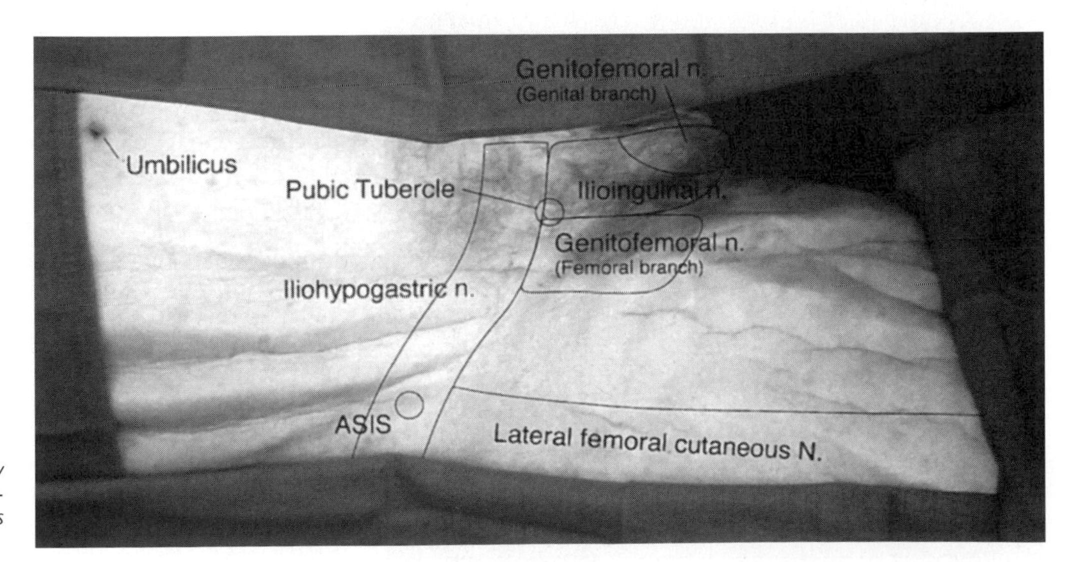

FIGURE 46-2 *Anterior view of right lower trunk, groin, perineum, and thigh shows cutaneous nerve distributions.*

steroid is usually used to prolong the therapeutic efficacy.[31, 32] It is also used for postoperative analgesia after hip surgery,[33] regional anesthesia for skin graft harvesting from the upper lateral thigh,[34] and muscle biopsy of vastus lateralis along with three-in-one block (lateral femoral cutaneous nerve, femoral, obturator nerves).[35, 36] Absolute contraindications to lateral femoral cutaneous nerve block are sepsis, local infection, and history of allergy to the injectate. One relative contraindication may be coagulopathy. In affected patients, and when there is a compelling clinical indication, the procedure should be done with extreme caution and with a 25-gauge needle.

TECHNIQUES

Classic Fan-wise Technique

The fan-wise technique was originally described by Labat,[6] and is described in Eriksson's and Bridenbaugh's books (Figs. 46–3, 46–4).[37, 38] The anterior superior iliac spine is identified with the patient lying in supine position. A point is marked on the skin 2 cm medial to and 2 cm caudad from the anterior superior iliac spine. The skin is prepared with povidone-iodine or alcohol, and a skin wheal is raised at the marked point with 1% lidocaine using a 25- or 27-gauge needle. A 22-gauge, 3.5-cm needle connected to the syringe containing 5 to 10 mL of 0.25% bupivacaine with 40 mg methylprednisolone is introduced through the wheal and advanced perpendicularly to until a sudden giving way, or pop, is felt. This indicates passage through the fascia lata. After that, the contents of the syringe are deposited with fan-wise needle movements above and below the fascia lata. A successful lateral femoral cutaneous nerve block may be confirmed by cutaneous analgesia to pinprick over the distribution of the nerve. Because of the significant individual variability in the course of the lateral femoral cutaneous nerve, the success rate with this technique is also quite variable. Different studies report success rates of 38% to 97%.[39, 40] In our experience, fan-wise technique has given consistently good results.

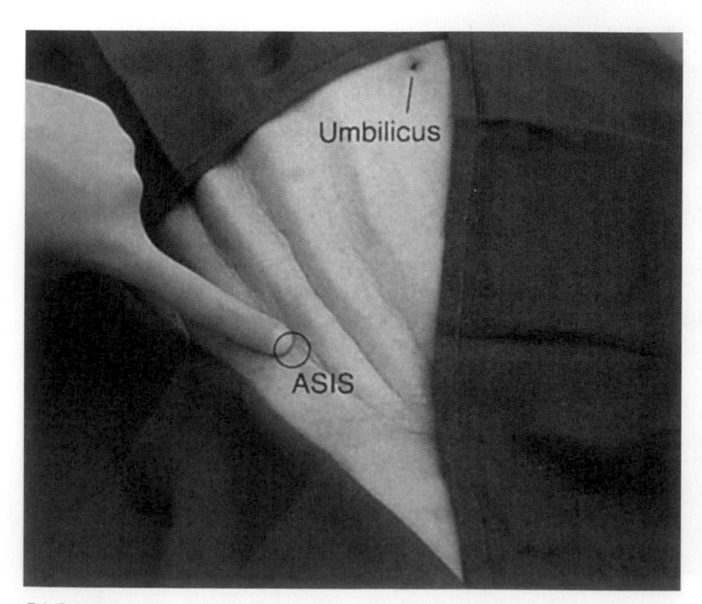

FIGURE 46–3 Palpating the important anatomic landmark, the anterior superior iliac spine (ASIS), before doing lateral femoral cutaneous nerve block.

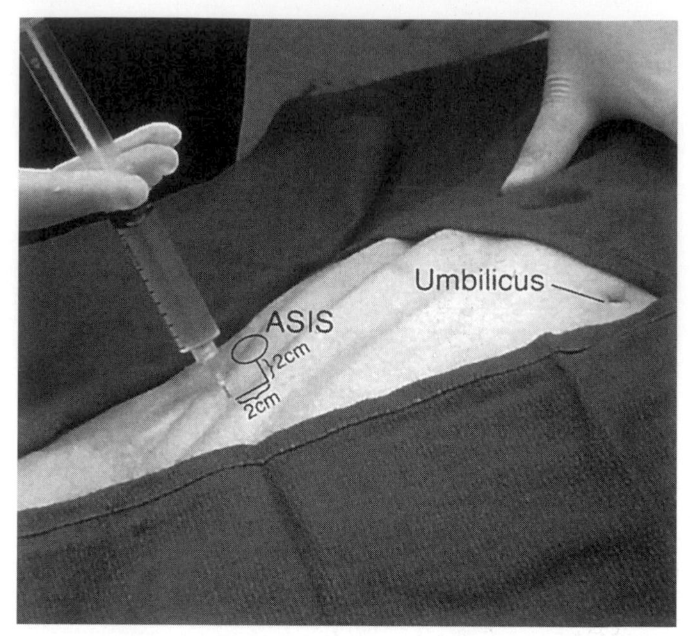

FIGURE 46–4 Technique of lateral femoral cutaneous nerve block. ASIS = anterior superior iliac spine.

Transinguinal Technique

In the transinguinal technique the needle is inserted above the inguinal ligament. This technique has no definite advantage over the classic fan-wise technique.[41]

Nerve Stimulator Technique

Shannon and coworkers reported improved success rates with the nerve stimulator technique for lateral femoral cutaneous nerve block.[42] In this technique, a hand-held, transdermal nerve stimulator is placed just below the inguinal ligament to elicit paresthesia referred to the lateral thigh. The point where the greatest paresthesia is elicited is marked, and this is assumed to be the approximate location of the nerve. A 26-gauge uninsulated needle attached to a nerve stimulator (Neurotechnology, Houston, Tex.; pulse width 100–200 μs: 1 Hz) is inserted at this point and used to localize the nerve more precisely. A paresthesia referred to the lateral aspect of the knee at 0.6 mA is used as an end point and, at that point, the injection is performed. A success rate of 100% was reported with this technique.[42] It has not been studied and is difficult to use in patients with meralgia paresthetica.

COMPLICATIONS

Complications are quite rare with lateral femoral cutaneous nerve block. Neuritis of the nerve secondary to needle trauma or drug toxicity is a potential, but unlikely, complication. There are no large blood vessels in the vicinity of this nerve; therefore, rapid systemic uptake or intravascular injection is rare. Local hematoma and infection may occur. Inadvertent femoral nerve block can occur in the course of lateral femoral cutaneous nerve block if the local anesthetic is injected farther medial and deeper.[43] Patients will have temporary quadriceps weakness until the effect of local anesthetic wears off.

SUMMARY AND CONCLUSION

Medical practitioners commonly encounter the diagnosis of meralgia paresthetica, which is a significant cause of pain and discomfort. Lateral femoral cutaneous nerve block is helpful in confirming the diagnosis. It is also a simple but effective method of management for this condition. The majority of patients can be managed by this conservative approach, with repeated lateral femoral cutaneous nerve blocks, which are done sparingly. Refractory cases may require surgery to decompress the nerve.

REFERENCES

1. Bernhardt M: Neuropathologische Beobachtungen. I. Periphere Laglungen. D Arch Klin Med 22:362, 1878.
2. Hegar W: Neuralgia femoris. Resection des Nerv. cutan. femoris anterior externus. Heilung Dtsch Med Wochenschr 11:218, 1885.
3. Roth VK: Meralgia paresthetica. Meditsinskoye Obozrainie Moskova 42:678, 1895.
4. Schiller F: Sigmund Freud's meralgia paresthetica. Neurology 35(4):557–558, 1985.
5. Hirschel G: Textbook of Local Anesthesia: For Students and Practitioners. New York, William Wood & Company, 1914, p 160.
6. Labat G: Regional Anesthesia: Its Technic and Clinical Application. Philadelphia, WB Saunders Company, 1922, pp 246–247.
7. Gray's Anatomy, The Anatomical Basis of Medicine and Surgery; Editor: William PL, Churchill Livingstone, ed 38. 1995, pp 1278–1280.
8. Hospodar PP, Ashman ES, Traub JA: Anatomic study of the lateral femoral cutaneous nerve with respect to the ilioinguinal surgical dissection. J Orthop Trauma 13(1):17–19, 1999.
9. Aszmann OC, Dellon ES, Dellon AL: Anatomical course of the lateral femoral cutaneous nerve and its susceptibility to compression and injury. Plast Reconstr Surg 100(3):600–604, 1997.
10. van-den-Broecke DG, Schuurman AH, Borg ED, Kon M: Neurotmesis of the lateral femoral cutaneous nerve when coring for iliac crest bone grafts. Plast Reconstr Surg 102(4):1163–1166, 1998.
11. Hogh J, Macnicol MF: Long term results following the Chiari osteotomy. J Bone Joint Surg 69B:365, 1987.
12. Thanikachalam M, Petros JG, O'Donnell S: Avulsion fracture of the anterior superior iliac spine presenting as acute-onset meralgia paresthetica. Ann Emerg Med 26(4):515–517, 1995.
13. Ferzli GS, Massaad A, Dysarz FA, Kopatsis A: A study of 101 patients treated with extraperitoneal endoscopic laparoscopic herniorrhaphy. Am Surg 59(11):707–708, 1993.
14. Parsonnet V, Karasakalides A, Gielchinsky I, et al: Meralgia paresthetica after coronary bypass surgery. J Thorac Cardiovasc Surg 101(2):219–221, 1991.
15. Kent KC, Moscucci M, Gallagher SG, et al: Neuropathy after cardiac catheterization: Incidence, clinical patterns, and long-term outcome. J Vasc Surg 19(6):1008–1013, 1994.
16. Suber DA, Massey EW: Pelvic mass presenting as meralgia paresthetica. Obstet Gynecol 53(2):257–258, 1979.
17. Rinkel GJ, Wokke JH: Meralgia paraesthetica as the first symptom of a metastatic tumor in the lumbar spine. Clin Neurol Neurosurg 92(4):365–367, 1990.
18. Nahabedian MY, Dellon AL: Meralgia paresthetica: Etiology, diagnosis, and outcome of surgical decompression. Ann Plast Surg 35(6):590–594, 1995.
19. Hutchins FL Jr, Huggins J, Delaney ML: Laparoscopic myomectomy: An unusual cause of meralgia paresthetica. J Am Assoc Gynecol Laparosc 5(3):309–311, 1998.
20. Brett A, Hodgetts T: Abdominal aortic aneurysm presenting as meralgia paresthetica. J Accid Emerg Med 14(1):49–51, 1997.
21. Yamout B, Tayyim A, Farhat W: Meralgia paresthetica as a complication of laparoscopic cholecystectomy. Clin Neurol Neurosurg 96(2):143–144, 1994.
22. Amoiridis G, Wohrle J, Grunwald I, Przuntek H: Malignant tumour of the psoas: Another cause of meralgia paresthetica. Electromyogr Clin Neurophysiol 33(2):109–112, 1993.
23. Pollen JJ: Chronic urinary retention masquerading as meralgia paresthetica. Br J Urol 68(5):554–555, 1991.
24. Suarez G, Sabin TD: Meralgia paresthetica and hypothyroidism. Ann Intern Med 112(2):149, 1990.
25. Rotenberg AS: Bilateral meralgia paresthetica associated with pelvic inflammatory disease. Can Med Assoc J 142(1):42–43, 1990.
26. Grace DM: Meralgia paresthetica after gastroplasty for morbid obesity. Can J Surg 30(1):64–65, 1987.
27. Kaufmann J, Canoso JJ: Progressive systemic sclerosis and meralgia paresthetica. Ann Intern Med 106(6):973, 1986.
28. Edelson JG, Nathan H: Meralgia paresthetica. An anatomical interpretation. Clin Orthop 122:255–262, 1977.
29. Williams PH, Trzil KP: Management of meralgia paresthetica. J Neurosurg 74(1):76–80, 1991.
30. Dureja GP, Gulaya V, Jayalakshmi TS, Mandal P: Management of meralgia paresthetica: A multimodality regimen. Anesth Analg 80:1060–1061, 1995.
31. Johnson A, Hao J, Sjolund B: Local corticosteroid application blocks transmission in normal nociceptive C fibers. Acta Anaesthesiol Scand 34:355–358, 1990.
32. Castillo B, Curley J, Holtz J, et al: Glucocorticoids prolong rat sciatic nerve blockade in vivo from bupivacaine microspheres. Anesthesiology 85(5):1157–1166, 1996.
33. Jones SF, White A: Analgesia following femoral neck surgery. Lateral cutaneous nerve block as an alternative to narcotics in elderly. Anaesthesia 40:682–685, 1985.
34. Karacalar A, Karacalar S, Uckunkaya N, et al: Combined use of axillary block and lateral femoral cutaneous nerve block in upper extremity injuries requiring large skin grafts. J Hand Surg Am 23(6):1100–1105, 1998.
35. Madej TH, Ellis FR, Halsall PJ: Evaluation of "3-in-1" lumbar plexus block in patients having muscle biopsy. Br J Anaesth 62:515–517, 1989.
36. Maccani RM, Wedel DJ, Melton A, Gronert GA: Femoral and lateral femoral nerve block for muscle biopsies in children. Paediatr Anaesth 5(4):223–227, 1995.
37. Eriksson E; Editor; Illustrated handbook in local anesthesia; Year Book Medical Publishers, Chicago; 1969, pp 103–104.
38. Bridenbaugh PO: The lower extremity: Somatic blockade. *In* Cousins MJ, Bridenbaugh PO (eds): Neural Blockade in Clinical Anesthesia and Management of Pain. Philadelphia, JB Lippincott, 1988, pp 429–439.
39. Hopkins PM, Ellis FR, Halsall PJ: Evaluation of local anesthetic blockade of the lateral femoral cutaneous nerve. Anesthesia 46:95–96, 1991.
40. Reyford H, Krivosic-Horber R, Adnet P, et al: Lateral cutaneous nerve of the thigh block—155 cases. Reg Anesth 17:S47, 1992.
41. Lang SA, Yip RW, Gerald M: The transinguinal approach to the lateral femoral cutaneous block. Anesth Analg 76:S208, 1993.
42. Shannon J, Lang SA, Yip RW, Gerald M: Lateral femoral cutaneous nerve block revisited. A nerve stimulator technique. Reg Anesth 20:100–104, 1995.
43. Konder H, Moysich F, Mattusch W: An accidental motor blockade of the femoral nerve following a blockade of the lateral femoral cutaneous nerve. Reg Anaesth 13(5):122–123, 1990.

CHAPTER • 47

Obturator Nerve Block

Somayaji Ramamurthy, MD

The obturator nerve originates from anterior primary rami of L2–L3 and L4 lumbar nerve roots. The contribution of L3 is the most predominant; contributions from L2 and L4 are small. The nerve passes through the psoas major muscle, emerging at its lateral border. It travels posterior to the iliac vessels and reaches the undersurface of the superior ramus of the pubis.[1] It passes through the obturator internus and externus muscles to emerge from the obturator foramen. Shortly thereafter, it divides into anterior and posterior branches. The anterior branch innervates the anterior adductor muscles and gives a branch to innervate the hip joint. The posterior branch innervates mainly the adductor magnus muscle. It travels down and communicates with the saphenous branch of the femoral nerve. It travels along the femoral vessels to the popliteal fossa and gives a branch to innervate the knee joint. The innervation of both the hip joint and the knee joint by obturator nerve can explain why a patient with a lesion in the hip joint sometimes complains of pain in the knee and *vice versa.* The obturator nerve is almost entirely a motor nerve. Sensory contribution to dermatomal distribution to the lower medial aspect of the thigh is variable and could be nonexistent.

INDICATIONS

The use of nerve stimulation has significantly improved the success of the obturator nerve block and has made it less uncomfortable for the patient.[2] Results of paresthesia techniques used before the days of the nerve stimulator or the multiple reinsertion and the infiltration technique were extremely unpredictable and very painful. This is because the obturator is predominantly a motor nerve and has little or no cutaneous innervation.

Surgical Anesthesia

The obturator nerve has to be blocked for any procedure above the knee or when a pneumatic tourniquet is placed over the thigh. It is blocked along with the femoral, lateral femoral cutaneous, and sciatic nerves for this purpose.[3] One of the most important surgical indications is due to the anatomic relationship of the obturator nerve as it runs close to the neck of the bladder and the prostate.[4–7] Because of the proximity of the nerve to the prostate, this nerve can be electrically stimulated during the transurethral resection. This stimulation can produce very significant contraction of the adductors, which can interfere with the surgical procedure, and on occasion can even result in the perforation of the bladder. This can occur even with adequate spinal analgesia that blocks the nerve roots proximal to the site of stimulation. Local anesthetic block of the obturator nerve has been well documented to abolish the spasms and facilitate the prostatic surgery.

Chronic Pain

Since the hip joint derives significant innervation from the obturator nerve, blockade of this nerve was one of the main indications in patients who had degenerative hip disease.[8] Since the advent of total joint replacement, however, the number of patients who require this type of block has significantly decreased. It still can be of use as a diagnostic block for a complex pain problem.[9, 10] Even under these circumstances, a direct hip joint injection provides more valuable diagnostic information than blockade of the obturator nerve.[11]

Obturator nerve entrapment has been described in athletes[12] and after pelvic surgery.[13, 14] The obturator nerve has been surgically released with good success. A diagnostic nerve block may help to make the diagnosis.

Spasticity

One of the most important nonsurgical indications was for adductor muscle spasticity. Obturator nerve block was used extensively to relieve adductor spasm to improve the personal hygiene of the patients with spasticity. Oral and intrathecal dosing with baclofen has very significantly reduced the use of neurolytic obturator nerve block for this purpose.

TECHNIQUE

Direct Approach

The direct approach (Fig. 47–1) blocks the nerve as it exits the obturator foramen underneath the superior ramus of the pubis. The patient is placed in the supine position. The thigh is slightly abducted. The pubic area is sterilized with a nonirritating antiseptic such as Betadine. The pubic tubercle, the most important landmark, is identified. The entry point is 1.5 cm lateral and inferior to the pubic tubercle. The skin is anesthetized with a 25- or 27-gauge short needle and a fast-acting local anesthetic such as 1% lidocaine. A 22-gauge (8-cm) spinal needle is advanced vertically downward. The needle usually contacts the bone of the upper third of the pubis. The negative electrode from a stimulator is attached to the needle, and the positive electrode is placed on the patient in an area where no paresthesia from the obturator nerve is expected. Over the bone 0.5 mL of 1% lidocaine is infiltrated to reduce the pain of walking the needle on the bone. The needle is redirected laterally and superiorly to induce contraction of the adductor muscles. When strong contractions are elicited the nerve stimulator is adjusted until good contractions are produced with current less than 1 mA with an uninsulated needle or less than 0.5 mA with an insulated needle. A 2-mL test dose of local anesthetic should abolish the contraction, confirming proximity of the needle tip to the obturator nerve. At this point, 7 to 12 mL of local anesthetic is injected. During the lateral and superior redirection, if the pubic ramus is encountered, the needle must be walked slightly inferiorly to enter the obturator foramen. The needle should not be advanced more than 2 to 3 cm into the obturator foramen lest it enter the pelvis and damage the bladder.

An alternative approach consists of identifying the adductor longus muscle and advancing the needle underneath the proximal end of the adductor longus muscle in a medial to lateral direction and looking for contraction of the other adductor muscles with nerve stimulation.[15] A successful block can be identified when the patient is asked to adduct the thigh against resistance. The accompanying dermatomal analgesia is very variable and could be nonexistent.

Neurolytic Block

The direct approach is the most suitable for neurolytic block of the obturator nerve. I use an insulated needle with a stimulator to ensure proximity of the needle tip to the nerve. Most clinicians use a 6% or higher concentration of phenol to block the nerve. Radiofrequency coagulation can also be utilized.

INDIRECT TECHNIQUE

Winnie and coworkers described a three-in-one block. During this technique the femoral nerve is identified and a volume of local anesthetic greater than 20 mL is injected, which is expected to spread to the lumbar plexus and block the obturator and the lateral femoral cutaneous nerves, in addition to the femoral nerve. This could be a significant advantage because the obturator nerve can be blocked easily without the pain of multiple injections. Whether the obturator nerve is consistently blocked is a matter of debate. The results of the three-in-one block were originally assessed by checking for cutaneous analgesia over the thigh. It was believed that analgesia over the anterior and lateral aspect of the thigh in the distribution of all three nerves indicated that the obturator nerve was also blocked. This may not be so when the obturator innervation of the skin is minimal or nonexistent. There have been cadaver studies[16] in which injection of methylene blue indicated that the dye does not spread to the lumbar plexus or to the obturator nerve. Studies compared three-in-one block with direct block of the obturator nerve with a nerve stimulator and assessed the results with motor evoked potentials.[17–21] It was clear that the three-in-one block did not produce consistent block of the obturator nerve.[17–20] Thus, if an obturator nerve block is needed to prevent abductor spasm during transurethral surgery or for neurolysis, the direct approach is preferred.

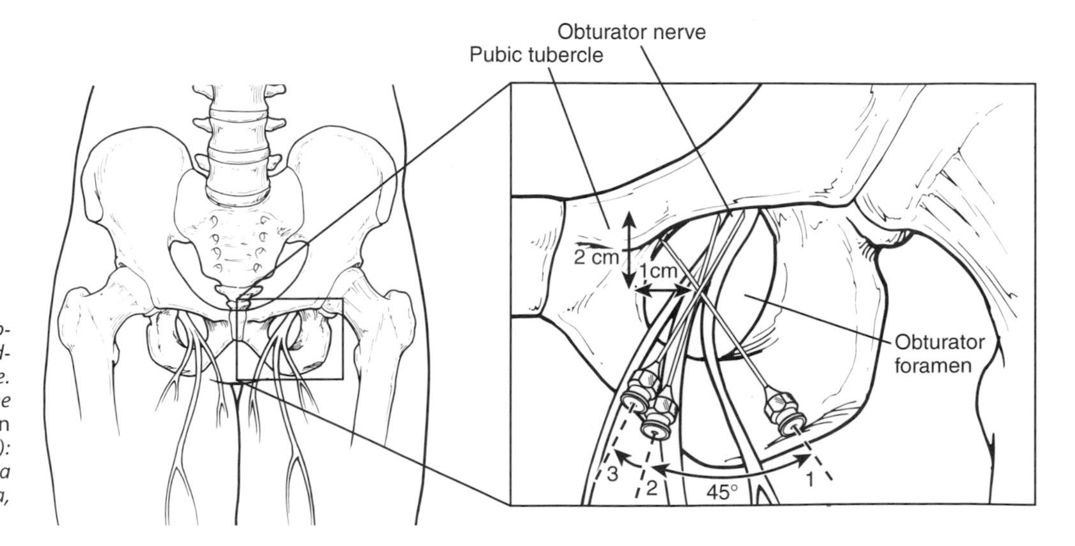

FIGURE 47–1 Anatomy of obturator nerve, showing bony landmarks used in nerve block technique. (Bridenbaugh PO, Wedel DJ: The lower extremity: Somatic blockade. In *Cousins MJ, Bridenbaugh PO (eds): Neural Blockade in Clinical Anesthesia in Management of Pain. Philadelphia, Lippincott-Raven, 1998, p 386.)*

COMPLICATIONS

Nerve block with a local anesthetic using the landmarks and techniques described here usually does not result in serious complications. The usual complications are infection, bleeding, and pain at the site of the injection, but usually they are not serious. If the needle is advanced more than 3 cm into the pelvis, it can damage pelvic organs including the bladder. Neurolytic blockade in a patient who has normal sensation can result in neuritis, which can produce severe burning pain along the inside of the thigh.

REFERENCES

1. R Warwick, PL Williams (eds): Gray's Anatomy, ed 35. Philadelphia, WB Saunders, 1973, pp 1052–1053.
2. Magora F, Rozin R, Ben-Menachem, et al: Obturator nerve block: An evaluation of technique. Br J Anaesth 41(8): 695–698, 1969.
3. Lim W, Kennedy N: Hemi-arthroplasty of the hip under triple nerve block. Anaesth Intensive Care 22(6): 722–723, 1994.
4. Deliveliotis C, Alexopoulou K, Picramenos D, et al: The contribution of the obturator nerve block in the transurethral resection of bladder tumors. Acta Urol Belg 63(3): 51–54, 1995.
5. Fujita Y, Kimura K, Furukawa Y, et al: Plasma concentrations of lignocaine after obturator nerve block combined with spinal anaesthesia in patients undergoing transurethral resection procedures. Br J Anaesth 68(6): 569, 1992.
6. Moulaert P, Verbaeys A, De Brock M: Obturator nerve block in preventing bladder perforation during endoscopic transurethral bladder surgery. Acta Urol Belg 56(4): 523–525, 1988.
7. Augspurger RR, Donohue RE: Prevention of obturator nerve stimulation during transurethral surgery. J Urol 123(2): 170–172, 1980.
8. James CD, Little TF: Regional hip blockade. A simplified technique for the relief on intractable osteoarthritic pain. Anaesthesia 31(8): 1060–1067, 1976.
9. Hong Y, O'Grady T, Lopresti D, et al: Diagnostic obturator nerve block for inguinal and back pain: A recovered opinion. Pain 67: 507–509, 1996.
10. Trainer N, Bowser BL, Dahm L: Obturator nerve block for painful hip in adult cerebral palsy. Arch Phys Med Rehabil 67(11): 829–830, 1986.
11. Edmonds-Seal J, Turner A, Khodadadeh S, et al: Regional hip blockade in osteoarthrosis. Effects on pain perception. Anaesthesia 37(2): 147–151, 1982.
12. Bradshaw C, McCrory P: Obturator nerve entrapment. Clin J Sports Med 7(3): 217–219, 1997.
13. Crews DA, Dohlman LE: Obturator neuropathy after multiple genitourinary procedures. Urology 29(5): 504–505, 1987.
14. Warfield CA: Obturator neuropathy after forceps delivery. Obstet Gynecol 64(3): 47S–48S, 1984.
15. Wassef MR: Interadductor approach to obturator nerve blockade for spastic conditions of adductor thigh muscles. Reg Anesth 18(1): 13–17, 1993.
16. Ritter JW: Femoral nerve "sheath" for inguinal paravascular lumbar plexus block is not found in human cadavers. J Clin Anesth 7(6): 470–473, 1995.
17. Atanassoff PG, Weiss BM, Brull SJ, et al: Compound motor action potential recording distinguishes differential onset of motor block of the obturator nerve in response to etidocaine or bupivacaine. Anesth Analg 82(2): 317–320, 1996.
18. Lang SA: Electromyographic comparison of obturator nerve block to 3-in-1-block (Letter). Anesth Analg 83(2): 436–437, 1996.
19. Atanassoff PG, Weiss BN, Brull SJ, et al: Electromyographic comparison of obturator nerve block to three-in-one block. Anesth Analg 81(3): 529–533, 1995.
20. Lang SA, Yip RW, Chang PC, et al: The femoral 3-in-1 block revisited. J Clin Anesth.

CHAPTER • 48

Caudal Epidural Nerve Block

Steven D. Waldman, MD, JD

Although the discovery of a practical way to administer drugs via the caudal approach to the epidural space preceded that for the lumbar approach by almost 20 years, the popularity of the caudal epidural nerve block has waxed and waned. There has been renewed interest in the caudal approach to the epidural space for a variety of applications, including surgical anesthesia, pediatric pain management, and the management of acute, chronic, and cancer-related pain. This interest has been further fueled by recent studies indicating that the caudal approach to the epidural space may in fact be more efficacious than the lumbar approach for many pain management applications. In this chapter I provide an overview of the current status of caudal epidural block in contemporary pain management.

HISTORICAL CONSIDERATIONS

In 1901, Cathelin[1] published the first accurate description of the caudal approach to the epidural space. In spite of the initial enthusiasm for the caudal approach after Cathelin's report, worldwide acceptance of the technique was inconsistent, at best. The reasons included lack of understanding of the clinical anatomy, overemphasis on the importance of the anatomic variations of the sacrum, and, perhaps most important, misapplication of the caudal approach for indications for which it was anatomically unsuited (i.e., to deliver drugs to the upper thoracic dermatomes). A tendency to compare the caudal epidural approach with the spinal and lumbar epidural approaches also contributed to misunderstanding of the appropriate role of this technique in surgical (and later in obstetric) anesthesia.

The description of the midline approach to the lumbar epidural space proposed by Pagés[2] in 1921 and refined by Dogliotti[3] and Gutierrez[4] in 1933 led to a further decline in use of the caudal approach. Just when it seemed that caudal nerve block was destined for extinction, in 1943, Hingson and Edwards[5] repopularized it for pain relief in childbirth. It was rapidly embraced by anesthesiologists, obstetricians, and patients alike. Unfortunately, this resurgence of interest was short-lived, owing in part to several widely publicized reports of fetal demise secondary to injection of local anesthetic into the fetus during caudal block and in part to the introduction of neuromuscular blocking agents in 1946.

Persistent ignorance of the detailed anatomy and technique of the caudal approach to the epidural space led to reported failure rates of 5% to 7%,[6] rates that did not compare favorably with the much lower ones of spinal and general anesthesia reported at the time.

Throughout the 1950s and 1960s, the caudal approach to the epidural space was left in the hands of a few enthusiasts, who, in the words of Bromage,[7] "somewhat inexplicably, made it their hobby." The second repopularization of the caudal approach to the epidural space occurred during the 1970s and 1980s, in tandem with the increasing interest in the role of neural blockade in pain management. The growing use of the caudal approach in the pediatric population and as a route for administration of opioids in anticoagulated patients has further enlarged use of this valuable technique.

INDICATIONS AND CONTRAINDICATIONS

Indications for caudal epidural nerve block are summarized in Table 48–1. In addition to applications for surgical and obstetric anesthesia, caudal epidural nerve block with local anesthetics can be utilized as a diagnostic tool when differential neural blockade is performed on an anatomic basis to evaluate pelvic, bladder, perineal, genital, rectal, anal, and lower extremity pain.[8, 9]

If destruction of the sacral nerves is being considered, caudal epidural nerve block is useful as a prognostic indicator of the extent of motor and sensory impairment that the patient may experience.[9]

Caudal epidural nerve block with local anesthetics may be utilized to palliate acute pain emergencies in adults and children—postoperative pain, pain secondary to pelvic and lower extremity trauma, pain of acute herpes zoster, and cancer-related pain—during the wait for pharmacologic, surgical, or antiblastic treatment to take effect.[10, 11] The technique is also valuable in patients with acute vascular insufficiency of the lower extremities secondary to vasospastic or vasoocclusive disease, including frostbite and ergotamine toxicity.[12] Caudal nerve block is also recom-

TABLE 48–1 **Indications for the Caudal Approach to the Epidural Space**

Surgical, obstetric, diagnostic, and prognostic
- Surgical anesthesia
- Obstetric anesthesia
- Differential neural blockade to evaluate pelvic, bladder, perineal, genital, rectal, anal, and lower extremity pain
- Prognostic indicator before destruction of the sacral nerves

Acute pain
- Palliation in acute pain emergencies
- Postoperative pain
- Pelvic and lower extremity pain secondary to trauma
- Pain of acute herpes zoster
- Acute vascular insufficiency of the lower extremities
- Hidradenitis suppurativa

Chronic benign pain
- Lumbar radiculopathy
- Spinal stenosis
- Low back syndrome
- Vertebral compression fractures
- Diabetic polyneuropathy
- Postherpetic neuralgia
- Reflex sympathetic dystrophy
- Orchalgia
- Proctalgia
- Pelvic pain syndromes

Cancer pain
- Pain secondary to pelvic, perineal, genital, or rectal malignancy
- Bony metastases to pelvis
- Chemotherapy-related peripheral neuropathy

Special situations
- Patients with previous lumbar spine surgery
- Patients who are "anticoagulated" or suffer from coagulopathy

mended to palliate the pain of hidradenitis suppurativa of the groin.[13]

Administration of local anesthetics or steroids via the caudal approach to the epidural space is useful in the treatment of a variety of chronic benign pain syndromes, including lumbar radiculopathy, low back syndrome, spinal stenosis, postlaminectomy syndrome, vertebral compression fractures, diabetic polyneuropathy, postherpetic neuralgia, reflex sympathetic dystrophy, phantom limb pain, orchalgia, proctalgia, and pelvic pain syndromes.[14–18] Because of the simplicity, safety, and patient comfort associated with the caudal approach to the epidural space, this technique is replacing the lumbar epidural approach for these indications in some pain centers.[15]

The caudal approach to the epidural space is especially useful in patients who have previously undergone low back surgery, which may make the lumbar approach to the epidural space less efficacious.[19] The caudal approach to the epidural space can be utilized in the presence of anticoagulation or coagulopathy, so local anesthetics, opioids, and steroids can be administered via this route, even when other regional anesthetic techniques, including the spinal and lumbar epidural approaches, are contraindicated.[20] This fact is advantageous for patients with vascular insufficiency who are fully anticoagulated and for cancer patients who have developed coagulopathy secondary to radiation or chemotherapy.

The caudal epidural administration of local anesthetics in combination with steroids or opioids is useful in the palliation of cancer-related pelvic, perineal, and rectal pain.[21] This technique has been especially successful in the relief of pain secondary to the bony metastases of prostate cancer and the palliation of chemotherapy-related peripheral neuropathy. Another benefit is that it can be used to administer local anesthetics, opioids, or steroids despite anticoagulation or coagulopathy.

Contraindications to the caudal approach to the epidural space are the following:
- Local infection
- Sepsis
- Pilonidal cyst
- Congenital abnormalities of the dural sac and its contents

Because of the potential for hematogenous spread via Batson's plexus, local infection and sepsis are absolute contraindications to the caudal approach to the epidural space. Pilonidal cyst and congenital anomalies of the dural sac and its contents are relative contraindications.

CLINICALLY RELEVANT ANATOMY

The Sacrum

The triangular sacrum consists of the five fused sacral vertebrae, which are dorsally convex (Fig. 48–1).[22] The sacrum inserts in a wedgelike manner between the two iliac bones, articulating superiorly with the L5 vertebra and caudally with the coccyx. On the anterior concave surface are four pairs of unsealed anterior sacral foramina that allow passage of the anterior rami of the upper four sacral nerves. It is the unsealed nature of the anterior sacral foramina that allows the escape of drugs injected into the sacral canal.[23]

The convex dorsal surface of the sacrum has an irregular surface, because the elements of the sacral vertebrae all fuse there. Dorsally, there is a midline crest called the *median sacral crest.* The posterior sacral foramina are smaller than their anterior counterparts. Leakage of drugs injected into the sacral canal is effectively prevented by the sacrospinal and multifidus muscles. The vestigial remnants of the inferior articular processes project downward on each side of the sacral hiatus. These bony projections, called the *sacral cornua*, represent important clinical landmarks for caudal epidural nerve block (see Fig. 48–1).[24]

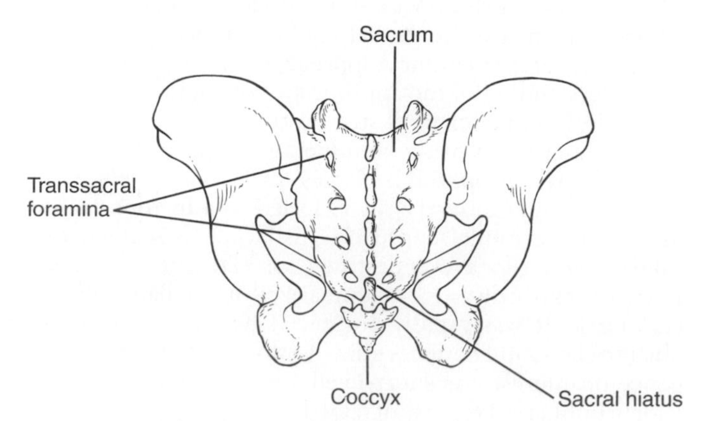

FIGURE 48–1 Anatomy of the sacrum and coccyx.

Although there are gender- and race-determined differences in the shape of the sacrum, they are of little importance relative to the ultimate ability to successfully perform caudal epidural nerve block on a given patient.[14]

The Coccyx

The triangular coccyx is made up of three to five rudimentary vertebrae (see Fig. 48–1). Its superior surface articulates with the inferior articular surface of the sacrum. Two prominent coccygeal cornua adjoin their sacral counterparts. The ventral surface of the coccyx is angulated anteriorly and superiorly. The tip of the coccyx is an important landmark for caudal epidural nerve block.[19]

The Sacral Hiatus

The sacral hiatus is the result of incomplete midline fusion of the posterior elements of the lower portion of the S4 and the entire S5 vertebrae. This U-shaped space is covered posteriorly by the sacrococcygeal ligament, which is also an important clinical landmark for caudal epidural nerve block (see Fig. 48–1). Penetration of the sacrococcygeal ligament provides direct access to the epidural space of the sacral canal.[22]

The Sacral Canal

A continuation of the lumbar spinal canal, the sacral canal continues inferiorly to terminate at the sacral hiatus (Fig. 48–2). The canal communicates with the anterior and posterior sacral foramina. The volume of the sacral canal, with all of its contents removed, averages approximately 34 mL in dried bone specimens.[14]

The Contents of the Sacral Canal

The sacral canal contains the inferior termination of the dural sac, which ends between S1 and S3 (Fig. 48–3).[23] The five sacral nerve roots and the coccygeal nerve all traverse the canal, as does the terminal filament of the spinal cord, the filum terminale. The anterior and posterior rami of the S1 through S4 nerve roots exit from their respective anterior and posterior sacral foramina. The S5 roots and coccygeal nerves leave the sacral canal via the sacral hiatus. These nerves provide sensory and motor innervation to their respective dermatomes and myotomes. They also supply partial innervation to several pelvic structures, including the uterus, fallopian tubes, bladder, and prostate.[19]

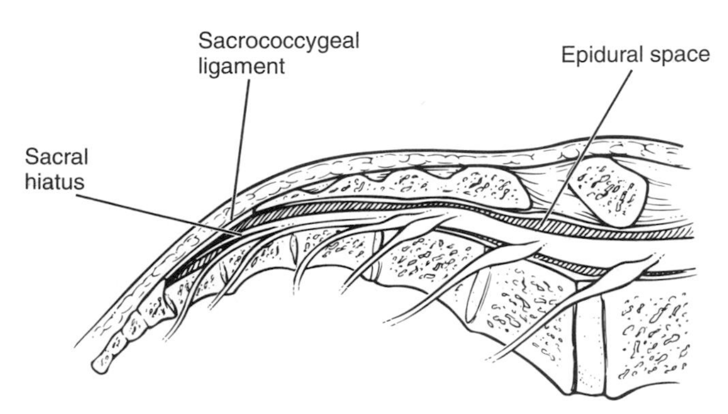

FIGURE 48–2 Lateral view of the sacral canal.

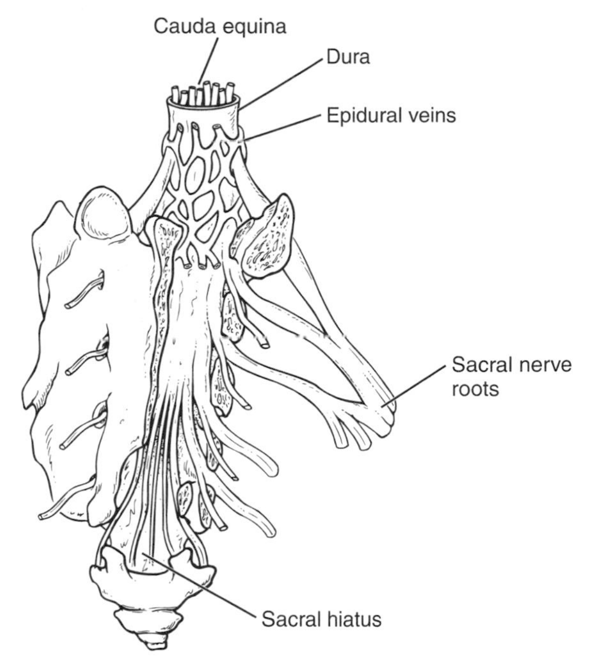

FIGURE 48–3 Sacral canal and its contents.

The sacral canal also contains the epidural venous plexus, which generally ends at S4 but may continue caudad (see Fig. 48–3). Most of these vessels are concentrated in the anterior portion of the canal.[23] Both the dural sac and the epidural vessels are susceptible to trauma during cephalad advancement of needles or catheters into the sacral canal.[24] The remainder of the sacral canal is filled with fat, which is subject to age-related increase in density. Some investigators believe that this change is responsible for the higher incidence of "spotty" caudal epidural nerve blocks in adults.[6]

TECHNIQUE

All equipment, including the needles and supplies for nerve block, the drugs, resuscitation equipment, oxygen supply, and suction, must be assembled and checked before beginning a caudal epidural nerve block.

Positioning the Patient

Caudal epidural nerve block is carried out with the patient in either the prone or the lateral position. Each position has its advantages and disadvantages. The prone position is easier for the pain management physician, but it may not be an option if the patient (1) cannot rest comfortably on the abdomen or (2) wears an ostomy appliance, such as

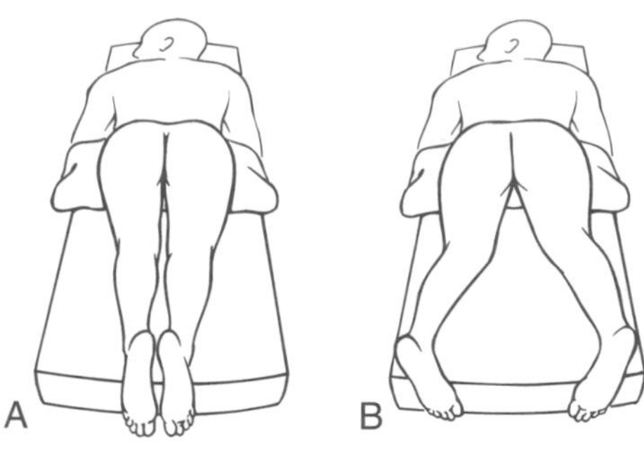

FIGURE 48–4 The prone position. A, Legs-together position causes contraction of the gluteus medius muscles. B, Legs-apart position with heels rotated externally allows relaxation of the gluteus medius muscles.

a colostomy or ileostomy bag. Furthermore, the prone position limits easy access to the airway, which might be needed if problems occur during the procedure. The lateral position affords better access to the airway but makes the approach technically more demanding.

The Prone Position

The patient is placed in the prone position, the head on a pillow and turned away from the operator. Another pillow is placed under the hips, to tilt the pelvis and make the sacral hiatus more prominent. The legs and heels are abducted to prevent tightening of the gluteal muscles, which could make identification of the sacral hiatus more difficult (Fig. 48–4).[8]

The Lateral Position

The patient is placed in the lateral position with the left side down for the right-handed pain management physician (Fig. 48–5). The dependent leg is slightly flexed at the hip and knee for the patient's comfort. The upper leg is flexed so that it lies over and above the lower leg and also in contact with the bed. This modified Sims's position separates the buttocks, making identification of the sacral hiatus easier. Because the buttocks sag in the lateral position, the gluteal fold is usually inferior to the level of the sacral hiatus and is therefore a misleading landmark for needle placement (see Fig. 48–5).[6]

Choice of Needle

A 1.5-inch, 22-gauge needle is suitable for the vast majority of adult patients. A 5/8-inch, 25-gauge needle is indicated for pediatric applications. A 1.5-inch, 25-gauge needle is utilized when caudal epidural nerve block is performed in the presence of coagulopathy or anticoagulation.[20] The use of longer needles, as advocated by some earlier investigators, increases the incidence of complications, including intravascular injection and inadvertent dural puncture. Furthermore, the use of longer needles contributes nothing to the overall success of this technique.

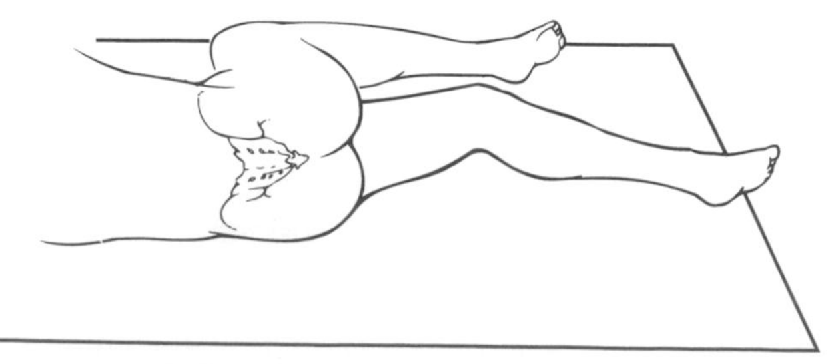

FIGURE 48–5 The lateral position.

Location of the Sacral Hiatus

Preparation of a wide area of skin with an antiseptic solution such as povidone-iodine is carried out, so that all landmarks can be palpated aseptically. A fenestrated sterile drape is placed to avoid contamination of the palpating finger.

The middle finger of the physician's nondominant hand is placed over the sterile drape into the natal cleft with the fingertip at the tip of the coccyx (Fig. 48–6). This maneuver allows easy confirmation of the sacral midline and is especially important when the patient is in the lateral position.

After careful identification of the midline, the area under the physician's proximal interphalangeal joint is located (Fig. 48–7). The middle finger is moved cephalad from the area that was previously located under the proximal interphalangeal joint (Fig. 48–8). This spot is palpated using a lateral rocking motion to identify the sacral cornua. If the operator's glove size is 7.5 or 8, the sacral hiatus is found at this level. If the operator's glove size is smaller,

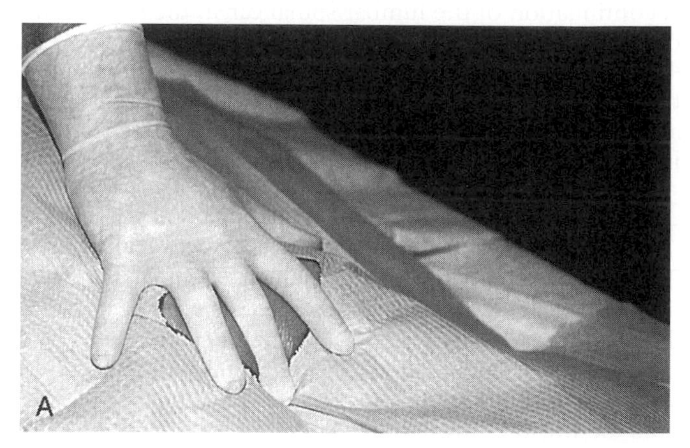

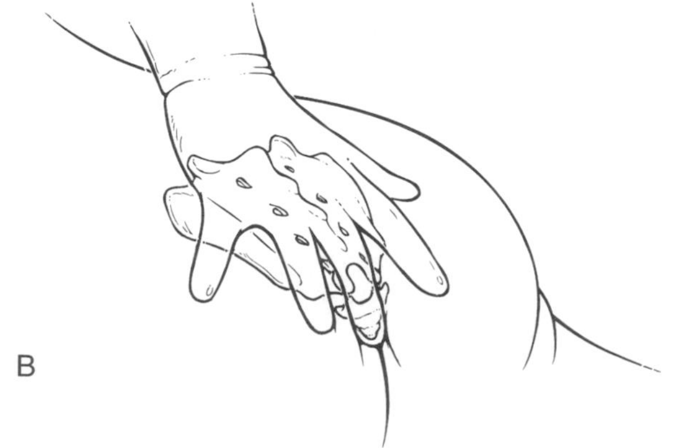

FIGURE 48–6 The operator's finger identifies the tip of the coccyx. A, Photograph. B, Line drawing.

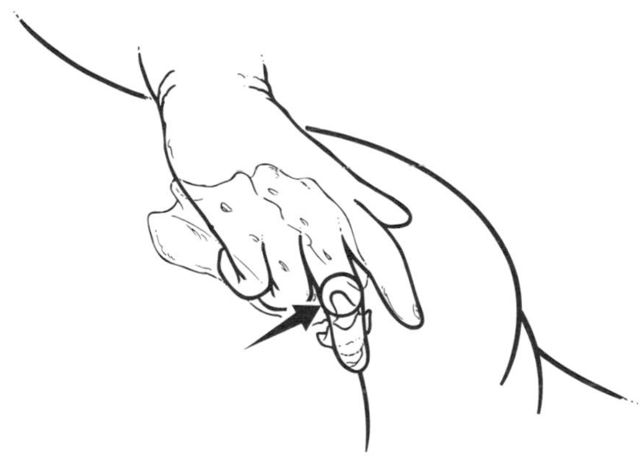

FIGURE 48–7 *Identification of the area under the operator's proximal interphalangeal joint (*arrow*).*

the sacral hiatus is located just superior to the area below the proximal interphalangeal joint when the fingertip is at the tip of the coccyx. If the operator's glove size is larger, the sacral hiatus is located just inferior to the area below the proximal interphalangeal joint when the fingertip is at the tip of the coccyx (Fig. 48–9).

Although significant anatomic variation of the sacrum and sacral hiatus is normal, the spatial relationship between the tip of the coccyx and the location of the sacral hiatus remains amazingly constant. When the approximate position of the sacral hiatus is located by palpating the tip of the coccyx, identifying the midline and locating the area under the proximal interphalangeal joint as just described, inability to identify and enter the sacral hiatus should occur in less than 0.5% of cases.

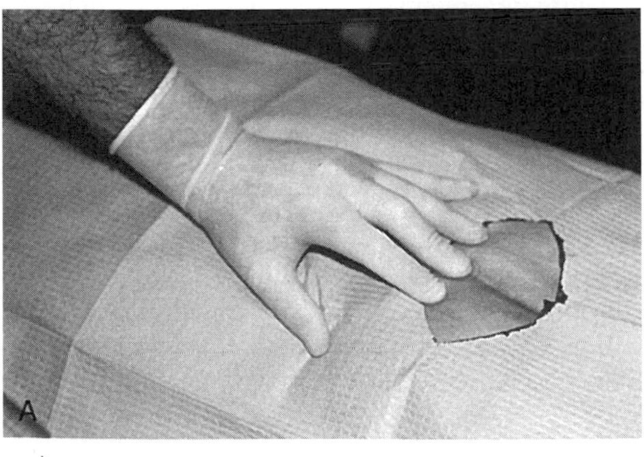

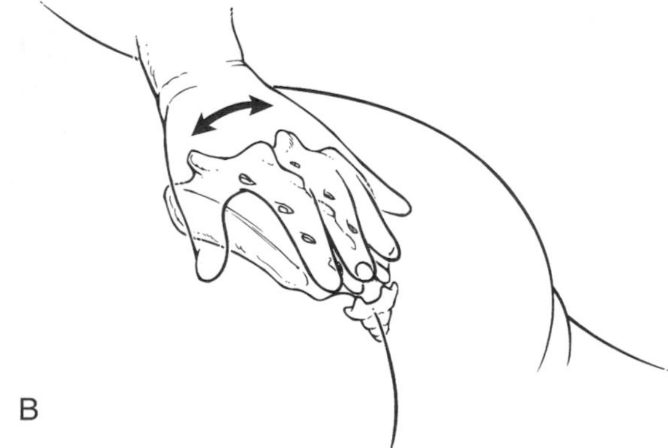

FIGURE 48–8 *Palpation of the sacral hiatus.* A, *Photograph.* B, *Line drawing.*

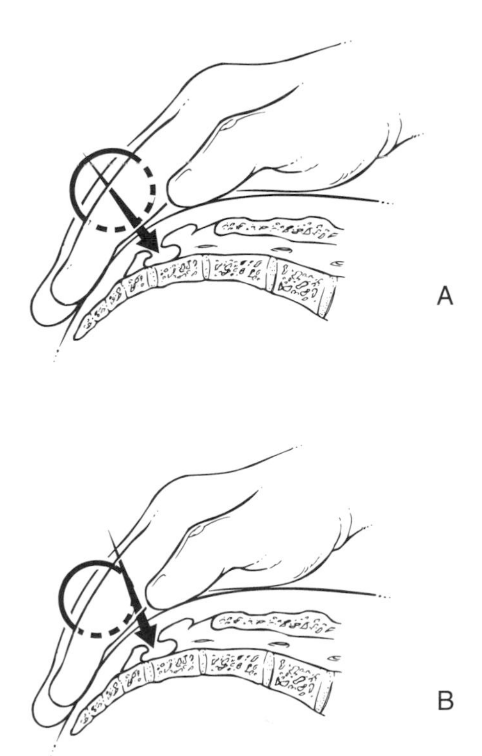

FIGURE 48–9 *Location of the sacral hiatus relative to glove size.* A, *Location of the sacral hiatus below the proximal interphalangeal joint for an operator with a size 8 glove.* B, *Location of the sacral hiatus above the proximal interphalangeal joint for an operator with a size 7 glove.*

After the sacral hiatus is located, 1 mL of local anesthetic is utilized to infiltrate the skin, subcutaneous tissues, and sacrococcygeal ligament (Fig. 48–10). Large amounts of anesthetic should be avoided, because the bony landmarks necessary for successful completion of this technique may be obscured.

The needle is inserted through the anesthetized area at a 45-degree angle into the sacrococcygeal ligament (Fig. 48–11). As the ligament is penetrated, the operator should feel a "pop" or "giving way." If contact with the interior bony wall of the sacral canal occurs, the needle should be withdrawn slightly, to disengage the needle tip from the

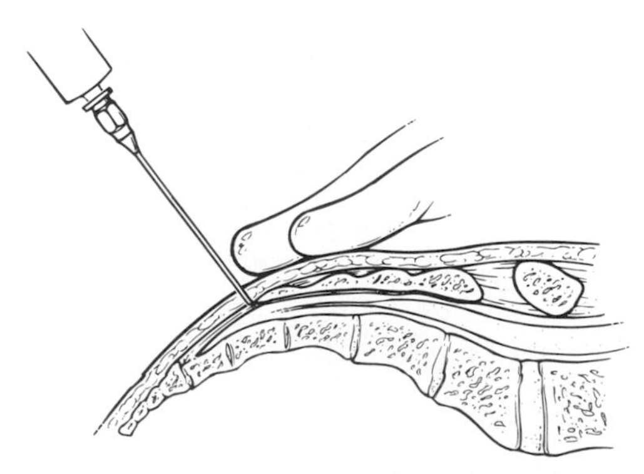

FIGURE 48–10 *Infiltration of the skin, subcutaneous tissues, and sacrococcygeal ligament.*

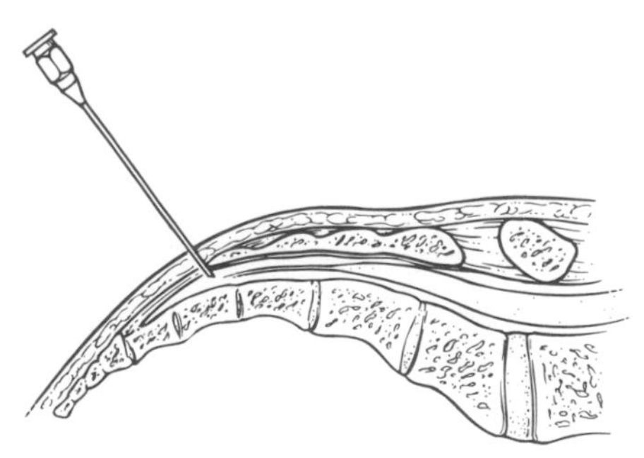

FIGURE 48-11 Needle through the sacrococcygeal ligament at a 45-degree angle.

periosteum. The needle is then advanced approximately 0.5 cm into the canal, to ensure that the entire needle bevel is beyond the sacrococcygeal ligament, to avoid injection into the ligament.

At this point, the needle should be held firmly in place by the bone ligament and subcutaneous tissues and should not sag if released by the pain management physician (Fig. 48-12). An air-acceptance test is performed by injecting 1.0 mL of air through the needle. There should be no bulging or crepitus of the tissues overlying the sacrum. The injection of air and the subsequent injection of drugs should feel to the operator like any other injection into the epidural space. The force required for injection should not exceed what was necessary to overcome the resistance of the needle. If there is initial resistance to injection, the needle should be rotated 180 degrees, as it might be correctly placed in the canal while the bevel is occluded by the internal wall of the sacral canal (Fig. 48-13). Any significant pain or sudden increase in resistance during injection suggests incorrect needle placement; the physician should stop injecting immediately and reassess the position of the needle.

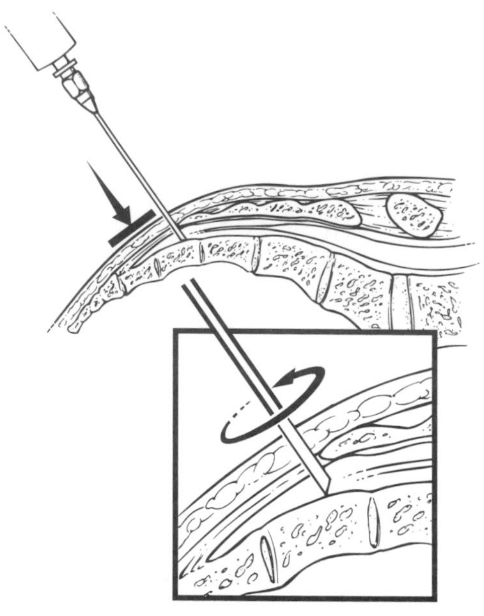

FIGURE 48-13 Rotation of the needle 180 degrees away from the canal wall.

Injection of Drugs

When the needle is satisfactorily positioned, a syringe containing the drugs to be injected is attached to the needle. Gentle aspiration is carried out to identify cerebrospinal fluid (CSF) or blood (Fig. 48-14). Although rare, inadvertent dural puncture can occur, and careful observation for spinal fluid must be carried out. Aspiration of blood occurs more commonly. It can be due either to damage to veins during insertion of the needle into the caudal canal or, less often, to intravenous placement of the needle.

If the aspiration test is positive for either CSF or blood, the needle is repositioned and the aspiration test is repeated. If the repeat test is negative, subsequent injection of 0.5-mL increments of local anesthetic is undertaken. Careful observation for signs of local anesthetic toxicity and subarachnoid spread of local anesthetic during the injection and after the procedure is indicated.

Choice of Local Anesthetic

The spread of drugs injected into the sacral canal depends on the volume and speed of injection, the anatomic variations of the bony canal, and the age and height of the patient.[14] A pregnant patient requires a significantly smaller volume to achieve the same level of blockade than do non-

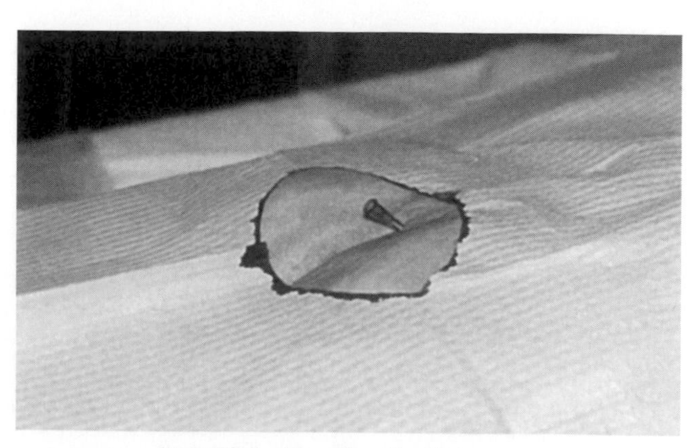

FIGURE 48-12 Needle in place.

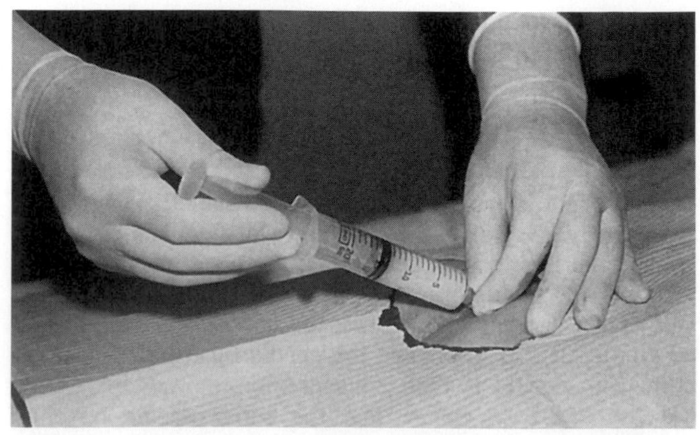

FIGURE 48-14 Gentle aspiration to identify cerebrospinal fluid or blood.

gravid controls.[6] As the injection proceeds, the drugs spread upward in the epidural space. There is a variable amount of leakage through the anterior sacral foramina, which can substantially alter the upward spread of the injected drugs. The onset of action is generally slower than with the lumbar approach to the epidural space.[14]

Local anesthetics capable of producing adequate sensory block of the sacral and lower lumbar nerve roots when administered via the caudal route include 1.0% lidocaine, 0.25% bupivacaine, 2% 2-chloroprocaine, and 1.0% mepivacaine.[14] The addition of epinephrine decreases the amount of systemic absorption and slightly lengthens the duration of action. Raising the concentration of drug increases the depth of motor block and speeds onset of action. A 20-mL volume of the drugs mentioned earlier, given in incremental doses, generally provides adequate sensory blockade of the sacral and lower lumbar dermatomes in most adults.[14] Significant intrapatient variability exists, however, and additional incremental doses of local anesthetic may have to be administered to ensure adequate anesthesia in adults. All local anesthetics administered via the caudal epidural route should be formulated for epidural use.[25]

In pediatric patients, there is a much greater correlation between the dose of local anesthetic and body weight. A dose of 1 mL/kg of 0.25% bupivacaine appears to be safe in children.[14] The established maximum for the total doses of each local anesthetic must always be observed, regardless of patient age, to avoid local anesthetic toxicity. For diagnostic and prognostic blocks, 1.0% preservative-free lidocaine is a suitable local anesthetic.[9] For therapeutic blocks, 0.25% preservative-free bupivacaine, in combination with 80 mg of depot methylprednisolone (Depo-Medrol), is injected.[10] Subsequent nerve blocks are carried out in a similar manner, but using only 40 mg of methylprednisolone. Daily caudal epidural nerve blocks with local anesthetic or steroid may be required to treat acute painful conditions.[10] Chronic conditions such as lumbar radiculopathy and diabetic polyneuropathy are treated daily to once a week, as the situation dictates.[9]

For selective neurolytic block of an individual sacral nerve, incremental 0.1-mL injections of either 6.5% phenol in glycerin or alcohol to a total volume of 1.0 mL may be utilized after the level of pain relief and potential side effects have been confirmed with local anesthetic blocks.[13]

If the caudal epidural route is chosen for administration of opioids, 4 to 5 mg of morphine sulfate formulated for epidural use is a reasonable initial dose.[20] More lipid-soluble opioids, such as fentanyl, must be delivered by continuous infusion via a caudal catheter.

Pitfalls in Needle Placement

It is possible to insert the needle incorrectly during performance of caudal epidural nerve block. The needle may be placed outside the sacral canal, resulting in the injection of air or drugs into the subcutaneous tissues (Fig. 48–15A). Palpation of crepitus and bulging of tissues overlying the sacrum during injection indicate needle malposition.[8] Greater resistance to injection accompanied by pain is also noted.

A second possible needle misplacement is into the periosteum of the sacral canal (Fig. 48–15B). This needle misplacement is suggested by considerable pain on injection, very high resistance to injection, and the inability to inject more than a few milliliters of drug.[22]

A third possibility for needle malposition is partial placement of the needle bevel in the sacrococcygeal ligament (Fig. 48–15C). There is significant resistance to injection and significant pain as the drugs are injected into the ligament.

A fourth possible needle malposition is to force the point of the needle into the marrow cavity of the sacral vertebra which results in very high blood levels of local anesthetic (Fig. 48–15D).[6] It can occur in elderly patients with significant osteoporosis. Such needle malposition is detected as initial easy acceptance of a few milliliters of local anesthetic followed by a rapid increase in resistance to injection, as the noncompliant bony cavity fills with local anesthetic. Significant local anesthetic toxicity can occur as a result of this complication.

The fifth and most serious needle malposition occurs when the needle is inserted through the sacrum or lateral to the coccyx into the pelvic cavity beyond (Fig. 48–15E),[23] where it could enter both the rectum or the birth canal, resulting in contamination of the needle. Repositioning of a contaminated needle into the sacral canal carries with it the danger of infection. Although in competent hands this complication is exceedingly rare, some investigators believe that caudal analgesia for obstetric applications is inadvisable once the baby's head has entered the pelvis, because inadvertent injection of local anesthetic into the head would cause fetal demise.

Caudal Epidural Catheters

An epidural catheter may be placed into the caudal canal through a Crawford needle, in a manner analogous to that for continuous lumbar epidural anesthesia.[6] The catheter is advanced approximately 2 to 3 cm beyond the needle tip.[26] The needle is then carefully withdrawn over the catheter. To avoid shearing of the catheter, under no circumstances is the catheter withdrawn back through the needle. After the injection hub is attached to the catheter, an aspiration test is carried out to identify the presence of blood or cerebrospinal fluid. A test dose of 3 to 4 mL of local anesthetic is then given via the catheter. The patient is observed for signs of local anesthetic toxicity or inadvertent subarachnoid injection. If no side effects are noted, a continuous infusion or intermittent boluses of local anesthetics or opioids may be administered through the catheter. Because of proximity to the anus, the risk of infection limits the long-term use of caudal epidural catheters.[14]

SIDE EFFECTS AND COMPLICATIONS OF THE CAUDAL APPROACH TO THE EPIDURAL SPACE

Local Anesthetic Toxicity

The caudal epidural space is highly vascular; therefore, the possibility of intravascular uptake of local anesthetic is

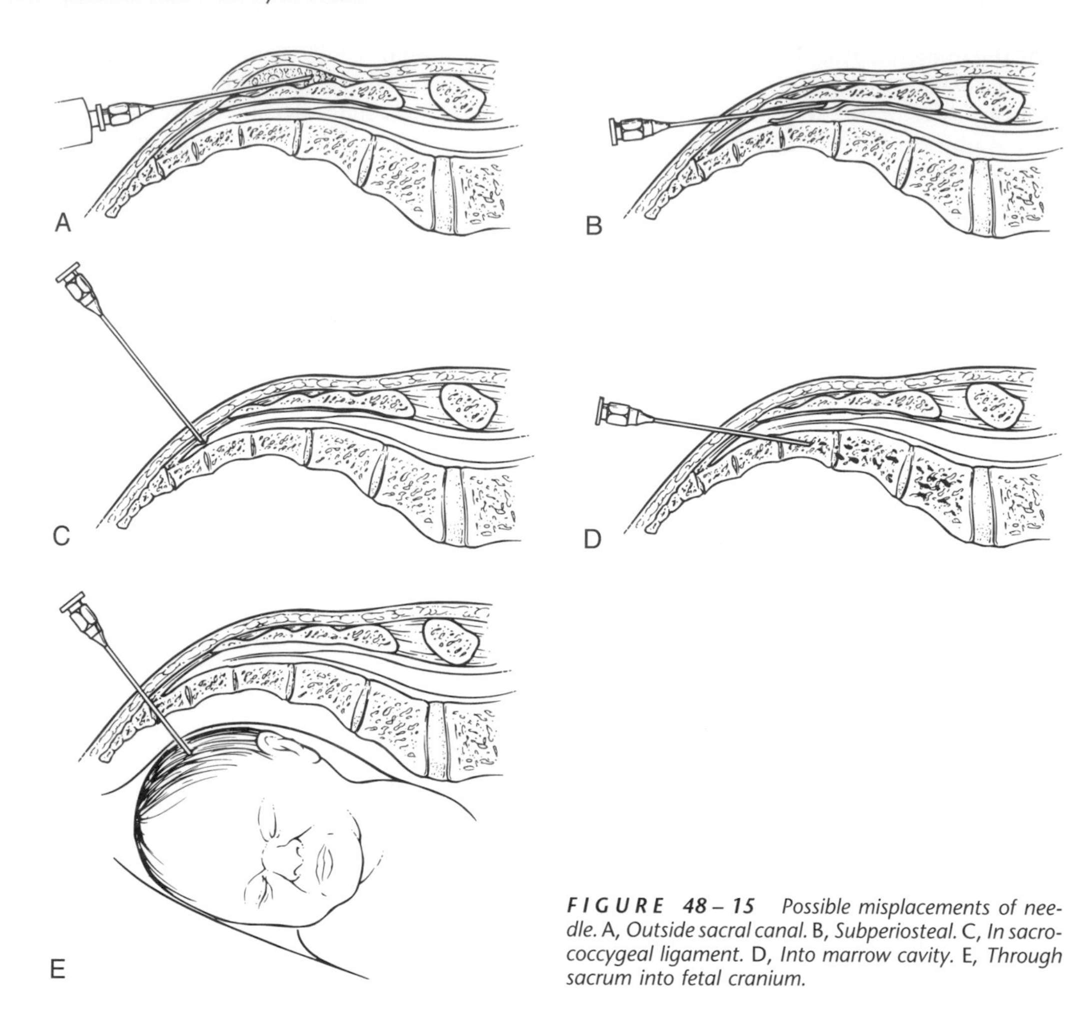

FIGURE 48–15 Possible misplacements of needle. A, Outside sacral canal. B, Subperiosteal. C, In sacrococcygeal ligament. D, Into marrow cavity. E, Through sacrum into fetal cranium.

significant with this technique.[14] Careful aspiration and incremental dosing with local anesthetic are important to allow early detection of toxicity. Careful observation of the patient during and after the procedure is mandatory.[9]

Hematoma and Ecchymosis

The epidural venous plexus generally ends at S4, but it may extend the entire length of the canal in some patients. Needle trauma to this plexus can result in bleeding and, thus, cause postprocedure pain. Subperiosteal injection of drugs, which may also result in bleeding, is associated with significant pain, both during and after injection. The chances of these two complications and the incidence of injection site eccyhmosis can be reduced by using short, small-diameter needles. Significant neurologic deficit secondary to epidural hematoma after caudal block is exceedingly rare.[14]

Infection

Although uncommon, infection remains an ever present possibility, especially in immunocompromised cancer patients.[23] Studies comparing cultures of the skin puncture sites of patients in whom lumbar and caudal epidural catheters were placed simultaneously for obstetric anesthesia have consistently demonstrated that the caudal sites produced a significantly larger number of positive results.[27] Early detection of infection is crucial to avoiding potentially life-threatening sequelae.

Neurologic Complications

Neurologic complications after caudal nerve block are exceedingly rare. Usually, they are associated with a preexisting neurologic lesion or with surgical or obstetric trauma, rather than with the caudal block itself.[14]

Urinary Retention and Incontinence

The application of local anesthetics and opioids to the sacral nerve roots results in a higher incidence of urinary retention.[14] This side effect of caudal epidural nerve block is seen more commonly in elderly males and multiparous females and after inguinal and perineal surgery. Overflow incontinence may occur in such patients if they are unable to void or if bladder catheterization is not utilized. It is advisable that all patients undergoing caudal epidural nerve block demonstrate the ability to void prior to discharge from the pain center.

SUMMARY

Caudal epidural nerve block is a simple, safe, and effective technique for a variety of surgical anesthetic applications. It is especially useful for outpatient surgery and in the pediatric population. The ability to perform caudal epidural nerve block in the presence of anticoagulation or coagulopathy is unique among the major neuroaxial regional anesthesia techniques. The utility of caudal epidural analgesia in the management of a variety of acute, chronic, and cancer-related pain syndromes makes the technique an excellent addition to the armamentarium of the pain management specialist.

REFERENCES

1. Cathelin MF: Une nouvelle voie d'injection rachidienne. Méthode des injections épidurales par le procedé du canal sacre. C R Soc Biol Paris 53:452, 1901.
2. Pagés E: Anestesia metamerica. Rev Sanid Mil Madr 11:351–385, 1921.
3. Dogliotti AM: Segmental peridural anesthesia. Am J Surg 20:107, 1933.
4. Gutierrez A: Valor de la aspiracion liquada en al espacio peridural en la anestesia peridural. Rev Circ 12:225, 1933.
5. Hingson RA, Edwards WB: An analysis of the first ten thousand confinements managed with continuous caudal analgesia with a report of the authors' first one thousand cases. JAMA 125:538, 1943.
6. Bromage PR: Caudal anesthesia. *In* Bromage PR (ed): Epidural Analgesia. Philadelphia, WB Saunders, 1978.
7. Bromage PR: Introduction. *In* Bromage PR (ed): Epidural Analgesia. Philadelphia, WB Saunders, 1978, p 2.
8. Moore DC: Single-dose caudal anesthesia. *In* Moore DC (ed): Regional Block, ed 4. Springfield, Ill, Charles C Thomas, 1965, p 439.
9. Waldman SD: The current status of caudal epidural nerve block in contemporary practice. Pain Digest 7:187–193, 1997.
10. Waldman SD: Management of acute pain. Postgrad Med 87:15–17, 1992.
11. Portenoy RK, Waldman SD: Alleviating cancer pain: A guide for urologists. Contemp Urol 6:40–59, 1994.
12. Waldman SD: Acute and postoperative pain management. *In* Weiner RS (ed): Innovations in Pain Management. Orlando, Fla, PMD Press, 1993, pp 12–13.
13. Gee WF, Ansell JS: Pelvic and perineal pain of urological origin. *In* Bonica JJ (ed): The Management of Pain. Philadelphia, Lea & Febiger, 1990, pp 1392–1393.
14. Willis RJ: Caudal epidural blockade. *In* Cousins MJ, Bridenbaugh DO (eds): Neural Blockade. Philadelphia, JB Lippincott, 1988, pp 376–377.
15. Waldman SD, Greek CR, Greenfield, MA: The caudal administration of steroids in combination with local anesthetics in the palliation of pain secondary to radiographically documented lumbar herniated disc—a prospective outcome study with six-month follow-up. Pain Clinic 11:43–49, 1998.
16. Waldman SD: Reflex sympathetic dystrophy. Intern Med 11:62–68, 1990.
17. Waldman SD: Acute herpes zoster and postherpetic neuralgia. Intern Med 11:33–38, 1990.
18. Wilson WL, Waldman SD: Role of the epidural administration of steroids and local anesthetics in the palliation of pain secondary to vertebral compression fractures. Pain Digest 1:294–295, 1992.
19. Katz J: Caudal approach—single injection technique. *In* Katz J (ed): Atlas of Regional Anesthesia. Norwalk, Conn, Appleton & Lange, 1994, p 129.
20. Waldman SD, Feldstein GS, Waldman HJ: Caudal administration of morphine sulfate in anticoagulated and thrombocytopenic patients. Anesth Analg 66:267–268, 1987.
21. Portenoy RK, Waldman SD: Managing cancer pain. Contemporary Oncology 13:33–41, 1993.
22. Brown DL: Caudal block. *In* Brown DL (ed): Atlas of Regional Anesthesia. Philadelphia, WB Saunders, 1999, pp 347–356.
23. Martin LV: Sacral epidural (caudal) block. *In* Wildsmith JAW, Armitage EN (eds): Principles and Practice of Regional Anesthesia. New York, Churchill Livingstone, 1987, pp 102–103.
24. Lofstrom B: Caudal anesthesia. *In* Eriksson E (ed): Illustrated Handbook of Local Anesthesia. Copenhagen, Sorensen & Co, 1969, pp 129–130.
25. Waldman SD: Issues in selection of local anesthetics. Hosp Formulary 26:590–597, 1991.
26. Katz J: Caudal approach—continuous technique. *In* Katz J (ed): Atlas of Regional Anesthesia. Norwalk, Conn, Appleton & Lange, 1994, pp 132–133.
27. Abouleish E, Orig T, Amortegui AJ: Bacteriologic comparison between epidural and caudal techniques. Anesthesiology 53:511, 1980.

CHAPTER • 49

Superior Hypogastric Plexus Block: A New Therapeutic Approach for Pelvic Pain

Richard B. Patt, MD • Ricardo Plancarte, MD

Anesthetic procedures have played an important historic role in the management of pain[1–3] and account for a large proportion of treatments rendered in contemporary practice. Despite such a strong focus, there are few new techniques. Advances have related mostly to modifications in accepted techniques, better integration in a multimodal matrix, and more sophisticated approaches to patient selection. The introduction of superior hypogastric plexus block in 1990 and its subsequent widespread acceptance represent a singularly important addition to the pain specialist's armamentarium.

DEVELOPMENT AND RATIONALE

The sympathetic nervous system has been implicated in the maintenance of numerous pain syndromes.[4–8] Historically, interruption of sympathetic pathways has been widely applied to relieve pain.[2, 9, 10] Neurolytic sympathetic block is often tolerated well, because numbness and motor weakness are uncommon and neuritis rarely develops. The classic targets for sympatholysis are the stellate or cervicothoracic ganglion for facial and upper extremity pain, celiac plexus for abdominal pain, and lumbar sympathetic chain for lower extremity pain (Fig. 49–1). In addition, the thoracic ganglion is occasionally blocked for the treatment of hyperhidrosis or of pain emanating from the pleura or esophagus. Even though a surgical technique has long been known for interrupting the superior hypogastric plexus (to treat pelvic pain),[11, 12] it was not until 1990 that a parallel anesthetic approach was described.

INVESTIGATIONS

In the first published study of superior hypogastric block, Plancarte and coworkers[13] reported on 28 patients with intractable pelvic pain secondary to neoplastic disease (cervical cancer, 20; prostate cancer, 4; testicular cancer, 1; radiation enteritis, 3). After treatment, all patients experienced significant reduction or elimination of pain, and no complications occurred. A mean reduction in pain of 70% was observed after neurolysis, and residual pain appeared to be predominantly somatic. Application of other treatments resulted in a global reduction in pain scores by 90%, and all but two patients with tumor-mediated pain reported no return of sympathetic-mediated symptoms until their demise (3 to 12 mo later). In another study of cancer patients with intractable pelvic pain, De Leon-Casasola and colleagues[14] achieved similar results. Of 26 patients with 10/10 pain intensity, 70% experienced satisfactory relief (to $< 4/10$) and the remaining patients, moderate relief (4/10–7/10). No complications were observed, and, at 6 mo, no patients with satisfactory relief had required a repeat procedure. The two groups of investigators used similar techniques.

ANATOMY

The superior hypogastric plexus is a bilateral retroperitoneal structure situated at the level of the lower third of the L5 vertebral body and the upper third of the S1 vertebral body, at the sacral promontory and close to the bifurcation of the common iliac vessels (Fig. 49–2).[15–18] This plexus (sometimes called the *presacral nerve*) is formed by the confluence of the lumbar sympathetic chains and branches of the aortic plexus, which contains fibers that have traversed the celiac and inferior mesenteric plexuses. In addition, it usually contains parasympathetic fibers that originate in the ventral roots of S2–S4 and travel as slender nervi erigentes (pelvic splanchnic nerves) through the inferior hypogastric plexus to the superior hypogastric plexus.

The superior hypogastric plexus divides into the right and left hypogastric nerves, which descend lateral to the sigmoid colon and rectosigmoid junction to reach the two

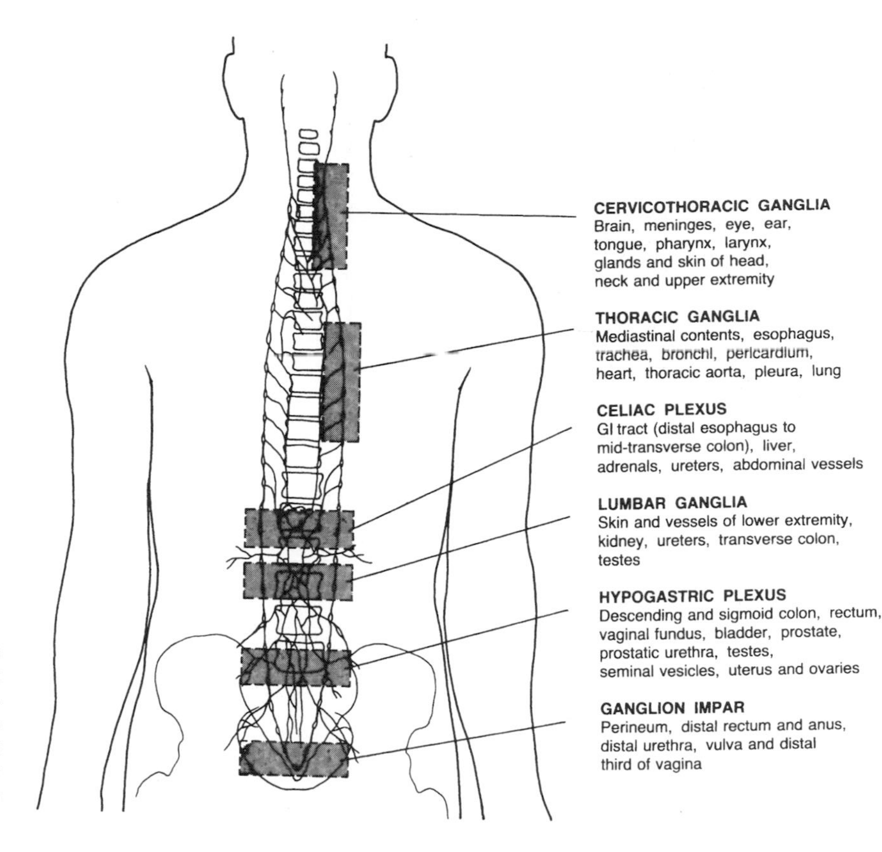

FIGURE 49–1 *Schematic outline of the sites for anesthetic blockade of the sympathetic nervous system and pertinent structures. The system is contiguous, and there is considerable overlap and variation of innervation. (From Plancarte R, Amescua C, Patt RB: Sympathetic neurolytic blockade.* In *Patt RB (ed): Cancer Pain. Philadelphia, JB Lippincott, 1993, pp 377–425.)*

inferior hypogastric plexuses. The superior plexus gives off branches to the ureteric and testicular (or ovarian) plexuses, the sigmoid colon, and the plexus that surrounds the common and internal iliac arteries. The inferior hypogastric plexus is a bilateral structure situated on either side of the rectum, the lower part of the bladder, and (in males) the prostate and seminal vesicles or (in females) the uterine cervix and vaginal fornices. In contrast to the superior hypogastric plexus, which is situated predominantly in a longitudinal plane, the inferior hypogastric plexus is oriented more transversely, extending posteroanteriorly and parallel to the pelvic floor. Because of its location and configuration the inferior hypogastric plexus does not lend itself to surgical or chemical extirpation.

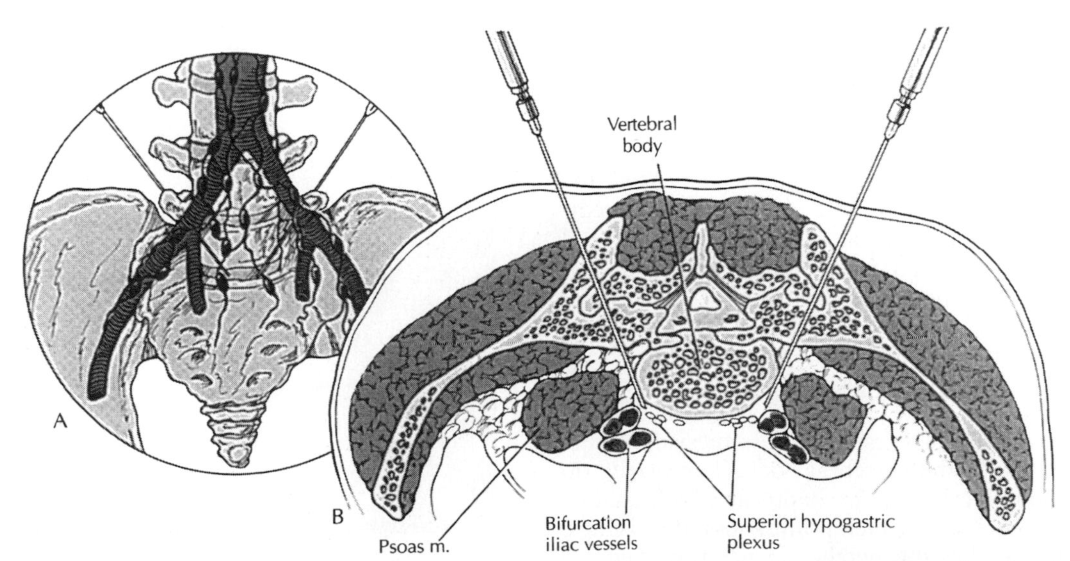

FIGURE 49–2 A, *Anterior schematic view of the pelvis demonstrates the approximate location of the superior hypogastric plexus and correct bilateral placement of needles.* B, *Cross-sectional schematic view illustrates bilateral superior hypogastric plexus block and regional anatomy. (From Plancarte R, Amescua C, Patt RB: Sympathetic neurolytic blockade.* In *Patt RB (ed): Cancer Pain. Philadelphia, JB Lippincott, 1993, pp 377–425.)*

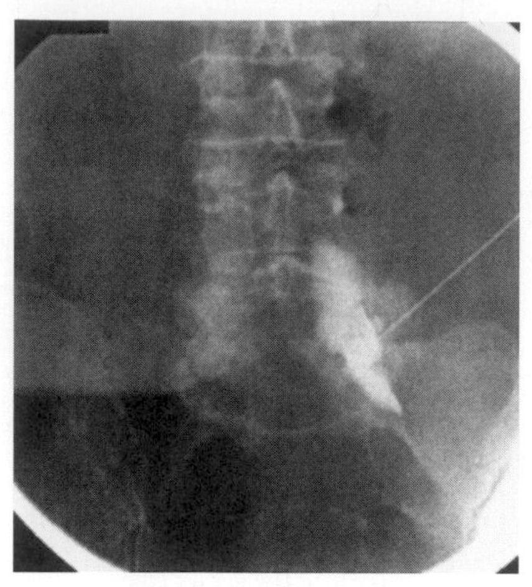

FIGURE 49–3 Posteroanterior radiograph demonstrates verification of correct needle placement for unilateral superior hypogastric plexus block. Note paravertebral disposition of contrast medium in the vicinity of the sacral promontory. (From Plancarte R, Amescua C, Patt RB: Sympathetic neurolytic blockade. In *Patt RB (ed): Cancer Pain. Philadelphia, JB Lippincott, 1993, pp 377–425.)*

TECHNIQUE

The patient assumes the prone position and padding is placed beneath the pelvis to flatten the lumbar lordosis. The lumbosacral region is cleansed aseptically. The location of the L4–L5 interspace is approximated by palpating the iliac crests and spinous processes and is then verified by fluoroscopy. Skin wheals are raised 5 to 7 cm bilateral to the midline at the level of the L4–L5 interspace. A 7-in, 22-gauge, short-beveled needle with a depth marker placed 5 to 7 cm along the shaft is inserted through one of the skin wheals with the bevel directed toward the midline. From a position perpendicular in all planes to the skin, the needle is oriented about 30 degrees caudad and 45 degrees mesiad, so that its tip is directed toward the anterolateral aspect of the bottom of L5 (see Fig. 49–2).

The iliac crest and the transverse process of L5 (which is sometimes enlarged) are potential barriers to needle passage, necessitating the use of the cephalolateral entrance site and oblique trajectory described. If the transverse process of L5 is encountered as the needle is advanced, the needle is withdrawn to the subcutaneous tissue and is redirected slightly caudad or cephalad. The needle is advanced again until the body of the L5 vertebra is encountered or until the needle tip is observed fluoroscopically to lie at the anterolateral aspect of the L5 vertebra. If the vertebral body is encountered, gentle effort may be made to advance the needle farther. If this is unsuccessful, the needle is withdrawn and, without altering its cephalocaudal orientation, is redirected in a plane slightly less mesiad, so that its tip is "walked off" the vertebral body. The needle tip is advanced about 1 cm past the depth at which contact with the body occurred, at which point a loss of resistance or "pop" indicates that the needle tip has traversed the anterior fascial boundary of the ipsilateral psoas muscle and lies in the retroperitoneal space. At this point, depending on the patient's body habitus, the depth marker often lies close to the level of the skin. The contralateral needle is inserted in a similar manner, using the trajectory and the depth of the first needle as a rough guide.

Biplanar fluoroscopy is utilized during needle passage and to verify needle placement. Anteroposterior views should demonstrate the needle tip at the level of the junction of the L5 and S1 vertebral bodies, and lateral views confirm placement of the tip just beyond the vertebral body's anterolateral margin. Water-soluble contrast medium, 2 to 4 mL, is injected through each needle to further verify accuracy of placement. In the anteroposterior view, the spread of the contrast medium should be confined to the midline or paramedian region. In the lateral view, a smooth posterior contour, corresponding to the anterior psoas fascia, indicates appropriate needle depth (Figs. 49–3, 49–4). Alternatively, computed tomography (CT) permits visualization of vascular structures.

Additional precautions include careful aspiration before injection and test doses of local anesthetic. Vascular puncture, with a risk of subsequent hemorrhage and hematoma formation, is possible because of the proximity of the bifurcation of the common iliac vessels. Intramuscular or intraperitoneal injection may result from an improper estimate of needle depth. These and less likely complications (subarachnoid and epidural injection, somatic nerve injury, renal or ureteral puncture) can be avoided by paying close attention to technique. For diagnostic blocks, 8 mL of 0.25% bupivacaine or 1% lidocaine is injected through each needle, and for neurolysis, 8 mL of 10% aqueous phenol is utilized bilaterally.

Modifications

Waldman and associates[35] observed bilateral spread of contrast medium injected through a single needle and have

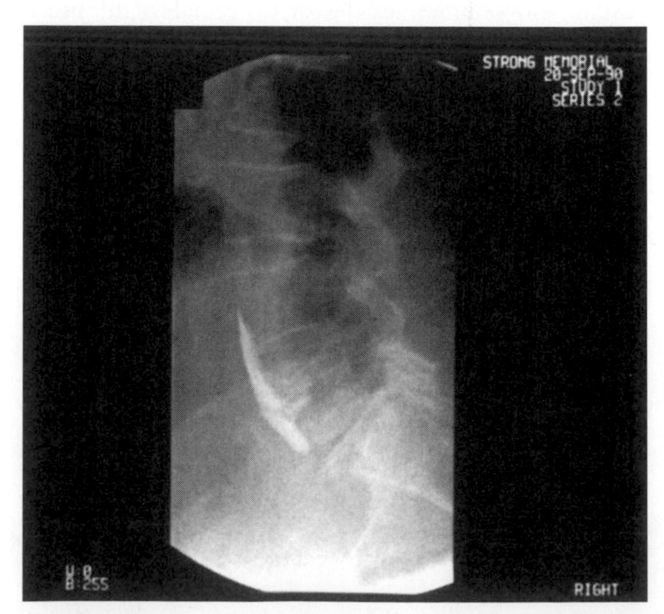

FIGURE 49–4 Lateral radiograph demonstrates verification of correct needle placement for unilateral superior hypogastric plexus block. Note smooth margins of opacity formed by contrast medium anterior to the psoas fascia, which suggests retroperitoneal placement. (From Plancarte R, Amescua C, Patt RB: Sympathetic neurolytic blockade. In *Patt RB (ed): Cancer Pain. Philadelphia, JB Lippincott, 1993, pp 377–425.)*

recommended CT-guided placement of a single needle, through which 10 mL of solution is injected. In a letter to the editor, De Leon-Casasola and colleagues[19] suggested avoiding a unilateral approach in patients with cancer, because the spread of injectate could be impeded and unpredictable owing to retroperitoneal infiltration by tumor. Ina and colleagues,[20] who advocate deliberate passage of needles through the L5–S1 disc for patients with anatomic anomalies, have reported on safe and successful use of this technique in eight patients. Our group has had good preliminary success with a transvascular approach (Patt RB, Plancarte R, De Leon-Casasola, unpublished data, 1995). A gynecologist-anesthesiologist investigator successfully used a transvaginal approach for local anesthetic blocks (J MacDonald, personal communication, 1994).

ALTERNATIVE TREATMENTS

In general, pharmacologic treatment is preferred for cancer pain, although even with optimal therapy, some 10% to 30% of patients require more invasive approaches.

The pelvis contains diverse, multiply, and complexly innervated structures that are potential sources of pain, particularly when the cause is cancer of the female reproductive system, which tends to spread locally by either direct invasion or metastases to regional lymph nodes. Pelvic pain is particularly difficult to manage, because it is often vague and poorly localized and tends to be bilateral or to cross the midline. Because of these properties of pelvic pain, neurosurgical interventions are not generally applicable. Of the various neurosurgical operations developed to control cancer pain, only percutaneous cordotomy is still in common use.[21, 22] Cordotomy produces analgesia that is strictly unilateral and therefore is a poor choice for pelvic pain. Bilateral cervical cordotomy is rarely elected because of the high associated risks of fatal sleep apnea (Ondine's curse) and bladder dysfunction. In selected patients, midline myelotomy may be appropriate, though results vary, and surgical recuperation is required.[23]

The proximity of the nerves that govern bladder, bowel, and lower extremity function and those that subserve pelvic sensation make subarachnoid and epidural neurolytic injections hazardous in this region. Except in patients who have had a colostomy or urinary diversion, neuroaxial blocks should be considered only as a last resort, and even then great care must be taken to avoid limb paresis. Of note is one study that combined unilateral cordotomy with contralateral subarachnoid neurolysis, with relatively good results.[24]

Intraspinal opioid therapy is an important option for certain patients with pelvic pain that is refractory to conventional pharmacologic management.[25] The utility of long-term intraspinal opioid therapy, though, is sometimes limited by factors such as unavailability of resources for maintenance of therapy, cost, the development of tolerance, and, in a proportion of patients, ineffectiveness.

Although no studies have been published, bilateral lumbar sympathetic block has been reported anecdotally to be an effective management tool for some patients with pelvic pain.[26, 27] The lumbar sympathetic chain does not directly innervate pelvic structures, but, because of its continuity with the superior hypogastric plexus, large volumes of solutions injected in this manner probably diffuse caudad. As noted, however, lumbar sympathetic block has yet to be studied systematically for this indication and may have a high failure rate in patients with large masses or retroperitoneal invasion, lesions that can restrict the caudal flow of neurolytic solution.

FUTURE DIRECTIONS

Superior hypogastric plexus block has proven utility for cancer-related pelvic pain that is refractory to more conservative management. Given the absence of reported complications, further studies are indicated in the affected population to determine whether earlier institution of this treatment might produce more rapid and complete pain control than standard pharmacotherapy does. Success may improve further if neurolysis is performed before extensive tumor infiltration shelters the targeted structures. Likewise, trials of surgical or chemical interruption of the plexus at the time of laparotomy are warranted.

Chronic pelvic pain not related to cancer is a common problem and is often refractory even to comprehensive multidisciplinary treatment.[28, 29] Although as many as half of patients' pain probably has nonnociceptive determinants,[30–33] pain secondary to a variety of nonneoplastic conditions (e.g., endometriosis, pelvic inflammatory disease, adhesions) may be amenable to treatment with superior hypogastric plexus block. Trials of this block in this population should include careful stratification of patients and measurement of psychological function, and sexual and functional capacity, in addition to pain.

INTERRUPTION OF THE GANGLION IMPAR (GANGLION OF WALTHER)

Pain arising from disorders of the viscera and somatic structures in the pelvis and perineum is a common cause of discomfort and disability, especially among women. The perineum, the anatomic area immediately below the pelvis, comprises diverse anatomic structures with mixed sympathetic and somatic innervation. Although various interventions have been proposed for the management of intractable perineal pain, their efficacy and applications are limited by the same factors that complicate the management of pelvic pain. In addition, historically, nerve blocks in this region have targeted somatic, rather than sympathetic, components. Blockade of the ganglion impar (ganglion of Walther) has been introduced as an alternative means of managing intractable neoplastic perineal pain of sympathetic origin.[34]

Characteristically, sympathetic-mediated pain in the perineal region has distinctive qualities: it tends to be vague and poorly localized and is commonly accompanied by sensations of burning and urgency. Although the anatomic interconnections of the ganglion impar are rarely described in any detail, even in the anatomic literature, it is likely that the sympathetic component of these pain syndromes derives, at least in part, from this structure. The ganglion impar is a solitary retroperitoneal structure located at the

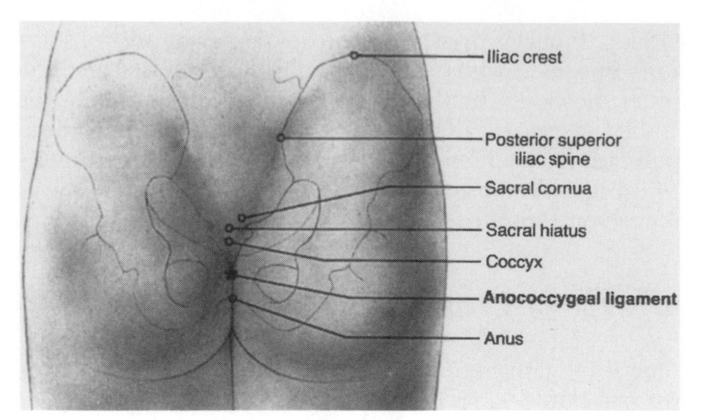

FIGURE 49–5 *Surface anatomy pertinent to blockade of the ganglion impar (see text for details). (From Plancarte R, Amescua C, Patt RB: Sympathetic neurolytic blockade.* In Patt RB (ed): *Cancer Pain. Philadelphia, JB Lippincott, 1993, pp 377–425.)*

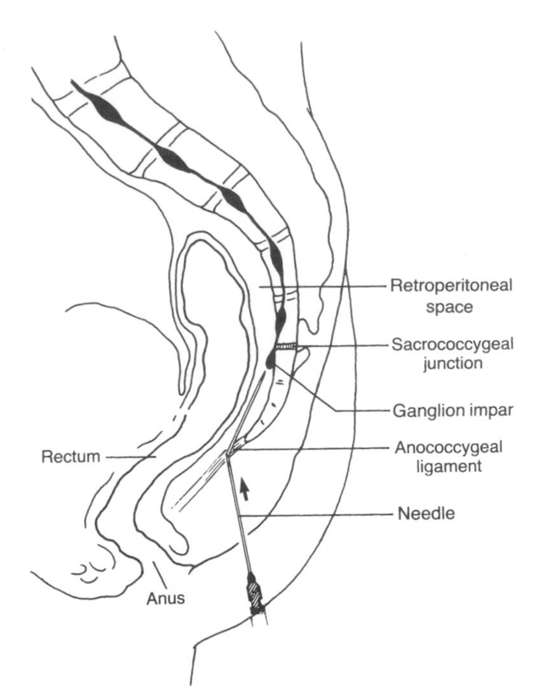

FIGURE 49–7 *Lateral schematic view demonstrates correct needle placement for blockade of ganglion impar and anatomic relations. (From Plancarte R, Amescua C, Patt RB: Sympathetic neurolytic blockade.* In Patt RB (ed): *Cancer Pain. Philadelphia, JB Lippincott, 1993, pp 377–425.)*

level of the sacrococcygeal junction that marks the termination of the paired paravertebral sympathetic chains.

The first report of interruption of the ganglion impar for relief of perineal pain appeared in 1990.[28] Sixteen patients were studied (13 women and 3 men aged 24 to 87 years, median age 48). All patients had advanced cancer (cervix, nine; colon, two; bladder, two; rectum, one; endometrium, two) and pain that persisted in all cases despite surgery or chemotherapy and radiation, analgesics, and psychological support. All had localized perineal pain that was characterized as burning and urgent by eight patients and of mixed character by eight others. Pain was referred to the rectum (seven patients), perineum (six), or vagina (three). After preliminary local anesthetic blockade and subsequent neurolytic block, eight patients experienced complete (100%) relief of pain, and the remainder experienced significant reductions (one

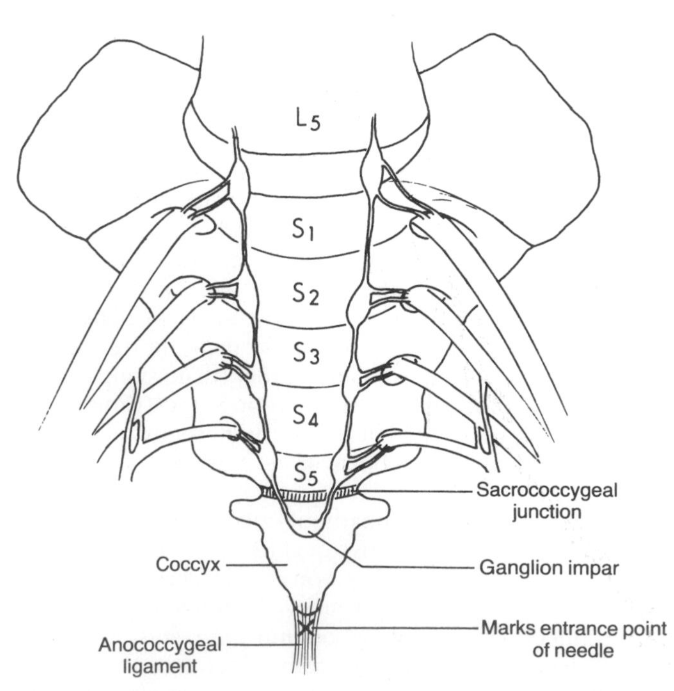

FIGURE 49–6 *Anterior schematic view through pelvis demonstrating location of ganglion impar and pertinent regional anatomy. (From Plancarte R, Amescua C, Patt RB: Sympathetic neurolytic blockade.* In Patt RB (ed): *Cancer Pain. Philadelphia, JB Lippincott, 1993, pp 377–425.)*

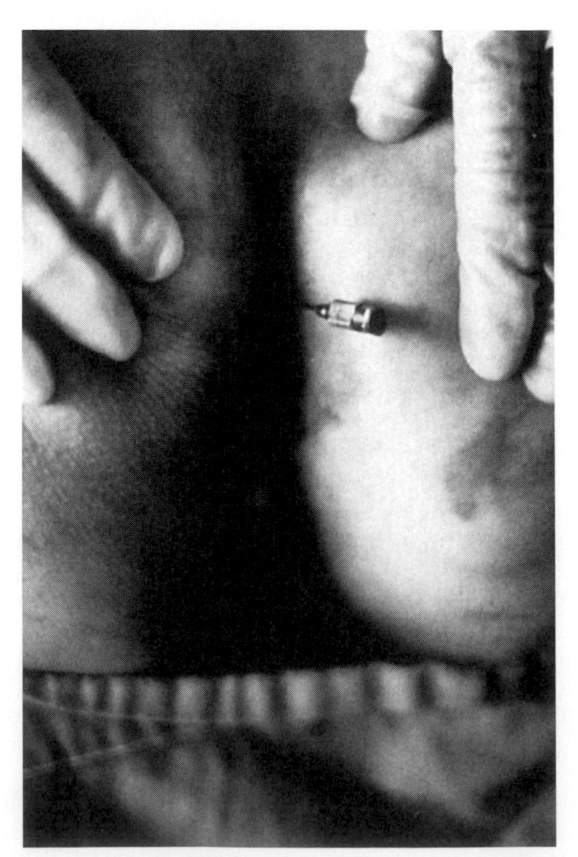

FIGURE 49–8 *Photograph demonstrates patient positioning and needle placement for blockade of the ganglion impar. (From Plancarte R, Amescua C, Patt RB: Sympathetic neurolytic blockade.* In Patt RB (ed): *Cancer Pain. Philadelphia, JB Lippincott, 1993, pp 377–425.)*

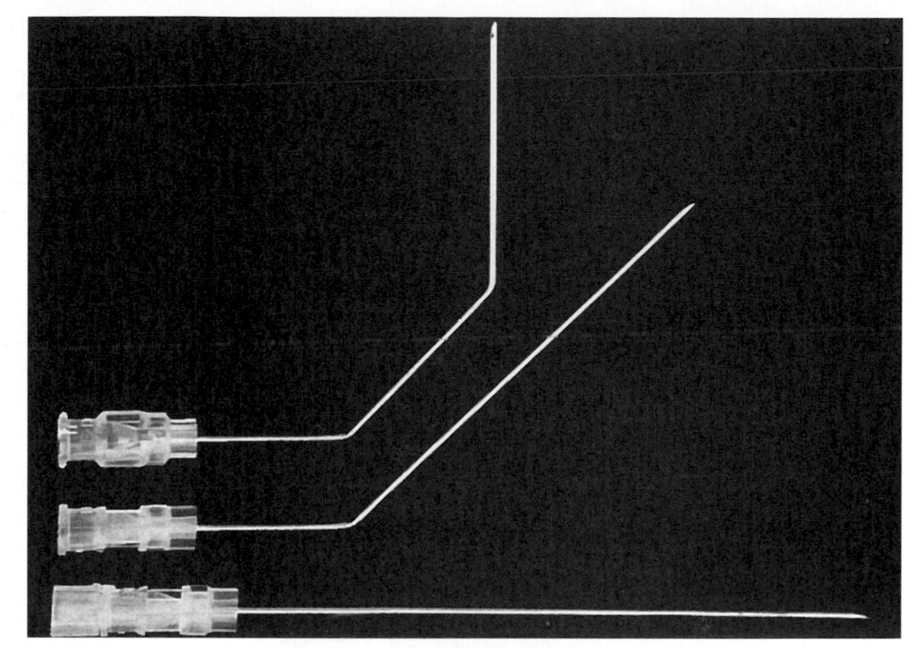

*FIGURE 49–9 Note difference between needles used for blockade of ganglion impar (*upper and middle needles*) and standard 20-gauge, 3.5-inch spinal needle (*lower needle*).* Middle *needle is bent manually to permit access to anterior surface of sacrum.* Upper *needle is doubly bent to permit access in patients with an exaggerated sacral concavity. (From Plancarte R, Amescua C, Patt RB: Sympathetic neurolytic blockade.* In *Patt RB (ed): Cancer Pain. Philadelphia, JB Lippincott, 1993, pp 377–425.)*

patient, 90%; two, 80%; one, 70%; four, 60%) as determined by the visual analogue scale (VAS). Repeated blocks in two patients yielded further improvement. The length of follow-up depended on the patient's survival and ranged from 14 to 120 days. In patients with incomplete relief of pain, residual somatic symptoms were treated with either epidural injections of steroid or sacral nerve blocks.

Technique

The patient lies in the lateral decubitus position, and a skin wheal is raised in the midline at the superior aspect of the intergluteal crease, over the anococcygeal ligament and just above the anus (Figs. 49–5 to 49–8). The stylet is removed from a standard 3.5-in, 22-gauge spinal needle, which is then manually bent about 1 in from its hub to an angle of 25 to 30 degrees (Fig. 49–9). This maneuver facilitates positioning of the needle tip anterior to the concave curvature of the sacrum and coccyx. The needle is inserted through the skin wheal with its concavity oriented posteriorly and, under fluoroscopic guidance, is directed anterior to the coccyx, passing close to the anterior surface of the bone, until its tip is observed to have reached the sacrococcygeal junction. Retroperitoneal positioning of the needle is verified by observation of the spread of 2 mL of water-soluble contrast medium, which typically produces a smooth-edged configuration resembling an apostrophe (Figs. 49–10, 49–11). Then, 4 mL of either 1% lidocaine or 0.25% bupivacaine is injected for diagnostic and prognostic

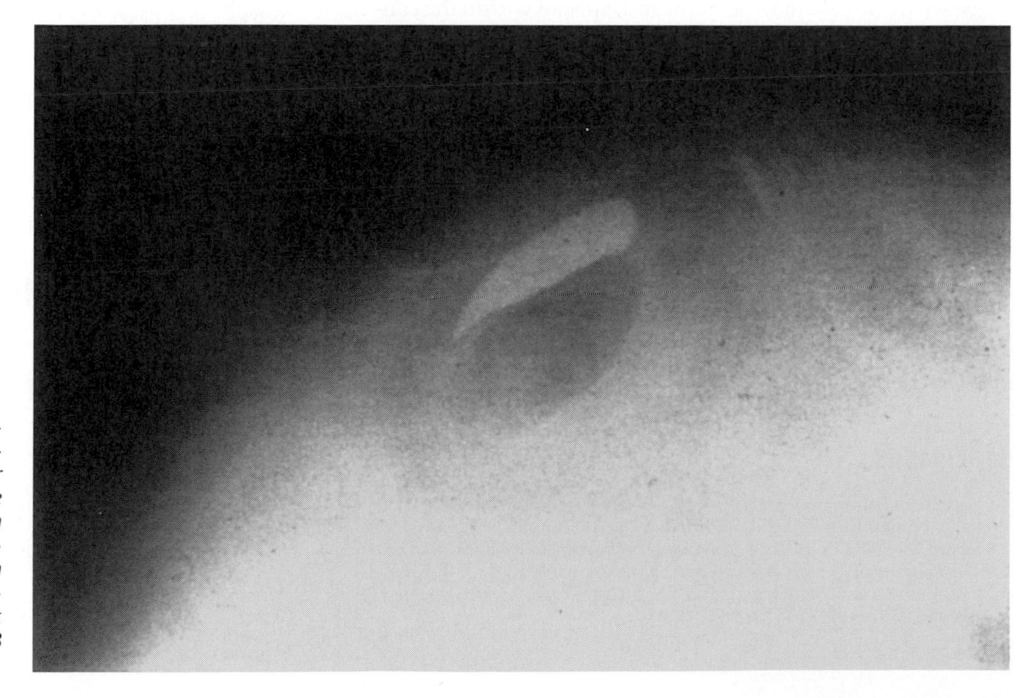

FIGURE 49–10 Lateral radiograph demonstrates placement of (intentionally) bent 22-gauge needle for block of the ganglion impar. Note smooth contours of contrast medium in retroperitoneum between sacrococcygeal region and rectal bubble. (From Plancarte R, Amescua C, Patt RB: Sympathetic neurolytic blockade. In *Patt RB (ed): Cancer Pain. Philadelphia, JB Lippincott, 1993, pp 377–425.)*

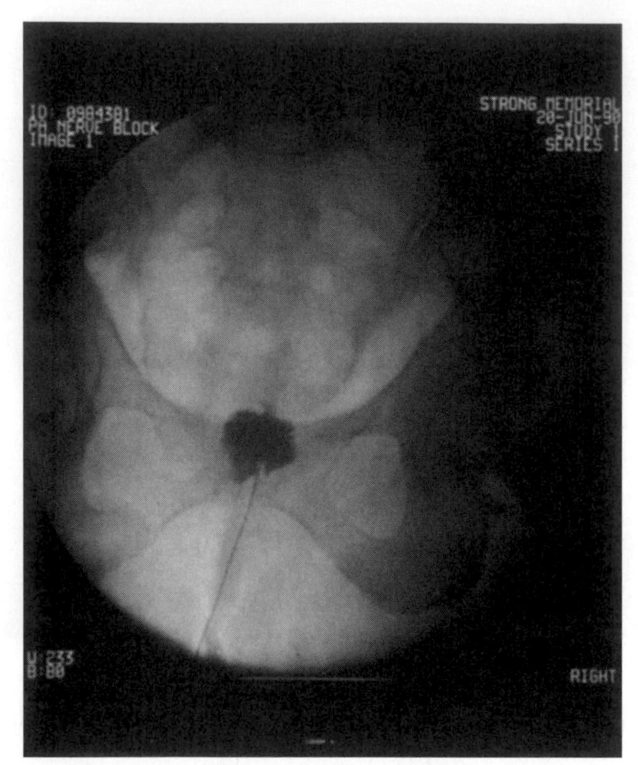

FIGURE 49–11 Posteroanterior radiograph after injection of contrast medium in the vicinity of ganglion impar. Note that contrast medium is confined to midline. (From Plancarte R, Amescua C, Patt RB: Sympathetic neurolytic blockade. In *Patt RB (ed): Cancer Pain. Philadelphia, JB Lippincott, 1993, pp 377–425.)*

purposes; alternatively, 4 to 6 mL of 10% phenol is injected for therapeutic neurolytic blockade.

Under most circumstances, needle placement is relatively straightforward. Local tumor invasion, particularly from rectal cancer, may block the spread of injected solutions. Observation is essential to ensure that the spread of contrast material is restricted to the retroperitoneum. We had experience with one case in which epidural spread within the caudal canal was evident. Also, unless care is taken to confirm the needle's posteroanterior orientation, perforation of the rectum or periosteal injection is possible. In addition, anatomic abnormalities of the sacrococcygeal vertebral column—specifically, exaggerated anterior curvature—may inhibit access, in which case the needle may be further modified with an additional bend (see Fig. 49–9).

ACKNOWLEDGMENT

The authors gratefully acknowledge the invaluable collaboration and contributions of Drs. Oscar De Leon-Casasola, Subhash Jain, and Mark Lema.

REFERENCES

1. Fink BR: History of neural blockade. *In* Cousins MJ, Bridenbaugh PO (eds): Neural Blockade, ed 2. Philadelphia, JB Lippincott, 1988, p 3.
2. Swerdlow M: The history of neurolytic blockade. *In* Racz GB (ed): Techniques of Neurolysis. Boston, Kluwer Academic, 1989, p 1.
3. Benedetti C: Intraspinal analgesia: An historical overview. Acta Anaesthesiol Scand 85:17–24, 1987.
4. Dargent M: Role of sympathetic nerve in cancerous pain. Br Med J 1:440, 1948.
5. Bonica JJ: Autonomic innervation of the viscera in relation to nerve block. Anesthesiology 29:793, 1968.
6. Tasker RR, Dostrovsky JO: Deafferentation and central pain. *In* Wall PD, Melzack R (eds): Textbook of Pain, ed 2. New York, Churchill Livingstone, 1989.
7. Cervero F: Mechanisms of visceral pain. *In* Persistent Pain, vol 4. New York, Grune & Stratton, 1983, p 1.
8. Haugen FP: The autonomic nervous system and pain. Anesthesiology 29:785, 1968.
9. DeBacker LJ, Kienzle WK, Keasling HH: A study of stellate ganglion block for pain relief. Anesthesiology 20:618, 1959.
10. Pereira AD: Blocking of the splanchnic nerves and the first lumbar sympathetic ganglion: Technique, accidents and clinical indications. Arch Surg 53:32, 1941.
11. Lee RB, Stone K, Magelssen D, et al: Presacral neurotomy for chronic pelvic pain. Obstet Gynecol 68:517–521, 1986.
12. Frier A: Pelvic neurectomy in gynecology. Obstet Gynecol 25:48, 1965.
13. Plancarte R, Amescua C, Patt R, et al: Superior hypogastric plexus block for pelvic cancer pain. Anesthesiology 73:236, 1990.
14. De Leon-Casasola OA, Kent E, Lema MJ: Neurolytic superior hypogastric plexus block for chronic pelvic pain associated with cancer. Pain 54:145–151, 1993.
15. Pitkin G: Autonomic Nervous System. *In* Southworth JL, Hingson RA, Pitkin WM (eds): Conduction Anesthesia, ed 2. Philadelphia, JB Lippincott, 1953.
16. Snell RS, Katz J: Clinical Anatomy for Anesthesiologists. Norwalk, Conn., Appleton and Lange, 1988, p 271.
17. Brass A: Anatomy and physiology: Autonomic nerves and ganglia in pelvis. *In* Netter FH (ed): The Ciba Collection of Medical Illustrations, vol 1. Nervous System. Summit, N.J., Ciba Pharmaceutical, 1983, p 85.
18. Woodburne RT, Burkel WE: Essentials of Human Anatomy. New York, Oxford Press, 1988, p 552.
19. De Leon-Casasola OA, Plancarte-Sanchez R, Patt RB, Lema MJ: Superior hypogastric plexus block using a single needle and computed tomography guidance (Letter to the Editor). Reg Anesth 18:63, 1993.
20. Ina H, Kobyashi MD, Imai S, et al: A new approach to the superior hypogastric plexus block: Trans-vertebral disc (L5–S1) technique. Reg Anesth 17(Suppl):123, 1992.
21. Patt RB: Neurosurgical interventions for chronic pain problems. Anesth Clin North Am 5:609, 1987.
22. Patt R: Pain therapy. *In* Frost EAM (ed): Clinical Anesthesia in Neurosurgery, ed 2. Boston, Butterworth, 1990, p 347.
23. Papo I: Spinal posterior rhizotomy and commisural myelotomy in the treatment of cancer pain. Adv Pain Res Ther 2:439–447, 1979.
24. Ischia S, Luzzani A: Subarachnoid neurolytic block (L5–S1) and unilateral percutaneous cervical cordotomy in the treatment of pain secondary to pelvic malignant disease. Pain 20:139, 1984.
25. Wang JK: Intrathecal morphine for intractable pain secondary to pelvic cancer of pelvic organs. Pain 21:99, 1985.
26. Cousins MJ: Anesthetic approaches in cancer pain. Adv Pain Res Ther 16:249, 1990.
27. Bonica JJ, Loeser DJ, Chapman RC, Fordyce EW (eds): The Management of Pain, ed 2. Philadelphia, Lea & Febiger, 1990.
28. Kames LD, Rapkin AJ, Naliboff BD, et al: Effectiveness of an interdisciplinary pain management program for the treatment of chronic pelvic pain. Pain 41:41–46, 1990.
29. Slocumb JC: Neurologic factors in chronic pelvic pain: Trigger points and the abdominal pelvic pain syndrome. Am J Obstet Gynecol 149:543, 1984.
30. Rapkin AJ, Kames LD, Darke LL, et al: History of physical and sexual abuse in women with chronic pelvic pain. Obstet Gynecol 76:92–96, 1990.
31. Milano R: Pelvic pain: Problems in diagnosis and treatment. *In* Bond MR, Charlton JE, Woolf CJ (eds): Proceedings of the VI World Congress on Pain. Amsterdam, Elsevier, 1991, pp 453–458.
32. Walker E, Katon W, Harrop-Griffiths J, et al: Relationship of chronic pelvic pain to psychiatric diagnoses and childhood sexual abuse. Am J Psychiatry 145:75–80, 1988.
33. Toomey TC, Hernandez JT, Gittelman DF, Hulka JF: Relationship of sexual and physical abuse to pain and psychological assessment variables in chronic pelvic pain patients. Pain 53:105–109, 1993.
34. Plancarte R, Amescua C, Patt RB, et al: Presacral blockade of the ganglion of Walther (ganglion impar). Anesthesiology 73:A751, 1990.
35. Waldman SD, Wilson WL, Kreps RD: Superior hypogastric plexus block using a single needle and computed tomography guidance: description of a modified technique. Reg Anesth 16:286–287, 1991.

CHAPTER • 50

Sacroiliac Joint Injection and Low Back Pain

Steven Simon, MD

The sacroiliac (SI) joint has been a source of pain to both sufferers of low back pain and those who refuse to recognize its contribution to this common problem.[1] Many of the frustrations experienced by those who hurt but continually have "negative" examinations and studies can be traced to this overlooked synovial joint and its unrecognized maladies. In this chapter I explore the anatomy, motion, pain generators, evaluation, and treatment of the SI joint and its relationship to low back pain.

ANATOMY

The axial spine rests on the sacrum, a triangular fusion of vertebrae arranged in a kyphotic curve and ending with the attached coccyx in the upper buttock. Iliac wings (innominate bones) attach on either side, forming a bowl with a high back and a shallow front. Three joints result from this union: the pubic symphysis in the anterior midline and the left and right SI joints in the back (Fig. 50–1). Multiple ligaments and fascia attach across these joint spaces, limiting motion and providing stability (Figs. 50–2, 50–3).[2] The hip joints are formed by the femoral heads and the acetabular sockets deep within the innominate bones. The hips create a direct link between the lower extremities and the spine, to relay ground reaction forces from weight bearing and motion. A physiologic balance between lumbar lordosis and sacral curvature exists both at rest and in motion. Changes of pelvic tilt and lumbar lordosis occur in the anteroposterior (AP) plane, relying on attached muscles and fascia, but do not have significant effect on the SI joints owing to a self-bracing mechanism. The sacrum positioned between the innominate bones functions as a keystone in an arch, allowing only cephalocaudad (CC) and AP motion.[3] Innervation is varied and extensive owing to the size of this joint, which includes outflow from anterior and posterior rami of L3–S1.[4]

The SI is a synovial (diarthrodial) joint that is more mobile in youth than later in life. The upper two thirds of the joint becomes more fibrotic in adulthood. The female pelvis is also more mobile to accommodate pregnancy and parturition. Ligament and muscle attachments help to maintain stability of the pelvic ring latissimus allowing movement within limits. Further motion is also limited by the irregular shape of the joint articulation, in which ridges and grooves increase resistance friction and add to the keystone arch structure. Prolonged loading (such as standing or sitting for long periods) and alterations of the sacral base (leg asymmetry or ligamentous injury) are associated with joint hypermobility and resultant low back pain.[3, 5, 6]

Multiple muscle attachments cross the SI joints and contribute to pelvic stability and force transfer.[3] The thoracolumbar fascia includes attachments to the 12th rib, lumbar spinous and lateral processes, and pelvic brim. Fascial and muscle attachments expand to include erector spinae, internal obliques, serratus posterior inferior, sacrotuberous ligament, dorsal SI ligament, iliolumbar ligament, posterior iliac spine, and sacral crest. Major muscles attached to the SI include the gluteus maximus, gluteus medius, latissimus dorsi, multifidus, biceps femoris, psoas, piriformis, obliquus, and transversus abdominis. Vleeming and coworkers concluded that the purpose of these muscles is not for motion but to confer stability for loading and unloading forces produced by walking and running.[7]

MOTION

Ligaments also limit mobility of the SI joint and functionally comprise the distal two thirds of the joint.[8] Motion is described in three-dimensions: AP, CC, and left-right (LR). The major ligaments and their actions are listed next (Figs. 50–2, 50–3).

1. The interosseous ligament resists joint separation and motion in the cephalad or AP directions.
2. Dorsal sacroiliac ligament covers and assists the interosseous ligament.
3. The anterior SI ligament, a thickening of the anterior inferior joint capsule, resists CC and LR motion.
4. The sacrospinous ligament resists rotational motion of the pelvis around the axial spine.

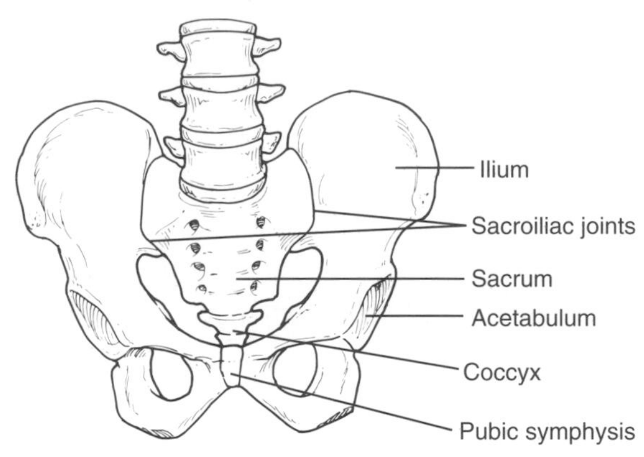

FIGURE 50–1 Anatomy of the bony pelvis.

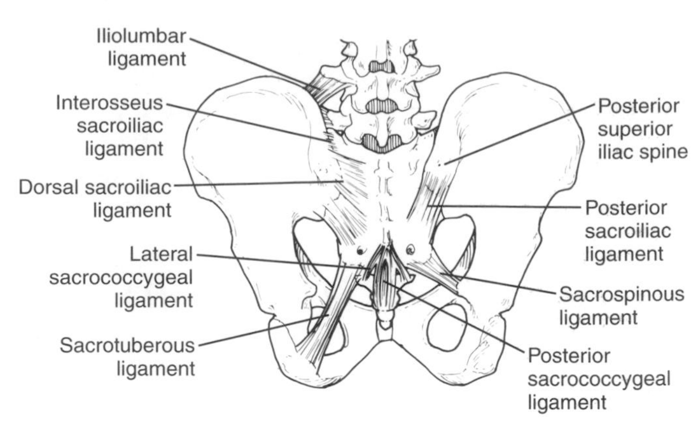

FIGURE 50–3 The posterior ligaments of the pelvis.

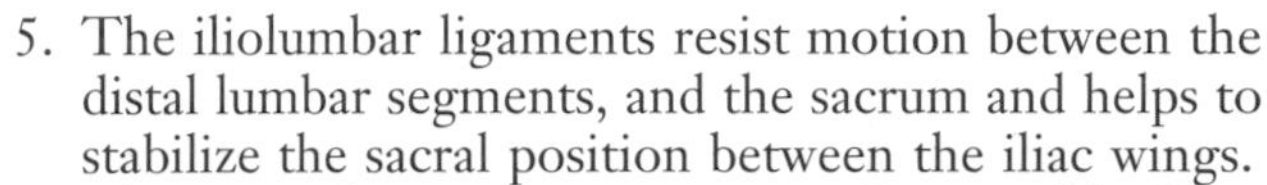

5. The iliolumbar ligaments resist motion between the distal lumbar segments, and the sacrum and helps to stabilize the sacral position between the iliac wings.
6. The sacrotuberous ligament resists flexion of the iliacs on the axial spine.
7. The pubic symphysis resists AP motion of the innominates, shear, and LR forces.

Next, actual movement of the pelvis and SI joints and their functions will be reviewed. We have already established that ground reaction forces from weight bearing pass through the legs and pelvis to the spine. The point in the body where these forces are in balance is termed the *center of gravity* and has been determined to be about 2 cm below the navel. Gravity can also be considered a force line that produces different effects on the pelvic girdle as it shifts from anterior to posterior relative to the center of the acetabular fossae.[9] Body posture and positioning, muscle strength, and weight distribution determine alterations in the force lines. An anterior force line produces anterior (downward) rotation of the pelvis, decreasing tension in the sacrotuberous ligament and maintaining tension in the posterior interosseous ligaments. As the line of gravity moves posterior to the acetabula, the pelvis rotates posterior (i.e., the anterior rim tilts upward), and the sacrotuberous and posterior interosseous ligaments tighten. This is easier to visualize if we imagine a line between the femoral heads on which the pelvis rotates. The vertical distance of motion is about 2.5 cm in each direction at L3.[10] The pelvis also rotates in relation to the spine during walking. As the legs alternately move forward, the pelvic innominate bones rotate forward and toward midline, but the spine and sacrum counterrotate, though to a lesser degree.[11] The SI joint lies between these moving planes and forces; central to vertical, horizontal, and rotational activity. Hula and belly dancers have perfected rhythmic pelvic motion, much to the delight of their audiences.

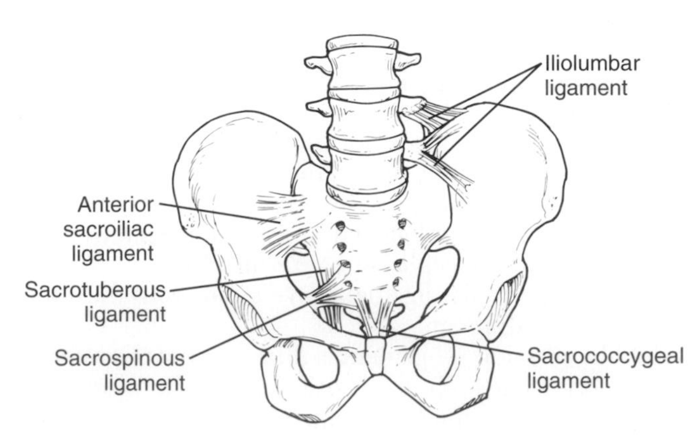

FIGURE 50–2 The anterior ligaments of the pelvis.

Dysfunction of the joint without direct trauma commonly arises from an imbalance in the anterior pelvis without adequate stabilization of posterior (sacrotuberous and interosseous) ligaments. Lifting or bending while leaning forward produces anterior pelvic tilt that slightly separates the innominates from the sacrum, making unilateral AP shift more likely, especially if proper ergonomic technique is not used.[12, 13] The net effect of such a unilateral anterior rotation on the ipsilateral side would be to raise the pelvic brim and posterior superior iliac spine (PSIS) and cause "apparent" leg lengthening in supine positions and shortening in long sitting. (By *apparent* means that the affected leg is not necessarily longer, but appears to be owing to its attachment to the hip socket, which is rotated forward, or caudad in a supine position. Long sitting in this situation positions the acetabulum posterior to the SI joint, resulting in apparent shortening.) Bilateral anterior SI rotation would not produce leg length asymmetry but would stretch the iliopsoas, simulating tight and tender hip flexors. Posterior unilateral rotation would produce ipsilateral PSIS and brim drop as well as a shortening of the supine leg and lengthening with long sitting.

PAIN GENERATORS

The net effect of this type of sustained unilateral force is to create an imbalance of attached myofascial insertions. Pain may result from periosteal irritation or circulatory congestion on the shortened side and loss of strength and tenderness on the elongated side. The joint line is stressed by the combined muscle and ligament pull, resisting resolution and normal positioning.

The SI joint line is densely innervated by several levels of spinal nerves (L3–S1) and may produce lumbar disc like symptoms when stimulated.[4] Muscle insertions near the area, such as the gluteus maximus and hamstrings, refer pain to the hip and ischial area, respectively, when stressed. Fortin and associates have examined normal and symptomatic patients to generate a pain map of SI symptoms. The most common discomfort was described as aching or hypersensitivity along the joint line to the ipsilateral hip and trochanter (Fig. 50–4).[1, 14]

Other pains, reported less frequently, occur about 2 inches lateral to the umbilicus on a line between the navel and anterior superior iliac spine (ASIS) or referred into the groins and testicles. Sitting can be painful when anterior rotation of the pelvis changes the relationship of acetabulum to femoral head. Because the ischial tuberosity cannot move while the subject is seated, balanced support for the pelvic "bowl" is lost, an effect aggravated by the tendency to sit lopsided. The resultant forces produce AP or LR torque on the SI joint. Standing decreases this pain because the femoral heads are repositioned and can in this fashion buttress the pelvis. Sciatic nerve stretch may also be relieved by allowing the pelvis to rotate, thereby shifting weight to the opposite leg.

EVALUATION

A thorough history must be taken to seek preexisting disease or injury, or new trauma, and to evaluate the patient's general health. Bladder, bowel, or sexual dysfunction or numbness often suggests an emergency that requires immediate care. The pain history should also include how long the problem has been present and treatments, including medications, injection, modalities, bracing, or manipulations and their outcomes. Provocative and palliative positions or activity can be guides to aid in treatment planning. Functional loss is significant, as it can be an indication of suffering and a measure of treatment success as the patient begins to resume activities.

Radiography is indicated to investigate fractures or lumbosacral lesions. Inflammatory changes in the SI joint are characteristic of rheumatoid spondylitis (Marie-Strümpell spondylitis) and can be verified with blood tests for HLA-B27. Males in their 20s to 30s generally present with atraumatic low back pain and stiffness. While films may be negative on initial view, and fuzziness over the SI region and stiffness in the lumbar spine may be the only early signs of this progressive disease, many of the tests listed below will still have positive results. Quantitative radionuclide bone scanning has also been helpful in early diagnosis.[15]

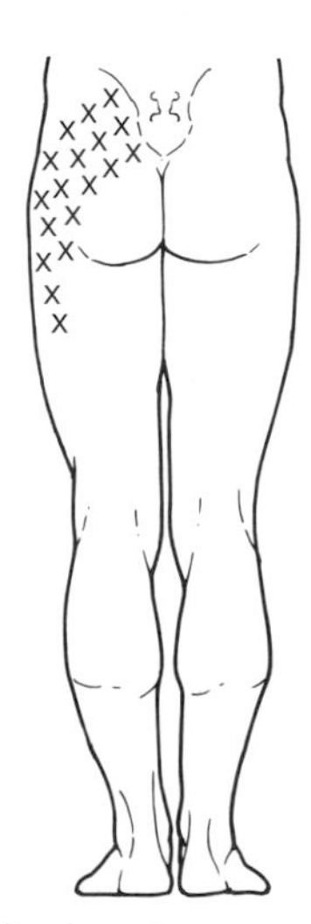

FIGURE 50–4 Distribution of pain emanating from the sacroiliac joint.

How the patient walks reveals important information on antalgic gait, weight shifting, and asymmetry of the pelvic brim or of shoulder height. Spinal examination for range of motion, scoliosis, myospasm, and ligamentous irritation will localize pain generators. Familiarity with the anatomy in this region (i.e., of muscle insertions and actions) is essential to understanding mechanical relationships to pelvic girdle positioning and the necessity of balancing forces to "cure," rather than just palliate, an SI syndrome. Various tests have been developed to detect SI dysfunction. Most can be performed simply during the regular examination and verified by provocation.

1. *Fortin's finger test:* The patient points to the area of pain with one finger. The result is positive if the site is within 1 cm of the PSIS, and generally inferomedial.
2. *Fabere maneuver* (*f*lexion, *ab*duction, *e*xternal *r*otation, and *e*xtension of hip, also known as *Patrick's test*): The patient lies supine. One heel is placed on the opposite knee and the elevated leg is guided toward the examining table. Result is positive if pain is elicited along the SI joint. (This also stresses the hip joint and may result in trochanteric pain.)
3. *Gaenslen's test:* The patient is supine. The hip and knee are maximally flexed toward the trunk, and the opposite leg is extended. Some examiners perform this with the extended leg off the examining table to force the SI joint through maximal range of motion. Finding is positive if pain is felt across the SI joint. This also stresses the hip joint, producing trochanteric pain.
4. *Compression test:* The patient lies on one side. The examiner applies pressure on one pelvic brim in the direction of the other. A positive result is pain across the SI joint.
5. *Compression test at SI joint:* The patient is prone. The examiner places a palm along the SI joint or on the sacrum and makes a vertical downward thrust. Discomfort along the joint line is positive.
6. *Pubic symphysis test:* The patient is supine. Pressure is applied with the examining finger at the left or right pubic bone adjacent to the symphysis. The result is positive if pain is felt at the site. (Most patients are not aware of this tenderness before it is elicited. The examiner should ask permission before applying pressure and might consider having a witness in the room to avoid the misconception of inappropriate sexual contract.)
7. *Distraction test:* The patient is supine. The examiner alternately presses each ASIS in a posterolateral direction. Result is positive if it produces pain or if movement is asymmetric.
8. *Fade test:* The patient is supine. The hip is flexed and adducted to midline. The examiner applies pres-

sure to the long axis of the femur to push the ilium posterior. A positive result is pain.

9. *Passive straight leg raising:* The patient is supine. The examiner grasps the heel and lifts the leg vertically from the examining table with the knee extended. The patient is asked to hold the leg elevated and then to slowly lower it. A positive result is ipsilateral pain, which suggests anterior rotation.
10. *One-legged stork test:* The patient stands with examiner behind. The examiner's thumbs are placed on one PSIS and on the sacrum at S2. The patient then flexes the palpated hip to 90 degrees. If the examiner's thumb moves upward instead of inferolaterally, as would be expected, the result is positive.
11. *Van Durson's standing flexion test:* The patient stands with examiner behind. The examiner's thumbs are placed just below each PSIS. The patient flexes the trunk forward without bending the knees. A positive sign is asymmetric motion (i.e., upward motion on the involved side).
12. *Piedallu's or seated flexion test:* The patient is seated with the examiner behind. The examiner's thumbs are placed just below each PSIS. The patient flexes the trunk forward. A positive result is asymetry of motion (i.e., upward motion on the involved side).
13. *Rectal examination:* Although it is not specific for SI involvement, a thorough rectal examination is necessary to search for referred pain from the prostate, uterus, or spasm in muscles of the pelvic floor. Piriformis muscle spasm can be localized at the end of the examiner's finger at the 2 or 10 o'clock position. Because this is associated with sciatic nerve entrapment, compression of this muscle reproduces painful symptoms.

TREATMENT

Recognition is the first part of treatment as it allows treatment to be directed toward the pain generator. Once the diagnosis is established, controlling the conditions for mechanical malpositioning can start with pain control and move on to education, modalities, and exercises.

Education

Mechanical descriptions of pelvic anatomy and rotations of the pelvic brim help the patient to understand what forces are continuing to stress the SI joint and cause pain. Proper ergonomic training for bending, lifting, and stretching prevents repeated injury from undermining the treatment program and increases the patient's interest and participation.

Modalities

Deep heat is tolerated better than ice and is more likely to reach affected areas. Hot packs feel good and may relax or "soften" muscles before stretching or massage. Ultrasound along the SI joint line is palliative. The addition of 10% steroid gel, which can replace electrode gel required for ultrasonography, can add some benefit by reducing inflammation.

Electricity can be curative by relaxing muscle spasm (electrogalvanic stimulation, functional electrical stimulation, electrical acupuncture) or palliative by blocking the pain signal (transcutaneous electrical nerve stimulation). The pain practitioner can choose from office-based units such as the Matrix, which offers 50 different electrical program choices for treatment, or portable transcutaneous nerve stimulator units such as PGS-3000 or RM-4, which are single-output units for directed treatment.

Traction for the pelvis has not been helpful for SI dysfunction but has proven helpful for some spine lesions. Bracing is a form of traction that applies direct pressure and stabilization over a movable area, which can be helpful in SI joint dysfunction. The SI belt should have a sacral pad directly over the sacrum and covering both SI joints. The belt should cross the pelvic brims, fasten in front, and fit tightly enough to resist AP motion. Ground reaction forces are very strong, however, and eventually will overcome most bracing attempts. Some argue that the real value of bracing is to remind the wearer to use proper body mechanics and limit rotational forces. Whatever the source of benefit, there seems to be some value in using bracing initially, especially if hypermobility exists.

Mobilization is helpful for restoring SI alignment and sacral position. There are many osteopathic, chiropractic, and physiotherapy techniques for restoring alignment. The reader is directed to other texts for full mechanical descriptions. Simple office manipulations are safe, effective, and immediately palliative for SI dysfunction but may be frustrated by muscle spasm along the pelvic floor or spinal attachments. One simple procedure that can be done in the office or by a helper at home is leg lengthening to correct anterior rotation shortening. The patient lies supine on the examining table with the examiner standing at the foot of the table and the examiner's thumbs placed over the medial malleoli to evaluate for leg length discrepancy. The patient is asked to sit up, and leg length is observed. If one leg appears to shorten, it can be grasped with the examiner's hands at the ankle and pulled gently toward the foot of the table. Leg length is checked again after this manipulation.

Self-mobilization is the key to giving the patient tools to correct recurrent malpositioning secondary to ligament laxity. Even proper seating can help to maintain a self-bracing system for the SI joint. A small cushion beneath the proximal thighs distributes weight directly on the ischium, and a second in the lumbar lordotic curve straightens the spine and allows even distribution of reaction forces.

Injections may be the best option for quickly reducing inflammation along the joint line.[16] Typical injections contain both analgesic and corticosteroid and are placed in the lower third of the joint (the true synovial portion) under computed tomographic or fluoroscopic guidance. Other "blind" injections with similar drugs to the upper two thirds of the joint line can also be very effective at reducing pain by reducing ligament irritation. We have substituted ketorolac for corticosteroids on repeated injections, with beneficial results.

The following procedure has been used successfully to inject the SI joint. The goals of this injection technique are first explained to the patient, who is placed in the supine position. The skin overlying the affected SI joint space is prepared with antiseptic solution. A sterile syringe containing the 4.0 mL of 0.25% preservative-free bipuvacaine and 40 mg of methylprednisolone is attached to a 3-in 25-gauge needle using strict aseptic technique. The PSIS is identified. At this point, the needle is then carefully advanced through the skin and subcutaneous tissues at a 45-degree angle toward the affected SI joint (see Fig. 50–1). If bone is encountered, the needle is withdrawn into the subcutaneous tissues and redirected superiorly and slightly more lateral. When the needle is correctly positioned the joint space, the contents of the syringe is gently injected. There should be little resistance to injection. If resistance is encountered, the needle is probably in a ligament and should be advanced slightly into the joint space until the injection can proceed without significant resistance. The needle is then removed, and a sterile pressure dressing and ice pack are placed on the injection site.

Proliferant injections instill an irritant (often dextrose) along the joint line, the desired result being thickening of ligaments or muscle attachments to stabilize a hypermobile joint. The operator should be familiar with technique and complications before attempting the procedure.[17]

Surgery should be considered only when pain is intractable and disabling and the patient has failed to respond to conservative treatments. Screw fixation of the ilium to the sacrum has been described.[18]

Exercises

The goals of an exercise program are to provide stretch and strength to connecting muscles, enhance posture, and a means of self manipulation for the patient. These can be done alone or with a helper.

Strengthening Exercises

We suggest a "6-pack" of repetitions of these isometric strengthening maneuvers: 6 sets of 6, 6 seconds on 6 seconds off, 6 times a day.

Abdominal crunches. The patient lies supine with hip and knee flexed and feet flat on the floor. A partial sit-up is performed and held as above for a 6 pack.

Hip Abduction, Adduction, and Extension. The patient may be standing, sitting, or lying down. Isometric exercises are performed by resisting the direction of motion, using furniture or hands.

Pelvic Tilt, Anterior and Posterior. The patient stands with hands on hips. The pelvis is tilted up (anterior) then back (posterior); held for 6 seconds, 6 times (a "6 pack").

Isometric Hip Extension. The patient may be sitting, lying down, or standing. The elevated foot must be braced on a pedestal in a vertical position. The hip and knee are flexed maximally against the trunk, held in the flexed position with both hands. Isometric extension is then resisted by the arms, as above for a 6 pack. Men especially seem to prefer a variation of this maneuver that involves standing against the inside of a door frame with one foot against the opposite side. Resisted extension of hip and knee from pressure against the sole of the foot produces a similar effect.

Posture Enhancement

Correct trunk posture enhances force distribution by maintaining correct spinal alignment. Holding the abdomen "in" (contracting the abdominal and rectus muscles) creates an internal brace against the lower back and helps to maintain adequate pelvic tilt and lumbar lordosis. Holding shoulders and head in proper alignment also enhances spinal positioning and distribution of forces.

REFERENCES

1. Fortin JD, et al: Sacroiliac joint: Pain referral maps upon applying a new injection/arthrography technique. Part I. Spine 19:1475–1482, 1994.
2. Willard FH: The anatomy of the lumbosacral connection. Spine 9:333–955, 1995.
3. Snijders CJ, et al: Transfer of lumbosacral load to iliac bones and legs. Part I: Biomechanics of self-bracing of the sacroiliac joints and its significance for treatment and exercise. Part II: Loading of the sacroiliac joints when lifting in a stooped posture. Clin Biomech 8:285–301, 1993.
4. Solonen KA: The sacroiliac joint in the light of anatomical, roentgenological and clinical studies. Acta Orthop Scand 27 (Suppl):27, 1957.
5. Simonian P, et al: Biomechical simulation of the anteroposterior compression injury of the pelvis. Clin Orthop 309:245–256, 1994.
6. Vrahas M, et al: Ligamentous contributions to pelvic stability. Orthopedics 18:271–274, 1995.
7. Vleeming A, et al: The posterior layer of the thoracolumbar fascia. Spine 20:753–758, 1995.
8. Vrahas M, et al: Ligamentous contributions to pelvic stability. Orthopedics 18:271–274, 1995.
9. DonTigny RL: Mechanics and treatment of the sacroiliac joint. J Manual Manip Ther 1:3–12, 1993.
10. Thorstensson A, et al: Trunk movements in human locomotion. Acta Physiol Scand 121:9–22, 1984.
11. Lavignolle B, et al: An approach to the functional anatomy of the sacroiliac joints in vivo. Anatomia Clinica 5:169–176, 1983.
12. Vlemming A, et al: Towards a better understanding of the etiology of low back pain. In Ref No. 1, pp 545–549.
13. Pierrynowski MR, et al: Three dimensional sacroiliac motion during locomotion in asymptomatic male and female subjects. Presented at the 5th Canadian Society of Biomechanics, Ottawa, Canada. August 1988.
14. Fortin JD, et al: Sacroiliac joint: Pain referral maps upon applying a new injection/arthrography technique, Part II: Clinical evaluation. Spine 19:1483–1449, 1994.
15. Maigne JY, et al: Value of quantitative radionuclide bone scanning in the diagnosis of sacroiliac joint syndrome in 32 patients with low back pain. Eur Spine J 7:328–331, 1998.
16. Maugars Y, et al: Assessment of the efficacy of sacroiliac corticosteroid injections in the spondylarthropathies: A double-blind study. Br J Rheumatol 35:767–770, 1996.
17. Reeves KD: Technique of prolotherapy. *In* Lennard TA (ed): Physiatric Procedures in Clinical Practice. Philadelphia, Hanley & Belfus, 1995, pp 57–70.
18. Matta JM, et al: Internal fixation of pelvic ring fractures. Clin Orthop 242:93, 1989.

CHAPTER • 51

Peripheral Neurolysis in the Management of Pain

P. Prithvi Raj, MD • Susan R. Anderson, MD

One option for prolonged interruption of nociceptive pathways involves the neurolysis of peripheral nerves by chemical, thermal, cryogenic, or surgical means. It is indicated for patients with limited life expectancy and patients who have recurrent or intractable pain after a series of analgesic blocks. Peripheral neurolysis has not become commonplace, for these reasons:

- It is not permanent.
- It can cause neuritis and deafferentation pain.
- It can produce motor deficit when mixed nerves are ablated.
- It has the potential to cause unintentional damage to nontargeted tissue.

The impact of each of these problems can be minimized by selecting patients carefully and performing the procedure with great care and technical expertise. The following conditions should be present before peripheral neurolysis:

- The pain is severe.
- The pain is expected to persist with less invasive alternative techniques.
- The pain is well-localized and in the distribution of an identifiable nerve.
- The pain is relieved by local anesthetic block.
- There are no undesirable deficits after the local anesthetic blocks.

ISSUES TO CONSIDER BEFORE NEUROLYSIS

The appearance of neuropathic pain (causalgia) is a feature common to most ablative procedures.[1, 2] It can be minimized by limiting the selection of patients to those with short life expectancy (i.e., a period unlikely to exceed the duration of pain relief). In the event that a patient does survive the duration of pain relief, the peripheral neurolysis should be repeatable at the same site or more proximally. The provision of neurolytic blockade in patients with chronic noncancer pain is controversial. Some believe that with proper informed consent it is acceptable practice in carefully selected patients with pain that is intractable but otherwise benign. The potential for damage to nontargeted tissue is a concern with any destructive procedure, but, in general, it is less likely to occur with peripheral neurolysis than when central or deep sympathetic neurolytic blocks are undertaken. This is particularly true when localization is facilitated by electrical stimulation, radiographic guidance, or test doses of a local anesthetic.[3–5]

Accurate localization and subsequent immobilization of the needle are critical to success. Most nerve blocks are performed percutaneously, without the benefit afforded by direct vision. A thorough knowledge of the pertinent regional anatomy is essential to make the best use of surface, vascular, and deep bony landmarks. Paresthesia, usually a sensitive guide to the proximity of the needle to the targeted nerve, is subject to differences in technique and in interpretation by the clinician and the patient. If paresthesia is to be relied upon, the patient must be oriented in advance and maintained in a cooperative, lucid state; the technique must be slow and deliberate, with maintenance of verbal contact throughout. Localization can be facilitated further by electrical stimulation, radiographic guidance, and observation for the spread of radiolographic contrast solution. These adjuncts are particularly useful when anatomic structures have been altered by tumor invasion, surgery, or radiotherapy. Unfortunately, it is often difficult to enlist the aid of a qualified radiologist. Although the preceding adjunctive techniques are useful, a preneurolysis test dose of local anesthetic should be regarded as essential (1) to rule out incorrect placement, (2) to guard against possible injury, and (3) to further confirm correct needle placement. Clearing the injecting needle with air or saline after administration of the neurolytic agent is another measure that may help to avoid skin slough and tissue injury from drug spilled on tissue during withdrawal of the needle. The reasons for the limited duration of analgesia are not known for certain, but it has been postulated to be related to the creation, by peripheral neurolysis, of an incomplete lesion of the targeted nerve.[6] Whereas local anesthetic injected in the general vicinity of a nerve trunk may diffuse through neighboring soft tissue and often results in effective neural blockade, neurolytic drugs spread poorly and require precise location of the needle on the targeted nerve. This means that best results are obtained when the neurolytic solution is deposited directly onto the nerve. To avoid complications, the volume and the concentration of the injected neurolytic must also be carefully controlled. Controlled comparisons between neurolytic agents in different concentrations and volumes have not been carried out. It may be that incomplete lesions and consequent return of partial function are influenced by those factors. Incomplete lesions may lead to the development of posttreatment neuritis.[6, 7] An association between the creation of incomplete or misplaced lesions and subsequent neuritis is supported indirectly by the work of Roviaro and colleagues,[8] who injected three neighboring intercostal nerves with 6% phenol in glycerine (1 mL per segment) under direct vision at thoracotomy. Of 32 patients treated, neither neuritis nor deafferentation pain was reported at 1-year follow-up, a finding in marked contrast to results of percutaneous neurolytic intercostal blocks.[9]

SELECTION OF A NEUROLYTIC AGENT

Early investigators used either absolute alcohol or 5% to 7% phenol for peripheral neurolysis. In an effort to improve the success rate, one used either absolute alcohol or higher than usual concentrations of phenol (10% to 12%).[10–14] Owing to limits in physical properties, a maximum of 6.7% phenol can be dissolved in water at room temperature, but the addition of a small amount of glycerine or water-soluble radiocontrast materials increase phenol's solubility to as much as 15%. Some workers are concerned that higher concentrations of phenol might predispose to vascular injury.[16] The effect of a neurolytic block is well known to be transient (2 weeks to 6 months). It is best to forewarn patients to expect that the procedure may need to be repeated as many as three times. In most clinical series, more than half the patients receive more than one neurolytic procedure.

Although alcohol and phenol are commonly used to produce chemical neurolysis in contemporary practice, ammonium sulfate and chlorocresol have occasionally been advocated. Compared with sympathetic and central sites, peripheral neurolysis is unique in that neuritis and dysesthesias follow treatment in 2% to 28% of patients.[7, 16] The incidence of neuritis after peripheral neurolysis with alcohol is widely held to be higher than with phenol, although this finding has not been documented in controlled studies.[17, 18]

Alcohol

Perineural injection of alcohol is followed immediately by severe burning pain along the nerve's distribution, which lasts about a minute before giving way to a warm, numb sensation. Pain on injection may be diminished by injecting a local anesthetic beforehand. Some authors enjoin against the injection of a local anesthetic and a neurolytic drug in succession because of theoretical concerns about dilution of the neurolytic and because pain on injection of alcohol serves to help confirm needle placement. To precede the injection of any neurolytic drug with an injection of local anesthetic optimizes comfort and serves as "test dose" to rule out incorrect needle placement, which could lead to irreversible side effects. Some burning or pain is still likely but is tolerated well when patients are forewarned. Extreme care must be taken to brace the needle to keep it immobile while syringes are changed.

Alcohol is commercially available in 1- and 5-mL ampules as a colorless solution that can be injected readily through small-bore needles and is hypobaric with respect to cerebrospinal fluid (CSF). Specific gravity is not a concern for injecting on the peripheral nerve, because injection takes place in a nonfluid medium. In the periphery, alcohol generally is used undiluted. Denervation and pain relief accrue over a few days after injection and are usually complete after a week. If pain relief has not occurred by 3 weeks, then neurolysis is incomplete and needs to be repeated.

Phenol

Injectable phenol requires preparation by a pharmacist. Various concentrations of phenol, ranging from 3% to 15% and prepared with saline, water, glycerine, and different radiocontrast solutions, have been advocated. Phenol is relatively insoluble in water, and at room temperature phenol concentrations in excess of 6.7% cannot be obtained without the addition of glycerine. Phenol mixed in glycerine is hyperbaric with respect to CSF but is so viscid that, even when warmed, injection is difficult through needles smaller in caliber than 20 gauge. Shelf life is said to exceed 1 year when preparations are refrigerated and are not exposed to light. Biphasic action observed clinically is characterized by an initial local anesthetic effect producing subjective warmth and numbness that gives way to neurolysis. It is our impression that the hypalgesia that follows phenol injection generally is not as dense as that after alcohol. Quality and extent of analgesia may fade slightly within the first 24 hours after administration, perhaps because of its local anesthetic action. The neurolytic action of phenol may be evident clinically only after 3 to 7 days. As with alcohol injection, if pain relief is inadequate at 2 weeks, neurolysis may be incomplete and another injection required.

Although some authors have suggested that alcohol and phenol are essentially interchangeable, neuritis is more likely with injections of alcohol. Most clinicians use phenol when a peripheral injection is indicated in patients with unknown life expectancy, to minimize the chance of neuritis. Typically, alcohol has been selected for injection of the cranial nerves.[19]

Alternative Techniques and Agents

Although alternatives for interrupting nerve transmission are less commonly applied, they warrant discussion here. Surgical interruption of peripheral nerves is rarely performed, in part because percutaneous nerve ablation is preferable to surgery, which is generally more invasive. Glycerol, noted only serendipitously to have neurolytic properties and used to treat idiopathic trigeminal neuralgia,[20] is being investigated for peripheral blocks. Butyl aminobenzoate (butamben), an anesthetic reported to have neurolytic characteristics, is expected to be a subject of further research.[21-24] Cryoanalgesia has its proponents,[25] but results have been disappointing, despite the theoretical advantage of producing reversible injury. Results of cryoanalgesia are often transient, the probes are bulky, and the technique requires exquisitely precise placement, which often necessitates the creation of lesions under direct vision. It probably should be reserved for patients with longer life expectancies, when it is essential to minimize the likelihood of neuritis. In contrast, thermal ablation by means of radiofrequency (RF) coagulation has numerous potential advantages over injection techniques and is increasing in popularity. RF probes are superior to those used for cryogenic lesioning, and the discrete, controllable lesion that results avoids the uncertainties associated with the spread of injected solutions. An RF lesion is produced within seconds, so great care must be taken to ensure that the probe is positioned properly. Unfortunately, neuritis can be a side effect with lesioning of peripheral nerves.

More recently, pulsed RF is being studied as a neuromodulatory technique. A pulsed RF lesion is achieved by applying RF energy with a pulsed time cycle of 2 × 20 msec/sec at temperatures not exceeding 42° C. This pulsing creates a silent phase that allows for the circulation and conductivity to heat or eliminate the heat that has been produced during the active phase.[26] While the effect is not neurodestructive, the electromagnetic field (EMF) created by traditional RF lesioning and thought to have clinical benefit is still present. The mechanism of the neuromodulation is unclear, but it could be due to the high current in the EMF that may disrupt the sodium or calcium pump in the ganglion, rendering the nerve less likely to transmit painful impulses and decreasing its capability to generate an action potential.[27] A preliminary study by Sluijter and colleagues compared the short-term clinical effects of a 42° C lesion made with conventional, continuous RF and a lesion made with pulsed RF. Among a total of 60 patients, the clinical effect of pulsed RF was superior to the conventional RF. More important, there was no neuritis-like reaction.[28] The merits of pulsed RF are these: It is a painless procedure (and does not require local anesthetic) because no depolarization takes place; it has no neuritis-like reactions or observed side effects, and clinically, it is not neurodestructive.[26] Pulsed RF may be used with clinical benefit for peripheral nerves such as peripheral nerve roots, the saphenous nerve, and the suprascapular nerve.

C3 Dorsal Root Ganglion Pulsed Radiofrequency

INDICATIONS

Pulsed RF may be applied to specific dorsal root ganglia in the cervical, thoracic, and lumbar regions.[1] These specific lesions may be used to palliate local pain due to postherpetic neuralgia, cancer pain, or failed neck surgery syndrome.[29]

ANATOMY

The cervical nerve roots exit their respective intervertebral foramina just below the transverse processes. The dorsal root of each spinal nerve has a dorsal root ganglion located in the intervertebral foramen, where it rests on the pedicle of the vertebral arch. Distal to the spinal ganglion and outside the intervertebral foramen, the dorsal and ventral nerve roots unite to form a spinal nerve. This nerve divides into a ventral ramus and a dorsal ramus.[30] The ventral ramus has motor innervation to the diaphragm (C3–C5), the neck muscles, the intercostal muscles, and the muscles of the upper extremity. The posterior division innervates the zygoapophyseal joints and certain posterior neck muscles.[31]

TECHNIQUE

C3–C7 Nerve Roots. The patient is placed in the prone position. The lateral aspect of the neck is prepared and draped using a sterile technique. The level of the cervical dorsal root ganglion (DRG) to be lesioned is identified in the anteroposterior (AP) and then the lateral view. The view is then changed to oblique to obtain the "string of pearls," the lateral mass of the cervical vertebra, posterior to the foramen. A skin wheal is raised over the targeted area using 1 mL of 1.5% lidocaine and a 25-gauge needle. A 16-gauge Angiocath is inserted through the skin wheal and directed at the pearl at the desired level (i.e., C2–3 for C2). A 5-cm, curved, blunt-tipped RF needle with a 5-mm active tip is directed through the angiocath to the middle of the pearl (Fig. 51–1). The needle is then checked in the AP view to ensure that it is at the "waist" of the articular pillar (Fig. 51–2).[32] Using the oblique view, the needle is then advanced to the anterior edge of the pearl (or lateral mass). This should be confirmed in the AP view to be at the midpoint (from lateral to medial) of the articular pillar. Needle placement may be confirmed with the spread of water-soluble, nonionic contrast medium demonstrating spread into the epidural space and out the desired nerve root sleeve. More specific placement can be obtained with sensory stimulation with the pulsed RF generator. The generator is set on 50 Hz, and paresthesia in the nerve root

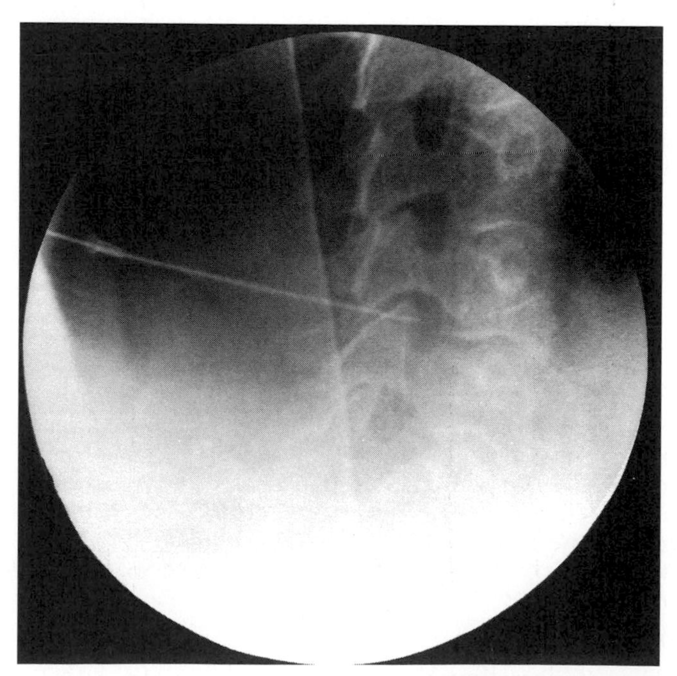

FIGURE 51–1 Lateral view of the radiofrequency needle directed through the angiocatheter to the middle of the pearl.

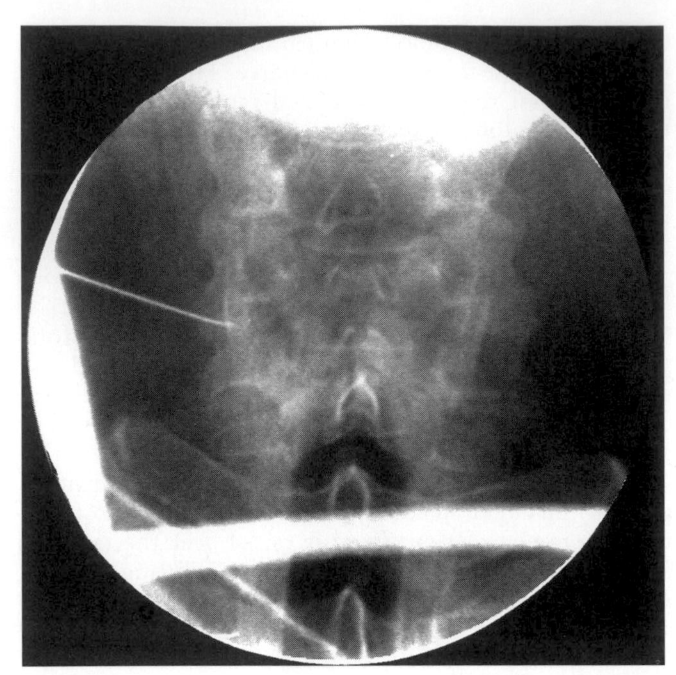

FIGURE 51-2 Anteroposterior view of the needle at the "waist" of the articular pillar. It is advanced to the midpoint of the pillar (from lateral to medial).

distribution between 0.3 and 0.7 V indicates satisfactory placement. Stimulation at 0.5 V is optimal. Stimulation with less than 0.3 V may indicate intraneural placement, so the needle must be retracted and redirected. Stimulation obtained with more than 0.7 V signifies that the needle is very near the desired ganglion, and minimal advancement will achieve optimal placement. After confirmation of the needle placement, the dorsal root ganglion undergoes pulsed RF at 42° C for 120 sec. This procedure is repeated twice, for a total of three applications. The needles are then withdrawn, and the site is covered with antibiotic and a Bandaid.

COMPLICATIONS

Potential risks of this procedure include entry into the epidural or subarachnoid space through the intervertebral foramen and injection into the nearby vertebral artery. Third occipital nerve blocks and C2 ganglion blocks may also be associated with unsteadiness and slight ataxia owing to interruption of the upper cervical proprioceptive afferents.[33, 34]

Suprascapular Nerve Pulsed Radiofrequency

INDICATIONS

Suprascapular nerve pulsed RF may be used as a palliative for chronic shoulder pain due to rotator cuff syndrome, frozen shoulder, chronic capsulitis, nerve entrapment secondary to scarring, or rheumatoid arthritis involving the glenohumoral joint.[35] The suprascapular nerve is the main sensory nerve to the shoulder and is easily accessed percutaneously.[36, 37]

TECHNIQUE

The patient is placed in the sitting position. The shoulder area is prepared and draped with sterile technique. The scapular spine is identified and bisected. A point is identified approximately one fingerbreadth superior to the midpoint of the spine of the scapula (Fig. 51–3).[37] A skin wheal is raised using 1 mL of 1.5% lidocaine and a 25-gauge needle. A 16-gauge angiocath is advanced through the skin wheal 1 to 2 cm. The upper extremity on the same side as the block is flexed at the elbow and rotated medially so that the hand is moved from the anatomic position to be placed on the opposite shoulder. This movement elevates the scapula away from the posterior wall and increases the potential distance the needle travels from the skin to the chest wall while searching for paresthesia.[38] A 10-cm curved, blunt RF needle with 10-mm active tip is advanced through the Angiocath to a total depth of 3 to 4 cm from the surface of the skin. Sensory stimulation is then tested with the pulsed RF generator at 50 Hz. A paresthesia in the distribution of the suprascapular nerve should be detected between 0.3 and 0.7 V for optimal placement. The nerve is then lesioned three times at 42° C for 120 sec. The needles are removed. The site is covered with antibiotic ointment and a Bandaid. The prone position may also be used with fluoroscopy as an alternative technique for pulsed RF. When using fluoroscopy, by directing the beam 30 degrees lateral to medial oblique with 5 degrees of caudocephalad rotation, the superior notch of the scapula is clearly visualized (Figs. 51–4, 51–5). The needle is directed

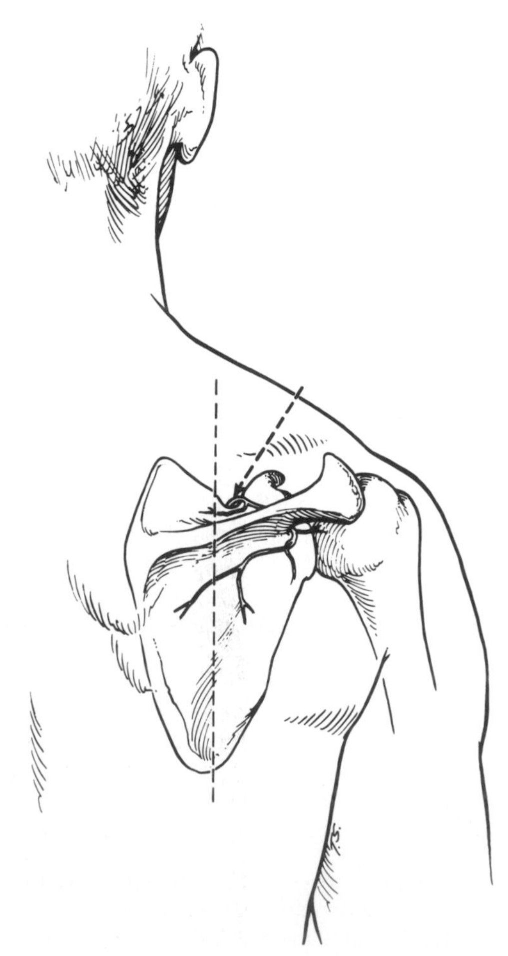

FIGURE 51-3 Drawing of the scapula illustrates the scapular spine and relation of the superior notch to the midpoint of the scapula.

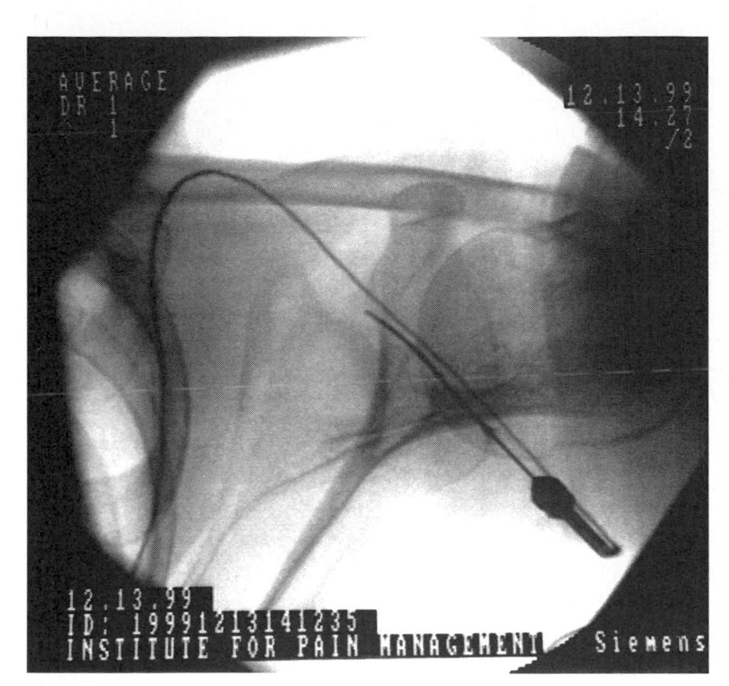

FIGURE 51–4 Oblique view of the scapula with the tip of the needle at the inferior aspect of the superior notch.

at the superior notch and "walked off." Motor and sensory stimulation may then be tested as above and the patient is then lesioned as previously discussed.

COMPLICATIONS

The most significant potential complication is inadvertent pneumothorax. A postprocedure chest film is mandatory.

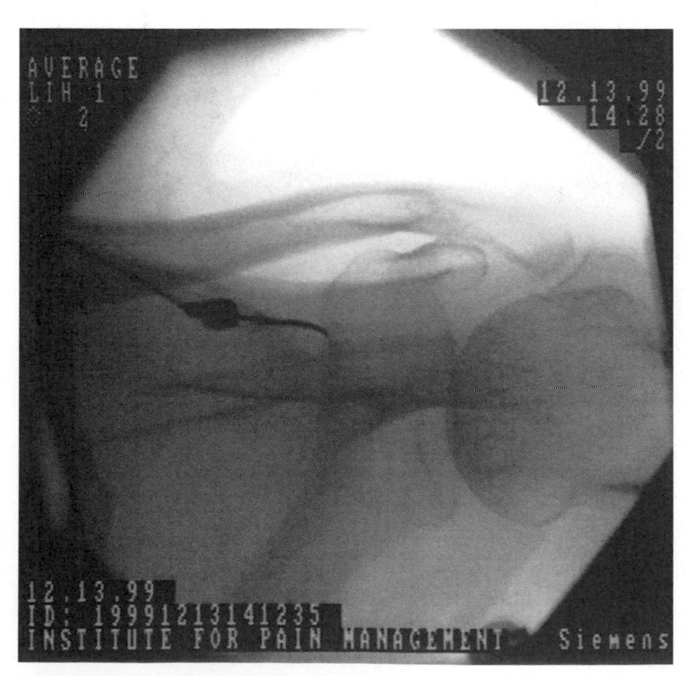

FIGURE 51–5 Anteroposterior view of the scapula with the tip of the needle in the superior notch.

Saphenous Nerve Pulsed Radiofrequency

INDICATIONS

Pulsed RF of the saphenous nerve may be used for neuritis in the distribution of the saphenous nerve secondary to scar entrapment from earlier injury or surgery. A successful diagnostic block should be performed before pulsed RF.

ANATOMY

The saphenous nerve is a purely sensory nerve that provides sensation to the anteromedial aspect of the lower leg from the knee to and including the medial malleolus.[39] It is located in the subsartorial canal, which extends from the apex of the femoral triangle, where the adductor longus meets the sartorius muscle, and continues distally under cover of the sartorius muscle in a triangular space bounded by the adductor longus and anteromedially by a strong apneurosis, which, under the sartorius, acts as a roof to the adductor canal. The subsartorial canal contains the femoral blood vessels and two nerves, the saphenous nerve and the nerve to the vastus medialis (before it enters the muscle), all of which run alongside each other maintaining a regular relationship lateral to the femoral artery in the proximal part of the adductor canal before the saphenous nerve crosses to the medial side of the artery. (Fig. 51–6)[40, 41]

TECHNIQUE

The technique as described by Mansour is performed by first palpating the groove between the vastus medialis and

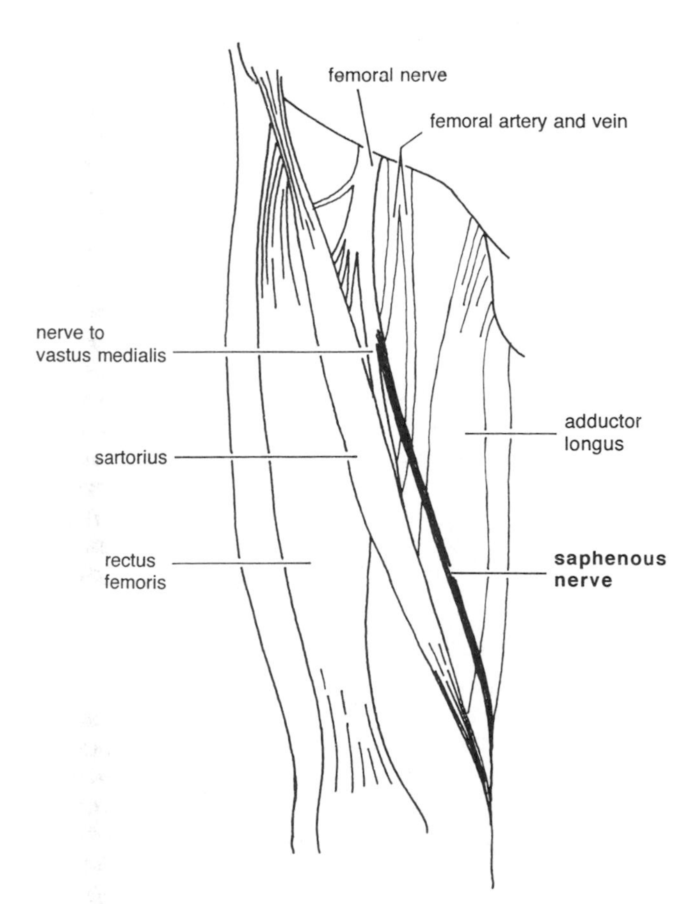

FIGURE 51–6 Drawing of the relationship of the sartorius to the saphenous nerve.

sartorius.[40] This is felt by gently rolling the finger from the lateral side medially. The sartorius muscle will be more prominent if the knee is flexed and the hip laterally rotated in semiflexion and abduction. This resembles the squatting position. The groove is most readily identifiable at the middle third of the thigh when the extremity is in this position, because the subsartorial (adductor) canal then faces forward more than medially, and the needle can be inserted at a right angle to the line of the thigh.[40] A skin wheal is raised using 1 mL of 1.5% lidocaine and a 25-gauge needle. A 16-gauge Angiocath is advanced through the skin wheal. Further penetration is made with a 10-cm, curved, blunt-tipped RF needle with a 10-mm active tip until a "click" is felt. This is the roof of the adductor canal. The needle is connected to the pulsed RF generator and is advanced until a paresthesia is detected in the distribution of the saphenous nerve with a stimulation of 50 Hz between 0.3 and 0.7 V (0.5 V being preferable). A motor stimulation test performed at 2 Hz and 2 V should be negative. A pulsed RF lesion should be performed three times at 42° C for 120 sec.

COMPLICATIONS

A potential complication specific to this procedure would be weakness secondary to lesioning of the nerve to the vastus medialis.

PERIPHERAL NEUROLYSIS IN THE HEAD AND NECK

The most common indication for neurolysis in the head and neck region is intractable pain due to cancer. Head and neck pain due to cancer remains a therapeutic challenge,[42] particularly when radiotherapy has proved ineffective or has already been maximized. Conventional analgesic therapy may be inadequate because of both the erosive nature of many tumors and the area's rich innervation. Furthermore, physiologic splinting, ordinarily an important protective reflex, is often ineffective for craniocervical pain, because it is aggravated by the relatively involuntary motion produced by swallowing, eating, coughing, talking, and other movements of the head. Despite overlapping contributions from cranial nerves V, VII, IX, and X and the upper cervical nerves, pain relief often can be obtained with carefully planned nerve blocks. Success of treatment may be affected adversely by anatomic distortion induced by previous surgery or radiotherapy and by the potential for tumor invasion or radiation fibrosis to reduce contact between the neurolytic and targeted nerve tissue, a so-called sheltering effect. Typically, there is considerable overlap among the sensory fields of neighboring nerves. For this reason and because of the influence of the cranial nerves on swallowing and breathing, neurolytic blocks should be preceded by diagnostic and prognostic local anesthetic injections. Despite these considerations, blockade of the cranial or upper cervical nerves is of great value in certain patients.

Trigeminal Ganglion and Nerve Neurolysis

Blockade of the trigeminal nerve within the foramen ovale at the base of the skull or of its branches may be adequate to relieve localized pain in the face. Lysis of the second or third division is usually performed via the extraoral route. Maxillary nerve block is indicated for pain involving the middle third of the face (i.e., the maxilla, cheek, nasal cavity, hard palate, and tonsillar fossa). Mandibular nerve block is indicated for pain involving the jaw and anterior two thirds of the tongue. Alcohol block of the mandibular nerve has occasionally caused skin slough.[9] Neurolytic blockade of the ophthalmic nerve is rarely used in contemporary practice.[43] If tumor progression is anticipated, it is preferable to extend the field of analgesia prophylactically by blocking the gasserian ganglion.[19]

Gasserian ganglion injection is considered for pain in the distribution of the second or third division when tumor growth or postsurgical changes block access to the maxillary or mandibular nerve. When pain extends cervically or to the angle of the jaw, supplementary paravertebral blockade of the second or third cervical nerve roots may be necessary for more complete relief of pain.[44] Blockade of the smaller branches of the trigeminal nerve has been described[7] and may be undertaken for well-localized pain in a confined distribution, particularly for pain due to a lesion that is more likely to erode than to spread or when anatomic distortion blocks access to the parent nerves (Figs. 51–7 to 51–9).

Glossopharyngeal and Vagal Neurolysis

For pain that is less well-localized or is concentrated near the base of the tongue, pharynx, or throat, blockade of

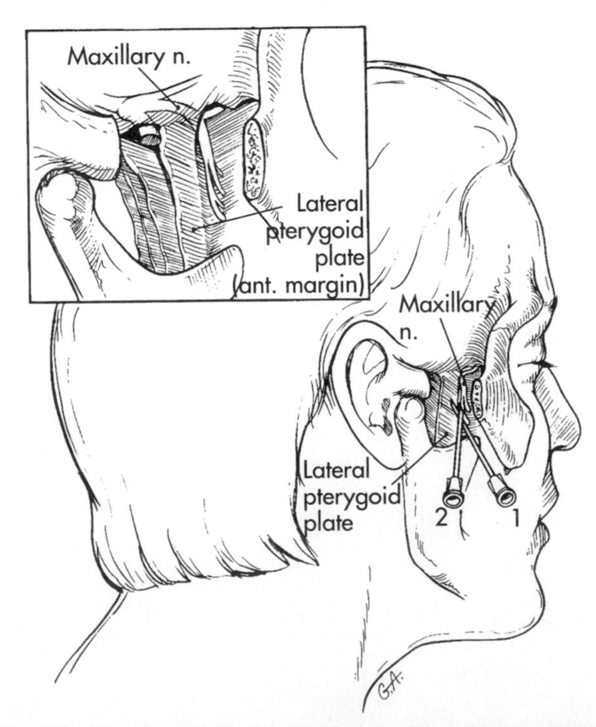

FIGURE 51–7 Maxillary nerve block. 1, The depth of needle entry necessary to reach lateral pterygoid plate; 2, the anterior direction of the needle required to slip off the pterygoid plate to reach the maxillary nerve. Inset, Magnification of pterygopalatine fossa through which the maxillary nerve travels. (From Katz J: Somatic nerve blocks. In Raj PP [ed]: Practical Management of Pain, 2nd ed. St. Louis, Mosby–Year Book, 1992.)

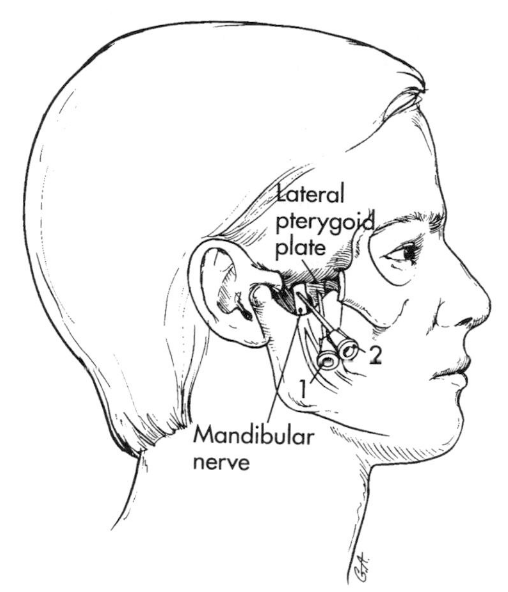

FIGURE 51–8 *Mandibular nerve block.* 1, *The initial needle direction needed to reach the lateral pterygoid plate;* 2, *the posterior direction of the needle required to reach the mandibular nerve at the base of the skull as it exits the foramen ovale. (From Katz J: Somatic nerve blocks.* In *Raj PP [ed:] Practical Management of Pain, 2nd ed. St. Louis, Mosby–Year Book, 1992.)*

C9 or C10 may be required to achieve more complete relief.[45, 46] The sensory field of the glossopharyngeal nerve includes the nasopharynx, eustachian tube, soft palate, uvula, tonsil, base of the tongue, and part of the external auditory canal. The vagus nerve subserves the larynx and contributes fibers to the ear, external auditory canal, and tympanic membrane. Bilateral destruction of the glossopharyngeal and vagus nerves is not recommended because of the potential for interference with swallowing mechanisms and protective airway reflexes.[7, 19] When available, RF coagulation is the preferred means of lesioning. Blockade of the superior laryngeal nerves has been described for laryngeal pain of tabetic, tuberculous, or malignant origin (Fig. 51–10).[14, 45, 47]

Phrenic Neurolysis

Intractable hiccups (singultus) also is amenable to nerve block therapy. Unilateral phrenic nerve block has been used under these circumstances, with excellent results, although conservative measures should be exhausted first.[7, 48] Before a neurolytic phrenic nerve block is performed, the results of a prognostic block with local anesthetic are evaluated to ensure that ventilatory function would not be compromised by a more permanent procedure.

When intractable craniocervical pain is not amenable to nerve block therapy, either intraspinal opioid therapy by means of an implanted cervical epidural catheter[49] or intraventricular opioid therapy may be considered.[49, 50] Numerous neurosurgical procedures have been devised to manage rostral pain, but they have limited practical value because they are invasive and have high rates of morbidity and mortality.[1]

Efficacy

In a series of 70 patients in pain from head and neck cancer treated with peripheral and cranial neurolysis, Bonica[45] achieved complete relief of pain for 63% of patients, moderate relief for 31%, and slight or insignificant relief for 6%. Similar results were obtained in an earlier study by Grant.[51] McEwen and associates[52] reported good or fair relief in 70% of cancer patients treated with gasserian ganglion block. Using RF thermocoagulation techniques, Siegfried and Broggi[53] reported lasting comfort in about 50% of 20 patients treated with percutaneous ablation of the trigeminal ganglion. The same authors reported good results in two patients treated with thermal ablation of the glossopharyngeal nerve.[54] Although one patient underwent

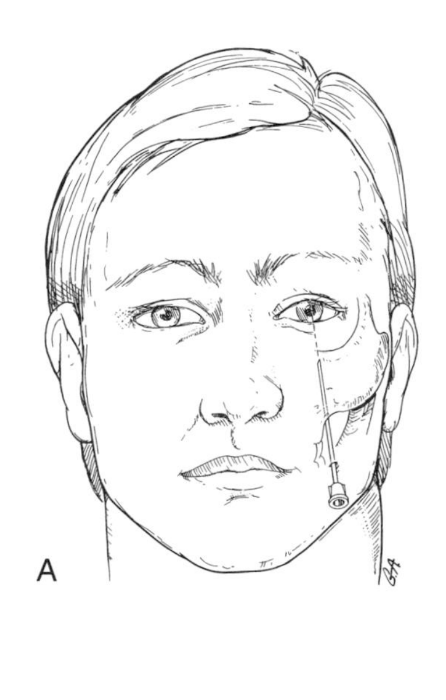

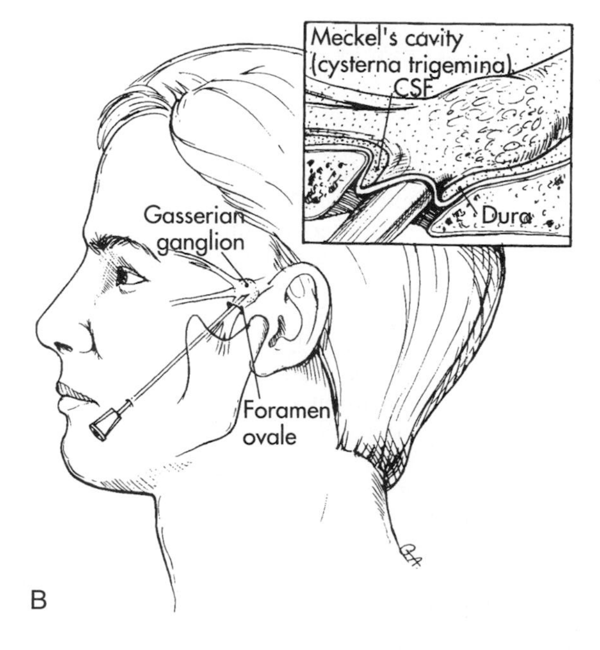

FIGURE 51–9 *Trigeminal (gasserian) ganglion block.* A, *The needle direction in the anterior view. The needle tip is in line with the pupil.* B, *Lateral view illustrates the posterosuperior direction of the needle tip, in front of the ear and at the superior edge of the coronoid notch. (From Katz J: Somatic nerve blocks.* In *Raj PP [ed]: Practical Management of Pain, 2nd ed. St. Louis, Mosby–Year Book, 1992.)*

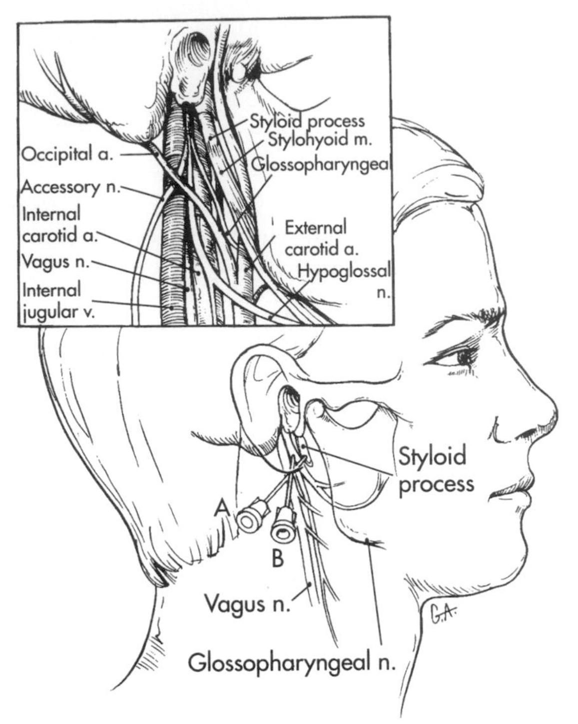

FIGURE 51–10 Glossopharyngeal and vagus nerve block. Needle direction for either glossopharyngeal, A, *or vagus,* B, *nerve block at the level of the styloid process.* Inset, *The relationships of important structures in that area. (From Katz J: Somatic nerve blocks.* In *Raj PP [ed]: Practical Management of Pain, 2nd ed. St. Louis, Mosby–Year Book, 1992.)*

a repeat procedure at 6 mo for recurrence of pain and the other had temporary dysphagia and permanent 12th nerve palsy, long-term results ultimately were gratifying. Using an anterior approach, Pagura and colleagues[55] reported good to excellent results in 15 cancer patients treated with thermocoagulation of the glossopharyngeal nerve. Treatment was supplemented by trigeminal thermoablation in eight patients because of overlapping pain.

PERIPHERAL NEUROLYSIS OF THE UPPER EXTREMITY

All neurolytic procedures that have the potential to relieve upper extremity pain carry the risk of producing weakness in the limb. Carefully performed, cervical subarachnoid neurolytic injections of phenol or alcohol are likely to relieve pain without affecting motor function, because the drug is deposited preferentially on the sensory rootlets. Paravertebral somatic block is applicable for localized pain, and, even then, because of sensory overlap, multiple nerves usually need to be blocked, and some motor dysfunction should be anticipated. Radiologic guidance is strongly recommended for neurolytic paravertebral block as is careful observation of the effects of preneurolytic test doses of local anesthetic and fractionated administration to avoid subarachnoid or epidural spread. The brachial plexus has a large proportion of motor fibers and therefore is not to be injected unless motor strength is already deficient (as in some cases of Pancoast's tumor) or unless the arm already is rendered useless by intractable pain (as with a pathologic fracture). Relatively little experience has been reported with neurolytic block of the more peripheral nerves of the upper limb (Fig. 51–11).

Efficacy

Bonica[7] infiltrated 20 mL of 95% alcohol on the brachial plexus, which did paralyze the upper extremity but relieved pain until death. Pain relief lasted from 3.5 wk to 3.5 mo after injections of 5% aqueous phenol on the brachial plexus. Kaplan and associates[56] reported on a single but well-documented case of phenol brachial plexus block in a patient with recurrent sarcoma involving the humeral head. After a successful prognostic local anesthetic block, 12.5 mL of 6% phenol in water injected by the supraclavicular route resulted in significant but incomplete pain relief. Residual pain was managed by supplementary paravertebral phenol blocks of C5 and C6, and later, in response to increased tumor growth, T1–T3 paravertebral blocks (0.5 to 1.0 mL of 6% aqueous phenol per segment). In another report of a single case, Neill[57] achieved excellent palliation of pain secondary to a pathologic fracture of the humerus in a man with multiple myeloma by means of two successive interscalene injections of 20 mL of 50% alcohol. In a report of five cases, Mullin[58] used an interscalene injection of 3% aqueous phenol to manage the pain of Pancoast's syndrome. Excellent short-term relief of pain was obtained in all patients and was sustained for as long as 7 mo in three, though only at the expense of relatively frequent repetition of the injections at 3- to 6-wk intervals. Absence of neurologic sequelae suggested that dilute phenol, although its effects are short lived, may be relatively safe for patients with normal motor function.

In response to concerns about reports of inadequate or short-lived analgesia after lytic brachial plexus block, Patt and Millard[10] elected treatment with a higher concentration of phenol than had been reported previously. Four patients underwent brachial plexus block with 10 to 20 mL of 10% to 12% aqueous phenol mixed with 20% glycerine to main-

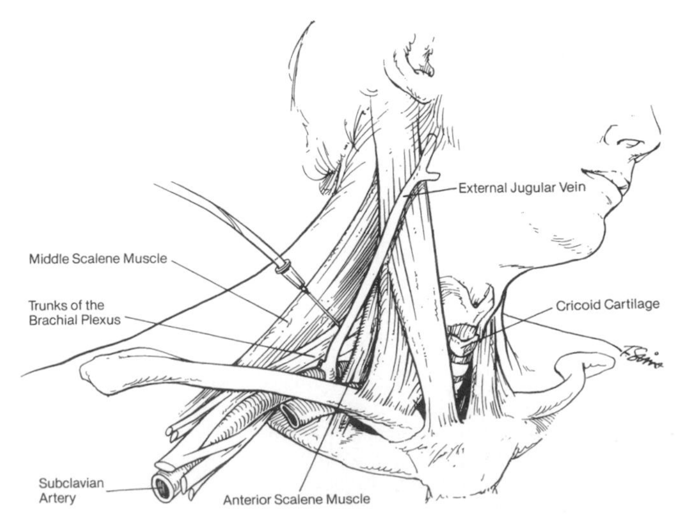

FIGURE 51–11 Brachial plexus block. (From Katz J: Somatic nerve blocks. In *Raj PP [ed]: Practical Management of Pain, 2nd ed. St. Louis, Mosby–Year Book, 1992.)*

tain the phenol's miscibility in water. The solution was mildly viscid and readily injectable through a 20- or 22-gauge needle. Three patients had pain and muscle weakness secondary to tumor invasion of the apex of the lung and brachial plexus, and one patient with breast cancer had painful metastases to the cervical spine. Pain persisted in the last patient, despite two cervical subarachnoid neurolytic blocks. One patient also had a pathologic fracture of the humerus, and all four had a useless limb because of either neurologic involvement or intractable pain. Patt and Millard[10] used an axillary approach in all patients. A paresthesia or positive response to electrical nerve stimulation was relied on for verification of needle placement in all but one procedure, which was conducted under fluoroscopy through a catheter. Good to excellent pain relief was obtained for all patients until they died—two patients at 12 weeks, one patient at 8 weeks, and the fourth at 5 weeks. No unexpected complications occurred. Increased motor weakness was observed in all cases but was tolerated well. Interestingly, in three of the four cases, relief of pain was not immediate but accrued over several days.

An additional patient with shoulder and upper arm pain was referred to Patt and Millard[10] for brachial plexus block but was found to have excellent upper limb strength. After a diagnostic and prognostic local anesthetic block, she was treated instead with 4 mL of 10% phenol injected in the vicinity of the suprascapular nerve, which was localized with a nerve stimulator. No loss of motor power occurred, and she had excellent pain relief until her death 8 weeks later. Another preterminal patient with shoulder pain secondary to multiple myeloma received a suprascapular nerve block with 4 mL of absolute alcohol, which resulted in moderate relief of pain without complications until his death 4 weeks later. A third patient with pain due to a parascapular soft tissue mass secondary to lung cancer experienced good pain relief for 4 weeks after a phenol suprascapular nerve block with 5 mL of 10% phenol. Pain gradually returned, and the patient was persuaded to undergo radiotherapy, which provided pain relief that lasted until his death.

PERIPHERAL NEUROLYSIS OF THORACIC AND ABDOMINAL WALL NERVES

Pain originating in the thoracic or abdominal wall or the parietal peritoneum can be treated with multiple intercostal[14, 59–61] or paravertebral blocks.[7, 62] Except after pneumonectomy, blocks performed in the thoracic region carry the risk of pneumothorax, although, when proper technique is observed, this complication should occur infrequently.[60] Use of radiologic guidance has been reported for intercostal block.[6] Most clinicians walk the needle off the rib, and paresthesias is usually relied on as a guide for placement. Localized bone pain associated with rib metastases may also respond to local infiltration around the bone with steroids, a technique that has produced good responses. Radiologic guidance is strongly recommended for neurolytic paravertebral block, as is careful observation of the effects of preneurolysis test doses of local anesthetic and fractionated administration to avoid subarachnoid, epidural, and intrapleural spread, all of which have been documented (Fig. 51–12).[63]

Efficacy

Doyle[59] reported on a series of 46 patients treated in a hospice environment with multiple phenol intercostal blocks. He used 1.0 to 1.5 mL of 6% phenol "in oil" per segment and obtained total relief of pain for a mean duration of 3 wk (range 1 to 6 wk). Radiologic guidance was not used, and no complications occurred. As an illustration that radiologic confirmation is advisable, a patient with adhesions experienced acute bronchospasm after presumed (unintentional) intrabronchial or intrapulmonary injection of 0.5 mL of 8% phenol in saline.[64]

Bonica[7] reported favorable results subsequent to the paravertebral injection of 1 mL of alcohol per involved segment in patients with abdominal and chest wall pain secondary to vertebral, paravertebral, and visceral neoplasms associated with peritoneal invasion. In an anecdotal report, Vernon[65] noted good relief of back pain of metastatic origin and no untoward effects after paravertebral injection of alcohol in two patients, although little detail was provided in the report.

Mehta and Ranger[66] reported on blocks of individual branches of the lumbar plexus in 103 patients with abdominal pain of unknown cause. The authors describe having blocked the iliohypogastric (65 patients), ilioinguinal (one patient), and upper and lower intercostal (two patients) nerves within the rectus sheath with 2 to 3 mL of aqueous

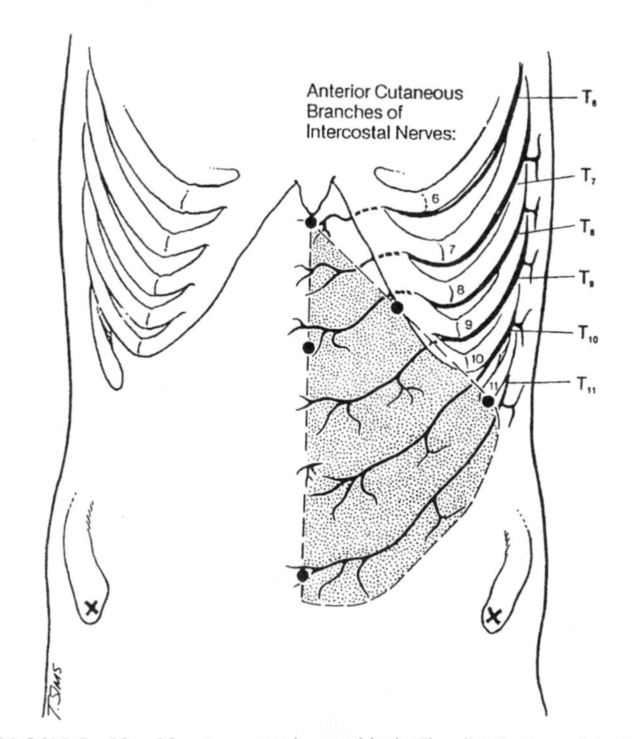

FIGURE 51–12 Intercostal nerve block. The distribution of the intercostal nerves T6 to T11 in the abdominal wall. They can be "neurolysed" for pain in the somatic structures of the abdomen. (From Raj PP, Pai U: Technique of nerve blocking. In *Raj PP, Pai U [eds]: Handbook of Regional Anesthesia. New York, Churchill Livingstone, 1985.)*

phenol. Follow-up at 3 weeks revealed complete and partial relief of pain in 58% and 32% of patients, respectively, and 70% of respondents and had no recurrence at 3-year follow-up.

PERIPHERAL NEUROLYSIS OF PERINEAL AND LOWER EXTREMITY NERVES

Treatment of intractable perineal and lower limb pain is difficult, because such pain is often bilateral or midline in distribution and the relevant neuroanatomy predisposes to paresis and incontinence when neurolytic techniques are applied. When bowel and bladder function are not of concern because of preexisting dysfunction or surgical diversion, neurolytic subarachnoid block should be considered.

Decision making is more difficult in a continent, ambulatory patient with intractable pain. Although neurolytic subarachnoid and epidural blocks can be performed relatively safely in the thoracic region, these techniques are hazardous in the lumbosacral region, even with careful attention to technique.

Blocks of the hypogastric plexus and ganglion impar have been introduced[67, 68] and can now be regarded as options for pelvic or rectal pain that is sympathetically mediated. The sacral roots are accessed readily as they emerge from the posterior plate of the sacrum, and injections here may relieve pelvic, rectal, and lower extremity pain. Selective sacral root block is preferable to spinal injections in this region for patients with normal urinary and bowel function, because, carefully executed, nerve blocks here do not affect continence.[69] A single sacral nerve, most often the third[70] but sometimes the fourth,[71] usually exerts a dominant influence on bladder musculature, and, as a result, blockade of the nondominant nerves based on trials of local anesthetic injections has little urodynamic effect. Radiologic guidance is a useful adjunct to sacral nerve block. The foramina are not well-visualized on anteroposterior views, but needle penetration of the posterior sacral plate is readily apparent on lateral views. Neurolytic injections of other peripheral nerves subserving the lower extremity are sometimes attempted, but generally only after local anesthetic injection has confirmed that pain reduction is possible without much affecting motor function (Fig. 51–13).

Efficacy

Robertson[69] described a series of nine patients with intractable perineal pain secondary to carcinoma of the rectum. After a test block with local anesthetic of the sacral nerves, he injected 2.5 mL of 6% aqueous phenol at the S4 foramen on the side of the greatest pain. Satisfactory analgesia was obtained in all cases and persisted in two patients for 202 and 414 days after single blocks. Duration was inadequate in the other patients, but after second or third injections, pain relief was maintained uniformly until death. In seven of the nine patients, duration of relief from the first neurolysis was less than 10 days, a finding that suggests that most patients require repeated treatment, but this limitation was mitigated by the ease of repetition. Motor and autonomic function were unaffected, and no other complications occurred. In a similar study on patients with bladder pain secondary to spasticity, Simon and colleagues[72] obtained an average of 26.5 mo of pain relief in patients after sacral injections of 2 mL of 6% aqueous phenol. Most patients had relief with unilateral blockade of the third sacral nerve, although preliminary local anesthetic blocks identified some patients whose pain was mediated by S2 and S4. Several patients required repeat treatment, and no lasting complications were observed.

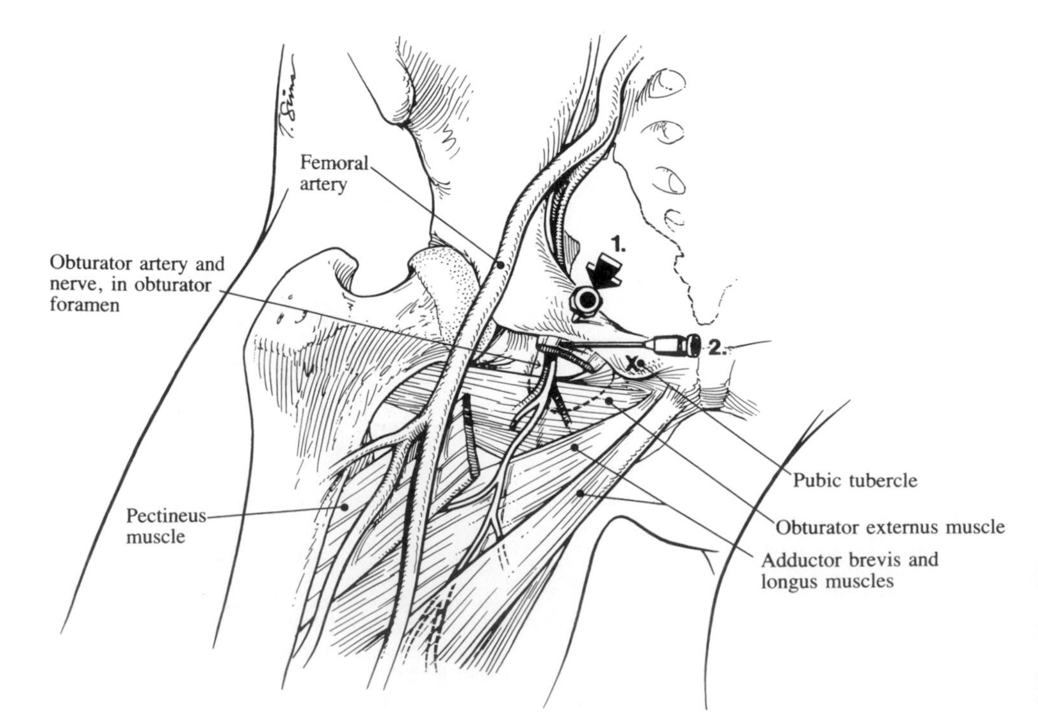

FIGURE 51–13 Anatomy of the technique of the obturator nerve block. The obturator nerve is shown to exit from the obturator foramen. The needle position, 1, on the superior ramus and, 2, in the obturator foramen. (From Raj PP, Pai U: Upper and lower extremity. In *Raj PP [ed]: Practical Management of Pain, 2nd ed. St. Louis, Mosby–Yearbook, 1992.)*

An isolated report of bladder atony after otherwise successful S3 and S4 alcohol block[73] emphasizes the need for careful observation of the results of preneurolysis prognostic blocks with local anesthetic. A well-designed study[69] assessed the spread of a mixture of radiopaque contrast solution and local anesthetic injected in 1- and 2-mL aliquots for sacral block. The authors demonstrated wider spread of solution with the larger volume and concluded that 1 mL of anesthetic is sufficient to produce a selective sacral nerve root block. They were able also to demonstrate that reflux into the sacral canal was much less likely when the needle tip was positioned at the anterior border of the sacrum rather than in the midportion of the sacral foramen. It is not certain, however, how these results apply to the spread of neurolytic solutions. Successful treatment of penile pain and malignant priapism secondary to venous obstruction from bladder cancer has been reported anecdotally with injections of 5% aqueous phenol near the dorsal nerves of the penis, close to the symphysis pubis.[74] Feldman and Yeung,[75] treating 26 patients for intractable claudication with paravertebral injections of lumbar somatic nerve using 5 to 10 mL of 7.5% phenol in myodil, reported good long-term improvement without negative sequelae. Doyle[59] mentioned performing two femoral nerve blocks with phenol in a patient with invasion of the femoral sheath area but provided no other details. Patt and Millard[10] performed alcohol injection of the sciatic nerve in a patient with preexisting motor weakness from invasion of the nerve by pelvic tumor, with good short-term results. They observed heightened distress and poor tolerance of resulting footdrop in other patients with less complete motor deficit, even though they had had prognostic local anesthetic sciatic nerve blocks. Rastogi and Kumar[5] make a brief mention of "successful" alcohol block of the sciatic nerve in three patients with cancer. Singler reported on a single case of successful sciatic and femoral neurolysis performed with 75% alcohol for intractable spasticity.[10] A few reports have appeared documenting the injection of the lumbar somatic nerves with phenol within the psoas sheath for the relief of ischemic pain.[75, 76] That 5 to 10 mL of 7% phenol[75] and 5 mL of 10% phenol[76] dissolved in contrast medium was injected without significant neurologic side effects is surprising but suggests potential applications in patients with cancer.

PERIPHERAL NEUROLYSIS FOR SPASTICITY

Peripheral nerve blocks with phenol have been advocated for spastic patients to improve balance, gait, self-care, and overall rehabilitation. An important distinction between peripheral neurolytic blocks for pain and for spasticity is that, in the latter, motor or mixed nerves are targeted preferentially. Nevertheless, given the paucity of data on peripheral neurolytic blocks for the management of pain, it is worthwhile to try to extrapolate from information obtained from work with spastic patients.

Moritz[77] reported on a series of 50 spastic patients who received a total of 90 peripheral nerve blocks (musculocutaneous, median, ulnar, tibial, obturator, femoral, and superior gluteal nerves) performed with either 2% phenol in saline or 3% aqueous phenol. A nerve stimulator was used for needle localization. Focal motor weakness lasted only about 1 wk in 15% of patients, but the average duration of effect was 8 mo. Moritz[77] noted transient dysesthesias (10%) that usually resolved in days or weeks with no sensory disturbances, a finding that is not surprising, given the dilute solutions used. Reporting on 521 blocks of peripheral nerves performed with 6% aqueous phenol, Gibson[78] noted one serious complication, in a 69-year-old hemiplegic patient, who, after five successful blocks, underwent a brachioradialis and musculocutaneous block and subsequently developed an arterial occlusion in the upper limb that required a high amputation.

LOCAL NEUROLYTIC INJECTION

Local anesthetic or steroid injection of "trigger points" is a well-accepted means of managing chronic myofascial pain. The clinical effects of locally injected neurolytics are unknown, and local infiltration generally is avoided because of concerns about skin slough and worsening of pain by local ischemia or necrosis. Cousins and associates[17] refer to the practice of injecting persistent trigger points with 5% to 6% aqueous phenol but caution that further research is needed to determine its safety and efficacy.

Ramamurthy and colleagues[2] mention having performed three "myoneural" blocks with 6% aqueous phenol but provide no further details. In a study of patients with painful palpable peripheral neuromas, local injections of 0.1 to 0.5 mL of 5% phenol in glycerine were performed.[79] Fifteen neuromas were treated in 10 patients with a total of 20 blocks. Complete relief was produced and sustained in all but one patient during the 8- to 22-month follow-up period, and no complications or neuritis was reported. In another series of patients with poststernotomy pain presumably due to scar neuroma,[80, 81] 17 patients were treated with multiple, serial local neurolytic injections of 2 to 3 mL of 6% aqueous phenol or 1.5 to 2.0 mL of absolute alcohol. Complete relief was obtained in most patients, and no complications referable to neurolysis were observed. Finally, Defalque[82] obtained complete relief in 63 of 69 patients by performing repeated trigger point injections near surgical scars with 1.0 mL of absolute alcohol and noted no complications other than localized numbness. The implications for the use of this treatment modality in patients with cancer pain are unclear.

Patt and Millard[10] have written of experiences with periosteal injections of dilute aqueous phenol (3%–5%) for persistent refractory bone pain, a technique mentioned by Swerdlow.[62] The two patients treated had minimal relief with periosteal injections of local anesthetic and steroid, and ultimately achieved lasting relief after two neurolytic injections.

Local subcutaneous infiltration with absolute alcohol for intractable anal and vulvar pruritus has been reported by several authors.[61, 83, 84] Although its applicability to cancer pain is indeterminate, the technique deserves mention, owing to its apparent safety in patients with nonmalignant pain and itch. In one series, more than two thirds of patients experienced complete symptomatic relief that persisted 1 to 5 years.[83] Complications were limited to local skin reactions that, although initially distressing, subsided over 2 to 3 weeks.

SUMMARY

Peripheral neurolysis has specific but important indications in the management of intractable cancer pain. It is inappropriate and inadequate for intractable pain of other causes. Careful consideration must be given to more conservative alternative techniques before peripheral neurolysis is attempted.

REFERENCES

1. Patt R: Neurosurgical interventions for chronic pain problems. Anesthesiol Clin North Am 5:609, 1987.
2. Ramamurthy S, Walsh NE, Schoenfeld LS, et al: Evaluation of neurolytic blocks using phenol and cryogenic block in the management of chronic pain. J Pain Symptom Manage 4:72, 1989.
3. Pender JW, Pugh DG: Diagnostic and therapeutic nerve blocks: Necessity for roentgenograms. JAMA 146:798, 1951.
4. Raj PP, Rosenblatt R, Montgomery S: Uses of the nerve stimulator for peripheral blocks. Reg Anesth 5:14, 1980.
5. Rastogi V, Kumar R: Peripheral nerve stimulator as an aid for therapeutic alcohol blocks. Anesthesiology 38:163, 1983.
6. Moore DC: Intercostal nerve block and celiac plexus block for pain therapy. Adv Pain Res Ther 7:309, 1984.
7. Bonica JJ: Management of Pain. Philadelphia, Lea & Febiger, 1953.
8. Roviaro GC, Varoli F, Fascianella A, et al: Intrathoracic intercostal nerve block with phenol in open chest surgery. Chest 90:64, 1986.
9. Moore DC: Regional Block, ed 4. Springfield, Ill. Charles C Thomas, 1965.
10. Patt RB, Millard R: A role for peripheral neurolysis in the management of intractable cancer pain. Pain Suppl 5:S358, 1990.
11. Szalados J, Patt R: Management of a patient with displaced orthopedic hardware. J Pain Sympt Manag 6:934–937, 1991.
12. Takagi Y, Kayama T, Yamamoto Y: Subarachnoid neurolytic block with 15% phenol glycerin in the treatment of cancer pain. Pain Suppl 4:133, 1987.
13. Ischia S, Luzzani A, Pacini L, et al: Lytic saddle block: Clinical comparison of the results, using phenol at 5, 10, and 15 percent. Adv Pain Res Ther 7:339, 1984.
14. Chrucher M: Peripheral nerve blocks in the relief of intractable pain. *In* Swerdlow M, Charlton JE (eds): Relief of Intractable Pain, ed 4. Amsterdam, Elsevier, 1989, p 195.
15. Swerdlow M: Spinal and peripheral neurolysis for managing Pancoast syndrome. Adv Pain Res Ther 4:135, 1982.
16. Mandl F: Paravertebral Block. New York, Grune & Stratton, 1947.
17. Cousins MJ, Dwyer B, Gibb D: Chronic pain and neurolytic neural blockade. *In* Cousins MJ, Bridenbaugh PO (eds): Neural Blockade, ed 2. Philadelphia, JB Lippincott, 1988, p 1053.
18. Katz J: Current role of neurolytic agents. Adv Neurol 4:471, 1974.
19. Madrid JL, Bonica JJ: Cranial nerve blocks. Adv Pain Res Ther 2:347, 1979.
20. Hakanson S: Trigeminal neuralgia treated by the injection of glycerol into the trigeminal cistern. Neurosurgery 9:638, 1981.
21. Shulman M: Treatment of cancer pain with epidural butylaminobenzoate suspension. Reg Anesth 12:1, 1987.
22. Shulman M: Intercostal nerve block with 10% butamben suspension for the treatment of chronic noncancer pain. Anesthesiology 71:A737, 1989.
23. Shulman M, Joseph NJ, Haller CA: Local effects of epidural and subarachnoid injections of butylaminobenzoate suspension. Reg Anesth 12:23, 1987.
24. Shulman M: Epidural butamben for the treatment of metastatic cancer pain. Anesthesiology 67:A245, 1987.
25. Evans PJD, Lloyd JW, Jack TM: Cryoanalgesia for intractable pain. J R Soc Med 74:804, 1981.
26. Sluijter ME, Van Kleef, M: Characteristics and mode of action of radiofrequency lesions. Curr Rev Pain 2:143–150, 1998.
27. Hammer M, Meneese, W: Principles and practice of radiofrequency neurolysis. Curr Rev Pain 2:267–278, 1998.
28. Sluijter ME, Cosman ER, Rittman WB, Van Kleef, M: The effects of pulsed radiofrequency fields applied to the dorsal root ganglion: A preliminary report. Pain Clinic 11:109–117, 1998.
29. Martin D: Failed neck surgery syndrome. Quarterly Grand Rounds presentation at Texas Tech University, Lubbock, Tex. September, 1999.
30. Moore KL: Clinically Oriented Anatomy, ed 2. Baltimore, Williams & Wilkins, 1985, p 606–608.
31. Bogduk N: The clinical anatomy of the cervical dorsal rami. Spine 7:319–330, 1982.
32. Bogduk N, Marsland A: The cervical zygapophysial joints as a source of neck pain. Spine 13(6):610–617, 1988.
33. Bogduk N: Local anesthetic blocks of the second cervical ganglion: A technique with an application in occipital headache. Cephalalgia 1:41–50, 1981.
34. Bogduk N, Marsland A: On the concept of third occipital headache. J Neurol Neurosurg Psychiatry 49:775–780, 1986.
35. Gado K, Emery P: Modified suprascapular nerve block with bupivacaine alone effectively controls chronic shoulder pain in patients with rheumatoid arthritis. Ann Rheum Dis 52:215–218, 1993.
36. Vecchio PC, Adebajo AO, Hazleman BL: Suprascapular nerve block for persistent rotator cuff lesions. J Rheumatol 20:453–455, 1993.
37. Moore DC: Regional Block, ed 4. Springfield: Charles C Thomas, 1979, pp 300–303.
38. Parris WCV: Suprascapular nerve block: A safer technique. Anesthesiology 72:580–581, 1990.
39. Van der Wal M, Lang SA, Yip RW: Transsartorial approach for saphenous nerve block. Can J Anaesth 40(6):542–546, 1993.
40. Mansour NY: Sub-sartorial saphenous nerve block with the aid of nerve stimulator. Reg Anesth 18:266–268, 1993.
41. Goss CM (ed): Gray's Anatomy of the Human Body, ed 37. Edinburgh, Churchill-Livingstone, 1989, p 1143.
42. Wilson PJEM: Neurosurgery and relief of pain associated with head and neck cancer. Ear Nose Throat J 62:250, 1983.
43. Pitkin GP: Blocking the trigeminal nerve. *In* Southworth JL, Hingson RA, Pitkin WM (eds): Conduction Anesthesia, ed 2. Philadelphia, JB Lippincott, 1953, p 360.
44. Patt R, Jain S: Management of a patient with osteoradionecrosis of the mandible with nerve blocks. J Pain Symptom Manage 5:59, 1990.
45. Bonica JJ, Buckley FP, Moricca G, et al: Neurolytic blockade and hypophysectomy. *In* Bonica JJ (ed): Management of Pain, ed 2. Philadelphia, Lea & Febiger, 1990, p 1980.
46. Montgomery W, Cousins MJ: Aspects of the management of chronic pain illustrated by ninth cranial nerve block. Br J Anaesth 44:383, 1972.
47. Labat G: Regional Anesthesia. Philadelphia, WB Saunders, 1922, p 114.
48. Twycross RG, Lack SA: Therapeutics in Terminal Care. Edinburgh, Churchill Livingstone, 1986.
49. Waldman SD, Feldstein GS, Allen ML, et al: Cervical epidural implantable narcotic delivery systems in the management of upper body pain. Anesth Analg 66:780, 1987.
50. Lobato RD, Madrid JL, Fatela LV, et al: Intraventricular morphine for intractable cancer pain: Rationale, methods, clinical results. Acta Anaesthesiol Scand 31:68, 1987.
51. Grant FC: Surgical methods for relief of pain. Bull NY Acad Med 19:373, 1943.
52. McEwen BW: The pain clinic: A clinic for the management of intractable pain. Med J Austr 1:676, 1965.
53. Siegfried J, Broggi G: Percutaneous thermocoagulation of the gasserian ganglion in the treatment of pain in advanced cancer. Adv Pain Res Ther 2:463, 1979.
54. Broggi G, Siegfried J: Percutaneous differential radiofrequency rhizotomy of glossopharyngeal nerve in facial pain due to cancer. Adv Pain Res Ther 2:469, 1979.
55. Pagura JR, Schnapp M, Passarelli P: Percutaneous radiofrequency glossopharyngeal rhizotomy for cancer pain. Appl Neurophysiol 46:154, 1983.
56. Kaplan R, Aurellano Z, Pfisterer W: Phenol brachial plexus bloc for upper extremity cancer pain. Reg Anesth 13:58, 1988.
57. Neill RS: Ablation of the brachial plexus. Anaesthesia 34:1024, 1979.
58. Mullin V: Brachial plexus block with phenol for painful arm associated with Pancoast's syndrome. Anesthesiology 53:431, 1980.

59. Doyle D: Nerve blocks in advanced cancer. Practitioner 226:539, 1982.
60. Moore D, Bridenbaugh DL: Intercostal nerve block in 4333 patients: Indications, techniques, complications. Anesth Analg 41:1, 1962.
61. Stone HB: A treatment for pruritus ani. Bull Johns Hopkins Hosp 27:242, 1916.
62. Swerdlow M: Rolc of chemical neurolysis and local anesthetic infiltration. *In* Swerdlow M, Ventafridda V (eds): Cancer Pain. Lancaster, MTP Press, 1987.
63. Conacher ID, Kokri M: Postoperative paravertebral blocks for thoracic surgery: A radiological appraisal. Br J Anaesth 59:155, 1987.
64. Atkinson GL, Shupack RC: Acute bronchospasm complicating intercostal nerve block with phenol. Anesth Analg 68:400, 1989.
65. Vernon S: Paralgesia: Paravertebral block for pain relief. Am J Surg 21:416, 1932.
66. Mehta M, Ranger I: Persistent abdominal pain. Anaesthesia 26:330, 1971.
67. Plancarte R, Amescua C, Patt R, et al: Superior hypogastric plexus block for pelvic cancer pain. Anesthesiology 73:236, 1990.
68. Plancarte R, Amescua C, Patt RB: Presacral blockade of the ganglion impar (ganglion of Walther). Anesthesiology 73:A751, 1990.
69. Robertson DH: Transsacral neurolytic nerve block: An alternative approach to intractable perineal pain. Br J Anaesth 55:873, 1983.
70. Clark AJ, Awad SA: Selective transsacral nerve root blocks. Reg Anesth 15:125, 1990.
71. Rockswold GL, Bradley WE, Chou SN: Effect of sacral nerve blocks on the function of the urinary bladder in humans. J Neurosurg 40:83, 1974.
72. Simon DL, Carron H, Rowlingson JC: Treatment of bladder pain with transsacral nerve block. Anesth Analg 61:46, 1982.
73. Goffen BS: Transsacral block. Anesth Analg 62:623, 1982.
74. Wilson F: Neurolytic and other locally acting drugs in the management of pain. Pharmacol Ther 53:431, 1981.
75. Feldman SA, Young ML: Treatment of intermittent claudication: Lumbar paravertebral somatic block with phenol. Anaesthesia 30:174, 1975.
76. Jack ED: Regional anaesthesia for pain relief. Br J Anaesth 47:278, 1975.
77. Moritz U: Phenol block of peripheral nerves. Scand J Rehabil Med 5:160, 1973.
78. Gibson IIJM: Phenol block in the treatment of spasticity. Gerontology 33:327, 1987.
79. Kirvela O, Nieminen S: Treatment of painful neuromas with neurolytic blockade. Pain 41:161, 1990.
80. Defalque RJ, Bromley JJ: Poststernotomy neuralgia: A new pain syndrome. Anesth Analg 69:81, 1989.
81. Todd DP: Poststernotomy neuralgia: A new pain syndrome. Anesth Analg 69:691, 1989.
82. Defalque RJ: Painful trigger points in surgical scars. Anesth Analg 61:518, 1982.
83. Woodruff JD, Babkinia A: Local alcohol injection of the vulva: Discussion of 35 cases. Obstet Gynecol 54:512, 1979.
84. Woodrull JD, Thompson B: Local alcohol injection in the treatment of vulvar pruritus. Obstet Gynecol 40:18, 1972.

RECOMMENDED READING

Patt R: Peripheral Neurolysis and the Management of Cancer Pain. Philadelphia, JB Lippincott, 1993, pp 359–376.

CHAPTER • 52

Subarachnoid Neurolytic Blocks

Alon P. Winnie, MD • Kenneth D. Candido, MD

Dogliotti first described the technique of subarachnoid chemical neurolysis using alcohol for the treatment of sciatic pain almost 70 years ago.[1] Suvansa in the same year described intrathecal carbolic acid for the treatment of tetanus.[2] A quarter of a century later Maher,[3, 4] in two landmark papers, described his experience with hyperbaric phenol and silver nitrate for subarachnoid neurolysis, stating, "It is easier to lay a carpet than to paper a ceiling." Over the ensuing years, however, lack of experience with either technique and fear of the anticipated complications have resulted in underutilization of this valuable modality. Furthermore, better understanding and increased use of neuraxial opiates for cancer pain over the last two decades has even further decreased the use of subarachnoid chemical neurolysis. Nonetheless, because of the physical separation of the sensory and motor roots of spinal nerves within the spinal canal, intrathecal dorsal rhizotomy (more appropriately called *rhizolysis*) is the only neurolytic procedure that allows sensory blockade without concomitant motor block. Because of this and because of the relative precision with which the affected nerve roots can be blocked, the technique is particularly useful for treating cancer pain in an extremity, where preservation of motor function is so important. In short, it is the physical separation of motor and sensory fibers in the subarachnoid space that preserves forever a small but unique role for subarachnoid neurolysis in the management of cancer pain in carefully selected patients.

SELECTION CRITERIA

Since the duration of action of neurolytic agents in the subarachnoid space is finite but unpredictable, great care must be exercised in choosing appropriate candidates for the procedure. Neurolytic blockade by this route is especially suited to patients in whom conventional treatment regimens have failed and who have a short life expectancy, usually less than a year. As with all neurolytic procedures, patients must be completely apprised of the possibility of debilitating side effects and other serious associated complications that can follow even a successful block, most notably, motor weakness and incontinence. The selection criteria for subarachnoid neurolysis include the following:

- The diagnosis is well-established.[5]
- The patient's life expectancy is short, usually 6 to 12 months.
- The patient's pain is unresponsive to antineoplastic therapy (chemotherapy, radiation).
- The patient's pain has failed to respond to adequate trials of analgesic agents and adjunctive drugs.
- The pain is localized to two or three dermatomes.
- The pain is predominantly somatic in origin.
- The pain is unilateral (neurolytic blocks for bilateral pain should be staggered).[6]

INFORMED CONSENT

It is crucial that not only the patient, but also the patient's family fully understand the anticipated procedure, its potential risks, the alternative forms of therapy available, and, most importantly, the possibility of serious complications. Furthermore, it is important that the patient and family understand that the procedure does not simply "take away pain," but rather substitutes numbness (loss of sensation) for the pain. So important is this concept that, with rare exceptions, before the decision is made to proceed with a subarachnoid neurolytic block, a prognostic subarachnoid block should be carried out using a local anesthetic, so that the patient can experience both the pain relief that may be anticipated after a neurolytic block and the accompanying sensory block. Although an occasional patient may decide that he or she cannot tolerate the numbness, the vast majority of patients certainly prefer this lack of sensation to the pain and choose to proceed with the neurolytic procedure.

TECHNIQUE

Because unfamiliarity with the details of this technique has been a major obstacle to its use and because it is proper execution of the technique that determines its success and safety, the focus of the present discussion is on the technical aspects of subarachnoid neurolysis. First of all, because of the "permanence" of the complications of this technique, subarachnoid neurolysis should be attempted only after careful review of a dermatome chart to determine precisely which nerve or nerves are subserving the patient's pain (Fig. 52–1). Furthermore, if the patient's pain is due to one or more metastases to bone, it may be useful to refer to a sclerotome chart, as the innervation of some parts of the skeleton differs from that of the overlying soft tissues (Fig. 52–2).

Secondly, because a neurolytic subarachnoid block must be carried out at the level where the dorsal root to be blocked leaves the spinal cord (to spare motor function), it is essential to determine which interlaminar foramen affords access to that root. Though the cervical nerves exit at a level higher than their respective vertebral bodies, all of the other nerves exit at a level below their respective vertebral bodies because of the differential growth of the spinal cord and vertebral column, both in utero and for the first few years of life (Fig. 52–3).[7] Finally, a choice must be made before the procedure is undertaken to determine whether a hyperbaric (phenol in glycerin) or hypobaric (absolute alcohol) technique is more appropriate. No controlled studies have compared the outcomes with subarachnoid alcohol and phenol, but in our experience hypobaric alcohol has been the technique of choice in the vast majority of cases, because most patients with severe, intractable pain cannot lie on the painful side, a requirement when using hyperbaric phenol. Although at one time clinicians believed that phenol might exert a preferential effect on the small fibers subserving pain, it has recently been determined that neither alcohol nor phenol is a selective neurolytic agent, thereby eliminating this as a rationale for choosing phenol over alcohol.[8–10]

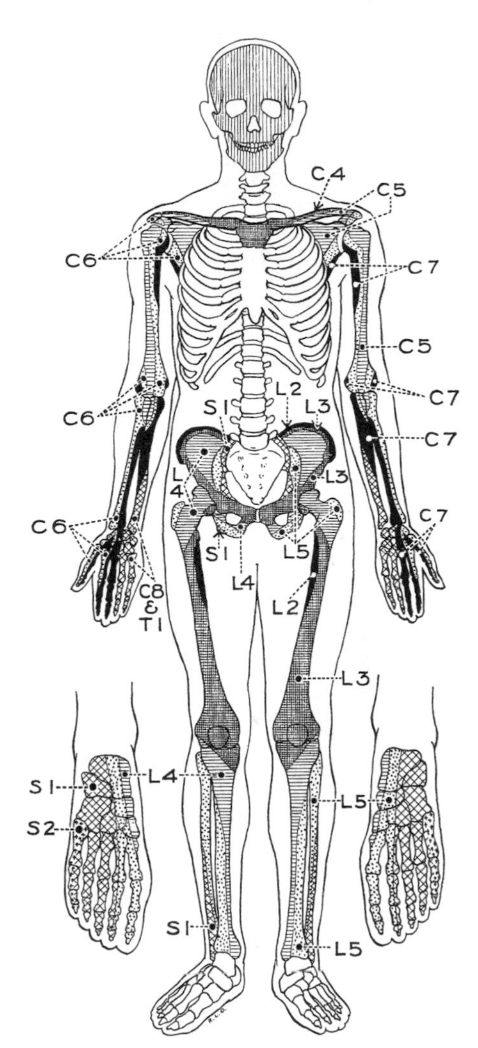

FIGURE 52–2 *The innervation of the skeleton by spinal segments from the anterior aspect. The various scelerotomes are indicated by the different styles of shading.* Insets *show scelerotomes of the dorsal aspect of the feet (modified after Dejerine). (Haymaker W, Woodhall B: Peripheral Nerve Injuries. Philadelphia, WB Saunders, 1945, p 41.)*

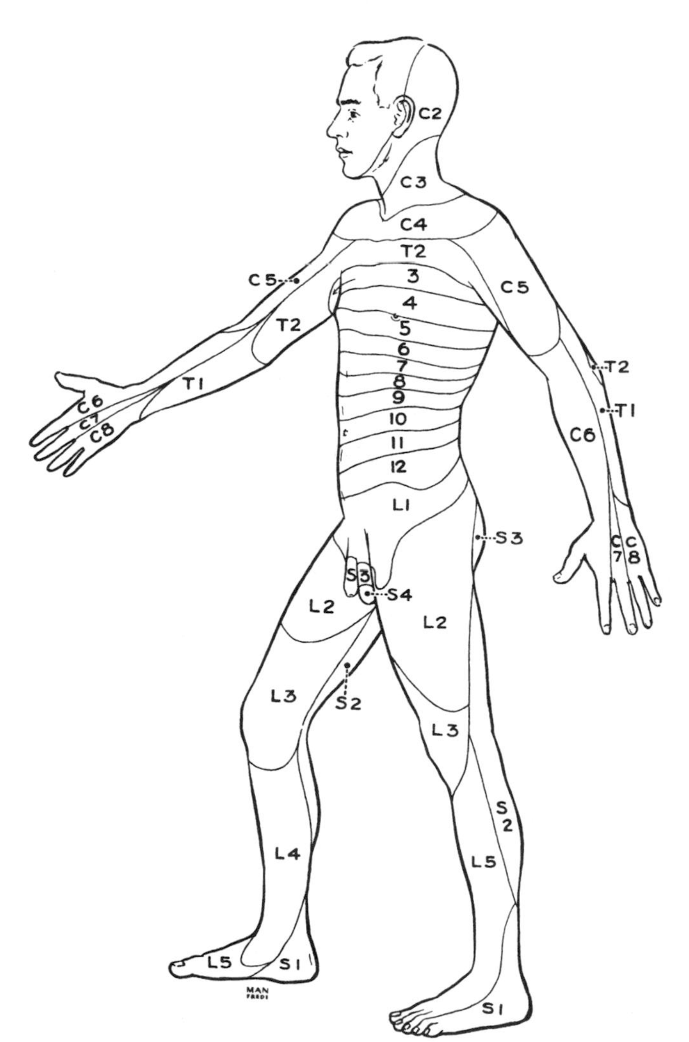

FIGURE 52–1 *A side view of the dermatomes (after Foerster). (Haymaker W, Woodhall B: Peripheral Nerve Injuries. Philadelphia, WB Saunders, 1945, p 20.)*

SUBARACHNOID NEUROLYSIS WITH ALCOHOL

Since absolute alcohol is extremely hypobaric, when this agent is utilized, the patient is first placed in the lateral decubitus position with the painful site uppermost and is then rolled anteriorly approximately 45 degrees to place

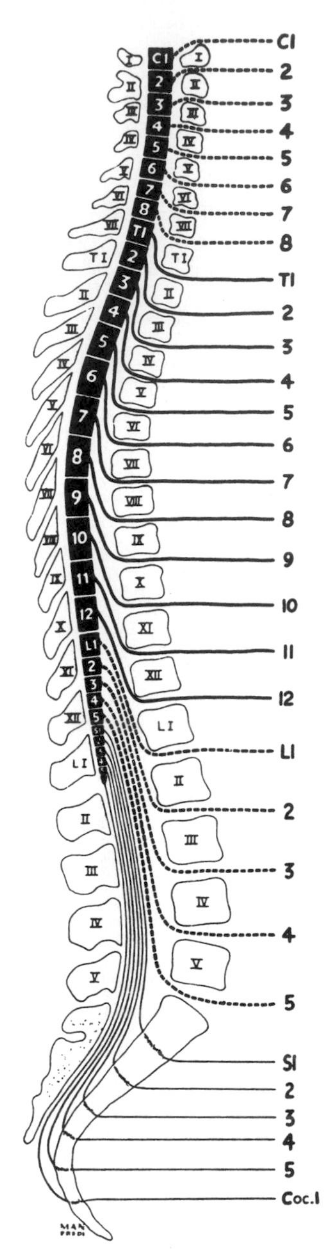

FIGURE 52–3 *The alignment of spinal segments with vertebrae. The bodies and spinous processes of the vertebrae are indicated by Roman numerals, the spinal segments and their respective nerves by Arabic. The cervical nerves exit through intervertebral foramina above their respective vertebral bodies, and the other nerves issue below those bodies. (Haymaker W, Woodhall B: Peripheral Nerve Injuries. Philadelphia, WB Saunders, 1945, p 24.)*

the dorsal (sensory) root uppermost (Fig. 52–4).[11] The patient is then stabilized with straps and made as comfortable as possible with pillows, since he or she will need to remain in this position throughout the procedure. An assistant is absolutely mandatory to stabilize the patient and to allay anxiety. After the patient has been properly positioned and the patient's role in the procedure has been reviewed, a 22-gauge spinal needle is inserted and advanced through the interlaminar space at the level of the dorsal root to be blocked. If the procedure is being carried out at a thoracic level, because of the long, caudally sloping spinous processes, a paravertebral approach is usually easier than a midline approach; but whatever the approach, the needle tip should penetrate the dura in the midline. Needles smaller than 22-gauge should not be selected for this technique, because the free flow of cerebrospinal fluid (CSF) is essential and because post–dural puncture headache is extremely rare after subarachnoid alcohol neurolysis. A prognostic block with local anesthetic should already have been carried out to determine whether the pain can, in fact, be relieved by the technique and, equally important, whether the patient can tolerate the numbness.

Contrary to the recommendation in many texts, a test dose of local anesthetic should *not* be given once the needle is in place for a neurolytic block. The reason is that none of the available local anesthetics can be made as hypobaric as absolute alcohol, so a hypobaric local anesthetic "test dose" would not find its way to and block the same nerve root as the much more hypobaric alcohol; resulting in misinformation as to the placement of the neurolytic solution. Furthermore, also contrary to the recommendation in most textbooks, a local anesthetic should not be administered before the injection of the alcohol because the pain produced by the injection of the alcohol is an essential indicator that enhances the accuracy and effectiveness of the procedure. Instead of preventing the burning pain caused by the alcohol, the physician must tell the patient *to expect* severe, localized, burning pain, *but only for a fraction of a second* after each injection, and to *focus attention* on whether that burning occurs *at*, *above*, or *below* the level of

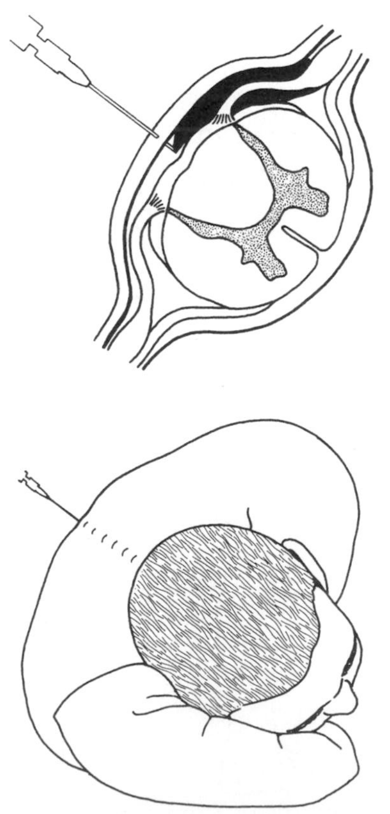

FIGURE 52–4 *Proper positioning of the patient with leftsided pain for intrathecal injection of alcohol. Note the 45-degree anterior tilt, intended to bathe the posterior (sensory) nerve roots with hypobaric alcohol while sparing the anterior (motor) roots. (Swerdlow M: Neurolytic blocks. In Patt RB (ed): Cancer Pain. Philadelphia, JB Lippincott, 1993, P 435.)*

the pain. The patient is also instructed to report any other sensations, such as tingling, warmth, or numbness.

Subarachnoid alcohol neurolysis is a very precise procedure, and to ensure efficacy and safety, the alcohol should be injected in 0.1-mL aliquots using a tuberculin syringe. The syringe containing the alcohol should not be attached to the needle until the free flow of CSF indicates that the needle is definitely in the subarachnoid space. Once the syringe has been attached to the needle, aspiration should *not* be carried out to verify proper needle placement, since alcohol causes the CSF to form a white coagulum within the syringe. When the syringe has been attached to the needle, the subjective experience of each injection and the importance of the brief burning sensation to the success of the technique are reiterated one more time, after which sequential injection of 0.1-mL increments of alcohol begins. The operator asks the patient the same questions about the presence and location of the burning after each aliquot. Actually, the first one or two increments of alcohol usually do not produce the expected burning pain, simply because this volume is just enough to fill the hub and shaft of the spinal needle. The third or fourth 0.1-mL increment, however, invariably produces the expected burning, and it reassures the patient as to how short-lived it is. More importantly, the level at which the burning is perceived in relation to the location of the pain serves as an indicator as to whether the needle has been placed at the proper level. If the burning occurs at precisely the level of the patient's pain, a total volume of absolute alcohol not greater than 0.7 mL is injected in 0.1-mL increments; and after about the fifth or sixth increment, there should be little or no additional burning. On the other hand, if the burning produced by the third or fourth increment of alcohol occurs *above* the site of the patient's pain, injections through that needle are discontinued, though the needle is left in place as a marker. A second needle (and if necessary even a third) must be inserted through progressively lower interspaces until the burning produced by the incremental injection of alcohol corresponds *exactly* to the distribution of the patient's pain. Likewise, if the initial injection of alcohol produces burning pain *below* the level of the patient's pain, a second needle (and if necessary a third) must be inserted through progressively higher interspaces until the injection of the 0.1-mL increments of alcohol produces burning in the precise distribution of the pain. At this point, the entire 0.7 mL is injected in 0.1-mL increments to produce the desired neurolysis. Once the total volume of alcohol has been injected through each needle, the stylet is replaced, and the needle is left in place until the entire procedure has been completed.

Once a nerve subserving a patient's pain has been identified and blocked by this process and a total of 0.7 mL of alcohol has been injected, the process is repeated above or below (or above *and* below) the level of the initial full injection to completely abolish the pain. No more than three or four nerves should ever be blocked at one session; but as indicated in the selection criteria above, this procedure is best reserved for patients with pain limited to two or three dermatomes. Unfortunately, in contrast to subarachnoid injections of local anesthetics for surgical anesthesia, the injection of alcohol for subarachnoid neurolysis must be made through a separate needle to block each nerve root. The reason that alcohol cannot be "floated" to a higher or lower level through a single needle, as is done when performing a hypobaric spinal for surgery, is that alcohol "fixes" too quickly and would not float far enough to block the adjacent dermatomes. Indeed, Matsuki et al showed that the CSF concentration of alcohol is rapidly reduced after intrathecal injection, a finding that implies rapid uptake by nerve tissue.[12] In short, for best results a separate needle *must* be placed at the level of each nerve root to be blocked. When the injections through the appropriate three or four needles are completed and before each needle is withdrawn (including those placed at inappropriate levels), 0.2 to 0.3 mL of air should be injected to clear the shaft and hub of alcohol to minimize the possibility that alcohol trickling from the needle as it is withdrawn from dura to skin will form a fistula. Fortunately, experience indicates that the 0.1 to 0.2 mL of alcohol injected at levels that turned out to be inappropriate does not cause any demonstrable neurologic damage.

SUBARACHNOID NEUROLYSIS WITH PHENOL

Intrathecal phenol in glycerin may be used as an alternative to alcohol for subarachnoid neurolysis. The technique is similar to that described earlier, except that the patient must be positioned with the painful side down, because phenol in glycerin is a *hyperbaric* solution. Since most patients with pain of malignant origin have difficulty lying on the painful side, in our experience alcohol remains the neurolytic of choice in most patients. If, however, phenol neurolysis is appropriate for a particular patient, the technique is similar to that utilized for alcohol neurolysis, except that the patient is positioned with the dorsal root lowermost and with the head of the bed slightly elevated (Fig. 52–5).[11] The patient must be tilted posteriorly with the back as close to the edge of the bed as possible, using bolsters, straps, or pillows to maintain the patient securely in position. Again, the presence of an assistant to hold the patient securely and provide emotional and physical reassurance is absolutely mandatory. For this technique a 22-gauge (or even better, a 20-gauge) spinal needle should be used because of the viscosity of the phenol-gylcerin mixture. In a manner essentially opposite to the technique of subarachnoid alcohol neurolysis, the bevel of the spinal needle should be directed inferiorly (laterally toward the table). Because of the viscosity of phenol in glycerin it takes significant pressure applied to the plunger of the syringe to force the phenol into the subarchnoid space, so the injection must be made slowly and carefully to prevent the escape of phenol from the syringe and onto the skin of the patient or the practitioner. Warming the phenol lessens its viscosity and makes it easier to inject. Because phenol has local anesthetic properties, its injection into the subarachnoid space is not accompanied by the burning pain produced by alcohol, though the patient may feel warmth, tingling, or even mild dysesthesia in the distribution of the nerve being injected. Like alcohol, the concentration of phenol in the CSF declines rapidly after the initial injection, again implying rapid absorption by neural tissues.[13] This has important implications as to how long *after* the neurolytic agent has been injected patients must remain as

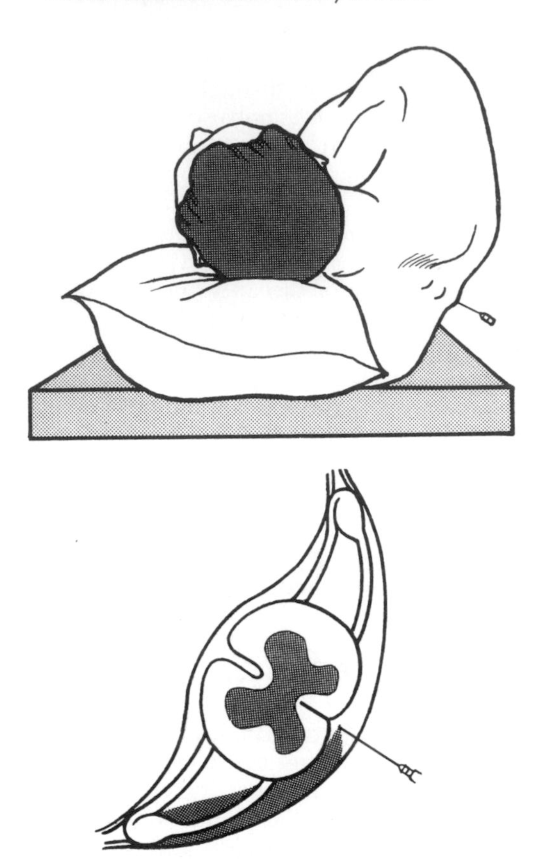

FIGURE 52–5 *Proper positioning of the patient with leftsided pain for intrathecal injection of phenol in glycerine. Note the 45-degree posterior tilt, intended to bathe the posterior (sensory) nerve roots with hyperbaric phenol while sparing the anterior (motor) roots. (Swerdlow M: Neurolytic blocks.* In *Patt RB (ed): Cancer Pain. Philadelphia, JB Lippincott, 1993, p 431.)*

originally positioned. Traditionally, they have been kept in these (obviously uncomfortable) positions for at least 30 min after the neurolytic injection, but probably patients can be allowed to assume a more comfortable posture after 15 to 20 min, keeping in mind the relative position of the dorsal roots in the spinal canal when doing so. As with alcohol, after the subarachnoid injection of phenol in glycerin, 0.1 to 0.3 mL of air is injected to flush the lytic solution from each needle before it is removed.

SUCCESS AND COMPLICATION RATES

Careful patient selection and equally careful technique are essential for successful subarachnoid neurolysis and for the prevention of complications. While subarachnoid neurolysis may be attempted at cervical, thoracic, or lumbosacral levels, the success rates and the incidence of complications vary somewhat, depending on the level of injection, primarily because of the anatomic differences at different levels. For example, the distance between the origins of nerve roots decreases progressively in the lumbosacral area, so that the lower an injection is made, the more difficult it becomes to block a single nerve root without involving adjacent roots. Yet cervical subarachnoid neurolytic blocks seem to be less successful than similar blocks carried out at thoracic or even lumbosacral levels.[14] To be sure, penetration of the spinal cord by the needle is a concern whenever these techniques are undertaken, especially at cervical or thoracic levels. Fortunately, this is a rare occurrence, but, when it does occur, Perese[15] has reported that no permanent injury results, only transient pain, which warns the clinician of the position of the needle and prevents subsequent injection into the cord. From the point of view of complications, neurolytic subarachnoid blocks may be safest when undertaken in the midthoracic region, since this region is relatively distant from the fibers that subserve limb, bowel, and bladder function,[16] so any motor loss would be of little consequence. Conversely, in the lumbosacral region, owing to the proximity of sensory and motor fibers to each other (because of the decreasing size of the conus medullaris the dorsal and ventral roots are very close together) and to the proximity of both to the autonomic fibers subserving bowel and bladder function, lumbar subarachnoid neurolysis is usually reserved strictly for very select individuals in whom the risk-benefit ratio has been clearly delineated. On the other hand, for patients who already have compromised sphincter function, lumbosacral subarachnoid phenol neurolysis has been advocated for rectal and pelvic malignancies because of the tendency of phenol to spare motor function.[17]

It is difficult to compare the success rates achieved with subarachnoid neurolysis by various investigators because of the different methods used to quantify pain and pain relief, but it would appear that one should expect a "beneficial effect" in about 75% of the patients, "excellent results" in 50%, and "fair results" in another 25%.[16] A review of the literature appears to indicate that the success rate is slightly greater with alcohol than with phenol, whereas the complication rate is slightly greater with phenol than with alcohol.[3, 4, 17–31] In assessing the success of a subarachnoid neurolytic procedure, it should be appreciated that even if a block produces only moderate pain relief, it may be sufficient to allow analgesic agents that could not previously control the pain to render the patient pain-free, or at least to make the patient very comfortable. Thus, one should not consider a neurolytic block to be successful *only* if the patient is rendered pain free without any supplemental analgesics, although such success is obviously very rewarding.

The impact of a complication, even a serious complication, on a patient and his/her family depends to a large extent on whether the patient has significant pain relief from the neurolytic procedure. If the patient and family have been properly apprised of all of the possible serious complications that can follow a subarachnoid neurolytic procedure, many find even the most serious and unexpected complications acceptable *if* the patient is pain-free or at least comfortable as a result of the procedure. On the other hand, if the patient and family are not told of the possible complications, even a fairly minor complication may upset them inordinately (but understandably), particularly if the block fails to produce the desired relief. Fortunately, the majority of the complications of neurolytic subarachnoid blocks are transient: Gerbershagen[32] reviewed reports that provided data on the duration of 303 complications of subarachnoid neurolytic procedures and found that 51%

of them disappeared within 1 week, 21% within 1 month, and 9% within 4 months, with only 18% lasting longer than 4 months. Interestingly, while post–dural puncture headache can follow any subarachnoid block, it is less frequent after neurolytic subarachnoid blocks than after subarachnoid blocks with local anesthetics for surgery, in spite of the fact that larger needles are used for neurolytic subarachnoid blocks.[33] Similarly, aseptic meningitis (and even septic meningitis) can develop after any subarachnoid block; but fortunately, it also is exceedingly rare after subarachnoid neurolytic blocks, presumably because the neurolytic solutions are self-sterilizing.

CONCLUSION

Because of the physical separation of the sensory and motor nerve roots in the spinal canal, intrathecal chemical dorsal rhizotomy is the only neurolytic procedure that allows sensory block without concomitant motor block. For this reason subarachnoid neurolysis is a unique, effective modality for the management of cancer pain in certain patients. If the patients are carefully selected and the technique carefully carried out, pain relief can be provided in the vast majority of cases without an excessive rate of complications.

REFERENCES

1. Dogliotti AM: Traitement des syndromes doloreaux de la peripherie par l'alcoholisation subarachnoidienne des racines posterieures à leur émergence de la moelle epineri. Presse Med 39:1249–1252, 1931.
2. Suvansa S: Treatment of tetanus by intrathecal injection of carbolic acid. Lancet 1:1075–1078, 1931.
3. Maher RM: Relief of pain in incurable cancer. Lancet 1:18–20, 1955.
4. Maher RM: Neurone selection in relief of pain. Further experiences with intrathecal injections. Lancet 1:16–19, 1957.
5. Katz J: Current role of neurolytic agents. Adv Neurol 4:471, 1974.
6. Hollis PH, Malis LI, Zappulla RA: Neurological deterioration after lumbar puncture below complete spinal subarachnoid block. J Neurosurg 64:253–256, 1986.
7. Haymaker W, Woodhall B: Peripheral Nerve Injuries. Philadelphia, WB Saunders, 1945.
8. Nathan PW, Sears TA: Effects of phenol on nervous tissue. J Physiol 150:565–580, 1960.
9. Nathan PW, Sears TA, Smith MC: Effects of phenol solutions on the nerve roots of the cat: An electrophysiological and histological study. J Neurol Sci 2:7, 1965.
10. Patt R, Jain S: Management of a patient with osteoradionecrosis of the mandible with nerve blocks. J Pain Symptom Mgt 5:59–60, 1990.
11. Swerdlow M: Neurolytic blocks. *In* Patt RB (ed): Cancer Pain. Philadelphia, JB Lippincott, 1993.
12. Matsuki M, Kato Y, Ichiyanagi K: Progressive changes in the concentration of ethyl alcohol in the human and canine subarachnoid spaces. Anesthesiology 36:617–621, 1972.
13. Ichiyanagi K, Matsuki M, Kinefuchi S, Kato Y: Progressive changes in the concentrations of phenol and gylcerine in the human subarachnoid space. Anesthesiology 42:622–624, 1975.
14. Swerdlow M: Spinal and peripheral neurolysis for managing Pancoast syndrome. Adv Pain Res Ther 4:135–144, 1982.
15. Perese DM: Subarachnoid alcohol block in the management of pain of malignant disease. Arch Surg 76:347–354, 1958.
16. Patt RB, Cousins MJ: Techniques for neurolytic neural blockade. *In* Cousins MJ, Bridenbaugh PO (eds): Neural Blockade. Philadelphia, JB Lippincott, 1998, pp 1007–1061.
17. Lifshitz S, Debacker LJ, Buchsbaum HJ: Subarachnoid phenol block for pain relief in gynecologic malignancy. Obstet Gynecol 48:316–320, 1976.
18. Stovner J, Endresen R: Intrathecal phenol for cancer pain. Acta Anaesth Scand 16:17–21, 1972.
19. Papo I, Visca A: Intrathecal phenol in the treatment of pain and spasticity. Proc Neurol Surg 7:56–130, 1976.
20. Papo I, Visca A: Phenol subarachnoid rhizotomy for the treatment of cancer pain: A personal account of 290 cases. Adv Pain Res Ther 2:339–346, 1979.
21. Ischia S, Luzzani A, Ischia A, et al: Subarachnoid neurolytic block (L_5–S_1) and unilateral percutaneous cervical cordotomy in the treatment of pain secondary to pelvic malignant disease. Pain 20:139–149, 1984.
22. Mark VH, White JC, Zervas NT, et al: Intrathecal use of phenol for the relief of chronic severe pain. N Engl J Med 267:589–593, 1962.
23. Hay RC: Subarachnoid alcohol block in the control of intractable pain: Report of results in 252 patients. Anesth Analg 41:12–16, 1962.
24. Bruno G: Intrathecal alcohol block—experiences on 41 cases. Paraplegia 12:305–306, 1975.
25. Tank TM, Dohn DF, Gardner WJ: Intrathecal injections of alcohol or phenol for relief of intractable pain. Cleve Clin Q 30:111–117, 1963.
26. Superville-Sovak P, Rasminsky M, Finlayson MH: Complications of phenol neurolysis. Arch Neurol 32:226–228, 1975.
27. Holland AJC, Youssef M: A complication of subarachnoid phenol blockade. Anaesthesia 34:260–262, 1978.
28. Totoki T, Kato T, Nomoto Y, et al: Anterior spinal artery syndrome—a complication of cervical intrathecal phenol injection. Pain 6:99–104, 1979.
29. Evans RJ, Mackay IM: Subarachnoid phenol nerve blocks for relief of pain in advanced malignancy. Can J Surg 15:50–53, 1972.
30. Derrick W: Subarachnoid alcohol block for the control of intractable pain. Acta Anesth Scand 24(Suppl):167–172, 1966.
31. Stern EL: Dangers of intraspinal (subarachnoid) injection of alcohol: Their avoidance and contraindications. Am J Surg 35:99–104, 1937.
32. Gerbershagen HU: Neurolysis: Subarachnoid neurolytic blockade. Acta Anaesth Belg 1:45, 1981.
33. Patt RB, Wu CL, Reddy S, et al: Incidence of postdural puncture headache following intrathecal neurolysis with large caliber needles. Reg Anesth 19(2S):86, 1994.

PART • IV

Neuroaugmentation

CHAPTER • 53

Mechanisms of Action of Spinal Cord Stimulation

Elliot S. Krames, MD

Chronic pain is a major cause of suffering for countless millions of people worldwide, represents a large proportion of American dollars spent for health care, and remains the leading cause of days lost and lost productivity from the industrial workforce. In fact, if left untreated, chronic pain will continue to be a burden on the economic well-being of the U.S. economy.

Only in the past 25 years, with a growing base of scientific and clinical information and understanding of the neurophysiologic, neuroanatomic, and neurochemical mechanisms of pain transmission and its modulation in the peripheral and central nervous system, have pain treatments that act on these systems been introduced. Based on electrical stimulation response studies in animal models, multiple and often conflicting mechanistic theories have been presented in the literature for one of these modalities for pain control—spinal cord stimulation (SCS). In this chapter we focus on and try to elucidate five broad theories for the mechanism or mechanisms of action of SCS and present some of the animal studies that support them. For ease of understanding, the theories will be grouped according to where in the ascending pain pathways or descending modulatory pathways they purport to impact. These five mechanistic theories for SCS will, therefore, be categorized broadly into *segmental* or *Supraspinal* inhibition (Table 53–1).

SEGMENTAL INHIBITION

SCS for clinical control of pain was first introduced in 1967 by Norman Shealy and colleagues,[1] in response to the publication of the gate control theory of pain by Melzack and Wall in 1965.[2] The gate control theory, as first published, without benefit of later refinements, proposed that painful "electrochemical" nociceptive information in the periphery is transmitted to the spinal cord in small-diameter, unmyelinated C fibers and lightly myelinated A-delta fibers. These fibers would also, in turn, terminate at the substantia gelatinosa of the dorsal horn, the gate, of the spinal cord. Likewise, other sensory information, such as touch or vibration, carried in large myelinated A-beta fibers, would also terminate at this gate of the spinal cord. The basic premise of this theory is that reception of large-fiber information such as touch or vibration would turn off or close the gate to reception of small-fiber information. The clinical result of this gate closure, these authors theorized, would be analgesia.

Shealy and associates theorized, as did Melzack and Wall, that, if the large A-beta fibers of the dorsal columns were electrically stimulated, the stimulated fibers would antidromically inhibit reception of painful small-fiber information at the substantia gelatinosa of the dorsal horn. Because these authors believed that electrical stimulation worked only at the dorsal horns of the spinal cord, they called this new stimulation treatment modality *dorsal column stimulation (DCS)*. Since it is now known that this electrical stimulation inhibition of nociception can occur with electrical stimulation almost anywhere in the spinal cord, this term has been supplanted in the literature by the more general, but accurate, term *spinal cord stimulation*.

Several studies supporting segmental antidromic inhibition of spinothalamic projection cells by electrically stimu-

TABLE 53–1 ***Spinal Cord Stimulation: Mechanisms of Action***

- Segmental, antidromic activation of A-beta afferents. (*gate control theory*)
- Blocking of transmission in the *spinothalamic tract*
- Supraspinal pain inhibition
- Activation of central inhibitory mechanisms influencing *sympathetic* efferent neurons
- Activation of putative *neurotransmitters* or *neuromodulators*

lating the dorsal columns (gate theory) soon appeared. R.D. Foreman and coworkers investigated the effects of dorsal column stimulation on spinothalamic tract cells in anesthetized monkeys.[3] Dorsal column stimuli were applied to midthoracic or cervical levels of the spinal cord while responses of spinothalamic cells to von Frey hair activation of the sural nerves were examined. These authors found that dorsal column stimulation depressed the activity of spinothalamic tract cells for about 150 msec and that the best points for stimulation producing inhibition were over the ipsilateral dorsal columns. Responses to electrical stimulation of peripheral nerves and mechanical stimulation of cutaneous nociceptors were similarly depressed by DCS. Lesioning the dorsal columns eliminated this depression of activity by DCS stimulation below the lesion. Lesioning the lateral columns in this model had no effects. Likewise, Handwerker, Iggo, and Zimmerman, and R.A. Feldman, in studies from single dorsal horn neurons in anesthetized cats, found that the discharges of class 2 cells, cells in the dorsal horn that respond to both noxious radiant heat stimulation and input from low-threshold cutaneous mechanoreceptors, were suppressed by electrical stimulation of cutaneous, myelinated, afferent nerve fibers and DCS of the collaterals of myelinated afferent fibers in the dorsal columns.[4, 5]

Another theory supporting the segmental effect of spinal cord stimulation is that SCS blocks actual transmission of electrochemical information anywhere in the spinothalamic tracts. In a study published in 1974, Larson and coworkers used averaged somatosensory recordings from scalp electrodes in 18 patients with cancer and intractable pain, before, during, and after application of current. Eleven patients reported decreased perception of touch and joint rotation and pain below the level of current. All neurologic changes returned to baseline 1 hour after discontinuation of the current. DCS was also applied to 15 monkeys over the lower, middle, and upper thoracic spinal cord, in nucleus ventralis posterior lateralis (VPL), and over the sensory motor cortex (SMC). Results of these studies suggested that applied currents blocked neuronal transmission by producing local changes in the cord. The authors suggest that, alternatively, this alteration of cerebral evoked potentials and relief of pain might be secondary to changes in supraspinal neurons.[6]

SUPRASPINAL EFFECTS

Alternatively, as suggested by Larson's group, DCS or SCS could produce changes in supraspinal neurons that affect either pain transmission or pain modulation. Saade and associates studied this effect, utilized a rat model of antinociception for two types of pain tests, the tail immersion test and the formalin test, respectively, to investigate two different putative neurophysiologic mechanisms—"phasic" and "tonic" pain. Dorsal column nuclei were stimulated through electrodes placed semipermanently rostrad to bilateral dorsal column lesions. Effects of dorsal column nucleus stimulation and DCS were then observed for the antinociception tests. The results showed a clear antinociceptive effect for dorsal column nucleus stimulation on both experimental models of phasic and tonic pain in awake animals. The authors attributed these effects to the activation of supraspinal pain-modulating centers, as antidromic activation of DCS was prevented by dorsal column cuts caudal to the stimulating electrodes.[7]

SCS AND THE SYMPATHETIC NERVOUS SYSTEM

A fourth mechanistic theory for SCS derives from the fact that vasodilatation is a consistent post-stimulation finding in animal models and humans alike: that SCS activates central inhibitory mechanisms that influence sympathetic efferent neurons. These effects might be secondary to the pain-relieving effect of SCS, might be secondary to antidromic effects on small afferent fibers, and might be secondary to direct effects of SCS on central neurophysiologic mechanisms controlling sympathetic efferent outflow from the spinal cord.

One hypothesis is that SCS antidromically activates primary afferent fibers, including unmyelinated, small-diameter fibers leading small fiber–activated, antidromic vasodilation. According to Linderoth and colleagues, this theory, based on the work of Bayliss[8] from experiments performed at the turn of the century, is unlikely to be valid, since this mechanism of action would require recruitment of high-threshold unmyelinated fibers not usually activated by SCS in clinical situations. In a study that tested this hypothesis of antidromic activation of small-diameter fibers, Linderoth and coauthors observed that vasodilatation, as measured by laser Doppler flowmetry, was present after DCS, and after stimulation of the proximal ends of cut dorsal roots innervating the hind limb, but not after stimulation of the distal ends of the same cut nerve roots. The conclusion drawn from the findings was that SCS antidromically activates a central "loop" and not small afferent fibers for poststimulation vasodilatation to occur.[9] Most

TABLE 53–2 ***Circulatory Effects of Epidural Spinal Cord Stimulation: Macrocirculatory Parameters Before and After Stimulation***

	Before	*After*	*Significance*
Systolic ankle/arm pressure index (%)	32 ± 14	37 ± 14	None
Systolic toe pressure (mm Hg)	9 ± 16	10 ± 23	None

TABLE 53–3 ***Circulatory Effects of Epidural Spinal Cord Stimulation: Microcirculatory Parameters Before and After Stimulation***

	Before	After	Significance
Skin capillary density (N/mm^2)	12 ± 6	30 ± 5	$p < .001$
Skin capillary diameter (μm)	15.7 ± 1.8	15.5 ± 1.5	None
Red cell velocity (mm/sec)	0.054 ± 0.014	0.762 ± 0.205	$p < .001$
Sodium fluorescein perfused capillaries (N/mm^2)	20 ± 4	44 ± 5	$p < .001$
Sodium flourescein appearance time (sec)	72.15	45 ± 9	$p < .001$

recently, Croom and associates proposed that the vasodilatory response to SCS, at least at high frequencies, is due to the fact that high-frequency stimulation releases vasoactive substances such as vasointestinal peptide, substance P, or calcitonin gene–related peptide. Studies to date of peptide release have been inconclusive.[10]

Linderoth and colleagues from the Karolinska Institute in Sweden, more than any other group, have helped to elucidate the autonomic effects of stimulation-induced vasodilatation. In his studies with the rat model, Linderoth has shown that high spinalization of rats before SCS, in and of itself, causes vasodilation, which increases more after SCS. This is taken as presumptive evidence that DCS-induced vasodilatation is not secondary to supraspinal autonomic centers. In the same rat studies, sectioning of the ventral roots, alpha-adrenergic blockade, and bilateral lumbar sympathectomy were found to abolish SCS-induced vasodilatation.[11] The study findings on the importance of the role of the spinal segmental autonomic nervous system have been corroborated, according to Linderoth's thesis, by other investigators.[12]

Since it was known that SCS caused vasodilatation in animal studies, clinicians have used this modality to treat pain secondary to peripheral vascular disease in humans. In fact, at one time, peripheral vascular disease was the leading indication in Europe for SCS.[13–16] Table 53–2, from the work of Jacobs' group, represents typical macrocirculatory parameters seen with SCS in human patients. Table 53–3, from the same authors, represents microcirculatory parameters before and after SCS. The reader can see that there are little, if any, macrocirculatory changes after SCS but a significant increase in skin capillary density, increase in red blood cell velocity, increase in the numbers of sodium fluorescein–perfused capillaries, and a decrease in sodium fluorescein appearance time after SCS. These changes reflect significant alterations in microcirculatory parameters after SCS.

Augustinsson and associates from the department of Neurosurgery at the University of Goteborg, Sweden published a paper in 1985 that reported significant pain relief and healing of painful ischemic ulcers in patients with both vasoocclusive and vasospastic disease (Table 53–4, 53–5).[17] In this study of 34 patients with severe limb ischemia with resting pain and ischemic ulcers in most, 26 had arteriosclerotic peripheral vascular disease, one had Buerger's disease, and seven had severe vasospastic disease. Of the entire group, 94% experienced pain relief and 50% experienced healing of their ulcers. Only 38% of the "stimulated" group subsequently had to undergo amputation, as compared with 90% of a comparative nonstimulated control group (mean follow-up of 16 months).

SCS RELEASES PUTATIVE NEUROTRANSMITTERS AND NEUROMODULATORS

A fifth (and final) theory of the mechanism of action of SCS is based on the clinical observation that pain relief often outlasts actual electrical stimulation of the spinal cord by minutes, hours, or even days. Proponents posit that stimulation must release putative neurotransmitters or neuromodulators, which effect this prolonged pain relief. This theory has been tested by numerous investigators, often

TABLE 53–4 ***Effects of Spinal Cord Stimulation on Pain Relief***

	Relief				
	None	Fair+	Good+	Excellent+	Total Improved (No)
Disease					
AS	2 (10%)	7 (33%)	9 (43%)	3 (14%)	19/21 (90%)
D	—	2 (40%)	2 (40%)	1 (20%)	5/5 (100%)
B	—	1	—	—	1/1
VSD	—	1 (14%)	1 (14%)	5 (72%)	7/7 (100%)
AS +D + B+ VSD	2 (6%)	11 (32%)	12 (35%)	9 (27%)	

AS, arteriosclerosis; D, diabetes; B, Buerger's disease; VSD, vasospastic disease (Reynaud's).

From Augustinsson LE, Holm J, Carl A, et al: Epidural electrical stimulation in severe limb ischemia. Ann Surg 202:104, 1985.

TABLE 53–5 ***Effects of Ischemic Ulcer Healing Within 12 months***

Disease	No Effect	Improved Healing	Ulcer Healed	Total Improved
AS	8 (50%)	4 (25%)	4 (25%)	8/16 (50%)
D	4 (80%)	0	1 (20%)	1/5 (20%)
AS + D	12 (57%)	4 (20%)	5 (23%)	9/21 (43%)
VSD	0	0	3	3/3 (100%)
AS + D + VSD	12 (50%)	4 (17%)	8 (33%)	12/24 (50%)

AS, arteriosclerosis; D, diabetes; VSD, vasospastic disease.

with confusing and conflicting results. Recently, however, Linderoth's laboratory in Sweden has shed significant light on our understanding of the effects of SCS on the release of neuromodulators within the substance of the spinal cord.

In 1980, Levin and coworkers found an increase in epinephrine in the CSF after SCS,[18] and Meyerson's group[19] found an increase in substance P–like immunoreactivity in the CSF after SCS. Naloxone, although it reverses the antinociceptive effects of deep-brain periaquaductal or periventricular stimulation, does not reverse the analgesic effects of SCS.[20] Tonelli and colleagues observed increases in beta-endorphin and beta-lipotropin in the CSF of some patients after SCS.[21] Broggi and coworkers studied spinal tissue of rats and DE Richardson and CW Dempsey the cerebrospinal fluid of humans. In both, after SCS, they found elevations in serotonin and 5-hydroxyindoleacetic acid (5-HIAA), the metabolite of serotonin.[22, 23] Likewise, Linderoth's group, using high-performance liquid chromatography for serotonin and radioimmunoassay for substance P, observed elevations of serotonin levels, but not 5-HIAA, after DCS was applied to the thoracic spinal cord of cats. These authors also found that substance P–like immunoreactivity did not increase in the dorsal horns after DCS of decerebrate animals but increased considerably after DCS in normal animals.[24] The clinical significance of these studies is yet to be determined.

Most recently, Cui and associates have looked at the role of both adenosine and gamma-aminobutyric acid (GABA) on the effects of SCS.[25, 26] Using dorsal horn microdialysis probes in rat models of neuropathic pain, they observed a decrease in GABA in the dorsal horn. After SCS, there was increased release of GABA in these rats. Psychophysiologic pain studies show improvement in pain behavior after SCS. In a separate study, in a group of rats that did not receive the analgesic benefit of SCS and who did not release GABA after SCS, the addition of Baclofen, a GABA-b agonist, leads to increased release of GABA and a return to antinociception.[27]

SUMMARY

In summary, I have presented the animal and human experimental evidence for five different mechanistic theories of the impact of SCS on either spinal or supraspinal levels: gate, segmental mechanisms, segmental blockade of neural transmission, activation of supraspinal inhibitory mechanisms by SCS, activation of inhibitory effects on the sympathetic nervous system, and release of putative neuromodulators and transmitters. To this day, the exact mechanism or mechanisms of action for this clinically effective, implantable, pain-relieving technology remain obscure. What is needed for future studies is an appropriate animal model for SCS testing neurophysiologic and psychophysical parameters similar to human experience. We have not, in this paper, tried to elucidate the actual electrical effects or varying stimulation parameters on the actual psychophysical clinical effects experienced by patients in a clinical setting. The reader is advised to investigate the many reviews on this subject.[28–30]

REFERENCES

1. Shealy CN, Mortimer JT, Reswick J: Electrical inhibition of pain by stimulation of the dorsal column: Preliminary clinical reports. Anesth Analg 46:489–491, 1967.
2. Melzack R, Wall P: Pain mechanisms: A new theory. Science 150:971–978, 1965.
3. Foreman RD, Beall JE, Applebaum AE, et al: Effects of dorsal column stimulation on primate spinothalamic tract neurons. J Neurophysiol 39:534–546, 1976.
4. Handwerker HO, Iggo A, Zimmerman M: Segmental and supraspinal actions on dorsal horn neurons responding to noxious and non-noxious skin stimuli. Pain 1:147–165, 1975.
5. Feldman RA: Patterned response of lamina V cells: Cutaneous and dorsal funicular stimulation. Physiol Behavior 15:79–84, 1975.
6. Larson SJ, Sauces A, Riegel DH, et al: Neurophysiological effects of dorsal column stimulation in man and monkey. J Neurosurg 41:217–223, 1974.
7. Saade NE, Tabet MS, Soueidan SA, et al: Supraspinal modulation of nociception in awake rats by stimulation of the dorsal column nuclei. Brain Res 36:307–310, 1986.
8. Bayliss WM: On the origin from the spinal cord of the vasodilator fibers of the hind-limb and on the nature of these fibers. J Physiol 382:173–209, 1987.
9. Linderoth B, Fedorcsak I, Meyerson BA: Is vasodilatation following dorsal column stimulation mediated by antidromic activation of small diameter fibers? Acta Neurochir 46(Suppl):99–101, 1989.
10. Croom JE, Foreman RD, Chandler M, Barron KW: Reevaluation of the role of the sympathetic nervous system in cutaneous vasodilation during dorsal spinal cord stimulation: Are multiple mechanisms active? Neuromodulation 1:91–101, 1998.
11. Linderoth B: Dorsal column stimulation and pain: Experimental studies of putative neurochemical and neurophysiological mechanisms. Published thesis. Karolinska Institute, Stockholm, 1992.
12. Fedorcsak I, Linderoth B, Bognar L, et al: Peripheral vasodilation due to sympathetic inhibition induced by spinal cord stimulation. Pro IBRO World Congress of Neuroscience 1991, p 126.
13. Jacobs MJHM, Jorning PJ, Joshi SR, et al: Spinal cord electrical stimulation improves microvascular blood flow in severe limb ischaemia. Ann Surg 207:179–183, 1988.

14. Robaina FJ, Dominguez M, Diaz M, et al: Spinal cord stimulation for relief of chronic pain in vasospastic disorders of the upper limbs. Neurosurgery 24:179–183, 1989.
15. Groth KE: Spinal cord stimulation for the treatment of peripheral vascular disease. Adv Pain Res Ther (9):861–870, 1985.
16. Tallis RC, Illis LS, Sedgwick C, et al: Spinal cord stimulation in peripheral vascular disease. J Neurol Neurosurg Psychiatry 6:478–484, 1983.
17. Augustinsson LE, Holm J, Carl A, et al: Epidural electrical stimulation in severe limb ischemia: Evidences of pain relief, increased blood flow and a possible limb saving effect. Ann Surg 202:104–111, 1985.
18. Levin BE, Hubschmann OR: Dorsal column stimulation: Effect on human cerebrospinal fluid and plasma catecholamines. Neurology 30:65–71, 1980.
19. Meyerson BA, Brodin E, Linderoth B: Possible neurohumoral mechanisms in CNS stimulation for pain suppression. Appl Neurophysiol 48:175–180, 1985.
20. Freemen TB, Campbell JN, Long DM: Naloxone does not affect pain relief induced by electrical stimulation in man. Pain 17:189–195, 1983.
21. Tonelli L, Setti T, Falasca A, et al: Investigation on cerebrospinal fluid opioids and neurotransmitters related to spinal cord stimulation. Appl Neurophysiol 51:324–332, 1988.
22. Broggi G, Franzini A, Parati E, et al: Neurochemical and structural modifications related to pain control induced by spinal cord stimulation. *In* Lazorthes Y, Upton ARM (eds): Neurostimulation: An Overview. New York, Futura, 1985, pp 87–95.
23. Richardson DE, Dempsey CW: Monoamine turnover in CSF of patients during spinal cord stimulation for pain control. Pain 2(Suppl):223, 1984.
24. Linderoth B, Gazelius B, Frank J, Brodin E: Dorsal column stimulation induces release of seratonin and substance P in the cat dorsal horn. Neurosurgery 31:289–296, 1992.
25. Cui JG, Sollevi A, Linderoth B, Meyerson BA: Adenosine receptor activation suppresses tactile hypersensitivity and potentiates effect of spinal cord in mononeuropathic rats. Neurosci Lett 223:173–176, 1997.
26. Cui JG, Meyerson BA, Sollevi A, Linderoth B: Effects of spinal cord stimulation on tactile hypersensitivity in mononeuropathic rats is potentiated by GABA-B and adenosine receptor activation. Neurosci Lett 247:183–186, 1998.
27. Meyerson BA, Cui JG, Yakhnitsa V, et al: Modulation of spinal pain mechanisms by spinal cord stimulation and the potential role of adjuvant pharmacotherapy. Stereotact Funct Neurosurg 68:129–140, 1997.
28. Holsheimer J, Struijk JJ, Tas NR: Effect of electrode geometry and combination on nerve fibre selectivity in spinal cord stimulation. Med Biol Eng Comp 33:676–682, 1995.
29. Wesselink WA, Holsheimer J, Nuttin B, et al: Estimation of fiber diameters in the spinal dorsal columns from clinical data. IEEE Trans Biomed Eng 45:1355–1362, 1988.
30. Wesselink WA, Holsheimer J, King GW, et al: Quantitative aspects of the clinical performance of transverse tripolar spinal cord stimulation. Neuromodulation 2:5–14, 1999.

CHAPTER • 54

Spinal Cord Stimulation and Intractable Pain: Patient Selection

Elliot S. Krames, MD

The costs of unrelieved pain and disability arising from it in the United States are, and will continue to be, a major problem until appropriate, cost-effective algorithms for the management of chronic pain are created and implemented. Chronic, unrelieved pain is not only a major drain on scarce healthcare resources but is the cause of untold suffering for millions of people worldwide. In a recent study of the general population of the state of Michigan, the Michigan Pain Study, it was found that one in five adults, or about 1.2 million people in Michigan, suffer from some form of chronic, ongoing or recurring pain.[1] In the workplace, in this population, pain is responsible for 400,000 workers' (12 percent of the state's workforce) failing to show up for work at some point in 1999. Of the pain sufferers surveyed, 35% missed more than 20 days of work during the year.

The direct, hard costs of unremitting pain to patients and their families are loss of job, loss of income, loss of savings (and therefore security), loss of insurance, and loss of self-esteem. More intangible results of unrelieved pain include depression, anger, frustration, and suffering, among others. The end result of all of this is staggering to society and to individuals unfortunate enough to suffer such pain. The Michigan Pain Study cited earlier surveyed 1500 Michigan residents aged 18 and older to determine the severity of the chronic pain problem, how people cope, access to treatment, and the effectiveness of available pain care. Of the 1.2 million people in Michigan who suffer from chronic pain, 42% say pain has affected their relationships with spouses, family members, and fellow workers. Nearly half (48%) experience depression; 18% have overdosed on pain medication; and 10%, about 120,000, have contemplated suicide. Looking for solutions for their pain has led 5% of them (approximately 60,000 adults) to drink alcohol, including 18% who admit to overdosing on their medication. Some 29% of the population felt that they were losing sleep because of their chronic pain. Indeed, these figures paint a gloomy and compelling picture of the true costs of chronic, unrelieved pain to our society.

In a 1999 survey cosponsored by The American Academy of Pain Medicine, The American Pain Society, and Janssen Pharmaceutica, it was found that 56% of all persons with chronic, moderate to severe pain had been suffering for more than 5 years, 47% of them had changed doctors at least once since their pain began (22%, three times or more), and for 48% the primary reason for changing physicians was persistent pain after treatment. The primary reasons for changing doctors included patients' continued suffering (42%), doctors' poor understanding of pain and its mechanisms (31%), doctors' not taking their pain seriously enough (29%), and doctors' unwillingness to treat it aggressively (27%).

Clearly, the problem of intractable chronic pain—whether related or unrelated to cancer—is, today, a major problem in the United States, if not in the world, because it is both a drain on scarce healthcare resources and it exacts a tremendous emotional and physical price, from patients and their families. It is my purpose in this chapter to present spinal cord stimulation as a viable and cost-effective intervention for the treatment of chronic, refractory pain when less invasive and less costly therapies have failed.

TOOLS OF THE TRADE

The physician who treats patients with chronic intractable pain should be familiar with the appropriate and accepted use of all "tools of the trade" that are considered acceptable for their treatment. The tools of the pain practitioner include all of the modalities and therapies, conservative and invasive, used for treating chronic and cancer-related pain syndromes. Implantable devices such as those for spinal cord stimulation also have a place in the management of chronic nonmalignant pain syndromes and in certain patients with prolonged life expectancy may have a role in cancer- and AIDS-related pain.

The physician treating chronic pain should know not only how and when to use treatment modalities but also the source of the pain and the psychological and behavioral factors operant in perpetuating the patient's pain. Because chronic pain is never solely a neurobiologic issue but almost always is multidimensional (involving neurophysiologic systems as well as emotional and behavioral ones), a multidisciplinary evaluation and treatment plan are essential for successful treatment. Once a pain syndrome–specific diagnosis is established, a treatment plan that addresses both the neurophysiologic process or processes operant in the patient's pain generation and the cognitive, emotional, and behavioral processes involved is created by the pain team, a group that includes experts in the fields of pain medicine, physical and occupational therapy, and cognitive and behavioral therapy.

Because multiple modality choices are available for the treatment of chronic pain, we suggest treating these patients according to a treatment algorithm that makes use of therapies in increasing order of invasiveness and cost. According to this pain treatment continuum, we first utilize therapies that are least invasive and least costly, in series or in combination, and then, when less invasive therapies fail to provide adequate analgesia, we utilize increasing levels of intervention until either a single therapy or a combination of therapies is found to be efficacious. Choices for the treatment of chronic pain utilizing multidisciplinary interventions include cognitive-behavioral psychological therapies, functional rehabilitation therapies, orthopedic and neurologic surgery, pharmacotherapy, anesthetic blocking techniques, neuromodulatory interventions such as spinal cord stimulation and spinally administered analgesia, and, finally, neurodestructive procedures. The therapies are listed in order, from the most conservative procedure to the most invasive one. This continuum might suggest that therapies are to be tried sequentially—that a new intervention is instituted when the previous one fails. The continuum, as presented here, merely lists therapies in order of increasing levels of invasiveness, and perhaps

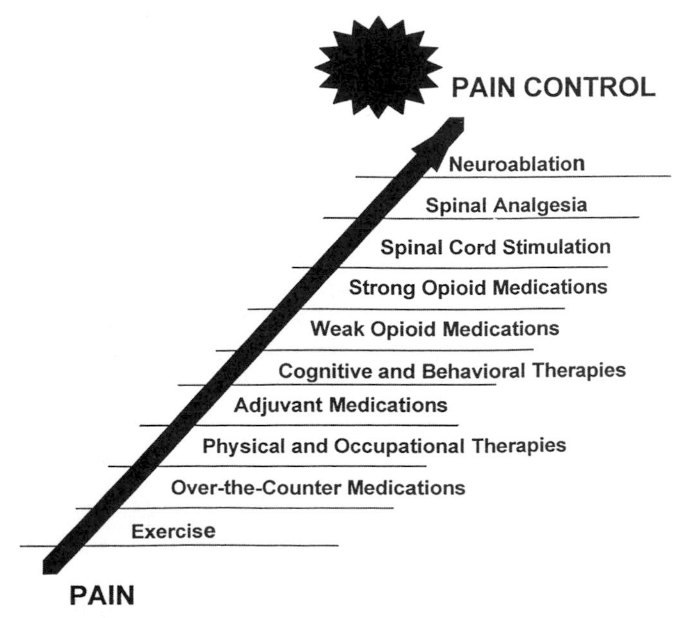

FIGURE 54–1 The Pain Treatment Continuum is a suggested algorithm for the appropriate use of possible pain management therapies. These therapies are listed in order of increasing invasiveness. The algorithm appears to suggest that therapies be used in series, abandoning therapies that don't work and enlisting more invasive therapies in sequential order. In actuality, these therapies can be used in parallel, with one or more therapies being tried at the same time.

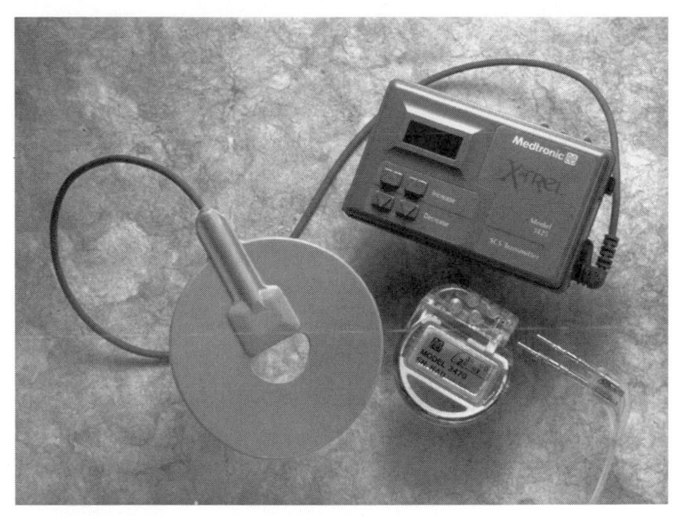

FIGURE 54–2 Medtronic Matrix implanted receiving device. (Courtesy of Medtronic, Minneapolis, Minn.)

cost. These therapies might be used in series, but, in fact, most often are used in parallel. For example, for failed back surgery syndrome in a patient who is taking nonsteroidal antiinflammatory drugs, weak opioids, tricyclic antidepressants, and membrane stabilizers and is participating in a cognitive-behavioral, functional restorative program, epidural analgesia is used to facilitate participation in the physical therapy. An example of a treatment continuum, one that the author uses and one certainly not based on clinical science, is found in Figure 54–1. This continuum is a *suggested* approach to treatments for intractable pain. Certainly, if the patient would benefit from a "surgical fix," that procedure should be performed before other pain-relieving modalities. As the reader can see from this algorithm, spinal cord stimulation is a technologic intervention that should be considered last resort therapy before neuroablative techniques. Some experts in the field would argue that radiofrequency ablative techniques should be used earlier, to obviate more costly "permanent" neuroaugmentation procedures.

SPINAL CORD STIMULATION: WHAT IS IT?

Spinal cord stimulation therapy for pain control applies an electrical field over the spinal cord, that, by some mechanism, blocks pain of neuropathic origin. It most successfully abolishes neuropathic appendicular pain, but it has also been shown to be successful in patients with neuropathic axial pain.[2] Except in the case of pain due to peripheral vascular disease, spinal cord stimulation is not effective for axial somatic, nociceptive pain. This therapy works by propagating an electrical pulse wave generated either (1) with an external neuropulse generator that transmits the electrical pulse via cable to an antenna worn externally that is radiocoupled to an implanted receiving device* (Fig. 54–2) or (2) with an implanted, programmable, neuropulse

* EXTREL or MATRIX, Medtronic, Minneapolis, Minn. or RENEW, Advanced Neuromodulation Systems, Plano, Tex.

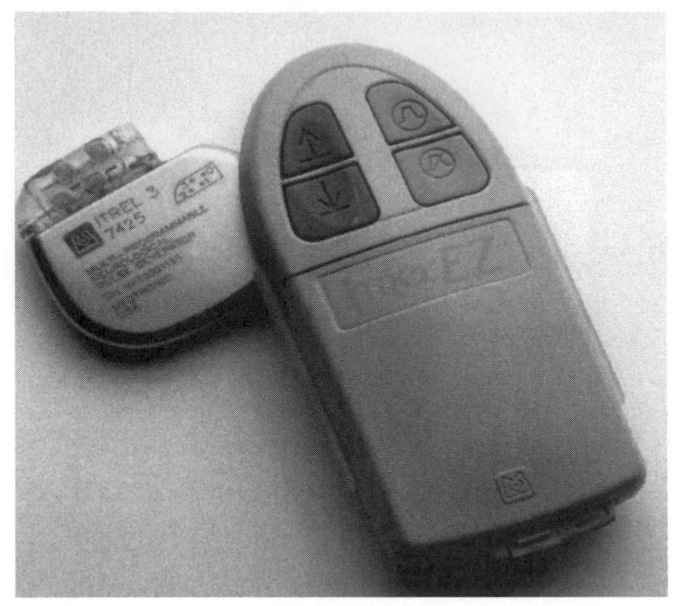

FIGURE 54–3 Medtronic Itrel 3 implanted, programmable neuropulse generator. (Courtesy of Medtronic, Minneapolis, Minn.)

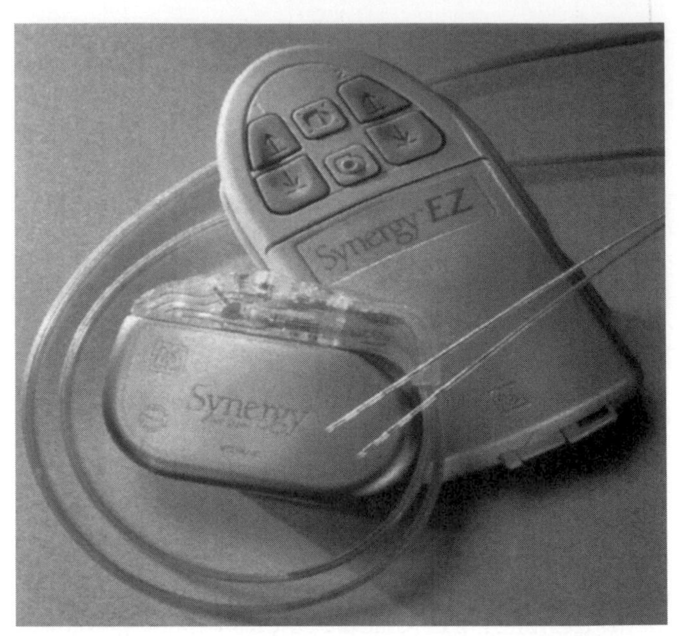

FIGURE 54–4 Medtronic Synergy implanted, programmable neuropulse generator. (Courtesy of Medtronic, Minneapolis, Minn.)

generator† that contains a battery pack, an antenna, and a computer module that allows external programming (Figs. 54–3, 54–4).

Whether the electrical pulse wave is generated by an implanted device or an external device through an implanted radiocoupled receiver, the pulse is transmitted to its intended target, the spinal cord, via an implanted electrical cable connected to an implanted array of electrodes placed percutaneously or surgically (Fig. 54–5).These electrode arrays are implanted in the epidural space overlying the spinal cord segment that is processing the patient's pain. In the early days of this therapy, unipolar electrodes were implanted surgically directly onto the dorsal columns. Later, thanks to advances in technology, multichannel quadropolar and octopolar leads utilizing bipolar stimulation were introduced and were superior to single-channel devices. Before the early 1990s, most, if not almost all, electrode arrays were single, quadropolar, electrodes implanted surgically or percutaneously.

IMPLANTATION OF ELECTRODE ARRAYS

Implantation of the electrode array or arrays into the epidural space is performed either percutaneously via a Tuohy epidural needle or directly through a minilaminotomy. For percutaneous implantation, an incision is made over the lumbar spine (for thoracic epidural placement) or over the thoracic spine (for cervical epidural placement). The incisions are carried down to the supraspinal fascia in the midline or, if off the midline, to the perispinal fascia. An epidural needle is placed at the cephalad apex of the incision and advanced anteriorly through the tissue planes of the back and cephalad from a paramedian position to the spinous processes and is introduced into the epidural space using a loss-of-resistance technique, to a point one to two segments above where the needle entered the incision. Once the needle is within the epidural space, the electrode array or dual arrays (advanced through two needles placed on either side of the epidural space) is advanced and steered within the epidural space. The target for electrode array placement is that segment of the spinal cord that, when electrically stimulated, produces a paresthesia perceived as comfortable that "covers" the patient's subjective pain complaint. This paresthesia (tingling) over the area of subjective pain complaint is called *the area of concordant paresthesia*. Because there is usually more than one area of the spinal cord that, when electrically stimulated, might produce concordant paresthesia, a second goal of stimulation

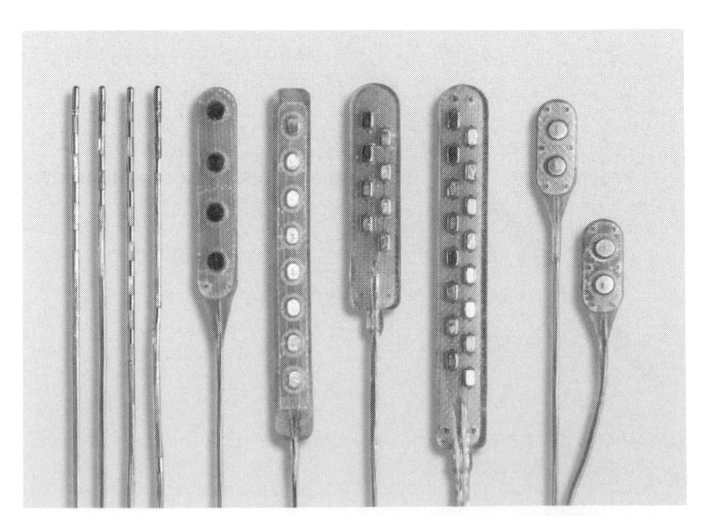

FIGURE 54–5 Grouping of electrodes from Advanced Neuromodulation Systems. (Courtesy of Advanced Neuromodulation Systems, Plano, Tex.)

† ITREL 3 or SYNERGY, Medtronic, Minneapolis, Minn.

is to produce this paresthesia with the least voltage, pulse width, or rate (battery drain) possible, and within a use range that is at least two to three times the perceptual threshold value. The ultimate goal, in addition to concordant paresthesia, is battery longevity.

Because this concordant paresthesia is subjective and perceptual, the patient must be awake while the operating surgeon locates the area. Patient participation is key—and fundamental—to the success of the procedure. During the placement phase, electrodes are programmed to generate an electric field. At the very least, one cathode (positive electrode) and one anode (negative) must be activated to generate an electrical field. The number of possible combinations of programming is directly proportional to the number of electrodes.

If implantation is performed directly through a laminotomy incision, the incision is usually placed directly over or slightly inferior or superior to the spinal cord segment that will be stimulated. The epidural space is entered directly through minilaminotomy, and a plate electrode array is placed over the area that produces concordant paresthesia. Usually, this area has been identified in a trial of spinal cord stimulation with percutaneously placed electrodes.

INDICATIONS AND EFFICACY

Single-electrode arrays are generally used successfully for stimulation of unilateral neuropathic pain of a lower or an upper extremity. The choice of single quadropolar leads or single octopolar leads depends on surgeon preference. Some investigators feel that the smaller interelectrode distances in octopolar leads have physiologic advantages[7] and the fact that octopolar arrays contain more electrodes than quadropolar arrays (eight instead of four) makes these leads more stable with gross cephalocaudad movement of the lead. If gross cephalocaudad movement of the array of electrodes outside the spinal target area should occur, concordant paresthesia (necessary for pain control) would be lost and might not be restored with simple reprogramming of different electrodes in a quadropolar array, whereas it might be recaptured by an octopolar array. If reprogramming is ineffective in recapturing concordant paresthesia, a costly surgical revision of electrode becomes necessary.

Although single-electrode arrays have been used successfully to produce concordant paresthesia (and therefore pain relief) for both unilateral and bilateral lower and upper extremity pain,[3–8] dual-electrode arrays, either dual quadropolar (MATRIX or RENEW) or dual octopolar (RENEW) percutaneously implanted arrays or surgically implanted arrays placed parallel to each other on either side of the midline of the spinal cord do this job more reliably, and better.[2,9,10] Single electrodes in the midline can produce this concordant paresthesia, but any slight movement off the absolute midline will shift more (sometimes all) paresthesia to the same side. This unfortunate complication demands costly replacement of the electrode array.

From recent computer modeling evidence from the University of Twente in the Netherlands[11–14] and from recent reports in the literature, it is becoming clear that patients with low back pain and bilateral leg pain, like those with chronic arachnoiditis or epidural fibrosis secondary to one or more back operations (failed back surgery syndrome), can obtain relief of not only their lower extremity pain but also their low back pain with dual quadropolar or octopolar lead arrays.[2, 9, 10, 15] Again, the choice of the appropriate system is left to the surgeon. As with single-lead systems a case could be made for greater stability of dual octopolar lead systems as compared with dual quadropolar systems.

Another indication for dual, triple, or even quadropolar electrode systems is nonmalignant pain at multiple sites. A good candidate would be a patient with both lumbar and cervical radiculitis who has upper and lower extremity pain. Because concordant paresthesia is necessary for pain relief, it would be necessary in such a patient to place single-lead (or even dual-lead) quadropolar or octopolar leads in the neck and the back.

In the United States, the primary indication for spinal cord stimulation is failed back surgery syndrome,[16] and both sympathetic pain and sympathetic-independent pain of complex regional pain syndrome.[7,8,17–19] In Europe, interest in spinal cord stimulation has been greatest in connection with treatment of chronic intractable angina[20–23] and pain and disability due to peripheral vascular disease.[24–28]

Mark Twain once said, "What a good thing Adam had when he said a good thing; he knew nobody had said it before." In the field of spinal cord stimulation there are numerous retrospective studies that tout the efficacy of spinal cord stimulation. These studies or reports usually lump together patients who have various pain syndromes of different kinds. The substance of many of these studies suggests that, for many such syndromes, efficacy is approximately 60% and relief lasts about 2 years. After 2 years, for whatever reason, in some patients efficacy seems to fall off. Spinal cord stimulation is effective not only for neuropathic pain of appendicular and axial origin but also for complex regional pain syndrome (CRPS), peripheral vascular disease, and in the pain of intractable angina.

CONCLUSION

In this chapter, I have introduced and summarized the present state of the knowledge on spinal cord stimulation and have introduced the reader to the concept of dual–spinal cord stimulation. Based on added movement stability, the advent of narrower, intralead distances, and the ability to enter multiple programs, these dual–spinal cord stimulation systems are adding significantly to our ability to control certain types of pain of neuropathic origin.

Spinal cord stimulation is cost-effective when used properly in appropriate patients, considering the staggering direct dollar costs of unrelieved pain and disability and the direct emotional costs to patients who suffer chronic unremitting pain and their families.

Spinal cord stimulation is efficacious, although the mechanism or mechanisms of action remain obscure to this day. More, however, is being learned each year about these mechanisms.

REFERENCES

1. The Michigan Pain Study. EPIC/MRA 4710 W. Saginaw Hwy. Lansing, Michigan 48917-2601, 1997.

2. Law JD: Spinal stimulation: Statistical superiority of monophasic stimulation of narrowly separated, longitudinal bipoles having rostral cathodes.
3. Long DM, et al: Electrical stimulation of the spinal cord and peripheral nerves for pain control: A ten year experience. Appl Neurophysiol 44:207–217, 1981.
4. Spiegelmann R, Friedman WA: Spinal cord stimulation: A contemporary series. Neurosurgery 28:65–70, 1991.
5. Barolat G, Ketchik B, He J: Long-term outcome of spinal cord stimulation for chronic pain management. Neuromodulation 1:19–30, 1998.
6. North RB, Roark GI: Spinal cord stimulation for chronic pain. Neurosurg Clin North Am 6:145–155, 1995.
7. Oakley JC, Weiner RL: Spinal cord stimulation for complex regional pain syndrome: A prospective study of 19 patients at two centers. Neuromodulation 2:47–51, 1999.
8. Bennett DS, Alo KM, Oakley J, Feler CA: Spinal cord stimulation for complex regional pain syndrome (RSD): A retrospective multicenter experience from 1995–1998 of 101 patients. Neuromodulation 3:202–210, 1999.
9. Alo KM, Yland MJ, Kramer DL, et al: Computer assisted and patient interactive programming of dual octrode spinal cord stimulation in the treatment of chronic pain. Neuromodulation 1:30–46, 1998.
10. Alo KM, Yland MJ, Charnov JH, Redko V: Multiple program spinal cord stimulation in the treatment of chronic pain: Follow-up of multiple program SCS. Neuromodulation 4:266–275, 1994.
11. Holsheimer J, Struijk JJ: How do geometric factors influence epidural spinal cord stimulation? Stereotact Funct Neurosurg 56:77–103, 1991.
12. Struijk JJ, Holsheimer J, van der Heide GG, Boorn HBK: Recruitment of dorsal column fibers in spinal cord stimulation: Influence of collateral branching. IEEE Trans Biomed Eng 39:903–912, 1992.
13. Holsheimer J, Struijk JJ, Wesselink WA: Analysis of spinal cord stimulation and design of epidural electrodes by computer modeling. Neuromodulation 1:30–46, 1998.
14. Holsheimer J, Barolat G: Spinal geometry and paresthesia coverage in spinal cord stimulation. Neuromodulation 1:129–137, 1998.
15. Van Buyten JP, Zundert JV, Milbouw G: Treatment of failed back surgery syndrome patients with low back and leg pain: A pilot study of a new dual lead spinal cord stimulation system. Neuromodulation 2:258–266, 1999.
16. North RB, Ewend MG, Lawton MT, Piantadosi S: Spinal cord stimulation for chronic, intractable pain: Superiority of "multi-channel" devices. Pain 44:119–130, 1991.
17. Broseta J, et al: Chronic epidural dorsal column stimulation in the treatment of causalgic pain. Appl Neurophysiol 45:190–194, 1982.
18. Barolat G, Schwartzman R, Woo R: Epidural spinal cord stimulation in the management of reflex sympathetic dystrophy. Stereotact Funct Neurosurg 53:29–39, 1989.
19. Stanton-Hicks M: Spinal cord stimulation for the management of complex regional pain syndromes. Neuromodulation 2:193–202, 1999.
20. Mannheimer C, Augustinsson LE, Carlsson CA, et al: Epidural spinal electrical stimulation in severe angina pectoris. Br Heart J 59:56–61, 1988.
21. Augustinsson LE: Spinal cord stimulation in severe angina pectoris: Surgical technique, intraoperative physiology, complications, and side effects. PACE 12:693–694, 1989.
22. Murphy DF, Giles KE: Dorsal column stimulation for pain relief from intractable angina pectoris. 3:365–368, 1987.
23. deJongste MJL, Hatvast RWM, Ruiters MHJ, ter Horst GJ: Spinal cord stimulation and the induction of c-*fos* and heat shock protein 72 in the central nervous system of rats. Neuromodulation 1:73–85, 1998.
24. Robaina FJ, et al: Spinal cord stimulation for relief of chronic pain in vasospastic disorders of the upper limbs. Neurosurgery 24:179–183, 1989.
25. Augustinsson LE, Holm J, Carl A, et al: Epidural electrical stimulation in severe limb ischemia: Evidences of pain relief, increased blood flow and a possible limb saving effect. Ann Surg 202:104–111, 1985.
26. Jacobs MJHM, et al: Spinal cord electrical stimulation improves microvascular blood flow in severe limb ischaemia. Ann Surg 207:179–183, 1988.
27. Groth KE: Spinal cord stimulation for the treatment of peripheral vascular disease. Adv Pain Res Ther 9:861–870, 1985.
28. Claeys LGY: Spinal cord stimulation and chronic critical limb ischemia. Neuromodulation 2:1, 1999.

CHAPTER • 55

Implantation Techniques for Spinal Cord Stimulation

Marshall D. Bedder, MD, FRCP(C)

Patients are selected for spinal cord stimulation (SCS) after more conservative treatment regimens and modalities have failed. A multidisciplinary approach that incorporates psychological screening is very important in ensuring appropriate patient selection.[1] Patients who exhibit mood disorders can be treated pharmacologically before a trial of SCS, to maximize its reliability. SCS has been used around the world for patients with angina, peripheral vascular disease, or a chronic pain syndrome.[2–4] In general, patients who present with neuropathic pain conditions are considered excellent candidates. These include diagnoses such as failed back surgery syndrome, arachnoiditis, perineural fibrosis, chronic regional pain syndrome (CRPS), phantom limb, and diagnoses subsumed under the rubric of *deafferentation pain*. Once the decision has been made to progress to SCS, the appropriate trial must be performed before implantation of the entire SCS system is undertaken.

TRIAL STIMULATION

Planning

The diagnosis and the location of the patient's pain dictate the choice and preference of leads and equipment for both the trial and final internalization of the complete system. The initial decision break point will determine if the patient will use a radiofrequency (RF)-coupled stimulator system (Fig. 55–1) or a totally implantable, programmable pulse generator (Fig. 55–2). For an RF system, the receiver portion is implanted subcutaneously and the pulse generator attached with adhesive to the skin. Because this type of system has external batteries, continual replacement of the implantable type of pulse generator when the batteries wear out is unnecessary. Another planning option is single leads (and number of contacts) or a multiple-lead array. Newer multiple-lead arrays with 16 contacts (Fig. 55–3) can be computer programmed for stimulation assessment and more complex program availability. Dual leads may be needed for certain patients whose pain is bilateral. Newer research indicates that failed–back surgery patients for whom low back pain (as opposed to radicular pain) is a major component of their complaint may do better with dual Octrodes.[5] Using eight-contact leads (Octrodes) instead of four (quad leads) may afford greater programming flexibility, so that lead revisions are minimized if lead migration occurs.[6]

Equipment

Two medical device manufacturers now dominate the field of SCS. Medtronic Inc. and Advanced Neuromodulation Systems (ANS) compete with devices that have different lead, generator, and programming capabilities. Traditionally, the strength of Medtronic has been its Itrel implantable pulse generators (see Fig. 55–2); ANS pioneered the development of multiple-lead arrays (Fig. 55–4) and computerized delivery of multiple stimulation programs (Fig. 55–5). The ANS PainDoc computerized support system has facilitated optimization of complex intraoperative and postoperative programming. The PainDoc is a comprehensive system for ongoing patient management. It has the capability to record pain maps, characteristics, and severity. It standardizes clinical data collection and documents outcomes, which then can be archived and managed. The Itrel generators must be programmed in a physican's office using a console programmer; although the patient does have limited control through an external unit that can control the ON-OFF function and pulse intensity and frequency (Fig. 55–6). The ANS Renew patient-controlled transmitter has three stimulation modes to increase the therapeutic options. Patients can manually select as many as 24 programs that were programmed earlier with the PainDoc system. The Multi-Stim feature automatically delivers multiple programs that allow stimulation of different anatomic segments for treatment of diffuse, multifocal pain patterns (Fig. 55–7).

This chapter is modified from Bedder M: Management of complications of spinal cord stimulation. Pain Rev 4:238–243, 1997, with permission.

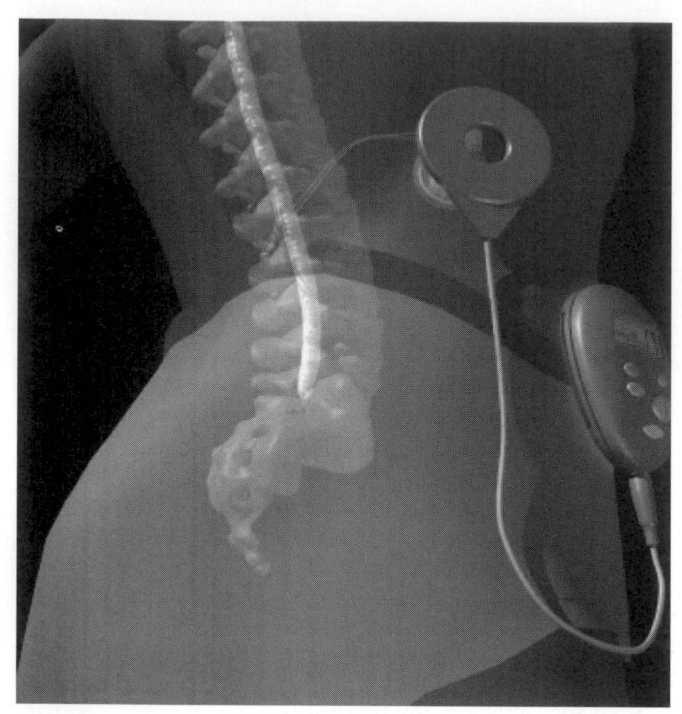

FIGURE 55–1 *Advanced Neuromodulation Systems (ANS) Renew Neurostimulation System. (Courtesy of Advanced Neuromodulation Systems, Plano, Tex.)*

Protocols

SCS trials are performed on an outpatient basis using either a percutaneous or a two-stage protocol. A simple percutaneous trial involves placing a separate trial lead, which is discarded after the trial. These trials can be performed in a fluroscopy suite (as opposed to an operating room) if desired. The procedure involves no cutdown or dissection, and the leads are not surgically anchored. New adhesive skin-anchoring systems are very effective in keeping the leads in place for the (traditional) 1-week trial period. One

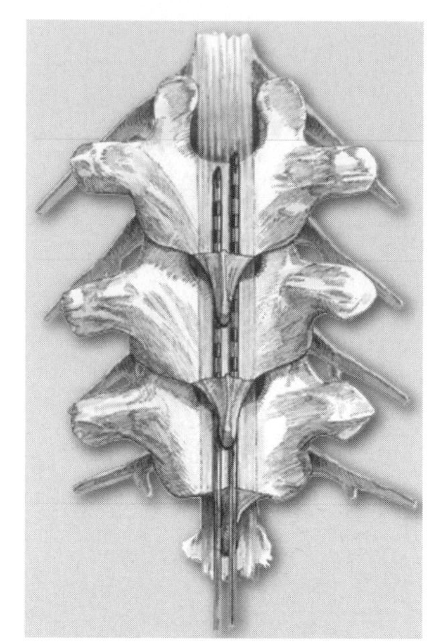

FIGURE 55–3 *ANS dual Octodes. (Courtesy of Advanced Neuromodulation Systems, Plano, Tex.)*

such system is the Percu-Stay percutaneous catheter fastener (Genetic Laboratories).

The benefits of the percutaneous trial add up to more than the cost savings. If a trial is unsuccessful, the lead can be removed without returning to the operating room, a step that would be necessary with a two-stage trial, when the lead is anchored after surgical dissection in anticipation of permanent implantation. One other major advantage is that the patient can experience trial SCS without the pain of a surgical incision. This can be important for an already sensitized chronic pain patient. Furthermore, many surgeons prefer a percutaneous trial, to avoid permanent implantation of an SCS system in a potentially contaminated

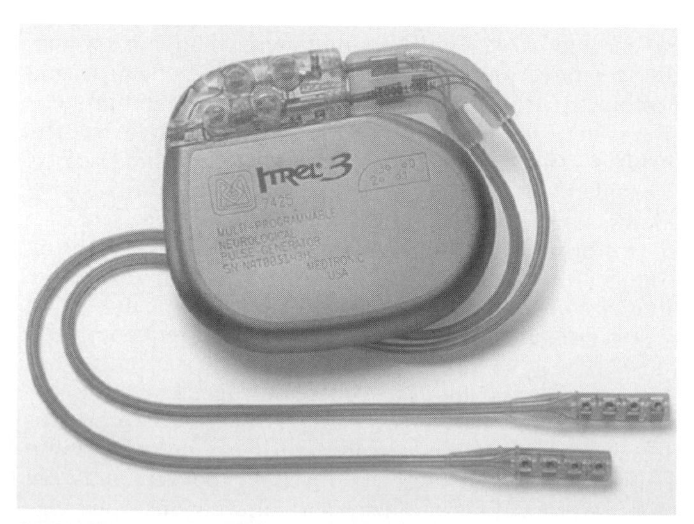

FIGURE 55–2 *Medtronic Itrel 3 implantable pulse generator. (Courtesy of Medtronic, Minneapolis, Minn.)*

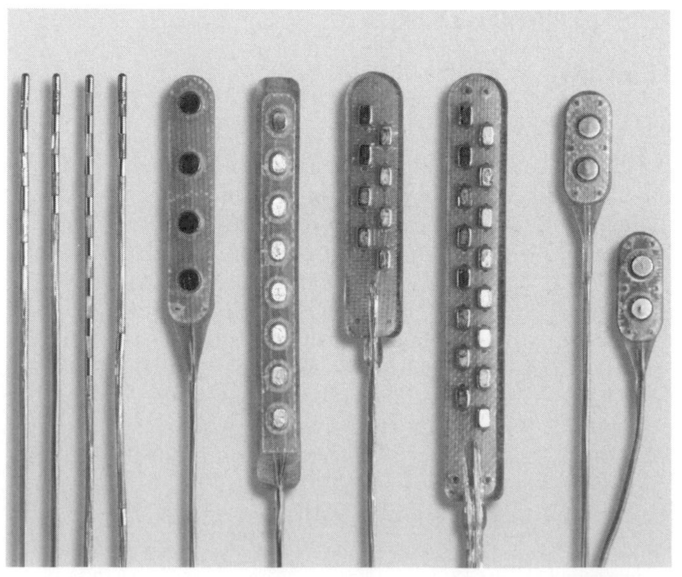

FIGURE 55–4 *ANS leads and arrays. (Courtesy of Advanced Neuromodulation Systems, Plano, Tex.)*

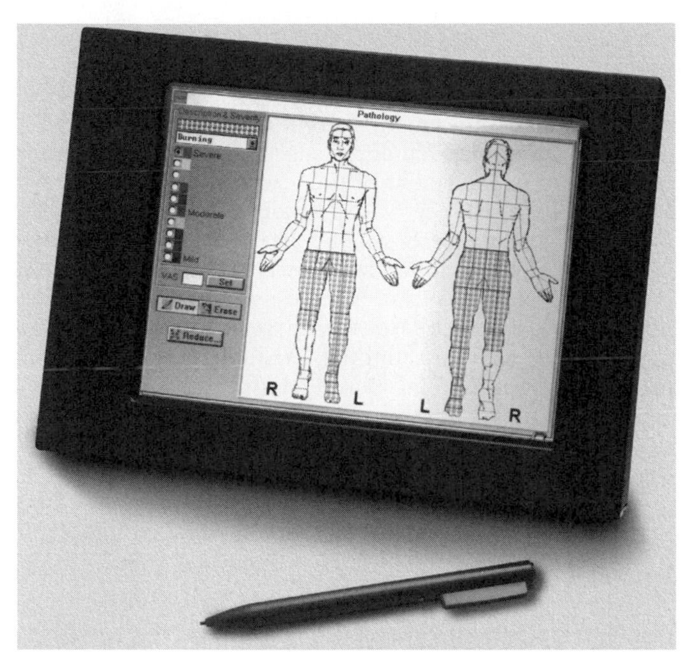

FIGURE 55–5 PAINDOC computerized support system. (Courtesy of Advanced Neuromodulation Systems, Plano, Tex.)

field (i.e., contamination through tunneled exteriorized trial connections).

Proponents of the two-stage approach argue that having to replace leads in the exact position where stimulation paresthesia was produced is time-consuming and costly. They also cite the added expense of using separate trial leads, which are discarded after the trial. To accurately analyze the cost-benefit ratio would require looking at the overall conversion rate from trials to full implantation. Which type of trial is utilized remains a matter of the physician's training, experience, access to resources, and type of pain practice.

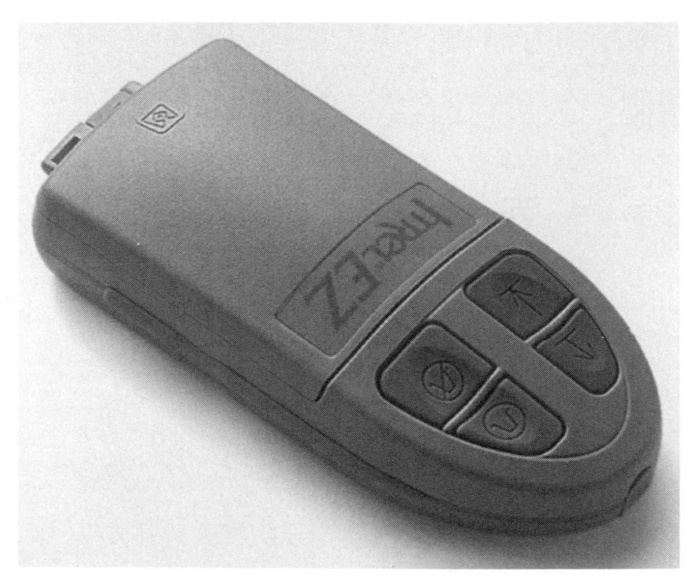

FIGURE 55–6 Medtronic Itrel EZ patient programmer. (Courtesy of Medtronic, Minneapolis, Minn.)

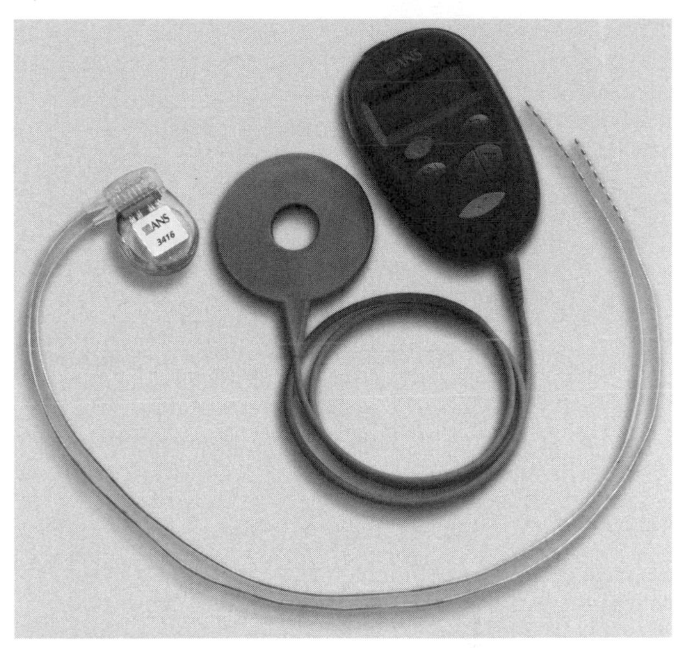

FIGURE 55–7 ANS Renew transmitter. (Courtesy of Advanced Neuromodulation Systems, Plano, Tex.)

Regardless of what trial protocol is utilized, the patient must be able to perform the usual activities of daily living (ADL) to fully assess its efficacy. A realistic assessment encompasses any enhancement of ADL coupled with medication and visual analogue pain scores. The assessment should last 1 week, to gain as objective an assessment as possible. It appears that trial durations are increasing worldwide.

SURGICAL TECHNIQUE

Once the type of lead and style of system have been chosen, the surgical techniques are basically similar. The practitioner must become familiar with the specific issues of each manufacturer's equipment and of the different models. ANS lead systems are available as one-piece units that, finally, must be connected in the generator pocket, although extensions are available and are used mainly for cervical implantation. All Medtronic lead systems utilize a lead extension, and the lead-lead extension connection is made at the spinal incision. A generator pocket of the correct depth is paramount. An RF receiver system must be implanted no deeper than 1 cm, whereas an Itrel implanted pulse generator is generally placed deeper, but no deeper than 1 inch (Fig. 55–8).

Lead Placement

For initial lead placement the patient can lie in the lateral decubitus position, but, increasingly, the prone position is being used and a bolster placed under the costal margin to promote adequate flexion of the spine and facilitate epidural lead placement. Whether for a simple percutaneous trial or a two-stage surgically anchored trial, the patient is prepared and draped in the usual manner for surgery,

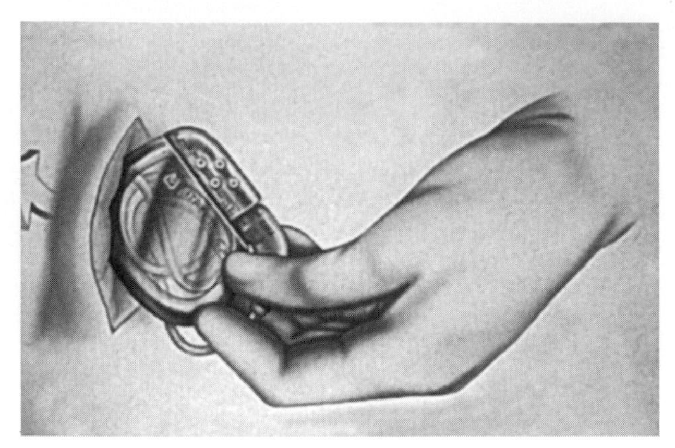

FIGURE 55–8 Subcutaneous pulse generator pocket. (Courtesy of Medtronic, Minneapolis, Minn.)

with strict aseptic technique. The usual entry level for patients with lower extremity, hip or back pain is L1–L2 (Fig. 55–9). Fluoroscopy is used to guide and confirm the midline and level of entry into the epidural space. Care must be taken to drape the fluoroscopy unit and to provide an extra side drape, to prevent contamination of the surgical field during cross-table views. Fluoroscopy will help to guide placement of two leads, if needed, for bilateral pain distribution. Local anesthetic with a vasoconstrictor is injected at the proposed insertion site. A combination of 1% lidocaine and 0.5% bupivacaine with epinephrine is a useful mixture for both short-term and postoperative analgesia.

Percutaneous trials are performed without skin incisions or dissection for anchoring. Two-stage initial lead placements or definitive placement of an SCS system after a successful trial will proceed with a midline or slightly paramedian skin incision after local anesthetic infiltration. Patients must be alert and responsive enough to report on stimulation coverage. Therefore, general anesthesia is contraindicated and appropriate and judicious sedation may be employed by the anesthesiologist. Entry into the epidural space, using the manufacturer's supplied modified Tuohy needle, is facilitated by a slightly paraspinal approach. It is important to keep the angle of entry as shallow as possible, to more easily advance the lead cephalad. With a shallower angle, steering of the lead is easier because of the mechanical advantage it affords.

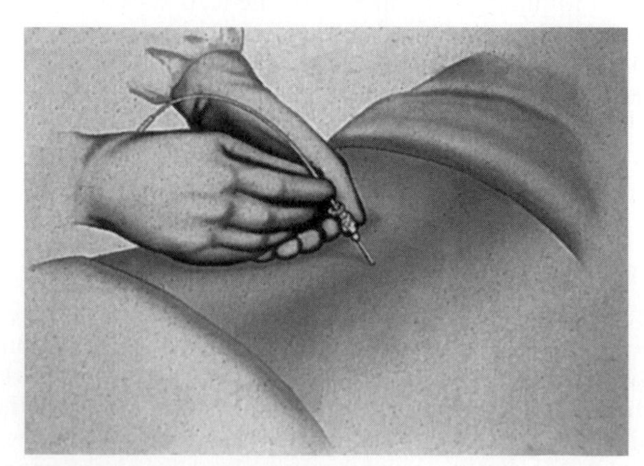

FIGURE 55–9 Surface anatomy with usual entry level at L1–L2. (Courtesy of Medtronic, Minneapolis, Minn.)

Fluoroscopy combined with the standard loss-of-resistance technique much increases the chance of atraumatic entry into the epidural space. Real-time imaging can often guide placement of the lead through (frequently encountered) resistance in the epidural space, along the way to final placement. Savolaine[7] has demonstrated, using CT epidurography, more fatty tissue, which produces a bulky, triangular structure. The resistance to, and deflections of, the trial leads seen with real-time fluoroscopy reinforce this anatomic finding. A single lead should be placed slightly ipsilateral to the painful side and as close as possible to the physiologic midline for bilateral pain coverage. Coverage of the painful region with stimulation paresthesia determines the final lead placement.

Anchoring and Tunneling

Ideally, dissection of subcutaneous tissue using combined blunt and sharp dissection with Metzenbaum scissors is targeted at exposing the supraspinous ligament, which is shiny and striated, in contrast to the fat and subcutaneous tissue. A dry sponge is very helpful in removing fatty tissue and exposing this target to fix the lead anchors. Failure to suture the anchors securely to the ligament and the lead to the anchor is the most common cause of lead migration. Traditional soft anchors have either a butterfly or a lead-through configuration. Medtronic has introduced a new rigid snap-close anchor that eliminates lead motion at the anchor (Fig. 55–10). This anchor still needs to be carefully attached to the ligament for long-term stabilization. Tunneling rods of various configurations are supplied in the SCS system surgical kits. Depending on the type, they have different end pieces for tunneling and pulling through leads or extensions. With the patient in the prone position many surgeons are placing Itrel generators in the posterior, superior aspect of the buttock. RF receivers can be placed in the midaxillary line, over the lower rib margin. Placement

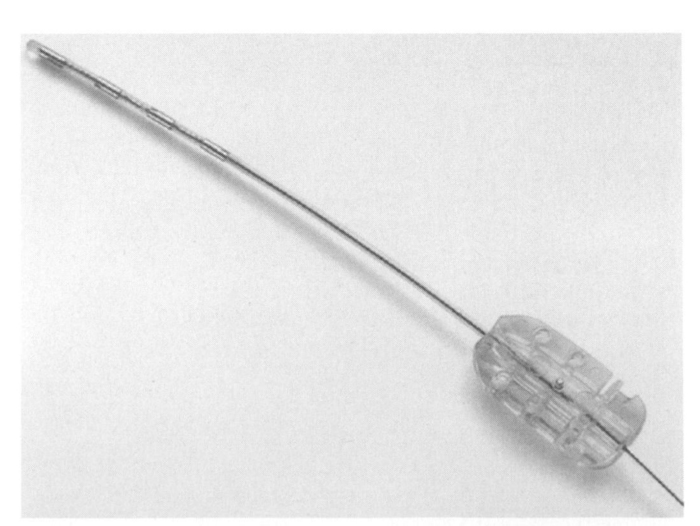

FIGURE 55–10 Medtronic rigid snap-lock lead anchor. (Courtesy of Medtronic, Minneapolis, Minn.)

in the buttock region, with the patient in the prone position, is also becoming more popular.

Pocket Formation

Preparing the pocket for either an RF receiver or an implanted pulse generator is a relatively straightforward and simple procedure. After infiltration of the proposed incision with local anesthetic, an incision of appropriate length is made, the goal being to produce a pocket that is the right size for the device and for any extra lead or extension that may be coiled behind it.

RF receivers must be no more than 1 cm from the skin surface and implanted generators, less than 1 in. Formation of these pockets can be accomplished mainly with blunt finger dissection accompanied, when necessary, by instrument dissection. General principles of tissue handling and hemostasis with electrocautery are standard. Pockets are best closed in two layers to prevent stress on the suture line from the implant. Integrity of the system should always be tested before the patient leaves the operating room, to detect easily correctable errors.

COMPLICATIONS*

Trial Complications

Trial protocols for percutaneous SCS have been well described and are important to (1) verify the efficacy of SCS for a particular patient, (2) screen out unsuitable candidates, and (3) effectively utilize healthcare resources.[8,9] Trials can be performed on outpatients with fluoroscopic guidance without anchoring the percutaneous lead, or, alternatively, in a sterile operating room to facilitate surgical anchoring of the percutaneously placed lead in anticipation of later internalization of the entire SCS system. Complications more unique and problematic to the trial period include (1) post–dural puncture headache (PDPH); (2) infection at the lead exit site; and (3) lead migration with subsequent change or loss of stimulation.

Post–Dural Puncture Headache

The incidence of PDPH during a trial varies with the training and experience of the practitioner. The use of fluoroscopy to help guide Tuohy needle placement, combined with the loss-of-resistance technique, should limit the incidence of PDPH to 1%. The modified Tuohy needles commonly used for percutaneous trial are approximately 14 gauge and produce significant cerebrospinal fluid loss and quite symptomatic spinal headaches. In patients with severe symptoms, assessing the response of a patient with PDPH to a trial of SCS may not prove reliable, or even possible. Abandoning the trial and providing standard therapy is often necessary until the symptoms abate and a new trial can be scheduled.

Infection at the Lead Exit Site

Percutaneous trial periods have increased in duration from 24 hours to weeks, depending on many variables. The object of prolonging trials is to continue to improve long-term outcome by fine-tuning patient selection based on response to trial stimulation. The major limiting factor on trial length is lead exit site induration or infection. Epidural abscess secondary to an SCS trial is extremely rare. The majority of epidural abscess reports continue to list spontaneous development as the major factor, usually secondary to seeding from a distant site. Prophylactic treatment with a first-generation cephalosporin (Ancef, 1 g) 1 hour before the procedure is routine. Neither continuing antibiotics for the duration of the trial or giving vancomycin has been shown to decrease the incidence of wound infections. If a superficial infection occurs, removal of the lead combined with appropriate antibiotic therapy usually results in resolution of the problem.

Lead Migration with Loss of Stimulation

The initial SCS trial will reveal any propensity for lead migration. If an unanchored percutaneous trial is utilized, this information may be exceedingly valuable for permanent lead implantation, if the trial is successful. Often, a lead that produces optimal stimulation paresthesia with the patient in the prone position for the trial proves to be less effective once the patient assumes the upright position and walks about.

A lead left with a gentle curve during the trial may straighten out and move slightly cephalad in an upright patient, thus changing stimulation parameters. This knowledge can lead to better positioning during permanent lead implant or to the decision to change to laminectomy placement of a platelike lead such as a Resume (Medtronic) or Lamitrode (ANS). Published reports document lead migration only after permanent implantation. The current trend toward longer SCS trials before permanent implantation allows for better assessment of early lead migration.

Surgical Complications

Like any surgical patient, SCS patients may develop the standard surgical complications: postoperative bleeding or hematoma, pocket seroma, cerebrospinal fluid hygroma, wound dehiscence, pocket infection, epidural abscess or meningitis, or cerebrospinal fluid leak or headache. Procedure-specific complications of SCS include lead migration; lead or extension fracture; lead or extension disconnection; receiver damage, rotation or failure; pulse generator battery or hardware failure; and lack of effect.

Postoperative Bleeding or Hematoma

For the physician, taking an adequate history and knowing what medications the patient is taking are crucial to avoiding bleeding complications. Correction of coagulopathy before surgery is medically recommended. Meticulous hemostasis and strict surgical technique during pocket prepa-

---

* Bedder M: Management of complications of spinal cord stimulation. Pain Rev 4:238–243, 1997.

ration reduce the incidence of postoperative hematoma. A hematoma deep in the wound can cause dehiscence or become infected secondarily. The skin incision should not be opened, except to drain the hematoma in the sterile environment of the operating room. A generator pocket with a tense hematoma may need to be reexplored to correct the bleeding problem. Drains are not recommended, as the implant can become contaminated.[10] Racz, in a series of 26 patients, reported one infected hematoma (3.8%); whereas Meglio reported three subcutaneous hematomas among 64 patients (4.6%).[11, 12] More recent studies, including a Medtronic-sponsored multicenter trial of 116 patients and North's study involving 50 patients, had no reports of pocket or wound hematomas.[6, 13–15]

Pocket Seroma or Hygroma

If, with implantation of the stimulator lead, dural puncture does not occur, collection of CSF or hygroma in the stimulator pocket is highly unlikely. Most patients (80%) have some degree of seroma formation, which is usually self-limiting and resolves in 4 to 8 weeks. Careful pocket preparation with minimal trauma to the tissues and judicious use of electrocautery can minimize seroma formation. On rare occasions, the operator may drain the seroma, observing strict aseptic technique. Aspiration of the serous fluid can lead to bacterial contamination.

Wound Dehiscence

Prevention of wound dehiscence begins with adequate communication with the patient both at the preoperative interview and during postoperative instruction. The patient must be aware of the physical restrictions after surgery and must be willing to comply with them. The patient should be available for follow-up and timely suture removal, if required, and for postoperative wound checks.

Closing with the appropriate suture materials and techniques is important, to avoid complications. Buried sutures hold wounds together and provide extra protection against tension along the wound for generator pockets. Monofilament sutures (Prolene, Ethilon) and Teflon-coated sutures may need extra instrument ties to increase security. Causes of wound dehiscence include errors in technique, poorly secured knots, excessive tension on the wound, infection, trauma to the suture line, tense fluid collections, and malnutrition and immunocompromise of patients.

Infections

Careful aseptic surgical technique combined with prophylactic antibiotics given 1 to 2 hours preoperatively has reduced the incidence of perioperative infections at the receiver or generator site or along the subcutaneous lead to about 4% to 5%.[6, 15] The most common wound infections are superficial *Staphylococcus aureus* or *Staphylococcus epidermidis* infections. Superficial infections of either the generator pocket or the back incision do not immediately necessitate hardware removal. Removal of sutures, if possible, replacement with Steri-Strips, and appropriate, culture-driven antibiotic treatment can resolve most infections. If the infection involves deeper tissue or the pocket itself and the implanted leads, all the implanted hardware must be removed to allow resolution of the infection. The infected wounds should be left open to drain and to heal by secondary intention. Keeping the wound moist with changes of wet-to-dry sterile saline dressings three times per day prevents dehydration and promotes epithelialization.

The most serious infections, of course, involve the epidural or intrathecal spaces.[16] Epidural abscess or meningitis is reported infrequently with SCS. The reported incidence of epidural abscess in hospitalized patients has been 1 in 100,000, and the cause most often is indeterminate but probably the result of seeding from distant sites. An epidural abscess can mimic an epidural hematoma, producing signs and symptoms consistent with spinal compression. Unexpected pain at the spine, paresis, or bowel or bladder dysfunction should be treated aggressively, with a high index of suspicion.

Contrast-enhanced computed tomography of the spine is the diagnostic test of choice, not magnetic resonance imaging (MRI). MRI would set up an electrical field surrounding the patient and the implanted SCS lead. This lead could act as an antenna toward the electrical field and damage tissues in contact with the electrode. Thus, MRI is contraindicated in patients implanted with SCS systems, regardless of which body region is imaged.

Equipment- and Technique-Related Complications

In the past, equipment-related complications that necessitated revision were fairly common.[17] Early studies documented 100% equipment failure rates, for reasons that ranged from dislocation of the electrode to cracks in the insulation of the lead or extension that caused leakage of electrical current. Equipment failures demand a second surgical procedure to correct the problem. Meglio's 1982 study reported an overall complication rate of 31%, of which 4 of 26 (15%) were device-related.[12] Kumar's 1986 study of 65 patients reported a total complication rate of 35%, of which 21% were lead-related.[18] His 1991 follow-up paper on 94 patients[4] (most treated with a Medtronic system) reported an overall complication rate of 46%: 25 electrode displacements, 4 lead fractures, 2 battery depletions, and 2 electrical leaks (equipment-related complication rate, 35%). North's 1991 report on 50 patients with failed back surgery syndrome reported that 48% of patients required some secondary procedure—most often repositioning because of lead migration, revision to enhance the stimulation pattern, lead fracture, or receiver failure.[14] An analysis of the subset of patients treated with multichannel devices showed that secondary surgical procedures were performed in only 34%. His follow-up report emphasized the superiority of multichannel devices: overall, the rate of revisions secondary to inadequate stimulation paresthesia was 23% for patients with bipolar systems, as compared with 16% for patients with multichannel systems.[15] The trend toward fewer complications and lower revision rates continued with Burchiel and colleagues' multicenter study of 70 patients (Medtronic equipment).

During the first year, 12 patients (17%) in Burchiel's group[16] required surgical procedures for revision or replacement of at least one component of the SCS system for some reason: lead migration (three), electrical shorting out (two), infection (three), lead fracture (one), decreased stimulation (one), change in pain topography (one), repositioning of the pulse generator (one), depleted battery (two), or ineffective pain control (one). It appears that the most common complication and need for second operation remains lead migration or change in stimulation paresthesia. Electrical shorting out can be caused by lead fracture or failure of technique in connecting the lead to the extension. Care must be taken to ensure that the boot covering the connection is watertight and secured with nonabsorbable suture material such as Ethibond or Prolene. Silk is a biologic suture that, in time, disintegrates. It should not be regarded as a permanent suture material. Newer lead improvements by ANS have decreased the incidence of lead and extension failures. The new leads incorporate polypropylene coatings instead of the older, stiffer bismuth-type leads.

Generators for SCS include internal pulse generators (Itrel, Medtronic) and external pulse generators utilizing RF receiver hookups (Extrel Mattrix, Medtronic and Renew, ANS). Battery life of any of these systems depends on the drain imposed on it. This can be affected by a number of variables, including, the use pattern (hours per day); the number of active electrodes; and the amplitude, pulse width, and frequency. Patients who have low power requirements, of course, have longer battery life with any system. A patient who requires high-amplitude stimulation with multiple leads and who uses the system continuously can deplete an internalized system within a year. Such patients are better candidates for an RF receiver system that allows them change or recharge the battery every day, if needed, to maintain efficacy.

An implanted pulse generator must be implanted in the pocket with the engraving on the case facing up so that it can easily be programmed. If the pocket is too large the generator may flip and the ability to program may be lost. This can sometimes be corrected by external rotation of the generator in the pocket without surgical correction.

CONCLUSION

Spinal cord stimulation continues to show significant improvements in pain and quality of life for patients with a variety of pain conditions that have not responded to conservative therapies. Advancements in both the hardware and surgical techniques are resulting in declining complication rates that make SCS an even safer and cost-effective treatment for long-term pain management.

REFERENCES

1. Olson KO, Bedder MD, Anderson VC, et al: Psychological variables associated with outcomes of spinal cord stimulation trials. Neuromodulation 1:6–13, 1998.
2. Vulink NC, Overgauuw DM, Jessurun GA, et al: The effects of spinal cord stimulation on quality of life in patients with therapeutically chronic refractory angina pectoris. Neuromodulation 2:33–40, 1999.
3. Claeys LG: Spinal cord stimulation and critical limb ischemia. Neuromodulation 2:1–3, 1999.
4. Kumar K, Toth C, Nath RK, Laing P: Epidural spinal cord stimulation for treatment of chronic pain—some predictors of success. A 15-year experience. Surg Neurol 50:110–121, 1998.
5. Alo KM, Yland MJ, Kramer DL, et al: Computer assisted and patient interactive programming of dual octrode spinal cord stimulation in the treatment of chronic pain. Neuromodulation 1:30–45, 1998.
6. North RB, Ewend MG, Lawton MT, et al: Spinal cord stimulation for chronic, intractable pain: Superiority of multichannel devices. Pain 44:119–130, 1991.
7. Savolaine ER, Pandya JB, Greenblatt SH, Conover SR: Anatomy of the human epidural space: New insights using CT epidurography. Anesthesiology 68:217–220, 1988.
8. Bedder MD: The anesthesiologist's role in neuroaugmentative pain control techniques: Spinal cord stimulation and neuraxial narcotics. Progr Anesthesiol 4:226–236, 1990.
9. Bedder MD: Spinal cord stimulation implant techniques. *In* Waldman SD, Winnie AP (eds): Interventional Pain Management. Philadelphia, WB Saunders, 1996, pp 419–422.
10. Complications. *In* Fewkes JL, Cheney ML, Pollack Fewkes JL, et al (eds): Illustrated Atlas of Cutaneous Surgery. Philadelphia, JB Lippincott, 1992, pp 14.1–14.7.
11. Racz GB, McCarron RF, Talboys P: Percutaneous dorsal column stimulator for chronic pain control. Spine 14:1–4, 1989.
12. Meglio M, Cioni B, Rossi GF: Spinal cord stimulation in the management of chronic pain. J Neurosurg 70:519–524, 1989.
13. Dooley DM, Heimburger RF, Hunter SE, et al: Medtronic Itrel Spinal Cord Stimulation System: Preliminary Clinical Results. Minneapolis, Minn., Medtronics Inc, 1984, pp 1–13.
14. North RB, Matthew GE, Lawton MT, et al: Failed back surgery syndrome: 5-year follow-up after spinal cord stimulator implantation. Neurosurgery 68:692–699, 1991.
15. Burchiel KJ, Anderson VC, Brown FD, et al: Prospective, multicenter study of spinal cord stimulation for relief of chronic back pain and extremity pain. Spine 21:2786–2794, 1996.
16. Darouiche RO, Hamill RJ, Greenberg SB, et al: Bacterial spinal epidural abscess. Review of 34 cases and literature survey. Medicine 71:369–385, 1992.
17. Meyerson BA: Electrical stimulation of the spinal cord and brain. *In* Bonica JJ (ed): The Management of Pain. 1st ed. Philadelphia, Lea & Febiger, 1990, pp 1862–1877.
18. Kumar K, Wyant GM, Ekong CEU: Epidural spinal cord stimulation for relief of chronic pain. Pain Clin 1:91–99, 1986.

CHAPTER • 56

Avoiding Difficulties in Spinal Cord Stimulation

K. Dean Willis, MD

Electrical neuromodulation has been providing relief for chronic pain sufferers for over 30 years. Estimates are that, worldwide, more than 250,000 neurostimulators have been surgically implanted since 1967.[1] It has been exciting for many of us to be a part of this remarkable evolution in pain management technology. Many advances have taken place in this field that have improved our ability to utilize technology with ever increasing success for an ever growing number of previously untreatable types of pain.[2–7] These advances have come from industry, with advances in equipment technology, and from physicians' becoming more skilled in selecting appropriate candidates, those whose pain is most likely to respond to electrical neuromodulation therapy.

CRITICAL OUTCOMES

Today we face a critical challenge to the future of electrical neurostimulation. With the recent surge in use of electrical neurostimulation to control pain combined with the relatively high cost of this equipment, outcomes not only must be tracked but must be exceptional. Research has been published that demonstrates the potential for this form of therapy to reduce long-term medical costs for chronic pain sufferers,[8, 9] but many insurance companies are fearful of the initial expense of the system and are skeptical about the present-day rate of success.

Bell and coworkers have shown that a reduction in the overall success rate for an individual procedure dramatically alters its cost effectiveness.[8] Poor patient selection, lead migrations requiring reoperation, postoperative infections requiring system explantation, and poor follow-up (failing to maximize both physical and psychological rehabilitation) are but a few of the difficulties an implant physician may face when trying to maintain a high success rate and long-term cost effectiveness.[8] Without cost-effectiveness data on both an individual and subsequently a global scale, reimbursement for neuromodulation therapy is and will continue to diminish. It is imperative for all implanting physicians to keep track of their personal outcomes data, both for personal use in maximizing their success rate and to enable them to provide that data to their third-party payors. The American Neuromodulation Society is currently involved with this process and assists private practitioners in this vital effort.

This chapter is devoted to the discussion of some of the difficulties that *every* implanter faces, regardless of level of training or experience. It is the hope of this author that these comments and literature citations will serve, not as an end, but rather as a beginning for the reader's never ending quest to perfect an evolving pain therapy. In this way, a therapy that for some patients is the *only hope* for long-term pain control and quality of life will remain readily available and become increasingly effective for years to come. That is a challenge each of us must meet.

COMMON DIFFICULTIES

There are six critical steps in the process of successful neuromodulation: (1) patient selection, (2) patient preparation, (3) pain practice organization, (4) surgical technique, (5) long-term follow-up, and (6) rehabilitation.

Each step has inherent difficulties that can lead to failure of therapy. Armed with knowledge of these difficulties and attention to the details of each of these steps, common difficulties can be largely eliminated. Emerging understanding of the intricacies of spinal cord stimulation therapy is making this technique progressively more useful.[10–12] After all, functionally the entire nervous system is an electrical circuit designed to transmit various impulses and signals for innumerable purposes. Transmission of pain is but one of these purposes. It is common sense to believe that neuromodulation of the electrical signals could be expected to provide safe and sustainable pain relief.

PATIENT SELECTION

Dan Doleys, a psychologist with 20 years' experience treating pain patients, lectures often on the difficulties of patient selection for implant therapy. He cites three broad elements that go into a successful implant: the right patient, the right therapy, and the right time. There are eight possible combinations of these three factors, but only one combination promises a successful implant. Chance would dictate one chance in eight of success, unless significant effort is devoted to recognizing, or creating, the right patient, therapy, and time. This exercise demonstrates the need for a multidisciplinary approach to neuromodulation, which helps to ensure proper patient selection and timing. Giving the right patient the right therapy at the wrong time will fail.

Accurate diagnosis begins the process of successful patient selection. Determination of the pathophysiologic mechanisms of the pain is essential. Pain can be broadly categorized as nociceptive or neuropathic. While most chronic pain patients have a combination of both types of pain, the astute diagnostician should be able to determine the relative elements of both pain types and their individual pattern distributions.

The patient most likely to respond to spinal cord stimulation is one with unilateral monoradicular pain. This type of neuropathic pain is generally easily covered by the distribution of paresthesias generated by a simple single-lead single-program spinal cord stimulator system.

More complex neuropathic pain patterns, such as axial and multiple extremity pain, can now be covered by dual-lead systems with more complex electrode array patterns.[13] These complex patterns of stimulation are much more difficult to maintain over the long term. New, advanced spinal cord stimulation (SCS) systems with patient-controlled multiple-program variability have largely solved this problem and have improved success rates.[14] These multiple-lead, variable-program systems now provide stimulation patterns that can cover the complex patterns of pain that single-lead, single-program systems cannot.

Nociceptive pain signals are transmitted to the brain by mechanisms different from those of neuropathic pain signals and thus are generally unresponsive to SCS therapy. Since many pain patients have a mixed pain syndrome, it must be remembered that SCS therapy may be only one element of the total pain therapy plan. Failure to recognize the input of multiple pain generators can lead to frustrating failure of SCS therapy.

Psychological evaluation of the potential implant patient should be done preoperatively, but not as the only mechanism for determining the patient's suitability for implant therapy. Published literature has demonstrated no consistent correlation between psychological factors affecting pain behavior and SCS failure.[15] In my own clinical experience, psychological factors have been more predictive of the difficulties one may face in dealing with an implant patient's follow-up than of outright therapeutic failure. Organic brain disorder, pathologic family dynamics, and secondary gain issues can contribute to patient dissatisfaction and continued dependency on medical resources, despite a "successful" physical result. In such cases, the implant becomes a vital step in the overall pain therapy plan, making success possible, though not inevitable. The multidisciplinary approach is necessary for implant pain therapy to succeed.[16]

Cancer patients are not generally considered good candidates for SCS therapy, owing to short life expectancy and the nociceptive nature of most malignant pain syndromes. The debilitated physical state of many end-stage cancer patients makes systemic narcotic therapy preferable in most cases. Spinal cord stimulation should still be considered when the underlying pain is neuropathic and when neurostimulating leads can be implanted quickly, safely, and inexpensively, regardless of the patient's life expectancy. Radiation neuritis and compression neuropathies are excellent examples of neuropathic pain that is unrelated to the malignancy and might be well-controlled with SCS therapy. Percutaneously implanted and tunneled leads used without pulse generators or receivers can be extremely cost-effective. When life expectancy is short, they can provide the same degree of pain relief as a fully implanted system for several weeks or months. It is not currently known precisely what the life expectancy must be to make a fully implanted spinal cord system a reasonable option.

PATIENT PREPARATION

Patient preparation is a step not often discussed and is easily confused with patient selection. I present it as a discrete process meant to help the physician select the appropriate therapy and establish the right time for SCS therapy.

To be an implant physician is to make claim to expertise in and ability to provide (or at least facilitate) delivery of *all* of the more conservative pain therapies. SCS therapy is still primarily considered an aggressive "salvage" procedure. Therefore, coordination of the delivery of a multidisciplinary approach to pain should be part of the implant physician's practice. The ability to coordinate the efforts of physical rehabilitation experts and psychologists with pharmacologic management, invasive interventional diagnostics, block therapy, and surgical therapeutics is prerequisite to implant therapy. The coordinated delivery of multidisciplinary care enhances conservative treatment outcomes and typically makes implant therapy unnecessary. SCS therapy is rarely needed but, when justified, is essential.

The algorithmic ladder of pain therapy is undergoing change,[17] but prospective, randomized, long-term outcome studies are needed if SCS therapy is to be established as a more conservative approach. Additionally, by working the patient through the earlier steps of care, they are adequately prepared for SCS therapy:

- Patients are taught coping skills and helped to establish reasonable expectations of their pain therapy.
- Accurate diagnoses are made and confirmed by various testing methods, including the patient's response to other pain therapies.
- Correctable lesions are identified, treated, and given ample time to heal, when possible.
- Physical function is maximized through consistent rehabilitative therapy, and drug use is stabilized.

By this point, the patient's level of commitment and compliance with the care plan will be well-known.

At the completion of this preparation, the physician has greater insight and can better evaluate the patient in light of both successful and failed therapies. A more intimate knowledge of the patient's physical and psychological status can be used to make decisions on the use of neuromodulation therapy. During this process many of the patient's "secondary" pain mechanisms may be brought under control or even resolved, in which case, the physician is afforded a clearer view of the refractory neuropathic pain, which may, indeed, respond best to electrical stimulation therapy. Without this patient preparation, the chances of success diminish precipitously and cost-effectiveness is lost. One can ill afford to "roll the dice" with such expensive therapy. This decision having been made, a patient is ready for trial SCS therapy.

Trial Stimulation Methods

Even the best and most experienced implant physician will have poor outcomes without an effective trial of SCS therapy. It is the decision to conduct a trial for *consideration* of permanent spinal cord stimulation therapy that is difficult, not the *decision* to permanently implant. A successful trial is what makes the decision to implant permanently. The key is an effective method of trial that minimizes false-positives (which lead to eventual implant failure) and, even worse, false negatives (eventual treatment failures). Several methods of trial stimulation have been proposed in the literature,[18] but selecting the best trial method should be an individual physician concern. It must take into consideration risk, cost, patient convenience and compliance, local politics, reimbursement issues, potential for malpractice litigation, and the comfort level of the implant physician who must use the information garnered from the trial to make a critical decision on long-term care for the patient. The one point that must be emphasized about this final step in patient preparation is that physical function must be validated *before* trial stimulation to provide a baseline for comparison *during* trial stimulation. Without this information the long-term results could be unexpectedly poor. The shorter the trial the more important this step becomes, owing to the potential for a placebo response and inconsistency in the patient's subjective pain reporting. A patient with pain who is physically able to function is more likely to have success with an implant than one who is pain-free but cannot function. A functional evaluation gathers objective and reproducible information that will seldom, if ever, mislead the specialist. Even severe deconditioning does not interfere with the ability of patients rendered significantly more comfortable to improve their function by 25% or more.

A percutaneous trial without tunneling can be done as an outpatient test and extended 3 to 5 days, with little risk of serious infection.[18] Oral and topical antibiotics are recommended during the trial period. To undergo an outpatient trial of any duration, the patient should be reasonably intelligent and have good home support. The advantage of this approach to a trial is the significant reduction in cost as compared with that of a surgically implanted lead with anchoring and tunneling. The obvious disadvantage is the short trial period and the increased likelihood of lead migration (since the lead is not anchored). This can produce a false-negative result if early lead migration is not recognized as the reason for failure to provide pain relief. If the distribution of paresthesias changes during the trial period, lead migration is the likely cause, and reprogramming with "electrical repositioning" of the electrode array is necessary. This consists of reprogramming the electrode array to reestablish proper stimulation coverage, rather than physically repositioning the lead.

A second method for trial is a percutaneously inserted but tunneled lead,[18] which can also be performed as an outpatient procedure. Percutaneous tunneling can be performed with a needle under local anesthetic and gives an additional degree of safety when a more prolonged trial is desired. Prophylactic antibiotics are still recommended throughout the trial. The appropriate interval is generally acknowledged to be no longer than 7 to 10 days. Close monitoring for signs of superficial or deep (intraspinal) infection is a must.

A third method of trial is a fully implanted, anchored, and tunneled lead that is externalized by using a temporary extension lead wire.[20] Theoretically, this type of trial could be maintained indefinitely with simple catheter care at the exit site. Some implanters have proposed that this can be used for rehabilitation purposes and for terminally ill cancer patients with short life expectancies. The cost is still substantially less than that of a fully implanted SCS system, which would include the pulse generator or receiver. There are cost savings if the trial is successful, because the lead does not require replacement at the time of permanent implantation, and revisions of the lead can be made, if necessary, at the time of pulse generator or receiver implantation. It is, however, significantly more expensive to remove than a percutaneously placed trial lead when the trial fails. Certainly, a more prolonged trial would afford time for a more complicated pain problem to reveal itself. For instance, there may be value in providing extensive physical rehabilitation during a trial, to verify success. During a prolonged trial, a placebo response essentially can be ruled out and secondary gain issues can be identified and addressed. Sometimes a more prolonged trial is advisable when some psychological instability is part of the patient's pain syndrome. Such psychological problems sometimes clear with good pain control, but they sometimes intensify unexpectedly, despite pain relief.

There is even an occasional implant physician who provides an "on the table" trial that, to declare a successful trial, requires only subjective patient verification of appropriate distribution of the stimulation pattern. While this author does not advocate this method of trial, current research cannot back an assertion that any particular method for trial is superior to any other. What the superior method is should emerge from the accrued long-term outcomes of the individual physician's practice. Once again, we see the need for outcome studies.

PAIN PRACTICE ORGANIZATION

Avoiding difficulties with SCS therapy requires a well-organized pain practice. This consists of three major components, multidisciplinary care, surgical facility, and implant coordination.

Multidisciplinary Care

Truly, the challenge of the day, for a pain practitioner and staff is to deliver multidisciplinary care in a coordinated fashion. "Multidisciplinary pain management" has become a catch phrase in our specialty and is widely acknowledged as the standard of care. Seldom is it actually delivered. Great difficulties are involved in developing this practice paradigm. The lack of available, qualified, dedicated, and experienced physical medicine experts, psychologists, and, even pain physicians, is discouraging. Convincing payors (third party or other) that the expense of such a program is cost-effective is another challenge. High overhead and the lack of available qualified staff make the temptation to develop a standardized "block shop" style of practice very compelling. It will remain an attractive option only until the outcomes of that type of practice are reported, and it will certainly lead to poor implant results.

Surgical Facility

The second critical component of pain practice organization relates to the resources needed to conduct the actual surgical procedure.

A supportive surgical facility suitable for both the trial and permanent implant procedures is a necessity. A stable, well-trained nursing staff must be available preoperatively, intraoperatively, and postoperatively to provide optimal care for patients with an intraspinal foreign body implant. This type of neurosurgical procedure tends to attract attention, especially when complications occur. A stable medical team of implant specialists minimizes these complications by maintaining consistency of care from admission to discharge and through the postoperative period. Simply opening the wrong device package can waste several thousands of dollars. Lack of careful attention to sterile technique can produce prolonged hospitalizations, emergency surgical procedures, paralysis, and even death.

Detailed knowledge of the charge and reimbursement issues for various surgical facilities is necessary for financial viability. This can be very complicated. The inability to control facility fees in some cases can make neurostimulation therapy unnecessarily costly and thus unlikely to win third-party payor approval.

Implant Coordinator

The third critical component of the pain practice organization is the role of the *implant coordinator*. This person's value cannot be overemphasized when developing an implant practice. Rosellen Lanning, an expert on the role of the nurse implant specialist, often speaks to the importance of designating a nurse specialist to handle such duties as patient education, ordering hardware, inservice training, intraoperative lead programming, and postoperative follow-up, to mention only a few.[20] Having these duties properly managed by an implant coordinator allows the implanting physician to concentrate more intensively on the duties that only he or she can manage. Without such support, an implant practice can quickly become overwhelming from the standpoint of the many critical details that must be handled for each case and the overall organization of the implant team.

Availability for postoperative management of "perceived" and real emergencies requires a commitment to a call schedule that must be maintained. Suffice it to say that any and all unexpected difficulties that arise after implantation of a neurostimulator are assumed to be a direct result of the stimulator in some way. The device will be blamed for everything from diarrhea to constipation, urinary tract infections to ringing in the ears. The implant physician will be required continually to educate and pacify the patient, other physician specialists, emergency room personnel, and family physicians about the device for many years to come, a charge that could become quite burdensome for a single-physician practice without expert help for covering emergency calls. This community educational effort can be facilitated by a qualified implant coordinator.

It is often said, "Once you implant a patient, you have married them." The physician should be very cautious when selecting a "marriage partner," as some can be extremely "high-maintenance" and attending to them very time-consuming.

SURGICAL TECHNIQUE

Innumerable pearls can be provided to enhance the skill of the implant physician in the surgical procedure itself. Each of these recommendations can help to lead to a successful implant rather than a failure.

In this section, I attempt a reasonably categorized presentation of some of the steps that can help to avoid difficulties with the spinal procedure and with subsequent management. It addresses three broad areas of concern: preoperative, intraoperative, and postoperative.

Preoperative

Patient Education

The patient should be well-informed about risks and reasonable expectations but should also be coached in anatomic labeling to reduce intraoperative confusion about which part of the body is being stimulated and whether it corresponds with the usual area of pain. It should not be surprising that many patients do not know their left from their right or their leg from their thigh when they are lying anxiously or partially anesthetized on an operating room table. Such circumstances are conducive to miscommunications. Clear, simple, and repetitive questions and instructions should be well-rehearsed before the surgical theater is entered.

Prophylactic Antibiotics

An intravenous dose of a cephalosporin given at least 45 minutes before the skin incision is made can help to avert disaster. Since no surgical procedure is totally safe from infection, all reasonable measures should be taken to avoid it. Patients with a depressed immune system and diabetic patients are at particularly high risk and might well be given dual-antibiotic prophylaxis, adding an aminoglycoside if no contraindication exists. All patients should be carefully screened and treated for any existing infection, obvious or occult. Urinary tract infections, otitis media, dental caries, and osteomyelitis are not infrequent occult infections that can easily seed a foreign body implant.

Implant Position Planning

The patient should be counseled about the options for positioning of the eventual permanent implant site. The most common sites for the receiver and pulse generator are the back upper buttock and the subcostal/flank area. After the patient selects the most agreeable implant site, the skin should be marked as the patient assumes multiple positions used every day, to ensure positioning of the implant. Lying in position for surgery, the skin and subcutaneous tissue can become quite distorted. A poorly placed pulse generator can be quite painful and may require surgical revision later.

Intraoperative

Anesthetic

Care should be taken not to obtund the patient if sedation is used, lest he or she give less than optimal responses during the testing phase when the proper lead position is being determined. With relaxation techniques and coping skills having already been maximized, most patients will be able to tolerate the percutaneous phase (lead placement) without any sedation at all. Intravenous sedation can be given freely after the lead position is finalized.

Equipment and Surgery Suite Layout

The room should provide ample space for all necessary equipment (anesthesia, fluoroscope, operating table, and sterile back table). The layout should allow for safe movement around the sterile fields and should minimize traffic in and out of the surgical suite during the open phase of implantation. This will minimize contaminated airflow. Comfortable viewing of the fluoroscopic monitor is important and requires planning, since many surgical suites are small and do not easily accommodate this much equipment.

Patient Positioning

The ideal patient position is one that gives easy access to all areas to be surgically incised without having to reposition, re-prep, and redrape the patient intraoperatively. This position should also afford the best fluoroscopic visualization of the spine. This best position is usually prone, although some prefer a lateral, or even a seated, position.

Fluoroscopic Visualization

The bony spine can be clearly visualized in most patients with a good C arm and can give the surgeon an idea of the bony, or "anatomic," midline, which is *not* identical to the "physiologic" midline. Proper positioning of the neurostimulating lead is dependent on the *physiologic* midline not the *anatomic* one. The anatomic midline gives a good reference point for initial lead placement. This could be misleading if the fluoroscopic view is in parallax, rather than truly anteroposterior. *Parallax* means the view is slightly oblique and misrepresents the midline. As a consequence, the lead could be misplaced. Many patients have mild to severe scoliotic deformities, an anomaly that requires correction of the C-arm angles every few segments as the lead is advanced. Lateral obliques and head-to-toe obliques are equally important. Pedicles should appear equally spaced, and vertebral body end plates should be superimposed one on another. Care should be taken to observe scrupulous sterile technique, particularly as the C arm is rotated to the table level, when contaminated drapes are brought up to the sterile field and contamination could occur.

Needle Placement

Only needles designed to be used with the neurostimulating leads are appropriate. Site of needle introduction into the skin is important and is determined by several important factors:

1. Anticipated final lead tip position: A maximum amount of lead wire should be inside the epidural space (minimum 15 cm) to minimize the chance of postoperative lead migration. Shorter epidural leads promote lead tip migration.
2. Vertebral interspace anticipated for needle entry: This space should be well below the intended final lead tip position to allow for an ample length of lead to be placed into the epidural space. A fairly immobile spinal segment (T1–T4 for cervical leads, L1–L4 for thoracolumbar leads) should be selected to minimize potential stress on the lead with the spinal motion of normal daily activities.
3. Initial puncture site: The level of the initial needle introduction through the skin should allow for a very shallow angle of advancement through the anticipated interspace, to minimize angular tension on the lead as it courses through the supraspinous ligament. A steep angle of entry makes inadvertent puncture of the dural membrane more likely. Puncture of the dural membrane does not necessitate termination of the procedure; however, it might be necessary to enter at another level. A shallow angle of entry also allows a more direct line to the eventual epidural "target" and affords easier steering of the lead tip. Final lead position is optimized in this manner. Needle entry should be just off the midline allowing for a straight-line approach to the epidural target. This minimizes the need for lead manipulation later and allows for anchoring to the supraspinous ligament by staying close to the midline.

Neurostimulator Lead Placement

Final lead position is based solely on the patient's perceived distribution of paresthesias. To be effective, this must cover the area of pain distribution as completely as possible. A good rule of thumb is to keep the lead 2 to 4 mm from the midline and to advance approximately to the T9 vertebral body level for lower extremity radicular pains. Anatomically, the cervical spine is highly variable, but generally, neck, shoulder, and radial stimulation coverage requires a C2–C3 lead tip position; median nerve distribution coverage is C3–C4; and ulnar nerve distribution requires a C5–C6 tip position. It is important to remember that here we are addressing spinal cord stimulation, *not* nerve root stimulation. The most distal and proximal electrodes may be left inactive in the final lead position to allow for "electrical reprogramming" postoperatively.

Anchoring

Several types of anchoring boots are available, from various manufacturers. These must be sutured to the supraspinous ligament to secure the lead as it exits the epidural space. Many leads have been known to fail because they migrated when anchored to a less firmly fixed tissue. An initial introducer needle position too far off midline requires the anchoring boot to be sutured to the posterior lumbar fascia. This tissue plane is unstable and the result is a much higher risk of lead migration.

Suture material should be of sufficient size (00 or 0) to provide the tensile strength necessary to anchor securely. It should be nonabsorbable and preferably braided, to minimize unraveling. A slipknot should be used to cinch down tight around the boot containing the lead to secure the lead in the boot. This is known as a *tie.* Multiple anchoring ties should be used, as slippage within the boot will most certainly result in migration of the lead with normal daily patient activity.

Tunneling

The extension lead should be long enough to allow a bit of slack so that normal body stretching will not pull unnecessarily on the lead at the site of the anchoring boot. A loop of extension deep to the receiver/pulse generator is advisable to allow for normal body movements. Taking care to pass the tunneling device through the subcutaneous tissues rather than piercing the muscle fascia puts less stress on the lead and creates less postoperative discomfort.

Placement Receiver/Pulse Generator

The position of the receiver and pulse generator should be planned and marked well in advance of the implantation. The site should be marked preoperatively with the patient in multiple positions to obtain the most desirable results. The surgical incision can then be made with confidence, regardless of patient's position on the surgical table. The depth of the subcutaneous pocket should be no more than 1 to 1.5 cm to allow the radiofrequency or programming signal to be picked up easily by the device yet deep enough to lie comfortably in the subcutaneous fat. The patient should participate in the final decision. The posterior upper buttocks and the subcostal abdomen are common placement sites. For the cervical leads, the anterior chest is commonly used for males, and the fatty tissue under the axilla is aesthetically ideal for most females.

Postoperative Period

The postoperative period consists of the time from day 1 until approximately 4 weeks after surgery. It is in this interval that most surgical complications occur.

Epidural Hematoma

The potentially devastating complication of epidural hematoma usually declares itself within the first 24 to 48 hours postoperatively. Early clinical signs are increased pain or focal neurologic deficit, often in areas not affected preoperatively by pain. Treatment should be quick and decisive, as delays in decompressive efforts can result in permanent neurologic deficit. Surgical evacuation of the hematoma with neural decompression is the treatment of choice when neurologic deficit develops. Otherwise, treatment can be conservative with the patient monitored closely. Diagnosis is made by magnetic resonance imaging with contrast. The rate of this complication is thought to be well below 1%, although exact statistics are not known.

Spinal Headache

Spinal headaches are very rare, because lead placement is epidural. Occasionally, the introducer needle inadvertently penetrates the arachnoid membrane during lead placement; then, a spinal headache can develop. It is always recognized by the second postoperative day, and conservative treatment should be initiated. An epidural blood patch is rarely necessary and is not advisable early in the postoperative period. Blood placed into a fresh healing wound containing a foreign body is a perfect culture medium for bacteria. Although this can be performed under sterile conditions (gown, gloves, mask, and drapes) with prophylactic antibiotics, it is more appropriate to place the patient in the traditional 10-degree Trendelenburg position or even more effectively a prone position for one or two consecutive 8-hour periods. This is generally successful. If an epidural blood patch becomes necessary, fastidious sterile technique is imperative. Prophylactic antibiotics should be utilized. Inserting the epidural catheter well below the site of the cerebrospinal fluid leak under fluoroscopic visualization and then guiding it carefully to the appropriate level minimizes potential damage or migration of the implanted lead system.

Infection

Infection can be superficial (e.g., an incisional infection) or a deep foreign body–related infection. Infections cannot always be avoided, but certainly they should be rare when all reasonable precautions are taken. The strictest of sterile technique should be observed at all times. The risk is highest for immunosuppressed patients. Special consideration should be given to elderly debilitated patients, diabetics, and patients with cancer or AIDS.

In immunosuppressed patients, occult infections can often seed the implanted hardware, even under optimal circumstances. The only protection is good preoperative screening for such things as urinary tract infections, severe dental caries, upper and lower respiratory tract infections, sinus infections, and otitis media. Infectious disease consultation may be beneficial in those cases. Two types of infections occur during the 4-week postoperative period: deep, hardware–related infections and superficial infections. The treatment for each is very different.

Hardware infections are processes in direct contact with any part of the implant and usually require removal of the implant. When the lead is involved, it is the general consensus to remove the lead immediately, débride the wound, and treat aggressively with intravenous antibiotics. The receiver/pulse generator can usually be spared if it is not directly infected, and this saves the high cost of replacement. When in doubt, it is always best to remove the entire system.

Superficial infections that do not directly communicate with any part of the hardware can be treated initially with oral antibiotics but with close observation for response to therapy. Intravenous antibiotics may be required. This type of infection usually involves the surgical wound or cellulitis of the skin overlying the subcutaneous implant. Surgical revision of the wound should be considered early if a positive response to aggressive antibiotic therapy is not seen within 48 to 72 hours, lest the infection progress to involve the hardware in the deep tissues and require explantation of the system.

Lead Migration

Lead migration should be regarded as inevitable, but it is not a matter of grave concern. The patient should be made aware of this prospect and of the virtual inevitability of postimplantation reprogramming. Reprogramming is usually necessary two or three times in the first 4 weeks after implantation, to keep stimulation patterns maximized. Lead migration so extensive as to render reprogramming of appropriate patterns of paresthesias impossible is rare.

Lead migration requiring surgical repositioning was a major deterrent to the use of SCS therapy until the late 1980s. At that time, the rate of lead migrations that required surgical revision was between 60% and 80%. Today, "electronic repositioning" can be performed by telemetry, activating different electrode arrays and thus altering the stimulation patterns without the need to physically move the lead. This advance in technology has greatly enhanced the cost efficiency of SCS therapy. The need for surgical repositioning should be less than 10% when leads are properly positioned initially to provide for maximal options for electrical reprogramming postoperatively.

Seroma or Stitch Abscess

The formation of a fluid collection around the implant is known as a seroma, and although it is a potential sight for infection, is usually sterile. This complication is common and almost always involves the receiver/pulse generator site. It is recognized by palpating slight to significant flocculence surrounding the hardware. It is apparent within 1 week postoperatively and resolves spontaneously, usually within the first 4 weeks. This fluid collection can prevent effective transmission of the radiofrequency signal driving the lead system or, in the case of a pulse generator, prevent reprogramming. Whether this fluid should be aspirated is the subject of debate. Percutaneous invasion of the implant pocket can introduce bacteria into a culture medium (serosanguineous fluid) containing a foreign body (the implant) and produce the perfect conditions for an abscess to develop. On the other hand, a large seroma can be painful and produce a permanent fibrous pocket much larger than the implant. This can allow movement of the implant within the pocket after sequestration of the seroma. Such movement can make transmission of radiofrequency or telemetry signals inconsistent over the long term. Should aspiration be attempted, strict sterile technique must be observed to minimize the risk of infection and potentially costly removal of the implant.

A stitch abscess, another sterile collection of fluid, is located in the subcutaneous tissues of the surgical wound. This can be a serious problem as it can cause breakdown of the surgical wound and exposure of the underlying hardware. It is usually apparent 1 to 2 weeks postoperatively and may resolve spontaneously. It may, however, require removal of the stitch that created the fluid collection. Close observation is required to prevent exposure of the implant, and revision of the surgical wound becomes necessary if hardware exposure becomes imminent.

LONG-TERM FOLLOW-UP

Once the patient has passed the 4th postoperative week, the system can be said to have *matured.* The body has now formed a fibrous capsule around the various components of the implant, which is less likely to migrate or produce any of the complications mentioned in the previous section. Several potential difficulties still lie in wait for the unsuspecting physician implanter.

Reprogramming

The ideal stimulation pattern—and resulting pain relief—are often lost within the first few weeks after implant, for several reasons. Periodic reprogramming becomes essential. As the fibrous tissue invests the lead electrodes, resistance to delivery of the electrical impulses increases. The result is the need to substantially increase the amplitude over time. This should be expected and the patient made aware that it is a normal occurrence. This maturation process can often require reprogramming of the electrode array, pulse width, and frequency. The three-dimensional space surrounding the lead can be altered by the natural process of healing in a manner that renders the stimulator system ineffective, despite a successful trial.

Migration of the lead after maturation is much less likely, but it still occurs with relative frequency. "Electrical repositioning" of the electrode array recovers the optimal stimulation pattern. Manipulation of the other parameters improves the *comfort* of the stimulator signal, which is a matter of individual patient preference.

I suggest routine clinic visits for stimulator reprogramming approximately every 3 to 6 months after the optimal stimulation programs have been initiated. This is essential in patients with stimulator systems that do not provide multiple patient-controlled programs. By varying the programs from time to time *accommodation* can be avoided. *Accommodation* describes the phenomenon by which the body comes to "ignore" a steady, unvarying electrical stimulus over time. Patients who leave their stimulator systems on continuously develop accommodation much more rapidly and this stimulation becomes ineffective, if not actually painful, over the long term. Most patients do best in a "cycling" mode; for example, 1 minute on, 1 minute off. This cycling mode also serves to prolong pulse generator battery life by relying on the "carryover" analgesic effect experienced by most SCS patients. This carryover effect can last seconds to hours.

Patient Compliance

Ultimately, patients are in charge of their own stimulator systems. Expert programming and superb patient education in the daily use of the stimulator system still demand that patients operate the system within recommended compliance limits. Patients must become expert with regard to the idiosyncrasies of the particular SCS system as it relates to their body. Changes in the patient's pain or stimulation pattern associated with changes of position and daily activities require system adjustments by the patient that cannot be taught. This *fine tuning* is quite difficult for some patients, such as those who have limited cognitive skills or are frightened. Simplification is sometimes in order to make the programs more user friendly. Industry is making systems simpler to understand and operate. Compliance with periodic long-term follow-up appointments is necessary to keep analgesic potential optimized. It can be said that a mature stimulator system is fairly constant, but the body is ever changing, and adjustments must therefore be made periodically to keep pain relief maximized. This makes long-term follow-up absolutely essential for reprogramming. Most chronic pain patients also need ongoing encouragement to follow lifelong physical and psychological rehabilitation recommendations.

Rehabilitation

Spinal cord stimulators are implanted for pain control. At least that is the prevailing notion. If we could begin to think of SCS implant therapy more in terms of *return of function*, our success rates would improve substantially. SCS is traditionally thought of as the *end* of therapy. It should be considered the *beginning*. For the patient with severe neuropathic pain, rehabilitation is often not possible without SCS implantation. After implantation, however, physical and psychological rehabilitation is possible. Although earlier attempts at rehabilitation may have failed, the newfound pain relief allows for physical and emotional recovery once seemingly impossible. *A thorough and consistent rehabilitation program should be at the heart of any quality implant program.*[20] Without such a program SCS will at best be a partial success, and most likely eventually a failure. Return of function is the most reliable measure of success and should help to keep us focused on the goal of implantation therapy, quality of life.

CONCLUSION

The information in this chapter highlights many of the difficulties that can be encountered with SCS therapy. Every potential problem could not possibly be addressed in such a short format as this chapter. It is the hope of this author that it will serve to identify SCS therapy as a technique that demands careful attention to detail at every step of the neuromodulation treatment process.

When SCS therapy becomes necessary, little or no alternative care is available. Therefore, it must be provided in such a way as to maximize the chances of success and minimize the likelihood of failure. Our chronic pain patients come to us with shattered lives and hopeless hearts. It is indeed an honor for us to be able to cross their paths and minister to their needs. As Albert Schweitzer once said, "*It is my ever greater privilege to care for those who are suffering—for pain is an even more terrible lord to man than death itself.*"

REFERENCES

1. Industry Estimates (Advanced Neuromodulation Systems and Medtronic Neurological), October 1999.
2. Petrakis IE, Sciacca V: Spinal cord stimulation in critical limb ischemia of the lower extremities: Our experience. J Neurosurg Sci 43:285–293, 1999.
3. Oosterga M, ten Vaarwerk IA, DeJongste M: Spinal cord stimulation in refractory angina pectoris—clinical results and mechanisms. Z Kardoil 86(Suppl 1):107–113, 1997.
4. Kumar K, Nath RK, Toth C: Spinal cord stimulation is effective in the management of reflex sympathetic dystrophy. Neurosurgery 40:503–508, 1997.
5. Feler C, Whitworth LA, Brookoff D, et al: Recent advances: Sacral nerve root stimulation using a retrograde method of lead insertion for the treatment of pelvic pain due to interstitial cystitis. Neuromodulation 2:211–216, 1999.
6. Burchiel K, Anderson C, Brown F, et al: Prospective, multicenter study of spinal cord stimulation for relief of chronic back and extremity pain. Spine 21:2786–2794, 1996.
7. DeJongste M: Efficacy, safety and mechanisms of spinal cord stimulation used as an additional therapy for patients suffering from chronic refractory angina pectoris. Neuromodulation 2:188–193, 1999.
8. Bell GK, Kidd D, North RB: Cost-effectiveness of spinal cord stimulation in treatment of failed back surgery syndrome. J Pain Symptom Manage 13:286–295, 1997.
9. Willis KD: Outcome assessment of the therapeutic cost benefit and combined success rates for spinal cord stimulation therapy. Proceedings of Worldwide Pain Conference 2000, San Francisco July 15–21, 2000.
10. Holsheimer J, Barolat G, Stnijk JJ, He J: Significance of the spinal cord position in spinal cord stimulation. Acta Neurochir 64 (Suppl):119–124, 1995.
11. Holsheimer J: Effectiveness of spinal cord stimulation in the management of chronic pain: Analysis of technical drawbacks and solutions. Neurosurgery 40:990–996, 1997.
12. Holsheimer J, Wesselink W: Effects of anode-cathode configuration on paresthesia coverage in spinal cord stimulation. Neurosurgery 41:1082–1087, 1997.
13. Barolat G: A Prospective multicenter study to assess the efficacy of spinal cord stimulation utilizing a multi-channel radiofrequency system for the treatment of intractable low back and lower extremity pain. Initial considerations and methodology. Neuromodulation 2:179–183, 1999.

14. Alo K, Yland M, Charnou JH, Redko V: Multiple program spinal cord stimulation in the treatment of chronic pain: Follow up of multiple programs SCS. Neuromodulation 2:266–275, 1999.
15. North RB, Kidd, DH, Wimberly RL, Edwin D: Prognostic value of psychological testing in spinal cord stimulation patients: A prospective study. Neurosurgery 39:301–311, 1996.
16. Doley DM, Olson K: Physiological Assessment and Intervention in Implantable Pain Therapies. Medtronic, 1997.
17. Wetzel FT, Hassenbusch S, Willis KD, et al. Treatment of chronic pain in failed back surgery patients with spinal cord stimulation: A review of current literature and proposal for future investigation. Neuromodulation 3:59–75, 2000.
18. Spinal Cord Stimulation, Implantation Technique Notebook. Medtronic, Minneapolis, MN, 1991, pp E1–E12 and pp E13–F9.
19. Lanning RM: The role of the clinical nurse coordinator. Presentation for the Dannemiller Interventional Techniques Workshop, Washington, D.C., January 1994.
20. Willis, KD. Rehabilitation: A key element to successful implantation therapy. In Synch Magazine. Vol 5:6–7, November 1994.

CHAPTER • 57

Peripheral Nerve Stimulation: Current Concepts

James E. Heavner, DVM, PhD • Gabor Racz, MD • P. Prithvi Raj, MD

Peripheral nerve stimulation (PNS) is an accepted modality for the treatment of pain. At the American Society of Neurosurgery National Pain Consensus meeting in 1999, the principle of PNS was embraced, with the provision that it is for mononeuropathy. This reflects favorable outcomes with this treatment at multiple centers. In this chapter we discuss various aspects of using electrical stimulation delivered via electrodes surgically implanted adjacent to peripheral nerves to treat painful conditions. The state of the art, from a clinical perspective (e.g., equipment, patient selection criteria, stimulation parameters), is presented, followed by a brief discussion of the evolution of the technique, and of mechanism(s) by which the therapy is thought to act.

STATE-OF-THE-ART TECHNIQUE AND EQUIPMENT

The technique of PNS is relatively simple: the nerve is exposed and an electrode is placed along the side of the nerve or beneath it (Fig. 57–1). The nerves commonly used for PNS are the median, ulnar, radial, common peroneal, and posterior tibial nerves.

The implantation is done by a qualified surgeon. Usually, a two-step surgical procedure is used, ending with both the peripheral nerve stimulator (programmable receiver, battery pack) and the electrodes totally implanted. The system is programmed by a portable transmitter that during programming is placed over the subcutaneously buried programmable receiver and battery pack. The first step of the procedure, implantation of the stimulating electrode, is followed by a trial period (usually about 3 days). An external battery pack is used during the trial period. If adequate pain relief is obtained during the trial, the second step of the surgery, implantation of the battery pack, is completed (Figs. 57–2 and 57–3).

A paddle-type electrode (e.g., Resumé, Medtronic, Inc.) used for spinal cord stimulation is also used for PNS. The electrode is usually placed proximal to the injury site. During implantation of the electrode, a thin layer of fascia is placed between the nerve and the electrode. The rationale for this maneuver is that fascia reduces irritation of the nerve by the electrode and discourages proliferation of fibrous tissue around the electrode. The resulting situation is considered to be analogous to the use of epidurally placed electrodes for spinal cord stimulation, where the electrode and the cord are separated by the meninges.

The electrodes usually have at least four contacts. Such a design allows selection of the optimal positive and negative electrode configuration using bipolar stimulation. The goal is to position the electrodes in a configuration such that, when stimulation is applied, the patient perceives sensation in the painful area.

With the programmable stimulating battery pack (e.g., Itrel, Medtronic, Inc.) the electrodes to be stimulated, pulse duration (μsec), and intensity (volts [V]), pulses per second, and on-and-off cycling can be selected. The usual initial settings are 190 to 400 μsec, 0.75 to 1.25 V, 65 to 85 pulses per sec, and 64 sec on, 2 min off. The appropriate voltage is determined by increasing the stimulus intensity by 0.25-V increments until the patient reports perception of stimulation. Optimal settings are then set by increasing or decreasing pulse duration. The reader may find further details on the implantation technique in the *Peripheral Nerve Stimulation Surgical Technique Notebook* available from Medtronic, Inc., Minneapolis, Minn.

NEW DEVELOPMENTS

Our clinical experience now includes more than 300 implants. There has been gradual improvement in our understanding and in the technology. For example, in the beginning, we approached pain in the sciatic nerve distribution by placing an electrode for tibial nerve stimulation above the ankle. For common peroneal nerve stimulation, electrode placement above the knee on the lateral side gave us good results; however, this approach required more than one implant in some of the patients whose foot injuries

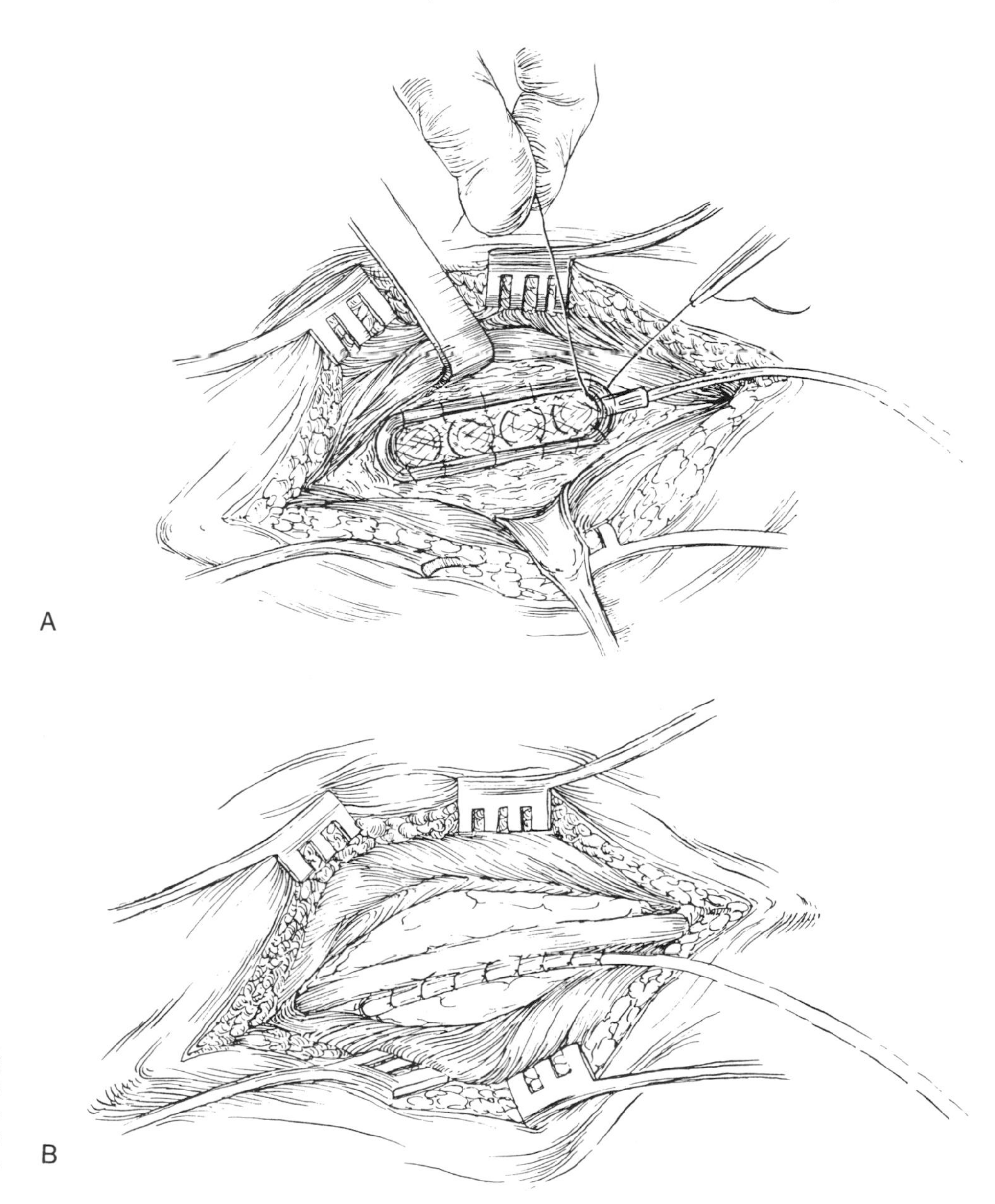

FIGURE 57–1 *Electrode implant.* A, *Fascia is sutured over the electrode and electrode is sutured in place.* B, *Nerve is allowed to fall into place over the electrode. (From Peripheral Nerve Stimulation Surgical Technique Notebook, Medtronic, Inc. Reproduced with permission.)*

involved both components of the sciatic nerve. Therefore, a new electrode is being explored that has a concavity. During the trial stimulation phase, tetanic stimulation is applied with patients under anesthesia without paralysis, and the grooved electrode is rotated so that motor contracture of the foot is first evident when it contacts the area of worst pain. Increasing the stimulus intensity covers the other part of the sciatic nerve and gives biphasic plantar flexion and dorsiflexion, evidence that the appropriate bundles in the sciatic nerve are being stimulated. It needs to be remembered, though, that the patient must not be given a muscle relaxant, which would render the test meaningless.

PATIENT SELECTION

Pain in the distribution of a single traumatized peripheral nerve is the best indication for PNS.[1] Good results have been reported with two nerve implants, however.[2] Good results have also been obtained when stimulation was applied to a nerve that, after injury, produced localized pain that subsequently spread to other areas of the body.[1] Patient selection criteria are listed in Table 57–1.

Pain reduction with a trial of transcutaneous electrical nerve stimulation (TENS) or with local anesthetic nerve block has been advocated as a screening procedure for PNS. Results from at least one study indicate that pain that is lessened by TENS is somewhat more likely to respond favorably to PNS.[3] A negative response to TENS, however, should not by itself eliminate a patient as a candidate for PNS. There are data that indicate that pain relief with nerve blockade does not ensure a favorable response to PNS, but continued pain despite a technically adequate nerve block makes it very unlikely that electrical stimulation of the same nerve will be successful.[4]

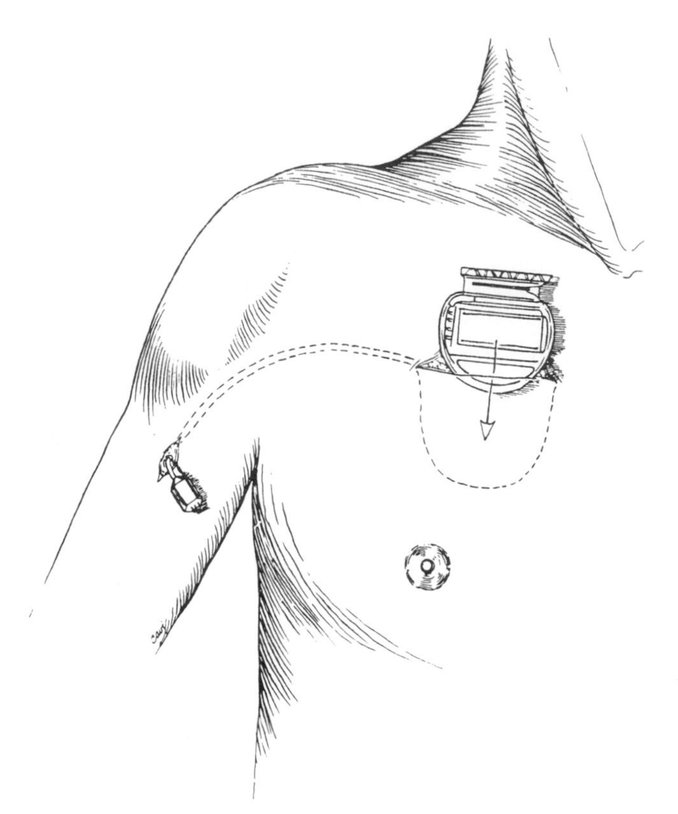

FIGURE 57–2 The pulse generator is implanted in the upper chest wall when the upper extremity is involved. (From Peripheral Nerve Stimulation Surgical Technique Notebook, Medtronic, Inc. Reproduced with permission.)

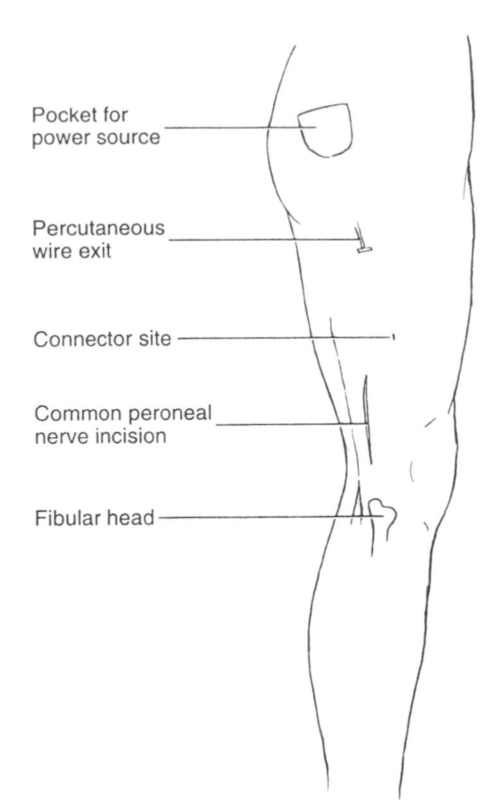

FIGURE 57–3 Incision sites for peripheral nerve stimulator implant. (From Peripheral Nerve Stimulation Surgical Technique Notebook, Medtronic, Inc. Reproduced with permission.)

COMPLICATIONS AND OUTCOMES

Complications of PNS are as follows:

- Infection
- Battery failure
- Broken wires
- Fluid shorting electrical connections
- Changing contact between electrodes and nerve
- Scarring between nerve and electrode
- No response to trial stimulation (leading to electrode removal)
- Interference with cardiac pacemakers
- Tissue damage when PNS equipment transmits output of radiofrequency devices (e.g., electrocautery, radiofrequency lesioning) to electrode contacts

Patients with implanted PNS systems should be given a medical card recommending exemption from x-ray security checks to avoid alterations of the PNS program by the x-ray equipment. They also should avoid areas where microwave ovens are in use. Reports indicate that success rates in excess of 80% (i.e., mild to marked relief of pain) can be achieved with PNS.[5–7] In our experience, adjunctive therapy may be needed. For instance, sympathetic nerve blocks may be required to deal with "sympathetic storms" during the first year after implantation. The general tendency over time is for patients who gain long-term benefit from PNS to improve progressively and then to become less reliant on PNS. Usually, however, PNS is a long-term commitment requiring good communication among the referring physician, the patient, and personnel at the center where the implantation is done.

Our 5-year follow-up[1] indicates dramatic improvement in patients returning to work to 54% in males, 35% in females and an 80% happiness rating in patients suffering from complex regional pain syndrome (CRPS) type II. More recently, in a combined series from Baylor University

TABLE 57–1 Patient Selection Criteria for Peripheral Nerve Stimulation

General criteria
Pathology for the pain complaint demonstrated
Cause of pain isolated to a single nerve (see text)
No demonstrable nerve abnormalities
Failure of more conservative therapies
No serious drug habituation problems
Psychological clearance
Successful trial stimulation
Correctable lesion (e.g., nerve entrapment) excluded
Causes of intractable pain for which PNS may be indicated
Direct or indirect nerve trauma
Reflex sympathetic dystrophy
Causalgia
Postherpetic neuritis
Conditions generally unresponsive to PNS
Sciatica
Pain associated with failed low back surgery
Cancer pain
Idiopathic pain
Pain due to nerve root injury

Medical Center in Houston and Texas Tech University: Health Sciences Center,[8] we found that CRPS responds well to spinal cord stimulation: visual analogue pain scores dropping from the 8 to 9 range to the 3 to 4 range at 36 months and staying down. PNS does uniformly better than spinal cord stimulation, but the best-sustained long-term effects came to patients who had both spinal cord and peripheral nerve stimulation.

The principle of the continuum of care is used to treat CRPS; that is, conservative measures are used first. Treatment modalities move to the next level if at approximately 3 months response is not appropriate and after sympathetically maintained and sympathetically independent pain have been addressed. If there is evidence of centralization of the pain or more than one nerve is involved, spinal cord stimulation is also effective, but the best results in this care come from simultaneous use of spinal cord and peripheral nerve stimulation.

EVOLUTION

Electricity was used empirically in medicine as early as the Socratic era (Table 57–2). The scientific basis for the use of PNS as pain therapy was provided by Melzack and Wall's[9] spinal gate control theory, first published in 1965. Wall and Sweet[10] conducted the first clinical test of the spinal gate control theory on eight patients with chronic cutaneous pain in 1967.

A number of groups reported their experience with PNS in the late 1970s and early 1980s. Little was published on the procedure over the next 10 years. The initial patient experiences helped to define patient selection criteria and to identify needed improvements in the technique and the equipment. Initially, circumferential cuff electrodes were used. In isolated instances, small electrodes were inserted directly into the nerve. Later, equipment originally designed for spinal cord stimulation was adapted for PNS. The number of centers reporting positive outcomes is increasing.[11–13]

MECHANISM(S) OF ACTION

What Is Stimulated?

The intensity of stimulation is adjusted so that the patient perceives a tingling sensation in the affected area. This is the first sensation elicited by the stimulation and is due to excitation of low-threshold sensory (afferent) nerve axons (e.g., A-beta). Under carefully controlled laboratory conditions, a reproducible strength-duration curve (a plot of volts against seconds, respectively) can be produced for different classes of nerve fibers (with different thresholds). A voltage below which axons cannot be activated, no matter how long the pulse duration, can be defined. Similarly, a pulse duration below which axons cannot be activated, no matter how great the voltage, can be determined. Between these extremes, combinations of pulse duration (width) and voltage that excite one or more populations of nerve fibers can be identified. This is the general basis for the selection of the initial voltage used for PNS and fine tuning of the stimulus by adjustment of pulse duration.

Current flow, not voltage, produces excitation and it may vary if resistance to current flow changes, but voltage is held constant, as with PNS stimulators. Resistance to current flow from the PNS electrodes to the nerve varies if, for example, the distance between the electrode and the nerve changes (decreases if closer, thus more current flow; increases if farther apart, thus less current flow). Obviously, decreasing current flow reduces intensity of stimulation (no sensation can be aroused), and increasing current flow increases stimulation intensity (the patient may have motor movements or experience sensations other than tingling, such as pain).

Stimulation frequency can also influence what voltage and duration are required to activate a nerve fiber population; lower values are needed as stimulation frequency increases. This is one reason why low-frequency stimulation may produce a tingling sensation and high-frequency stimulation with the same voltage and pulse duration produces pain.

TABLE 57–2 Evolution of Peripheral Nerve Stimulation (PNS)

Socratic era
Electrogenic torpedofish to treat pain of arthritis and headache (Scibonius Longus).
Middle Ages
Electrostatic generators combined with Leyden jars.
19th century
Discovery of electric battery led to continued investigation of electroanalgesia.
Modern era (beginning in 1965)
Melzack and Wall's spinal gate control theory provided scientific basis for use of PNS.
First clinical test by Wall and Sweet in 1967.

How Does Stimulation of Low-Threshold Afferent Axons Produce Analgesia?

The most widely accepted explanation of how low-threshold afferent activation produces pain relief involves activation of local inhibitory circuits in the dorsal horn of the spinal cord. These inhibitory circuits act to diminish nociceptive transmission through the spinal cord. Another proposed mechanism is production by PNS of an indecipherable code, thereby "jamming" sensory input into the central nervous system. What must be kept in mind is that electrical stimulation of a peripheral nerve delivers a synchronous volley of activity to the spinal cord from a large number of axons, something that usually does not happen in everyday life. For discussion of investigations that attempted to define the mechanisms of action of peripheral nerve stimulation, the reader should see the paper by Calvillo and coworkers.[8]

SUMMARY

PNS has found a niche in contemporary pain management. Current concepts have been discussed here. Our understanding of how PNS acts to relieve pain, however, is still evolving, as are improvements in the technique and equipment.

REFERENCES

1. Shetter AG, Racz GB, Lewis R, Heavner JE: Peripheral nerve stimulation. *In* North RB, Levy RM (eds): Neurosurgical Management of Pain. New York, Springer-Verlag, 1997, pp 261–270.
2. Racz GB, Lewis R, Laros G, Heavner JE: Electrical stimulation analgesia. *In* Raj PP (ed): Practical Management of Pain, ed 2. St Louis, Mosby–Year Book, 1992, pp 922–933.
3. Picaza JA, Hunter SE, Cannon BW: Pain suppression by peripheral nerve stimulation. Appl Neurophysiol 40:223–234, 1977/78.
4. Sweet WH: Control of pain by direct electrical stimulation of peripheral nerves. Clin Neurosurg 23:103–111, 1976.
5. Cooney WP: Chronic pain treatment with direct electrical nerve stimulation. *In* Gelberean RH (ed): Operative Nerve Repair and Reconstruction. Philadelphia, JB Lippincott, 1991, pp 1551–1561.
6. Hassenbusch SJ, Stanton-Hicks M, Walsh J, et al: Effects of chronic peripheral nerve stimulation in a stage III reflex sympathetic dystrophy (RSD). Presented at the Congress of Neurological Surgeons, 42nd Annual Meeting, Washington, DC, November 4, 1992.
7. Racz GB, Lewis R, Heavner JE, Scott J: Peripheral nerve stimulation implant for treatment of causalgia. *In* Stanton-Hicks M (ed): Pain and the Sympathetic Nervous System. Boston, Kluwer, 1990, pp 225–239.
8. Calvillo O, Racz G, Diede J, Smith K: Neuroaugmentation in the treatment of complex regional pain syndrome of the upper extremity. Acta Orthop Belg 64:57–63, 1998.
9. Melzack R, Wall PD: Pain mechanisms: A new theory. Science 150:971–978, 1965.
10. Wall PD, Sweet WH: Temporary abolition of pain in man. Science 155:108–109, 1967.
11. Stanton-Hicks M, Salamon J: Stimulation of the central and peripheral nervous system for the control of pain. J Clin Neurophysiol 14:46–62, 1997.
12. Long DM: The current status of electrical stimulation of the nervous system for the relief of chronic pain. Surg Neurol 49:142–144, 1998.
13. Cooney WP: Electrical stimulation and the treatment of complex regional pain syndromes of the upper extremity. Hand Clinics 13:519–526, 1997.

BIBLIOGRAPHY

Campbell JN, Long DM: Peripheral nerve stimulation in the treatment of intractable pain. J Neurosurg 45:692–699, 1976.

Campbell JN, Taub A: Local analgesia from percutaneous electrical stimulation: A peripheral mechanism. Arch Neurol 28:347–350, 1973.

Chung JM, Fang ZR, Hori Y, et al: Prolonged inhibition of primate spinothalamic tract cells by peripheral nerve stimulation. Pain 19:259–275, 1984.

Chung JM, Lee KH, Hori Y, et al: Factors influencing peripheral nerve stimulation produced inhibition of primate spinothalamic tract cells. Pain 19:277–293, 1984.

Ignelzi RJ, Nyquist JK: Excitability changes in peripheral nerve fibers after repetitive electrical stimulation: Implications in pain modulation. J Neurosurg 51:824–833, 1979.

Law JD, Sweet J, Kirsch WM: Retrospective analysis of 22 patients with chronic pain treated by peripheral nerve stimulation. J Neurosurg 52:482–485, 1980.

Long DM, Erickson DL, Campbell JN, North RB: Electrical stimulation of the spinal cord and peripheral nerves for pain control: A 10-year experience. Appl Neurophysiol 44:207–217, 1981.

Nashold BS, Goldner JL, Mullen JB, Bright DS: Long-term pain control by direct peripheral nerve stimulation. J Bone Joint Surg 64A:1–10, 1982.

PART • V

Spinal Administration of Opioids and Other Analgesic Compounds

CHAPTER • 58

When All Else Fails: A Role for Implantable Pain Management Devices

Elliot S. Krames, MD

The rational and appropriate use of interventional pain management techniques—and specifically the use of implantable technologies for pain management such as spinal cord stimulation and infusional intraspinal analgesia—should be solidly grounded on thorough knowledge of the neurobiology of pain, its endogenous modulation, and the clinical presentations of different pain syndromes. The treating physician who chooses to use implantable devices for pain control should also know (1) the appropriate and accepted use of all of the "tools of the trade" for managing chronic cancer pain and other pain syndromes and (2) proper temporal use of these tools. The tools of the pain practitioner include all of the modalities and therapies, conservative and invasive, for chronic and cancer-related pain syndromes. Implantable technologies that deliver spinal cord stimulation and infusional, intraspinal analgesia also have their places in the management of chronic and cancer-related pain. It is my purpose in this chapter to guide practitioners of pain medicine in the rational use of all therapies for the relief of cancer-related pain and other chronic pain, and, more specifically, in the rational use of implantable devices, including spinal cord stimulation and spinal analgesics.

In the United States, the costs of chronic pain and the disability it causes are, and will continue to be, a major problem until appropriate, cost-effective algorithms for the management of chronic pain are created and implemented. Chronic, intractable pain is not only a major drain on scarce healthcare resources but is the cause of untold suffering of millions of people worldwide. It is estimated that approximately 30% of the general U.S. population suffer from chronic pain.[1] In a recent study of the general population of the state of Michigan, the Michigan Pain Study, it was found that one adult in five, or about 1.2 million people in Michigan, suffer from some form of chronic, ongoing or recurring pain.[2] In the workplace, in this population, pain was responsible for 400,000 workers' (12% of the Michigan workforce) failing to show up for work at some point in 1999. Of the pain sufferers surveyed, 35% had missed more than 20 days of work in the past year.

The direct, "hard" costs of intractable pain to patients and their families are loss of job, loss of income, loss of savings (and therefore security), loss of insurance, and loss of self-esteem. More subjective results of unrelieved pain include depression, anger, frustration, and suffering. The end result of all this is staggering to society and to persons who suffer relentless pain. The Michigan Pain Study, cited earlier, surveyed 1500 Michigan residents aged 18 and older to determine the severity of the chronic pain problem and how people coped, their access to treatment, and the effectiveness of available pain care. Of the 1.2 million people in Michigan who suffer from chronic pain, 42% said that pain had affected their relationships with spouses, family members, and fellow workers. Nearly half (48%) experienced depression; 18% had overdosed on pain medication; and 10% (about 120,000) had contemplated suicide. Looking for solutions for their pain led 5% of chronic pain sufferers in this population (approximately 60,000 adults) to drink alcohol, and 18% of them admit to overdosing on their medication. Some 29% of the population felt that they were losing sleep because of their chronic pain. Indeed, these figures paint a gloomy—and compelling—picture of the true costs of chronic, unrelieved pain to our society.

In a recent 1999 survey cosponsored by The American Academy of Pain Medicine, The American Pain Society, and Janssen Pharmaceutica, it was found that 56% of all persons with chronic, moderate to severe pain had been suffering for more than 5 years; that 47% of these sufferers had changed doctors at least once since their pain began (22%, three times or more), and that 48% stated that their primary reason for changing physicians was persistent pain after treatment. The primary reasons for changing doctors included patients' continued suffering (42%), their doctors' lack of knowledge about pain (31%), their doctors' not taking their pain seriously enough (29%), and their doctors' unwillingness to treat it aggressively (27%).

Clearly, the problem of intractable chronic pain (whether cancer-related or not) in terms of its drain on scarce healthcare resources and the emotional and physical price exacted of patients and their families, today is a major problem in the United States, if not in the world. In years past, there was, in terms of treatment, little to offer sufferers of chronic pain. There had been an overwhelming belief among the medical community, government regulators, and the general population alike, that potent opioid analgesics used for chronic intractable pain would most probably lead to addiction, tolerance, and loss of personal control. To fill this therapeutic void for the treatment of chronic pain, many neurosurgical procedures were developed to destroy pain-generating nerve tissue. Because of unexpected complications such as exacerbation of pain after some neurodestructive procedures, early enthusiasm, based on early successes, gave way to skepticism and avoidance of these procedures. All too often, patients and their families would hear the same frustrating and exasperating words from their physicians: "You must learn to live with your pain; there is nothing more that I, or medicine, can do for you."

Compounding this lack of effective treatment for chronic pain was a fundamental ignorance of the neuropathophysiologic mechanisms that cause it. There was a strong belief among those in the medical and psychological communities that chronic pain must, in fact, be a behavioral disorder and should be treated as one. Again, such thinking was based on ignorance of the mechanisms of chronic pain and on probability theory. It seemed likely that, since, statistically, most people heal and do not end up with chronic, persistent pain after physical injury, when such pain develops, the precipitant is some underlying unresolved emotional issue or behavioral cause. In newly established pain clinics, behavioral and cognitive principles became the basis for treating these patients, who were often regarded by the medical community as deranged or simply engaged in drug seeking. The underlying philosophy of the pain clinic was that chronic pain was a disorder of behavior and that medical intervention for a behavior disorder was counterproductive and contraindicated. Patients with chronic pain were thought to derive some subconscious gain from their pain. Treatment for chronic pain in these pain clinics therefore relied on changing pain behaviors and reinforcing "healthy" behaviors. Treatment relied on detoxification of patients from their "addictive" medications, treatment with intensive group and individual cognitive and goal-oriented behavioral therapies, and restoration of muscles (and therefore function) deconditioned by months or years of inactivity through intensive physical rehabilitation. Because these early pain-relieving interventions often failed in the long run and because these chronic pain patients would often rely solely on healthcare providers and not on themselves for relief of their pain, all pain interventions were thought to be counterproductive and reinforcing of abnormal pain behavior.

Only in the last 25 years, thanks to growing scientific understanding of the neurophysiologic, neuroanatomic, and neurochemical mechanisms of pain transmission and its modulation in the peripheral and central nervous systems, were clinical pain treatment modalities developed that directly address these systems. Now, we are also beginning to understand that chronic, persistent pain may be the result of pain-processing changes in a plastic central nervous system in response to an initial injury or to repeated injuries.

Persistent pain can also be a disorder of behavior or a disorder of both physiology and emotions or behavior. Today, pain management specialists recognize that chronic, persistent pain is never unidimensional but rather is a multidimensional mix of pain generation, either nociceptive or neuropathic, and disordered emotions and social relationships. In multidisciplinary pain care services, therefore, treatments for chronic pain address both the neurophysiologic and nociceptive dimensions and the affective and cognitive-behavioral dimensions of pain.

TREATING CANCER AND AIDS-RELATED PAIN

Albert Schweitzer once said, "Pain is a greater lord of mankind than even death itself." The treatment of pain and suffering of the dying, provided all available tools are used, is rewarding and truly a privilege for those who care for terminal cancer and AIDS patients.

It has been suggested that 90% to 95% of cancer or AIDS-related pain syndromes can be well controlled using guidelines established by the World Health Organization (WHO; Fig. 58–1).[3] The pharmacologic tailoring approach of these guidelines groups cancer and AIDS-related pain syndromes by severity and intensity—mild, moderate, or severe—and suggests tailoring the potency of medications to the severity of the pain. Nonopioid medications

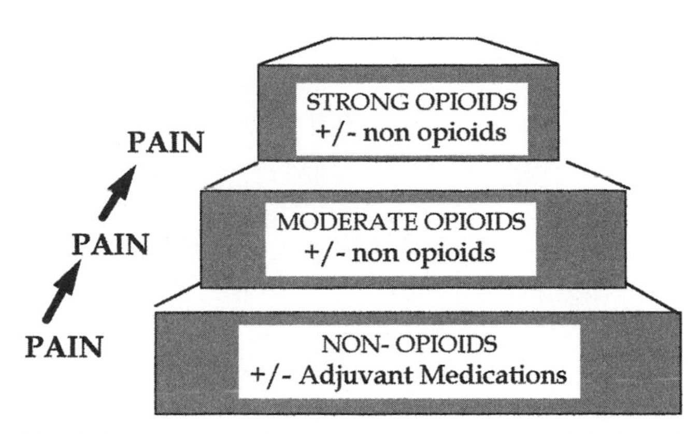

FIGURE 58–1 World Health Organization narcotic ladder. The WHO ladder is an attempt by the WHO Committee on Cancer Pain Management to suggest an algorithm for pain management for patients with cancer pain that both developed and Third World countries could easily implement. These guidelines suggest tailoring pharmacologic therapy to the level of pain that the patient is experiencing. For mild pain the guidelines suggest using nonopioid analgesics, with or without adjuvant medications. If pain persists, the guidelines suggest adding a mild opioid to the therapy. If pain still persists, a strong opioid should be added to the previous doses.

such as the nonsteroidal antiinflammatory drugs and adjuvant medications are suggested for mild to moderate cancer or AIDS-related pain. Adjuvant medications might include heterocyclic antidepressants, anticonvulsants, steroids, sodium and calcium channel–blocking agents, $alpha_2$ agonists, $alpha_1$-blocking agents, beta-blocking agents, and gamma-aminobutyric acid agonists. Weak to medium-strength opioids such as codeine and hydrocodone, along with appropriate nonopioid and adjunctive medications, are suggested for moderately severe cancer pain. Potent opioids such as morphine, hydromorphone, and methadone, together with nonopioids and adjuvants, are suggested for severe cancer pain. Guidelines for dose increases, sequential drug trials, and management of medication-related side effects and symptoms are also provided in the guidelines.

If only 90% to 95% of patients respond to the treatments set forth in the WHO guidelines, 5% to 10% do not. Why do some patients fail to respond? Portenoy believes that the reasons for opioid therapeutic failure in cancer patients may vary widely and may include not only the development of opioid-unresponsive pain syndromes (such as neuropathic pain) or of pain of variable intensity (such as incident pain syndromes like pain with movement) but also clinician- and patient-related factors.[4] Clinician factors include uncertainty about the role of opioid therapy for patients with early-stage, indolent metastatic, or treatment-related disease. Undertreatment, another clinician factor, can result from misinformation about opioid therapy, failure of assessment, overestimation of the risks of addiction, pharmacologic outcomes, or fear of sanctions by regulatory agencies. Patient-related factors in opioid therapeutic failure can include ineffectual pain reporting, misguided fear of addiction or the belief that opioids are inherently harmful, or noncompliance with the dosing schedule.

When implementation of the WHO guidelines fails to provide pain relief for the patient suffering from a cancer-related pain syndrome, it is imperative that caregivers not give up seeking alternative pain control techniques. All too often, caregivers rely only on familiar therapies for pain control, even when those fail to provide analgesia, and they are unaware of alternatives. Sometimes, because alternative therapies are unavailable, patients pass the last weeks of their lives in unnecessary suffering. This need not be.[5]

Available therapies when all else fails include alternative opioid delivery systems such as transdermal fentanyl patches or epidural and intrathecal opioid infusion systems, local anesthetic somatic or sympathetic nerve blocks, intraspinal conduction blockade with local anesthetics, intrapleural analgesia, and neurolytic blocks with alcohol or phenol (including trigeminal neurolysis, celiac plexus neurolysis, paravertebral gangliolysis or rhizolysis, lumbar sympathetic neurolysis, superior hypogastric plexus neurolysis, epidural neurolysis, subarachnoid neurolysis, among others). Neuroaugmentative and some neurodestructive surgical procedures may also be of use in caring for the patient suffering from intractable cancer or AIDS-related pain. Neuroaugmentative procedures include implantation of intraspinal infusional analgesic systems such as the Medtronic Synchromed (Fig. 58–2) or Arrow International Model 3000 (Fig. 58–3) implantable drug delivery systems or implantation of spinal cord– or peripheral nerve–stimulating devices such as equipment provided by Medtronic (Minneapolis, Minn.) (Fig. 58–4) and Advanced Neuromodulation Systems (Plano, Tex.; Fig. 58–5). Some examples of appropriate neurodestructive surgical procedures of last resort for terminal cancer or AIDS patients are cordotomy, pituitary alcohol ablation, rhizotomy, celiac plexus surgical ablation, and myelotomy.

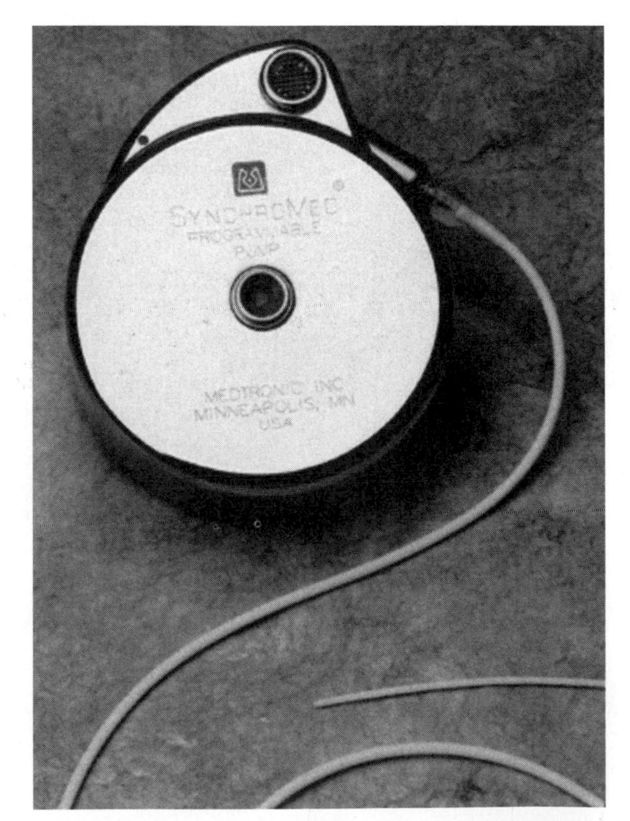

FIGURE 58–2 Medtronic Synchromed pump. (Courtesy of Medtronic, Minneapolis, Minn.)

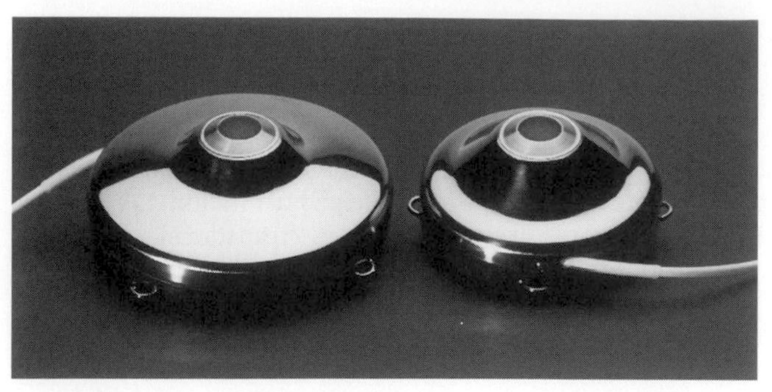

FIGURE 58–3 Arrow models 3000 and 3000-16 implantable pumps. (Courtesy of Arrow International, Reading, Pa.)

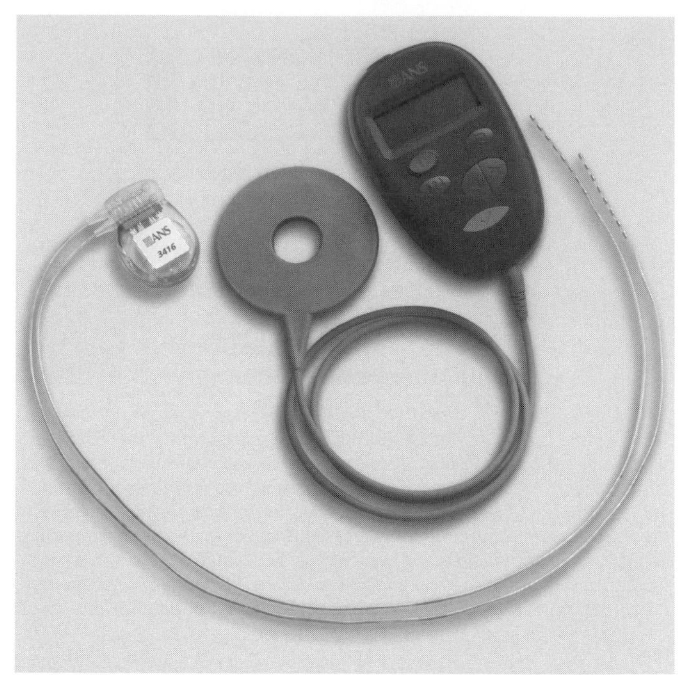

FIGURE 58–5 Advanced Neuromodulation Systems spinal cord stimulation products. (Courtesy of Advanced Neuromodulation Systems, Plano, Tex.)

TREATMENT OF CHRONIC PAIN USING A PAIN TREATMENT CONTINUUM: MULTIPLE CHOICES

The treatment of chronic pain not related to cancer or AIDS, like the treatment of cancer-related pain, requires that the pain treatment physician understand the mechanisms of the patient's pain, the psychological and behavioral factors operant in perpetuating the pain, and which treatment modalities are appropriate for the specific pain syndrome. Because chronic pain almost always involves neurophysiologic systems and emotional and behavioral systems (i.e., is multidimensional), multidisciplinary evaluation and treatment planning is usually warranted. Once a diagnosis is made, after a thorough multidisciplinary evaluation, a parallel treatment plan is created that addresses both the neurophysiologic process or processes involved in the patient's pain and the cognitive, emotional, and behavioral processes. Because multiple modalities are available for the treatment of chronic pain, we treat such patients according to a treatment continuum of therapies of increasing degrees of intervention or invasiveness. According to this algorithm we first choose therapies that are least invasive, and then, as less invasive therapies fail to provide adequate analgesia, we try more invasive ones until either a single treatment or a combination is effective. Treatment modalities for chronic pain not related to cancer or AIDS include cognitive-behavioral psychotherapy, functional rehabilitation, orthopedic and neurologic surgery, pharmacotherapy, anesthetic blocking techniques, neuroaugmentative procedures, and, finally, neuroablative procedures. An example of a treatment continuum is found in Fig. 58–6.

The psychological evaluation and treatment plan should address certain key issues in chronic pain patients. Psychological components of pain must be sought; psychological barriers to successful medical management of pain identified; coping strategies for pain control maximized; and loss issues addressed.

Chronic pain may involve, to some degree, the emotional and cognitive life of the patient. At the very least, some

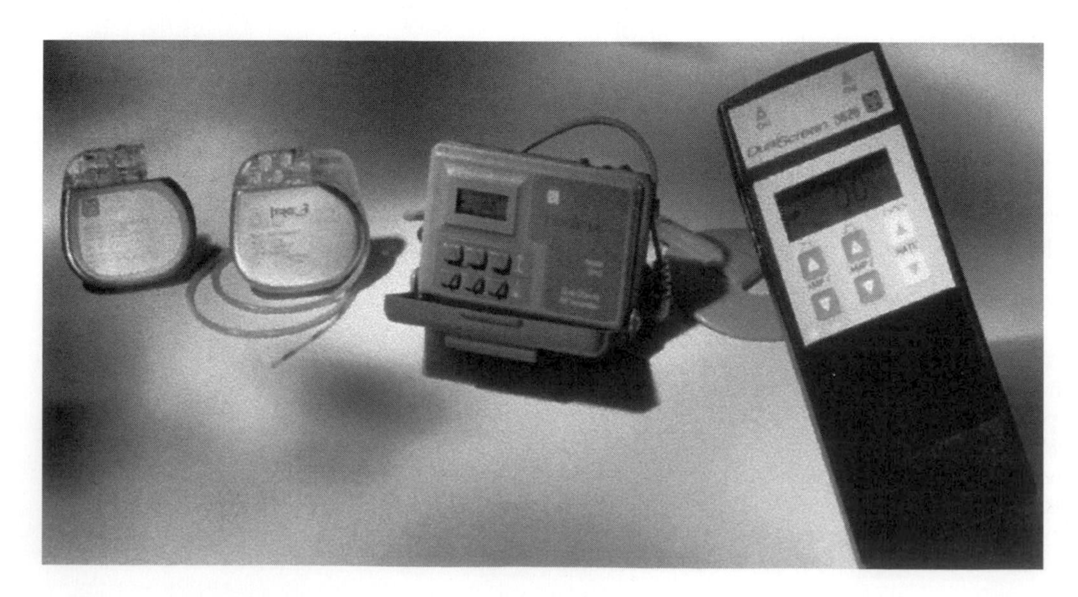

FIGURE 58–4 Medtronic spinal cord stimulation products. (Courtesy of Medtronic, Minneapolis, Minn.)

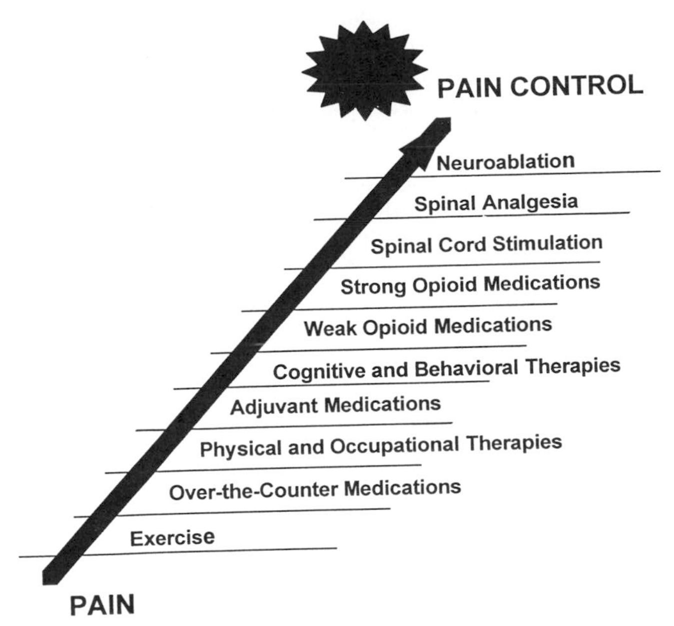

FIGURE 58–6 The Pain Treatment Continuum is a suggested algorithm for appropriate use of possible pain management therapies. These therapies are listed in order of increasing invasiveness. The algorithm appears to suggest that the therapies be used in series, abandoning therapies that do not work and enlisting more invasive therapies in sequential order. In actuality, these therapies can be used in parallel, trying with one or more at the same time.

chronic pain patients merely lack coping skills necessary for internal, self-directed pain modulation and some unconsciously derive secondary gain from their persistent pain. Some patients may have personality disorder or neurosis that frustrates successful pain management, including addictive personality, hysteria, hypochondriasis, or depression. At the other extreme, persistent, chronic pain may be a somatiform disorder; that is, a patient who is unable to deal with unresolved emotional pain finds it easier to unconsciously create somatic pain. In psychobehavioral terms, somatic pain becomes the focus for emotional pain that is "too hot to handle." Rather than addressing the emotional conflicts directly by seeking the help and support of a psychiatrist or a clinical psychologist, the patient seeks a "quick fix," in the form of a pill or a medical intervention. These pain patients are the rare extremes of cases, but are the hardest to treat. They are convinced that they have a physical, somatic illness and they are focused on the body. They tend to deny any problems in their life aside from their "painful illness" and they certainly deny any psychological component to their pain. All medical interventions are doomed to fail until the patient understands, accepts, and addresses the issues that are really causing the underlying emotional pain. Psychological pain interventions include long-term psychotherapy; goal-directed, short-term psychotherapy; operant reconditioning; conjoint, interrelational therapies; chronic pain group therapy; biofeedback; teaching relaxation and distraction techniques; hypnosis; and self-hypnosis.

Medical management of these patients should muster the skills of a wide variety of healthcare professionals, including anesthesiologists, neurologists, surgeons, physiatrists, nurses, physical therapists, occupational therapists, psychologists, psychiatrists, addiction specialists, and vocational rehabilitation specialists.

Chronic pain patients, because of the inactivity brought on by their pain, are generally in bad physical shape. They protect their bodies to the extreme and do not use their muscles appropriately. The role of functional rehabilitation in the treatment of chronic pain is to recondition deconditioned muscles through physical therapy, occupational therapy, and physical and rehabilitation medicine and to provide retraining in activities of daily living or vocational rehabilitation.

Pharmacologic management of the patient with chronic pain utilizes medications that have been shown to be efficacious for either nociceptive or neuropathic pain syndromes. Nociceptive pain most often responds to nonsteroidal antiinflammatory drugs (NSAIDs) or opioids. Non-opioid NSAIDs should be tried before opioids, although the long-term use of these drugs could damage the liver or the kidneys. There is, however, no physiologic down side to the long-term use of strong opioid medications. If an opioid is to be used, its strength should be tailored to the intensity of the pain. Doses should be established empirically rather than from some fictitious published "average dose." Weak opioids should be given for mild pain and strong opioids should be given for intense pain. For constant pain, opioids should be given on a schedule consistent with the pharmacokinetics of the drug rather than as needed (p.r.n.). Since some chronic pain is constant, it may also be desirable to reduce the dosing intervals by choosing an opioid that is relatively longer-lasting. Longer-acting opioids include methadone, levorphanol (Levo-Dromoran) long-acting, slow-release morphine preparations, and transdermal fentanyl. There is a ceiling effect with NSAIDs that is not shared by opioid medications. Once the ceiling dose for a given NSAID is reached, increasing the doses will not increase analgesia but may only increase undesirable side effects. Dosages of opioids can be increased repeatedly to meet the increasing requirement of the patient's pain. If side effects do not develop, more opioid might be better. Side effects of opioid medications include inanition, loss of appetite, nausea and vomiting, sedation, constipation, urinary retention, depression of the hypothalamic-pituitary axis, hallucinations, dry mouth, sweating, and respiratory depression. Not all patients have the same intolerance to opioids. Some patients tolerate one or more of them but not all; some do not tolerate any; and others tolerate all of them. If a patient fails to tolerate one opioid, another should be tried until one produces analgesia without undue side effects. These sequential drug trials should be performed before opioid therapy is abandoned.

Other nonopioid medications, beside the NSAID, that have some degree of analgesic efficacy for chronic pain syndromes are called, as a group, *adjunctive medications*. These adjunctive medications are the same ones suggested for cancer pain and include the heterocyclic antidepressants; the nonheterocyclic, serotonin-enhancing antidepressants; the anticonvulsant medications; GABA analogues, sodium channel–blocking, membrane-stabilizing agents; calcium channel–blocking agents; alpha- and beta-adrenergic agents; $alpha_2$ analogues, substance P–depleting agents; steroids; and the psychogenic amines and their analogues. As with opioids, correct doses should be established through sequential drug trials, as single agents or in combination with other active agents. Doses of these drugs should be increased slowly to enhance patient acceptance, and the doses should be "pushed" until pain is relieved or side effects develop. If side effects develop before analgesia, other drugs of the same class should be tried before the whole class is abandoned. This trial-and-error process of finding an effective analgesic agent takes time, and patients should be counseled to have patience.

As one can see from the treatment continuum, interventional pain management—and certainly the implantable technologies for pain control—should be therapies of last resort that are used before neuroablative and neurodestructive procedures. Implantable technologies are more recent developments for the treatment of chronic pain. They are invasive and relatively expensive as compared with nonsurgical interventions for pain control. They are to be used when more conservative, noninvasive therapies fail to provide analgesia. As we will see, these therapies, when used appropriately in the right patients, add immeasurably to the aforementioned tools of the trade for the pain care team.

INFUSIONAL SPINAL ANALGESIA AND DRUG ADMINISTRATION SYSTEMS

The discovery of opioid receptors and endogenous opioid compounds in the spinal cord[6–8] provided a rationale for early attempts to deliver opioid drugs intraspinally, first in experimental animals[9, 10] and then in patients with chronic pain.[11, 12] This experience with "selective spinal analgesia"[13] appeared to offer specific benefits to some patients and was followed by trials of continuous subarachnoid opioid infusions using implanted pumps with factory preset flow rates.[14, 15] During the past decade, published reports and abstracts in the United States literature have repeatedly documented the safety and efficacy of implanted nonprogrammable and programmable pumps for long-term subarachnoid delivery of opioids for the management of cancer pain[16–19] and other pain.[20–25]

This documented efficacy, however, may be specific to certain opioid-responsive pain syndromes.[26–28] Nociceptive pain—defined as pain produced by damage or insult to the body and mediated by mechanical, thermal, or chemical nociceptors—is responsive to opioid analgesics (Table 58–1). Neuropathic pain—pain produced by damage to or pathologic changes in central or peripheral pain-processing mechanisms—on the other hand, may be less responsive to opioid analgesics or may require higher doses than those used clinically for nociceptive pain to be effective (see Table 58–1).[29, 30]

Although some chronic neuropathic pain syndromes may be resistant to intraspinal opioid infusion, these syndromes may respond to other intraspinal agents, for example, $alpha_2$ agonists, somatostatin[31] and its analogues,[32] intrathecal NSAID, *N*-methyl-D-aspartate–receptor antagonists, gangliosides, neurotropic factors, neuron-specific calcium channel–blocking agents,[33] or midazolam.[34, 35] Except for opioid and local anesthetic combinations, most of these agents, today, are experimental and not available for widespread clinical use.

TABLE 58–1 Characteristics of Nociceptive and Neuropathic Pain

Nociceptive pain
- Mediated by nociceptors throughout the body
- Nociceptors are chemical, thermal, and mechanical
- Nociceptors transduce noxious information into electrical information for transmission to the central nervous system
- Pain of trauma, tissue injury, surgery
- Opioid-responsive pain syndrome

Neuropathic pain
- Not mediated by nociceptors
- Due to peripheral or central nervous system damage or abnormal pain-processing mechanisms in the peripheral or central nervous system
- Abnormal pain processing mechanisms due to toxicity of the nervous system or unrelieved nociception which activates the *N*-methyl-D-aspartate (NMDA) receptor system
- NMDA receptor system opioid-responsive, -resistant, or unresponsive pain syndrome

Recently, several clinical reports on the use of local anesthetic–opioid intraspinal mixtures for the treatment of cancer-related and other severe pain were published.[11, 36–39] Animal toxicity and human post-mortem studies suggest that long-term infusion of intrathecal bupivacaine in low doses is clinically safe.[40, 41] Other reports, however, in both the animal and human clinical literature cite the potential neural toxicity of local anesthetic agents when used over the long term. One study showed neurotoxicity after long-term subarachnoid infusions of bupivacaine, lidocaine, and 2-chloroprocaine in a rat model.[42] These neurotoxic effects, however, were both dose- and duration-dependent, and bupivacaine appeared to have a less extensive effect than either lidocaine or tetracaine. There are also recent clinical reports in the anesthesia literature of permanent neurologic damage and sequelae, specifically cauda equina syndrome, when 5% lidocaine was used in concentrations needed to produce spinal anesthesia, particularly when delivered through small-bore intrathecal catheters.[43] It is not clear whether this significant clinical complication was drug related, catheter related, technique related, or a combination of these. One report suggests that no tachyphylaxis occurred with prolonged continuous spinal infusions of bupivacaine.[44]

SPINAL CORD STIMULATION

Spinal cord stimulation for the clinical control of pain was introduced in 1967 by Norman Shealy and colleagues[45] in response to the publication of the gate control theory of pain by Melzack and Wall in 1965.[46] The gate control theory, as first published (without benefit of later refinements), held that painful "electrochemical" nociceptive information from the periphery is transmitted to the spinal cord via small-diameter, unmyelinated C fibers and "lightly" myelinated A-delta fibers. These fibers, in turn, terminate at the dorsal horn, the "gate," of the spinal cord. Likewise, other sensory information such as touch or vibration carried in large myelinated A-beta fibers would also converge at this gate. The basic premise of the gate control theory is that reception of large-fiber information, such as touch or vibration would "turn off" or close the gate to reception, or more appropriately, to transmission, of small-fiber information, and, therefore, pain. The clinical result of this gate closure, these authors theorized, would be analgesia.

Shealy and colleagues extrapolated from the gate control thesis that, if the large A-beta fibers of the dorsal columns were electrically stimulated by currents applied over the dorsal columns, the stimulation would antidromically inhibit reception of afferent, painful, small-fiber information at the segmental level of the spinal cord.[45] In fact, these authors presented the first clinical evidence of efficacy of electrical stimulation analgesia in their paper. Because they believed that electrical stimulation worked only at the dorsal columns of the spinal cord, they called this treatment modality *dorsal column stimulation*. Since it is now known that this inhibition of nociception can occur with electrical stimulation almost anywhere in the spinal cord, the term has been supplanted in the literature with the more general but accurate term, *spinal cord stimulation*.

The actual mechanism or mechanisms of action of spinal cord stimulation are not known, but there are several theories. Each one is supported by abundant animal data, but, until animal models of chronic pain are created that are germane to the human experience, they will remain just theories. Theories include the spinal, segmental theories of gate blocking or tractal, conductance blocking; the supraspinal theory of blocking or activating supraspinal pain processing nuclei; activation of sympathetic blocking mechanisms; and release of putative neuromodulatory chemicals.

Since these first clinical reports on spinal cord stimulation for the relief of intractable pain in humans, multiple reports have been published on the efficacy of spinal cord stimulation for widely different chronic pain syndromes[47–55] and for clinical pain due to peripheral vascular disease in humans. In fact, peripheral vascular disease is the leading indication for spinal cord stimulation in Europe today.[56–60] Besides peripheral ischemic vascular disease, spinal cord stimulation has also been used effectively to treat the pain of intractable angina.[61–63]

Because of differences in hardware technologies used and different criteria for patient selection and trials for efficacy, it is difficult to know from these published reports on the efficacy of spinal cord stimulation what is, and what is not, true. What has become clear from these studies, however, is that spinal cord stimulation is effective to some degree for pain states of neuropathic origin and for pain of ischemic origins but is not effective for acute pain or pain of nociceptive origin.

RATIONAL USE OF IMPLANTABLE TECHNOLOGY: WHEN TO PUMP AND WHEN TO "STIM"

The abundant information on patient selection and efficacy of the two implantable treatment modalities (spinal cord stimulation and implantable drug delivery systems) notwithstanding, little, if anything, has been written about decision making. How, in practice, does the clinician choose one modality over the other? Based on my own review of the literature and on clinical "art" developed from 20 years' experience with these modalities, in this section, I will suggest an algorithm for such decision making.

A rational approach for deciding on appropriate therapy for chronic pain starts with a complete multidisciplinary workup, including complete pain and medical histories and complete physical, psychologic, and functional examinations. Once a diagnosis is derived from these evaluations, rational and complementary medical and psychosocial intervention plans are created. Such a plan might include, as later resort therapies, implantable devices.[64] Considerations in the choice of one of the implantable technologies over another include the type of pain syndrome and the distribution of the pain. Fundamental to the choice of one modality over the other is the understanding that not all pain is the same and that different implantable neuromodulatory modalities work for different pain syndromes. Spinal cord stimulation is effective in treating neuropathic pain and the pain of peripheral vascular disease (which might be nociceptive), but it is not effective for acute or nociceptive pain syndromes. Spinally administered opioids are effective for nociceptive syndromes, because the drug is delivered directly to the opiate receptors in the spinal cord. Because the response to opioids of neuropathic pain may be variable, it is imperative to confirm responsiveness before an expensive intraspinal drug delivery system is implanted. This point cannot be emphasized enough. If neuropathic pain fails to respond to systemic opioids after an appropriate trial, it is doubtful that it will respond to intraspinal opioids alone; although it might respond to admixtures of agents, including opioids and/or local anesthetics and/or clonidine. If these agents fail, the pain might respond to one of the experimental agents cited earlier that have proven analgesic efficacy when given intraspinally. For emphasis, and because this is a key issue in the rational use of these modalities, I will again define nociceptive and neuropathic pain.

Nociceptive pain, defined as pain mediated by nociceptors widely distributed in the soma of the body, is often characterized by patients in such terms as *dull*, *aching*, *sharp*, or *throbbing*. Nociceptors respond to mechanical, thermal, and noxious chemical stimuli and "transduce" this noxious information into electrical information for transmission to the central nervous system. At the spinal cord level, this nociceptive pain is modulated pre- and postsynaptically, at the dorsal horn, by endogenous and exogenous opioids acting at opiate receptors. Therefore, nociceptive pain is usually responsive to opioid therapy, whether delivered orally, parenterally, or spinally. Examples of nociceptive pain include postsurgical pain, trauma pain, vertebrogenic pain, and cancer pain emanating from bone, connective tissue, or viscera.

Neuropathic pain, on the other hand, is not mediated by nociceptors in the periphery but is caused by damage to the peripheral or central nervous system or by pathologic changes in neurofunctional relationships in these pain-processing systems. Examples of these pathologic changes in functional relationships causing chronic persistent pain include sensitization of nociceptors, central sensitization or "windup," abnormal sympathetic and somatic nervous system interactions, and abnormal activation of NMDA

TABLE 58–2 ***Criteria for Implantable Technologies***

- Establish a diagnosis
- Use of a pain treatment continuum
- Failure of conservative therapies
- No psychological impediments to a successful implantation after trial
- Trial for efficacy; rule out toxicity and powerful placebo effects of therapy

receptors. These pains, unlike nociceptive pain, are most often described by patients in terms of electric-like sensations such as *tingling*, *burning*, *shooting*, and *lightninglike*. Examples of neuropathic pain include the monoradiculopathies, "sciatica," trigeminal neuralgia, phantom limb pain, postherpetic neuralgia, causalgia, reflex sympathetic dystrophy, and peripheral neuropathies. Neuropathic pain is thought to be opioid resistant and, unlike nociceptive pain, may respond to higher than "normal" opioid doses, or may not respond to opioid therapy at all.

Spinal Cord Stimulation

After the patient's pain syndrome has been identified, and before the appropriate implantable modality is chosen, it is also essential to understand that distribution of pain is an important issue when considering implantable technologies for the control of pain. Efficacy of spinal cord stimulation is directly related to concordance of paresthesia coverage to the area of subjective pain complaint. In the past, stimulation was fairly limited by technology to unilateral, single-focus, neuropathic pain. However, in the last decade, advances in our understanding of appropriate stimulation programming, lead placement, and technology[65–67] has made possible multisite stimulation and stimulation with different programs. In the past, low back, axial, neuropathic pain was inaccessible to stimulation, but, today, with dual-electrode arrays and hardware that support dual stimulation, relief of this pain is possible.[68–71] Because of advances in technology that allow for multisite stimulation, alternating programs of stimulation, steering of stimulation paresthesia, and computer programming of stimulation parameters, spinal cord stimulation has, indeed, become a truly versatile mode of analgesia that is accessible to more patients today than in the past. Still, because of proven efficacy, this modality is most appropriate for neuropathic pain of appendicular origin and less efficacious for axial neuropathic pain.

Spinally Administered Analgesia

Success of infusional spinal analgesia depends on the physicochemical properties of the drug being infused by the implanted delivery system in relation to the tip of the implanted intrathecal catheter connected to the pump.[72] If the patient has pain at multiple sites subserved by large areas of the spinal cord, it might be essential to use hydrophilic agents, which disseminate far in cerebrospinal fluid. If the patient has a single pain focus and a lipophilic agent such as fentanyl, meperidine, bupivacaine or even clonidine is desired, the spinal catheter tip connected to the pump must be positioned as close as possible to the spinal cord segment that is mediating the patient's pain.

Implantable Selection Criteria

Even though there may be syndrome-specific indications for preferring one implantable pain-relief modality over another, certain basic criteria for all implantables must be met before implantation is undertaken. Whether the choice is spinal cord stimulation or spinally administered opioids, certain criteria for implantation must be met (Table 58–2). The "implantables selection criteria" include a psychological evaluation (psychological interview and appropriate psychometric testing with psychological clearance for implantation), failure of accepted and recognized, more conservative therapies, and, most important, a successful preimplantation trial of the modality under consideration. Again, it should be fundamental to any pain practice that invasive therapies for pain management be used only in the proper place in the treatment continuum for each pain syndrome, utilizing less invasive therapies before more invasive ones.

To Choose

Once interventional, implantable pain therapy is considered appropriate, and after all selection criteria have been met, it is appropriate to choose one of the two implantable therapies. For neuropathic pain, either appendicular or axial, unilateral or bilateral, that is amenable to stimulation (that is, the spinal cord area subserving the pain can be effectively stimulated with either single or dual, quadripolar or octipolar electrodes) and is unchanging, spinal cord stimulation should be tried before spinal administration of analgesics is considered. If a trial for spinal cord stimulation is not successful, then a trial of spinal analgesics should be considered (Fig. 58–7). If a patient has principally somatic, nociceptive, opioid-responsive pain, at a single focus or

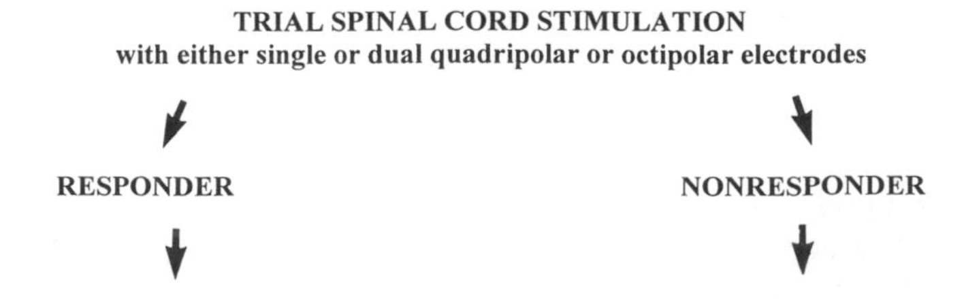

FIGURE 58–7 Algorithm for the management of patients with neuropathic pain. If the physical site of pain is amenable to stimulation of the spinal cord, the disease process is static, and the pain is radicular or appendicular, a trial of spinal cord stimulation may be tried.

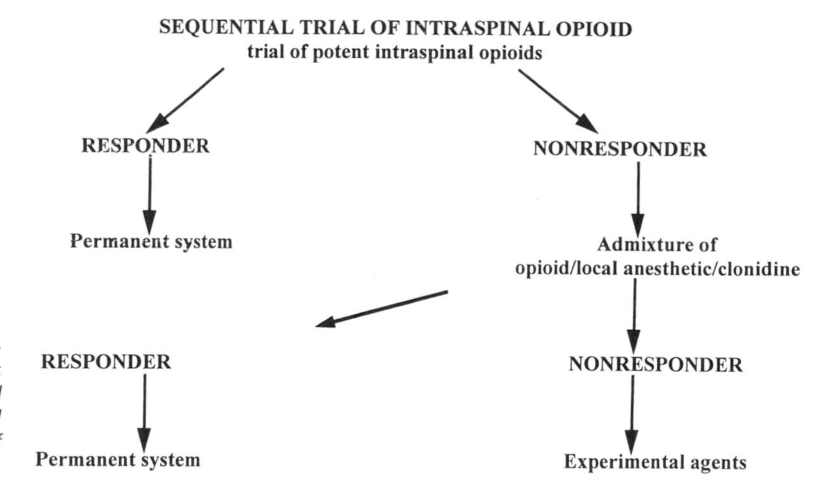

FIGURE 58–8 Algorithm for the management of patients with nociceptive pain. If the pain is responsive to opioids but administration of potent, long-acting opioids has failed (i.e., if side effects developed before the analgesic effects) and the disease process is static or changing, a sequential trial of intraspinal opioid is given.

multiple foci, and possibly spreading disease, a trial of spinally administered opioids is warranted after systemic administration of opioids fails (*failure* being defined as too many side effects before desired analgesia with all potent, long-acting opioids trialed) before resorting to more invasive and irreversible procedures such as neuroablative surgery (Fig. 58–8).

Certain pain syndromes clearly fall into one treatment category or the other. For these syndromes, the indications for spinal cord stimulation and spinally administered opioids are clear and thoroughly described in the literature. Patients with single monoradicular pain such as lumbar monoradiculopathy are clearly the best candidates for spinal cord stimulation; although with the newer technologies and our greater understanding of how stimulation works, more patients with different neuropathic pain syndromes (such as neuropathic, axial back pain) are also having good results. Patients with pure visceral pain that is responsive to opioids and patients with metastatic cancer or undisputed nociceptive, nonmalignant pain are the most appropriate candidates for spinal opioids.

Many patients have mixed nociceptive and neuropathic pain syndromes that fall into "gray" zones and that might respond to one or both treatment modalities (Fig. 58–9). Patients with mixed nociceptive and neuropathic pain should, when appropriate, undergo a trial of spinal cord stimulation before a trial of infusional spinal analgesia. Of course, common sense dictates the appropriate course of action. Patients with equal and multiple foci of pain, though it be mixed pain, are not going to be adequately treated with spinal cord stimulation via a single electrode array and may need multiple electrodes. These patients may need combination therapy or may benefit from an experimental therapy. Infusional analgesia with combined opioids and local anesthetics has been shown to be efficacious for neuropathic and nociceptive pain.

Spinal cord stimulators have been implanted in tens of thousands of people worldwide, and, to my knowledge, no one has been injured by electrical fields over the spinal cord. However, because spinally administered analgesics may produce unfortunate neurologic sequelae,[73] a trial of spinal cord stimulation should be conducted before spinal

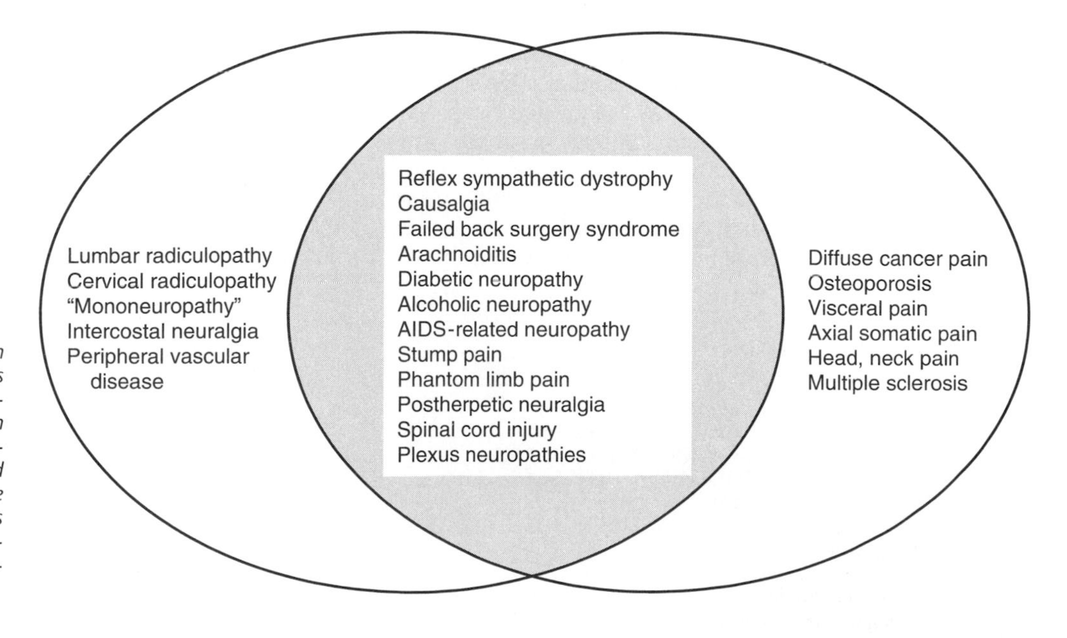

FIGURE 58–9 The circle on the left lists chronic pain syndromes that respond to spinal cord stimulation. The circle on the right lists pain syndromes that respond to the intraspinal administration of opioid medications. The shaded area in the middle of the overlapping circles lists pain syndromes that respond to either spinal cord stimulation or spinally administered opioids.

administration of opioids, if appropriate, is considered. If a trial of spinal cord stimulation fails or if the patient develops tolerance to its antinociceptive effects, a trial of spinal analgesics, with opioids alone or in combination with local anesthetics and/or clonidine, is in order.

SUMMARY

In summary, a decision tree has been presented for the selection of appropriate therapies for cancer- and AIDS-related pain and other chronic pain syndromes. For cancer pain syndromes, pharmacologic tailoring using the WHO guidelines for the management of cancer-related pain should be the initial therapy of choice. Provided that caregivers use these guidelines, understand what syndromes are responsive to systemic opioid therapy, and are guided by knowledge of the pharmacokinetics and pharmacodynamics of the drugs, 90% to 95% of patients will obtain adequate pain control. The 10% of the patients whose cancer pain is unresponsive to such therapy or who develop intolerable side effects, in spite of sequential trials of opioids, are still a significant number of patients in pain. They should not be abandoned; more invasive therapies should be tried.

Rational use of a treatment continuum approach to chronic nonmalignant pain has been presented. This algorithm is also a rational guide to the use of more invasive therapies—and, specifically, to implantable technologies, when all else fails. Both spinal cord stimulation and spinally administered opioids should be used in the context of this treatment continuum but only after syndrome-specific, conservative therapies have failed. All patients considered for implantable pain technologies should meet appropriate selection criteria: no untreated drug habituation, psychological interview and clearance, a trial for efficacy, and no surgical contraindications. Clearly, spinally administered opioids are more appropriate for opioid-responsive nociceptive pain syndromes and spinal cord stimulation is the better choice for mononeuropathic pain syndromes, pain of ischemic origin, and pain due to intractable angina pectoris. Patients whose pain might respond to both technologies should have a trial of spinal cord stimulation before spinal opioids are considered. We consider spinal cord stimulation a known entity, totally reversible, and one with very few reported complications. Spinal administration of opioids, on the other hand, is a newer procedure with scant information on the complications of long-term infusion of opioids into the spinal canal. Both technologies, however, should be given a trial before more invasive pain treatments such as neuroablative surgical procedures are contemplated.

REFERENCES

1. Bonica JJ: Chronic non-cancer pain. *In* Anderson S, Bond M, Mehta M, et al (eds): Lancaster, UK, MTP Press, 1987.
2. The Michigan Pain Study. EPIC/MRA 4710 W. Saginaw Hwy. Lansing, Michigan 48917-2601, 1997.
3. World Health Organization: Cancer Pain Relief, ed 2. Geneva, World Health Organization, 1989.
4. Portenoy RK: Inadequate outcome of opioid therapy for cancer pain: Influences on practitioners and patients. *In* Patt RB (ed): Cancer Pain. Philadelphia, JB Lippincott, 1993, pp 119–128.
5. Krames ES: Cancer pain management, practical issues when using neuraxial infusion. Oncology 13 (Suppl 2):37–44, 1999.
6. Pert CB, Snyder S: Opiate receptors—demonstration in nervous tissue. Science 179:1011, 1973.
7. Hughes J, Smith TW, Kosterlitz HW, et al: Isolation of two related pentapeptides from brain with potent opiate activity. Nature 258:577, 1975.
8. Terenius L, Wahlstrom A: Morphine-like ligand in opiate receptors in human CSF. Life Sci 16:1759–1764, 1975.
9. Yaksh TL, Rudy TA: Studies on the direct spinal action of narcotics in the production of analgesia in the rat. J Pharmacol Exp Ther 202:411–428, 1977.
10. Yaksh TL: Analgetic actions of intrathecal opiates in cat and primates. Brain Res 153:205–210, 1978.
11. Wang JF, Nauss LA, Thomas JE: Pain relief by intrathecally applied morphine in man. Anesthesiology 50:149–151, 1979.
12. Behar M, Olshwang D, Magora F, et al: Epidural morphine in treatment of pain. Lancet 1:527, 1979.
13. Cousins MJ, Mather LE, Glynn CJ, et al: Selective spinal analgesia. Lancet 1:1141–1142, 1979.
14. Onofrio BM, Yaksh TL, Arnold PG: Continuous low dose intrathecal morphine administration in the treatment of chronic pain of malignant origin. Mayo Clin Proc 55:469, 1981.
15. Coombs DW, Saunders RL, Gaylor M, et al: Epidural narcotic infusion: implantation technique and efficacy. Anesthesiology 55:469, 1981.
16. Harbaugh RE, Coombs DW, Saunders RL: Implanted continuous epidural morphine infusion system. J Neurosurg 56:803–806, 1982.
17. Krames, ES, Gershow J, Glassberg A, et al: Continuous infusion of spinally administered narcotics for the relief of pain due to malignant disorders. Cancer 56:696–702, 1985.
18. Shetter AG, Hadley MN, Wilkinson E: Administration of intraspinal morphine for the treatment of cancer pain. Neurosurgery 18:740–747, 1986.
19. Brazenor GA: Long-term intrathecal administration of morphine: A comparison of bolus injection via reservoir with continuous infusion by implanted pump. Neurosurgery 21:484–491, 1987.
20. Hassenbusch SJ, Stanton-Hicks MD, Soukup J, et al: Sufentanil citrate and morphine/bupivacaine as alternative agents in chronic epidural infusions for intractable non-cancer pain. Neurosurgery 29:76–82, 1990.
21. Goodman RR: Treatment of lower extremity reflex sympathetic dystrophy with continuous intrathecal morphine infusion. Appl Neurophysiol 50:425–426, 1987.
22. Krames ES, Lanning RM: Intrathecal infusional analgesia for nonmalignant pain: Analgesic efficacy of intrathecal opioid with or without bupivacaine. J Pain Symptom Manage 8(8):539–548, 1993.
23. Krames ES: Intraspinal opioids for non-malignant pain. Curr Rev Pain 1:198–211, 1997.
24. Schuchard MS, Krames ES, Lanning RM: Intraspinal analgesia for nonmalignant pain. Neuromodulation 1:46–56, 1998.
25. Krames ES, Olson K: Clinical realities and economic considerations: Patient selection in intrathecal therapy. J Pain Symptom Manage 14:S3–S12, 1997.
26. Arner S, Arner B: Differential effects of epidural morphine in the treatment of cancer related pain. Acta Anaesthesiol Scand 29:332–336, 1989.
27. Arner S, Meyerson B: Lack of analgesic effect of opioids on neuropathic and idiopathic forms of pain. Pain 33:11–23, 1988.
28. Vecht CJ: Nociceptive nerve pain and neuropathic pain (Letter to Editor). Pain 39:243–244, 1989.
29. Portenoy RK, Foley KM, Inturrisi CE: The nature of opioid responsiveness and its implications for neuropathic pain: New hypothesis derived from studies of opioid infusions. Pain 43:273–286, 1990.
30. Hammond DL: Do opioids relieve pain? *In* Casey KL (ed): Pain and Central Nervous System Disease: The Central Pain Syndromes. New York, Raven Press, 1991, pp 233–241.
31. Meynadier J, Chrubasik J, Dubar M, Wunsch E: Intrathecal somatostatin in terminally ill patients: A report of two cases. Pain 23:9–12, 1985.
32. Penn RD, Paice JA, Kroin JS: Intrathecal octreotide for cancer pain. Lancet: 738, 1990.
33. Bowersox SS, Gadbois T, Singh T, et al: Selective N-type neuronal voltage-sensitive calcium channel blocker, SNX-111, produces spinal

antinociception in rat models of acute, persistent and neuropathic pain. J Pharm Exp Ther 279:1243–1249, 1996.
34. Bahar M, Cohen ML, Grinshpon Y, Chanimov M: Spinal anesthesia with midazolam in the rat. Can J Anaesth 44:208–215, 1997.
35. Goodchild CS: Nonopioid spinal analgesics: Animal experimentation and implications for clinical developments. Pain Rev 4:33–58, 1997.
36. Coombs DW, Pageau MG, Saunders RL, et al: Intraspinal narcotic tolerance: Preliminary experience with continuous bupivacaine HCl infusion via implanted infusion device. Int J Artif Organs 5:379–382, 1982.
37. Berde CB, Sethna NF, Conrad LS, et al: Subarachnoid bupivacaine analgesia for seven months for a patient with a spinal cord tumor. Anesthesiology 72:1094–1096, 1990.
38. Nitescu P, Lennart A, Linder L, et al: Epidural versus intrathecal morphine-bupivacaine: Assessment of consecutive treatments in advanced cancer pain. J Pain Symptom Manage 5:18–26, 1990.
39. Van Dongen RTM, Crul BJP, de Bock M: Long-term intrathecal infusion of morphine and morphine/bupivacaine mixtures in the treatment of cancer pain: A retrospective analysis of 51 cases. Pain 55:107–111, 1993.
40. Kroin JS, McCarthy RJ, Penn RD, et al: The effect of chronic subarachnoid bupivacaine infusion in dogs. Anesthesiology 66:737–742, 1987.
41. Sjoberg M, Karlsson PA, Nordborg C, et al: Neuropathologic findings after long-term intrathecal infusion of morphine and bupivacaine for pain treatment in cancer patients. Anesthesiology 76:173–186, 1992.
42. Li DF, Hahar M, Cole G, et al: Neurological toxicity of the subarachnoid infusion of bupivacaine, lignocaine, or 2-chloroprocaine in the rat. Br J Anaesth 57:424–429, 1985.
43. Rigler ML, Drasner K, Krejcie TC, et al: Cauda equina syndrome after continuous spinal anesthesia. Anesth Analg 72:275–281, 1991.
44. Raj PR, Denson DD, de Jong RH: No tachyphylaxis with prolonged, continuous bupivacaine. *In* Wust HJ, Stanton-Hicks M (eds): New Aspects in Regional Anaesthesia 4: Major Conduction Block: Tachyphylaxis, Hypotension, and Opiates. New York, Springer-Verlag, 1986, pp 10–18.
45. Shealy CN, Mortimer JT, Reswick J: Electrical inhibition of pain by stimulation of the dorsal column: Preliminary reports. Anesth Analg 46:489–491, 1967.
46. Melzack R, Wall PD: Pain mechanisms: A new theory. Science 150:971–978, 1965.
47. Long DM, et al: Electrical stimulation of the spinal cord and peripheral nerves for pain control: A ten-year experience. Appl Neurophysiol 44:207–217, 1981.
48. Broseta J, et al: Chronic epidural dorsal column stimulation in the treatment of causalgic pain. Appl Neurophysiol 45:190–194, 1982.
49. Meglio M, Cioni B, Rossi GF: Spinal cord stimulation in management of chronic pain: A 9-year experience. J Neurosurg 70:519–524, 1989.
50. Spiegelmann R, Friedman WA: Spinal cord stimulation: A contemporary series. Neurosurgery 28:65–70, 1991.
51. Barolat G, Schwartzman R, Woo R: Epidural spinal cord stimulation in the management of reflex sympathetic dystrophy. Stereotact Funct Neurosurg 53:29–39, 1989.
52. North RB, Kidd DH, Zahurak M, et al: Spinal cord stimulation for chronic intractable pain: Experience over two decades. Neurosurgery 32:384–395, 1993.
53. Kumar K, Toth C, Nath RK, Laing P: Epidural spinal cord stimulation for treatment of chronic pain: Some predictors of success. A 15-year experience. Pain 50:110–121, 1998.
54. Segal R, Stacey BR, Rudy TE, et al: Spinal cord revisited. 20:391–396, 1998.
55. Barolat G, Ketcik B, Jiping H: Long-term outcome of spinal cord stimulation for chronic pain management. Neuromodulation 1:19–29, 1998.
56. Jacobs MJHM, et al: Spinal cord electrical stimulation improves microvascular blood flow in severe limb ischaemia. Ann Surg 207:179–181, 1988.
57. Robaina FJ, et al: Spinal cord stimulation for relief of chronic pain in vasospastic disorders of the upper limbs. Neurosurgery 24:179–183, 1989.
58. Groth KE: Spinal cord stimulation for the treatment of peripheral vascular disease. Adv Pain Res Therapy 9:861–870, 1985.
59. Tallis RC, Illis LS, Sedgwick C, et al: Spinal cord stimulation in peripheral vascular disease. J Neurol Neurosurg Psychiatry 46:478–484, 1983.
60. Augustinsson LE, et al: Epidural electrical stimulation in severe limb ischemia: Evidences of pain relief, increased blood flow and a possible limb-saving effect. Ann Surg 202:104–111, 1985.
61. Murphy DF, Giles KE: Dorsal column stimulation for pain relief from intractable angina pectoris. Pain 3:365–368, 1987.
62. Mannheimer C, Augustinsson LE, Carlsson CA, et al: Epidural spinal electrical stimulation in severe angina pectoris. Br Heart J 59:56–61, 1988.
63. DeJongste MJJ: Efficacy, safety and mechanisms of spinal cord stimulation used as an additional therapy for patients suffering from chronic refractory angina pectoris. Neuromodulation 2(3):188–193, 1999.
64. Krames ES: Interventional pain management: Appropriate when less invasive therapies fail to provide adequate analgesia. Med Clin North Am 83:787–808, 1999.
65. Holsheimer J, Struijk JJ: How do geometric factors influence epidural spinal cord stimulation? A quantitative analysis of computer modeling. Stereotact Funct Neurosurg 56:234–249, 1991.
66. Holsheimer J, Struijk JJ, Tas NR: Effects of electrode geometry and combination on nerve fibre selectivity in spinal cord stimulation. Med Biol Eng Comput 33:676–682, 1995.
67. Holsheimer J, Barolat G: Spinal geometry and paresthesia coverage in spinal cord stimulation. Neuromodulation 1:128–136, 1998.
68. Law JD: Spinal stimulation: Statistical superiority of monophasic stimulation of narrowly separated, longitudinal bipoles having rostral cathodes. Appl Neurophysiol 46:129–137, 1983.
69. Law JD: Targeting a spinal stimulator to treat the "failed back surgery syndrome." Appl Neurophysiol 50:437–438, 1987.
70. Alo KM, Yland MJ, Kramer DL, et al: Computer assisted and patient interactive programming of dual octrode spinal cord stimulation in the treatment of chronic pain. Neuromodulation 1:30–46, 1998.
71. Van Buyton JP, Van Zundert J, Milbouw G: Treatment of failed back surgery syndrome patients with low back and leg pain: A pilot study of a new dual lead spinal cord stimulation system. Neuromodulation 2:258–266, 1999.
72. Krames ES, Schuchard M: Implantable intraspinal infusional analgesia: Management guidelines. Pain Rev 2:243–267, 1995.
73. Schuchard M, Lanning R, North R, et al: Neurologic sequelae of implantable drug delivery systems: Results of neurologic sequelae survey of implanters of implantable drug delivery systems. Neuromodulation 1:137–149, 1998.

CHAPTER • 59

Spinal Administration of Opioids for Pain of Malignant Origin

Lowell Reynolds, MD • Divakara Kedlaya, MD

HISTORICAL ASPECTS

Although use of opium for analgesia has been reported since the 9th century, the analgesic action of intrathecal morphine in experimental animals was first reported in 1976.[1] In 1979, intrathecal[2] and epidural[3] use of morphine in humans were both shown to control pain effectively. Spinal administration of morphine for pain control in cancer patients was first reported by Wang and colleagues,[2] and it was well-documented by Ventafridda's group.[4] The World Health Organization in 1986 developed a three-step approach to managing cancer-related pain, which works very well in treating the vast majority (about 90%) of patients. For patients who do not receive pain relief from the three-step approach, intraspinal opioids can be a fourth step in attacking pain of malignant origin. Studies on the use of intraspinal opioids for cancer pain are summarized in Table 59–1.[5–17]

CLINICAL PHARMACOLOGY

Opioid analgesics reduce pain by binding to opioid receptors in the spinal cord. Taken orally, the dose must be relatively large to achieve therapeutic benefit at the spinal level. This approach, while usually successful in controlling cancer pain, can lead to side effects such as constipation, sedation, and respiratory depression (to name a few). For this reason, intrathecal or epidural administration of opioids has been used to provide quality analgesia and to avoid some of the systemic side effects of high-dose narcotics given by more indirect routes. This may include single-shot opioids for initial pain relief, but more frequently it involves continuous infusions or patient-administered dosing.

Opioid Receptors

The primary opioid analgesic receptors are the mu receptors located in the spinal cord. These generally are thought to be in the substantia gelatinosa of the dorsal horn. Other receptors include kappa and delta, among others. Unfortunately, binding to these secondary opioid receptors can lead to dysphoria, respiratory depression, and other side effects.

Choice of Opioid

Many different opioid analgesics are used intraspinally, including morphine, hydromorphone, fentanyl, sufentanil, meperidine, and methadone. The choice of the agent frequently is determined by the unique properties of the medication and the goal of each particular situation (Table 59–2).

Route of Administration

Whether given intrathecally or epidurally, the opioid must eventually bind to the mu receptor in the substantia gelatinosa. This means that, to work, an opioid given epidurally must pass through the dura. Intrathecal and epidural opioids for pain control are compared in Table 59–3.[18] Inappropriate use of the epidural route for treating cancer pain should be avoided.[19] A lipophilic agent will cross this barrier much more easily than a hydrophilic one; however, a lipophilic medication might be significantly absorbed by the fat and other tissues in the epidural space and surrounding structures, resulting in reduced action.[20]

INDICATIONS AND CONTRAINDICATIONS

Intrathecal and epidural opioids administered for the management of cancer pain may be indicated when the WHO three-step approach has failed to achieve analgesia or when the side effects are significant. The most widely accepted indication is for patients treated with systemic opioids with effective pain relief but with unacceptable side effects or unsuccessful treatment with sequential strong opioid drug

TABLE 59–1 **Studies on Use of Spinal Opioids in Cancer Pain**

Investigators, Year	Number of Patients/Route	Follow-up Duration	Results	Adverse Effects/Complications
Penn et al, 1984[5]	8/Epidural 6/Intrathecal	≤2152 days	8 Excellent 5 Good 1 Poor	Not reported
Krames et al, 1985[6]	16/Intrathecal	97 mo	3 Excellent 7 Good 6 Fair	Catheter dislodgement, urinary retention, constipation
Shetter et al, 1986[7]	14/Intrathecal-epidural	≤23 mo	7 Excellent 4 Good 3 Fair	Cerebrospinal fluid fistula
Penn and Paice, 1987[8]	35/Intrathecal	5.4 mo	17 Excellent 11 Good 4 Poor 3 Failure	Transient urinary retention
Onofrio and Yaksh, 1990[9]	53/Intrathecal	Mean 4 mo	34 Excellent/good 19 Fair/poor	Not reported
Hassenbusch et al, 1990[10]	41/Epidural	≤27 mo	41 Excellent	Wound infection, catheter migration, voiding problems, etc
Anderson et al, 1991[11]	9/Intrathecal	2 mo	9 Significant reduction in VAS	Catheter kinking
Waterman et al, 1991[12]	33/Epidural	≤8 mo	18 Excellent 5 Good 6 Fair 4 Poor	Respiratory depression, urinary retention, seroma, etc
Follett et al, 1992[13]	35/Intrathecal	≤44 mo	35 Good	Spinal headache, nausea, lethargy, etc
Paice et al, 1996[14]	133/Intrathecal	≤24 mo	52% Excellent 43% Good 5% Poor	Delivery system problems, nausea and vomiting, pruritus, edema, etc
Erdine et al, 1996[15]	54/Intrathecal	≤24 mo	49 Satisfactory 5 Poor	44% Adverse effects, PDH in 16 patients
Smitt et al, 1998[16]	91/Epidural	Median 38 days	Adequate pain relief 73–76%	Technical complications in 43%
Gilmer et al, 1999[17]	9/Intrathecal	≤354 days	9 Good/excellent	Not reported

TABLE 59–2 **Comparison of Opioids for Spinal Use (Epidural)**

Morphine	Hydromorphone	Fentanyl, Sufentanyl	Meperidine	Methadone
Hydrophilic, lipid solubility 1	Intermediate, lipid solubility 1.4	Lipophilic, lipid solubility 580, 1270	Lipophilic, lipid solubility 28	Lipophilic, lipid solubility 82
Long duration (12–24 hr)	Intermediate duration (6–12 hr)	Short duration (2–4 hr)	Short duration (4–8 hr)	Short duration (4–8 hr)
Slow onset (30–60 min)	Intermediate onset (20–30 min)	Rapid onset (5–15 min)	Rapid onset (10–20 min)	Rapid onset (10–20 min)
High CSF solubility and spread	Intermediate CSF solubility and spread	Low CSF solubility and spread	Low CSF solubility and spread	Low CSF solubility and spread
5–10 Times more potent than IV	5 Times more potent than IV	Equipotent to IV	1–2 Times more potent than IV	Less potent than IV

TABLE 59–3 **Comparison of Intrathecal and Epidural Opioids**

Factors	Intrathecal	Epidural
Infection rate	Same as epidural	Same as intrathecal
Pain relief	Better for long term	Good only for short term
Dose	Lower	Higher
Pump refills	Less frequent	More frequent
Side effects	Fewer	More
Technical complication (first 20 days)	25%	8%
(Long term)	5%	55%
Catheter occlusion and fibrosis	Minimal	High
Epidural metastasis	Less affected	More affected

TABLE 59–4 **Comparison of Continuous and Intermittent Bolus Spinal Opioids**

Factor	Continuous	Intermittent Bolus
Dose escalation	Higher	Lower
Analgesic quality	Better	Fair
Bupivacaine combinations	Minimal motor or hemodynamic complications	Higher motor or hemodynamic complications

TABLE 59–5 **Adverse Effects Attributable to Spinal Opioids**

1. Minor sedation
2. Persistent nausea
3. Urinary retention
4. Pruritus
5. Hyperalgesia (higher doses)
6. Myoclonus (higher doses)
7. Respiratory depression

TABLE 59–6 **Technical Complications of Spinal Therapy**

Mechanical problems
Skin breakdown at insertion site
Local infection, catheter infection, epidural abscess, meningitis, systemic infection
Cerebrospinal leak, headache, cerebrospinal fluid seroma
Hematoma
Catheter withdrawal, occlusion, leak

trials despite escalating doses.[21] Contraindications include coagulopathy, local infection, and sepsis.

TECHNIQUES

Single-shot epidural and intrathecal opioids can be helpful in providing short-term relief of pain. It may also serve as an indicator of future success of continuous infusions or patient-controlled analgesia using opioids. A comparison between continuous and intermittent bolus treatment is shown in (Table 59–4).[22] Adequate relief of pain with trial spinal opioids is mandatory before more permanent procedures or long term treatment. Options for delivering this form of pain relief include percutaneous catheters, tunneled catheters, and implantable programmable pumps. If the patient has only a few days to live, placement of a simple percutaneous catheter may be the easiest and most cost-effective option. Unfortunately, the risk of infection and high failure rate limit their use. A tunneled catheter can be very helpful, providing months of effective and cost-effective analgesia. If spinally administered opioids are to be given for 3 months or more, an implantable, programmable infusion pump is the most cost-effective.[23] It may also provide better quality of life by allowing patients to participate in more activities.

ADVERSE EFFECTS AND COMPLICATIONS

Adverse effects of spinally administered opioids include the problems associated with other routes of administration, such as sedation, nausea, itching, urinary retention, constipation, and respiratory depression (see Table 59–5). However, the degree of these problems may be significantly less severe than those associated with systemic use. Other complications unique to these invasive techniques include infection, bleeding, and catheter problems (Table 59–6).[24]

SUMMARY AND CONCLUSION

For patients who do not obtain adequate pain relief with the WHO three-step approach, a fourth step—intraspinally administered opioids—can improve pain management and quality of life. Future studies on different new agents and combinations with opioids will optimize the use of this advanced mode of pain control in cancer patients.

REFERENCES

1. Yaksh TL, Rudy TA: Analgesia mediated by a direct spinal action of narcotics. Science 192:1357–1358, 1976.
2. Wang JK, Naus LA, Thomas JE: Pain relief by intrathecally applied morphine in man. Anesthesiology 50:149–151, 1979.
3. Behar M, Olshwang D, Magora F, Davidson JT: Epidural morphine in treatment of pain. Lancet 1979; I:527–528.
4. Ventafridda V, Figliuzzi M, Tamburini M, et al: Clinical observation on analgesia elicited by intrathecal morphine in cancer patients. *In* Bonica JJ, Ventafridda V (eds): Advances in Pain Research and Therapy, vol 2. New York, Raven, 1979, pp 559–565.
5. Penn RD, Paice JA, Gottschalk W, Ivankovich AD: Cancer pain relief using chronic morphine infusion. Early experience with a programmable implanted pump. J Neurosurg 61:302–306, 1984.
6. Krames ES, Gershow J, Glassberg A, et al: Continuous infusion of spinally administered narcotics for relief of pain due to malignant disorders. Cancer 56:696–702, 1985.
7. Shetter AG, Hadley MN, Wilkinson E: Administration of intraspinal morphine sulfate for the treatment of intractable cancer pain. Neurosurgery 18:740–747, 1986.
8. Penn RD, Paice JA: Chronic intrathecal morphine for intractable pain. J Neurosurg 67:182–187, 1987.
9. Onofrio BM, Yaksh TL: Long-term pain relief produced by intrathecal morphine infusion in 53 patients. J Neurosurg 72:200–209, 1990.
10. Hassenbusch SJ, Pillay PK, Magdinec M, et al: Constant infusion of morphine for intractable cancer pain using an implanted pump. J Neurosurg 73:405–409, 1990.
11. Anderson PE, Coher JI, Everts EC, et al: Intrathecal narcotics for relief of pain from head and neck cancer. Arch Otolaryngol Head Neck Surg 117:1277–1280, 1991.
12. Waterman NG, Hughes S, Foster WS: Control of cancer pain by epidural infusion of morphine. Surgery 110:612–614, 1991.
13. Follet KA, Hitchon PW, Piper J, et al: Response of intractable pain to continuous intrathecal morphine: A retrospective study. Pain 49:21–25, 1992.
14. Paice JA, Penn RD, Shott S: Intraspinal morphine for chronic pain: A retrospective, multicenter study. J Pain Symptom Manage 11:71–80, 1996.
15. Erdine SS, Yucel A: Intrathecal morphine delivered by implanted manual pump for cancer pain. Pain Digest 6:161–165, 1996.
16. Smitt PS, Tsafka A, Teng-van-de-Zande F, et al: Outcome and complications of epidural analgesia in patients with chronic cancer pain. Cancer 83:2015–2022, 1998.
17. Gilmer HS, Boggan JE, Smith KA, et al: Intrathecal morphine delivered via subcutaneous pump for intractable pain in pancreatic cancer. Surg Neurol 51:6–11, 1999.
18. Crul BJ, Delhaas EM: Technical complications during longterm subarachnoid or epidural administration of morphine in terminally ill cancer patients: A review of 140 cases. Reg Anesth 16:209–213, 1991.
19. Mercadante S, Agnello A, Armata MG, Pumo S: The inappropriate use of the epidural route in cancer pain. J Pain Symptom Manage 13:233–237, 1997.
20. Rawal N: Spinal opioids. *In* Raj PP (ed): Practical Management of Pain. St. Louis, Mosby–Year Book, pp 829–851.
21. Krames ES: Intrathecal infusional therapies for intractable pain: Patient management guidelines. J Pain Symptom Manage 8:36–46, 1993.
22. Gourlay GK, Plummer JL, Cherry DA, et al: Comparison of intermittent bolus with continuous infusion of epidural morphine in the treatment of severe cancer pain. Pain 47:135–140, 1991.
23. Hassenbusch SJ, Paice JA, Patt RB, et al: Clinical realities and economic considerations: Economics of intrathecal therapy. J Pain Symptom Manage 14:S36–S48, 1997.
24. Nitescu P, Sjoberg M, Applegren L, Curelaru I: Complications of intrathecal opioids and bupivacaine treatment of refractory cancer pain. Clin J Pain 11:45–62, 1995.

CHAPTER • 60

Intraspinal Analgesia for Nonmalignant Pain

Elliot S. Krames, MD

Chronic pain, in addition to causing untold suffering for millions of patients worldwide, tears at the very economic and social fabric of our culture. It is estimated that approximately 30% of the general population of the United States suffers from chronic pain—some 70,000,000 people.[1] According to Lemrow and coworkers, in the United States, back pain is the second leading reason for physician office visits and the third most common reason for hospital admissions.[2] In a recent study testing the relationship of low back pain to cardiovascular mortality in a representative sample of persons older than 29 in Finland, 76% of 8000 persons in the sample stated that they had experienced back pain.[3] In 1992, in a study on the dollar impact on 12 diverse, large American businesses, it was shown that disability cost these businesses an average of $2500 per employee.[4] For the period from 1980 to 1990, temporary disability cost the federal government $6.5 billion. The cost to state governments for temporary disability during the same period was $4.5 billion. Combined costs to both the federal and state governments during this period was a staggering $11 billion.[5]

In a recent study of the general population of the state of Michigan, The Michigan Pain Study, one in five adults, or about 1.2 million people, suffer from some form of chronic (ongoing or recurring) pain.[6] Pain was responsible for 400,000 workers' (or 12% of the Michigan workforce) failing to show up for work at some point during the past year. Of the pain sufferers surveyed, 35% had missed more than 20 days of work in the last year.

The direct, hard costs of unrelieved pain to patients and their families are loss of job, loss of income, loss of savings and therefore security, loss of insurance, and loss of self-esteem. More intangible results of unrelieved pain include depression, anger, frustration, and suffering. The end result of all this is staggering to society and to persons unfortunate enough to suffer unrelieved pain. The Michigan Pain Study surveyed 1500 Michigan residents aged 18 and older, to determine the severity of the chronic pain problem, how people cope, access to treatment, and the effectiveness of available pain care. Of the 1.2 million people in Michigan who suffer from chronic pain, 42% say pain has affected their relationships with spouses, family members, and fellow workers. Nearly half (48%) experience depression, 18% have overdosed on pain medication, and 10%, about 120,000 persons, have contemplated suicide. Looking for solutions for their pain has led 5% of the chronic pain sufferers in this population (~60,000 adults) to drink alcohol, and 18% of those admitted to overdosing on their medication. Some 29% of the population felt that they were losing sleep from their chronic pain. Indeed, these figures paint a gloomy and compelling picture of the true costs of chronic, unrelieved pain to our society.

Clearly, the problem of intractable chronic pain of nonmalignant origin, because of both its drain on scarce healthcare resources and the emotional and physical price exacted of patients and their families, is a major problem in the United States, if not the world, today. It is my purpose in this chapter to present the delivery of intraspinal analgesic as a viable and cost-effective intervention for the treatment of chronic, unrelieved pain when less invasive and less costly therapies have failed.

MULTIDIMENSIONALITY OF PAIN

Chronic pain of nonmalignant origin not only is costly but is a multidimensional disorder of combined neurophysiologic, cognitive, behavioral, cultural, social, and economic causes. The appropriate, cost-effective treatment of chronic nonmalignant pain should call on the expertise of different health care professionals, including, but not limited to, physicians, psychologists, physical therapists, occupational therapists, and nurses who are specifically trained to treat patients with chronic pain. Because of the multiple causes of chronic pain, the treatment options are many.

Cost-effective treatment of chronic nonmalignant pain should obey the KISS principle ("Keep it simple and safe"). Accordingly, the available interventions for syndrome-specific chronic pain problems should be applied in order of increasing invasiveness and, in a cost-conscious society, by cost. This listing of interventions by increasing order of complexity and cost is called a *pain treatment continuum.* Less invasive and less expensive treatments are tried before more invasive and more expensive interventions and are discarded based on failure of response for more complex and costly interventions until an intervention is found that is efficacious. The appropriate use of this continuum does not mandate a sequential series of interventions by order of increasing invasiveness and cost but allows for intercurrent interventions. An example is a patient with complex regional pain syndrome type 1, who is taking an anticonvulsant and antidepressants for allodynia but also requires opioids and a continuous epidural to facilitate physical and occupational therapy.

Spinal analgesia does have a rational place in this treatment continuum for some chronic nonmalignant pain states. It is my purpose in this chapter to outline appropriate patient selection and to discuss rational therapy and management of complications of intraspinal analgesia for such pain while defining its place in the pain treatment continuum.

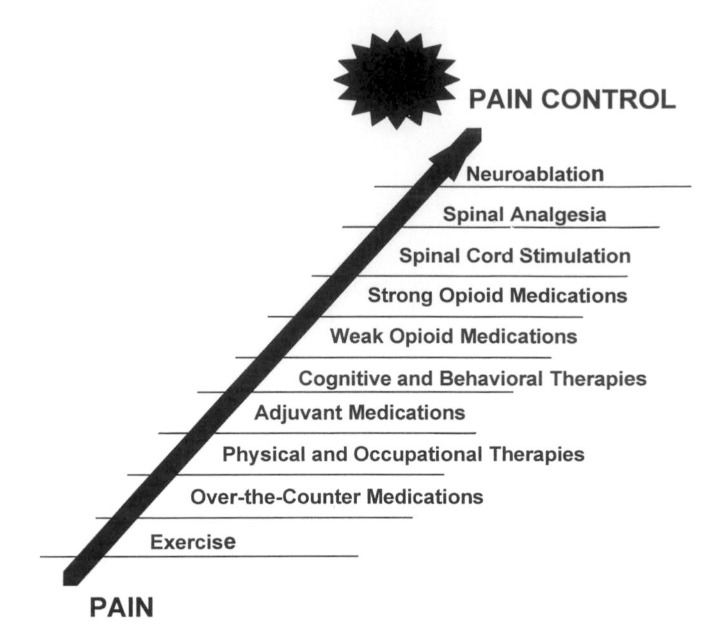

FIGURE 60–1 The pain treatment continuum is a suggested algorithm for the appropriate use of possible pain management therapies. These therapies are listed in order of increasing invasiveness. The algorithm appears to suggest that the therapies be used in series, abandoning therapies that don't work and enlisting more invasive therapies in sequential order. In actuality, these therapies can be used in parallel, trying one or more at the same time.

THE TREATMENT OF CHRONIC PAIN: MULTIPLE CHOICES

The treatment of chronic noncancer pain, like the treatment of cancer-related pain, requires the pain treating physician to understand the source of the pain, the psychological and behavioral factors operant in perpetuating it, and the treatment options available for the particular pain syndrome. Because chronic pain is almost always multidimensional (involving neurophysiologic systems and emotional and behavioral ones), a multidisciplinary evaluation and treatment plan is usually warranted. Once a diagnosis is made, after a thorough multidisciplinary evaluation, a parallel treatment plan is developed that addresses both the neurophysiologic process or processes and the cognitive, emotional, and behavioral and functional processes involved in generating the pain. Because multiple modalities are available for the treatment of chronic pain, we use a treatment continuum (i.e., increasing levels of intervention and complexity). Choices for the treatment of chronic nonmalignant pain, utilizing multidisciplinary interventions, include cognitive/behavioral psychological therapies, functional rehabilitation therapies, orthopedic and neurologic surgery, pharmacotherapies, anesthetic blocking techniques, neuroaugmentative procedures, and finally neurodestructive procedures (Fig. 60–1).

A psychological evaluation and treatment plan must address certain issues in chronic pain patients, including ferreting out psychological causes of pain, identifying any addictive tendencies, identifying psychological barriers to successful medical management of pain, maximizing coping strategies for pain control, and addressing loss issues. At the very least, some chronic pain patients may merely lack the coping skills necessary for internal, self-directed pain modulation, whereas others may derive unconscious secondary gain from persistent pain. Some patients have personality or neurotic barriers to successful pain management, including addictive personality, hysteria, hypochondriasis, or depression. At the other extreme, persistent, chronic pain can be a somatiform disorder, a manifestation of the patient's inability to deal with unresolved emotional pain, which results in subconscious creation of somatic pain. In psychobehavioral terms, somatic pain is the manifestation of emotional pain that is "too hot to handle." Rather than addressing the emotional conflicts directly by seeking psychiatric or psychological support, the patient subconsciously seeks a quick fix in the form of a pill or a medical intervention. These patients are the rare extreme of pain patients and are the hardest to treat. They tend to deny that there are any problems in their life beside their "painful illness" and certainly deny any psychologic component to the pain. All medical interventions are doomed to fail until the patient understands, accepts, and addresses the real issues causing the underlying emotional pain. Psychological interventions for pain include long-term psychotherapy; goal-directed, short-term psychotherapy; "operant reconditioning"; conjoint, interrelational therapies; group therapy; biofeedback; relaxation and distraction techniques; hypnosis; and self-hypnosis.

Pharmacologic management of the patient with chronic pain utilizes medications that have been shown to be efficacious for either nociceptive or neuropathic pain. Nociceptive pain—pain mediated by chemical, thermal, or mechanical nociceptors (found throughout the body except in nerve tissue)—most often responds to nonsteroidal anti-inflammatory drugs (NSAIDs) or opioids. Nonopioid NSAIDs should be used before opioids, although long-term use could damage the liver or renal system. There is no physiologic downside to the long-term use of strong opioid medications. If opioids are to be used, the strength of the drug should be tailored to the intensity of pain. Dosages should be determined empirically and not depend on some arbitrary "average dose." Weak opioids should be given for mild pain and strong ones for intense pain. For constant pain, opioids should be taken according to a schedule consistent with the pharmacokinetics of the drug prescribed, not as needed. Since chronic pain is often constant, it may also be desirable to increase dosing intervals by choosing an opioid that is longer lasting over one that has a shorter duration of action. Longer-acting opioids include methadone, levorphanol, long-acting, slow-release morphine preparations, and transdermal fentanyl. A ceiling is associated with NSAIDs that is not shared by opioids. Once the ceiling dose for a given NSAID is reached, adding more will not produce more profound analgesia; it can only lead to an increase in undesirable side effects. Doses of opioids can be repeatedly elevated to control increasing pain. If side effects do not occur, more drug may be better. Side effects of opioid medications include inanition, loss of appetite, nausea and vomiting, sedation, constipation, urinary retention, depression of the hypothalamic/pituitary axis, hallucinations, dry mouth, sweating, and respiratory depression. Not all patients can take all opioids. Some tolerate one or more of them but not all; some do not tolerate any; and some tolerate all. If a patient cannot tolerate one opioid, others should be tried sequentially until one produces analgesia without undue side effects. Sequential drug trials should be performed before opioid therapy is abandoned.

Nonopioid medications other than NSAIDs that have been shown to have some degree of analgesic efficacy for chronic pain syndromes are called, as a class, adjuvant medications. They include the heterocyclic antidepressants, nonheterocyclic, serotonin-enhancing antidepressants, anticonvulsant medications, GABA analogues, sodium channel–blocking, membrane-stabilizing agents, calcium channel–blocking agents, alpha- and beta-blocking agents, $alpha_2$ analogues, substance P–depleting agents, steroids, and the psychogenic amines and their analogues. These medications, like the opioids, should be prescribed using sequential drug trials as single agents or in combination with other active agents. Doses should be slowly titrated to enhance patient acceptance, and doses should be "pushed" until efficacy or side effects develop. If side effects develop before analgesia, a different drug of the same class should be tried before the whole class of drugs is abandoned. This trial-and-error process takes time, and patients should be counseled to have patience.

As one can see from the treatment continuum, interventional pain management, and certainly intraspinal analgesics for pain control, should be therapies of last resort before neuroablative and neurodestructive procedures. These therapies, when used appropriately in an appropriate patient, add immeasurably to the aforementioned tools of the trade of the pain care team.

ORAL OPIOIDS FOR NONMALIGNANT PAIN

Opioid therapy for noncancer pain, though once very controversial, is becoming in many of the United States a useful and necessary agent for this application. Unfortunately, many U.S. government regulators still consider opioids inappropriate for nonmalignant pain,[7] fearing that patients who are not terminally ill will invariably develop tolerance, drug abuse, and addiction. These fears, once pervasive, were engendered by unscientific data obtained by questioning a population of addicts about how they became addicted to opioids. These data suggested a causal relationship between addiction and the prescription by physicians of opioid medications for pain control. Unfortunately, the studies were biased by the fact that the sample population were all addicts; their findings reflected no input from nonaddicted patients who had been given opioid medications for their pain problems (i.e., the study was not controlled).

In the past 10 years, however, many retrospective and prospective studies of samples of patients given opioids for noncancer pain or for disorders not associated with pain, actually suggest a low incidence of tolerance, few if any pharmacologic adverse consequences, and a low incidence of iatrogenic addiction.[8–11] In fact, some studies suggest that opioids may actually increase function in patients with debilitating nonmalignant pain.[12, 13] Because of this new information, more and more pain practitioners are prescribing opioids for patients who continue to suffer after failure of more conservative interventions.

If oral opioids are appropriate for chronic nonmalignant pain syndromes, then, certainly, there is a rational place for intraspinal opioid therapies for such pain. This rational and appropriate use of infusional intraspinal analgesia should be well-founded on a thorough knowledge of the neurobiology of pain generation, its endogenous modulation, and the clinical presentations of different pain syndromes. The treating physician who chooses an implantable device for pain control should also know the appropriate and accepted use of all of the tools of the trade—all of the available modalities and therapies, conservative and invasive, for treating chronic pain syndromes.

INTRASPINAL ANALGESIC THERAPY FOR CHRONIC PAIN

To answer the question why the opium poppy exists in nature to provide mankind with substances to relieve pain, researchers sought endogenous substances in animals and humans that have similar effects.[14, 15] Further studies elucidated the role of these substances, given intraspinally, in providing analgesia in animals[16, 17] and humans.[18, 19] These early studies of intraspinal opioids in animals and humans alike appeared to offer specific benefits to some patients and was followed by trials of continuous subarachnoid opioid infusions using implanted pumps that had factory-preset flow rates.[20, 21] During the past years, published reports and abstracts in the U.S. literature have repeatedly documented the safety and efficacy of implanted nonprogrammable and programmable pumps for long-term subarachnoid delivery of opioid drugs for pain of terminal illness[22–30] and for nonmalignant pain.[31–39]

This documented efficacy of both the systemic and spinal delivery of opioids, however, may be variably subject to specific opioid responsive or opioid resistant pain syndromes.[40–42] Opioid-responsive nociceptive pain, mediated by nociceptors widely distributed in the body, is often described in terms such as *dull*, *aching*, *sharp*, or *throbbing*. Nociceptors respond to noxious mechanical, thermal, and chemical stimuli and transduce this noxious information into electrical information for transmission to the central nervous system. At the first-order neuron of the dorsal horn of the spinal cord, nociceptive pain is modulated both presynaptically and postsynaptically by endogenous and exogenous opioids acting at opiate receptors. Nociceptive pain is most usually responsive to opioid therapies, whether delivered orally, parenterally, or spinally. Examples of nociceptive pain include postsurgical pain, the pains of trauma, vertebrogenic pain, and cancer pain emanating from bone, connective tissue, and viscera (Table 60–1).

Neuropathic pain, on the other hand, is not mediated by nociceptors in the periphery but is caused by damage to the peripheral or central nervous system or by pathologic changes in neurofunctional relationships within these pain-processing systems. Some examples of the pathologic changes in functional relationships causing chronic persistent pain are peripheral sensitization of nociceptors, central sensitization (or "spinal windup"), abnormal sympathetic-somatic nervous system interactions, and abnormal activation of *N*-methyl-D-aspartate (NMDA), receptors. Neuropathic pain, unlike nociceptive pain, is most often described in terms of "electrical" sensations such as *tingling*, *burning*, *shooting*, and lightninglike. Examples of neuropathic pain are the monoradiculopathies, "sciatica," trigeminal neuralgia, phantom limb pain, postherpetic neuralgia, causalgia, reflex sympathetic dystrophy, and peripheral neuropathies (See Table 60–1). Neuropathic pain is thought to be opioid resistant, and, unlike nociceptive pain, may respond to higher than "normal" opioid doses or may not respond to opioid therapy at all. Although these neuropathic pain syndromes may be resistant to intraspinal opioid infusions, they might respond to other intraspinally administered, nonopioid, agents such as alpha$_2$ agonists, somatostatin and its analogues, intrathecal NSAIDs, NMDA-receptor antagonists, gangliosides, neurotrophic factors, neuron-specific calcium channel blockers, and local anesthetic-opioid combinations.

TRIAL OF SPINALLY ADMINISTERED OPIOIDS

Once it has been established that the patient who has undergone a sequential trial of systemically administered opioids and, because of either the development of toxic side effects with each and every agent tried or because the patient has opioid unresponsive pain within nontoxic levels of opioid, the patient is a candidate for a trial of intraspinal analgesia. I prefer using the term *intraspinal analgesia*, rather than *intraspinal opioid*, because we do have nonopioid agents for intraspinal use that might be effective for opioid-unresponsive pain. Agents that have been shown to be efficacious for opioid unresponsive pain and are being used clinically include the local anesthetic bupivacaine and the alpha$_2$ agonist clonidine. Other agents that might be used but are considered experimental include somatostatin[43] and the somatostatin analogues, octreotide,[44] SNX-111 (an *N*-channel calcium blocker),[45] and midazolam.[46, 47]

All patients who are candidates for intraspinal delivery of analgesics should have failed more conservative therapies tried and there should be no contraindications to implanting a drug delivery system and intrathecal catheter, such as allergy to the agents trialed, localized infection in the areas where surgery is necessary, sepsis, and coagulopathy.

It cannot be stressed strongly enough how important it is when intraspinal opioids are considered for a patient who has failed to respond to opioid sequential systemical trials and all other conservative therapies, to establish opioid responsiveness or, for opioid-unresponsive pain, to conduct trials of other drugs. There really is no magic to the intraspinal route of delivery for opioids. If patients do not respond to oral or systemic opioids, intrathecal opioid is not magically going to provide analgesia. Should it do so during the trial, the effect is short-lived and most probably due to nonspecific placebo effects. Clinically useful agents that have shown efficacy in patients with neuropathic, opioid-unresponsive pain syndromes include the local anesthetic bupivacaine and the alpha$_2$ agonist clonidine.

Any trial should prove both analgesic and functional efficacy, rule out toxicity, and eliminate so far as is possible nonspecific, placebo effects of the drug. Trials for intraspinal opioids and nonopioids alike have been performed with single-shot epidural or intrathecal infusion of one or more drugs, repeat single-shot epidural or intrathecal infusions, and, finally, continuous drug delivery via the epidural or intrathecal route using an external pump.

Because any analgesic intervention, and most important, last resort interventions like intraspinal analgesia, produce very strong placebo responses in patients suffering from intractable noncancer pain, trials for efficacy must also mitigate against these strong responses. The only way to do this, in any given patient, is to extend the trial as long as possible. Giving a single patient a single-blinded or even a double-blinded placebo and deciding whether that patient is or is not a "placebo responder" makes no sense or science at all. To withhold therapy from a "placebo responder" because that patient responded to the inactive placebo or to implant an expensive drug delivery system in a patient who responded positively to a single-shot active agent makes no sense at all. Since all people react to both the specific and the nonspecific effects (placebo responses) of the agent, we cannot tell, from any given patient's response to a single encounter with a single agent, whether the resultant effect is specific or nonspecific. In effect, we are all placebo responders, and patients suffering unremitting pain, given a chance at last resort therapies, are going to be a population with very strong placebo responses. During

TABLE 60–1 Characteristics of Nociceptive and Neuropathic Pain

Nociceptive Pain
- Mediated by nociceptors throughout the body
- Nociceptors are chemical, thermal and mechanical
- Nociceptors transduce noxious information into electrical information for transmission to the central nervous system
- Pain of trauma, tissue injury, surgery, etc.
- Opioid-responsive pain syndrome

Neuropathic Pain
- Not mediated by nociceptors
- Due to damage to peripheral or central nervous system or due to abnormal pain processing
- Mechanisms in the peripheral or central nervous system
- Abnormal pain processing mechanisms due to toxicity of the nervous system or unrelieved nociception which activates the *N*-methyl-D-aspartate receptor system
- Opioid-responsive, -resistant, or -unresponsive pain syndrome

the trial the placebo response is heralded by a decreasing analgesic response over time when pain was well-controlled at the start of the trial. The only way to mitigate against the placebo response is to design a trial that mimics as closely as possible the final intended delivery system and to deliver the intended agent as long as is logistically possible.

Over the years, we have come to realize that a continuous intrathecal trial extended as long as possible is the one trial that allows for both sequential trials of intrathecal agents and extended trials to identify potent placebo responses. Although not perfect, since placebo responses can occur and last longer than 12 months, our trials are usually performed with the patient at home. At present, for intrathecal trials we are surgically implanting an intrathecal catheter (Model #8709, Medtronic, Minneapolis, Minn.) and attaching it to a tunneled, externalized subcutaneous DuPen Epidural Catheter System (Bard Access Systems, Salt Lake City, Ut.). All of our patients are given intravenous, preoperative antibiotics to prevent what, statistically, would be a *Staphylococcus aureus* or *Staphylococcus epidermidis* infection, if it developed, and are sent home with oral antibiotics to cover these same bacteria for the length of the trial. The catheter system exit site is covered with a clear plastic dressing, and the patient is discharged home and instructed to lead as normal a lifestyle as they usually do. The entire system is attached to an external pumping system. Enough medication is prepared for a 1- to 2-week trial. During the trial, if the patient tolerates the initial drug, dosing is adjusted by reprogramming the pump to accelerate delivery. When a patient does not tolerate a drug, only the drug reservoir and tubing are changed proximal to the .22-μm filter, which is outside the clear dressing. Then, and only then, is the tubing changed during the trial. Since it has become clear to most that the rate of delivery system infections is directly related to the number of times that the system is "fiddled with," our protocol calls for a hands-off policy with tubing, drug, and dressing changes.[48] The only time the dressing is changed is within the first 48 hours, and all dressing changes are performed by the physicians who implanted the catheters or by nurses who are quite familiar with the system.

During the trial of an agent, a 50% reduction in pain intensity, improvement in function, and a concomitant significant reduction in oral or systemic analgesic requirements is usually indicative of analgesic effectiveness. Clearly, we would like to show improvement in physical functioning for patients when opioids are prescribed. The final evaluation of efficacy of a trial of intraspinal opioids must be individualized, weighed carefully against the risks of the procedure or changes in the lifestyle of the patient or burden of care on the family. Patient and family input is essential to deciding whether a result is positive or not. During the trial, because the equianalgesic dose of spinally administered opioid is significantly smaller than the systemic dose, it is important to prevent acute withdrawal when giving intraspinal opioid. To prevent acute withdrawal during the trial for intraspinal opioid delivery, we suggest that 50% of the orally administered opioid dose be given as an intrathecal equivalent during the first day of the trial and that the patient be allowed to swallow the other 50% of the dose. Each subsequent day, the oral dose should be decreased by 20% and the intrathecal dose increased by 20%.

PHARMACOLOGIC MANAGEMENT

Morphine remains the "gold standard" of spinally administered opioid therapy because of its long duration of action and relative ease of use. Morphine has an extensive history; more is published in the literature on the use of intraspinal morphine than on any other opioid available. In the United States, only morphine has been approved for clinical intraspinal, intrathecal analgesia. However, based on the literature and sound clinical judgment, other opioids, such as hydromorphone, fentanyl, meperidine, and methadone, have been used intraspinally when patients did not tolerate intrathecal morphine. Although physicians do use these drugs intraspinally, they are not labeled for this use and have not been approved by the FDA for it.

Time to onset of action of opioid given spinally, duration of action, uptake and distribution, availability to supraspinal centers, and central nervous system side effects are all governed by the opiate's lipid solubility and opiate receptor affinity (Table 60–2).[49] Opioids such as morphine, with low lipid solubility, enhanced hydrophilia, and high receptor affinity, cross the dura and enter the lipid substance of the spinal cord slowly but remain bound for a prolonged time. Thus, the onset of analgesic action for hydrophilic opioids is slow, but analgesia is generally prolonged. Because of its low lipid solubility or avid hydrophilia, more drug remains in the cerebrospinal fluid (CSF) and therefore is available to ascend to supraspinal centers through bulk flow of CSF. Because of the hydrophilic property of drugs such as morphine, placement of a catheter for intrathecal infusion of the drug anywhere in the thecal sac ensures analgesia anywhere in the body. Risks of CSF side effects such as sedation, nausea and vomiting, and respiratory depression are greater with this hydrophilic group of opioids than with those with higher lipid solubility and higher receptor affinity, such as fentanyl or sufentanil.

As expected from their physicochemical properties, lipophilic drugs such as sufentanil have rapid onset and prolonged duration of action. Once receptors are saturated with sufentanil, drug becomes available for redistribution through spinal vessel uptake and CSF bulk flow. Overesedation then can become a problem. Because lipophilic agents enter the substance of the lipid-containing spinal cord rapidly and are quickly eliminated from the CSF, catheter tip placement is essential for optimal analgesia. If lipophilic agents are to be used to reduce supraspinal opioid effects—and this eventuality should always be planned for—the

TABLE 60–2 ***Receptor Affinity and Solubility of Opioid Drugs****

		Solubility	
Drug	**Affinity**	**Lipid**	**Water**
Morphine	High	Low	High
Dilaudid	High	Low	High
Fentanyl	Low	High	Low
Sufentanil	High	High	Low
Lofentanil	Complete	High	Low

* S. DuPen, unpublished observations.

intraspinal catheter tip should always be placed as close as possible to the spinal cord segment processing and modulating the patient's pain.

The appropriate dose of opioid for epidural or intrathecal use is highly individualized and depends on the patient's age and pain syndrome and the systemic dose of the drug needed for analgesia before the decision to move to intraspinal delivery. As a general rule, patients with neuropathic pain may require higher doses than are usual for nociceptive pain, and elders usually require less drug than patients who are younger. However, dosing should be individualized for each patient. For clinical purposes we use the following formula when converting systemic morphine to spinal morphine.

300 mg oral morphine =
100 mg parenteral morphine =
10 mg epidural morphine =
1 mg intrathecal morphine.

Some patients do not tolerate morphine but do tolerate other hydrophilic, though more lipophilic, agents such as hydromorphone. Sometimes, we may want to use more lipophilic agents such as fentanyl, sufentanil, or meperidine to decrease supraspinal effects such as severe nausea. Table 60–3 contains a suggested chart for converting a dose of morphine to equianalgesic doses of other opioid agents.

SIDE EFFECT STRATEGIES FOR INTRASPINAL OPIOIDS

Patients who tolerate a drug well during the screening trial may at some time during infusional therapy develop intolerance or tolerance to the drug or may in fact develop an opioid-resistant pain syndrome. These problems can be categorized into *side effects of* and *decreasing analgesic effects of* the drug. Should the known side effects of therapy develop (e.g., nausea and vomiting, urinary retention, generalized pruritus, constipation, oversedation, confusion) or other complications of intraspinal opioid therapy (e.g., paranoia,[50] hyperalgesia/myoclonus syndrome,[51–55] Ménière's-like symptoms,[56] nystagmus,[57, 58] herpes reactivation),[59–62] an attempt should be made to manage the symptoms pharmacologically before switching to some other spinal agent. Although respiratory depression is a known consequence of the use of intrathecal opioids in the opiate-naive patient,[63, 64] it is rarely seen in patients who are tolerant to the effects of the opioids because of extended systemic or intraspinal use. Because there is incomplete cross-tolerance of one opioid agonist to other opioid agonists, patients who have side effects from one drug may not have the same effects with another drug in equivalent doses.

Over time, some patients become tolerant to the agent being infused. Tolerance to one opioid analgesic, however, does not necessarily mean tolerance to all. Again, taking advantage of incomplete cross-tolerance, analgesia can be restored by switching to a different opioid at a lower dose (usually half the expected equivalency).

INTRASPINAL ADMIXTURES FOR THE TREATMENT OF CHRONIC PAIN

If patients do not respond to sequential intraspinal opioid trials with different opioids, a strategy using the pharmacologic property of synergy of drugs of two distinctly different classes has been effective in animals.[65–69] Several recent clinical reports show positive analgesic response to admixtures of opioids with either local anesthetics or alpha-adrenergic agents for the treatment of pain, both cancer-related and other pain.[70–79] Admixtures of morphine hydrochloride, bupivacaine hydrochloride, and clonidine hydrochloride have been shown to be stable in reservoir bags for up to 90 days.[80]

In our clinic, when patients no longer receive analgesia with ever-increasing doses of intraspinal opioids, to an arbitrary ceiling of 20 mg morphine intrathecal equivalent, we add the local anesthetic bupivacaine to the opioid. Our starting dose of bupivacaine is 5 to 10 mg/day of the highest available concentration of bupivacaine to ensure relatively long intervals between refills. (In our clinic, we are able to get bupivacaine made up to 3% using bupivacaine powder.) This dose of bupivacaine is increased by 20% per week until analgesia or side effects occur. According to van Dongen and coworkers, neurologic side effects to intrathecal bupivacaine do not occur before 25 mg/24 hours are infused.[78]

COMPLICATIONS

During and after implantation of a pump for intraspinal opioid therapy, the physician must be prepared for problems, which do arise. These complications can be broadly categorized as surgical, mechanical, or pharmacologic.

Bleeding

Bleeding occurs naturally with all surgical incisions and dissections. The avoidance and control of surgical bleeding

TABLE 60–3 ***Equianalgesic Opioid Conversion (mg)***

	Oral	Parenteral	Epidural	Intrathecal
Morphine	300	100	10	1
Hydromorphone	60	20	2	0.25
Meperidine	3000	1000	100	10
Fentanyl	2—	1	0.1	0.01
Sufentanil	2—	0.1	0.01	0.001

require that surgeons screen their patients appropriately for coagulopathies, especially cancer patients undergoing chemotherapy (who may have low platelet counts) and patients who take excessive amounts of NSAIDs. Patients who are anticoagulated are not candidates for these procedures until the clotting time returns to normal. In spite of good surgical evaluation and technical skills, surgical bleeding is often unavoidable. A good rule is never to close a wound while there is active uncontrolled bleeding. Collections of blood are a good medium for growth of bacteria, which can lead to postoperative infections.

Because the technique for implantation of drug delivery systems most often uses Tuohy needles to "blindly" position intrathecal drug catheters into the thecal sac, bleeding can occur within the epidural space without the surgeon's being aware of it. This bleeding, if significant, could lead to epidural hematoma, spinal cord compression, and the cauda equina syndrome of paresis, which is associated with paralysis and bowel and bladder dysfunction. The surgeon should expect this complication if the patient complains of persistent, exquisite back pain and tenderness, develops extremity paresis, complains of urinary retention (neurogenic bladder), or complains of anal sphincter tone weakness and fecal incontinence. The diagnosis is confirmed with emergency spine imaging with magnetic resonance (MRI) or computed tomography with contrast medium. Epidural hematoma is a neurosurgical emergency only when it leads to neurologic impairment.

Infections

To prevent surgical infections, it is wise to use preoperative antibiotics and intraoperative antibiotic irrigation. Strict adherence to sterile technique is mandatory. Because these procedures consist of implantation of costly foreign bodies, any break in good sterile technique could lead to disastrous—and quite costly—consequences. Since most operative infections are caused by *S. aureus* and *S. epidermidis*, either a cephalosporin or vancomycin is used preoperatively by most surgeons.

Although all wound infections can be serious, some are more serious, in terms of significance and outcome, than others. Not all require removal of implanted hardware. Superficial wound infections should be treated with appropriate antibiotics. If the infection involves the implanted catheter or the pocket for placement of the implant, it is imperative that all implanted material be removed. Failure to do so often leads to persistent infection and spread of infection. Once implanted material is removed, it is also wise to leave wounds open and packed to close by themselves. Wet-to-dry dressing changes with sterile saline three times per day support good wound care and allow healing and closure of almost all infections. When the source or the extent of the infection or what treatment is most appropriate is in doubt, we strongly recommend a consultation with an infectious disease expert.

Other, more serious infections, involving implantable devices include epidural and intrathecal infections. These infections demand immediate removal of all foreign body material and appropriate intravenous antibiotic therapy. Again, consultation with an infectious disease expert is recommended.

Intrathecal infections are rare. The diagnosis should be expected if the patient presents with fever, stiff neck, and positive stretch signs, including Kernig's and Brudzinsky's sign. Diagnosis is confirmed by CSF findings consistent with bacterial infection; however, the diagnosis should be confirmed conclusively before action (surgical removal of hardware) is taken. In my experience, a large percentage of patients with newly implanted intrathecal catheters develop a fever spike (≤ 38.5° C) within the first 72 hours of implantation. These noninfectious fever spikes may be associated with a slight stiff neck owing to CSF leak from the dura around the newly implanted catheter and sometimes by postspinal headache. The complete blood count is often normal. CSF drawn from the pump side port, if analyzed, often reveals only leukocytosis and elevated protein while Gram stain or culture for bacteria is negative. This leukocytosis is common and presumably due to spinal tissue reaction to the implanted intrathecal catheter. The fever always abates within 48 to 72 hours. It is important, here, to remember that this picture may be similar to that of meningitis and does not require removal of the hardware. CSF analysis must be the guide.

Epidural infections, left untreated, progress to epidural abscesses. Like epidural hematomas, epidural abscesses are expanding epidural masses that may compress the thecal sac and damage sensitive intrathecal neural tissues. Also like epidural hematoma, abscesses can lead to the cauda equina syndrome of paresis with paralysis and bowel and bladder dysfunction. The diagnosis is suspected from clinical signs and symptoms and confirmed by MRI or computed tomography, with contrast, of the spine. Treatment consists of removal of all foreign material and appropriate antibiotic therapy.

Damage to Vital Tissue

Implantation of the spinal catheter for drug delivery into the spinal canal is usually performed with blind needle techniques. Placement of these needles, though performed under fluoroscopy, could lead to damage to nerve roots or the spinal cord itself. Damage to nerve roots could result in paresis or radiculitis with resultant neuropathic pain in the distribution of the damaged nerve root. Damage to the spinal cord could also lead to painful dysesthesias or myelopathic pain below the level of the damaged spinal cord.

Because mixing and spread in CSF of the drug depends on its lipid and water solubility, it is good to place the drug delivery intrathecal catheter tip as close to the pain-mediating spinal segment as possible. This ensures that more lipophilic agents such as sufentanil could be used should more hydrophilic ones such as morphine or hydromorphone cause intractable supraspinal side effects. Placing the catheter tip close to the mediating spinal segment requires advancement of the catheter rostrally from the lumbar segments.

Advancement of the catheters intrathecally for delivery of opioids could also lead to subarachnoid complications, such as damage to the nerve rootlets, the conus medullaris, or the spinal cord itself. Damage to these tissues could lead to radiculitis, myelitis, paralysis, paresis, loss of bowel and bladder control, or myelopathic pain.

Long-term catheter placement close to the substance of the spinal cord could produce a nonspecific reaction around the catheter tip. This reaction could lead to an expanding, sterile, mass at the tip, and, over time, to cord compression with signs of myelopathy. Several reports in the literature document just such an event.[81, 82] Why some patients develop this reaction, while most patients with pumps and catheters do not, is not known.[83] In a patient with an implanted spinal catheter development of new pain or of neurologic deficits over time should suggest this possibility. An early magnetic resonance study that demonstrates a mass around the tip of the catheter confirms the diagnosis. Failure to diagnose the problem correctly could lead to permanent neurologic sequelae. Once the diagnosis is confirmed, rapid surgical decompression of the spinal cord, removal of the mass, and removal of the spinal catheter is essential. If intraoperative culture suggests the mass is sterile, the pump could be salvaged for use later, should another catheter placement be deemed appropriate.

Besides possible damage to vital spinal tissue, tunneling catheters subcutaneously, if performed hastily or incorrectly, can perforate an abdominal viscus, a retroperitoneal viscus such as the kidney, or even the lung (from chest wall tunneling). The surgeon must exercise great caution when tunneling these devices across the subcutaneous tissues of the abdomen, flank, or chest wall. Perforation of small or large bowel could lead to peritonitis and should be suspected if the patient complains of severe postoperative abdominal pain associated with signs of peritonitis. These signs include ileus, splinting of the abdominal muscles, rigidity of the abdominal wall with rebound tenderness, and nausea and vomiting. Peritonitis is associated with postoperative fever, elevated sedimentation rate, and leukocytosis. Abdominal plain films show signs of bowel obstruction, including air-fluid levels and dilated loops of bowel. Perforation of the lung itself results in hemoptysis and obvious pneumothorax. Perforated viscus is a surgical emergency and should be handled as such. Perforation of a catheter into bowel, since there is gross contamination, requires removal of the catheter.

Cerebrospinal Fluid Leaks

The placement of an intrathecal drug delivery catheter through a Tuohy needle involves placing the needle through the back incision, the intraspinous ligament, the ligamentum flavum, and the epidural space before puncturing the dura. A catheter smaller than the needle is then placed through the needle into the thecal sac and advanced to the desired spinal level. When the needle is removed, it leaves a hole in the dural sac surrounding the catheter that is larger than the catheter itself. A CSF leak into the epidural space is therefore inevitable. Persistent CSF leak leads to postspinal headache in many patients. The treatment of postspinal headache is autologous epidural blood patching, which should be performed with careful attention to sterile technique and under fluoroscopic guidance to avoid injuring the spinal catheter. In our clinic, the rate of postspinal headache approaches 20%. Of course, these headaches usually disappear over time, and temporizing may be all that is necessary. It is my experience, however, that patients feel that these headaches are worse than the primary pain syndrome being treated. This complication should be treated aggressively.

CSF can leak anywhere along the catheter. A subcutaneous collection of CSF is called a *CSF hygroma.* Most of these are self-limiting. Their size is limited by the size of the subcutaneous pocket, the expansibility of the tissue, and the actual duration of healing around the catheter hole in the dura. Healing most often takes place within 1 to 2 weeks; however, hygromas have been known to persist for months. These hygromas are usually only annoying to the patient and are otherwise of no consequence. Care must be taken to avoid contaminating these fluid collections, since they are contiguous with the CSF in the thecal sac. Surgical intervention is warranted only if the fluid continues to leak through the skin incision suture line. Then wound takedown and resuturing are in order.

Pump Pocket Seroma

After surgery, and because the body abhors a vacuum, newly created pump pockets sometimes develop a fluid collection, or seroma, that can last 1 to 2 months after implantation. Such collections are self-limiting and usually are of no clinical significance. Patient reassurance is usually the only treatment necessary. If the fluid collection is excessive and bothersome to the patient, an abdominal binder might help to shrink the seroma and promote healing. If infection is suspected, aspiration should be performed for Gram stain, and culture and sensitivity specimens. Gram stain must show bacteria to distinguish infection from simple seroma. All seromas contain large numbers of white blood cells. If bacterial contamination of the wound is proven, the patient should be given intravenous antibiotics. Antibiotic irrigation of the pocket itself is recommended. Conservative management at this point would consist of removing the pump and all catheters, although some infections have been managed with appropriate antibiotic therapy. If the physician elects to "treat and watch," puncture of the pump refill or side ports is contraindicated for fear of contaminating the pump itself. If there are any signs of spread of infection along the catheter at this time or if the infection does not resolve, the pump and catheter must be removed.

Mechanical Drug Delivery System Catheter Complications

Mechanical catheter complications include breaking, kinking, disconnection of the various necessary connections, obstruction at the catheter tip, and dislodgement of the catheter. These complications terminate analgesia, owing to failure of the pumped analgesic to reach the target organ, the spinal cord. Loss of analgesia, however, can also be caused by disease progression (i.e., spread of cancer), tolerance formation, exacerbation of pain necessitating higher medication doses, or a change in the pain syndrome leading to cessation of opioid response. Clinically, over time, the patient experiences loss of good analgesic control, in spite of increasing doses of the drug.

Mechanical catheter problems are easily confirmed with imaging. A simple radiograph including the spine and pump tells whether the catheter has dislodged, has broken completely, is disconnected from the pump, or has been disconnected from the larger pump catheter. Unfortunately, plain films will not demonstrate obstruction at the catheter tip, a minor break with leakage of analgesic to "non–target" tissues, or kinks in the system. If the pump has a side port, simple injection of nonionic radiographic dye under fluoroscopic visualization will allow correct diagnosis of major or minor catheter breakage, kinking, disconnection of necessary connections, obstruction at the catheter tip, and dislodgement of the catheter; although the physician must understand that this maneuver could have dire consequences. Injection of the dye through the side port of a pump could lead to an overdose of medication, especially if there is a high concentration of the medication in the dead space of the catheter system. If the dead space is not aspirated before contrast material is injected, the patient receives an extremely high dose of medication in a single bolus.

If the pump does not have a side port, the task of diagnosing the problem becomes more difficult. In this instance it is recommended that radiolabeled technetium be used as a tracer. The recommended procedure is to empty the pump, fill it with technetium, then program it to deliver a bolus injection of the tracer. After some time, the catheter tip is scanned for radionuclide to ensure normal technetium flow into the CSF and to verify that the catheter is indeed in the intrathecal space.

The treatment of mechanical catheter complications requires the removal and reimplantation of catheters that are obstructed at the tip, reimplantation of dislodged ones, or reconnection of disconnected ones. Surgical correction of kinked catheters might require simple freeing up of some minor scarring around the catheter causing the kink or might require removal and replacement of the catheter if extensive scar formation makes dissection and freeing of the catheter impossible.

Drug Delivery Pump Complications

Programmable pump complications include overfilling of the pump, battery failure, pump failure, hybrid failure, and torsion or flipping of a freely movable pump. Like catheter problems, battery failure or pump failure for any reason is heralded by loss of analgesia. The normal life of a programmable pump battery depends on the programmed flow rate and may be as long as 3 to 5 years. Pumps can be damaged by overpressurization from overfilling or by incompatible drugs placed in the pump. Overpressurization may lead not only to pump damage and failure but also to overdosing. It is strongly suggested that only Medtronic refill kits be used to refill these programmable pumps. These kits contain a manometer system that tells the physician or nurse if the system is overpressurized.

Drug and pump incompatibility may lead to breakdown of the internal catheter system and corrosion of the internal workings of the pump. Hybrid failure—failure of the electronic telemetric receiving module—prevents the pump from receiving programmed instructions. The pumps will continue to function, but, in fact, become constant–flow rate pumps, delivering drug at the last rate programmed. Battery failure or pump failure requires explantation of the old pump and implantation of a new one. Hybrid failure, however, may not require a pump change. The decision depends on the importance of programmability to the physician and the patient.

Free movement of the pump within its pocket not only may be uncomfortable to the patient but can also cause torsion of the pump and tension on the catheter system, or actual flipping of the pump. Because of this complication catheters have actually been pulled directly out of the intrathecal space, another event heralded by loss of analgesia. When a pump flips over on itself because of free movement in the pocket, it becomes impossible to refill it. This problem is usually noticed when it is time to refill. Failure of telemetry with programmable pumps suggests this possibility. Pump flip is confirmed by radiography or image-intensified fluoroscopy. Surgical revision of the pump pocket and anchoring of the pump is the suggested remedy.

Refilling and Programming Errors

Refilling errors—which can lead to disaster—include reprogramming errors, dosing errors, and errors in the refilling procedure itself. Pumps contain drug reservoirs that need to be filled every so often, depending on the concentration of the drug and the daily dose. Each refilling is hazardous and risky for the patient.

Any injection of drug into the catheter side port could lead to an overdose of the drug, morbidity, and even death. The morbidity associated with massive overdoses of intrathecal opiates is well described in the literature; signs include muscle rigidity, severe myoclonus, seizure activity, hypertension, cardiovascular collapse, and severe respiratory depression.[84,85] Animal studies have shown some severe neurotoxicity with overdoses of intraspinal opioids.[86,87]

If the person refilling the pump is aware of the possible complications, proceeds with caution, and follows the guidelines described earlier, these complications can be avoided. Some physicians, however, do not take the risk of using pumps with side ports. They feel that the risks of the side port are too great when weighed against its benefits—easy solving of catheter problems. Therefore, they implant only pumps without side ports.

Like refilling the pump, reprogramming a programmable pump can have dire or even disastrous consequences. These pumps are telemetrically instructed to perform according to the physician's wishes within the constraints of the software in the programmer. Programming for a drug concentration higher or lower than the actual concentration of the drug contained in the pump could lead to underdosing, leading to increasing pain, or even abstinence syndrome, or overdosing leading to morbidity or even death. Likewise, programming for higher or lower doses than the refiller intended could also lead to morbidity or death. Newer software that is available with the Medtronic programmable pumps and programmers does ask the programmer if he or she has made the right choices and is thus safer for the patient. Still, the programmer should check and recheck his or her work before discharging the patient.

Should an overdose occur from either a refilling error or a reprogramming error and the physician be aware of it, it is recommended that CSF be removed immediately and replaced with saline. Venous access should be obtained, and the patient should be moved immediately to the hospital, preferably the intensive care unit, for observation. Should there be signs of respiratory depression, naloxone should be given immediately by bolus injection and then by continuous infusion. Because naloxone may increase the hypertension produced by massive doses of opioids,[88] it is preferable to observe the patient for signs of developing respiratory depression before starting infusion of naloxone. Other signs of central nervous system toxicity, including seizure activity and myoclonus, should be treated symptomatically in the intensive care unit.

CONCLUSION

Over the last 15 years a great deal has been said and written about the use of intraspinal opioids for nonmalignant pain. It has been my purpose in this chapter to address some of the key issues surrounding the use of this therapy. A rational approach to the use of intraspinal opioids has been presented. Patient selection for intraspinal opioids should obey the KISS principle and follow a pain treatment continuum. Once a decision has been made to use this therapy some pharmacologic and management guidelines and the management of complications have been presented. If the physicians who choose to use this therapy understand appropriate patient selection, know how to use the drugs for intraspinal use wisely, and manage complications expertly, this therapy will add immeasurably to the tools of the trade for the management of nonmalignant pain.

REFERENCES

1. Bonica JJ: Chronic non-cancer pain. In Anderson S, Bond M, Mehta M, Swerdlow M (eds): Lancaster, UK, MTP Press, 1987, p 13.
2. Lemrow N, Adams D, Coffey R, et al: The 50 most frequent diagnosis-related groups, diagnoses, and procedures: Statistics by hospital size and location. DHHS Publication No. (PHS) 90-3465, Hospital Studies Program Research Note 13, Agency for Health Care Policy and Research. Rockville, Md., Public Health Service, September 1990.
3. Heliovaara M, Makela M, Aromaa A, et al: Low back pain and subsequent cardiovascular mortality. Spine 20:2109–2111, 1995.
4. Chelius J, Galvin D, Owens P: Disability: It's more expensive than you think. Business Health 10:80, 1992.
5. United States Department of Commerce, Statistical Abstracts, 113th ed., Tables 579 and 587, 1993.
6. The Michigan Pain Study. EPIC/MRA 4710 W. Saginaw Hwy. Lansing, Michigan, 48917-2601, 1997.
7. Joranson D: Intractable pain treatment laws and regulations. Bull Am Pain Soc 5:2:1–17, 1995.
8. Kolb L: Types and characteristics of drug addicts. Mental Hygiene 9:300, 1925.
9. Porter J, Jick H: Addiction rare in patients treated with narcotics. NEJM 302:123, 1980.
10. Perry S, Heidrick G: Management of pain during debridement: A survey of US burn units. Pain 13:267–280, 1982.
11. Portenoy RK, Foley KM: Chronic use of opioid analgesics in nonmalignant pain: Report of 38 cases. Pain 25:171–186, 1986.
12. Zenz M, Sturmpf M, Tryba M: Long-term oral opioid therapy in patients with chronic nonmalignant pain. J Pain Symptom Manage 7:69–77, 1992.
13. Schofferman J: Long-term opioid analgesic therapy for severe refractory lumbar spine pain. Clin J Pain 15:136–140, 1999.
14. Pert CB, Pasternack G, Snyder S: Opiate antagonists discriminate by receptor binding in brain. Science 82:1359–1361, 1973.
15. Terenius L, Wahlstrom A: Morphine-like ligand in opiate receptors in human CSF. Life Sci 16:1759–1764, 1975.
16. Yaksh TL, Rudy TA: Studies on the direct spinal action of narcotics in the production of analgesia in the rat. J Pharmacol Exp Ther 202:411–428, 1977.
17. Yaksh TL: Analgetic actions of intrathecal opiates in cat and primates. Brain Res 153:1978.
18. Wang JF, Nauss LA, Thomas JE: Pain relief by intrathecally applied morphine in man. Anesthesiology 50:149–151, 1979.
19. Bahar M, Olshwang D, Magora F, et al: Epidural morphine in treatment of pain. Lancet.
20. Onofrio BM, Yaksh TL, Arnold PG: Continuous low dose intrathecal morphine administration in the treatment of chronic pain of malignant origin. Mayo Clin Proc 56:516–520, 1981.
21. Coombs DW, Saunders RL, Gaylor M, Pageau RN: Epidural narcotic infusion: Implantation technique and efficacy. Anesthesiology 56:469–473, 1982.
22. Harbaugh RE, Coombs DW, Saunders RL: Implanted continuous epidural morphine infusion system. J Neurosurg 56:803–806, 1992.
23. Krames ES, Gershow J, Glassberg A, et al: Continuous infusion of spinally administered narcotics for the relief of pain due to malignant disorders. Cancer 56:696–702, 1985.
24. Coombs DW, Saunders RL, Gaylor MS: Relief of continuous chronic pain by intraspinal narcotics infusion via an implanted reservoir. JAMA 250:2336–2339, 1983.
25. Shetter AG, Hadley MN, Wilkinson E: Administration of intraspinal morphine for the treatment of cancer pain. Neurosurgery 18:740–747, 1986.
26. Penn RD, Paice JA: Chronic intrathecal morphine for intractable pain. J Neurosurg 67:182–186.
27. Dennis GC, DeWitty RL: Management of intractable pain in cancer patients by implantable morphine infusion systems. J Natl Med Assoc 79:939–944, 1987.
28. Brazenor GA: Long-term intrathecal administration of morphine: A comparison of bolus injection via reservoir with continuous infusion by implanted pump. Neurosurgery 21:484–491, 1987.
29. Onofrio BM, Yaksh TL: Long-term pain relief produced by intrathecal infusion in 53 patients. J Neurosurg 72:200–209, 1990.
30. Spaziante R, Cappabiance P, Ferone A, et al: Treatment of chronic cancer pain by means of continuous intrathecal low dose morphine administration with a totally implantable subcutaneous pump. J Neurosurg Sci 29:143–151, 1985.
31. Follett KA, Hitchon PW, Piper J, et al: Response of intractable pain to continuous intrathecal morphine: A retrospective study. Pain 49:21–25, 1992.
32. Auld AW, Maki-Jokela A, Murdock DM: Intraspinal narcotic analgesia in the treatment of chronic pain. Spine 10:777–781, 1984.
33. Hadley MN, Shetter AG: Intrathecal opiate administration for analgesia. Contemp Neurosurg 8:1–6, 1986.
34. Hassenbusch SJ, Stanton-Hicks MD, Soukup J, et al: Sufentanil citrate and morphine/bupivacaine as alternative agents in chronic epidural infusions for intractable non-cancer pain. Neurosurgery 29:76–82, 1991.
35. Goodman RR: Treatment of lower extremity reflex sympathetic dystrophy with continuous intrathecal morphine infusion. Appl Neurophysiol 50:425–426, 1987.
36. Jacobson L: Clinical note: Relief of persistent postamputation stump and phantom limb pain with intrathecal fentanyl. Pain 37:317–322, 1989.
37. Prager JP, DeSalles A, Wilkinson A, et al: Loin pain hematuria syndrome: Pain relief with intrathecal morphine. Am J Kidney Dis 25:629–631, 1995.
38. Kanoff RBL: Intraspinal delivery of opiates by an implantable, programmable pump in patients with chronic, intractable pain of nonmalignant origin. J Am Osteopathic Assoc 94:487–493, 1994.
39. Schuchard M, Lanning R, Krames ES: Intraspinal analgesia for nonmalignant pain: A retrospective analysis for efficacy, safety, and feasibility in 50 patients. Neuromodulation 1:46–56, 1998.

40. Arner S, Arner B: Differential effects of epidural morphine in the treatment of cancer related pain. Acta Anaesthesiol Scand 29:332–336, 1989.
41. Arner S, Meyerson B: Lack of analgesic effect of opioids on neuropathic and idiopathic forms of pain. Pain 33:11–23, 1988.
42. Vecht CJ: Nociceptive nerve pain and neuropathic pain (Letter to Editor). Pain 39:243, 1989.
43. Meynadier J, Chrubasik J, Dubar M, Wunsch E: Intrathecal somatostatin in terminally ill patients: A report of two cases. Pain 23:9–12, 1985.
44. Penn RD, Paice JA, Kroin JS: Intrathecal octreotide for cancer pain. Lancet 738, 1990.
45. Bowersox SS, Gadbois T, Singh T, et al: Selective *N*-type neuronal voltage-sensitive calcium channel blocker, SNX-111, produces spinal antinociception in rat models of acute, persistent and neuropathic pain. J Pharmacol Exp Ther 279:1243–1249, 1996.
46. Bahar M, Cohen ML, Grinshpon Y, Chanimov M: Spinal anesthesia with midazolam in the rat. Can J Anaesth 44:208–215, 1997.
47. Goodchild CS: Nonopioid spinal analgesics: Animal experimentation and implications for clinical developments. Pain Rev 4:33–58, 1997.
48. Van Dongen RTM, Crul BJP, de Bock M: Long-term intrathecal infusion of morphine and morphine/bupivacaine mixtures in the treatment of cancer pain: A retrospective analysis of 51 cases. Pain 55:107–111, 1993.
49. Cousins MJ, Cherry DA, Gourlay GK: Acute and chronic pain: Use of spinal opioids. *In* Cousins MJ, Bridenbaugh PO (eds): Neural Blockade in Clinical Anesthesia and Management of Pain, ed 2. Philadelphia, JB Lippincott, 1988, pp 955–1029.
50. Christie JM, Meade WR, Markowsky S: Paranoid psychosis after intrathecal morphine. Anesth Analg 77:1298–1299, 1993.
51. Shohami E, Evron S: Intrathecal morphine induces myoclonic seizures in the rat. Acta Pharmacol Toxicol 56: 50–54, 1985.
52. Ali NMK: Hyperalgesic response in a patient receiving high concentrations of spinal morphine. Anesthesiology 65:449, 1986.
53. Arner S, Rawal N, Gustafsson LL: Clinical experience of long-term treatment with epidural opioids—a nationwide survey. Acta Anaesthesiol Scand 32:253–259, 1988.
54. De Conno F, Caraceni A, Martini C, et al: Hyperalgesia and myoclonus with intrathecal infusion of high-dose morphine. Pain 47:337–339, 1991.
55. Parkinson SK, Bailey SL, Little WL, Mueller JB: Myoclonic seizure activity with chronic high-dose spinal opioid administration. Anesthesiology 72:743–745, 1990.
56. Linder S, Borgent A, Biollaz J: Meniere-like syndrome following epidural morphine analgesia. Anesthesiology 71:782–783, 1989.
57. Fish DJ, Rosen SM: Epidural opioids as a cause of vertical nystagmus. Anesthesiology 73:785–786, 1990.
58. Ueyama H, Nishimura M, Tashiro C: Naloxone reversal of nystagmus associated with intrathecal morphine administration. Anesthesiology 76:153, 1992.
59. Crone LA, Conly JM, Storgard C, et al: Herpes labialis in patients receiving epidural morphine following caesarean section. Anesthesiology 73:208–213, 1990.
60. Pennant JH, Wallace D: Intrathecal morphine and reactivation of oral herpes simplex. Anesthesiology 75:919, 1991.
61. Carden E: Herpes simplex after spinal morphine. Anaesthesia 39:938, 1984.
62. Ross A, Hill A: Intrathecal morphine and herpes reactivation. Anaesth Intensive Care 21:126, 1993.
63. Bailey PL, Rhondeau S, Schafer PG, et al: Dose-response pharmacology of intrathecal morphine in human volunteers. Anesthesiology 79:49–59, 1993.
64. Nichols DG, Yaster M, Lynn AM, et al: Disposition and respiratory effects of intrathecal morphine in children. Anesthesiology 79:733–738, 1993.
65. Yaksh TL, Reddy SVR: Studies in the primate on the analgesic effects associated with intrathecal actions of opiates, alpha adrenergic agonists and baclofen. Anesthesiology 54:451–467, 1981.
66. Drasner K, Fields HL: Synergy between the antinociceptive effects of intrathecal clonidine and systemic morphine in the rat. Pain 32:309–312, 1988.
67. Omote K, Kitahata LM, Collins JG, et al: Interaction between opiate subtype and alpha$_2$-adrenergic agonists in suppression of noxiously evoked activity of WDR neurons in the spinal dorsal horn. Anesthesiology 74:737–743, 1991.
68. Maves TJ, Gebhart GF: Antinociceptive synergy between intrathecal morphine and lidocaine during visceral and somatic nociception in the rat. Anesthesiology 76:91–99, 1992.
69. Fraser H, Chapman V, Dickenson A: Spinal local anaesthetic actions on afferent evoked responses and wind-up of nociceptive neurones in the rat spinal cord: Combination with morphine produces marked potentiation of nociception. Pain 49:33–41, 1992.
70. Coombs DW, Pageau MG, Saunders RL, et al: Intraspinal narcotic tolerance: Preliminary experience with continuous bupivacaine HCl infusion via implanted infusion device. Int J Artif Organs 5:379–382, 1982.
71. Coombs DW, Saunders RL, Lachance D, et al: Intrathecal morphine tolerance: Use of intrathecal clonidine, DADLE, and intraventricular morphine. Anesthesiology 62:358–363, 1985.
72. Tanelian DL, Cousins MJ: Failure of epidural opioid to control cancer pain in a patient previously treated with massive doses of intravenous opioid. Pain 36:359–362, 1989.
73. Berde CB, Sethna NF, Conrad LS, et al: Subarachnoid bupivacaine analgesia for seven months for a patient with a spinal cord tumor. Anesthesiology 72:1094–1096, 1990.
74. Nitescu P, Lennart A, Linder L, et al: Epidural versus intrathecal morphine-bupivacaine: Assessment of consecutive treatments in advanced cancer pain. J Pain Symptom Manage 5:18–26, 1990.
75. DuPen SL, Williams AR: Management of patients receiving combined epidural morphine and bupivacaine for the treatment of cancer pain. J Pain Symptom Manage 27:125–127, 1992.
76. Krames ES, Lanning RM: Intrathecal infusional analgesia for nonmalignant pain: Analgesic efficacy of intrathecal opioid with or without bupivacaine. J Pain Symptom Manage 8:539–548, 1993.
77. Motsch J, Graber E, Ludwig K: Addition of clonidine enhances postoperative analgesia from epidural morphine: A double-blind study. Anesthesiology 73:1067–1073, 1990.
78. van Dongen RTM, Crul BJP, van Egmond J: Intrathecal coadministration of bupivacaine diminishes morphine dose progression during long-term intrathecal infusion in cancer patients. Clin J Pain 15:166–172, 1999.
79. Lundborg CN, Nitescu PV, Appelgren LK, Curelaru ID: Long-term intrathecal administration of opioid and bupivacaine relieved intractable pain in a patient with familial amyloidosis polyneuropathy: A case report. Neuromodulation 1:199–208, 1998.
80. Wulf H, Gleim M, Mignat C: The stability of mixtures of morphine hydrochloride, bupivacaine hydrochloride, and clonidine hydrochloride in portable pump reservoirs for the management of chronic pain syndromes. J Pain Symptom Manage 9:308–311, 1994.
81. North RB, Protagoras NC, Epstein JA, et al: Spinal cord compression complicating subarachnoid infusion of morphine. Neurosurgery 29:778–784, 1991.
82. Aldrete JA, Vascello LA, Ghaly R, Tomlin D: Paraplegia in a patient with an intrathecal catheter and a spinal cord stimulator. Anesthesiology 81:1542–1545, 1994.
83. Schuchard M, Lanning R, North R, et al: Neurologic sequelae of intraspinal drug delivery systems: Results of a survey of American implanters of implantable drug delivery systems. Neuromodulation 1:137–148, 1998.
84. Bowdle TA, Rooke GA: Postoperative myoclonus and rigidity after anesthesia with opioids. Anesth Analg 78:783–786, 1994.
85. Groudine SB, Cresanti-Daknis C, Lumb PD: Successful treatment of a massive intrathecal morphine overdose. Anesthesiology 82:292–295, 1995.
86. Coombs DW, Colburn RW, DeLeo JA, et al: Comparative spinal neuropathology of hydromorphone and morphine after 9 and 30-day epidural administration in sheep. Anesth Analg 78:674–681, 1994.
87. Rawal N, Nuutinen L, Raj PP, et al: Behavioral and histopathological effects following intrathecal administration of butorphanol, sufentanil, and nalbuphine in sheep. Anesthesiology 75:1025–1034, 1991.
88. Sauter K, Kaufman HH, Bloomfield SM, et al: Treatment of high-dose intrathecal morphine overdose. J Neurosurg 81:143–146, 1994.

CHAPTER • 61

Spinal Administration of Nonopiate Analgesics for Pain Management

Jason E. Garber, MD •
Samuel J. Hassenbusch III, MD, PhD

HISTORY OF INTRATHECAL ADMINISTRATION

Pain remains one of the most frequent causes of disability that reduces the quality of life for many people. Pain crosses all cultural, racial, and religious barriers. Consequently, people have utilized a number of methods to treat acute and chronic pain. Two of the most important advances in the long-term management of severe pain have been the refinement of opioid administration via the intraspinal (intrathecal, epidural) route and the development of better devices for successful intrathecal administration.

Goldstein and colleagues discovered opioid receptors in 1970.[1] They were first isolated in nerve tissue in 1973,[2] discovered in the brain in 1974,[3] and subsequently reported in the spinal cord in 1976.[4] As a result, opioid administration has evolved to include both epidural and intrathecal administration for human pain modulation. The management of postraumatic, postoperative, cancer-associated, and other types of acute and chronic pains has been extensively reported in the literature.

In the United States, there are only two Food and Drug Administration (F.D.A.)–approved drugs for long-term intrathecal administration: preservative-free morphine and preservative-free baclofen (Table 61–1). Preservative-free morphine, given via the intraspinal route, classically has been the first choice in the treatment of acute and chronic pain. Other opioid compounds can be used for intrathecal administration, such as hydromorphone, sufentanil, and fentanyl. Paice and Penn, in a retrospective survey, determined that the most common agent for intraspinal infusion in the United States was morphine; however, hydromorphone and sufentanil were also frequently used for intrathecal pain management.[5] Although meperidine (Demerol, pethidine) has also been used with success in long-term intrathecal infusions, a number of concerns have been raised. Long-term use of meperidine is thought possibly to cause damage to implantable pumps, although whether it does remains indeterminate.

The combination of bupivacaine with either morphine or hydromorphone has also been reported in the literature[6–8]; however, the maximum commercially available concentration of bupivacaine that is used in the United States for intrathecal administration (0.75%, or 7.5 mg/mL) is generally thought to be less effective than an adjunctive opioid.[9, 10] Tetracaine, also a local anesthetic, is cautioned strongly for intrathecal use, because some evidence indicates that it might cause spinal cord damage or toxicity.

Side effects can occur with use of intrathecal opioids. The potential side effects commonly include nausea, vomiting, pruritis, sedation, respiratory depression, gastrointestinal hypomotility or constipation, and urinary hesitancy. A number of less common, somewhat idiosyncratic reactions also can occur with opioids, headache, anaphylaxis, dysphoria, agitation, and even seizures among them. The addition of a local anesthetic agent to opioids carries the risk of sensory or motor changes at the spinal level of administration.

The other F.D.A.–approved long-term intrathecal therapy is preservative-free baclofen. Baclofen is used primarily for the treatment of spasticity, but it does have limited application for pain management. Specifically, its analgesic effect is related to the pain generated by the spasticity itself.

NONOPIOID ANALGESIC ADMINISTRATION

Nonopioid intrathecal analgesic infusion remains at the forefront of pain research and clinical investigation. There are a number of reasons for exploring alternative, nonopioid medications for intrathecal administration. The development of innovative, intrathecal analgesic therapies is based on several principles:

1. Intrathecal opioids may not be effective in every patient.
2. Intrathecal opioids can cause systemic side effects.
3. The increasing doses of opioids needed over time might require increasing infusion rates, consequently reducing the battery life of implantable pumps.[11]
4. A number of spinal cord receptor types other than opioid receptors are known to modulate pain transmission.

TABLE 61–1 **Intraspinal Agents Currently Utilized with Implantable Devices**

Opioids	Local Anesthetic	Antispasmodic
Morphine Hydromorphone Sufentanil Fentanyl	Bupivacaine	Baclofen

For these reasons, an alternative intrathecal medication may be an option to replace or supplement opioid infusion therapy, especially when the infusions cause side effects. Furthermore, the nonopioid agents might provide improved treatment for various pain conditions. This raises the possibility of better pain relief for certain conditions, particularly neuropathic pain.

The pain research community has focused great interest and research on the development of alternative agents for intrathecal infusion. The major classes of compounds currently under investigation include acetylcholinesterase inhibitors, benzodiazepines, cells in matrix, adrenergic agonists, long-acting local anesthetics, *N*-methyl-D-aspartate (NMDA) antagonists, somatostatin analogues, and calcium channel blockers (Table 61–2).

Several other groups of compounds remain experimental at this time. These include the tricyclic antidepressants, prostaglandin synthesis inhibitors, neuropeptides, beta blockers, nitric oxide synthase inhibitors, and adenosine.

The role of alternative and innovative intrathecal analgesics centers around five principles:

1. The exploration of new receptors that modulate pain.
2. Demonstrating efficacy in pain treatment (analgesia).
3. Addressing the potential side effects that may develop with long-term use of opioids.
4. Employing clinically useful solubility and pump compatibility profiles.
5. Formulating a viable plan for commercial development and distribution.

ACETYLCHOLINESTERASE INHIBITORS—NEOSTIGMINE

Acetylcholine is a neurotransmitter used by certain interneurons at the level of the dorsal horn. These interneurons provide inhibitory input to the second-order nociceptor neurons. It appears that outflow axons from the rostroventral medulla (RVM) stimulate the acetylcholine-containing interneurons, potentially through the use of a neurotransmitter such as serotonin or norepinephrine.

Neostigmine is one of the primary examples of an acetylcholinesterase inhibitor that has been studied for intrathecal analgesia. Since it is an inhibitor of cholinesterase, it prevents or slows down the resorption of acetylcholine. This results in an increase in the quantity of acetylcholine in the synaptic junctions and serves to prolong the effect of the ongoing inhibitory neurotransmission at the level of the second-order nociceptor neurons. Therefore, the effectiveness of neostigmine relies on preexisting activation of the descending antinociceptive system, whose activation results in increased release of acetylcholine from inhibitory interneurons in the dorsal horn. Neostigmine prolongs the half-life of the released acetylcholine and thus serves as a mechanism potential for pain modification with intrathecal administration.

The antinociceptive effects of spinal cholinergic stimulation and possible interactions with substance P have been well-described.[12] Furthermore, use of intrathecal neostigmine for postoperative analgesia has been reported in a sheep model.[13]

Intrathecal neostigmine has also been examined in human volunteers. It appears to produce antinociception to cold, painful stimuli in a dose-dependent manner. Studies of the safety of intrathecal administration of neostigmine were first conducted in dogs and rats.[14] Phase I safety trials of intrathecal neostigmine methylsulfate have also been reported in humans.[15] The side effects noted include nausea, emesis, and, rarely, paresis.[15] Acetylcholine receptors have also been found in the inferomediolateral cell column and the ventral horn of the spinal cord. These two sites probably account for the side effects of nausea, emesis, and paresis.

The reported preliminary data suggest that neostigmine is a relatively safe drug for intrathecal delivery in humans. This is a novel mechanism, because neostigmine accentuates a normal body's response to ongoing chronic pain. Its efficacy, however, remains under investigation.

BENZODIAZEPINES—MIDAZOLAM

Midazolam hydrochloride (Versed), though not currently available in the United States as a preservative-free, liquid

TABLE 61–2 **Alternative Intraspinal Agents Used with Implantable Drug Administration Devices**

New Agents	Possible Future Agents
Alpha$_2$-adrenergic agonists (clonidine) Somatostatin analogues (octreotide, vapreotide) Neuron-specific calcium channel blockers (SNX-111 [Ziconotide]) *N*-methyl-D-aspartate antagonists (dextromethorphan, dextrorphan, memantine, MK-801) Acetylcholinesterase inhibitors (neostigmine) Gamma-aminobutyric acid–responsive agonists (benzodiazepines [e.g., midazolam]) Long-acting local anesthetics (Butambin) Bioactive implants (adrenal medullary cells in matrix)	Tricyclic antidepressants Nitric oxide synthase inhibitors Liposomal encapsulation of local anesthetics

formulation suitable for intraspinal infusion, is one of the more interesting compounds that may prove promising in the future for intrathecal delivery. This compound acts directly on gamma-aminobutyric acid receptors. There is some reported experience with this drug in Australia for acute postoperative pain, but solid data and detailed clinical trials have yet to be produced. Current investigation in the United States focuses on the efficacy and toxicity of intrathecal delivery in animals. A possible human phase I clinical trial of intrathecal infusion of the drug is being planned.

CELLS IN MATRIX

Adrenal medullary cell transplantation into catheter delivery systems and direct subarachnoid adrenal medullary transplantation are novel alternatives for pain management. There have been reports of subarachnoid adrenal medullary transplantation for the treatment of terminal cancer pain. The investigations have yielded promising preliminary results.[16] Other clinical studies focus on direct release of catecholamines into the cerebrospinal fluid. This method of delivery could provide a unique mechanism for pain relief that depends on living cells for the delivery of intrathecal analgesia.[17]

CLONIDINE-ALPHA-2 ADRENERGIC AGONISTS

Mechanism of Action

The only commercially approved, nonopioid, non–local anesthetic intraspinal analgesic available in the United States is clonidine. It represents a major advance and has been shown to be effective in the treatment of both cancer and neuropathic pain. Siddall and coworkers also described the use of intrathecal clonidine in the treatment of spinal cord injury pain.[18] Their single case report is important because it demonstrates that the combination of morphine and clonidine was successful in treating a very difficult central pain pain syndrome. It also supports the use of clonidine combined with morphine for the treatment of neuropathic, sympathetic-independent pain not related to cancer.

Clonidine is an alpha2-adrenergic agonist and appears to act at the level of the spinal cord, although action at higher levels cannot be ruled out. Clonidine appears to inhibit the release of substance P and acts on nociceptive neurons. It acts postsynaptically, between the first-order and second-order nociceptive neurons. This suggests synergy with the spinal opioid receptor, which is often considered to be presynaptic. One of the major side effects of clonidine, however, is systemic hypotension. This has been observed with local injections at the thoracic level and involves cholinergic preganglionic sympathetic neurons. There may also be a supraspinal effect related to the hypotensive effects, since the sympathetic nervous system still must be intact.

A review of neuromodulation from both the ascending and descending spinal antinociceptive systems suggests that norepinephrine appears to be the outflow transmitter from the rostroventral medulla (RVM) to the dorsal horn via the dorsal lateral funiculus (DLF). Subsequently, the norepinephrine either directly inhibits the second-order nociceptor or stimulates a local interneuron at the level of the dorsal horn. This local interneuron, in turn, directly inhibits the second-order nociceptor. Thus, norepinephrine is an important inhibitory neurotransmitter for pain transmission at the dorsal horn level.

Norepinephrine may also serve as a local inhibitory neurotransmitter at the level of the RVM. If this hypothesis is correct, norepinephrine may have effects paradoxical to the ones described earlier; however, this mechanism does not appear to be clinically significant. This possible RVM effect does suggest less profound analgesia with the intraspinal infusion of clonidine if it were to have significant brain stem exposure instead of spinal cord contact only.

Formulations and Other Adrenergic Agonists

Clonidine is moderately lipophilic. It is commercially available in the United States for spinal delivery at a concentration of 100 mg/mL. It is commercially labeled for epidural, medium-term use for cancer pain. In Europe and Australia, a commercial preparation is available for intravenous use (150 mg/mL) that might also prove suitable for intrathecal use. One study of the stability of the mixture of morphine, bupivacaine, and clonidine in a portable pump has been reported.[19] The stability of the mixture was documented over a period up to approximately 90 days.

Tizanidine is another experimental adrenergic agonist that has been used in the treatment of chronic pain. Dexmetomidine is another alternative that has been studied only in animals but was found to be safe. When injected into the locus ceruleus, dexmetomidine has produced pain relief. The commercial availability of clonidine in the United States, however, seems to make alternative adrenergic agonists unnecessary.

Animal Studies

Clonidine is perhaps the agent best studied for safety of intraspinal delivery. The intrathecal and epidural use of clonidine has been studied for spinal toxicity in six different non-human species. These animal models have shown no pathologic changes in neurologic status or histopathologic examination.

Human Studies

The use of clonidine, by epidural or intrathecal routes, has been widely reported in the medical literature for more than 2000 patients.[20–24] Although two thirds of these patients received clonidine via the epidural route, an increasing number of patients are now taking this drug in long-term intrathecal infusions. Clonidine has been reported in a multicenter study for epidural delivery in the treatment of cancer pain.[25, 26] Eighty-five patients with intractable cancer pain received either epidural clonidine or a placebo, in addition to epidural patient-controlled morphine analgesia (PCA). The addition of clonidine appeared to reduce the pain intensity as compared with a placebo. This study suggested that clonidine was effective in improving pain relief for patients with severe, cancer-related pain.

Epidural clonidine has also been reported in the treatment of complex regional pain syndrome (CRPS), also known as reflex sympathetic dystrophy (RSD).[27] Twenty-six patients were divided into study groups that received (1) placebo (saline), (2) various epidural doses of clonidine, or (3) a continuous epidural infusion of clonidine at rates ranging from 10 to 15 μg/hr. The results indicated that clonidine provided better analgesia compared to the control group. Side effects of the clonidine included bradycardia, systemic hypotension, and sedation. Pain relief was significantly poorer with boluses of 300 and 700 μg of epidural clonidine. Nineteen patients received a continuous infusion for an average of 6.1 weeks at an average dose of 32 μg/hr. Thirty-five percent of the patients who were placed on a continuous-rate clonidine infusion reported significant improvement in their pain.

Thirty-two patients at the M.D. Anderson Cancer Center have been treated over the long term with intrathecal clonidine. The majority of these patients had CRPS, and clonidine was the only analgesic used in these trials. The average follow-up was 4.9 months. Fifty-six percent of patients reported improvements not only in their pain scale rating but also in their CRPS symptoms. Systemic hypotension was the major side effect with medium-sized doses (15–23 μg/hr) but was eliminated at the highest doses of about 40–50 μg/hr. Three patients described generalized malaise, and two had to discontinue the medication because of it. Headaches were also noted in three patients but were significant in only one of them. The dose range was 100 to 960 μg/day, although most patients' doses were in the range of 480 to 900 μg/day. It should be emphasized, however, that the major potential side effect is systemic hypotension and there is not yet long-term (>5 years) human experience with continuous intrathecal infusions.

LONG-ACTING LOCAL ANESTHETICS—BUTAMBIN

Butambin is an analgesic agent that was developed as a single epidural injection for the treatment of chronic pain. Its pharmacologic action centers on its function as a local anesthetic; possibly, it affects the nerve roots themselves. Butambin is formulated as a semiliquid paste that can applied directly to the epidural space or a nerve root sleeve via a catheter or needle. Initial reports indicate that butambin provides pain relief on a medium- or long-term basis. A multicenter study of this chemical is currently being conducted, and its safety and long-term efficacy are still being evaluated. The long-term local side effects, and the possibility of nerve root scarring, are not known. This is an especially important consideration in view of its pasty consistency.

N-METHYL-D-ASPARTATE ANTAGONISTS

The classic NMDA antagonist is ketamine. MK801 has been studied for many years from a more research-oriented viewpoint, but we have yet to identify its clinical utility. Clinical compounds currently under investigation include dextrorphan, dextromethorphan, and memantine. Two major functions of these compounds appear to be the prevention of opioid tolerance and the treatment of neuropathic pain.

NMDA antagonists block the NMDA receptor, one of several involved in the transmembrane facilitation of calcium ion influx into the cell. Substance P also appears to facilitate calcium ion influx. The accumulation of intracellular calcium facilitates the expression of oncogenes such as c-*fos*, which, in turn, appear to contribute heavily to the development of chronic pain at the cellular level.

The NMDA antagonist decreases calcium flux into the cell and, therefore, decreases the "vicious cycle" of the neuropathic pain syndrome. Intrathecal delivery of ketamine has been described in the literature for perioperative and postoperative pain control. No extensive studies focused on the long-term usage of ketamine for pain control exist. One very limited report did demonstrate reduction of morphine requirements in patients with terminal cancer.[28] In this double-blind crossover study comparing intrathecal ketamine and intrathecal morphine, patients who received ketamine required less morphine. Pain scores, however, did not significantly vary. With a 1-mg intrathecal bolus of ketamine given twice daily, no serious side effects were noted. It should be emphasized, however, that long-term human intrathecal use of ketamine is not supported by any significant toxicity studies and should be avoided until such data become available.

Another report regarding the use of an intrathecal *N*-methyl-D-aspartate antagonist, CPP, suggested that it may eliminate neurogenic pain.[29] The patient described in this report had unilateral, lower extremity, continuous deep pain and allodynia with secondary generalized radiation of the pain. The patient received 200- and 500-nmol intrathecal injections of CPP and the secondary, generalized pain appeared to have been eliminated. There was, however, no change in the deep pain or the allodynia.

Animal toxicology testing has been performed with memantine, dextrorphan, and dextromethorphan. Testing of all three compounds demonstrated histologic evidence of toxicity, specifically, the development of inflammation and necrosis within the spinal cord in a dose-related manner.[30] Furthermore, there appears to be clinical evidence of motor dysfunction and even paralysis in the animal model.

NMDA antagonists are not without potential side effects. Well known side effects include psychiatric disease, specifically dissociative feelings, and even hallucinations. Central effects include drowsiness, dizziness, and nystagmus. There have also been reports of sensory blockade with the intrathecal use of ketamine.

SOMATOSTATIN ANALOGUES—OCTREOTIDE

Octreotide and vapreotide are the two most studied somatostatin analogues. Both have been tested on patients with cancer pain, and both have yielded promising clinical results. Animal toxicology is currently being studied, although commercial development is unclear. At the pharmacologic level, there is an interneuron in the dorsal horn that uses somatostatin as a neurotransmitter. These central neurons are inhibitory on the pre- and postsynaptic junctions between the first-order and second-order nociceptive neurons. Somatostatin analogues appear to act on the same inhibitory receptors. The somatostatin receptor has been localized in the periaqueductal gray matter (PAG), the substantia gelatinosa, descending pathways for the antinociceptive system, and primary afferent nerve terminals. In human trials, six of eight patients experienced pain relief, although two of them had demonstrable histopathologic changes at autopsy.[31] Octreotide has been described in several articles for its intrathecal analgesic effects and may prove promising in the future as a possible alternative to intrathecal opioids.[32, 33]

SNX-111-CALCIUM CHANNEL BLOCKERS

SNX-111 (brand name Ziconotide) is the best-studied calcium channel blocker and the closest to clinical approval. This compound was originally isolated as a small–molecular weight protein, which occurs naturally in a giant cone snail of the South Pacific. SNX-111 is a neuron-specific compound that blocks presynaptic calcium influx at the presynaptic terminal. This action serves to prevent neurotransmitter vesicle fusion with the presynaptic membrane. The net effect is prevention of vesicular release of a neurotransmitter into the presynaptic junction and, thus, prevention of neurotransmission from the first-order to the second-order neuron.

Three different types of calcium channels are involved in pain:

1. The L calcium channel is affected by verapamil and similar agents.
2. The P calcium channel is affected by a toxin from the funnel web spider.
3. The T calcium channel is affected by SNX-111 and related compounds.

SNX-111 is a small–molecular weight protein that is now synthesized. It has been studied in both rats and dogs with both the Chung and Bennett and the hotplate models.[34] Furthermore, it has been given intravenously in high doses to humans to treat stroke and brain trauma. At this time, the long-term effects (e.g., 5 years) in humans are unknown, although a multicenter, randomized study of the long-term intrathecal infusion of SNX-111 is being completed.

TRICYCLIC ANTIDEPRESSANTS

Tricyclic antidepressants have also been studied for the intrathecal management of chronic pain. The mechanism of action focuses on reuptake inhibition of norepinephrine and serotonin. Rat models have been developed to analyze the modulation of hyperalgesia and allodynia. Early experimental results have been promising to the extent that they suggest that the intrathecal administration of tricyclic antidepressants may attenuate chronic pain in these models. In the clinical setting, however, the application of tricyclic agents is somewhat limited because of the unavailability of a preservative-free solution and the possibility of extremity weakness with large doses. Toxicologic assessment remains inconclusive, and for long-term intraspinal use in humans tricyclics should be considered investigational.

OTHER POSSIBLE AGENTS FOR FUTURE USE

Intrathecal nitric oxide synthase inhibitors have also been studied for chronic pain management. Their pharmacologic effects appear to be centered in the dorsal root ganglion and in postsynaptic junctions, where nitric oxide synthase has been found. Nitric oxide moves extracellularly and facilitates neurotransmitter release; however, intracellular nitric oxide is toxic to cells. Although there are three types of nitric oxide synthase, there are no published clinical trials of pain modulation and these inhibitors.

The liposome encapsulation of local anesthetics has also been reported in the literature and is of interest for management of chronic pain. Research trials include analysis of the anesthetic activity of bupivacaine when placed in lipospheres and delivered by intrathecal injections in rats. Preliminary results indicate that liposome encapsulation appears to increase the anesthetic duration of bupivacaine sixfold.[35] The clinical use of liposome-associated bupivacaine has also been described and appears to prolong action as much as twofold as compared with bupivacaine alone for epidural analgesia.[36]

Liposome encapsulation of tetracaine, lidocaine, and procaine anesthetics has also been described. Encapsulation appears to increase the duration of action of each of these compounds by a factor of 2 to 3.[37, 38]

Another innovative concept is the use of a biodegradable polymer matrix as a carrier for local anesthetics. Cylindrical pellets have been developed with bupivacaine hydrochloride and implanted along the sciatic nerve in the rat. The results have demonstrated sensorimotor blockade that lasts between 2 and 6 days.[39] Nonbiodegradable polymers are also currently under investigation for sustained delivery of various analgesic compounds. Sustained-release of local anesthetics may provide adequate analgesia with smaller doses of opioids.

SUMMARY

Nonopioid intrathecal analgesics remain in the vanguard of pain management as we enter the 21st century. They are important alternatives to opioids for treatment of chronic cancer pain and other pain. Clonidine is currently commercially available in the United States, both as a liquid preparation and, now, a preservative-free powder. Clonidine remains clinically useful and is palliative for approximately 50% to 60% of patients who do not respond favorably to opioids.

There is the potential for various combinations of intrathecal analgesic agents, as they would allow the pain specialist to customize medications to the specific type, quality, and location of an individual patient's pain.

Several issues must be emphasized with regard to the intrathecal administration of pain medication (Table 61–

TABLE 61–3 Six Criteria for Successful Intrathecal Drug Clinical Availability

Proven antinociceptive effect
Safe based on animal toxicology studies
Drug must be stable both in shelf solution and at body temperature
Must be compatible with long-term spinal infusion pump
Sufficiently high potency and solubility in drug preparation
A pharmaceutical company must be willing to develop commercially

3). Efficacy of pain relief is obviously the most important, and the first, step. Equally important, however, are the short-term and long-term effects on the spinal cord and potential toxicities. The stability of an individual drug or of a combination of drugs in the spinal fluid must be researched. Compatibility with implantable pump delivery systems is an area that must be investigated. The aforementioned issues, however, should first be examined in the laboratory and in animal models. These issues should be carefully translated into protocols that can be incorporated into human trials. To be practical for clinical use, the drug must have sufficient potency and solubility to be useful in the finite volume of an implanted infusion pump. Finally, there must be some hope of commercial development of the drug, (i.e., a pharmaceutical company willing to pursue full F.D.A. approval). In the United States, researchers need to work under F.D.A. approval to help to identify potentially successful medications that might ultimately become commercially available.

This background of research and knowledge, coupled with the many compounds currently in development for intrathecal analgesia, will ultimately provide this field with numerous opportunities to develop commercially available analgesic agents that will, indeed, make a difference.

REFERENCES

1. Goldstein A, Lowney LI, Pal PK: Stereospecific and nonspecific interactions of the morphine congenitor levorphanol in subcellular fractions of mouse brain. Proc Natl Acad Sci USA 68:1742–1747, 1971.
2. Pert C, Snyder S: Opiate receptor: Demonstration in nerve tissue. Science 48:1011–1014, 1973.
3. Kuhar MH, Pert CB, Snyder SH: Regional distribution and opiate receptor binding in monkey and human brain. Nature 245:447–450, 1973.
4. Lamotte C, Pert CB, Snyder SH: Opiate receptor binding primate spinal: Distribution and change after dorsal root section. Brain Res 11:407–412, 1976.
5. Paice A, Penn R: Intraspinal morphine for chronic pain: A retrospective multicentered study. J Pain Symptom Manage 11:71–80, 1996.
6. Hardy P, Wells JC: Continuous intrathecal lidocaine infusion analgesia: A case report of a nine week spinal. Pallative Med 3:23–25, 1989.
7. Sjoberg M, et al: Long-term intrathecal morphine and bupivacine in "refractory" cancer pain. Results from the first series of 52 patients. Acta Anaesth Scand 35:30–43, 1991.
8. Berde CB, et al: Subarachnoid bupivacaine analgesia for seven months for a patient with a spinal cord tumor. Anesthesiology 72:1094–1096, 1990.
9. Krames ES, Lanning RM: Intrathecal infusional analgesia for nonmalignant pain: Analgesic efficacy of intrathecal opioid with or without bupivacaine. J Pain Symptom Manage 8(8):539–548, 1993.
10. Appelgren L, et al: Continuous intracisternal and high cervical intrathecal bupivacaine analgesia in refractory head and neck pain. Anesthesiology 84:256–272, 1996.
11. Hinnerk W, et al: The stability of mixtures of morphine hydrochloride, bupivacaine chloride, and clonidine hydrochloride in portable pump reservoirs for the management of chronic pain syndromes. J Pain Symptom Manage 9:308–311, 1994.
12. Smith MD, et al: Antinociceptive effect of spinal cholinergic stimulation: Interaction with substance P. Life Science 45(14):1255–1261, 1989.
13. Bouaziz H, et al: Postoperative analgesia from intrathecal neostigmine in sheep. Anesth Analg 80(6):1140–1144, 1995.
14. Yaksh TL, et al: Intraspinal Drugs. Anesthesiology 82(2):412–427, 1995.
15. Hood DD, et al: Phase I safety assessment of intrathecal neostigmine methylsulfate in humans. Anesthesiology 82(2):331–343, 1995.
16. Winnie AP, et al: Subarachnoid adrenal medullary transplants for terminal cancer pain. A report of preliminary studies. Anesthesiology 79(4):644–653, 1993.
17. Wu HH, et al: Antinociception following implantation of mouse B16 melanoma cells in mouse and rat spinal cord. Pain 56(2):203–210, 1994.
18. Siddall SD, et al: Intrathecal clonidine and the management of spinal cord injury pain: A case report. Pain 59:147–148, 1994.
19. Wulf H, et al: The stability of mixtures of morphine hydrochloride, bupivacaine hydrochloride, and clonidine hydrochloride in portable pump reservoirs for the management of chronic pain syndromes. J Pain Symptom Manage 9:308–311, 1994.
20. Coombs DW, Saunders RL, Fratkin JD, et al: Continuous intrathecal hydromorphone and clonidine for intractable cancer pain. J Neurosurg 64(6):890–894, 1986.
21. Coombs DW, Saunders RL, Lachance D, et al: Intrathecal morphine tolerance: Use of intrathecal clonidine, DADLE, and intraventricular morphine. Anesthesiology 62(3):358–363, 1985.
22. Malinovsky JM, Lepage JY, Cozian A, et al: Intrathecal clonidine as sole anesthetic agent for surgery. Reg Anesth 18:(Suppl):15. 1993.
23. Filos KS, Goudas LC, Patroni O, Polyzou V: Dose-related hemodynamic and analgesic effects of intrathecal clonidine after cesarean section. Reg Anesth 18:(Suppl):18. 1993.
24. Van Essen EJ, Bovill JG, Ploeger EJ, Beerman H: Intrathecal morphine and clonidine for control of intractable cancer pain: A case report. Acta Anaesthesiol Belg 39(2):109–112, 1988.
25. Fibuch EE: Uncommon applications for continuous spinal anesthesia. Regional Anesth 18(6):419–423, 1993.
26. Abram SE: Continuous spinal anesthesia for cancer and chronic pain. Regional Anesth 18(6):406–413, 1993.
27. Rouck RL et al: Epidural clonidine treatment for refractory reflex sympathetic dystrophy. Anesthesiology 80(5):1181–1182, 1994.
28. Yang CY: Intrathecal ketamine reduces morphine requirements in patients with terminal cancer pain. Can J Anesth 43(4):379–383, 1996.
29. Kristensen JD, et al: The NMDA-receptor antagonist CPP abolishes neurogenic 'wind-up pain' after intrathecal administration in humans. Pain 51(2):249–253, 1992.
30. Hassenbusch SJ, Satterfield WC, Gradert TL, et al: Preclinical toxicity study of intrathecal administration of the pain-relievers dextrorphan, dextromethorphan and memantine in the sheep model. Neuromodulation 1999 (In press).
31. Mollenholt P, et al: Intrathecal and epidural somatostatin for patients with cancer. Analgesic effects and postmortem neuropathologic investigations of spinal cord and nerve roots. Anesthesiology 81:534–542, 1994.
32. Penn RD, et al: Octreotide: A potent new non-opioid analgesic for intrathecal infusion. Pain 51(2):261–262, 1992.
33. Penn RD: Intrathecal octreotide for cancer pain. Lancet 335 (8691):738, 1990.
34. Malmberg AB, Yaksh TL: Effect of continuous intrathecal infusion of omega-conopeptides, N-type calcium-channel blockers, on behavior and antinociception in the formalin and hot-plate tests in rats. Pain 60(1):83–90, 1995.
35. Hersh EV, et al: Anesthetic activity of the lipospheres bupivacaine delivery system in the rat. Anesth Progr 39(6):197–200, 1993.
36. Boogaerts JG, et al: Epidural administration of liposome-associated bupivacaine for the management of postsurgical pain: A first study. J Clin Anesthesiol 6(4):315–320, 1994.
37. Langerman L, et al: Prolongation of spinal anesthesia. Differential action of a lipid drug carrier on tetracaine, lidocaine, and procaine. Anesthesiology 77:475–481, 1992.
38. Langerman L, et al: Spinal anesthesia: Significant prolongation of the pharmacologic effect of tetracaine with lipid solution of the agent. Anesthesiology 74(1):105–197, 1991.
39. Masters DB, et al: Prolonged regional nerve blockade by controlled release of local anesthetic from biodegradable polymer matrix. Anesthesiology 79(2):340–346, 1993.

CHAPTER • 62

Tunneled Epidural Catheters: Practical Considerations and Implantation Techniques

Stuart L. Du Pen, MD • Anna Du Pen, ARNP, MN

Intraspinal opioid analgesia represents a major advance in the management of pain.[1-10] The intraspinal delivery of opioids adds a new dimension to opioid therapy by allowing prolonged analgesia through the use of significantly lower doses than those required for systemic administration. Intraspinal opioid analgesia gained immediate popularity in the management of both postoperative and obstetric pain; however, owing to the late introduction of suitable long-term implantable drug delivery systems, the use of intraspinal analgesia for the treatment of cancer and nonmalignant pain has lagged behind. The introduction and ongoing research into new epidural and intraspinal drugs has enhanced interest in epidural analgesia.

Epidural percutaneous catheters have long been utilized for the administration of local anesthetics for surgical and obstetric anesthesia. With the advent of spinal opioid analgesia, the use of these short-term percutaneous catheters was extended to the administration of intraspinal opioids to provide analgesia for the immediate postoperative period. The clinical results of this application were so encouraging that these temporary epidural catheters were placed through short subcutaneous tunnels to improve their stability and durability. This allowed the pain specialist to provide prolonged postoperative analgesia.[4] Zenz[11] reported a technique of catheter fixation that further extended the useful life of the temporary epidural catheter. This technique was successful in maintaining some catheters as long as 1.5 years for the management of cancer-related pain.[11] Maintaining temporary catheters for long-term use is an ongoing problem for clinicians. Tape and dressings used for fixation of the catheters have improved over time, but dislodgement and local infections at the exit site remain limiting factors for a long-term solution.

In 1981, Poletti and associates[12] reported successful placement of silicone rubber Broviac catheters using a laminectomy to gain permanent access to the epidural space.[12] The required laminectomy and the duration of postoperative recovery limited the usefulness of the technique. Racz and colleagues[8] introduced a silicone-coated, wire-reinforced epidural catheter in 1982, which for the first time allowed accurate percutaneous placement of a nonreactive catheter. In 1986, a silicone rubber epidural catheter, modeled after the Hickman catheter, was introduced by Du Pen for long-term use in the epidural space.[6] The Du Pen catheter featured a Dacron cuff for fixation and later a Vitacuff for antimicrobial protection. In 1991, Yue and coworkers[13] reported experience with a new epidural catheter that combined a Racz epidural catheter and a silicone rubber segment for subcutaneous tunneling. The technology was further advanced by the introduction in 1993 of a subcutaneously implanted port system. The anesthesiologist today has a choice of several devices to access the epidural space for either short- or long-term implantation. The selection of the device is usually based on the expected duration of use and whether bolus or continuous infusions will be used.

WHERE THE TUNNELED EPIDURAL CATHETER FITS ON THE CONTINUUM OF PAIN TREATMENT MODALITIES

Cancer-related pain and some pain states not related to cancer may require interventional pain management techniques to achieve functional analgesia. The decision to consider interventional techniques is based on failure to achieve functional analgesia after maximization of oral opioid analgesia with the development of unacceptable side effects. Neuropathic pain is generally less responsive to aggressive opioid analgesia and usually requires the use of adjunctive analgesics. Opioid analgesia should be tried first, before interventional procedures are considered. Continuous pain assessment allows for continuous fine tuning of pain management techniques and drug choices to ensure optimal pain relief. Pain assessment should include not only the pain intensity, which dictates dosages of opioids, but both pain character and pain pattern, which drive the decision process in determining both adjunctive drugs and the use of short-acting opioids.

The medical management of intractable pain should follow the World Health Organization (WHO) ladder for cancer pain relief, using continuous pain assessment and aggressive treatment of side effects to optimize therapy.[14–17] The intensity of pain is determined from the patient's rating of pain on a scale from 1 to 10. Pain intensity drives the choice of opioid therapy. The use of long-acting opioids (LAO) to control constant pain and short-acting opioids (SAO) for episodic pain is driven by the pattern of pain. LAO and sustained-release opioids are used to treat continuous pain, whereas the rapid-acting and SAO are used to treat episodic pain. Before consideration is given to a tunneled epidural catheter, patients suffering from cancer-related pain should be treated aggressively with standard therapies, and optimization of systemic opioid therapy utilizing sustained-release opioid preparations with rescue doses of SAO to control episodic pain. Intravenous and subcutaneous infusions with patient-controlled analgesia capability are also appropriate modalities in the initial management of cancer pain. Patients receiving traditional opioid therapy who either do not achieve analgesia or experience side effects that do not respond to appropriate treatment may require more invasive analgesic techniques. Invasive techniques should be considered carefully and thoughtfully before one is implemented. The practice of intraspinal analgesia is not limited to the placement of an intraspinal device. The "art" of intraspinal analgesia begins with appropriate patient and device selection.

Pain assessment, with particular attention to the character of the pain, is a critical component of the early diagnosis.[3, 17–20] Intensity of pain, pain character, and pain pattern identification allow the clinician more completely to determine the severity and potential response to therapy of a specific kind of pain. The choice of a delivery system is based on many factors, including the expected duration of therapy, pain sources, and planned drug therapy. Both subarachnoid drug delivery systems and tunneled epidural catheters have distinct advantages and disadvantages.[1, 5, 6, 9, 10, 20, 21] Implantation of an epidural catheter may be as simple as placement of a temporary catheter at the patient's bedside or as complicated as operative placement of a totally implantable drug delivery system in the surgical suite.[5, 6, 9, 12, 13, 22, 23] The importance of appropriate patient and device selection and of technical mastery of implantation cannot be overstated. Ongoing management of patients after implantation of a drug delivery system is equally important; therefore, educating the patient and family in the techniques of epidural catheter care and drug administration is paramount to the long-term success of implantable drug delivery systems.[24] Close patient follow-up with frequent reassessment and timely dose and drug adjustments is also essential. A strong outpatient clinic and home care component to the program help to ensure good outcomes.

This chapter contains a comprehensive discussion of the issues commonly encountered by clinicians managing tunneled epidural catheters. Patient and device selection, implantation, epidurograms, and postoperative care are described. Content covering clinical monitoring, dose adjustment, home care, and complications is intended to assist the clinician in the treatment phase of the practice.

PATIENT SELECTION

General Considerations

A comprehensive consultation and assessment of the patient can greatly affect the successful outcome of treatment and patient and provider satisfaction with the technique. The American Pain Society[25] and the Agency for Health Care Policy and Research of the U.S. Public Health Service[26] have developed clinical practice guidelines, professional and public education, and quality assurance mechanisms to define and evaluate the appropriate use of "high-tech" therapies.[25, 26]

Seven areas are important to explore in considering appropriate patient selection criteria for long-term epidural opioid analgesia:

- Presence of pain despite aggressive systemic opioid therapy
- Presence of treatment-resistant side effects
- Presence of significant neuropathic and/or incident pain
- Pain pattern (particularly mild baseline pain with severe episodic pain)
- Patient/caregiver ability to manage the technology
- A successful trial of epidural analgesia
- Ruling out of neurodestructive blocks and surgery as options

Intractable Pain

Moderate to severe pain that persists despite aggressive dosing of conventional systemic opioids and adjuvant drugs is considered *intractable*. It is important to remember that, in general, there is no "ceiling" for oral opioids and that persistent pain may be the result of failure to maximize opioid therapy, to treat side effects, or to combine opioids with appropriate adjuvant drugs. More recent research indicates that in some cases high doses of systemic opioids (either directly or via metabolites) can be toxic, most often by causing hyperalgesia or myoclonic activity. These situations are clearly indications for spinal delivery to achieve dose reduction. Moderate side effects should be treated to allow optimal use of systemic opioid analgesics, and some severe side effects may require a sequential trial of opioids for relief.[16] Pain patterns include constant, constant with breakthrough, and episodic pain. *Episodic pain* is pain of sudden onset, and often short duration, that can be motion related. The pain's character (neuropathic, somatic, visceral, mixed) is important in choosing adjunctive drug therapy and epidural drug therapy. Examples of syndromes of episodic pain are pain associated with pathologic fractures, nerve root impingement by tumor, and plexopathy-associated pain. In the majority of patients suffering from this type of pain, relief can be achieved with the skillful use of an immediate-release oral opioid for the incident-related events. The best possible use should be made of adjuvant analgesics before resorting to invasive therapy.

The use of nonsteroidal antiinflammatory drugs (NSAIDs) for the treatment of metastatic bone pain and tricyclic antidepressants and anticonvulsant therapy for neuropathic pain is well-established in the literature.[27] These adjuvant therapies may be effective enough to obviate or delay the need for invasive therapy. Gabapentin has gained widespread use as an adjuvant drug for neuropathic pain. Minimal side effects and proven efficacy have led to its widespread use.

Management of Side Effects

Patients with a history of persistent side effects from systemic opioid therapy may be considered for long-term epidural opioid therapy. Patients with proven opioid sensitivity and unmanageable side effects can benefit from the relatively smaller amount of drug that reaches the central nervous system with epidural opioid therapy than with the systemic route of administration. Sedation, nausea, and vomiting are common severe side effects of systemic opioids that often resolve after a period of stable dosing and side effect treatment. Persistent sedation can be managed with stimulant drugs, including coffee and tea. Methylphenidate in daily doses ranging from 5 to 30 mg can reverse drowsiness. Strong antiemetics should be given routinely for 48 to 72 hours for opioid-related nausea. Sequential trials of other opioids should first be conducted before systemic opioid therapy is abandoned and an interventional technique attempted. Constipation frequently accompanies opioid therapy and must be managed with regular bowel care. Some authors recommend that the doses of stool softener and laxative be adjusted according to the dose of opioid, but any clinician prescribing opioids should always address the issue of constipation (i.e., 1 stool softener for each 30 mg of oral morphine).[27] Maximizing and individualizing systemic therapy is an important prerequisite, but, when pain or side effects nevertheless persist, the intraspinal route should be considered.

Patient and Caregiver Support

The patient's and caregiver's ability to cope with the technology and perform tasks associated with drug administration must be considered. For any patient expecting to function independently and return home, this criterion takes priority over the other issues. For example, patients may have functional handicaps such as chemotherapy-induced peripheral neuropathy in the hands and fingers, which may limit their ability to care for a delivery system. Hygiene is an important consideration. For example, a patient with a colostomy who fails to consistently observe hygienic practices is a poor candidate for an implantable drug delivery system. The patient's cognitive function may be an issue. Mental retardation or changes in cognitive function may lead to impairment in the patient's ability to take oral medication to control pain. The level of cognitive deficit may not require assistance in daily living, yet the patient may not be able to take SAO pain medication safely without over using it. Implantable devices, may allow these patients to achieve consistent functional analgesia without the risk of overdose. Patients with a history of drug abuse may respond in a similar way.

A caregiver partner is very desirable if an externalized drug delivery system is being considered. The absence of a proficient caregiver should prompt the practitioner to consider a totally implantable system or, in some cases, to completely reconsider the use of the spinal route. A partner to help monitor care, assist in maintaining aseptic technique, and assume responsibility for drug administration if the patient should become less functional enhances the likelihood of a good outcome. The responsibilities and potential strain on this person should be discussed and factored into the decision. Some family members may be reluctant to undertake such responsibilities. Other caregivers are often eager and willing to do whatever they can to help their loved ones obtain pain relief. Early identification and incorporation of a caregiver helps to ensure a good postdischarge course. In this world of managed care, authorization must be obtained before considering implantation and infusions. These procedures are expensive and require long-term care. Most insurers approve the devices when prior approval is requested.

Nonmalignant Pain: Special Considerations for Patient Selection

Patients suffering from nonmalignant pain require special consideration. In general, these patients are best treated with a multidisciplinary approach. The treatment team need to evaluate each candidate in the following areas: (1) coping mechanisms and psychological stability, (2) potential for drug abuse or misuse, (3) opioid-responsive pain syndrome, and (4) expected length of drug therapy. Long-term opioid therapy should be used cautiously in patients with significant concurrent psychosocial deficits. Preliminary data and clinical experience suggest that patients with chronic nonmalignant pain who demonstrate successful coping skills can be treated with opioid therapy. A structured treatment and follow-up plan, designed with the patient as an active participant, should be established and then monitored regularly. The use of a treatment plan with an opioid treatment contract gives the practitioner and the patient a clear understanding of expectations for both as treatment progresses. Nonmalignant pain patients are good candidates for long-term opioid pain treatment when expectations are well outlined.

Preliminary data and clinical experience suggest that intraspinal opioids may be considered for patients with opioid-responsive nonmalignant pain who are likely to need long-term therapy.[28] This determination should be based on a risk-benefit analysis, by which the benefits are determined by a trial of intraspinal opioid. A typical trial of therapy utilizes a temporary epidural or intrathecal catheter to deliver intraspinal analgesic. The duration of the test period is determined by the response of the patient to therapy. If an intrathecal delivery system is being considered, measurable changes in pain intensity, use of pain medication, and/or improved functional capacity should be demonstrated. The tools used to determine functional capacity have been developed for injured workers but have not been adapted to patients with cancer-pain or to disabled patients. Therefore their application in this population requires practitioners to develop their own tools. The best tool seems to be a determination of what the patient *cannot do* before the test as compared with their capabilities at its end. It is important to get the patient out of the hospital or clinic environment to determine the efficacy of the technique instead of using a bolus test in that environment. Cost-effectiveness of interventional procedures needs to be addressed; however, no good tools are available to apply to this clinical situation that give a reliable and realistic picture of the cost or cost-benefit ratio of aggressive pain management.

Clinical applications of tunneled epidural catheters in the control of nonmalignant pain include the use of these catheters for intermediate- and long-term treatment. Intermediate-duration treatment may be applied for testing for intrathecal pump placement, treatment of moderate-duration pain states, and clinical problems for which precise catheter tip placement allows short-term targeted therapy. Pain associated with compression fractures from osteoporosis or secondary to long-term steroid therapy can be treated with short-term epidural infusions of opioid, with or without bupivacaine. With relief of pain, affected patients can be mobilized, facilitating the healing of the fractures, which in turn effectively eliminates the pain source and the need for the epidural catheter. Cervical and thoracic compression fractures may require precise catheter tip placement, which may not be achievable using temporary catheters. A long-term opioid-responsive pain syndrome (i.e., longer than 6 months) should prompt the clinician to consider a totally implantable drug delivery system.[29] Implanted pump placement is probably more cost-effective and theoretically carries a lower risk of infection.[29]

In general, owing to the risk of infection and the cost associated with epidural infusions, externalized devices should be reserved for use of short or intermediate duration.[30] Preliminary studies from Europe indicate that externalized subarachnoid catheters may be used safely for long-term pain therapy,[31–33] but these reports are few and require replication and validation before any meaningful conclusions may be drawn.

The Preimplantation Assessment

Patient Factors

The preoperative assessment provides the clinician valuable information about pain intensity and character, the patient's physical status, and status of the epidural space. These patient-specific data are necessary for proper device selection and implantation. The targeted pain history, physical examination, radiographic examination, and chart review contribute to the comprehensive preoperative pain assessment. This assessment incorporates the patient's report of pain character, intensity, location, and temporal quality. The character of pain provides important information that can affect catheter positioning and drug choices.[17, 19, 20, 33–35] Motion-related or incident pain is analyzed, because it plays a role in treatment planning. This critical self-report information is then correlated with findings of the physical examination. Skin anesthesia, motor function, and reflexes are determined to assess cord function. Patient-reported assessment data, physical findings, and radiographic studies are analyzed together to establish a relationship between objective and subjective findings. This preoperative assessment is critical for implantation planning as well as general treatment outlook.

Pain Assessment

Patient report of pain intensity is the best clinical measure available to the practitioner. Pain levels should be recorded in consistent, objective terms in all hospital records, giving hospital personnel an outcome measure of treatment response. The visual analogue scale (VAS), which has been shown to be a reproducible and accurate representation of pain intensity, is the standard for pain intensity reporting in publications and research projects.[14, 36] The patient verbal numeric rating scale (0–10 or 0–5), which is more practical for clinical use, has been shown to be an accurate representation of pain intensity as compared with the VAS.[14, 36] This scale incorporates the use of colors or words with the numeric scale to give patients an alternative method of measuring their pain. This tool allows the clinicians to record and compare an accurate report of the patient's pain intensity over time and should become a common language for pain-related record keeping in all settings (hospital, clinic, home care). Consistent use of a standard assessment format allows clinicians to communicate accurately the intensity of a patient's pain for ongoing evaluation of analgesic management.

Mental Status

Mental status evaluation is another important factor in device selection and implantation. Cognitive performance allows an estimation of the patient's self-care capability. The patient may be incapable of self-care after discharge and may require home care support or a skilled nursing facility. Strong family or caregiver support facilitates successful home care, and those whose support is inadequate often must be placed in a nursing facility. Some nursing facilities do not accept patients receiving epidural analgesia, possibly a limitation on the patient's options for postdischarge care. This problem can usually be corrected through education of caregivers at the nursing facilities. The patient's psychosocial status is equally important to address. Routine use of psychological consultation should be entertained for patients who are deemed to be implantation candidates. Tunneled catheters are less invasive and may not require consultation in all patients, but the clinician should be aware of the psychosocial impact of any implantation.

Laboratory Parameters

The patient's general preoperative status merits review. Hematology and chemistry profiles with a comparative record review help to avoid intraoperative problems. Radiation therapy and chemotherapy may result in bone marrow suppression, which may increase the risk of infection or intraoperative bleeding into the epidural space. Most reports of postoperative epidural hematoma formation are associated with surgery and procedures being done while patients are taking anticoagulants. Most recently, the use of oral heparin preparations have been associated with spinal cord compression. A survey of the patient's preoperative medication is important. Coagulation ratios below 1.2 are not considered suitable for operative candidates. Platelet counts below 30,000 are common and may be associated with increased operative bleeding.[3] Rather than assigning a specific platelet count as a minimum for elective surgery, the quality of the platelets must be determined by obtaining a coagulation screening or by performing a simple Lee-White whole blood clotting time at the bedside.[3] This information helps the clinician to ascertain the actual risk of bleeding complications. Electrolyte studies determine the patient's renal and general metabolic status and anesthetic risks.

Anesthesia and Patient Positioning

Anesthetic risk is often a major concern, because a majority of cancer patients have extensive multisystem disease. The implantation is normally accomplished with local anesthesia with intravenous sedation and monitored anesthesia care. Some patients require general anesthesia because of pain secondary to pathologic fractures or direct invasion of tumor. For example, breast cancer patients may have extensive skin or chest wall invasion that makes lateral positioning painful. A position of comfort and safety, with support for all extremities, allows less anesthetic and more patient comfort.

Infection

The risk of infection associated with long-term externalized epidural catheterization is not only real but predictable.[30, 37] In our experience, patients with gastrointestinal tumors and enterostomies appear to have a higher incidence of epidural infections. Patients with systemic infections or chronic cutaneous infections also appear to be at higher risk. The path of the tunneled catheter should be planned to limit the risk of infection by avoiding stomas and other devices (e.g., percutaneous endoscopic gastrostomy, [PEG], nephrostomy). Risk of infection must be weighed against the benefits of epidural analgesia for each patient, because there may be no alternative therapies.[30, 37, 38] The use of a double-filter technique, in our experience, has decreased the rate of epidural infections to less than 1%. The inner filter is never changed unless damaged, and the outer filter and pump tubing are changed only once a month. This protects the patient from contamination of the infusion solution during bag changes.[39]

Assessment of the Epidural Space

Preimplantation assessment of all patients should include a complete neurologic examination and review of relevant previous radiologic studies and scans.[16] The placement of an epidural catheter without radiographic guidance is acceptable in patients suffering from postoperative pain or for those with cancer pain when significant spinal metastatic disease is unlikely. In cancer patients with epidural space compromise from severe vertebral compression or tumor invasion, preimplantation assessment of the epidural space by computed tomography, magnetic resonance imaging, myelography, or epidurography should be strongly considered. These studies help to determine the best epidural entry site and the optimal terminus for the catheter tip. The correlation of pain symptoms with the neurologic findings assists with future estimates of analgesic requirements.[40] If no pain sources have been identified, further studies are required to determine the source of the pain (i.e., new metastatic sites or acute disc disease). Additional diagnostic studies, such as electromyography, discography, and myelography, may be indicated, but cost and patient discomfort should be considered. A simple spine film may be adequate to identify extension of metastatic sites or new acute vertebral compression.[41]

The risk of passing an epidural catheter through areas of epidural compromise (secondary to tumor or another lesion), have to be considered[42]; however, disease in the spinal canal is not necessarily a contraindication to epidural catheterization. The majority of metastatic lesions in the spinal column are located in vertebral bodies. The epidural catheter position is generally in the dorsal epidural space, away from vertebral body tumors. Epidural invasion (without cord compression) can be effectively "bypassed," to avoid complications and loss of analgesia. When obstruction of the epidural space is evident, entry into the epidural canal and anticipated location of the catheter tip may require modification. In patients with significant epidural space obstruction from tumor (multiple myeloma, epidural melanoma) the catheters may need to be placed above and below the area of tumor involvement to achieve adequate analgesia. Patients with extensive epidural space involvement may benefit from intrathecal catheter placement.[5, 38, 43–45]

Location of Catheter Placement

Once the epidural space has been assessed, the location of the epidural entry site and catheter tip can be planned. The character of the pain (neuropathic, somatic, visceral) may further modify the catheter tip location.[19] Neuropathic pain requires the catheter tip to be near the affected dermatomal level to allow effective use of local anesthetic agents or clonidine through the catheter.[46] Visceral pain usually responds to opioids alone, and thus, catheter tip location can be less of an issue.[34, 47, 48]

Selection of the Tunneling Path

The viability and comfort of the tunneled catheter track depend on the condition of the skin over the catheter tunnel and the depth of the tunnel. Changes in the skin blood supply due to radiation, previous surgery, and tumor invasion all influence location of the catheter track. Nephrostomies, gastrostomies, and enterostomies must be considered potential sources of infection that are to be avoided. A distant thoracic catheter exit site may be selected to protect the tunneled catheter from possible contamination. The placement of the catheter tunnel must be planned as carefully as the placement of the epidural catheter tip. The patient's body image, sexual activity, age, vision compromise, and limitations of dexterity may further influence the placement of the catheter track and exit site. In some cases, patient preference may determine the exit site.

DEVICE SELECTION

Selection of implantable drug delivery systems is much influenced by the clinician's experience, training, and personal preference and, to a lesser degree, by the medical literature. Well-designed, randomized clinical trials are desperately needed to evaluate the various access devices for efficacy, safety, and cost. Bedder and colleagues[29] attempted to compare costs of permanent exteriorized epidural catheters and subarachnoid pump systems. Carefully controlled studies are needed to give the clinician a clear algorithm for device selection.[14, 49]

Preoperative assessment of the patient, including expected prognosis or expected duration of care, home care support, and outcome expectations, is important to device selection.[24, 50, 51] Decisions about a temporary or permanent epidural catheter, the best catheter exit site, and the ideal catheter tip position are based on a comprehensive evaluation.[52] Patients who are likely to remain in the hospital can easily be treated with temporary epidural catheters. Patients expected to be discharged home for prolonged treatment may better be treated with a permanent epidural catheter. Patients receiving epidural local anesthetic or alpha$_2$-agonist infusions may also be better served with a permanent device because of the risk of migration of temporary catheters.[53, 54]

Temporary Epidural Catheters

Temporary catheters designed for short-term use are generally made of inexpensive materials that can easily be passed into the epidural space. Polytetrafluoroethylene catheters allow visualization of aspirated fluid but eventually become stiff and may migrate into the intravascular or subarachnoid spaces.[53] Nylon catheters may induce a significant tissue reaction when used for long periods.[32] Polyurethane and polyamide catheters produce the least tissue reaction and maintain enough rigidity to be passed through a needle into the epidural space.[32] Table 62–1 lists some of the commercially available temporary epidural catheters by material.

The increased utilization of epidural catheters in the management of postoperative pain led many manufacturers to search for less reactive and softer materials. Coupled with this search was an effort to correct the ongoing problem of failure of the catheter adapter or connector. A connector may become dislodged or the catheter may break near a connector. Tunneling a temporary catheter may add stability, but the durability of both catheter and connector are major determinants of the catheter's suitability for long-term use.[52]

Permanent Epidural Access Devices

Currently two long-term epidural devices are commercially available and approved by the U.S. Food and Drug Administration (FDA)—the Du Pen silicone rubber epidural catheter and the Port-A-Cath epidural port system.[6] Other products are in development and still others are being sold commercially that have not received FDA approval for long-term use (S.K. Yue, personal communication, 1994). Table 62–1 also lists some of the commercially available permanent epidural catheters by catheter material.

TABLE 62–1 **Commercially Available Epidural Catheters**

Material	Manufacturer
Temporary catheters	
Polyurethane	Arrow International, Inc., Reading, Pa.
	Abbott Laboratories, North Chicago, Ill.
	Pharmacia Deltec, Inc., St. Paul, Minn.
Nylon	Concord/Portex, Keene, NH
Polytetrafluoroethylene	Abbott Laboratories, North Chicago, Ill.
Polyamide	B. Braun Medical, Inc., Bethlehem, Pa.
	Abbott Laboratories, North Chicago, Ill.
Permanent catheters	
Silicone rubber	CR Bard, Inc., Salt Lake City, Ut.
Du Pen catheter	
Silicone rubber–coated	
SKY catheter	PMT, Inc., Chanhassen, Minn.
Polyurethane epidural port catheter system	
Port-A-Cath	Pharmacia Deltec, Inc., St. Paul, Minn.

As for a temporary epidural catheter, the selection of a long-term device is based on clinical experience, clinician and patient preferences, and reported complications associated with each device.[37] There are basically two similar externalized, tunneled catheters and a totally implanted epidural Port-A-Cath system.[37, 55, 56] Device selection can be based on the same criteria used to determine selection of vascular access devices. Long-term intermittent use favors the Port-A-Cath system, whereas continuous infusion favors externalized systems. Infection rates for externalized and port systems have not been adequately studied.[37] In the future, better data on the incidence of infection with each type will allow accurate assessment of the risk-benefit ratio.

CONSIDERATIONS PRIOR TO IMPLANTATION

The implantation of a permanent epidural catheter is a simple surgical procedure within the capability of most pain specialists. Assistance by a surgeon may be helpful for the first few implantations when the specialist is not comfortable with the surgical techniques required.

Preoperative antibiotics are commonly given to most patients receiving implanted devices. Standard therapy includes administration of a broad-spectrum antibiotic 1 hour before surgery and two doses 8 hours apart postoperatively.[6] The implantation technique described utilizes the Du Pen catheter, although the techniques for the other implantable devices are very similar. The clinician should review the instructions supplied by the manufacturer before

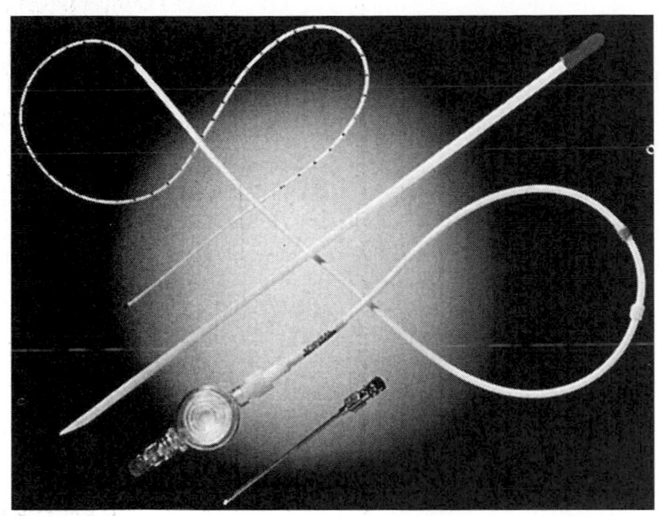

FIGURE 62–1 Permanent catheter tray supplies. The Du Pen catheter kit includes the two-part catheter, needle, connector, wire stylet, and filter. (C.R. Bard, Salt Lake City, Ut.)

proceeding. The Du Pen catheter is constructed from radiopaque silicone rubber with an obstructed distal tip and five side-holes for gentle infusion of drug into the epidural space. The barium content of the catheter allows visualization of the catheter over the vertebra, without the use of contrast medium.[6] The tunneled portion of the catheter has a Dacron cuff for anchoring by tissue ingrowth and a Vitacuff as an antibacterial barrier.[57] The two-part catheter and connector system is designed to allow a single catheter set to be adapted to all patients. The system kit contains the catheter (small-diameter epidural catheter and larger tunneled catheter), a polytetrafluoroethylene-coated flexible wire stylet, needle, tunneling device, connector, and filter (Fig. 62–1). The surgical instrumentation required for epidural catheter implantation is contained in a small plastic surgery set. Surgical assistance from both a circulating nurse and a scrub nurse is desirable. Radiographic guidance via a C-arm fluoroscopy unit may aid in placement of the proximal catheter. Full sterile surgical precautions should be taken with all implantation procedures, including skin preparation, drapes, and sterile surgical gown and gloves.

IMPLANTATION

Patient Positioning and Operative Preparation

The lateral patient position is used for catheter placement to allow both the posterior incision and the tunneling of the catheter to the anterior abdominal wall without repositioning. Individual patients may require modification of the position to satisfy special needs and personal preferences for catheter tunnel and exit sites. During the preoperative assessment, the optimal catheter tip position is determined, along with the level of the epidural space entry and the location of the catheter exit site. Left or right lateral position is selected, according to whether the patient is left-handed or right-handed. The patient is placed in a "tuck" position with the knees drawn up to a 110-degree angle with the trunk, which still allows easy access to the upper abdominal wall. The arms are supported and angled upward to allow free access to the abdominal wall for the catheter exit site. Arm boards are not used unless required because of the patient's size, as they can obstruct the free use of the C-arm fluoroscopic unit. Two pillows are placed between the legs to prevent rotation of the thoracic spine. The operating table should be positioned to allow easy access for the C-arm for use in two planes while maintaining the sterile field. This can be accomplished in a small surgical suite by positioning the table parallel to the outer door of the operating room with the surgical field away from the doors (Fig. 62–2). The patient is prepared and draped with a transverse drape to expose the surgical site, catheter tunnel, and exit site with a single drape. An adhesive 50-cm sterile drape is used to secure the drapes along the planned tunnel track and maintain a sterile visible surgical field.

The Surgical Procedure

The incision is made perpendicular and lateral to the dorsal spine, 2 to 3 cm long, and down into the subcutaneous fat but not into the paraspinous muscle fascia. A pocket is created in the subcutaneous fat by blunt dissection. The

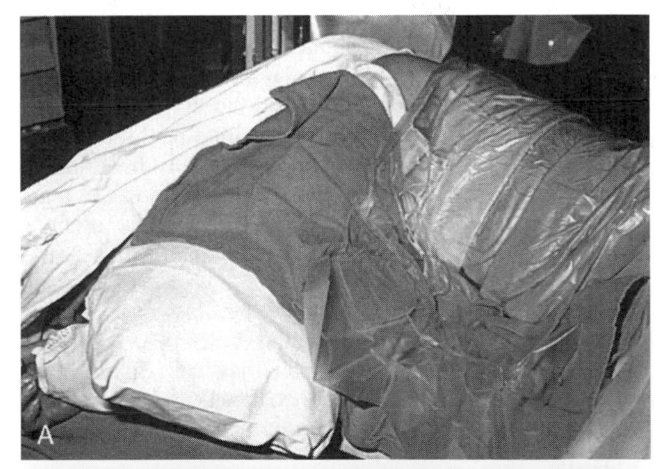

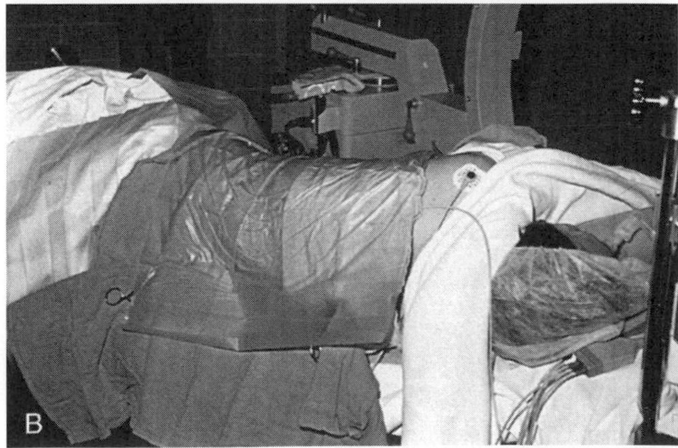

FIGURE 62–2 Patient position, sterile drapes, and room setup for surgery. A, Front view; B, Back view. The lateral position with adhesive drapes allows surgical access to both the posterior incision and the exit site.

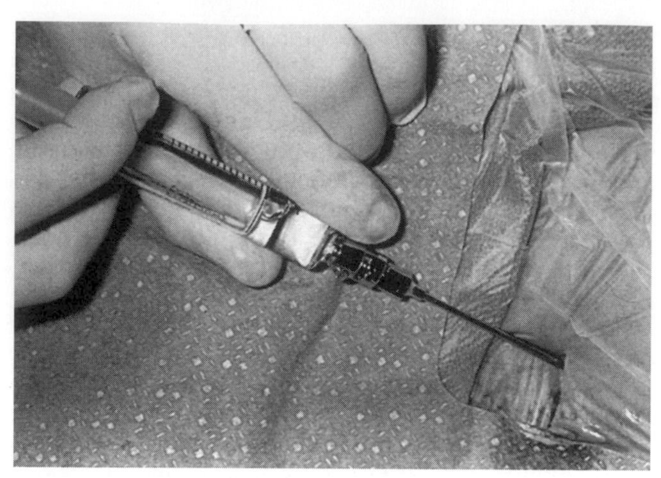

FIGURE 62–3 *Epidural needle placement using a "flat" paramedian approach.*

dorsal spine and lamina are palpated through the incision to locate the intervertebral opening to the epidural space (Fig. 62–3). A paramedian approach to the epidural space allows easier catheter threading than a midline approach.[6, 50, 51, 58] The paramedian approach results in a catheter angle greater than 130 degrees, which is less traumatic to the structures of the epidural space and is more apt to allow the catheter to pass easily into the dorsal epidural space. If the catheter-needle angle is less than 120 degrees, the catheter may deflect off the vertebral body and pass up the ventral epidural space. The greater angulation of the catheter allows it to be withdrawn with less risk of shearing.

Figure 62–4 shows the fluoroscopic needle-catheter angle view encountered with the traditional midline (versus the angulated paramedian) approaches. Intraoperative fluoroscopy is useful during permanent epidural catheter placement to avoid catheter malpositioning during the procedure.

Through a paramedian approach from one level below the dorsal spine of the planned entry site, the 14-gauge Hustead needle is angled cephalad and medially to facilitate midline entry into the epidural space. The needle should enter the paravertebral tissue 1.5 cm lateral to the dorsal spine. Once the ligamentum flavum is encountered, the loss-of-resistance technique is used to enter the epidural space.[58] The size of the 14-gauge Hustead needle opening is half that of the similar-sized Tuohy needle, facilitating easy entry into the epidural space and lessening the risk of dural puncture.[6] The large size of the needle allows early recognition of subarachnoid positioning and avoids subdural positioning. To verify entry into the epidural space, the epidural catheter with stylet is passed 1 cm into the space to "feel" it. Once the epidural space is entered, the space may be dilated using 10 to 15 mL of saline solution. Dilating the epidural space with saline makes it easier to thread the catheter into the epidural space. Local anesthetic may be utilized instead of saline to provide segmental anesthesia and facilitate catheter tunneling, provided that the patient is monitored properly for hypotension and for inadvertent subarachnoid, intravascular, or subdural injection of the anesthetic.[6] The silicone rubber epidural catheter is prepared for threading by first wetting its inside so that the polytetrafluoroethylene-coated wire stylet slides easily into and out of it. This is accomplished by first identifying the open end of the catheter. The catheter is marked with a large black mark on the end that is obstructed and where the sideholes are located. There are centimeter marks along the catheter to indicate length, starting 10 cm from the catheter tip. Once the open end of the catheter is identified, a 20-gauge intravenous polytetrafluoroethylene catheter is placed 2 to 4 mm inside the catheter and, 1 to 2 mL of saline is injected to "wet" the inside of the catheter. The polytetrafluoroethylene-coated wire stylet is relatively stiff on one end and has a very flexible tip on the other. If the stiff end is passed first into the catheter, it stiffens the catheter tip and may increase the risk of perforating the dura. The flexible end enables greater manipulation of the catheter as it is passed in a caudal direction or directed around areas of epidural space compromise.

Threading of the epidural catheter is facilitated both by entering the space in the midline (from a paramedian approach) and by dilating the space with normal saline or local anesthetic agent (Fig. 62–5). The high barium content of the catheter allows easy fluoroscopic visualization during

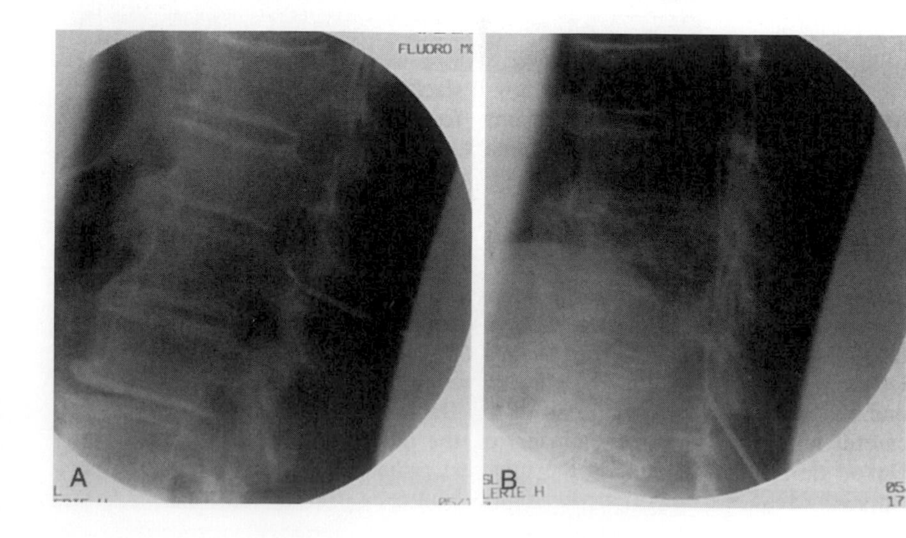

FIGURE 62–4 *Fluoroscopy showing epidural catheter and needle position with a traditional midline approach, A, and a paramedian approach, B.*

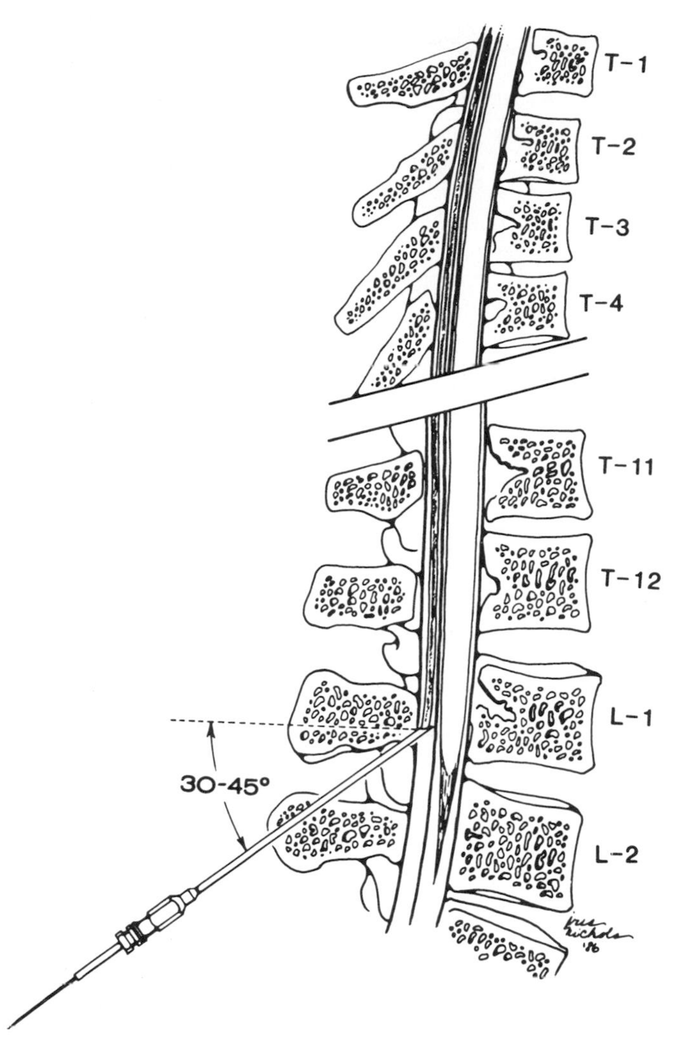

FIGURE 62-5 Insertion of catheter and wireguide stylet. Paramedian epidural needle position facilitates epidural catheter threading.

catheter passage within the epidural space (Fig. 62–6). Difficulty gaining the desired catheter position may be overcome by withdrawing the catheter and changing the needle bevel direction. The needle and catheter should be removed together to avoid catheter damage.

The epidural catheter should be advanced to two vertebral levels above the planned catheter tip position, for two reasons. First, it allows the catheter to be withdrawn by one vertebral segment during positioning. Second, it affords additional catheter movement that can occur with normal patient activity. A review of epidurograms demonstrated a one-segment withdrawal in most patients during the first year of catheter use, whereas later, no catheter movement was noted.[59]

Position of the epidural catheter must be checked in two radiographic planes (anteroposterior and lateral) to be sure that it has not passed through an intervertebral foramen and up along the paravertebral muscles. The catheter should also be checked for inadvertent subarachnoid or intravascular placement by aspiration and irrigation of the catheter. This step can be accomplished by placing a 20-gauge intravenous polytetrafluoroethylene catheter into the distal end of the epidural catheter. If a constant flow of clear fluid greater than the amount used for irrigation is encountered, it should be tested for glucose. If subarachnoid placement is identified, the catheter should be replaced. A constant flow of blood from the catheter indicates intravenous catheter placement, and the catheter should be replaced. A return of blood-tinged irrigation fluid is normal. The cause is either the trauma of catheter positioning or epidural tumor.

After the clinician is satisfied that good positioning of the catheter has been achieved, the catheter is transected 2 to 3 cm beyond the skin edge to allow slack in the line that will be needed when attaching the proximal and distal catheter segments. Now the exteriorized segment of the catheter can be placed.

Catheter Tunneling and Exit Site Selection

The exteriorized portion of the epidural catheter is prepared for tunneling by sliding the free end of the catheter over the tunneling device. It is helpful to use a 60-cm length of 20 Dexon to secure the catheter to the tunneling instrument on one end and to the proximal end of the Dacron cuff (being careful not to occlude the catheter) on the other end. The Dexon tie remains alongside the tunneled catheter and can be secured to the subcutaneous fascia when the posterior incision is closed, as an extra measure of support until the tissue grows into the Dacron cuff (Fig. 62–7).

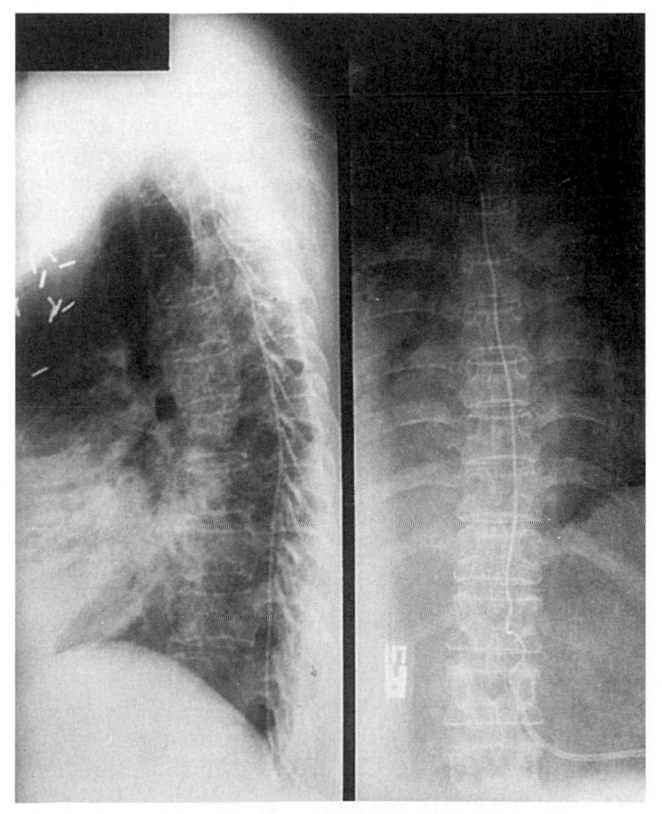

FIGURE 62-6 Thoracic spine plain films show the opaque epidural catheters in place. (From Du Pen SL, Peterson DG, Bogosian AC, et al: A new permanent externalized epidural catheter for narcotic self-administration to control cancer pain. CANCER, 59, pp 986–993, 1987. Copyright © 1987 American Cancer Society. Reprinted by permission of Wiley-Liss, a subsidiary of John Wiley & Sons, Inc.)

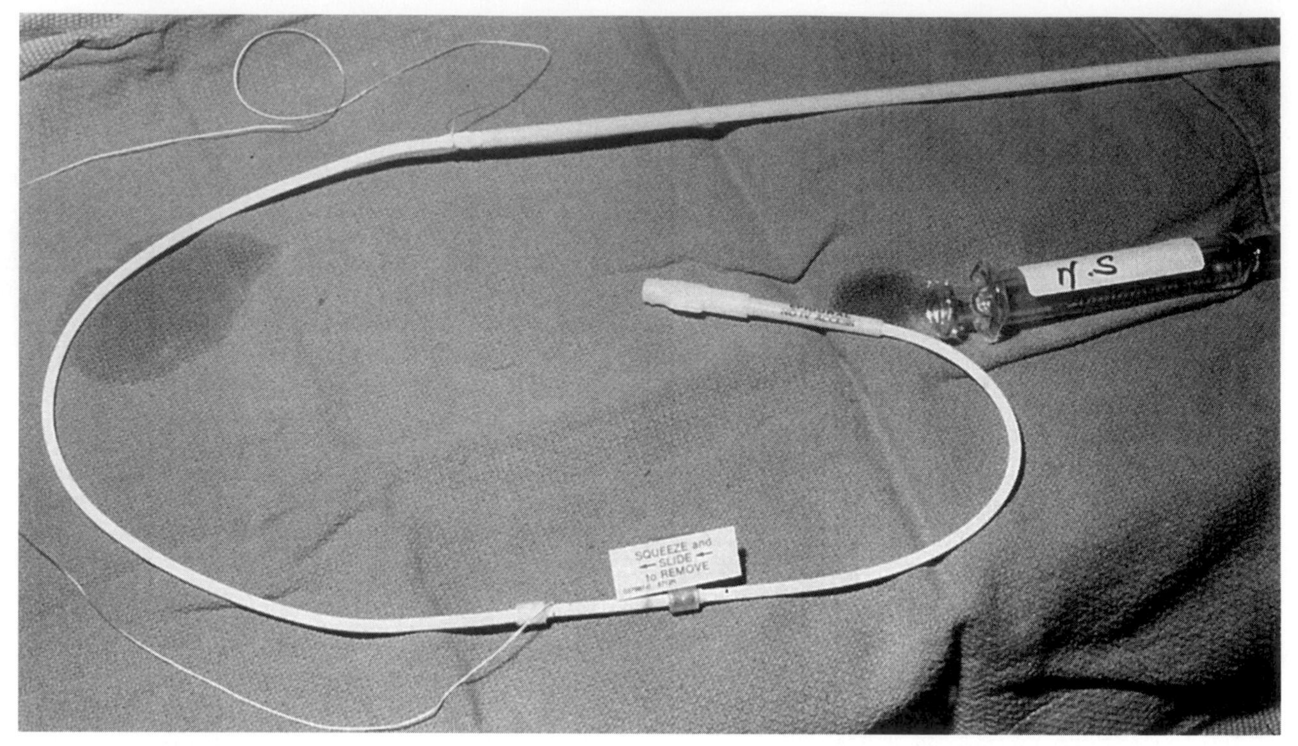

FIGURE 62–7 The tunneled catheter has been prepared for tunneling with a long Dexon tie secured to the tunneler and to the Dacron cuff.

The tunneling process starts with the creation of an exit site. For female patients the site should be in the midline, below and between the breasts, to ensure visualization, prevent pressure from clothing, and avoid skinfolds where chronic yeast infection could be harbored. The site should be selected with an eye to the potential for future abdominal or thoracic surgery. PEG tube gastrostomy placement in the upper left quadrant may pass near the catheter track, making a right-sided track preferable in patients likely to need PEG support. Patient preference must be considered and should be discussed during the consultation and informed consent discussion.

A 6-mm incision is made at the planned exit site through the skin and into the subcutaneous fat tissue to allow passage of the Dacron cuff. The tunneling tool is advanced through the incision into the fat tissue plane and is tunneled posteriorly to the posterior midline incision. The clinician should constantly palpate the tunneling tool with the nondominant hand as the dominant hand advances it posteriorly through the tissues (Fig. 62–8).

The tunneling tool usually allows tunneling to occur in a single step, but in larger patients, a single midtrack exit and reinsertion site may be used. To avoid passing the tunneling tool under the ribs and into the thoracic cavity, its tip *must be palpated* during the tunneling procedure. As the tunneling tool exits the posterior incision, care must be taken not to dislodge the proximal epidural segment of the catheter.

The desired length for the exteriorized segment of the catheter is calculated by first pulling the catheter into its final position, with the Vitacuff just inside the anterior exit site. When the exteriorized catheter is situated in the tunnel, the two catheters are connected. The catheter connector is a simple piece of 20-gauge stainless steel needle stock with an etched center for identification. Two 20 silk ties are used to secure each catheter to the connector. The outer ties ensure that pressure within the catheter will not dilate the catheter off the connector, and the inner ties on each side are secured together, thus holding the catheter ends together over the connector.

The extra 2 to 3 cm of slack that was left on the internalized segment of the epidural catheter enables the joined catheter to be pulled forward slightly through the abdominal exit site. This is accomplished by grasping the external catheter connection at the exit site and pulling it while supporting the catheter connection with smooth forceps. The operator continues to pull the external catheter segment until the connection lies within the tunnel. The final catheter connector position within the tunnel track helps to avoid catheter kinking, which can occur if the connector segment is unsupported in the subcutaneous pocket. No securing sutures are used to connect the catheter junction to the intraspinous ligaments. Earlier, such a suture was recommended, but it was found to be a site of catheter kinking. The catheter is better left free in the subcutaneous fat tissue. The posterior wound and anterior exit site are irrigated with 1 : 50,000 units of bacitracin in 10 to 15 mL of normal saline. Tunneling is a blind procedure that may result in bleeding and subsequent hematoma formation under the posterior incision. A drain is placed in the posterior incision to avoid this complication. A 10-cm section of the epidural catheter is saved and used as a drain, each end being passed into the subcutaneous tissue and the middle closed in the incision (Fig. 62–9). During closure, the 20 Dexon tie that was secured distally to the Dacron cuff is now secured to the subcutaneous fascia in the first layer

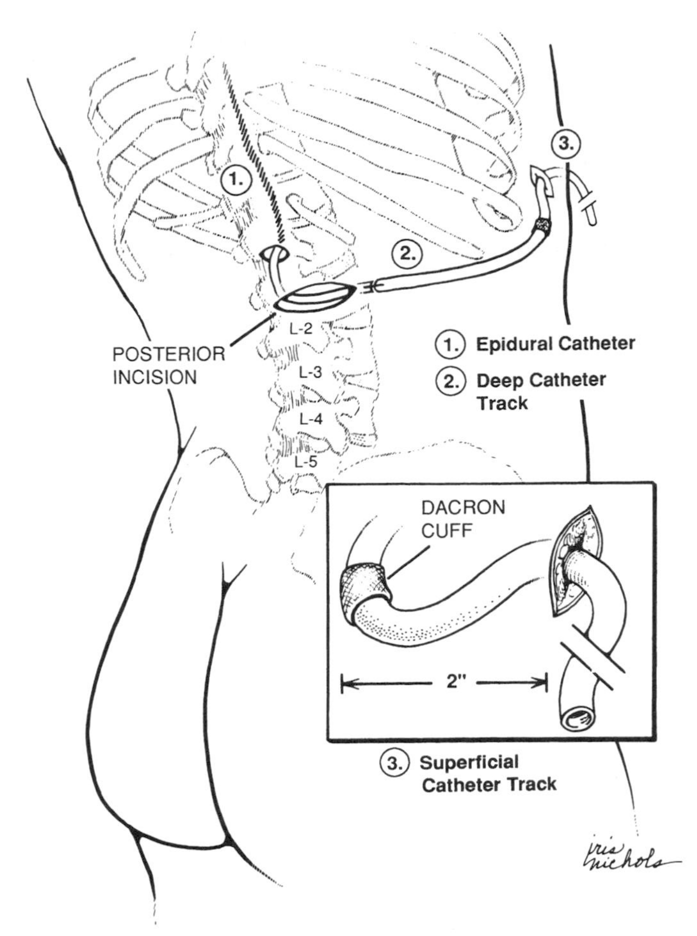

FIGURE 62–8 The epidural catheter tunnel track from the anterior abdominal exit site to the epidural insertion site. (From Du Pen SL, Peterson DG, Williams AR, et al: Infection during chronic epidural catheterization: Diagnosis and treatment. Anesthesiology 73:905–909, 1990.)

of the closure. The posterior incision is closed in two layers: the subcutaneous fascia with Dexon and the skin with nylon. Skin sutures are left in place for 10 to 14 days.

If epidural analgesia was used during the procedure, the patient is taken to the recovery room to be monitored for hypotension from the sympathetic blockade. Postoperative orders consist of antibiotics, epidural analgesia, fluids, diet, and decreasing doses of oral or intravenous opioids.

Double Epidural Catheter Placement

Double epidural catheter placement may be indicated when there is significant compromise of the epidural space. The epidural space may be compromised by epidural tumor mass or by compression from vertebral fractures. It may occur at any time and can be demonstrated by one of several radiologic studies. Magnetic resonance or contrast computed tomography may delineate space obstruction before catheter placement. Epidurography delineates the extent of epidural space obstruction after catheter placement. Known space compromise may be compensated for by placing the epidural catheter above or below the obstruction, depending on the pain source.[20] When the origin of pain is both above and below the obstruction, the patient may require two catheters, one above and one below the obstruction, to obtain adequate pain relief.

Double catheter placement may be done in one session when obstruction is recognized before catheter placement. In this case, catheter epidural entry sites are selected so that the catheter tips can be located around the obstruction. The tunnel track and exit sites are selected so that the epidural catheter position is easy to distinguish. We have found that placing the two exit sites in a vertical row with the upper epidural catheter exit site above the lower catheter exit site allows for differentiation between catheters. Also, a single dressing can be placed for both catheter exit sites. The two catheters may require different infusions, or one may be accessed for bolus injection and the other used for infusion. If the patient suffers from neuropathic pain below the obstruction and somatic pain above it, the solutions selected may be an opioid-bupivacaine infusion for the catheter below the obstruction and opioid alone for the other. To help avoid accidental cross-use of the catheters, a cassette-style pump system may be used for the upper opioid infusion (low volume and high concentration) and a similar pump for the lower catheter using an intravenous bag reservoir and a larger infusion volume to effectively benefit from the bupivacaine infusion.

EPIDUROGRAMS

The use of local anesthetic agents to test for subarachnoid catheter positioning and of epinephrine to determine intravascular position are accepted standard practice for pain management. Long-term cannulation of the epidural space, however, may require more definitive verification. Radiographic verification utilizing dye flow not only verifies placement but also gives the clinician valuable information about catheter position, flow dynamics, and space continuity. The epidural space may be compromised by spinal stenosis, intrinsic tumor, or external compression.

Using information gained from the epidurogram, the clinician can choose the most effective infusion rate to manage the patient's pain. The use of contrast radiography to predict the level of anesthetic blockade has been the

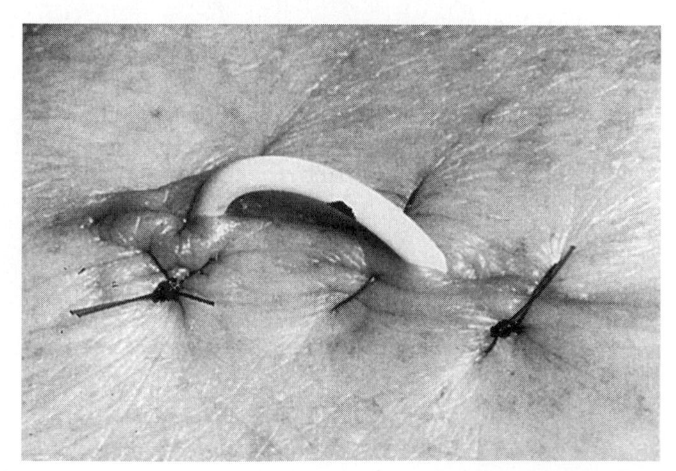

FIGURE 62–9 Drain placement in the posterior insertion site. A 9-cm section of the epidural catheter may be placed in the wound as a drain.

subject of some discussion in the literature.[60, 61] Sjögren and associates[61] studied the extent of dermatomal block after epidural bupivacaine and its correlation with contrast radiographs when 8-mL epidurograms (group I, 10 patients) were compared with 16-mL epidurograms (group II, 11 patients). They reported a statistically significant correlation between the extension of epidural block and the spread of contrast medium in group II.[61]

Information from epidurograms definitely assists in treatment planning with respect to volume of bolus injection or rate of infusion. Patients with very large, open epidural canals may be able to benefit from high-volume injectate, particularly when there are multiple levels of nociceptive input. Alternatively, patients with spinal stenosis, degenerative changes, or tumor may require low-volume therapy with more concentrated drug. Individualizing flow rates of epidural drug on the basis of the known spread of injectate becomes more important when combinations of opioid and local anesthetics are utilized. Epidurography is best done with a series of two 5-mL injections of water-soluble contrast medium suitable for myelography. This procedure gives an indication of the volume required to achieve analgesia, depending on the locus of pain and the catheter tip location. The study should include anteroposterior and lateral scout films, followed by similar views after each of two 5-mL doses of a nonionic dye, such as iohexol (Omnipaque 180). The resulting films and fluoroscopy views show the catheter, the catheter tip location, dye flow after 5-mL and 10-mL injections, distribution of dye in the epidural space, and the highest and lowest extents of dye flow in both anteroposterior and lateral views. Information of the following categories is reported by the radiologist reviewing the study:

- General radiographic review of normal and abnormal anatomy
- Comparison with previous films to determine change over time
- Space where Omnipaque 180 is present (intravascular, subarachnoid, subdural, or epidural space, or outside the epidural space)
- Epidural catheter tip location (vertebral level) and position in the epidural space (anterior or posterior)
- Volume flow after 5 mL of Omnipaque 180; upper and lower extents of flow as described by vertebral level
- Volume flow after 10 mL Omnipaque 180 and comparison with the 5-mL injection
- Abnormalities and/or obstruction of flow and level
- Flow of Omnipaque 180 outside the epidural space

The epidurograms are a valuable resource to review if the quality of the analgesia changes during therapy (Fig. 62–10). The epidurogram obtained after catheter placement can be used as a standard for comparison.[62] A comparison of contrast flow helps the clinician to plan treatment when new tumor spread or vertebral body compression occurs in the epidural space. Obstruction may be overcome by surgical or radiation intervention or may be bypassed by placing a second epidural catheter above or below it. Increasing pain on injection may indicate epidural infection or epidural compromise, which an epidurogram may help to ascertain. A positive culture of fluid from the epidural space with an epidurogram showing catheter encapsulation is diagnostic of an epidural space infection. Loss of analgesia may be due to coiling of the catheter out into the subcutaneous tissue or outward migration of the catheter through an intervertebral foramen. These changes in catheter position can be identified on a simple spine radiograph.[62]

POSTOPERATIVE CARE

Postoperative care includes local care of the device to avoid damage or infection and aseptic procedures required for administration of medication. Patient care may be seri-

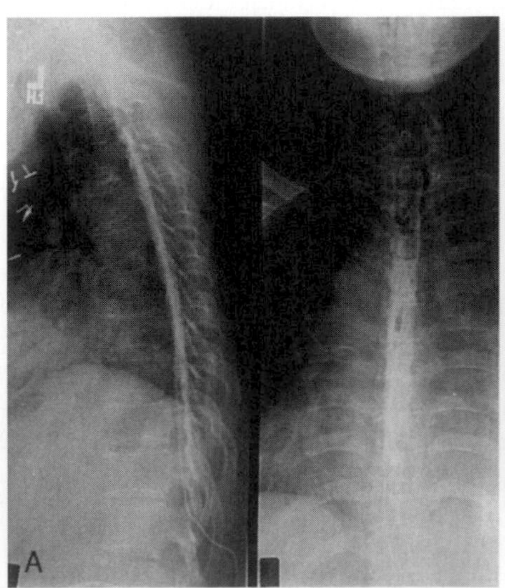

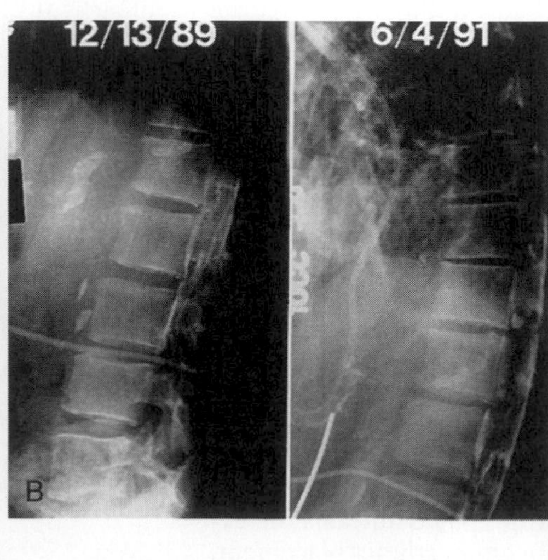

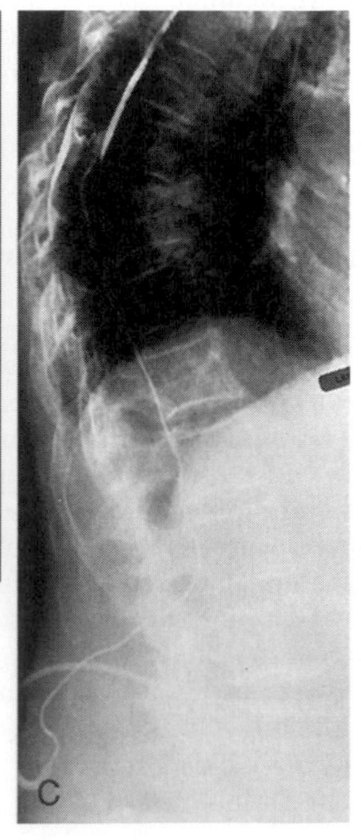

FIGURE 62–10 A, Normal postoperative epidurograms. B, Comparative epidurograms show no change in dye flow over 1.5 years. C, Epidurogram shows dye flow above an area of epidural space compression.

ously—and permanently—compromised by complications resulting from poor postoperative care.

Catheter care consists of (1) immediate postoperative care and (2) ongoing follow-up. Sterile precautions should be used whenever the catheter is manipulated or cleansed. Most patients have little understanding of aseptic technique, so instruction in this is critical to avoiding postoperative complications. During the postoperative period (the first 2 weeks after placement), while the catheter exit site is healing and the skin sutures may still be in place, catheter care consists of daily cleansing of the exit site with hydrogen peroxide and povidone-iodine and coverage with a light 2 × 2-inch dressing.[6, 13] The incisions are cleansed and new dressings applied daily until the sutures have been removed. The mature catheter exit site may be cleaned with soap and water as long as there is no inflammation. When inflammation is identified, exit site care should include a daily hydrogen peroxide and povidone-iodine wash. If exit site inflammation persists, addition of a triple antibiotic ointment or oral antibiotics should be considered.[30]

Long-term dressing procedures for catheter exit sites vary with clinician preference, but strict aseptic technique should be practiced consistently by both patient and caregiver(s). Weekly or biweekly changes of occlusive dressings have been recommended by some practitioners, whereas others prefer daily changes of gauze dressings. Patients with enterostomies or other infection risk factors may require the added protection afforded by a chlorhexidine-impregnated product such as the BIOPATCH dressing (Johnson & Johnson) changed weekly. This patch can be covered with a moisture vapor–permeable transparent dressing such as MVP dressing (Johnson & Johnson) to ensure that the wound stays dry. Constant observation of the exit site guarantees early detection of any inflammation.

Several other factors are important for ongoing follow-up. Using a hot tub or swimming requires added protection, but normal showers may be taken without protection. A simple mini- or "traveling" colostomy bag may be designed to protect the catheter and exit site from contamination while allowing the patient to continue to use a hot tub. Changing of epidural infusion tubing, filters, or reservoir bags requires careful aseptic technique. Many catheter-related infections are isolated to the epidural space, indicating contamination through the injectate.[30] Any manipulation of the catheter system should be considered a potential risk for contamination. Thorough patient teaching and verification of patient or caregiver competence are vital before this responsibility is turned over to either person. All system connections should be cleansed liberally with povidone iodine before the line is opened.[30] Home care nurses have traditionally taken the lead in teaching patients the care of these devices. The nurse may determine that the patient and available caregivers are incapable of providing consistent aseptic care. In these situations, alternative care may need to be arranged. Daily home nursing visits may be provided if the patient's insurance coverage is adequate; otherwise, placement in a skilled nursing facility may be necessary.

CLINICAL MONITORING AND INITIATION OF CARE

Clinical monitoring of patients receiving long-term epidural analgesia is a continuous process. Pain sources and levels of pain perception change constantly for cancer patients. The patient with chronic pain not related to cancer may experience similar exacerbations in the relatively constant pain. Constant communication among the patient, home caregiver(s), and clinician is required to provide a constant level of analgesia. Pain assessment using a patient report pain scale is key to that communication. Patients receiving epidural analgesia should be monitored for analgesic level, sedation, and side effects. Those receiving infusions containing bupivacaine are also monitored for postural hypotension. When clonidine is added to the epidural infusion, blood pressure is closely monitored.[63, 64]

Mechanical complications related to the device can also occur—migration, withdrawal, or compression of the catheter, among them. Patency of the catheter may be affected by kinking, vertebral compression, tumor, or fibrosis. Infection or epidural tumor can cause sequestration of drug flow around the catheter and failure of drug to diffuse to the spinal receptors. The viability and integrity of the device require vigilant monitoring by competent caregivers and frequent evaluation by the clinician.

Initiation of Epidural Opioid Therapy

A starting epidural drug dose is selected by the clinician. Much disagreement surrounds equianalgesic conversion from systemic to intraspinal opioid. For example, some authors suggest that 10 mg of parenteral morphine is equivalent to 1 mg of epidural morphine (10:1), whereas others suggest ratios as high as 10:5.[22, 35, 65] Highly lipid soluble drugs such as fentanyl may have 1:1 equivalency when parenteral administration is compared with epidural.[5] The starting dose selected by the clinician reflects the previous systemic opioid dose adjusted for such things as age of the patient, level of pain intensity, presence of opioid-resistant pain, and character of pain.[66]

Because the starting epidural opioid dose cannot be relied on for complete analgesia, a systemic opioid should always be available to "rescue" the patient in the event that the starting dose is suboptimal. Pain intensity and level of sedation should be monitored. The frequency of monitoring should be based on the onset and duration of action of the agent. For example, evaluation of epidural morphine bolus therapy may be indicated every 4 hours during the first 24 hours, with appropriate dose increases or decreases no more often than every 8 hours. The efficacy of epidural fentanyl infusions can be evaluated continuously, with increases or decreases in the dose every 3 to 4 hours during the initial trial. During the initiation of epidural therapy, systematic diminution of oral or parenteral opioids is necessary to prevent withdrawal symptoms. Withdrawal may occur when systemic opioids are stopped, even when epidural opioids are being given concomitantly. To avoid withdrawal symptoms, the systemic opioid dose may be reduced by 20% to 50% every 24 hours; a transcutaneous clonidine patch may assist with symptom suppression.

The optimal volume and concentration of drug to be administered into the epidural space remain controversial.[28] Waldman[67] recommended a standard dilution of 7 mL as a single dose for lumbar epidural administration and 5 mL for single-dose cervical administration. Others have discussed volume as it pertains to drug lipophilia and segmental spread in the cerebrospinal fluid.[4, 68] The addition of a local anesthetic to the epidural infusion would argue in favor of more dilute solutions, particularly when multiple nerve root sites are targeted for analgesia.

Clinical monitoring during initial empirical dosing should reflect pain and sedation levels and vital signs. Respiratory depression is not generally a concern in opioid-tolerant patients. Some centers utilize orders reflecting "respiratory rate less than 8 and sedation level less than 1" as prerequisites for the administration of naloxone. The rationale for these orders is that oversedation and a concomitant decrease in respiratory rate are the most reliable signs of opioid overdose. Reserving naloxone for these situations prevents the unfortunate opioid reversal that accompanies opioid antagonism in opioid-tolerant patients.

Initiation of Epidural Bupivacaine

When indicated, bupivacaine added to an epidural opioid regimen can provide dramatic relief. Several key nursing implications exists for the safe initiation of this therapy, however, including the requirement that it be started in the hospital. Outpatient initiation of therapy may be done only for well-hydrated patients for whom nursing monitoring is available for the first 8 hours of therapy. Additional daily or twice daily home nursing visits may be necessary, after the first 8 hours of monitoring, at the initiation of therapy. Before therapy begins, a set of postural blood pressures should be obtained and intravenous hydration started. A dehydrated patient is at high risk for the hypotension associated with the sympathetic blockade that accompanies initial administration of epidural bupivacaine.[69] Pretreatment or concurrent intravenous fluid therapy helps to prevent hypotension. Starting infusion doses of epidural bupivacaine are generally in the range of 0.08% to 0.12%.[69] Infusion rates vary from 3 to 10 mL per hour, depending on the spread of drug desired to achieve analgesic blockade of the affected nerve roots. Clinical monitoring of patients receiving epidural opioid-bupivacaine infusions consists of pain and sedation levels, vital signs, and evaluation of skin anesthesia and postural hypotension. Postural blood pressure checks are done every nursing shift until pressures are stable, then every day or every home visit.[69]

Initiation of Epidural Clonidine

Clonidine is added to an epidural infusion to treat neuropathic pain that does not respond to opioid alone. Clonidine is synergistic when added to either opioid or bupivacaine. The average therapeutic dose of clonidine is 700 to 900 mg/day, but our average starting dose is 300 g per day. Add clonidine to the infusion solution and decrease both the opioid and bupivacaine by 10%. Hypotension and bradycardia are noted side effects of clonidine and may be limited by slow titration and hydration.[63, 64]

Dose Titration

With accurate pain assessment, incremental opioid dosing can be done. Bolus injections of epidural opioid can be increased in dose or in frequency. Infusions can be increased by raising either the concentration or the infusion rate. The same principles that apply to titration of oral or systemic opioids apply to epidural administration: increase gradually to effect (the only dose ceiling is untreatable side effects).

For titration of opioid-bupivacaine combinations, a bit more deductive assessment is necessary. Assessment of pain relief must be balanced with the side effects of both the opioid and the bupivacaine. One drug may be increased or decreased in relation to the other drug to obtain the best balance between analgesia and side effects. For example, for a patient with increasing pain who is experiencing sedation but no numbness, the opioid dose may be reduced and the bupivacaine dose increased. Another way to minimize side effects of drugs, particularly with patients who have a significant component of movement-related pain, is by adding a patient-controlled epidural analgesic component to the infusion. The patient's baseline infusion can be a relatively lower dose, and bolus doses of drug are utilized during periods of higher activity.

The use of "titration parameters" for hospital and home can be extremely helpful in ensuring rapid and effective dosing for escalating pain. Changes in the treatment plan should be dictated by pain assessment. For example, for a hospitalized patient, the physician may leave the following orders:

For pain rated below 3 on the VAS, make no change in therapy.
For pain rated 3 to 5, increase epidural morphine dose 20%.
For pain 6 to 7, increase epidural morphine dose 30%.
For pain greater than 8, increase epidural morphine dose 50% to 80% and call for assistance.

Severe pain (>8) is considered a medical emergency and should be treated as such. In home care, a standing order to increase the opioid dose by 25% in any given 24-hour period for uncontrolled pain allows fast response while maintaining a safe range of dose escalation. These parameters are best utilized with an experienced and well-trained nursing staff.

HOME CARE ISSUES

Home care must be a major concern in the choice not only of a delivery system but also of the technique of administration.[24, 70] These considerations are relevant:

What is the social structure of the home?
Is it possible for someone to be at home to help the patient?
Can opioids be stored in the home, and will the patient have access to them?
What are the sanitary conditions?

Successful home care plans generally begin with predischarge teaching. Home visits are scheduled frequently during the first week for patients with externalized self-care systems. Reinforcement of teaching for site care and drug administration should be a priority, as should pain assessment and side effect management. For less proficient caregivers, weekly transparent dressing changes and pump reservoir changes can be done by the home care nurse.

The availability of experienced nurses, in both the hospital and the home care setting, much enhances the success of an epidural pain management program. Initial orientation to nursing care of the epidural catheter should cover basic anatomy and physiology, drug administration by bolus and infusion methods, appropriate monitoring, exit/insertion site care, and filter maintenance and general principles of pain management.[24]

Patient and caregiver teaching on both drug administration and catheter care are critical to a successful outcome. Filters that may act as barriers should be changed according to manufacturer's recommendations. Rescue medications must always be available to the patient. Instruction in when and how rescue medications are to be used is another important item for discussion with patient and family. Patients receiving epidural infusions should have an alternative plan in case of pump failure or failure of delivery of infusion supplies. Sublingual morphine tablets and oral morphine solution are examples of rescue medications. The progressive nature of cancer dictates that every patient have a rescue plan, no matter how far from the hospital he or she lives or what the treatment is. Communication is essential for home care to be a successful continuation of the pain management program started in the hospital. Weekly conference calls among the clinician, nurse, and pharmacist allow the pain service to keep in touch with both the family and the home care team.

COMPLICATIONS

Complications associated with long-term epidural catheters separate into three major groups: mechanical problems, drug-related side effects and complications, and infections. Patients, caregivers, and professionals offering home care services must stay in constant touch to identify and treat these problems as they arise.

Mechanical problems may be associated with the pump, the filter, or the implanted device. The most common cause of loss of analgesia during epidural infusion is failure of the infusion pump owing to program input errors or an air bubble in the pump system. Filter failure should be ruled out first when catheter obstruction is encountered. Catheter obstruction may be further investigated by lumbar spine radiography or epidurography. Acute loss of analgesia with a subcutaneous swelling at the insertion site may occur if the catheter has slipped and is infusing subcutaneously; this problem is easily diagnosed with a simple spine radiograph.

Drug side effects include both drug toxicity and other drug-related side effects. Opioid side effects, such as nausea or vomiting, urinary retention, constipation, myoclonic activity, and sedation, may be seen, but respiratory depression is rare in opioid-tolerant patients. These side effects should be treated aggressively, but if they are unresponsive to treatment, a change in opioid should be considered.[16] Intravascular catheter migration and drug preparation errors should be considered when toxicity becomes clinically apparent.[69] Local anesthetic toxicity is rare when analgesic concentrations are used.[20] Side effects of local anesthetics include postural hypotension, skin anesthesia, and motor loss. They are treated by vascular volume replacement and drug concentration adjustments.[20] Once normovolemia is achieved, postural hypotension is rarely a problem unless the patient becomes dehydrated.[20]

Epidural catheter–related infections may occur at any time during therapy and are associated with both temporary and permanent tunneled epidural catheters.[30, 71] Early diagnosis and treatment are key to a successful outcome. The source of infection may be one of three: the drug infusate, the catheter track, or local abscess. The signs of epidural infection are acute loss of analgesia, fever, and elevated white blood cell count.[30, 71] Epidural infection and catheter encapsulation are manifested in three signs: (1) pain on injection, (2) retrograde flow of infusate with pooling in the paravertebral tissues, and (3) loss of analgesia. In an immunosuppressed cancer patient, fever and white blood cell elevation may be delayed. Diagnosis can be determined by obtaining an epidural aspirate sample for Gram stain and culture.[30] Culturing material from the catheter tip after removal may sample the catheter track and may miss an epidural infection. Appraising the epidural space for response of the abscess to treatment is best done with magnetic resonance imaging or contrast-enhanced computed tomography.[30]

FUTURE DEVELOPMENTS AND RESEARCH

Developments in pharmacology will determine the future role of chronic epidural analgesia. Basic pain researchers will discover more sites in the central nervous system that are amenable to new drug development. New epidural drug formulations will be developed to offer the clinican more treatment options. Clonidine will become a standard part of therapy and other alpha$_2$ agonists will be developed. Spinal drug treatment algorithms will be developed to help clinicians to optimize intrapinal therapy. Long-acting local anesthetic agents, opioids, and additional analgesic agents will encourage the use of epidural ports. The introduction of new alpha$_2$ agonists and *N*-methyl-D-aspartate antagonists will support intraspinal analgesia in general. Concern about infections and tissue reactions will be attenuated with new catheter materials that will inspire new catheters and new techniques for percutaneous catheterization. New catheter coatings will discourage infection, thrombosis, and tissue reactions. New filters and a better understanding of the causes of epidural infections will make the procedure safer for all patients. Finally, the introduction and refinement of epiduroscopy will create additional tools with which to achieve difficult epidural space catheterizations, noninvasive neurodestructive procedures, and diagnostic visualization of epidural space impingement.

REFERENCES

1. Coombs DW, Saunders RL, Harbaugh R: Relief of continuous chronic pain by intraspinal narcotic infusion via an implantable reservoir. JAMA 250:2336–2338, 1983.
2. Cousins MJ: Anesthetic approaches in cancer pain. Adv Pain Res Ther 16:249, 1990.
3. Cousins MJ, Bromage PR: Epidural neural blockade. *In* Cousins MJ, Bridenbaugh PO (eds): Neural Blockade in Clinical Anesthesia and Management of Pain, ed 2. Philadelphia, JB Lippincott, 1988, pp 253–360.

4. Cousins MJ, Cherry DA, Gourlay GK: Acute and chronic pain: Use of spinal opioids. *In* Cousins MJ, Bridenbaugh PO (eds): Neural Blockade in Clinical Anesthesia and Pain Management, ed 2. Philadelphia, JB Lippincott, 1988, pp 955–1029.
5. Cousins MJ, Mather LE: Intrathecal and epidural administration of opioids. Anesthesiology 61:276, 1984.
6. Du Pen SL, Peterson DG, Bogosian AC, et al: A new permanent externalized epidural catheter for narcotic self-administration to control cancer pain. Cancer 59:986–993, 1987.
7. Malone BT, Beye R, Walker J: Management of pain in the terminally ill by administration of epidural narcotics. Cancer 55:438, 1985.
8. Racz GB, Sabonghy M, Gintautes J, Klein WM: Intractable pain therapy using a new epidural catheter. JAMA 248:646–647, 1982.
9. Zenz M: Epidural opiates long term experiences in cancer pain. Klin Wochenschr 63:225, 1985.
10. Zenz M, Schappler Scheele B, Neuhans R, et al: Long-term peridural morphine analgesia in cancer pain. Lancet 1:91, 1981.
11. Zenz M, Piepenbrock S, Husch M, et al: Erfahrungen mit langerliegenden Periduralkathetern: Peridurale Morphinanalgesie bei Karzinompatienten. Reg Anesth 5:26, 1981.
12. Poletti CE, Cohen AM, Todd DP, et al: Cancer pain relieved by long-term epidural morphine with permanent indwelling systems for self-administration. J Neurosurg 55:581, 1981.
13. Yue SK, St. Marie B, Henrickson K: Initial clinical experience with the SKY epidural catheter. J Pain Symptom Manage 6:107–114, 1991.
14. Portenoy R: Cancer pain: General design issues. Adv Pain Res Ther 18:233–266, 1991.
15. World Health Organization: Cancer Pain Relief, ed 2. Geneva, World Health Organization, 1989.
16. Foley K: The treatment of cancer pain. N Engl J Med 313:84, 1985.
17. Portenoy R, Foley K, Inturrisi C: The nature of opioid responsiveness and its implications for neuropathic pain: New hypotheses derived from studies of opioid infusions. Pain 43:372–386, 1990.
18. Arner S, Arner B: Differential effects of epidural morphine in the treatment of cancer related pain. Acta Anaesthesiol Scand 19:32, 1985.
19. Samuelsson H, Hedner T: Pain characterization in cancer patients and the analgetic response to epidural morphine. Pain 46:3–8, 1991.
20. Du Pen S, Williams A: Management of patients receiving combined epidural morphine and bupivacaine for the treatment of cancer pain. J Pain Symptom Manage 7:56–58, 1992.
21. Eisenach JC, Rauck RL, Buzzanell C, Lysak C: Epidural clonidine analgesia for intractable cancer pain. Phase I. Anesthesiology 71:647–652, 1989.
22. De Castro J, Zenz M: Cancer pain. *In* De Castro J, Meynadier J, Zenz M (eds): Regional Opioid Analgesia: Developments in Critical Care Medicine and Anesthesiology. Boston, Kluwer Academic, 1991, pp 363–424.
23. Waldman SD, Feldstein G, Allen ML, et al: Cervical epidural implantable narcotic delivery systems in the management of upper body cancer pain. Anesth Analg 66:780, 1987.
24. Williams AR, Beaulaurier KL, Seal DL: Chronic cancer pain management with the Du Pen epidural catheter. Cancer Nurs 13:176–182, 1990.
25. American Pain Society: Principles of Analgesic Use in the Treatment of Acute Pain and Cancer Pain, ed 3. Skokie, Ill., American Pain Society, 1992.
26. Agency for Health Care Policy and Research: Clinical Guideline: Cancer Pain Management. Bethesda, Md., US Public Health Service, 1993.
27. Levy M: Oral controlled release morphine: Guidelines for clinical use. Adv Pain Res Therapy 14:285–295, 1990.
28. Cousins MJ, Plummer JL: Spinal opioids in acute and chronic pain. Adv Pain Res Ther 18:457–473, 1991.
29. Bedder MD, Burchiel K, Larson A: Cost analysis of two implantable narcotic delivery systems. J Pain Symptom Manage 6:368–373, 1991.
30. Du Pen SL, Peterson DG, Williams AR, et al: Infection during chronic epidural catheterization: Diagnosis and treatment. Anesthesiology 73:905–909, 1990.
31. Sjoberg M, Nitescu P, Appelgren L, Curelaru I: Long-term intrathecal morphine and bupivacaine in patients with refractory cancer pain. Anesthesiology 80:284–297, 1994.
32. Crul BJ, Delhaas E: Technical complications during long-term subarachnoid or epidural administration of morphine in terminally ill cancer patients. Reg Anesth 16:203–213, 1991.
33. Nitescu P, Appelgren L, Hultman E, et al: Long-term, open catheterization of the spinal subarachnoid space for continuous infusion of narcotic and bupivacaine in patients with "refractory" cancer pain. Clin J Pain 7:143–161, 1991.
34. Patt R, Jain S: Long term management of a patient with perineal pain secondary to rectal cancer. J Pain Symptom Manage 5:127, 1990.
35. Warfield C: Role of epidural and intraspinal opioids in the management of cancer pain. *In* Current Concepts in Cancer and Acute Pain Management: Proceedings of Annual Symposium: New York, Memorial Sloan–Kettering Cancer Center, Dec., 1992.
36. Wallenstein SL: The VAS relief scale and other analgesic measures. Adv Pain Res Ther 18:97–103, 1991.
37. DeJong PC, Kansen PJ: A comparison of epidural catheters with or without subcutaneous injection ports for treatment of cancer pain. Reg Anesth 78:94–100, 1994.
38. Ali N, Hoffman J: Tolerance during long-term administration of intrathecal morphine. Conn Med 53:266–268, 1989.
39. Du Pen S: Impantable spinal catheters and drug delivery systems: Complications. Techniques Reg Anesth Pain Manage 2:152–160, 1998.
40. Cherry DA, Gourlay GK, Cousins MJ: Extradural mass associated with lack of efficacy of epidural morphine, and undetectable CSF morphine concentrations. Pain 25:69, 1986.
41. Williams MP, Cherryman GR, Husband JE: Magnetic resonance imaging in suspected metastatic spinal cord compression. Clin Radiol 40:286, 1989.
42. Findlay GFG: Adverse effects of the management of malignant spinal cord compression. J Neurol Neurosurg Psychiatry 47:761, 1984.
43. Cramond T, Stuart G: Intraventricular morphine for intractable pain of advanced cancer. J Pain Symptom Manage 8:465–473, 1993.
44. Lenzi A, Galli G, Gandolfini M, et al: Intraventricular morphine in paraneoplastic painful syndrome of the cervicofacial region: Experience in 38 cases. Neurosurgery 17:6, 1985.
45. Ventafridda V, Spoldi E, Caraceni A, et al: Intraspinal morphine for cancer pain. Acta Anaesthesiol Scand Suppl 85:47, 1987.
46. Asari H, Inove K, Shibata T, Soga T: Segmental effect of morphine injected into the epidural space in man. Anesthesiology 54:75, 1981.
47. Hugenholtz H, Nelson R, Dehoux E: Intrathecal baclofen: The importance of catheter position. Can J Neurol Sci 20:165–167, 1993.
48. Hunt R, Massolino J: Spinal bupivacaine for the pain of cancer. Med J Austr 150:350, 1989.
49. Stambaugh JE: Issues for chronic pain models with specific emphasis on the chronic cancer pain model. Adv Pain Res Ther 18:287–290, 1991.
50. Denobile J, Chester W, Etienne H, Ghosh B: Long-term epidural pain relief using a totally implantable access system. J Surg Oncol 43:92–93, 1990.
51. Driessen J, deMulder P, Claessen J, et al: Epidural administration of morphine for control of cancer pain: Long-term efficacy and complications. Clin J Pain 5:217–222, 1989.
52. Ali N, Hanna N, Hoffman J: Percutaneous epidural catheterization for intractable pain in terminal cancer patients. Gynecol Oncol 32:22–25, 1989.
53. Bames RK: Delayed subarachnoid migration of an epidural catheter. Anaesth Intensive Care 18:564–566, 1990.
54. Hatrick CT, Pither CE, Paj V, et al: Subdural migration of an epidural catheter. Anesth Analg 64:175, 1985.
55. Cherry DA, Gourlay GK, Cousins MJ, Gannon BJ: A technique for the insertion of an implantable portal system for the long-term epidural administration of opioids in the treatment of cancer pain. Anaesth Intensive Care 13:145, 1985.
56. deJong P, Kansen P: A comparison of epidural catheters with or without subcutaneous injection ports for treatment of cancer pain. Anesth Analg 78:94–100, 1994.
57. Wright BD: The use of an attachable silver impregnated cuff on chronically implanted epidural cathers for infection prophylaxis. Reg Anesth 15(Suppl):38, 1990.
58. Moore DC: Epidural Block. *In* Moore DC (ed). Regional Block, ed 4. Springfield, Ill., Charles C Thomas, 1967, pp 427–438.
59. Du Pen S, Williams A, Feldman R: Epidurograms in the management of longterm epidural catheters. Reg Anesth 21(1):61–67, 1996.

60. Asato F, Goto F: What caused the unilateral epidurogram and bilateral epidural analgesia? Anesth Analg 75:303–313, 1992.
61. Sjogren P, Gefke K, Banning A, et al: Lumbar epidurography and epidural analgesia in cancer patients. Pain 36:305–309, 1989.
62. Du Pen SL, Williams AR: Epidurograms in the management of patients with longterm epidural catheters. Submitted for publication 1995.
63. Eisenach JC, Du Pen S, Dubois M, et al: Epidural clonidine analgesia for intractable cancer pain. Pain 61(3):391–399, 1995.
64. Grace D, Bunting H, Milligan KR, Fee JPH: Postoperative analgesia after co-administration of clonidine and morphine by the intrathecal route in patients undergoing hip replacement. Anesth Analg 80:86–91, 1995.
65. Rocco AG, Chan V, Iacobo C: An algorithm for the treatment of pain in advanced cancer. Hospice J 5:93–103, 1989.
66. Du Pen SL, Williams AR: The dilemma of conversion from systemic to epidural morphine: A proposed conversion tool for the treatment of cancer pain. Pain 56:113–118, 1994.
67. Waldman S: The role of spinal opioids in the management of cancer pain. J Pain Symptom Manage 5:163–168, 1990.
68. Bromage P, Camporesi F, Durant P, Niclsen C: Rostral spread of epidural morphine. Anesthesiology 56:431–436, 1982.
69. Du Pen SL, Kharasch ED, Williams AR, et al: Chronic epidural bupivacaine-opioid infusion in intractable cancer pain. Pain 49:293–300, 1992.
70. Smith DE: Spinal opioids in the home and hospice setting. J Pain Symptom Manage 5:175–181, 1990.
71. Schoeffler P, Pichard E, Ramboatiana R, et al: Bacterial menengitis due to infection of a lumbar drug release system in patients with cancer pain. Pain 25:75, 1986.

CHAPTER • 63

Implantation Techniques for Totally Implantable Drug Administration Systems

Elliot S. Krames, MD, FACPM

Interest in the safety, efficacy, and relative ease of delivery of intraspinal opioids and other analgesics for the control of intractable pain is ever increasing. Recent technologic advances have provided clinicians with accurate devices for the intraspinal long-term infusion of drugs.

Because of these advances, interest in intraspinal infusional therapy for the control of chronic pain is still growing. The use of long-term oral opioid therapy for chronic nonmalignant pain remains a controversial issue, although growing evidence supports it as a viable treatment for certain unfortunate patients.[1-7] If oral and systemic administration of opioids have a place in the treatment continuum for chronic pain, then certainly the intraspinal delivery of opioids and nonopioid analgesics has a place.[8-11] It is my belief and practice that spinal administration of opioids should be reserved for those patients who develop intractable side effects to treatment with oral or parenteral therapies. It is my purpose in this chapter to broadly outline the safe and successful techniques for implantation of spinal analgesic infusion devices. The Medtronic Synchromed totally programmable pump systems (Medtronic, Minneapolis, Minn.; Fig. 63–1) and the Arrow factory-preset flow rate pumps (Arrow, Walpole, Mass.; Fig. 63–2) are two different implantable systems that have been approved by the U.S. Food and Drug Administration for clinical use.

TRIAL OF INTRASPINAL ANALGESICS

Before implantation of a system for delivery of intraspinal analgesics, a trial with the agents that are intended for long-term use is suggested. *Trials should not only verify the efficacy of the intended agent but should also rule out toxicity and mitigate against strong placebo influences.* Trials may be performed either epidurally or intrathecally and may be (1) single-shot trials performed by placing the test agent intraspinally through a needle or (2) continuous trials by placing catheters epidurally or intrathecally and infusing the intended agents over some period of time. I recommend that the decision to implant be made, not on the basis of a single-shot trial, but on the basis of the results of multiple single-shot interventions or of continuous infusion of the agents via an intraspinal catheter.

I also recommend that single, "n-of-one" placebo trials with saline not be factored into the decision of whether to implant. A positive response to a single-blinded or even a double-blinded placebo by any one patient does not conclusively and scientifically identify that patient as a placebo responder who, consequently, is not a candidate for intraspinal dosing. All patients, especially patients who are appropriate candidates for intrathecal delivery are placebo responders. Since a positive response to an active agent is either a specific response (response to the agent) or a nonspecific response (placebo response), for any single patient, what constitutes a positive response cannot be known. Accepting a patient for intrathecal therapy based on a positive response to the intended agent or ruling out a patient based on their positive response to a blinded saline injection is unscientific and makes no sense. In fact, if decisions are based on response to placebos, some patients will be ruled out unfairly and others ruled in because of a specific positive response to an active agent, when, in fact, those patients are simply strong placebo responders. The only way to minimize false-positive placebo responses is to extend trials out over time.

In our practice, we believe that a continuous intrathecal trial, by virtue of its mimicking the intended final delivery system, is the best trial for intrathecal therapy. A continuous intrathecal trial, not only allows for sequential trials of different agents and combinations of agents, but also allows for a prolonged trial to ferret out powerful placebo responders. It is currently our practice to surgically implant a permanent Medtronic No. 8709 intrathecal, Silastic catheter (Medtronic Inc., Minneapolis, Minn.; Fig. 63–3) and tunnel and connect that catheter to the tunneled distal subcutaeous arm of a DuPen Long Term Epidural Catheter (Bard Access Systems, Salt Lake City, Ut.). The catheter

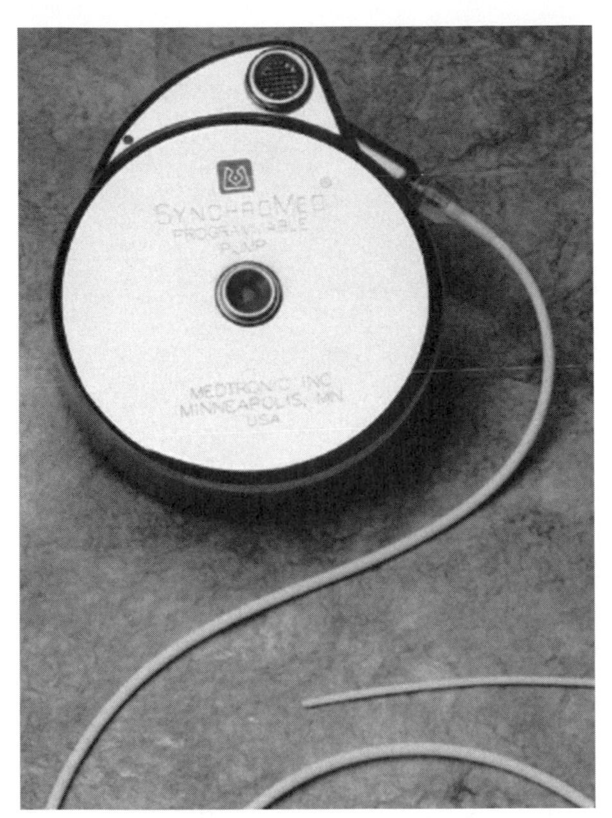

FIGURE 63–1 *Medtronic Synchromed pump. (Courtesy of Medtronic, Minneapolis, Minn.)*

system is then connected to an external drug delivery pump that continuously delivers the intrathecal agent. To prevent infection, all patients take antibiotics and an in-line, 22-μm filter is placed between the drug pump and the intrathecal catheter system. After some length of time—enough to (1) identify that an agent or agents are appropriate or inappropriate for intrathecal delivery and (2) to detect placebo responders—the permanent catheter is either removed or connected to an implanted drug delivery system. A successful trial in our clinical practice is one in which the patient has greater than 50% improvement in subjective pain complaint and some improvement in physical functioning.

If the successful trial is performed either with multiple, single-shot injections of agent or by placement of a temporary catheter, permanent implantation of pump and cathe-

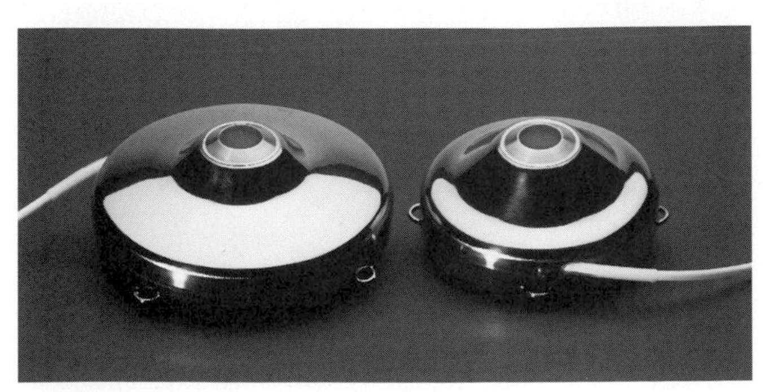

FIGURE 63–2 *Arrow model 3000 implantable pumps. (Courtesy of Arrow International, Reading, Pa.)*

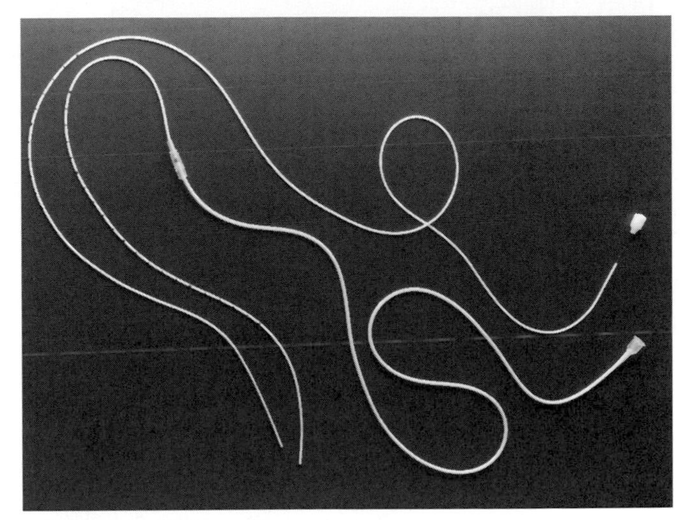

FIGURE 63–3 *Medtronic Silastic intrathecal catheters. (Courtesy of Medtronic, Minneapolis, Minn.)*

ter must be performed during the same operation. If the trial was performed via a permanently implanted catheter, as just described, the intrathecal catheter is disconnected from the tunneled subcutaneous Dupen arm and tunneled to the surgically prepared pump pocket and pump.

SURGICAL PLACEMENT OF PUMP AND CATHETER IN ONE SESSION

For the purposes of this chapter, the procedure for placement of both permanent catheter and pump during a single operation will be described. After induction of anesthesia, correct positioning of the patient, and preparation and draping, the first step is making the incision for and placement of an intrathecal spinal catheter via a Tuohy intraspinal needle. The catheter, once placed and anchored, is then tunneled subcutaneously and connected to a subcutaneously placed totally implanted drug delivery system. Because these procedures are relatively lengthy and because patients with chronic pain do not tolerate lying in one position for prolonged periods of time, we choose, in our clinic, whenever possible, to perform these procedures under general anesthesia. Some implanters believe that general anesthesia is contraindicated because sleeping patients cannot give feedback to alert the implanter to impending insult or damage to neural tissues such as nerve rootlets or the spinal cord itself by either the blindly placed needle into the thecal sac or advancement of the intrathecal catheter or both. In our hands, however, performing these procedures under general anesthesia has proven to be safe and humane to the great majority of our patients.

It is our practice to always perform this operation under fluoroscopic guidance. Placing a catheter anywhere into the thecal sac suffices if the patient is to receive only hydrophilic opioid agents such as morphine and hydromorphone. Continuous infusion of these hydrophilic opioids is accompanied by general mixing of the agents throughout the cerebrospinal fluid. Over time, these agents, if infused anywhere into the cerebrospinal fluid, "bubble up" to higher spinal segments and supraspinal centers. At some later time, because of either poor analgesia or side effects of the hydrophilic drug, it may become necessary to use lipophilic opioids (e.g., meperidine, fentanyl, sufentanil, methadone, or even bupivacaine or clonidine). To facilitate this, it is important to place the catheter tip as close as possible to the spinal segment mediating patient's pain. *An ounce of prevention is worth a pound of cure.* Lipophilic agents diffuse directly into the lipid substance of the spinal cord around the tip of the intraspinal catheter and usually do not bubble up in the cerebrospinal fluid to higher spinal segments or supraspinal centers. For all these reasons, it is important to use fluoroscopic guidance to place the spinal catheter tip as close as possible to the target spinal segment.

After antibiotic prophylaxis and induction of general anesthesia, the patient is positioned in the left lateral decubitus position if the operative surgeon is right handed or in the right lateral decubitus position if the surgeon is left handed. These positions facilitate the surgeon's comfort during placement of the Tuohy needle from the caudal to the rostral plane. The C arm of the fluoroscopic unit is then placed across the table from the surgeon. In our practice, before prepping and draping, the vertebral "midline" between T12 and L4 is identified, using the C arm oriented in the anteroposterior direction, and marked on the patient's back with an indelible marking pen (Fig. 63–4).

After the anatomic midline has been identified and marked on the skin of the patient, the patient is prepared for surgery and draped in the usual manner. Because this operation necessitates a middle lower-back incision for placement of the intraspinal catheter and a low abdominal incision for placement of the totally implanted subcutaneous drug administration system, both areas must be "draped out" for surgical access. In our operating room, this is accomplished with a split drape system. Split drapes are placed above and below the prepped back, flank, and lower quadrant of the abdomen with the flanges of the split drape system outlining the back and abdomen.

The first task of this operation is intrathecal placement of the spinal catheter via a 16-gauge Touhy epidural needle. It is standard procedure for some surgeons to place the intrathecal needle through the skin with fluoroscopic guidance before making an incision (Figs. 63–5, 63–6). Once the catheter has been advanced to the spinal "target" (as determined by the dermatome of origin of the patient's pain) and in place (Fig. 63–7), these surgeons make an incision around the needle and carry it down to the supraspinous fascial plane (Fig. 63–8). It is our practice, however, to make an incision from the skin to the supraspinous fascia before placing the Touhy needle, which is then advanced through the most cephalad apex of the incision. Our usual location for this skin incision is between L2–3 and L4. In my opinion, the needle should never be introduced into the thecal sac above L2, for fear of its damaging the spinal cord. The incision is then carried down through the subcutaneous tissues to the supraspinous fascia.

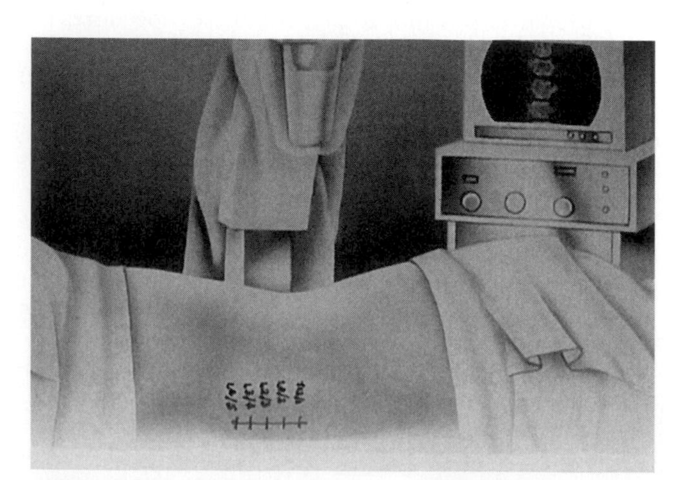

FIGURE 63–4 Locations of lumbar spines between L1 and L4 are marked on patient's skin. (Courtesy of Medtronic, Minneapolis, Minn. Reprinted with permission from Medtronic, Inc. ©Medtronic, Inc. 1996.)

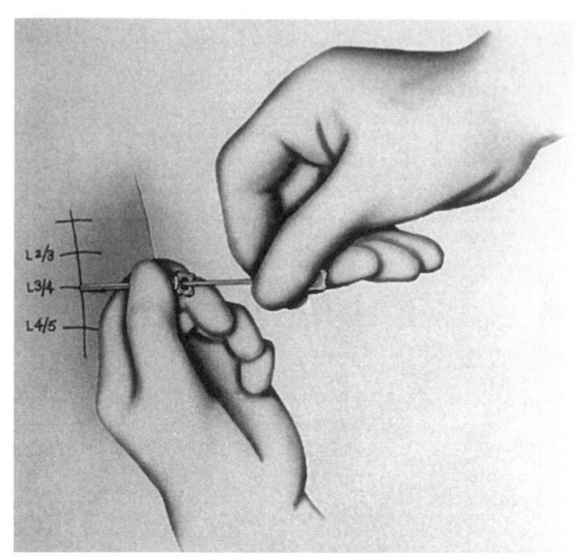

FIGURE 63–5 Tuohy needle is placed with fluoroscopic guidance. (Courtesy of Medtronic, Minneapolis, Minn. Reprinted with permission from Medtronic, Inc. ©Medtronic, Inc. 1996.)

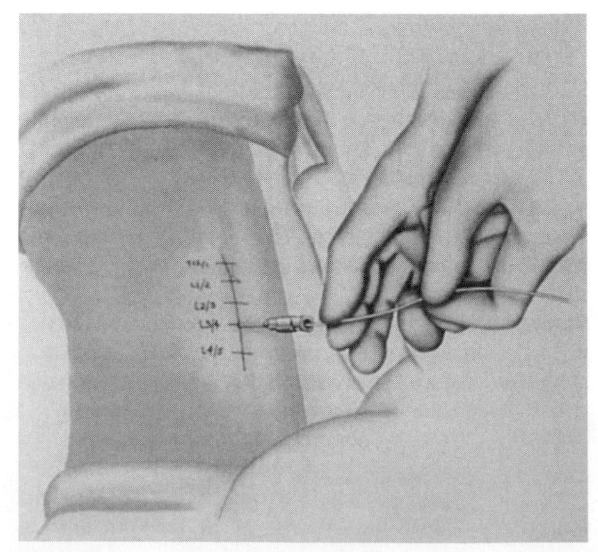

FIGURE 63–6 A radiopaque catheter is advanced through the needle. (Courtesy of Medtronic, Minneapolis, Minn. Reprinted with permission from Medtronic, Inc. ©Medtronic, Inc. 1996.)

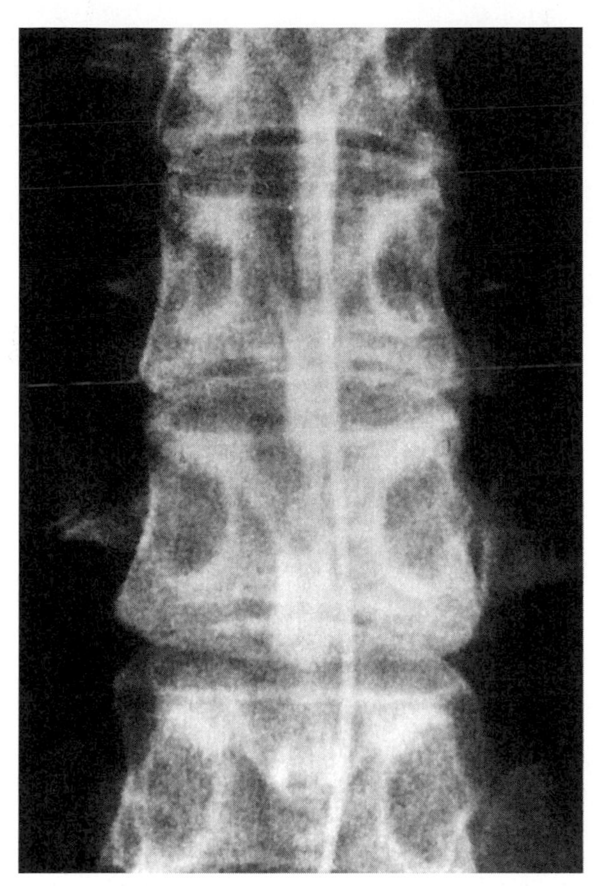

FIGURE 63-7 The catheter tip is advanced to the dermatomal level of pain.

to 90 degrees) as it often does with a midline needle approach, the catheter, when advanced, tends to abut the anterior thecal sac, making it somewhat difficult to advance it rostrally. It is clear that the shallower and less acute the angle of the needle tract is the easier it is to advance the catheter centrally and rostrad. Using a shallow angle but one greater than 45 degrees, our needle tip usually enters the supraspinous fascia from a paramedian approach at L3 or L3–4 and finally enters the thecal sac below L2. This paramedian approach also precludes tenting or sandwiching of the posterior dural sac against the anterior dural sac by the advancing Touhy needle, a complication sometimes seen with the midline approach. When sandwiching of the posterior to anterior dural membranes occurs, cerebrospinal fluid flow is obstructed, making it difficult to confirm correct placement of the needle into the sac.

Whether the surgeon chooses to introduce the needle before making an incision or afterward, it is very important to ensure that adequate hemostasis is accomplished before closing these incisions. Direct pressure on bleeding points or electrocautery is mandatory to ensure that proper hemostasis is accomplished. Closure of wounds on active bleeding may lead to hematoma formation and increase the risk of postoperative infection. To prevent infection, it is our practice to copiously irrigate all wounds with an antibiotic solution before closing them.

Once the catheter tip is placed at the spinal segment "responsible" for the patient's pain, it is the practice of some surgeons to place a purse-string, 2-0 silk suture into the supraspinous fascia, either around the Touhy needle

Meticulous hemostasis is provided by electrocautery, and the wound is copiously irrigated with an antibiotic solution before the intraspinal Touhy needle is placed into the wound. The appropriate length of the incision depends upon the amount of subcutaneous fat and varies from patient to patient. A small 1- to 1.5-in incision usually suffices in patients who are extremely thin. A larger incision may be required for patients who are obese. Before the needle is placed, a small subcutaneous, undermined "shelf" is created at the base of the wound at the level of the supraspinous fascia using a combination of sharp and blunt dissection. This shelf, underlying the subcutaneous tissues at the base of the wound, permits excess intraspinal catheter exiting the fascia to have a gentle curve and sweep for connection to the pump catheter. It is likewise important that the needle enter the supraspinous fascia at the most rostrad apex of the incision, not the midportion or caudal end. This maneuver also ensures that the intraspinal catheter, exiting the supraspinous fascia, has sufficient room caudally for a gentle and not too abrupt sweep for connection to the pump catheter. If careful attention is not paid to these two maneuvers, kinking of the catheter system may occur.

To facilitate safe, easy, and relatively unobstructed catheter placement, we recommend shallow, angled, paramedian placement of the Tuohy needle below the L2 spinal level. This maneuver allows easy rostrad advancement of the intraspinal catheter in the intrathecal space. If the needle enters the intrathecal space at an acute or steep angle (45

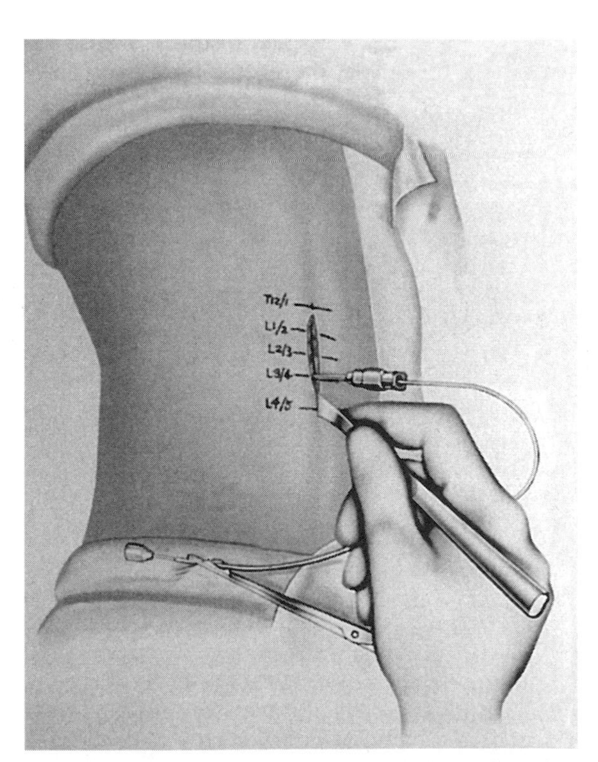

FIGURE 63-8 An incision is made around the needle to the supraspinous fascial plane. (Courtesy of Medtronic, Minneapolis, Minn. Reprinted with permission from Medtronic, Inc.)

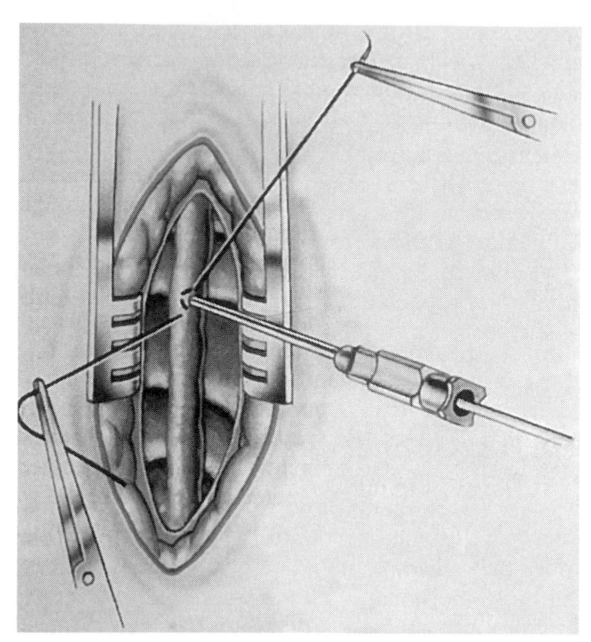

FIGURE 63–9 A pursestring suture is placed around the Tuohy needle. (Courtesy of Medtronic, Minneapolis, Minn. Reprinted with permission from Medtronic, Inc. ©Medtronic, Inc. 1996.)

before removing it (Fig. 63–9) or directly around the catheter after removing the needle (Fig. 63–10). If the surgeon chooses to place the purse-string suture directly around the catheter, the suture should not be cinched too tight lest it block the flow of cerebrospinal fluid. After this suture is placed, it is imperative that cerebrospinal fluid flow be checked and be unobstructed. The purpose of the purse-string suture is to prevent back-flow of cerebrospinal fluid from the catheter's dural entry site along the spinal catheter track. If this were to occur, a subcutaneous collection of fluid might form that is called a *hygroma*. Cerebrospinal fluid hygromas are usually self-limiting and of no serious consequence unless the fluid leaks through the cutaneous suture line. This unfortunate event might require takedown and resuturing of the wound. I suggest that, if a hygroma develops, the treating physician should take a wait-and-see attitude toward it. Unnecessary draining of the hygroma could lead to infection or leakage of cerebrospinal fluid.

After the Tuohy needle is removed and after the purse-string suture is placed around the catheter exit site from the supraspinous fascia, the catheter is then anchored to the supraspinous fascia with one of several types of Silastic anchors provided by the manufacturer. These anchors are placed around and over the catheter and sutured to the supraspinous fascia with interrupted 2-0 or 3-0 silk sutures. Caution must be taken to avoid damaging the catheter with the sharp needle or occluding it by cinching the sutures too tight around it. Before the next step in this operation is taken, the exiting spinal catheter tip should be gently clamped and secured to the drapes, to prevent excessive loss of cerebrospinal fluid or inadvaertent dislocation.

Before the second part of the operation—incision for and implantation of the drug infusion device—the pump must be prepared and primed for placement according to the manufacturer's specifications and instructions. If a programmable Medtronic Synchromed pump is to be implanted, the implant coordinator or nurse technician, before removing it from its packaging, must "read" the pump telemetrically to ensure that the pump calibration constant is consistent with the calibration constant printed on the package. This calibration consistency is necessary to ensure correct dosing when programming the pump (Fig. 63–11). This step is not necessary with nonprogrammable, rate-specific pumps. The internal sterile packaging containing the pump is then handed off to the scrub nurse, who removes it from the package. The Silastic covering

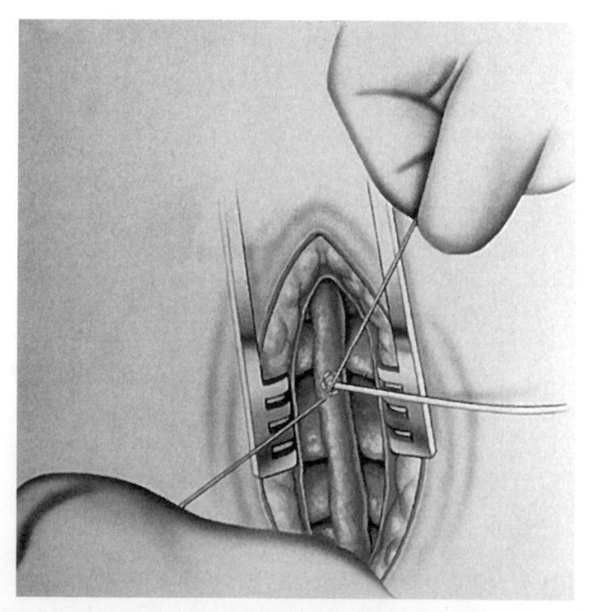

FIGURE 63–10 A pursestring suture is placed around the catheter after the Tuohy needle has been removed. (Courtesy of Medtronic, Minneapolis, Minn. Reprinted with permission from Medtronic, Inc. ©Medtronic, Inc. 1996.)

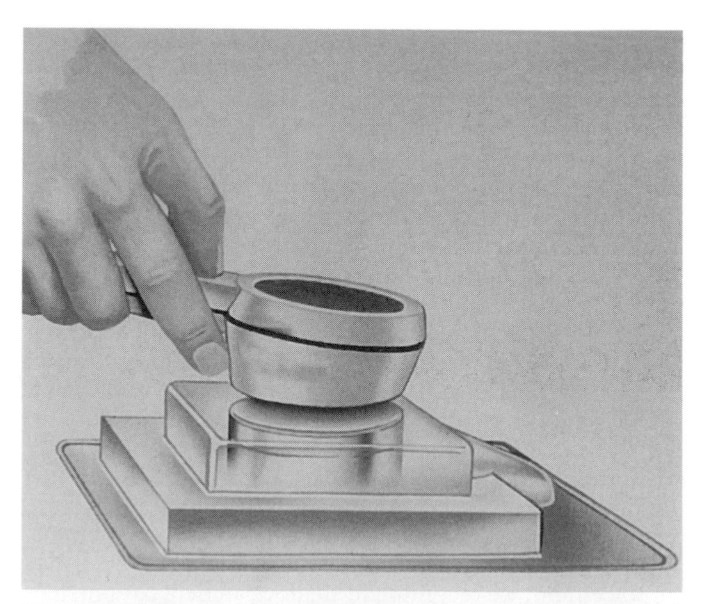

FIGURE 63–11 The pump is programmed via telemetry through a sterile package to begin a 360-μl purge to verify pump function and to purge air and fluid from internal pump tubing. (Courtesy of Medtronic, Minneapolis, Minn. Reprinted with permission from Medtronic, Inc. ©Medtronic, Inc. 1996.)

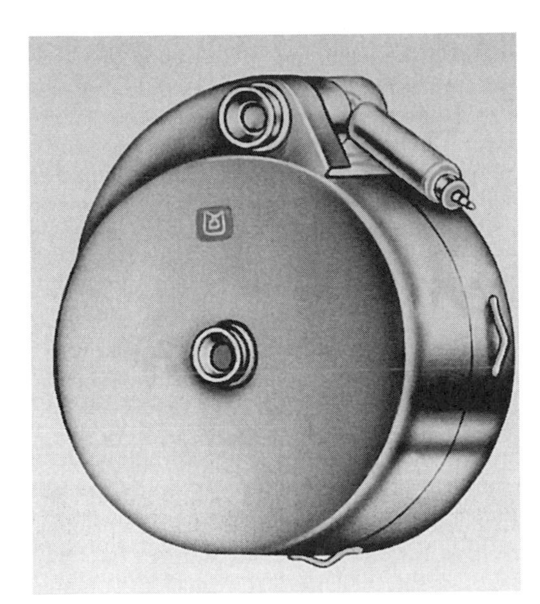

FIGURE 63–12 Type of pump with loops provided to suture pump to fascia. (Courtesy of Medtronic, Minneapolis, Minn. Reprinted with permission from Medtronic, Inc. ©Medtronic, Inc. 1996.)

over the nipple outlet of Synchromed pumps should be removed, to allow free flow of the purged contents of the pump, and a Dacron pouch (provided by Medtronic, if applicable) placed over the pump. According to the implanter's choice, programmable pumps are programmed to purge either before the sterile water (contained in all Medtronic Synchromed pumps) is removed or after it has been removed and replaced in the reservoir with the analgesic drug. Arrow, nonprogrammable, rate-specific pumps also contain water that must be removed and replaced with drug before implantation.

Some of the Medtronic Synchromed pumps and all Arrow pumps are provided with suture loops to stabilize the pump and prevent it from moving in its pocket (Fig. 63–12). Some Synchromed pumps are provided with a Dacron pouch, which is carefully placed over the pump (Fig. 63–13). The Dacron pouch serves the same anchoring function as the suture loops. Over time, fibroblasts invade the fabric to form a tight fibrous capsule around the pump that prevents its moving in its pocket.

All pumps, whether programmable or nonprogrammable, should be placed into a warmer at least 30 min before surgery and into a basin containing warm water during surgery. With a 22-gauge Huber-type needle and syringe provided with the implant kits, the reservoir is emptied of its water and filled with approximately 10 mL of the opioid or analgesic solution to be infused (in the case of a programmable pump) or the entire volume (if a nonprogrammable one is used; Figs. 63–14, 63–15). Although the Synchromed pump reservoir holds approximately 18 mL, it is the manufacturer's recommendation that the first volume of solution not exceed 10 mL.

After placement of the intrathecal catheter, anchoring the catheter and after preparation and filling of the pump, the second part of the operation—creation of a pocket for the pump—begins. An incision is made at or about the umbilical level, in the right lower quadrant of the abdomen if the operating surgeon is right-handed or in the left lower quadrant if the surgeon is left-handed. If the patient is thin, this incision is carried down to the rectus fascia to create a pocket above the fascia. Because of refilling and programming requirements, if the patient is obese the incision should not be carried down to the fascia but only to the mid-fat plane of the lower quadrant of the abdomen. Before making the incision, the surgeon should be cognizant of the aesthetic result the patient desires and, when possible, should "design" the operation accordingly. The pump must not be placed too close to the iliac crest or the inferior rib cage, lest it cause the patient discomfort. After the incision is carried down to either the rectus fascia or the

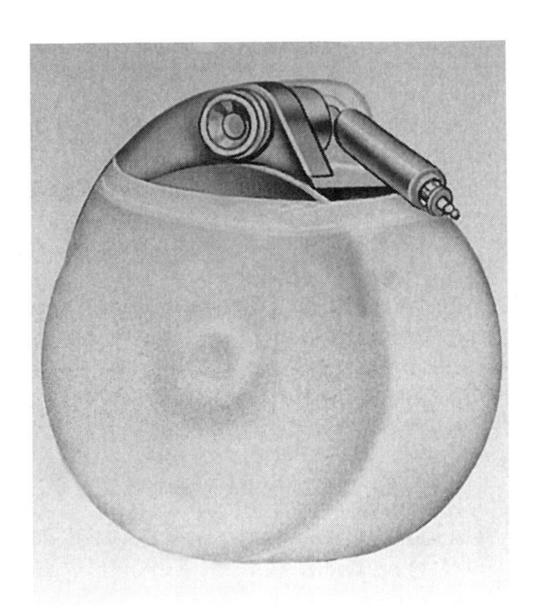

FIGURE 63–13 SynchroMed pump with Dacron pouch. (Courtesy of Medtronic, Minneapolis, Minn. Reprinted with permission from Medtronic, Inc. ©Medtronic, Inc. 1996.)

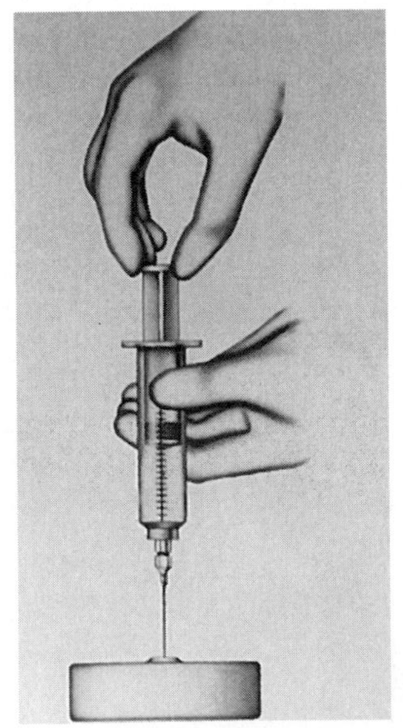

FIGURE 63–14 The warmed pump is accessed and its contents totally removed. (Courtesy of Medtronic, Minneapolis, Minn. Reprinted with permission from Medtronic, Inc. ©Medtronic, Inc. 1996.)

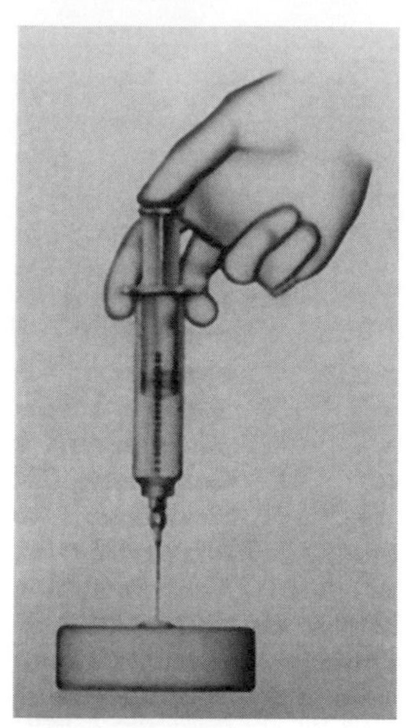

FIGURE 63–15 Ten milliliters (10 mL) of drug is slowly introduced into the reservoir of the pump. (Courtesy of Medtronic, Minneapolis, Minn. Reprinted with permission from Medtronic, Inc. ©Medtronic, Inc. 1996.)

mid-fat plane, a pocket just large enough to accommodate the pump is created using a combination of sharp and blunt dissection working from the incision in a caudal direction (Fig. 63–16). A 1- to 2-cm portion of this pocket should be created rostral to the incision to ease pump placement and refilling. With placement of the catheter, once the pocket is formed, meticulous hemostasis must be achieved with electrocautery, and the pocket should be copiously irrigated with antibiotic solution. Any large bleeders that are not adequately coagulated with electrocautery must be suture ligated.

Once the pump pocket has been created, tunneling of the catheter system and connection to the pump is the next, and final, step in this operation. Tunneling can be accomplished with either a neuro-shunt tunneling device or a tunneling device provided by the manufacturer. The surgeon must always take care to ensure that the tunneling device remains just under the skin and is not forcefully pushed (1) through muscle and the abdominal wall into the peritoneal cavity or (2) under the ribs, through the diaphragm, into the intrapleural space. Gentle subcutaneous guidance of the tunneling device with gently applied pressure on the skin over the device usually suffices to ensure safe tunneling (Fig. 63–17). Tunneling proceeds either from the pocket to the back incision or from the back incision to the pocket, depending on what catheter system is used. If the implanter uses the Medtronic, one-piece No. 8709 catheter (see Fig. 63–3) or the Arrow one-piece, all-flex catheter system (Fig. 63–18), tunneling proceeds from back to abdominal wall pocket and is facilitated by a small midflank incision. For the Medtronic two-piece system (e.g., No. 8703 W; see Fig. 63–3) tunneling of the subcutaneous portion of the pump catheter proceeds from the abdominal incision and pocket to the back incision, again facilitated by a midflank incision. Once tunneled the pump catheter is connected to the intrathecal catheter in the prescribed manner with a titanium catheter connector and a strain-release Silastic covering is placed over the connection (Fig. 63–19). Before this connection is made, any extra length of spinal or pump catheter is cut and

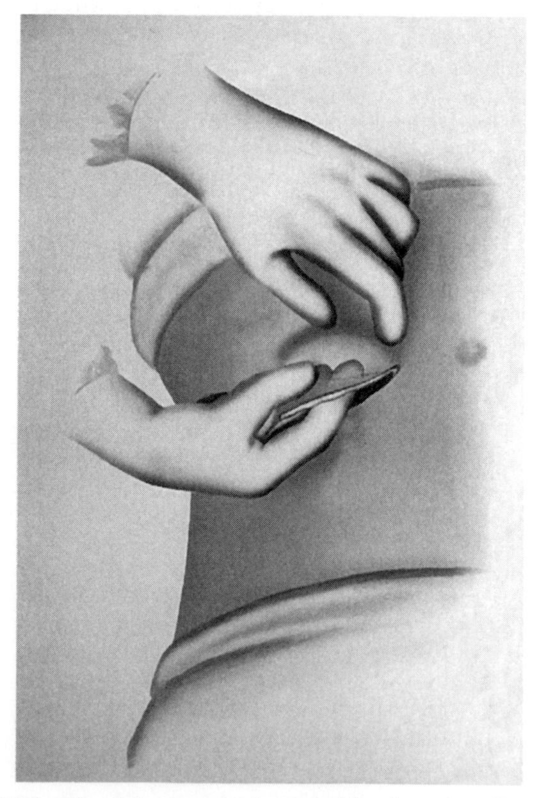

FIGURE 63–16 A pocket is created for the pump. (Courtesy of Medtronic, Minneapolis, Minn. Reprinted with permission from Medtronic, Inc. ©Medtronic, Inc. 1996.)

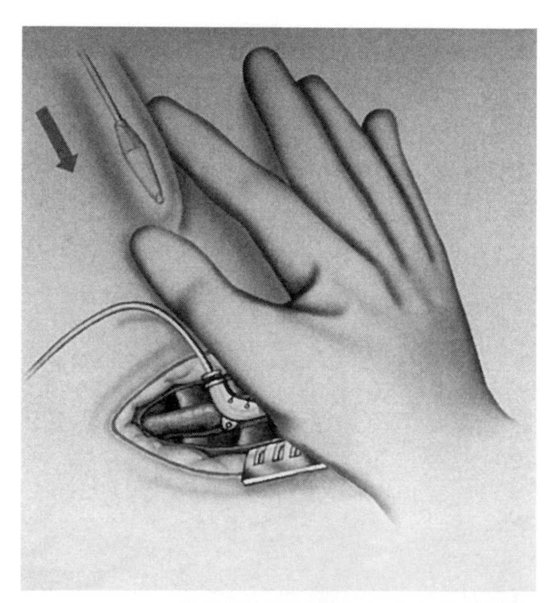

FIGURE 63–17 The arrow tip of the tunneling device is guided under the subcutaneous tissue. (Courtesy of Medtronic, Minneapolis, Minn. Reprinted with permission from Medtronic, Inc. ©Medtronic, Inc. 1996.)

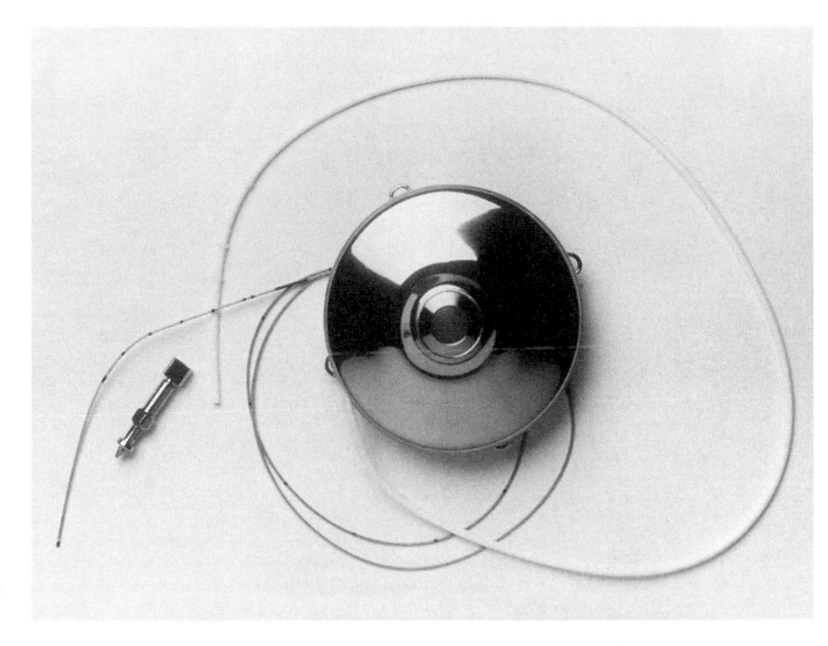

FIGURE 63–18 Arrow all-flex catheter system. (Courtesy of Arrow International, Reading, Pa.)

discarded. The pump catheter, with its swedged-on connector, is now secured to the pump.

At all points in the operation it is essential to ascertain free flow of cerebrospinal fluid out of the catheter system. If a two-piece catheter system is used, once the two catheters are connected and before the spinal catheter is connected to the pump, it must be ascertained that cerebrospinal fluid flow is unimpeded. Likewise, if a single-catheter system is used, after tunneling and before connecting to the pump, free flow of fluid must be confirmed (Fig. 63–20). If free flow cannot be confirmed, there may be some obstruction to flow. Any such obstruction must be identified, localized, and repaired before all incisions are closed.

After the catheter system has been connected to the pump, the pump is carefully placed into its pocket (Fig. 63–21). Any redundant catheter material is placed behind the pump, well away from where it might be punctured by a needle during refilling procedures. The back wound and the pump pocket wound are once again copiously irrigated with antibiotic solution and closed in a two layer closure according to the preference of the surgeon (Fig. 63–22).

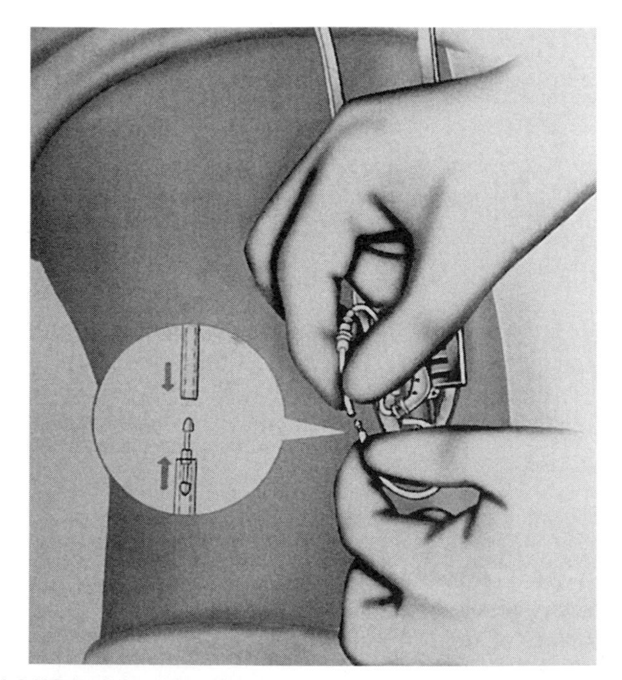

FIGURE 63–19 The spinal catheter and the pump catheter are connected with a titanium connector. (Courtesy of Medtronic, Minneapolis, Minn. Reprinted with permission from Medtronic, Inc. ©Medtronic, Inc. 1996.)

CONCLUSION

In this chapter, I have provided the reader an outline for pump implantation of two different totally implanted drug infusion systems, Medtronic Synchromed programmable systems and nonprogrammable, factory-preset flow rate Arrow systems.*

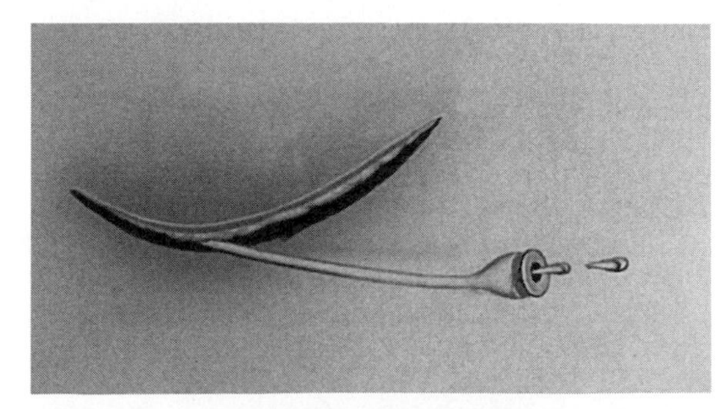

FIGURE 63–20 Catheter is checked for free flow of cerebrospinal fluid. (Courtesy of Medtronic, Minneapolis, Minn. Reprinted with permission from Medtronic, Inc. ©Medtronic, Inc. 1996.)

* The figures representing surgical technique in this article were created by and provided by Medtronic Corporation of Minneapolis, Minn.

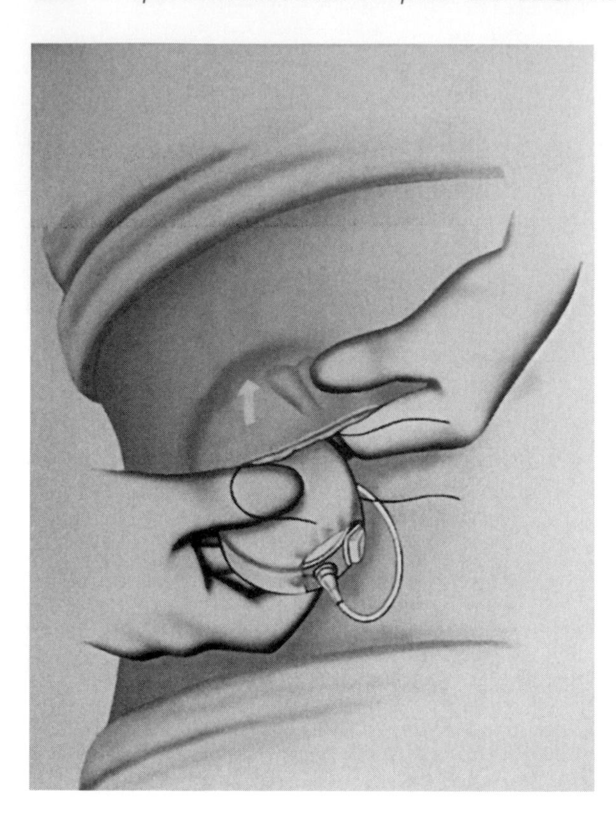

FIGURE 63-21 *After the catheter is connected, the pump is placed into the subcutaneous pocket. (Courtesy of Medtronic, Minneapolis, Minn. Reprinted with permission from Medtronic, Inc. ©Medtronic, Inc. 1996.)*

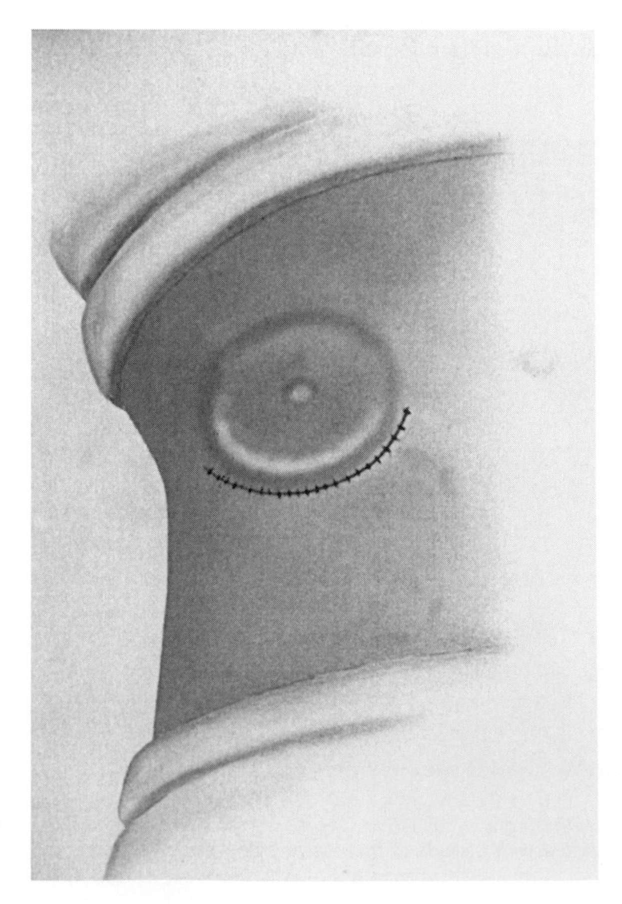

FIGURE 63-22 *The pump pocket is closed with a two-layer suture enclosure. (Courtesy of Medtronic, Minneapolis, Minn. Reprinted with permission from Medtronic, Inc. ©Medtronic, Inc. 1996.)*

REFERENCES

1. Kolb L: Types and characteristics of drug addicts. Ment Hygiene 9:300, 1925.
2. Porter J, Jick H: Addiction rare in patients treated with narcotics. N Engl J Med 302:123, 1980.
3. Perry S, Heidrick G: Management of pain during debridement: A survey of US burn units. Pain 13:267–2, 1982.
4. Portenoy RK, Foley KM: Chronic use of opioid analgesics in nonmalignant pain: Report of 38 cases. Pain 25:171–186, 1986.
5. Zenz M, Sturmpf M, Tryba M: Long-term oral opioid therapy in patients with chronic nonmalignant pain. J Pain Symptom Manage 7:69–77, 1992.
6. Joranson, D: Intractable pain: Treatment laws and regulations. Bull Am Pain Soc 5:2:1–17, 1995.
7. Medical Board of California: New, Easy Guidelines on Prescribing. Action Report of the Medical Board of California 51:8, 1994.
8. Auld AW, Maki-Jokela A, Murdock DM: Intraspinal narcotic analgesia in the treatment of chronic pain. Spine 10:777–781, 1984.
9. Hassenbusch SJ, Stanton-Hicks MD, Soukup J, et al: Sufentanil citrate and morphine/bupivacaine as alternative agents in chronic epidural infusions for intractable non-cancer pain. Neurosurgery 29:76–82, 1991.
10. Barolat G, Schwartzman RJ, Aries L: Chronic intrathecal morphine infusion for intractable pain in reflex sympathetic dystrophy. *In* Sessle B, Anderson K, Burchiel KJ (eds): Proceedings, Combined American/Canadian Pain Society Meeting. November 10-13, 1988. Toronto, Canada. New York, Raven Press, 1999.
11. Schuchard M, Lanning R, Krames ES: Intraspinal analgesia for nonmalignant pain: A retrospective analysis for efficacy, safety and feasibility in 50 patients. Neuromodulation 1:46–56, 1998.

CHAPTER • 64

Implantable Technology for Pain Control: Identification and Management of Problems and Complications

Richard B. Patt, MD •
Samuel J. Hassenbusch III, MD, PhD

The use of implantable technology for controlling pain is new enough that data are still insufficient to make authoritative statements about the incidence and nature of complications and the definitive means of their prevention and management. The content of this review is derived in large part from clinical experience, a comprehensive review chapter,[1] and lecture notes from symposia sponsored by Medtronic, Inc., and the Danemiller Education Foundation. Although we anticipate that, over time, standardized protocols will emerge, recommendations provided here, unless stated otherwise, should be considered, at most, guidelines intended to assist the clinician in decision making.

DEFINITION OF TERMS

At the outset, it is useful to make a distinction among side effects, corollary effects, and complications.[2] Side effects and corollary effects are similar phenomena and differ from complications in that they are anticipated, at least in a large proportion of cases. According to Webster's Dictionary,[3] a *corollary effect* is one that "follows as a normal result," and a *side effect* is a "secondary and usually adverse effect." In contrast, although the risk of a *complication* may be known, it is unanticipated, it is a "difficult factor or issue, often appearing unexpectedly."[3] The term *complication* further implies an adverse outcome, which may or may not apply to a corollary effect or side effect.

It is important that the distinction between anticipated and unanticipated events (corollary and side effects versus complications) be appreciated, so that the outcome can be characterized accurately. Furthermore, this distinction is important to invoke in discussions with patients, their families, and referring physicians, to ensure they understand the potential risks and benefits of a treatment and its alternatives.

The term *complication* implies an unanticipated adverse outcome. Although complications are by definition iatrogenic (caused by treatment), the occurrence of a complication or of an adverse outcome does not, in and of itself, imply negligence. An injury due to *negligence* is one caused by a breach of duty, by a preventable error associated with poor outcome.[4] A variety of factors predispose to such outcomes, independent of physician competence. Such factors include passage of sharp needles through tissue, the potential for movement of the needle or of the patient, dependence on some degree of inference to determine actual needle placement (even with the benefit of radiologic guidance), normal anatomic variations, distortion of normal tissues by tumor mass, failure of mechanical devices, and normal incidences of perioperative infections and other complications. Because of such factors, even independent of any contribution from physician error, if a sufficient number of procedures are undertaken, some complications are inevitable.

Regrettably, in addition to the factors just listed, physician error contributes to many adverse outcomes, although the actual incidence is not known. Given the potentially serious nature of complications, every conceivable effort obviously should be made to eliminate preventable errors. In addition, it is essential that, once a complication has occurred, it be recognized promptly, so treatment or rehabilitation can be instituted. To achieve the most successful outcome, a fundamental knowledge of the pertinent anatomy, physiology, and pharmacologic effects related to the procedure is essential. A thorough understanding of the possible complications of a given procedure and of strategies aimed at their prevention is also essential. Access to monitoring and resuscitation equipment and knowledge of their use are required. A comprehensive quality-assurance program that includes a process for credentialing physicians and nurses, establishing protocols, monitoring outcome, and providing in-service training workshops is an essential component of any implantation program.

Unfortunately, standards of training for pain specialists have not been established. Some level of experience with the given procedure or a related one is assumed. Physicians with limited or accruing experience do well to consult with a more expert authority. Even with ample experience, a review of reference materials is prudent before undertaking a procedure.

COMPLICATIONS ASSOCIATED WITH IMPLANTABLE DEVICES

Technical Problems Common to Implantable Infusion and Stimulation Technology

Bleeding

Bleeding may occur intraoperatively or postoperatively, may be superficial or deep, and may be due to mechanical or systemic factors.

INTRAOPERATIVE BLEEDING

Systemic Sources of Bleeding

Systemic factors may produce diffuse bleeding in the surgical field that is difficult to control until the factors that predisposed to bleeding are identified and corrected. It is essential that patients scheduled for surgery (particularly that involving the central nervous system) undergo screening for risk factors for bleeding of systemic origin. There is considerable debate about what screening methods strike a reasonable balance between clinical prudence and cost-effectiveness. There is no doubt that a careful interview is a sensitive screening tool and should be conducted in every case. The history taking should include eliciting easy bruising, difficulty in stopping bleeding once it has started, epistaxis, rectal bleeding, use of anticoagulants including aspirin and nonsteroidal antiinflammatory drugs (NSAID), and a family history of bleeding disorders. Some authorities argue that such a history is sufficient to rule out systemic factors that might predispose to surgical bleeding, especially in young patients. Given that implantation of pain control devices involves the potential for occult central nervous system hemorrhage, however, it may be prudent to require laboratory tests (prothrombin time, partial thromboplastin time, platelets, and bleeding time) for all surgical candidates.

In summary, the strategy for the management of bleeding induced by systemic factors is prevention. The management of intraoperative bleeding suspected to be related to systemic factors is reviewed elsewhere. Krames[5] recommends discontinuing anticoagulants 3 to 7 days before surgery and insisting on an increase in prothrombin time to 75% of normal before surgery is undertaken.[5]

Intraoperative Bleeding due to Mechanical Causes

Superficial Bleeding. Intraoperative bleeding is most often due to simple mechanical factors (i.e., ineffective local hemostasis). The requisites for the management of superficial bleeding related to mechanical causes are vigilance, patience, and experience. Excessive bleeding is uncommon, because implantation of pain control devices does not require extensive surgery, nor are the contiguous anatomic areas densely vascular.

Regardless of the type of anesthesia that is chosen, infiltration with a local anesthetic containing 1:200,000 epinephrine is strongly recommended to reduce the risk of surgical bleeding. An important technical means of reducing the likelihood of bleeding is using electrocautery instead of sharp surgical instruments. A sharp scalpel should be used to incise the skin; after that, electrocautery may be used extensively. When further dissection is needed, blunt dissection is preferred. When sharp dissection is required, scissors are preferable to the scalpel, and care must be taken to spread the blades beneath each tissue plane before cutting and to keep the tips of the scissors constantly in view.

When bleeding does occur, the field should be kept as dry as possible with suction and dry gauze wielded by an assistant while the source is calmly identified. The most effective method of identifying the source of bleeding and reducing or eliminating it is firm pressure applied with dry gauze pads. The pads should be pressed directly onto the surface of the wound and never rubbed, as rubbing increases bleeding. An initial trial of simple pressure applied for 30 to 60 secs may be all that is required to stop bleeding by promoting local vasoconstriction and clot formation. If bleeding persists, the area should be irrigated, and, when a source of bleeding is identified, the coagulation mode of the electrocautery should be applied, but sparingly. The current should not be so high as to create an arc between the cautery tip and tissue. Extensive cauterization distorts anatomic detail, creates friable tissue, and, by generating a large area of devitalized tissue, may create a nidus for infection. Rarely, a larger vessel is incised or transected, in which case it may be ligated with an absorbable suture or metal clip.

Deep Bleeding. Bleeding into the subarachnoid or epidural space is a more worrisome problem, because such bleeding is often occult and may be associated with neurologic morbidity. Fortunately, the incidence of clinically significant neuroaxial hemorrhage after implantation is extremely low. The key strategy is again prevention: (1) identifying and correcting systemic factors that might predispose to bleeding; (2) utilizing good surgical technique; and (3) promptly recognizing the problem and applying aggressive intervention.

Access to the epidural or subarachnoid space should be gained with as few passages of the large Tuohy needle as possible. This is facilitated by the judicious use of fluoroscopy. Periosteum is an important potential source of hemorrhage, so contact with bone should be appreciated immediately to minimize trauma. If access is difficult, a 22-gauge pilot needle may be used to identify an appropriate trajectory. Tumor is another important source of potential hemorrhage, so particular caution should be exercised in patients with bony metastases. In our experience, it is not uncommon to encounter frank bleeding from the epidural or subarachnoid space when entry has been difficult, particularly when multiple passages of a guidewire have been necessary to clear a tract for the catheter or lead. Although this incident has not been associated with postoperative problems in our experience, it calls for careful postoperative observation. Bleeding is usually sparse and ultimately ceases after irrigation with saline through the Tuohy needle. Patients should be observed particularly carefully for new back pain and neurologic abnormalities (altered sensation, motor or sphincter weakness) in the postoperative period. If bleeding persists, it is prudent to obtain an intraoperative consultation with a neurosurgeon for consideration of laminotomy to identify and eliminate the source of hemorrhage.

POSTOPERATIVE BLEEDING

Deep Bleeding: Subarachnoid or Epidural Hemorrhage
In the rare instance when a clinically significant subarachnoid or epidural hemorrhage occurs, it is usually manifested in the onset of back pain and rapidly progressive neurologic abnormalities in the postoperative period. To identify such changes, it is essential that the results of a careful neurologic examination be documented preoperatively. Patients should routinely have a neurologic examination during the recovery phase. Subjective complaints of new back pain, weakness, and sensory changes should be elicited and taken seriously. New neurologic abnormalities (subjective or objective) suggest a space-occupying collection of blood and warrant further investigation. Fever and nuchal rigidity may result from blood in the subarachnoid space. The results of closely spaced, serial neurologic examinations determine whether these findings are transient. If they persist or progress, urgent consultation with a neurologist or neurosurgeon should be sought, and patients should undergo urgent radiologic screening—with magnetic resonance imaging (MRI), computed tomography (CT), or myelography, depending on the clinical scenario. MRI is contraindicated in the case of a spinal stimulator and requires that special precautions be exercised if a drug-infusion device has been implanted. Testing of the implanted device may provide indirect evidence of a fluid collection. Clotted blood may interfere with function by impeding flow through an infusion device (tested by accessing the side port) or by a reduction in electrical contact manifested as a loss of stimulation or increased impedance.

Epidural or subarachnoid hemorrhage is a surgical emergency. Symptoms (back pain, altered sensation, bowel or bladder incontinence) characteristically progress over a period of hours, and permanent neurologic injury is likely if decompressive surgery is delayed.

Superficial Bleeding: Wound Hematoma or Seroma
Superficial bleeding is manifested as a *hematoma*, a collection of coagulated blood, or a *seroma*, a collection of serum. The incidence of these problems can be reduced by meticulous attention to maintaining intraoperative hemostasis. The first sign of such problems is usually a sensation of local pressure or pain during the recovery period, with or without the leakage of sanguineous or serosanguineous material from the wound edges. This ordinarily resolves with the application of local pressure and ice but occasionally requires reexploration or reversal of systemic clotting abnormalities.

Often, hematoma or seroma is not identified until after the immediate postoperative period, in which case it manifests as a diffuse bruise or a fluctuant collection, respectively. Both conditions are usually self-limited and resolve with time, during which analgesics may be provided and hot packs applied for comfort. Some authorities believe that a pocket seroma may occur in as many as 80% of patients, whereas others report seroma in fewer than 10% of cases. Generally, seromas are a self-limited problem that resolve over time and that should be managed with simple observation and reassurance. Treatment of excessive or chronic collections is controversial. Because a chronic seroma or hematoma is an ideal medium for infection, conventional surgical texts recommend fine-needle aspiration, and even insertion of a polyethylene catheter when collections repeatedly re-form. Others caution that aspiration may result in bacterial contamination.[6] Large postoperative seromas and liquefied hematomas should probably be aspirated, but under strict sterile conditions. Early and frequent pump refills should be minimized when such a collection is present, to reduce the risk of contamination. In addition, such collections may increase the difficulty of accurately locating the access port of an infusion device,[7,8] an obstacle that predisposes to accidental subcutaneous or intrathecal deposition of drug during attempts at pump refilling.

Infection

Fortunately, the incidence of infection after implant surgery for pain and spasticity is low. Most authorities advocate the use of prophylactic antibiotics. The most common recommendation is vancomycin, 500 mg, 2 hours before surgery, and copious irrigation of all wounds with irrigation fluid containing antibiotics. The same fluid may be used to bathe hardware before insertion. Other authorities recommend intravenous cephalothin, 2 g preoperatively and then every 6 hours for 24 hours. The incidence of infection is probably highest in the immediate postoperative period, which is when vigilance should be greatest. Problems range from local infections of the pocket or subcutaneous tract to meningitis and epidural abscess.

LOCAL INFECTION

Local subcutaneous infection is usually heralded by fever, leukocytosis, and inflammatory skin changes (erythema, tenderness, fluctuance, drainage) overlying the infected region. Leukocytosis is often observed in Gram stains of fluid aspirated from the subcutaneous pocket in patients with simple seroma (see earlier), so a pathogen should be sought if infection is suspected.

When infection is suspected, concerns relate both to resolving the local process and to guarding against extension of the infectious process to the central nervous system. What is the best treatment is controversial. Some authorities advocate vigorous conservative management for 1 to 2 weeks with intravenous antibiotics and local wound care while observing for signs of central nervous system involvement. Local ("intrapocket") deposition of antibiotics has also been advocated. Others believe that removal of all hardware is always indicated. An infectious disease consultation may be warranted, although the implant surgeon should be aware that such a consultation is usually accompanied by the recommendation that hardware be removed.

CENTRAL NERVOUS SYSTEM INFECTION

Meningitis

Meningitis is inflammation of the meninges of the brain or spinal cord. After surgical implantation, meningitis is more likely to be a relatively focal process involving the spinal cord, although, with encephalitis, more diffuse involvement is a possibility.

Meningitis is usually heralded by fever, chills, leukocytosis, malaise, headache, vomiting, and back or neck pain and stiffness, and it tends to be accompanied by signs of meningeal irritation. Kernig's sign is pain associated with simultaneous flexion of the hip and extension of the knee in a supine patient. Brudzinski's sign is involuntary flexion of the knee when the supine patient's neck is abruptly flexed. Although it is difficult to quantify, a key diagnostic finding is that affected patients tend to look extremely ill, or "septic." Progression of signs and symptoms is typically rapid. Patients may become confused, stuporous, and dehydrated and may develop unstable hemodynamics. Classically, cerebral involvement is manifested by cranial nerve abnormalities (including loss of auditory acuity), seizures, focal cerebral signs (hemiparesis, visual field defects), and signs of elevated intracranial pressure, although this presentation is unusual in patients with infection due to implanted intraspinal devices.

Early recognition is essential, and consultation with a neurologist or infectious disease specialist is recommended. Laboratory examinations of the blood and cerebrospinal fluid (CSF) help to confirm a diagnosis, although culture results are affected if empirical antibiotic treatment has already been instituted. Recovery is usually complete when a diagnosis and treatment with intravenous antibiotics are rendered promptly. Removal of all implanted hardware is necessary. The only possible exception to this dictum involves the patient with imminently terminal cancer whose pain is well-controlled. In this case, considerations of comfort may prevail, and treatment with intrathecal antibiotics may be considered.

Epidural Abscess

Signs and symptoms of epidural abscess are similar to those described for epidural hematoma, but, if the abscess is allowed to progress, symptoms and signs consistent with meningitis may become more prominent. The presenting signs are usually localized back pain and deep tenderness. Symptoms may be radicular in nature and, depending on the size and location of the lesion, may be associated with neurologic abnormalities (focal weakness, sensory abnormalities, incontinence). Progression of symptoms, especially weakness in a paraplegic or root distribution, generally occurs over a course of hours or days with a slower progression of symptoms than that seen with postoperative hemorrhage. Fever and meningeal signs may be present but are less prominent than with frank meningitis. Laboratory studies should include blood work and examination of the CSF, but, ultimately, myelography is required for diagnosis and localization. Treatment is prompt surgical decompression and removal of all implanted hardware. Ideally intravenous antibiotics should be started after specimens for cultures and Gram stain have been obtained. *Staphylococcus aureus* is often the infecting bacteria; therefore, the initial antibiotic should be effective against it.

Postoperative Fever

Postoperative fever should always generate concern and a high index of suspicion of underlying local or systemic infection, especially considering the serious consequences of the conditions already described, though they are relatively uncommon. It should be recognized that, in the initial days after implantation (particularly of an intrathecal catheter), a large proportion of patients develop fever in the absence of signs of local, systemic, or meningeal infection. In this scenario, low-grade fever (38° to 38.5° C) is usually associated with a normal white blood cell (WBC) count and CSF that is remarkable only for pleocytosis and elevated protein content. Treatment is conservative, and administration of antibiotics is unwarranted. Indiscriminate early use of antibiotics later makes the selection of effective therapy much more problematic if cultures eventually yield positive results.

Cerebrospinal Fluid Leak, Postdural Puncture Headache, and Hygroma

CSF leak is definitely a risk after puncture of the dura with a large (15-gauge) Tuohy needle. It can occur during placement of a spinal cord stimulator if the dura is accidentally punctured during efforts to identify the epidural space or if the guidewire or lead pierces the dura. CSF leak may occur after subarachnoid catheter placement under two circumstances. First, leakage can occur by the same mechanism cited earlier if successful dural puncture is followed by inability to advance the catheter, and a second puncture becomes necessary. Second, CSF leakage can occur around the implanted catheter, because the track created by the needle slightly exceeds the caliber of the catheter. Many surgeons routinely create a purse-string suture in the ligament surrounding the catheter's entrance into the dura, usually with absorbable material. In addition to possibly reducing the risk of CSF leak, this measure may also discourage catheter extrusion. If a purse-string suture is chosen, care must be taken to ensure that (1) the needle does not damage the catheter and (2) the suture is not pulled so tight as to occlude the lumen of the catheter. The risk of catheter occlusion may be reduced by creating the purse-string suture when the catheter is still within the needle and by periodically verifying free flow of CSF.

CSF leak is usually heralded by a classic postural postdural puncture headache, although other causes of headache should still be considered. Many headaches resolve with conservative management. Although what constitutes proper conservative management of postdural puncture headache is still debated, several days' bed rest, fluids, and an abdominal binder is recommended. Persistent postural headache may be treated with an epidural blood patch, using 5 to 15 mL of autologous blood. Blood patch should be performed under the strictest of aseptic conditions and with fluoroscopy, to avoid damaging the catheter or lead. Rarely, when headaches persist, surgical exploration and placement of a fat graft may be necessary.

Hygroma typically refers to a benign, distended, lymph-filled cavity, usually in a child, but the word is also used for a postoperative collection of CSF. Hygroma can develop after a large CSF leak and eventually is manifested as a subcutaneous bulge near the dorsal incision. The mechanism may even be disruption of the pia arachnoid membrane and formation of a subdural collection through a ball-valve effect. Theoretically, such a collection may produce focal neurologic deficits in the same way an epidural abscess does, but, in general, such signs have little clinical significance. Diagnosis is based on clinical findings and radiologic studies. Most authorities recommend that such collections not be aspirated owing to the risk of infection; rather they advise waiting for it to resolve or reoperating. Large collections occasionally require aspiration, although care must be taken to avoid damaging the underlying apparatus. An infected hygroma should be treated in the same way as meningitis is. Frank percutaneous CSF leak requires revision of the wound with primary closure.

Malposition of the Subcutaneous Pocket

Care should be taken to ensure that the subcutaneous position of the infusion device or pulse generator does not impinge on the ribs superiorly or the iliac crest inferiorly. Such bony impingement is a cause of chronic postoperative pain and usually requires reoperation. It can usually be avoided by marking the patient's skin before surgery and observing where the marks fall when the patient is supine, standing, and sitting. A pocket positioned too far cephalad or caudad or too close to the skin surface can also impair wound healing and predispose to erosion through the skin. Patients who are cachectic, diabetic, or taking steroids are at increased risk for these complications. A pocket placed too deep (>2.5 cm) also can create problems during refills.

When implanting a spinal cord stimulator, it should be ascertained that the pulse generator is placed with the Medtronic trademark facing outward, to avoid problems with programming. Care should be taken to tighten set screws snugly, to avoid disconnection but not so tight as to strip the threads. With an infusion device, care must be taken to properly anchor the Dacron sleeve, to avoid rotation of the pump, which could put enough traction on the catheter to cause it to withdraw from the intrathecal space.

Technical Problems Specific to Implantable Infusion Devices

Contamination of Pump Reservoir

The pump reservoir can be contaminated by seeding by skin flora during refills. Although the Medtronic's 0.22-μm filter would be expected to prevent extension of an infection from the reservoir to the CNS, prudence dictates that documentation of infected aspirate be followed by removal of the system.

Catheter Care

Silastic catheters are extremely fragile and ideally should be handled only with the fingers. If such a catheter must be manipulated with forceps, rubber shods should be used. The catheter may become difficult to manipulate owing to the lubricity of body fluids, in which case the field should be irrigated. Dry gauze also provides excellent traction and causes no trauma. The catheter should never be forced into the epidural or subarachnoid space, because the guidewire would develop a "memory" that would make further passage difficult. The catheter should be stabilized with an anchoring sleeve and should not be sutured directly. Nicking or cutting of the catheter should be avoided. Excess length of catheter should be coiled behind the infusion device, well away from the access port.

Pump Care

The pump reservoir should be emptied before instillation of drug (10 mL) and should be programmed to deliver at least 0.096 mL/day. The necessity initially to fill the reservoir only partially cannot be overemphasized, because overpressurization can be associated with erratic infusion rates (Total reservoir capacity is 18 mL.) The incision for the subcutaneous pocket should be positioned eccentrically, so that it is not directly over the access port.

Failure of Analgesia in Patients with Infusion Devices

IMMEDIATE POSTOPERATIVE FAILURE

Failure of mechanical causes is most often occurs in the immediate postoperative period. Uncontrolled postoperative (nonsurgical) pain in a patient who previously was comfortable during a trial of intraspinal opioids suggests some error during implantation. Such difficulties may relate to failure to cannulate the epidural or subarachnoid space; a disconnected, kinked, or leaking catheter; or programming or pharmacy error. Problems can usually be avoided by careful confirmation of the location of the catheter tip, gentle handling of the catheter, careful suturing, and confirmation of the accuracy of the program and the prescription. Before the spinal catheter is connected to the infusion device, if it is intrathecal, free flow of CSF should be confirmed, and if it is epidural, the catheter should be checked for obstruction or occlusion. The same procedures should be performed through the infusion device's side port once the catheter has been connected.

LATE FAILURE

Failure of analgesia after apparently successful implantation is not uncommon, but it is usually due to the development of anesthetic tolerance or new foci of pain and rarely to mechanical malfunction. Because physiologic, rather than mechanical, causes are most often responsible, it is reasonable to respond initially by increasing the rate of the infusion to determine whether pain control can be regained. Although often this is ultimately a correct and effective approach, intervention should be individualized and predicated on the findings of a careful history and examination.

DIFFERENTIAL DIAGNOSIS

The differential diagnosis of late failure of analgesia includes development of tolerance, new foci of pain, an incorrect prescription, failure to properly load the pump, pump malfunction,[9] disconnection, and obstruction or migration of the catheter system.[10] A careful history and physical examination should be performed and, when indicated, should be supplemented with communication with the family, primary care physician, oncologist, and home nursing and pharmacy services. Assessment is undertaken to rule out a new pain-generating lesion or extension of underlying disease. Pain is multifactorial; because the pain threshold is influenced by a variety of factors, new psychosocial causes should be sought as well.

Progression of Disease. Local extension, distant metastases, or an unrelated pain problem should be confirmed or excluded by the history and physical examination findings, appropriate laboratory and radiologic investigations, and, when indicated, consultation.

Tolerance. *Tolerance* is manifested as the need for progressively higher doses of a drug over time to achieve a given degree of effect. If problems related to the integrity of the delivery system and demonstrable new underlying disease (physical and psychological) have been excluded, the most likely explanation for increased pain is tolerance. In the past, loss of analgesia had been assumed to be rather uniformly related to the development of tolerance. More recently, it has been accepted that loss of analgesia is more often related to undetected progression of cancer and more extensive tissue damage.[11] Nerve injury of new onset often produces neuropathic pain, which may be less opioid responsive. Tolerance remains an important cause of failed analgesia. Tolerance does not usually develop equally to all effects of a drug at the same rate, and, fortunately, tolerance to a drug's undesirable effects can also develop.[12] The management of tolerance is discussed later.

Mechanical Failure. Examination of the infusion system is approached logically and simply, working sequentially from the periphery of the system toward the center:

1. Examination of the drug prescription and confirmation of its accuracy.
2. Examination of the infusion device and verification that the program and prescription are correct. Verification of proper battery function and that the volume in the reservoir corresponds to the expected and actual volume of drug delivered (≤15%).
3. Examination of external portions of the system for kinking and to confirm that the drug is actually exiting the pump tubing.
4. Examination of the tunneled portion of the catheter to detect kinks or rents in the tubing or evidence of infection or subcutaneous drug deposition.
5. In the absence of demonstrable defects in the integrity of the delivery system, injection of radiopaque contrast medium and radiography. The results of these studies provide more definitive data on the system's integrity and help to identify catheter migration or diminished drug delivery due to tumor or deposition of fibrous tissue around the catheter outlet. MRI is a potentially useful adjunct to assessment, although the device may create artifacts. MRI is not contraindicated, but it requires that the device first be emptied and turned off. Myelography may be performed after injection of contrast medium through the device's access port, and, subsequently, CT can be performed.

Radiography, Myelography, and Epidurography or Test Doses

The radiopacity of the system's catheter facilitates radiologic visualization, although filling the catheter lumen with contrast medium is often useful to enhance image quality. The model 8615 device (Medtronic, Minneapolis, Minn.) has a second port that is eccentrically located and bypasses the pump for myelography or epidurography. If a model without a bypass port (Medtronic 8611–H) has been implanted, the reservoir may be filled with contrast medium, and the rate of infusion can be increased, after which films can be obtained. A water-soluble, nonionic contrast medium should be used in all cases,[13] and the patient should first be screened for a history of allergy. If further information is needed, postcontrast CT may be performed. Although their use is not encouraged owing to considerations of safety, the same means can be utilized for the administration of test doses of local anesthetics.

Treatment Strategies for Opioid Tolerance

Tolerance is implied by failure of analgesia in the absence of new disease or equipment failure. Obviously, the approach to tolerance depends on the baseline treatment protocol. In general, a reasonable approach when tolerance is suspected involves sequentially increasing the dose by 10% to 30% per day. If this strategy would require administering excessive volumes of drug, the solution may need to be reformulated. What constitutes an excessive flow rate still is not known, although Leak and colleagues[14] offer 10 to 15 mL/hr for epidural infusion and a daily rate that does not exceed 10% of a given patient's calculated CSF volume for intrathecal devices. Morphine can readily be concentrated to 50 mg/mL and hydromorphone to about 200 mg/mL.[15] Long-term infusions of high concentrations of morphine have not been associated with neurotoxicity or central nervous system lesions, although collection of more animal and human data is warranted before definitive conclusions can be drawn about neurotoxicity.[16] Maximum daily doses cited in the literature range from 60 to 480 mg for epidural morphine[17] and to 150 mg for intrathecal morphine.[18]

TITRATION-RESISTANT TOLERANCE

Tolerance may make it impossible to regain analgesia by simple dose titration, although it is not clear to what extent titration-resistant tolerance represents tolerance per se or the emergence of a relatively opioid-resistant neuropathic focus of pain.

PREVENTING TOLERANCE

The emergence of true, pharmacodynamically based tolerance can be managed in several ways, none entirely satisfactory. One approach is prophylaxis. It has been suggested that tolerance appears to be less troublesome when intraspinal opioids are administered by continuous infusion rather than intermittent boluses,[19–22] although this theory has not been proven conclusively. It has also been suggested that the use of a more potent opioid, such as sufentanil, may result in slower receptor downregulation.[23–25]

USE OF NONOPIOID SUBSTANCES

Once tolerance develops, theoretically, other spinal antinociception-modulating systems can be employed, either temporarily, to "rest" and "recruit" receptors (a drug holiday) or over the long term as an alternative or supplement to opioid therapy. A variety of disparate substances have been administered intraspinally in efforts to produce safe, reliable analgesia. Even encouraging reports warrant cautious interpretation, because animal and human studies of toxicology and efficacy are inadequate in many cases. No substances other than morphine and baclofen are currently approved for administration via an implanted Medtronic infusion device.

Clonidine. The alpha$_2$-adrenergic agonist clonidine is perhaps the best-studied of these agents. Successful management of both cancer pain and postoperative pain has been reported with epidural and intrathecal clonidine.[26–28] Clonidine appears to produce spinally mediated antinociception by its action on postsynaptic receptors in the dorsal horn, activating descending noradrenergic inhibitory systems.[29] Analgesia is reversible with alpha-antagonist agents but is not affected by naloxone. Hypotension is the main potential adverse effect. When clonidine is used in combination with opioids, opioid-mediated respiratory depression may be potentiated, especially in opioid-naive patients. Clonidine appears not to cause local toxicity.[30] Reporting on 52 patients with chronic cancer pain, Glynn and associates[28] observed consistently adequate analgesia in 20 patients with a low incidence of side effects, and Eisenach and colleagues[26] treated patients successfully with intrathecal clonidine and morphine for as long as 5 months. It has been suggested that intraspinal clonidine may have a particularly important role in the management of opioid-resistant neuropathic pain syndromes. Preliminary evaluations of the alpha-adrenergic agonists tizanidine and dexmedetomidine are ongoing.

Droperidol. Droperidol appears to be a safe and effective adjunct to intraspinal opioid therapy. Animal experiments have demonstrated that intrathecal morphine analgesia is prolonged and potentiated by the addition of droperidol and that tolerance is delayed.[31] The pooled results of clinical series suggest that the addition of 2.5 mg of droperidol to epidural or intrathecal morphine may potentiate analgesia, reduce a range of side effects (nausea, vomiting, pruritus, urinary retention, hypotension), and delay tolerance, although sedative effects may occur.[32, 33]

Somatostatin and Calcitonin. Chrubasik and coworkers[34, 35] have reported that somatostatin, an endogenous neuropeptide, when injected intrathecally, epidurally, or intraventricularly, produces analgesia equal to that of intrathecal morphine in persons with postoperative or cancer pain. On the basis of these findings, somatostatin is another potential means of limiting or managing opioid tolerance, although expense and suggestions of local neurotoxicity are barriers to more widespread trials.[36, 37] Octreotide, a synthetic somatostatin analogue, may ultimately prove to be a safer and more useful compound.[38, 39] Intrathecal salmon calcitonin, although probably ineffective alone as an analgesic agent, has an opioid-sparing effect when used in conjunction with morphine.[36, 40] The currently available data from animal research are insufficient to recommend routine clinical use of intrathecal or epidural calcitonin.[41]

Antinociceptive Agents. Stein and Brechner[42] administered epidural norepinephrine, 50 to 250 μg, combined with morphine in a tolerant patient and consequently were able to reduce the dose of opioid by 50% without altering analgesia. Russell and Chang demonstrated in rats that alternating administration of relatively receptor-specific agent modifies tolerance favorably.[43] (Morphine affects predominantly mu receptors; D-Ala2-D-Leu5-enkephalin [DADL] predominantly delta receptors.) Anecdotal reports of analgesia in morphine-tolerant patients given intrathecal DADL, a synthetic enkephalin analogue, have also appeared in the literature.[44, 45] Other substances with potential antinociceptive activity at the level of the neuraxis are ketamine,[46] midazolam,[47] baclofen,[48] an injectable form of aspirin (lysine acetylsalicylate), and various alpha-adrenergic adenosine analogues.[36]

USE OF A DIFFERENT OPIOID

Cross-tolerance is the phenomenon whereby tolerance to one drug induces tolerance to another. The issue of cross-tolerance among the various subsets of opioid receptors and different receptor systems is an important one. There is some evidence for incomplete cross-tolerance,[39, 49, 50] and that is a rationale for substituting one opioid for another, although additional research is required to gain a better understanding of the nature of incomplete cross-tolerance among otherwise similar drugs.

SUBSTITUTION OF LOCAL ANESTHETICS

An alternative strategy for reversing tolerance or delaying its development involves the administration of epidural, or even intrathecal, local anesthetic. Local anesthetic may be substituted for opioids to provide an opioid-free interval (a drug holiday), during which receptor activity may revert toward normal, once again rendering the patient opioid sensitive.[51] This strategy should be employed only in a closely supervised setting to monitor for adverse sequelae of opioid withdrawal (abstinence syndrome) or of the local anesthetics (hypotension).

COMBINING OPIOID WITH OTHER AGENTS

Alternatively, dilute concentrations of local anesthetic (0.012%–0.25% bupivacaine) can be added to an epidural opioid infusion. Such combinations are often employed successfully to manage acute pain and have well-established safety profiles in the acute-care setting. Du Pen[52] has demonstrated the safety of administering a combination of epidural morphine and dilute bupivacaine to patients in their homes. In a series of 105 patients treated with epidural morphine, 0.75% (8 patients) required further analgesia with bupivacaine for new bone or nerve pain. In addition to epidural morphine, these patients received epidural bupivacaine, 0.125% to 0.5%, with epinephrine, administered at 6 mL/hr. Clinically significant hypotension did not develop, and many patients remained ambulatory. Patients receiving this treatment should be well-hydrated and should be restricted to bed rest during the initial stages of therapy. Such combination therapy may minimize the adverse side effects of each type of agent[53] and may be particularly efficacious for sharp, incident pain due, for example, to a pathologic fracture or a neurogenic process. Animal evidence for synergistic effects after the administration of combinations of opioids with distinctive receptor affinities[54] or an opioid and alpha agonist[55] suggest that combining such agents is another means of reducing or offsetting opioid tolerance.

SUMMARY

Careful assessment helps to determine the relative contributions of each of the factors that might be responsible for loss of analgesia during previously reliable intraspinal opioid therapy. The system's integrity and the patient's physiologic and psychological status should be evaluated. Subsequent management must be expressly individualized.

Psychological and emotional adjustments to progressive cancer, disability, and impending death sometimes color subjective reports of pain and must be addressed. Increased complaints of pain may signal the need for counseling or treatment with psychotropic agents, including antidepressants and sleep-restoring medications. Any new lesions (bowel obstruction, pathologic fracture, spinal cord compression) should be identified and, when appropriate, managed with alternate palliative interventions (e.g., radiation therapy, surgery, steroids). Neuropathic pain is often resistant to intraspinal opioid therapy but may be effectively managed with oral adjuvants (antidepressants, anticonvulsants, sodium channel blockers) or local anesthetic blockade. Intermittent regional blocks or the addition of a local anesthetic to the intraspinal opioid infusion may be particularly efficacious when symptoms are sympathetically maintained. Incident pain can often be effectively managed by supplementing the continuous intraspinal opioid infusion with oral opioids. Depending on the system in use, patient-controlled analgesia (PCA) or the addition of a preprogrammed bolus schedule may be useful. As clinical experience with new agents and methods of administration accrues, better-defined roles for these interventions are anticipated.

Problems with Refills of Infusion Devices

Accidental overdose of morphine in the course of refilling an intrathecal infusion device is an uncommon event but has been known to occur (Medtronic, Personal communication, 1991). The potential for accidental overdose due to equipment malfunction or human error has been cited as a possible disadvantage of implantable systems.[56] Accidental massive overdoses of opioids in other settings have been reported, including malfunction of a PCA device (administration of 495 mg meperidine within 20 mins, resulting in respiratory arrest),[57] and with epidural[58] and intrathecal morphine.[59] Independent of route of administration, excessive doses of opioids may result in a variety of adverse outcomes, including respiratory depression, hypothermia, myoclonic seizures, pulmonary edema, coma, and death.[36, 60]

ACCIDENTAL SUBCUTANEOUS ADMINISTRATION

In a case reported in 1992, a patient accidentally received a subcutaneous bolus injection of 480 mg morphine that was supposed to be instilled into the reservoir of an infusion pump and administered continuously over 6 to 8 weeks.[7] Mild respiratory depression and confusion developed approximately 2 hours afterward, but no significant cardiovascular effects or lasting neurologic deficits resulted. The patient was treated with 0.16 mg of naloxone intravenously, predominantly for diagnostic purposes. After 20 hours of observation, the patient was discharged without sequelae. The relatively innocuous outcome was probably related to a constellation of factors, including opioid tolerance, early recognition, and prompt management. Given the patient's stable course, the Emergency Medicine housestaff involved in the case were reluctant to believe that such an overdose actually occurred, but tolerance to high doses of opioids after long-term exposure to these drugs is well-known in the cancer pain literature.[61] Reversal of respiratory depression with an opioid antagonist is warranted in such cases, but it should be accomplished with small, incremental doses to avoid severe hypertension, dysrhythmias, and pulmonary edema, which presumably result from the rapid increases in sympathetic tone that may accompany the sudden return of pain when opioid effects are antagonized too rapidly.[62]

The Medtronic SynchroMed infusion pump is a titanium device about the size of a hockey puck that is usually implanted in the subcutaneous tissue of the flank. In the center of the pump's ventral surface is a small silicone injection port that must be palpated through intact skin. Identification of the septum may be difficult shortly after surgery because of swelling and inflammation. Passage of a 22-gauge, eccentrically tipped needle is marked by a characteristic giving way and ready return of clear fluid. Postoperative edema, obesity, or a deep implant may interfere with easy palpation of the port. It is possible that in the case just cited, the curved tip of the Huber needle slid over the pump's metal surface, mimicking the anticipated "give." Serous extravasation or seroma (usually clear) has been noted as one of the most common complications after surgery on subcutaneous tissue[63]; thus, in the postoperative patient described in this case, aspiration of a seroma mimicked return of drug.

ACCIDENTAL INTRATHECAL BOLUS ADMINISTRATION DURING INTENDED REFILL

Two models of the Medtronic SynchroMed infusion pump are currently available. The older, Model 8611H pump has a single refill port located centrally and no accessory port, whereas the newer Model 8615 has a central port for refill and an eccentric accessory port. The accessory port bypasses the reservoir and pump mechanism and is intended to facilitate myelography and to allow for planned intraspinal bolus or test doses of drug. At least four cases of accidental administration of large doses of morphine into accessory ports have been reported; two were fatal.[8] Accidental administration of baclofen into accessory ports has also been reported. These prompted issuance of an FDA-required "Urgent Medical Device Safety Alert" (June 15, 1992) by Medtronic that should be required reading for all healthcare professionals involved in the maintenance of implantable intraspinal infusion systems.

AVOIDING AND MANAGING PROBLEMS DURING REFILL OF A MEDTRONIC RESERVOIR

The potentially devastating events just described seem not to be the result of faulty design or system malfunction; rather, they are directly attributable to human error. Thus, they should be reliably preventable by careful observation of the precautions and guidelines related to replenishing the pump as they are set forth in the SynchroMed pump and refill kit technical manuals and reviewed here. The most important and essential precautionary measure is to use the Medtronic Model 8551 refill kit *each time* a pump's reservoir is replenished. The pump model is first identified, so that the proper template[7] will be used to locate the refill port, which is located centrally. A Huber needle is then inserted, using sterile technique, through the template's center hole and is advanced through the skin, subcutaneous tissue, and pump septum until the rigid needle stop arrests the needle's progress. The reservoir's residual volume should be emptied by applying continuous, gentle negative pressure to the plunger of the syringe. Proper needle placement is evidenced by air bubbles, which normally are not seen if the accessory port has accidentally been entered. Tubing and a three-way stopcock are provided in the kit to avoid entraining air into the reservoir. Resuscitation equipment, including naloxone (for morphine infusions) and physostigmine (for baclofen infusions), should be immediately available. Algorithms for both contingencies are included in the FDA-mandated safety alert already cited. Guidelines call for support of the airway, breathing, and circulation; serial intravenous administration of naloxone or physostigmine (when indicated); and (when not contraindicated) withdrawal of CSF.

Risk factors for problems during refilling include obesity, a "deep" implant, and, particularly early after implantation, local edema. If needed, fluoroscopy may be used to locate the proper port. Air bubbles normally are not obtained when the accessory port has been entered accidentally (CSF is returned). If a question remains about which port has been entered, CSF can be identified by chemically testing the aspirate for glucose. Given the serious nature of an error, a routine dipstick examination would not be imprudent. Our report recommends that, during refilling of the reservoir, its entire volume be intermittently aspirated to verify that the residual volume is equal to that that has been instilled during intended refill.

An alternative safety measure that we recently adopted is to empty the pump and then inject preservative-free saline and aspirate it before loading the reservoir with fresh morphine. We believe that the theoretical disadvantage of diluting the ultimate dose of morphine slightly (by mixing saline within the pump's dead space volume) is offset by the reduced risk of injecting even a few milliliters of concentrated morphine (25–50 mg/mL) intrathecally.

A final precaution concerns pump selection. Although an accessory port is often desirable, the option of the Medtronic Model 8611H (without accessory port) should be seriously considered for patients who are likely to be followed outside the geographic area of the implanting physician.

SUMMARY

Although several regrettable incidents of patient injury have occurred in association with the use of the intraspinal infusion pump, it appears to be a reliable and safe device. More such incidents can be prevented by the institution of several simple precautions and the implementation of pump training programs for all involved healthcare professionals.

Physiologic and Pharmacologic Side Effects

Unlike their opioid-naive counterparts, cancer patients with long-term exposure to systemic opioids rarely have dose-limiting side effects.[64, 65] This distinction provides a tremendous measure of safety. Because a cardinal rule for instituting intraspinal therapy is documented failure of conservative pharmacotherapy, it would be unusual to institute long-term intraspinal therapy in an opioid-naive patient.

Potential side effects of intraspinal opioids that occur with clinically significant frequency include respiratory depression, gastrointestinal hypomotility, inhibition of micturition, nausea, vomiting, pruritus, and central nervous system toxicity (usually manifested as sedation).[66] DeCastro and colleagues[64] list a multitude of other side effects that occur much more rarely or have been reported only anecdotally but of which the clinician should be aware. They include dysphoria, hypothermia, oliguria, failure of ejaculation, headache, erythema, agitation, miosis, muscle weakness, hallucinations, catatonia, abdominal spasm, diarrhea, shivering, hypotension, abstinence syndrome, and (in a patient with intracranial hypertension) seizure.[67] Treatment of side effects is generally symptomatic, but persistent or severe ones can usually be countered with intravenous or intramuscular naloxone, often with preservation of analgesia.[68, 69]

RESPIRATORY DEPRESSION

Of all potential complications, the risk of respiratory depression generates the most clinical concern. Respiratory depression may be an early (<2 hours from initial administration) or late (4–24 hours after administration) phenomenon.[25, 70–72] Activity at both the mu and delta receptors has been demonstrated to be associated with both types of respiratory depression.[73, 74] Kappa receptor activation may not be associated with significant respiratory depression,[75] but a pure kappa agonist with reliable analgesic properties is not yet available.[25, 71]

Management of Respiratory Depression

Factors that predispose to respiratory depression include accidental overdose, absence of severe pain, advanced age or debility, coexisting pulmonary disease, sleep apnea, inter-current opioid analgesic dosing by alternate routes, and opioid naivete.[36] Respiratory depression is significantly more likely to occur in opioid-naive patients, and there are few or no reports of late respiratory depression in patients previously maintained on systemic opioids for even short periods. Reversal of respiratory depression can be accomplished with the administration of a mu antagonist (naloxone) or the kappa agonist–mu antagonist nalbuphine.[64, 76–80] Oral naltrexone administered (prophylactically) in surgical patients reduces pruritus, nausea, and somnolence but may be associated with a decrement in analgesia.[81] That these agents must be administered cautiously and in small increments is supported by reports of cardiogenic shock, irreversible ventricular fibrillation, and pulmonary edema associated with the sudden reversal of systemic and intraspinal opioids.[53, 73, 82, 83] A report of the successful reversal of respiratory depression by the replacement of aspirated CSF with normal saline suggests another intriguing therapeutic approach.[84]

GASTROINTESTINAL SIDE EFFECTS

Constipation. Maintenance of gastrointestinal motility and avoidance of constipation are of particular concern in cancer patients. Systemic opioids delay gastric emptying and decrease lower gastrointestinal tract motility, presumably by their action on opioid receptors in the gut. Experimental work suggests that intrathecal morphine does not decrease peristalsis,[85, 86] but systematic studies in humans have not been reported.[53] Clinically, gastrointestinal motility seems to be better preserved with intraspinal than with systemic opioids but may still be adversely affected as intraspinal doses increase. Studies in postoperative patients do, however, confirm that postoperative ileus persists longer when pain is treated with epidural morphine than with bupivacaine.[22]

Management of Constipation. Constipation in a cancer patient is commonly multifactorial. Reversible causes should be identified and treated, and, in addition, a prophylactic symptomatic approach using a sliding-scale regimen of cathartics should be adopted. The pharmacology of these agents and a rationale for their use is reviewed elsewhere.[87] The tendency toward less constipation with intraspinal opioids may provide a rationale for a transition from systemic to intraspinal therapy when intractable constipation complicates management with systemic opioids.[88]

Nausea and Vomiting. Epidural morphine has been observed to reduce gastric emptying and small intestinal transit in volunteers.[89] The incidence of nausea and vomiting associated with the administration of intraspinal opioids may range as high as 25% to 30% in opioid-naive subjects but is very low in patients with prior long-term exposure to opioids. Like nausea and vomiting induced by oral opioids, these effects generally resolve rapidly with continued administration.[90, 91] Nausea and vomiting are believed to be related to activity at the chemoreceptor trigger zone and vomiting center: That the vestibular system is often involved as well is suggested by a higher incidence of nausea and vomiting in ambulatory patients than in bed-bound ones.[92]

Management of Nausea and Vomiting. Nausea and vomiting may be reversed with the administration of nalbuphine or naloxone (see earlier), but this therapy is usually unnecessary because symptoms generally subside with time. If symptoms persist, patients should first be treated symptomatically with standard antiemetics, such as a phenothiazine, a butyrophenone, hydroxyzine, metoclopramide, or dexamethasone. Alternatively, patients may benefit from a trial of a more lipophilic opioid.[36] In a double-blind, placebo-controlled study that targeted patients receiving epidural morphine (postoperatively), transdermal scopolamine was shown to be more effective than either placebo or a combination of metoclopramide and droperidol.[93]

URINARY SIDE EFFECTS

Intraspinally administered morphine may be associated with naloxone-reversible urinary retention, owing principally to decreased detrusor muscle tone and detrusor–urethral sphincter dyssynergia.[61, 94, 95] Such effects on the urinary tract appear to be mediated by mu and delta, but not kappa, receptors.[96] Urinary retention has not been reported after intraventricular administration of morphine, which suggests that a spinally mediated mechanism is responsible. Despite incidences of 20% to 40% and higher in male patients after an initial dose of intraspinal opioids,[97] retention is rarely observed in opioid-tolerant cancer patients or in women.

Management. Tolerance often develops after 24 to 48 hours of continued treatment, during which time treatment with small doses of an opioid antagonist[93] or intermittent bladder catheterization may be undertaken. Alternative approaches include conversion to treatment with a more lipid-soluble opioid (especially methadone, which has been observed to actually increase detrusor tone, or buprenorphine, which seems to have little or no effect) and a trial of phenoxybenzamine.[98–101]

PRURITUS

Pruritus can be very disturbing to patients. Fortunately, although extremely common in opioid-naive subjects, especially after intrathecal administration, pruritus is extremely uncommon in cancer patients. Treatment with diphenhydramine, antihistamines, opioid antagonists,[76] and droperidol all have been recommended, but all interventions yield, at best, mixed results.[36, 61] The best solution may be to embark on a therapeutic trial of alternative opioids, seeking to find a compatible agent based on incomplete cross-tolerance.

OPIOID WITHDRAWAL (ABSTINENCE SYNDROME)

The abrupt conversion from systemic to intraspinal administration of opioids may result in opioid withdrawal with its classic signs and symptoms,[102] such as lacrimation, rhinorrhea, mydriasis, diaphoresis, pilomotor erection, restlessness, irritability, tremor, nausea, vomiting, diarrhea, and abdominal cramping.[12] Episodes of heightened pain, pulmonary edema, and cardiovascular collapse have also been reported.[82, 103] The development of this syndrome is attributed to reductions in the total dose of drug and subsequent delivery of reduced quantities of opioid to rostral central nervous system sites. The administration of an opioid antagonist or agonist-antagonist drug to an opioid-dependent patient, systematically or at the neuraxial level, can also induce profound withdrawal, and even shock.[61, 104] Prevention of this syndrome is facilitated by tapering systemic opioids and cautious introduction of drugs with antagonist properties, should they be indicated. Guidelines for these procedures have been published.[105]

ANAPHYLAXIS

Despite a high incidence of patients with so-called morphine allergy, true allergic reactions to morphine and its congeners are rare.[106, 107] Such a history is usually more consistent with an unpleasant side effect.

Miscellaneous Problems

MISINJECTIONS

There is no question that a fully internalized system that needs to be replenished only from time to time reduces the likelihood of accidental injection of other drugs. Various substances have been accidentally injected through (mostly externalized) epidural and intrathecal catheters, including thiopental, methohexital, diazepam, pancuronium, gallamine, potassium chloride, magnesium sulfate, ephedrine, ranitidine, cephazolin, paraldehyde, total parenteral nutrition solutions, hypertonic contrast medium, hypertonic saline, and collodion.[108] Most cases involved infusion of dilute solutions that resulted in self-limited back pain and spasm, although severe permanent neurologic injury has occurred in several cases.[104] Prevention of such incidents by applying special care in affixing distinctive labels to intraspinal catheters, lines, and infusion devices, occluding accessory ports, and reducing the proximity of ports by thoughtful routing cannot be overemphasized. Various interventions have been undertaken once an injection error has occurred, including injection of epidural steroids, dilution with epidural saline, and aspiration and dilution of the injectate via an intrathecal catheter.

TRAVEL, SECURITY SYSTEMS, AND HIGH ALTITUDES

Patients should be provided with identification cards to alert security personnel to the probability that their implanted drug delivery systems will activate metal detectors. These systems may also trigger some of the newer antitheft detectors. Neither high altitude within a pressurized cabin nor relocation to areas up to 10,000 feet above sea level should affect flow rates.

MAGNETIC RESONANCE IMAGING AND OTHER THERAPIES

Despite early controversy about the safety of MRI in patients with implanted drug delivery systems, most authorities now agree that, because the only portions of the Synchro Med pump that are ferrous are the rotors, MRI can safely be performed. Current recommendations call for turning the device off before the examination. Although it is probably unnecessary, it may also be prudent to empty the reservoir, too. Once the examination has been completed, the reservoir should be refilled and the pump carefully reprogrammed. There is still the potential for a poor image due to artifact. MRI should not be used for patients with spinal cord stimulators, because of the potential for lead movement and consequent trauma.

Certain physical therapy devices (diathermy and ultrasound) should not be permitted near the site of the device. The lithotripter should be directed away from the device.

ALARMS

The infusion device has alarms that signal low battery reserve and low capacity (recommended setting 2 mL). The infusion rate may decrease spontaneously when the 2-mL limit is reached (by $\leq$ 15%), and, as a result, devices should be refilled before that point.

HYPERBARIC THERAPY, HOT TUBS, AND SCUBA DIVING

Hyperbaric therapy may lead to underinfusion and should not be carried out while an infusion pump is operational. Hot tubs (temperature $\leq$ 110° F or 43° C) do not the affect infusion rate, but scuba diving to depths greater than 20 feet may be associated with underinfusion.

DISPOSITION AFTER PATIENT'S DEATH

Because of the risk of explosion, implanted drug infusion devices should be removed by funeral personnel prior to cremation. Explanted pumps should *not* be resterilized and reused.

Technical Problems Specific to Spinal Cord Stimulation

Surgical Complications

Many of the potential complications related to the surgical implantation of spinal cord stimulators are similar to those encountered with pump implantation. They are intraoperative bleeding, epidural hematoma, wound hematoma, seroma, wound infection, meningitis, epidural abscess, CSF leak, post–dural puncture headache, and malposition of the subcutaneous pocket, all of which have been described in the preceding section.

Failed Analgesia

Failed analgesia may be due to myriad causes. Problems may be patient related, disease related, mechanical, or a combination of any. Patient selection, education, and preparation are key issues that must be addressed to avoid difficulties. Considerations related to the patient's psychological status and the nature of the disease that is causing the pain are discussed in depth elsewhere in this volume. The emphasis here is on mechanical problems and how to avoid them.

Preoperative Check of Equipment to Be Implanted

Before implantation, the surgeon or pain management specialist should take these measures:

- Confirm that a screening device with a fresh battery is available and functional
- Ensure that the proper equipment is available and that the lead and extension match. It is wise to have additional stock of each item in case of contamination, damage, or defects. (If the equipment budget is tight, additional units should be ordered just before surgery; any that are not used can replace those utilized for surgery.)
- Ascertain that the patient has been properly oriented to the procedure to maximize compliance
- Obtain informed patient consent
- Discuss the procedure with the anesthesiologist to ensure that the patient will be both comfortable and cooperative

Difficult Lead Placement

Although not a complication per se, difficulty in placing leads is a potentially troublesome and critical problem that may ultimately be a source of complications. Positioning of the patient is often overlooked but is key to facilitating lead placement. Before the patient is prepared for surgery, the surgeon should verify that fluoroscopic access is not impaired by radiolucent components of the operating room table and that mechanical passage of the C arm is unimpeded. Fluoroscopy is an essential adjunct to placement and should be utilized freely throughout the procedure rather than being reserved until the conclusion. Nonionic contrast medium should be available to confirm localization of the epidural space and to distinguish between subarachnoid and epidural lead placement. Whether a prone or lateral position is selected, patients should be positioned precisely, so that true anteroposterior and lateral films are obtained. Most clinicians prefer the prone position, in which case the table should be flexed and padded to minimize lumbar lordosis. The back should be flexed, and consideration should be given to securing the patient in position with adhesive tape and a safety belt.

During needle placement, care should be taken to think three-dimensionally, particularly if a slightly paramedian approach is selected, which is preferred by most physicians. A steep angle in the cephalocaudad plane should be adopted to facilitate the lead's passage. Ten milliliters of preservative-free saline may be injected before passage of the lead to expand the epidural space. If advancing the lead is difficult, epidural positioning should be verified. Passage may be facilitated by rotating the bevel of the needle carefully up to 45 degrees to either side (with the lead retracted), and the lead may be gently rotated between the thumb and forefinger while it is advanced, in an effort to "steer" its tip. Finally, if problems persist, a guidewire may be gently advanced under fluoroscopic guidance to create a track, or alternatively, another needle trajectory or interspace may be selected. Occasionally, the entry point is too far from the pain-generating site, so that the electrode portion of the lead does not extend to the intended target and the boot cannot be placed. In implantation planning, the guidelines shown in Table 64–1 may be useful. The lead, and, indeed, all component parts, should be handled carefully. Kinking, bending, and tension on the lead should be avoided. The lead should not be forced into the epidural space against resistance, and sutures should not be tied directly to it. Extreme caution should be exercised when sharp instruments are used around the lead. The lead should be handled only with the fingers; when it is necessary to manipulate it with instruments, rubber shods should be used.

If, once it has been inserted, the lead needs to be repositioned. Care should be taken to withdraw it gently and carefully through the needle, to avoid damaging the lead. If resistance is met, the lead and needle should be removed simultaneously and the epidural space should approached anew. Once the lead is optimally positioned, it must be stabilized while the needle is removed. Intermittent or continuous fluoroscopy is useful to confirm that the tip of the lead does not move during this process.

TABLE 64–1 ***Spinal Levels for Catheter Entry and Lead Tip Location According to Pain Distribution***

Pain Distribution	Entry Level	Lead Tip Level
Foot only	L2–L3	T11–T12
Lower extremity w/hip and back involvement	T12–L1	T9–T10
Upper chest wall (intercostals)	T4–T6	T1–T2
Upper extremity	T1–T3	C3–T5

Accidental Dural Puncture

Dural puncture is usually heralded by a frank flow of CSF. If this occurs, a neighboring interspace should be selected, and treatment of post–dural puncture headache should be anticipated.

Subarachnoid Lead Placement

Occasionally, dural puncture occurs in the absence of obvious CSF leakage, owing to either the catheter or guidewire's breaching the dura or altered CSF mechanics secondary to scarring from earlier surgery. Dural puncture usually is manifested as unexpectedly low stimulation thresholds (often ≤ 1 V) and can be confirmed if anterior displacement of the lead is noted on fluoroscopy and if injection of contrast material through the needle produces a radiographic image more characteristic of a myelogram than an epidurogram. Even if adequate stimulation is obtained, the risk of migration and scarring requires that the lead be removed and reinserted at another interspace.

Neurologic Injury

Significant neurologic injury is unusual. Occasionally, patients experience radicular pain coincident with advancement of the lead, in which case it should be withdrawn. If new pain or new neurologic signs emerge in the immediate postoperative period, the patient should be investigated for epidural hematoma. If signs and symptoms occur later in the postoperative period, infection must be ruled out. It is not uncommon for new, well-localized paresthesias to develop with minor nerve root injury, but they usually resolve over days or weeks. Lead removal usually is not necessary, although CT may be indicated.

Lead Migration and Positional Stimulation

When a patient describes a change in the stimulation pattern that consists of either the perception of adequate stimulation in a body part other than the painful area or a stimulation pattern that changes with posture, lead migration is probably responsible. Unfortunately, this complication occurs with some frequency. It is inherent to the procedure, because adequacy of pain relief depends in large part on localization of the lead within a living, moving human being. A process of "scarring down" is generally thought to occur during the first weeks after surgery; restricting movements (bending, reaching) during this period may promote immobilization of the lead. Some clinicians require a short period of bed rest or even a soft cervical collar as a reminder to patients to limit their activity.

Stimulation can often be recaptured by meticulous reprogramming. Problems may, to an extent, be forestalled by initially locating the lead directly over the involved dermatomes, to give some margin for readjustment on either side. A change in stimulation pattern warrants anteroposterior and lateral radiographs, which should be compared with postoperative films to document lead movement. If proper stimulation cannot be recaptured, elective surgical revision is indicated, with consideration of substituting a plate-type (Resume) electrode for the original lead.

Truncal Stimulation

Occasionally, patients experience truncal stimulation either in addition to or in place of the topically desired therapeutic stimulation. This complication is manifested by paresthesias and muscle twitching, usually along the myotomes of the flank. It may be related to current leak or to stimulation of a nerve root owing to a lateral shift in lead position. It can often be averted by reprogramming but sometimes requires surgical revision.

Insulation Failure, Fracture or Disconnection

Failure of insulation or fracture or disconnection of wires may manifest itself as total loss of stimulation or a combination of loss of the usual stimulation pattern or intermittent stimulation coupled with focal pain that, ultimately, corresponds to the site of the short circuit. Some authorities advocate applying either bone wax or cyanoacrylate to connections prophylactically. In cases of suspected electrical leak or discontinuity, an electronic survey should be performed to exclude pulse generator failure and to detect abnormally high impedance. A battery-operated portable radio may be used as an adjunct; an AM radio, tuned between stations to produce static, is applied to the skin overlying the system. The radio is then passed gently over the skin along the path of the system from the pocket to the back, over the lead tips. Increased static usually correlates with a site of current leakage. Radiographs should be reviewed to detect disconnection or a break in wiring, although such films usually look normal. Elective revision is indicated. At surgery, the system can be tested sequentially, usually starting at the pocket and moving proximally.

Painful Connector or Transmitter Site

Pain at the site of a connector or transmitter may be due to mechanical causes, as when a generator impinges on the ribs or iliac crest, or to electrical leakage, in which case patients typically complain of a local sensation of burning.

Pacemakers, MRI, and Security Systems

Insertion of a spinal cord stimulator may be contraindicated in patients with pacemakers. Demand pacemakers may mistake the pulse generator's impulses for those originating in the heart. Theoretically, patients with fixed-rate devices do not have problems, although consultation with the stimulator manufacturer is recommended before considering implantation in a patient with any type of pacemaker. Although infusion devices need only to be emptied and turned off, MRI is still contraindicated for patients with stimulators, because of the potential for damage to the device and for electrical and mechanical injury to the patient. A stimulating system may also activate airport boarding-gate alarms and certain other alarms intended to detect theft.

Published Data on Complications

Spinal Cord Stimulation

Regrettably, there is a paucity of good, controlled studies that provide detailed descriptions of patient selection, outcome, and morbidity. This status is characteristic of interventions for pain in general and should not be regarded as an indictment of spinal cord stimulation. The quality of later literature is markedly superior to that associated with earlier eras. It is essential that this literature be scrutinized extremely carefully. The reader must bear in mind that data from earlier studies are influenced by less sophisticated patient selection methods and equipment that was far cruder and more prone to failure than contemporary systems. In addition there is a considerable delay between submission of a study and its publication; thus, a large study population usually means that the data were collected over several years before the paper was submitted. There is also widespread agreement that the results of treatment are very specific to the practitioner, the technique, and the disorder being treated, so the reader should be aware that outcome reflects the skill and experience of the implant surgeon and the technique and the study population.

The following brief review of the literature is, admittedly, incomplete, but it gives a sense of the variety and incidences of the complications that have been reported for spinal cord stimulation (SCS). In a 1982 European study, Siegfried and Lazorthes[109] reported on 191 patients with chronic low back pain who underwent trials of SCS, of whom 89 had an implant. It is noteworthy that the study population was characterized by patients with histories of long-standing pain, multiple laminectomies, and oil-based myelography. Most systems were placed via laminectomy, and it is again noteworthy that a proportion of them underwent deliberate subarachnoid, subdural, and endodural placement of leads. At 1 year, among the 89 patients, 21 failures (24%) were attributed to nonmechanical failure—"psychiatric causes" in nine cases, "narcotic dependency" in five, and idiopathic in seven. Another 21 failures (24%) were due to mechanical causes—electrode migration in nine cases, defects in the stimulating system in three, necrosis and infection in seven, and receiver rejection in two.

In 1983, de La Porte and Siegfried[110] reported on 94 patients who underwent trials of SCS for "lumbosacral spinal fibrosis (spinal arachnoiditis)," 38 of whom (40%) underwent implantation. In these 38 patients, 50 more procedures were performed owing to problems with wound healing (10 cases), removal or reimplantation (5 cases), and other complications (23 cases). Only 12 of the implanted devices were Medtronic systems, and these were implanted by laminectomy. A total of 26 complications occurred in this subgroup (skin erosion, seven; incisional pain, three; receptor site pain, two; lead migration, six; electrode malfunction, two; and system malfunction, cable or connection disruption, and antenna malfunction, one each). In this admittedly antiquated study, no complications were encountered in 50% of patients and no reintervention was required for 60% of patients. An interesting conclusion was that the occurrence of postoperative problems increased the chances of further problems enormously. Again, the study's vintage must be taken into account, as must its population (patients with pain from failed back surgery).

In a brief report that lacks detailed descriptions, Romy and Sussman[111] described 19 patients who underwent implantation of Cordis SCS systems. Of these, two systems were removed (11%) and 11 (58%) required at least one revision for reasons that were not reported. Murphy and Giles,[112] reporting on implantation of Medtronic systems in a group of 10 patients treated for angina, fared considerably better. A faulty signal receiver was replaced in one patient, and another required revision owing to posturally related changes in stimulation.

Meglio and Cioni[113] reported on 26 patients who received permanent percutaneous implants (Medtronic, Sigma lead) between 1978 and 1981. Thirteen of their patients (50%) had vascular disease, only 6 had arachnoiditis, and the rest had other problems (e.g., herpes zoster, cancer). Eight patients (31%) experienced complications, of whom seven required corrective procedures. Reported complications were subcutaneous hematoma (3), inadequate paresthesia (2), receiver malfunction (1), subcutaneous lead rejection (1), and aseptic meningitis (1). Side effects that did not require reoperation included headache, asthenia, dizziness, and radicular muscle twich.

Meglio and colleagues[114] reported on 64 patients who underwent implantation with Medtronic systems. Low back pain was the indication for treatment in only a small proportion of patients, and in all but 5, a percutaneous approach was utilized. These authors reported complications in 26 patients and side effects in 11, although it is not clear whether the problems occurred in the implanted group only (64) or in the larger group who underwent trials (109). Complications included four cases of aseptic meningitis (two of which resolved within days without system removal), bacterial infection at the electrode site (2) and pocket (1), lead rejection (2), CSF leak (3), subcutaneous hematoma (3), pain at the electrode site (2), accidental removal of the system by the patient (1), and "suspected system failure" (4). One of the patients with bacterial infection at the lead site developed paraplegia within a few days, despite removal of the system and treatment with antibiotics. Reexploration revealed an extradural-intradural bacterial abscess and the result was "good but incomplete" recovery.

Krainick and associates[115] reported on 84 patients implanted between 1972 and 1974, 64 of whom were amputees with lower extremity pain. Four patients experienced partial transverse spinal lesions, three of which resolved after system removal. Disagreeable thoracic radicular paresthesias were "common," especially with unipolar systems, but they usually improved after alteration of the stimulation parameters. Interestingly, CSF leakage occurred in three patients who were among the first few to undergo subdural placement, and this complication did not recur once the protocol was altered to one of exclusive epidural placement, suggesting the superiority of the latter approach. Removal of the system due to technical failure was necessary in three cases, but the exact causes were not specified (because of lead damage during removal). One patient with cervical placement experienced symptoms consistent with spinal cord compression 2 years after surgery and, during system removal, was found to have a severe tissue reaction.

In 1986, Kumar and colleagues[116] reported on the implantation of 65 Medtronic systems, most in patients with back pain. Complications were reported in 23 cases (35%): wound infection (3, only 1 requiring removal), CSF leak (1, resolved with bed rest), electrode displacement (12), electrode fracture (2), lead fibrosis (3), and a sensation of burning over the receiver site (2). In a 1991 follow-up study reporting on 94 patients (60% with back problems) who had implants (mostly Medtronic systems), the same group reported 43 complications (46%).[117] They were electrode displacement (25), infection (8, with 7 requiring system removal), lead fracture (4, usually at the entrance to the epidural space), battery depletion (2), electrical leak (2, usually at junction of extension and receive), and CSF leak (2, resolved with bed rest). Patients with scoliosis or "similar spinal deformities" were found to have a threefold greater increase in rate of electrode displacement.

A group of Spanish investigators reported, in abstract form, on a single case of transient tetraplegia after implantation in a patient with mediastinal sarcoma and herpes zoster.[118] The system was removed, and the authors concluded that, under certain circumstances (osteolytic metastases), the lead and associated edema could act like a space-occupying lesion. Preliminary results of a Medtronic-sponsored multicenter trial of their original Itrel system were published in 1984.[118a] They reported on 116 implants in patients with low back pain, leg pain, or both. Twenty-three systems (20%) were explanted for various reasons. Problems at implantation included a malfunctioning portable programmer (1), stripped set screw (1), ineffective stimulation (1), "medicine reaction" (1), device accidentally removed by patient (1), and electrode failure (1). Subsequent problems were infection at the site of the pulse generator (6, 4 requiring surgery), burning near generator site (3), radicular stimulation (3), positional stimulation (2), dislodged leads (6), difficulty with programming (3, requiring replacement), and flank pain (1). In one of the cases of infection, the generator was sterilized and reimplanted without apparent problems, although this procedure is not recommended by Medtronic.

In 1991, North and colleagues[119] reported on implantation (64% percutaneous, mostly Medtronic) in 50 patients with failed back surgery (average 3.1 operations) with 2-year and 5-year follow-up. All together, 48% of patients required some secondary procedure (mostly repositioning). Six patients (12%) developed superficial *Staphylococcus* infection that required system removal. Other problems were spontaneous migration (1, or 0.5%), revision to enhance the stimulation pattern (14, or 28%), lead fracture (7, or 14%), and receiver failure (4, or 8%). Of note is that secondary procedures were required in only 34% of the subset of patients treated with four-channel systems. In a follow-up report, North and colleagues[120] documented similar findings that emphasized the superiority of multichannel systems. Of patients treated with multichannel systems, only 16% required revision because of inadequate topographic stimulation, as compared with 23% of patients who had bipolar systems.

In a 1989 study, Racz and associates[121] reported on 26 patients (predominantly with back pain and having undergone an average of 21 prior procedures) who received Medtronic SCS implantation. Twenty-seven complications occurred: lead migration (18), lead fracture (6), infected hematoma (1), and wound infection (2). The authors observed that electrode migration was far more likely to occur early, "probably before fibrous tissue was able to form," and that it was usually from a dorsal to a more anterolateral position. Migration was usually manifested by the appearance of a radicular, intercostal pattern of stimulation and little change in electrode position on radiographs.

Infusion Systems

Because of the relatively new technology with narrow indications, the data available on problems related to the implantation of long-term drug infusion systems are even more meager than those for spinal cord stimulation. In a series of 18 patients undergoing implantation for baclofen infusion,[122] there were three instances of extrusion of the intrathecal portion of the Silastic catheter. One instance of device malfunction resulted in an overdose in a system that had been operable for 1 year. Interestingly, there were seven infectious complications (four cases of local sepsis and three of transient meningitis) in patients treated with an implanted port that required regular percutaneous access, and none in patients who received a SynchroMed implant. Similarly, in Penn and Kroin's[123] series of 7 spastic patients treated with the SynchroMed system, no infectious complications occurred. Two devices were explanted for apparent malfunction (overdose and beeping) but were subsequently found to be functional ex vivo. Two catheters were replaced, one for a kink that occurred at its junction with the pump and a second for a nick produced during surgery. One incidence of erosion of the pocket incision occurred, and there were several instances of self-limited (7–10 days) seroma.

SUMMARY

If one uses a broad definition of *complication*, spinal cord–stimulating systems are subject to a relatively high rate of complications that, although often requiring another intervention, tend by far to be benign. Implanted infusion devices are associated with a relatively low incidence of such problems.

REFERENCES

1. Waldman S, Leak D, Kennedy D, Patt RB: Intraspinal opioid analgesia in the management of oncologic pain. *In* Patt RB (ed): Cancer Pain. Philadelphia, JB Lippincott, 1993, pp 285–328.
2. Bridenbaugh PO: Complications of local anesthetic neural blockade. *In* Cousins MJ, Bridenbaugh PO (eds): Neural Blockade, ed 2. Philadelphia, JB Lippincott, 1988, p 695.
3. Webster's Dictionary.
4. Quimby CW: Medicolegal hazards of destructive nerve blocks. *In* Abram SE (ed): Cancer Pain. Boston, Kluwer Academic, 1989, p 137.
5. Krames E: Faculty Handbook. Minneapolis, Minn., Medtronic, 1992.
6. Hahn M: Faculty Handbook. Minneapolis, Minn., Medtronic, 1992.
7. Wu C, Patt RB: Accidental overdose of systemic morphine during intended refill of intrathecal infusion device. Anesth Analg 75:130–132, 1992.
8. Patt RB, Wu C, Bressi J, Catania J: Accidental intraspinal overdose revisited. Anesth Analg 76:202, 1993.
9. Penn RD, Paice JA, Gottschalk W, et al: Cancer pain relief using chronic morphine infusions: Early experience with a programmable implanted drug pump. J Neurosurg 61:302, 1984.
10. Hirsch LF, Thanki A, Nowak T: Sudden loss of pain control with morphine pump due to catheter migration. Neurosurgery 17:965, 1985.
11. Portenoy R: Practical aspects of pain control in the patient with cancer. CA: Cancer J Clin 38:327, 1988.
12. Jaffe JH, Martin WR: The opioid analgesics and antagonists. *In* Gillman AG, Rall TW, Nies AS, et al: The Pharmacologic Basis of Therapeutics, ed 8. New York, Pergamon, 1980.
13. Catania JA, Patt RB: Radiologic guidance, contrast medium and untoward reactions. *In* Patt RB (ed): Cancer Pain. Philadelphia, JB Lippincott, 1994, pp 616–624.
14. Leak WD, Kennedy LD, Graef W: Clinical experience with implantable, programmable pumps: The Medtronic SynchroMed pump. Clin J Pain 7:44, 1991.
15. Swenson C, Patt RB: Manufacturing processes. *In* Patt RB (ed): Cancer Pain. Philadelphia, JB Lippincott, 1994, pp 612–615.
16. Yaksh TL, Onofrio BM: Retrospective consideration of the doses of morphine given intrathecally by chronic infusion in 163 patients by 19 physicians. Pain 31:211, 1987.
17. Amer S, Rawal N, Gustafsson LL: Clinical experience of long-term treatment with epidural and intrathecal opioids, a nationwide survey. Acta Anaesthesiol Scand 32:253, 1988.
18. Ventafridda V, Spoldi E, Caraceni A, et al: Intraspinal morphine for cancer pain. Acta Anaesthesiol Scand 85:47, 1987.
19. Coombs DW, Saunders RL, Harbaugh R, et al: Relief of continous chronic pain by intraspinal narcotics infusion via an implanted reservoir. JAMA 250:2336, 1983.
20. Shetter AG, Hadley MH, Wilkinson E: Administration of intraspinal morphine sulfate for the treatment of intractable cancer pain. Neurosurgery 18:740, 1986.
21. Pasqualucci V: Advances in the management of cardiac pain. *In* Benedetti C, Chapman RC, Moricca G (eds): Advances in Pain Research and Therapy. Vol. 7. New York, Raven, 1984.
22. Sundberg TT, Wattwil M, Garvill JE, et al: Effects of epidural bupivacaine and epidural morphine on bowel function and pain after hysterectomy. Acta Anaesthesiol Scand 33:181, 1989.
23. Stevens CW, Yaksh TL: Potency of spinal antinociceptive agents is inversely related to magnitude of tolerance after continuous infusion. J Pharmacol Exp Ther 250:1, 1989.
24. Sosnowski M, Stevens CW, Yaksh TL: Comparison of magnitude of tolerance development observed after continuous spinal intrathecal infusions in rats. Reg Anesth 14:76, 1989.
25. Baskoff JD, Watson RL, Muldoon SM: Respiratory arrest after intrathecal morphine. Anesthesiology 7:12, 1980.
26. Eisenach JC, Rauck RL, Buzzanell C, et al: Epidural clonidine analgesia for intractable cancer pain: Phase I. Anesthesiology 71:647, 1989.
27. Coombs DW, Saunders RL, LaChance D, et al: Intrathecal morphine tolerance: Use of intrathecal clonidine, DADL and intravenous morphine. Anesthesiology 62:358, 1985.
28. Glynn CJ, Jamous A, Dawson D, et al: The role of epidural clonidine in the treatment of patients with intractable pain. Pain Suppl 4:45, 1987.
29. Yaksh TL, Reddy SV: Studies in the primate on the analgesic effects associated with intrathecal actions of opiates, alpha-adrenergic agonists and baclofen. Anesthesiology 54:451, 1981.
30. Coombs DW, Allen C, Meier FA, et al: Chronic intraspinal clonidine in sheep. Reg Anesth 9:47, 1994.
31. Kim KC, Stoelting RK: Effect of droperidol on the duration of analgesia and development of tolerance to intrathecal morphine. Anesthesiology 35(Suppl):S219, 1980.
32. Naji P, Farschtschian M, Wilder-Smith O, et al: Epidural droperidol and morphine for postoperative pain. Anesth Analg 70:583, 1990.
33. Bach V, Carl P, Ravlo ME, et al: Potentiation of epidural opioids with epidural droperidol. Anaesthesia 41:1116, 1986.
34. Chrubasik J, Meynadier J, Blond S, et al: Somatostatin, a potent analgesic. Lancet 2:1208, 1984.
35. Meynadier J, Chrubasik J, Dubar M, Wünsch E: Intrathecal somatostatin in terminally ill patients: A report of two cases. Pain 23:9, 1985.

36. Bruera E: Narcotic-induced pulmonary edema. J Pain Symptom Manage 5:55, 1990.
37. Gaumann DM, Yaksh TL, Post C, et al: Intrathecal somatostatin in cat and mouse studies on pain, motor behavior and histopathology. Anesth Analg 68:623, 1989.
38. Penn RD, Paice JA, Kroin JS: Octreotide: A potent new non-opiate analgesic for intrathecal infusion. Pain 49:13–19, 1992.
39. Candrina R, Galli G: Intraventricular octreotide for cancer pain. J Neurosurg 336–337, 1992.
40. Fiore CE, Castolina F, Malatino LS, et al: Antalgic activity of calcitonin: Effectiveness of the epidural and subarachnoid routes in man. Int J Clin Pharmacol Res 3:257, 1983.
41. Eisenach JC: Demonstrating safety of subarachnoid calcitonin: Patients or animals. Anesth Analg 67:298, 1988.
42. Stein C, Brechner T: Epidural morphine tolerance: Use of norepinephrine. Clin J Pain 2:267, 1987.
43. Russell RD, Chang KJ: Alternated delta and mu receptor activation: A strategy for limiting opioid tolerance. Pain 36:381, 1989.
44. Krames ES, Wilkie DJ, Gershow J: Intrathecal D-ala^2-D-leu^5-enkephalin (DADL) restores analgesia in a patient analgetically tolerant to intrathecal morphine sulfate. Pain 24:205, 1986.
45. Onofrio BM, Yaksh TL: Intrathecal delta-receptor ligand produces analgesia in man. Lancet 2:1386, 1983.
46. Naguib M, Adu-Gyamfi Y, Absood GH, et al: Epidural ketamine for postoperative analgesia. Anesth Analg 67:798, 1988.
47. Cripps TP, Goodchild CS: Intrathecal midazolam and the stress response to upper abdominal surgery. Br J Anaesth 58:1324, 1986.
48. Wilson PR, Yaksh TL: Baclofen is anti-nociceptive in the spinal intrathecal space of animals. Eur J Pharmacol 51:323, 1978.
49. Yaksh TL: Spinal opiates: A review of their effect on spinal function with an emphasis on pain processing. Acta Anaesthesiol Scand Suppl 85:25, 1987.
50. Coombs DW: Effect of spinal adrenergic analgesia on opioid resistant pain. Acta Anaesthesiol Scand 91:37, 1989.
51. Coombs DW: Intraspinal narcotics for intractable cancer pain. *In* Abrams S (ed): Cancer Pain. Boston, Kluwer Academic, 1989, p 82.
52. Du Pen SL: After epidural narcotics: What next? Anesth Analg 66(Suppl):S46, 1987.
53. Taff RH: Pulmonary edema following a naloxone administration in a patient without heart disease. Anesthesiology 59:576, 1983.
54. Omote K, Nakagawa I, Kitahata LM, et al: The antinociceptive role of mu and delta opiate receptors and their interactions in the spinal dorsal hom of cats. Anesth Analg 68(Suppl):S215, 1989.
55. Omote K, Nakagawa I, Kitahata LM, et al: Spinal delta but not mu opiate receptors appear to interact with noradrenergic systems in the cat's spinal dorsal hom. Anesth Analg 68(Suppl):S216, 1989.
56. Waldman SD, Coombs DW: Selection of implantable narcotic delivery systems. Anesth Analg 68:377–384, 1989.
57. Kreitzer JM, Kirschenbaum LP, Eisenkraft JB: Safety of PCA devices. Anesthesiology 70:881, 1989.
58. Dahl JB, Jacobsen JB: Accidental epidural narcotic overdose. Anesth Analg 70:321–322, 1990.
59. Kaiser KG, Bainton CR: Treatment of intrathecal morphine overdose by aspiration of cerebrospinal fluid. Anesth Analg 66:475–477, 1987.
60. Parkinson SK, Bailey SL, Little WL, Mueller JB: Myoclonic seizure activity with chronic high-dose spinal opioid administration. Anesthesiology 72:743–745, 1990.
61. Ventafridda V, Spoldi E, Caraceni A, et al: Intraspinal morphine for cancer pain. Acta Anaesthesiol Scand Suppl 85:47, 1987.
62. Flacke JW, Flacke WE, Williams GD: Acute pulmonary edema following naloxone reversal of high-dose morphine anesthesia. Anesthesiology 47:376–378, 1977.
63. Gurdin MM, Carlin GA: Aesthetic surgery of the breast. *In* Masters FW, Lewis JR (eds): Symposium on Aesthetic Surgery of the Face, Eyelid, and Breast, vol 4. St Louis, CV Mosby, 1972, p 160.
64. De Castro J, Meynadier J, Zenz M: Regional opioid analgesia. Dordrecht, Kluwer Academic, 1991.
65. Cousins MJ, Mather LE: Intrathecal and epidural administration of opioids. Anesthesiology 61:276–310, 1984.
66. Ventafridda V, Spoldi E, Caraceni A, et al: Intraspinal morphine for cancer pain. Acta Anaesthesiol Scand Suppl 85:47, 1987.
67. Arai T, Dote K, Senda T, et al: Convulsion after epidural injection in a patient with increased intracranial pressure. Pain Clinic 3:195, 1987.
68. Korbon GA, James DJ, Verlander JM, et al: Intramuscular naloxone reverses the side effects of epidural morphine while preserving analgesia. Reg Anesth 10:16, 1985.
69. Rawal N, Schott U, Dahlstrom B: Influence of naloxone infusion on analgesia and respiratory depression following epidural morphine. Anesthesiology 64:194, 1986.
70. Davies GK, Tolhurst-Cleaver CL, James TL: CNS depression from intrathecal morphine. Anesthesiology 52:280, 1980.
71. Glynn CJ, Mather LE, Cousins, MJ, et al: Spinal narcotics and respiratory depression. Lancet 1:356, 1979.
72. Christensen V: Respiratory depression after extradural morphine. Br J Anaesth 52:841, 1980.
73. Sosnowski M, Yaksh TL: Spinal administration of receptor-selective drugs as analgesics: New horizons. J Pain Symptom Manage 5:204, 1990.
74. Pazos A, Florez J: Interaction of naloxone with agonists on the respiration of rats. Eur J Pharmacol 87:309, 1983.
75. Abboud TK, Moore M, Zhu J, et al: Epidural butorphanol or morphine for the relief of post cesarean section pain: Ventilatory responses to carbon dioxide. Anesth Analg 66:887, 1987.
76. Latasch L, Probst S, Dudziak R: Reversal by nalbuphine of respiratory depression caused by fentanyl. Anesth Analg 63:814, 1984.
77. Baise A, McMichan JC, Nugent M, et al: Nalbuphine produces side effects while reversing narcotic induced respiratory depression. Anesth Analg 65(Suppl):S19, 1986.
78. Hammond JE: Reversal of opioid associated late onset respiratory depression by nalbuphine hydrochloride. Lancet 2:1208, 1984.
79. Schmauss C, Doherty C, Yaksh TL: The analgesic effects of an intrathecally administered partial opiate agonist, nalbuphine hydrochloride. Eur J Pharmacol 86:1, 1983.
80. Wakefield RD, Mesaros M: Reversal of pruritus secondary to epidural morphine with a narcotic agonist/antagonist nalbuphine (Nubain). Anesthesiology 63(Suppl):A255, 1985.
81. Abboud TK, Lee K, Zhu J, et al: Prophylactic oral naltrexone with intrathecal morphine for cesarean section: Effects on adverse reactions and analgesia. Anesth Analg 71:367, 1990.
82. Prough BS, Roy R, Bumgamer J, et al: Acute pulmonary edema in healthy teenagers following conservative doses of intravenous naloxone. Anesthesiology 60:485, 1984.
83. DesMarteau JK, Cassot AL: Acute pulmonary edema resulting from nalbuphine reversal of fenatnyl-induced respiratory depression. Anesthesiology 65:237, 1986.
84. Kaiser KG, Bainton CR: Treatment of intrathecal morphine overdose by aspiration of cerebrospinal fluid. Anesth Analg 66:475, 1987.
85. Cousins MJ, Cherry DA, Gourlay GK: Acute and chronic pain: Use of spinal opioids. *In* Cousins MJ, Bridenbaugh PO (eds): Neural Blockade, ed 2. Philadelphia, JB Lippincott, 1988, p 955.
86. Yaksh TL, Noueihed R: The physiology and pharmacology of spinal opioids. Annu Rev Pharmacol Toxicol 25:433, 1985.
87. Twycross RG, Harcourt JMV: The use of laxatives at a palliative care center. Palliat Med 5:27, 1991.
88. Patt R, Jain S: Long term management of a patient with perineal pain secondary to rectal cancer. J Pain Symptom Manage 5:127, 1990.
89. Thom T, Tanhhoj H, Jarnerot G: Epidural morphine delays gastric emptying time and small intestinal transit in volunteers. Acta Anaesthesiol Scand 33:174, 1989.
90. Benedetti C: Intraspinal analgesia: An historical overview. Acta Anaesthesiol Scand 85:17–24, 1987.
91. Watson RL, Rayburn RL, Muldoon SM, et al: The mechanism of action and utility of epidurally administered morphine. *In* Wain HJ (ed): Treatment of Pain. New York, Aaronson, 1982.
92. Calvey TN: Side effect problems of the mu and kappa agonists in clinical use. Update Opioids 1:803, 1987.
93. Loper KA, Ready LB, Dorman BH: Prophylactic transdermal scopolamine patches reduce nausea in postoperative patients receiving epidural morphine. Anesth Analg 68:144, 1989.
94. Rawal N, Mollefors K, Axelsson K, et al: An experimental study of urodynamic effects of epidural morphine and of naloxone reversal. Anesth Analg 62:641, 1983.
95. Dray A: Epidural opiates and urinary retention: New models provide new insights. Anesthesiology 68:323, 1988.
96. Durant PAC, Yaksh TI: Drug effects on urinary bladder tone during spinal morphine–induced inhibition of the micturition reflex in unanesthetized rats. Anesthesiology 68:325, 1988.

97. Rawal N, Mollefors K, Axelsson K, et al: Naloxone reversal of urinary retention after epidural morphine. Lancet 2:1411, 1981.
98. Evron S, Samueloff A, Simon A, et al: Urinary function during epidural analgesia with methadone and morphine in post-cesarean section patients. Pain 23:135, 1985.
99. Drenger B, Magora F, Evron S, et al: The action of intrathecal morphine and methadone on lower urinary tract in dog. J Urol 135:852, 1986.
100. Drenger B, Pikarsky AJ, Magora F: Urodynamic studies after intrathecal fentanyl and buprenorphine in the dog. Anesthesiology 67(Suppl):A240, 1987.
101. Evron S, Magora E, Sadovsky E: Prevention of urinary retention with phenoxybenzamine during epidural morphine. Br Med J 288:190, 1984.
102. Messahel FM, Tomlin PJ: Narcotic withdrawal syndrome after intrathecal administration of morphine. Br Med J 283:471, 1981.
103. Delander GE, Takemori AE: Spinal antagonism of tolerance and dependence induced by systemically administered morphine. Eur J Pharmacol 94:35, 1983.
104. Christensen FR, Anderson LW: An adverse reaction to extradural buprenorphine. Br J Anaesth 54:476, 1982.
105. American Pain Society: Principles of Analgesia Use in the Treatment of Acute and Chronic Cancer Pain: A Concise Guide to Medical Practice, ed 2. Skokie, Ill., American Pain Society, 1989.
106. Fisher MM: The diagnosis of acute anaphylactoid reactions to drugs. Anaesth Intensive Care 9:234, 1981.
107. Zucker-Pinchoff B, Ramanathan S: Anaphylactic reaction to epidural fentanyl. Anesthesiology 71:599, 1989.
108. Kopacz DJ, Slover RB: Accidental epidural cephazolin injection: Safeguards for patient controlled analgesia. Anesthesiology 72:944, 1990.
109. Siegfried J, Lazorthes Y: Long-term follow-up of dorsal cord stimulation for chronic pain syndrome after multiple lumbar operations. Appl Neurophysiol 45:201–204, 1982.
110. deLaPorte C, Siegfried J: Lumbosacral spinal fibrosis (spinal arachnoiditis): Its diagnosis and treatment by spinal cord stimulation. Spine 8:593–603, 1983.
111. Romy M, Sussman M: Intraspinal neural stimulation for relief of intractable pain: Introduction and technique of insertion. J Neurol Orthop Med Surg 5:33–42, 1984.
112. Murphy DF, Giles KE: Dorsal column stimulation for pain relief from intractable angina pectoris. Pain 28:365–368, 1987.
113. Meglio M, Cioni B: Personal experience with spinal cord stimulation in chronic pain management. Appl Neurophysiol 45:195–200, 1982.
114. Meglio M, Cioni B, Rossi GF: Spinal cord stimulation in the management of chronic pain. J Neurosurg 70:519–524, 1989.
115. Krainick JU, Thoden U, Traugott R: Pain reduction in amputees by long-term spinal cord stimulation. J Neurosurg 52:346–350, 1980.
116. Kumar K, Wyant GM, Ekong CEU: Epidural spinal cord stimulation for relief of chronic pain. Pain Clinic 1:91–99, 1986.
117. Kumar K, Nauth R, Wyant GM: Treatment of chronic pain by epidural spinal cord stimulation: A 10 year experience. J Neurosurg 75:402–407, 1991.
118. Miranda-Casas JA, Garcia-Ferrando V, Seller-Losada JM: Transitory tetraplegia after electrocatheter implantation in the cervical epidural space. World Congress of Pain, November 1990, Adelaide.
118a. Dooley DM, Heimburger RF, Hunter SE, et al: Medronic Itrel Spinal Cord Stimulation System: Preliminary Clinical Results. Minneapolis, Minn., Medtronics, 1984, pp 1–13.
119. North RB, Ewend MG, Lawton, MT, et al: Failed back surgery syndrome: 5 year follow-up after spinal cord stimulator implantation. Neurosurgery 28:692–699, 1991.
120. North RB, Ewend MG, Lawton MT, Piantadosi S: Spinal cord stimulation for chronic, intracatable pain: Superiority of multichannel devices. Pain 44:119–130, 1991.
121. Racz GB, McCarron RF, Talboys P: Percutaneous dorsal column stimulator for chronic pain control. Spine 14:1–4, 1989.
122. Lazorthes Y, Sallerin-Caute B, Verdie JC, et al: Chronic intrathecal baclofen administration for control of severe spasticity. J Neurosurg 72:393, 1990.
123. Penn RD, Kroin JS: Long-term intrathecal baclofen infusion for treatment of spasticity. J Neurosurg 66:181, 1987.

PART • VI

Neurosurgical Techniques in the Management of Pain

CHAPTER • 65

The Role of Neurosurgery in the Management of Intractable Pain

Michael S. Yoon, MD • Michael Munz, MD, FRCS-C

The neurosurgeon can play a vital role in the team approach to the management of chronic intractable pain. A number of procedures are available to assist the anesthesiologist or other caretaker in treating the patient when other measures have failed. This introductory chapter to the neurosurgical techniques will briefly cover a number of the more common procedures that neurosurgeons have in their armamentarium to combat pain refractory to conservative therapies.

TECHNIQUES FOR THE TREATMENT OF TRIGEMINAL NEURALGIA

For medically refractory trigeminal neuralgia, three basic options are now available: percutaneous techniques, microvascular decompression, and stereotactic radiosurgery. The choice of the procedure to use depends on the surgeon's preference and experience, as all have advantages and disadvantages. In general, the less invasive procedures are used for older, less healthy patients owing to life expectancy and the likelihood of medical complications.

Percutaneous techniques involve lesioning the trigeminal ganglion with glycerol, radiofrequency electrocoagulation, or balloon compression. For a glycerol rhizotomy, the patient is given mild sedation and local anesthesia is administered. A 20-gauge spinal needle is placed through the patient's cheek under fluoroscopic guidance into the foramen ovale, where the mandibular branch of the trigeminal nerve exits (Fig. 65–1). Cerebrospinal fluid is obtained once the dural sleeve is pierced, and intrathecal contrast medium is then injected to fill the trigeminal cistern. The appropriate divisions of the trigeminal nerve are then lesioned by injecting a controlled amount of anhydrous glycerol into the cistern.

A similar approach is used for the radiofrequency technique, except a 19-gauge needle is used. Once cerebrospinal fluid is encountered, the stylet is replaced with a radiofrequency electrode thermistor. The ultimate position of the needle is determined by stimulating the patient and evaluating the sensory response. When motor responses alert the surgeon to the proximity of the electrode to the motor root, the electrode should be repositioned. A lesion is made by heating the electrode tip with the generator to 75° C for 90 sec. This is considered the procedure of choice for trigeminal neuralgia secondary to multiple sclerosis.

Percutaneous balloon compression of the trigeminal ganglion requires general anesthesia and a 14-gauge needle. A No. 4 Fr Fogarty catheter is then advanced into the needle and inflated with contrast to achieve a pear shape within Meckel's cave. The balloon is inflated and allowed to compress the ganglion for approximately 1 min. Reflex hypertension and bradycardia typically occur during this procedure.

Microvascular decompression requires general anesthesia and a lateral suboccipital craniectomy to access the posterior fossa of the skull. With the use of a microscope, a

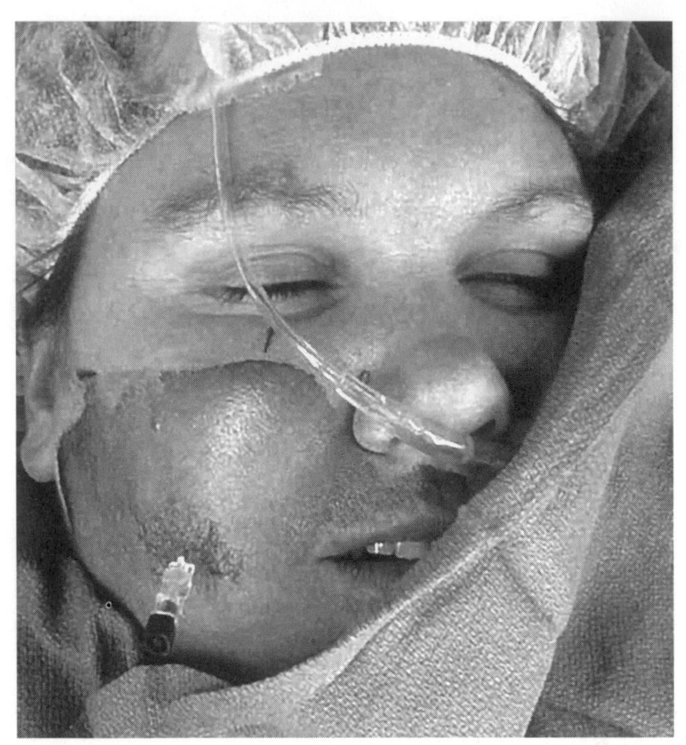

FIGURE 65–1 A percutaneous glycerol rhizotomy for trigeminal neuralgia involves placing a spinal needle through the patient's cheek into the foramen ovale.

piece of teased Teflon felt is placed between the trigeminal nerve and a loop of the superior cerebellar artery, which is most often the offending lesion as it pulsates against the nerve (Fig. 65–2). This technique has also been found to be effective in treating vascular compression of other cranial nerves in disorders such as hemifacial spasm and glossopharyngeal neuralgia.

More recently, stereotactic radiosurgery has come into use as a noninvasive procedure to treat trigeminal neuralgia. This technique requires that the patient be placed into a stereotactic head frame using local anesthesia and mild sedation. An MRI is then obtained to identify the trigeminal nerve as it exits the pons and enters Meckel's cave. A neurosurgeon, radiation oncologist, and medical physicist then plan the radiosurgery and select the proper dose. Typically, 70 to 90 Gy is focused on the target site with a gamma knife. A few patients with refractory cluster headaches have also been treated with radiosurgery targeted at the trigeminal nerve root entry zone, with good results.[1]

In a recent article that combined the results of a number of series, initial pain relief was found to be 98% for successfully completed procedures with both microvascular decompression and radiofrequency rhizotomy, 93% with balloon compression, and 91% with glycerol rhizotomy.[2] With stereotactic radiosurgery, initial complete pain relief was reported at 60% and an additional 17% experienced significant reduction in their pain.[3] It should be noted that 15% of patients who intended to have a microvascular decompression underwent open partial rhizotomy instead because significant vascular compression was not seen or adequate decompression was not considered safe. Six percent of glycerol rhizotomies are not completed owing to failure to locate the needle site, and 1% of balloon compressions are incomplete because of failure to cannulate the foramen ovale. Radiofrequency rhizotomy was completed in all patients in the series reviewed.

Long-term pain recurrence is 54% with glycerol rhizotomy, 21% with balloon decompression, 20% with radiofrequency rhizotomy, and 15% with microvascular decompression. Stereotactic radiosurgery has a reported recurrence rate of 10% in short-term follow-up (mean 18 months) of those who initially reported complete pain relief.

Facial numbness was experienced by 98% after radiofrequency rhizotomy, 72% after balloon compression, 60% after glycerol rhizotomy, and 10% after stereotactic radiosurgery. Only 2% experienced facial numbness after microvascular decompression, but this rate should be considered in light of the fact that 15% of patients who intend to

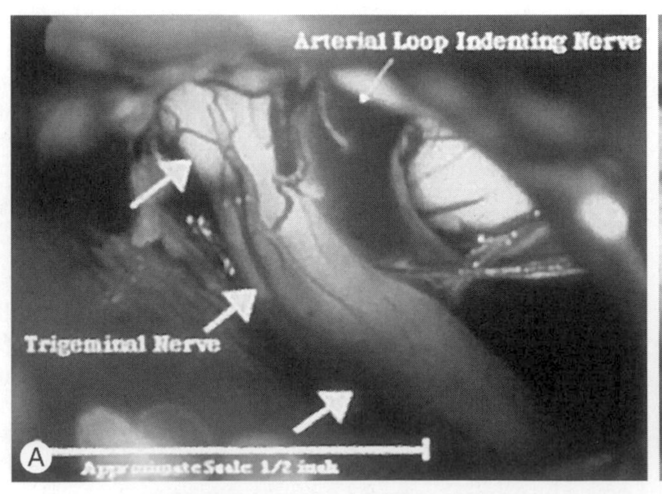

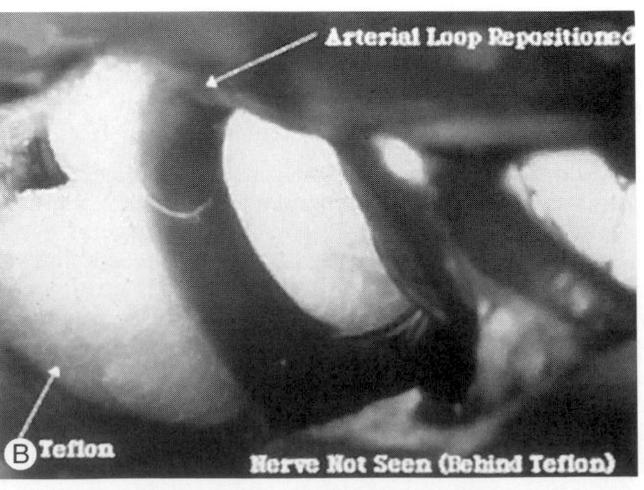

FIGURE 65–2 A microvascular decompression for trigeminal neuralgia as seen under an operating microscope. A, The trigeminal nerve, as it exits the brain stem, is being compressed by a loop of the superior cerebellar artery. B, The same view after a piece of Teflon has been placed between the nerve and the artery. (Courtesy of Peter J. Jannetta, M. D.)

undergo microvascular decompression receive a partial rhizotomy, for the reasons mentioned earlier; 100% of patients experience facial numbness after partial rhizotomy. Nevertheless, most facial numbness is mild and limited in severity. Major dysesthesia occurs in 2% to 10% of the percutaneous procedures but in only 0.3% of patients undergoing microvascular decompression. Anesthesia dolorosa occurs in 0.1% to 1.8% after the percutaneous techniques and not at all after microvascular decompression or stereotactic radiosurgery.

The prevalence of corneal anesthesia after radiofrequency rhizotomy is 7%, after glycerol rhizotomy 3.7%, after balloon compression 1.5%, and after microvascular decompression 0.05%. The rate of trigeminal motor dysfunction after balloon compression is 66% and after radiofrequency rhizotomy 23%, but it is very low after glycerol rhizotomy (1.7%) and does not complicate microvascular decompression.

Permanent cranial nerve deficit occurs in 3% of patients who undergo posterior fossa exploration for microvascular decompression and does not occur after the percutaneous techniques. Perioperative complications such as wound infection and meningitis are highest (10%) with posterior fossa exploration for microvascular decompression and less likely in the percutaneous techniques (≤ 1.7%). Posterior fossa exploration is also associated with a 1% rate of major intracranial hemorrhage or infarction and a 0.6% rate of death. These complications did not occur after the percutaneous procedures in the series reviewed. There are rare reports of temporal lobe hemorrhage, seizure, stroke, and death after percutaneous techniques.[4]

CORDOTOMY

Patients who suffer from intractable cancer pain can benefit quite a bit from a percutaneous or open cordotomy. The percutaneous approach is performed under local anesthesia and mild sedation. Using the guidance of fluoroscopy or computed tomography, a 20-gauge spinal needle is introduced through the neck, contralateral to the affected region, into the spinal canal at the C1–C2 interspace. Once cerebrospinal fluid is encountered, contrast medium is injected to delineate the cord and the dentate ligament. A second needle with a stylet is then introduced ventral to the ligament where the lateral spinothalamic tract is located (Fig. 65–3). After the stylet is removed, a radiofrequency electrode is introduced through the needle and, after physiologic data are gathered from the electrode within the cord and anatomic data from radiography, a thermal lesion is generated by heating the electrode to 80° C for 10 sec. The open cordotomy requires general anesthesia and a laminectomy to gain access to the spinal cord. Using microsurgical technique, a small part of the lateral cord is exposed and then divided.

A recent study of percutaneous cordotomy performed for malignant pain found that 87% were completely relieved of pain after a unilateral procedure.[5] Complications included severe motor deficit (8.1%), urinary retention (6.5%), and mirror-image pain (6.5%). The incidence of complications was higher after bilateral cordotomy and the success rate much lower (50%). Bilateral cordotomy has been reported

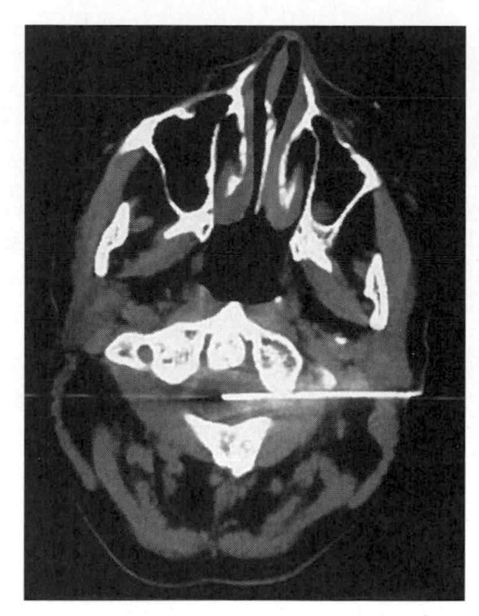

FIGURE 65–3 A CT view through the level of C1 demonstrates the placement of the radiofrequency needle in a percutaneous cordotomy. The needle has entered the spinal canal and pierced the spinal cord.

to cause sleep-induced apnea (Ondine's curse) and severe hypotension.[6]

DEEP BRAIN STIMULATION

With the proven effectiveness and more widespread use of spinal cord stimulation and intrathecal pumps, which are both discussed elsewhere in this textbook, deep brain stimulation (DBS) certainly is not considered an early-line treatment for chronic pain, but it can be very useful in certain patients. The technique involves placing the patient in a stereotactic head frame under local anesthesia and mild sedation. Magnetic resonance or computed tomography images are then obtained to stereotactically localize the target sites, typically the periventricular and periaqueductal gray matter of the mesencephalic-diencephalic transition area, the specific sensory thalamic nuclei, the internal capsule, and the motor cortex. Once the coordinates for the target site are obtained, an electrode is placed into the brain via a burr hole under local anesthesia and sedation (Fig. 65–4). Electrophysiologic recording and motor and sensory responses with a stimulating electrode guide the neurosurgeon to the ultimate placement of the permanent DBS electrode. After the electrode is placed in the appropriate position, the patient is given general anesthesia and the proximal lead is tunneled in the subcutaneous space to the infraclavicular space of the chest, where it is attached to a pulse generator, much as a cardiac pacemaker is implanted. The pulse generator can be programmed to various settings by external interrogation.

A long-term follow-up study found DBS to be most effective for failed back syndrome, trigeminal neuropathy, and peripheral neuropathy, whereas patients with thalamic pain, spinal cord injury, and postherpetic neuralgia did poorly.[7] Nociceptive pain was relieved in 71%, whereas neuropathic pain was relieved in only 44%. The majority of the patients in this study had failed back syndrome, and of these 91% had early pain relief and 74% continued to have long-term relief. Overall complications included

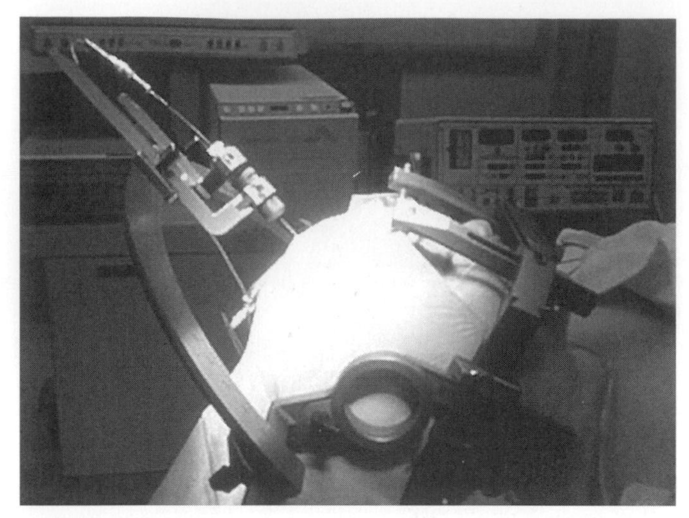

FIGURE 65–4 This photograph shows the stimulating and testing phase of the placement of a deep brain stimulator. The patient's head is in a stereotactic head frame.

headachy pain (22%), infection (6%), fractured electrode (3%), hardware malfunction (3%), postoperative seizures (3%), blurred vision with stimulation (3%), electrical leak (1%), and intracerebral hematoma (1%). The pulse generator battery has to be replaced approximately every 3 to 5 years. A distinct advantage of DBS over ablative procedures is that it is potentially nondestructive and reversible.

DORSAL ROOT ENTRY ZONE LESIONING

A dorsal root entry zone (DREZ) lesion destroys nociceptive secondary neurons in the spinal cord. It is useful for refractory phantom limb, postherpetic, and reflex sympathetic pain; in the partially damaged dorsal horn associated with paraplegia, with or without syringomyelia; or in the completely denervated dorsal horn of brachial plexus avulsion injuries. The technique involves laminectomy and intradural exposure of the spinal cord. With an operating microscope, the dorsal roots are identified, and then a small radiofrequency electrode is placed into the dorsal horn of the affected side. A contiguous series of lesions is made by heating the electrode tip with a generator to 75° C for 15 seconds. For avulsion injuries, the pain relief from the DREZ operation is often immediate, although in a rare patient the pain initially is worse. In a series of more than 100 patients with brachial plexus avulsion, 70% have experienced good pain relief that lasted longer than 5 years after a DREZ operation.[8] The major complication, weakness in the ipsilateral leg (5% overall rate), is due to involvement of the adjacent pyramidal tract. This complication occurs most frequently in patients with postherpetic chest or abdominal pain, for which lesions are made in the thoracic spinal cord. Leg weakness after cervical DREZ lesioning is rare.

SYMPATHECTOMY

Surgical procedures to disrupt the sympathetic nervous system can be used to treat causalgia, reflex sympathetic dystrophy, Sudeck's atrophy, and painful ischemic states such as Raynaud's phenomenon or angina pectoris. To determine which patients might be good candidates for sympathectomy, a temporary sympathetic blockade can be performed, most commonly by injecting local anesthesia into the stellate ganglion or into the region of the lumbar sympathetic ganglia. If the patient responds favorably, an ablative sympathectomy can be performed open via a posterior costotransversectomy approach, percutaneously, or endoscopically. Recently, the transthoracic endoscopic approach has gained favor for upper thoracic ganglionectomy

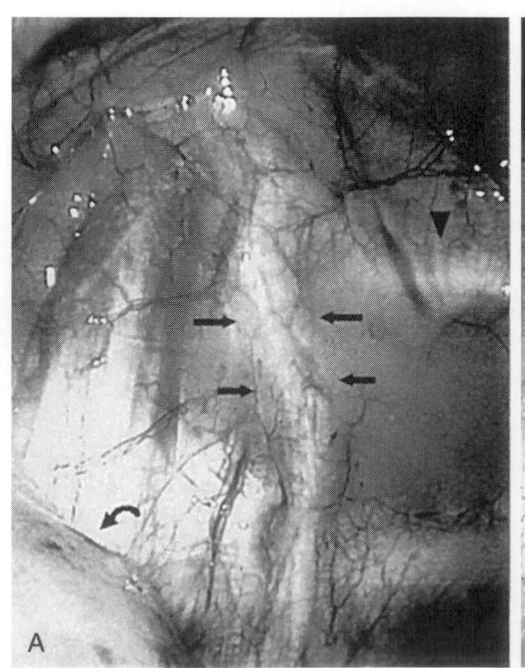

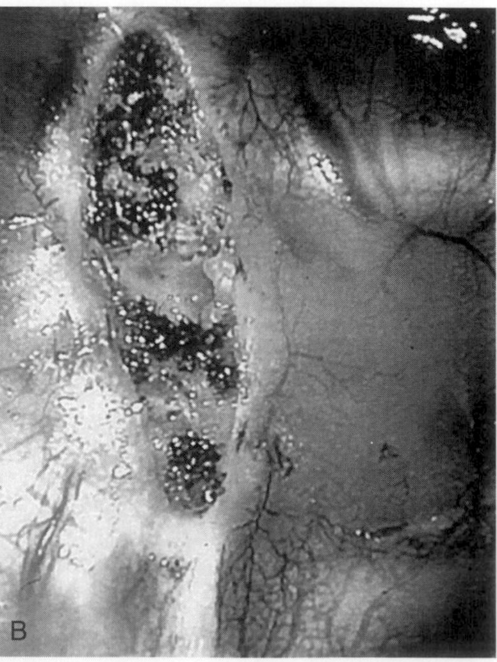

FIGURE 65–5 The view from a left-sided endoscopic transthoracic sympathectomy. A, The arrows delineate the sympathetic chain indenting the pleura. The arrowhead points to the superior portion of the second rib, and the curved arrow points to the collapsed lung. B, A slightly more magnified view after the sympathetic chain has been ablated by thermal coagulation. (Courtesy of Raj K. Narayan, M. D.)

thanks to improved instrumentation and minimal invasiveness. It is actually very effective for the treatment of hyperhidrosis. This particular approach involves collapsing the lung on the affected side with a double-lumen endotracheal tube. Through small lateral chest incisions, the endoscopic instruments are introduced through the pleural cavity, and the thoracic sympathetic chain is clearly identified and thermally coagulated (Fig. 65–5). As many as 95% of patients with causalgia obtain significant pain relief after sympathectomy[9]; however, only about 50% apparently receive lasting relief.[10] Complications from sympathectomies include Horner's syndrome and tension pneumothorax. The major complication associated with lumbar sympathectomy is loss of male sexual function (when sympathectomy is bilateral).

CONCLUSION

Certainly, a wide range of techniques are available to the neurosurgeon to treat a variety of intractable pain entities, including the benign pain of trigeminal neuralgia and the pain of many cancers. The newly reported success of stereotactic radiosurgery in alleviating trigeminal neuralgia and cluster headaches is an encouragement, as it adds yet another tool for neurosurgeons to fight severe pain. Better equipment and instrumentation are also making procedures such as the endoscopic sympathectomy more likely to be technically successful and better tolerated by patients. As the field of pain management and the specialty of neurosurgery continue to evolve, many more options should become available to treat patients who otherwise have little hope of relief.

REFERENCES

1. Ford RG, Ford KT, Swaid S, et al: Gamma knife treatment of refractory cluster headache. Headache 38(1):3–9, 1998.
2. Taha JM, Tew JM: Comparison of surgical treatments for trigeminal neuraglia: Reevaluation of radiofrequency rhizotomy. Neurosurgery 38(5):865–871, 1996.
3. Kondziolka D, Perez B, Flickinger JC, et al: Gamma knife radiosurgery for trigeminal neuralgia: Results and expectations. Arch Neurol 55(12):1524–1529, 1998.
4. Sweet WH, Poletti C: Complications of percutaneous rhizotomy and microvascular decompression operations for facial pain. *In* Schmidek HH, Sweet WH (eds): Operative Neurosurgical Techniques: Indications, Methods, and Results, ed 3. Philadelphia, WB Saunders, 1995, pp 1543–1546.
5. Sanders M, Zuurmond W: Safety of unilateral and bilateral percutaneous cervical cordotomy in 80 terminally ill cancer patients. J Clin Oncol 13(6):1509–1512, 1995.
6. Tranmer BI, Tucker WS, Bilbao JM: Sleep induced apnoea following percutaneous cervical cordotomy. Can J Neurol Sci 14:262–267, 1987.
7. Kumar K, Toth C, Nath RK: Deep brain stimulation for intractable pain: A 15-year experience. Neurosurgery 40(4):736–747, 1997.
8. Nashold BS, Nashold JRB: The DREZ operation. *In* Tindall GT, Cooper PR, Barrow DL (eds): The Practice of Neurosurgery. Baltimore, Williams & Wilkins, 1996, pp 3129–3151.
9. Ochoa JL: The newly recognized painful ABC syndrome: Thermographic aspects. Thermology 2:65–107, 1986.
10. Young RF: Sympathetic nervous system and pain. *In* Tindall GT, Cooper PR, Barrow DL (eds): The Practice of Neurosurgery. Baltimore, Williams & Wilkins, 1996, pp 3129–3151.

CHAPTER • 66

Neuroadenolysis of the Pituitary: Indications and Technique

Steven D. Waldman, MD, JD

HISTORY

Surgery has been used to palliate pain secondary to hormone-dependent tumors since the late 1800s. Early surgical efforts were directed primarily at surgical castration.[1] The addition of adrenalectomy followed, as the importance of this gland in the secretion of sex hormones became better understood.[2] Advances in the field of endocrinology in the 1950s led to an increasing focus on the pituitary gland. To this end, transcranial hypophysectomy was performed in an effort to induce regression of hormone-dependent tumors and to palliate symptoms. Investigators became aware that pain relief was a more consistent finding than actual tumor regression.[3]

Unfortunately, transcranial hypophysectomy was a major procedure with significant surgical risk that precluded its use in many of the patients who could most benefit; namely, patients suffering from advanced malignancy. Consequently, less invasive means of pituitary destruction were undertaken. These attempts included radiation therapy, implantation of radon seeds, and, ultimately, chemical neurolysis of the pituitary.[4]

Neuroadenolysis of the pituitary (NALP) was first described by Moricca in 1958, as a technique to relieve pain of malignant origin by placing multiple needles into the pituitary gland and then injecting small amounts of absolute alcohol.[5] Moricca's early reports led other investigators to adopt and modify this procedure. To date, more than 14,000 patients suffering from intractable pain have been treated with NALP.[6]

INDICATIONS AND CONTRAINDICATIONS

Indications for NALP are as follows:

- Failure of all antiblastic treatments
- Failure of all other appropriate pain-relieving measures
- Bilateral facial or upper body cancer pain
- Bilateral diffuse cancer pain
- Intractable visceral pain
- Pain secondary to compression of neural structures
- Loss of hormonal control of pain

NALP is an appropriate treatment for patients who suffer from bilateral facial or upper body cancer pain, bilateral diffuse cancer pain, intractable visceral pain, or pain secondary to compression of neural structures after all antiblastic methods and other analgesic measures have been exhausted. When medical hormonal control of pain no longer works, patients may also benefit from the procedure.[4] Most investigators observe better results in patients whose pain is secondary to hormone-dependent tumors, although the procedure is also effective for palliation of pain from hormone-unresponsive malignancies.[7] Contraindications to neuroadenolysis of the pituitary are summarized in Table 66–1. Local infection, sepsis, coagulopathy, significantly increased intracranial pressure, and empty sella syndrome are absolute contraindications to NALP.[4,7] Relative contraindications to NALP include poor anesthesia risk, disulfiram therapy, and significant behavioral abnormalities. Obviously, owing to the desperate circumstances of most patients considered for NALP, the risk-benefit ratio is shifted toward performing the procedure on both ethical and humanitarian grounds.

CLINICALLY RELEVANT ANATOMY AND TECHNIQUE

In an effort to improve on Moricca's original technique, Corssen and associates[8] and other investigators have modified it by decreasing the number of needles used. Levin and colleagues[9] further modified the technique by utilizing a stereotactic head frame. Attempting to reduce the incidence of postoperative cerebrospinal fluid leakage, these investigators suggested initially placing an 18-gauge, 6-inch spinal needle through the floor of the sphenoid sinus. The needle was then removed, and a smaller, 20-gauge, 6-inch spinal needle was placed through the hole left by the 18-gauge needle. The 20-gauge needle was then advanced into the sella turcica. On occasion, these investigators found it necessary to drill through the floor of the

TABLE 66–1 **Contraindications to Neuroadenolysis of the Pituitary**

Absolute contraindications
- Local infection
- Sepsis
- Coagulopathy
- Significantly increased intracranial pressure
- Empty sella syndrome

Relative contraindications
- Poor anesthesia risk
- Disulfiram therapy
- Significant behavioral abnormalities

sella turcica with a Kirschner wire because the needle would not pass through dense bone. They also noted the occasional occurrence of cerebrospinal fluid (CSF) leakage until they instituted the injection of ethyl alphacyanomethacrylate resin through the spinal needles.

Waldman and Feldstein[10] further modified NALP by using a needle-through-needle technique, thus eliminating the need for the stereotactic frame or drilling. These modifications made the procedure more suitable for use in the community hospital.

Phenol, cryoneurolysis, radiofrequency lesioning, and electrical stimulation in place of alcohol all have been advocated for NALP.[11–13] More experience is needed with each of these modalities to determine whether some of the theoretical advantages and disadvantages of each modification translate into clinically relevant benefits.

Preoperative Preparation

Screening laboratory tests, consisting of a complete blood count, chemistry profile, electrolyte determination, urinalysis, coagulation profile, chest radiography, and electrocardiography, are performed as for any other patient undergoing general anesthesia. Anteroposterior and lateral skull films are also obtained to evaluate the size and relative position of the sella turcica and to rule out sphenoid sinus infection, which may be clinically silent.[4, 10]

Preoperative treatment of all patients with an intravenous dose of a cephalosporin and aminoglycoside antibiotic 1 hour before induction of anesthesia is indicated to reduce the risk of infection in these immunocompromised patients.[10] Most investigators perform NALP with the patient under general endotracheal anesthesia, although, because the procedure is relatively painless, it can be performed with local anesthesia.[14] Opioids are avoided before and during the operation to avoid pupillary miosis, which might obscure the pupillary dilatation observed when alcohol spills out of the sella onto the oculomotor nerve (see later).[7, 10]

Technique of Neuroadenolysis of the Pituitary

With the intubated patient in the supine position on a biplanar fluoroscopy table, the nose is packed with pledgets soaked in 7.5% cocaine solution to provide vasoconstriction and shrinkage of the nasal mucosa (Fig. 66–1). After 10 minutes, the packs are removed and the anterior nasal mucosa and face are prepared with povidone iodine solution. Sterile drapes are placed over the nose and face. The anterior medial mucosa and deep tissues are infiltrated with a solution of 1.0% lidocaine and 1 : 200,000 epinephrine. During infiltration and subsequent needle placement, care must be taken to avoid Kesselback's plexus lest vigorous bleeding ensue. It is imperative that the head be kept precisely in the midline to allow accurate needle placement.

A 17-gauge, 3.5-inch spinal needle with the stylet in place is advanced under biplanar fluoroscopic guidance, care being taken to ensure that the needle remains exactly in the midline to avoid trauma to the adjacent structures, including the carotid arteries (Fig. 66–2). The needle is advanced until its tip rests against the anterior wall of the sella turcica (Fig. 66–3). At this point, plain radiographs are taken to confirm needle position (Fig. 66–4). After satisfactory positioning is verified, the stylet is removed from the 17-gauge needle. A 20-gauge, 13-cm, styleted Hinck needle (Cook Incorporated, Bloomington, Ind.) is placed through the 17-gauge needle and is carefully advanced through the anterior wall of the sella turcica (Fig. 66–5). This process feels like passing a needle through an eggshell. The Hinck needle is then further advanced under biplanar fluoroscopic guidance through the substance of the pituitary gland, until the tip rests against the posterior wall of the sella turcica (Fig. 66–6). Needle position is again confirmed with plain radiographs (Fig. 66–7).

The patient's eyes are then exposed, and alcohol in aliquots of 0.2 mL is injected as the Hinck needle is gradually withdrawn back through the pituitary gland (Fig. 66–8).

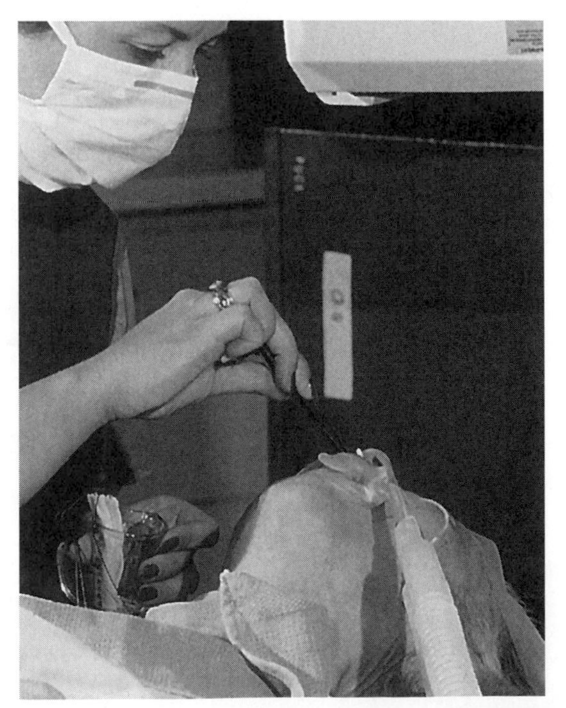

FIGURE 66–1 *The nose is packed to provide vasoconstriction and mucosal shrinkage.*

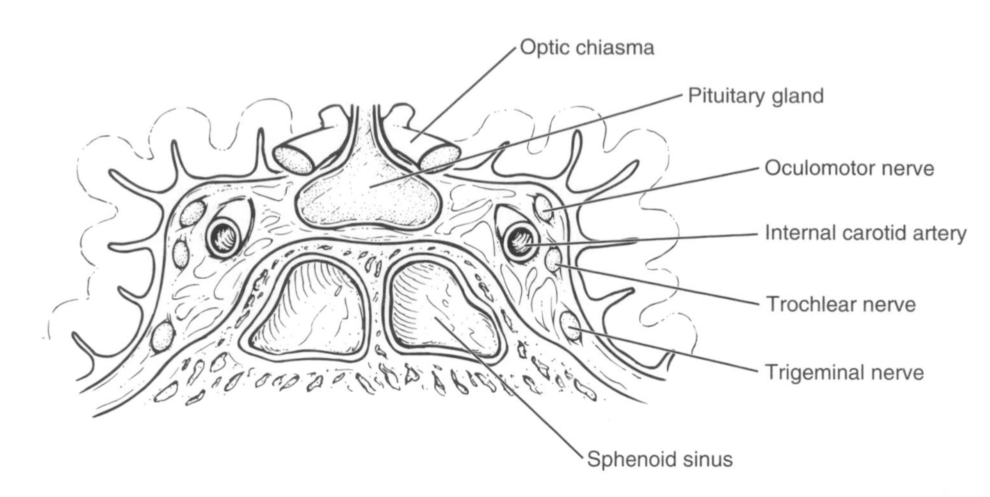

FIGURE 66–2 Lateral view of the sphenoid sinus, sella turcica, and pituitary, and of the relationship of the carotid arteries and oculomotor nerve.

Depending on the size of the sella, a total of 4 to 6 mL of alcohol is injected. During the injection process, the pupils are constantly monitored for dilatation. Pupillary dilatation indicates that the alcohol has spilled outside the sella turcica and has come in contact with an oculomotor nerve. If pupillary dilatation is observed, injection of alcohol is discontinued and the needle is withdrawn to a more anterior position. The injection process then resumes. In most instances, if the alcohol injection is discontinued at the first sign of pupillary dilatation, any resultant visual disturbance is transitory.[15] It has been suggested that monitoring with visual evoked responses during alcohol injection may be a more sensitive test for visual complications than pupillary dilatation is.[4]

After the injection of alcohol is completed, 0.5 mL of cyanamethacrylate resin is injected via the Hinck needle to seal the hole in the sella turcica and to prevent CSF leakage. Both needles are removed. The nasal mucosa is

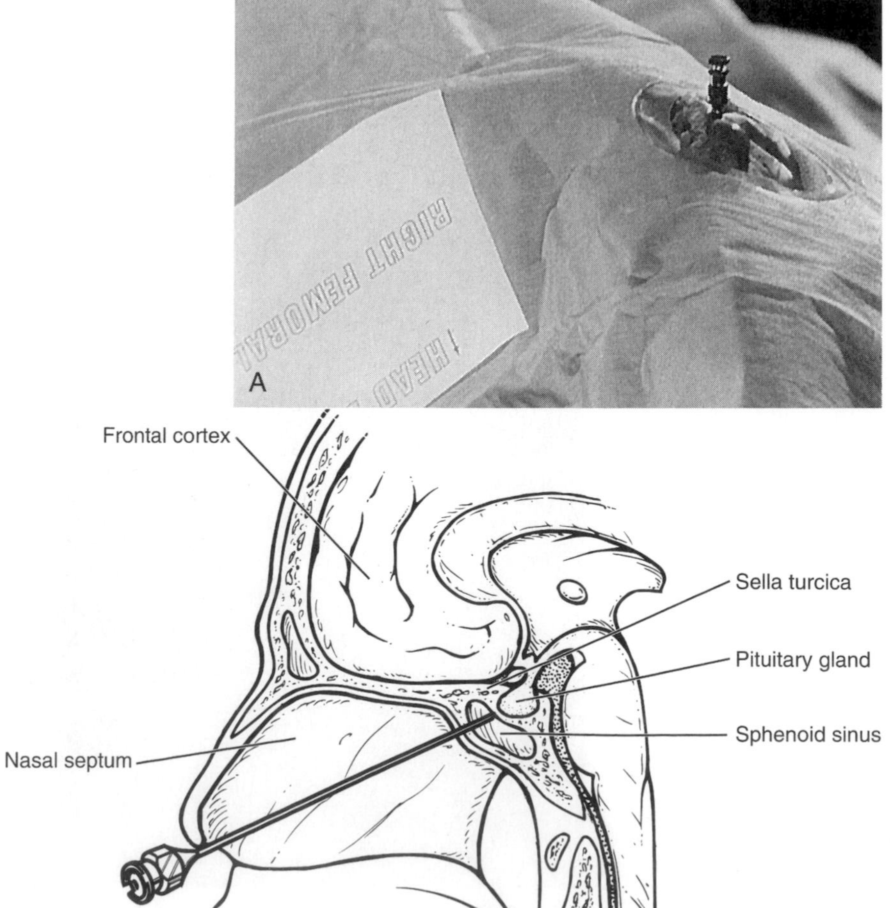

FIGURE 66–3 A, *A 17-gauge, 3.5-inch needle is in midline position with the tip resting against the anterior wall of the sella turcica.* B, *Drawing of a lateral view of the needle trajectory with the tip of a 17-gauge spinal needle against the anterior wall of the sella turcica.*

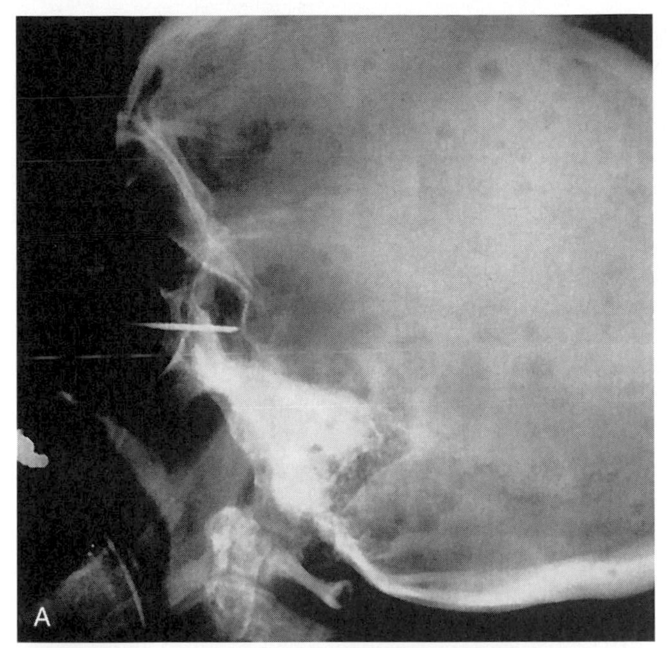

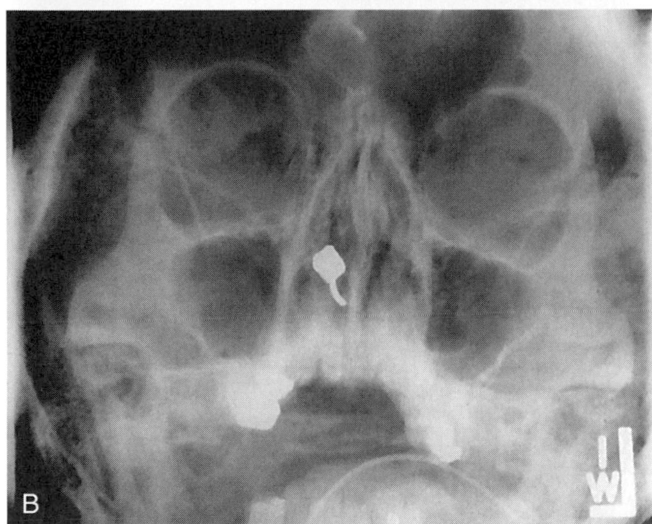

FIGURE 66–4 Plain radiographs confirming placement of the 17-gauge, 3.5-inch needle in a midline position with the tip resting against the anterior wall of the sella turcica. A, *Lateral view.* B, *Anteroposterior view.*

observed for bleeding or CSF leakage. Nasal packing is not generally required with this modified procedure. The patient is then extubated and taken to the recovery room. Approximately 30 min is required to perform NALP.

Postoperative Care

All patients are continued on antibiotics for 24 hours. Endocrine replacement, consisting of 15 mg prednisone and 0.15 mg levothyroxine sodium (Synthroid) every morning is required for every patient.[10]

Accurate monitoring of intake and output is mandatory, as transient diabetes insipidus occurs in approximately 40% of patients undergoing NALP.[16] In most instances, the diabetes insipidus is self-limited, but vasopressin administration should be considered for patients who are unable to drink as much as they excrete or whose urinary output exceeds 2.5 L per day.[4] Failure to identify and treat diabetes insipidus is the leading cause of morbidity and mortality in patients who undergo NALP.

All patients are continued on preoperative levels of oral narcotics for 24 hours, and then doses are tapered. Patients generally resume their normal diet and activities the day of the procedure.

MECHANISMS OF PAIN RELIEF

Levin, Ramirez,[15] and Bonica[7] have reviewed the proposed mechanisms of pain relief after NALP. Early investigators centered their theories on the concept of pain relief secondary to elimination of the pituitary hormones responsible for enhancement of nocioceptive transmission. Later, Yanagida and colleagues[11] suggested that pain appears to be independent of the extent of pituitary damage and may be caused by reactionary hyperactivity of the hypophyseal system exerting inhibitory influences on the pain pathways of the brain. In spite of extensive research, the exact mechanism of pain relief after NALP remains unclear, as does whether the procedure produces pain relief by neurodestruction or neuroaugmentation.[13]

RESULTS

Incidence of Pain Relief

In 1990, Bonica[7] reviewed the world literature on NALP and summarized the data and conclusions. The world literature suggests a success rate (pain relief rated complete to

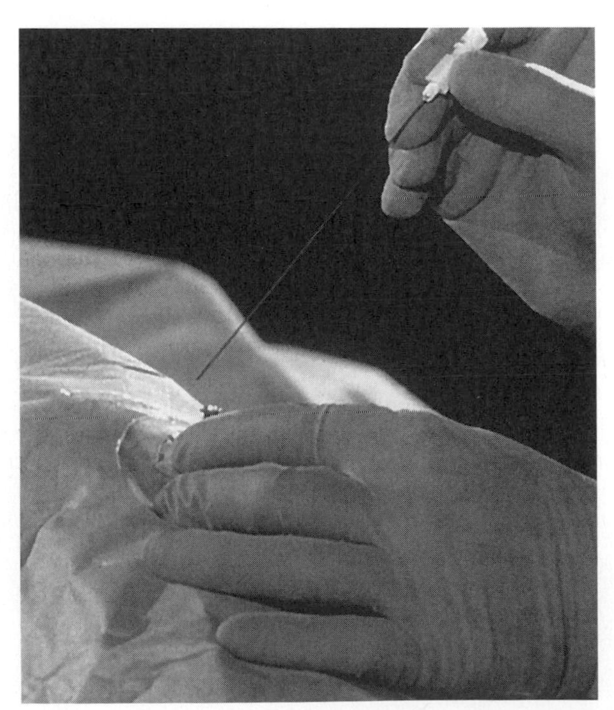

FIGURE 66–5 A 20-gauge, 13-cm Hinck needle is introduced through the 17-gauge needle.

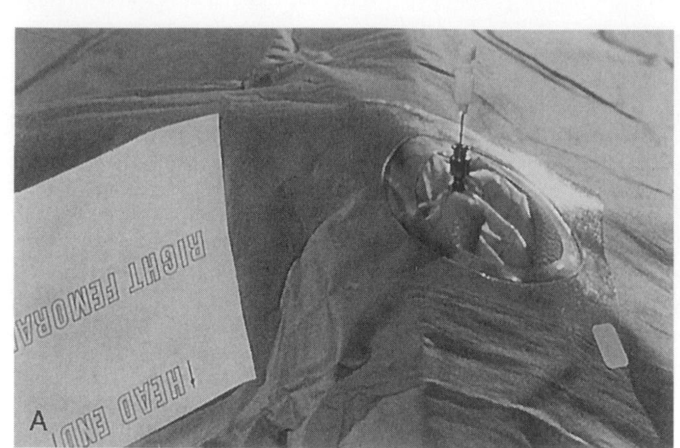

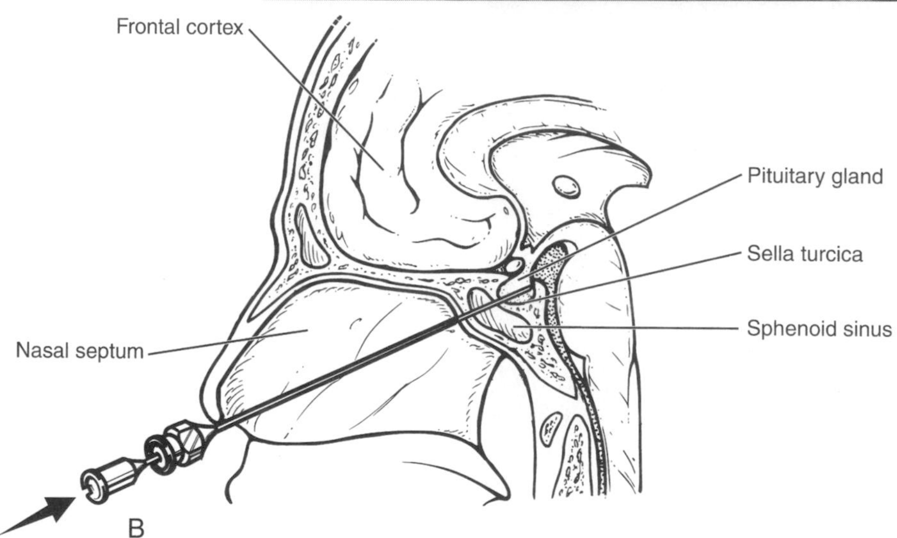

FIGURE 66–6 A, *The Hinck needle has been placed through the 17-gauge needle, and the Hinck needle's tip is resting against the posterior wall of the sella turcica.* B, *Drawing of a lateral view of the needle trajectory with the tip of the 17-gauge spinal needle against the anterior wall of the sella turcica and the Hinck needle through it into the substance of the pituitary.*

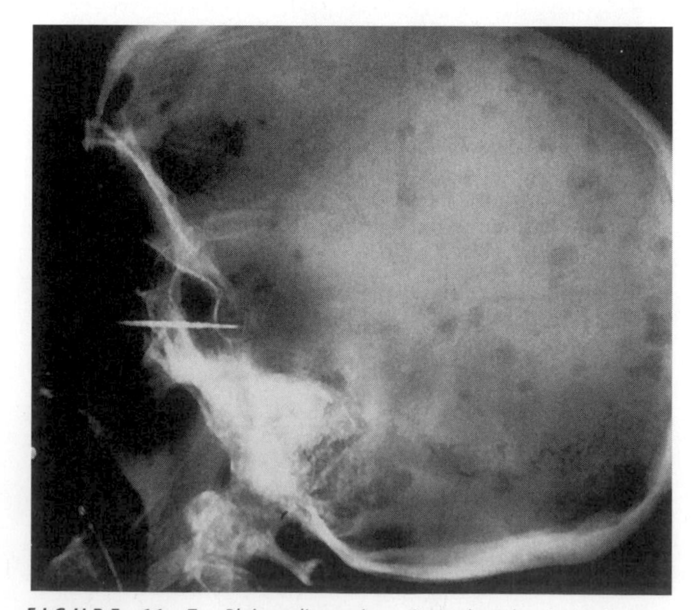

FIGURE 66–7 *Plain radiograph confirms that the tip of the Hinck needle is resting against the posterior wall of the sella turcica.*

good) of approximately 63%. An additional 23% of patients described their pain relief as fair. Fourteen percent of patients reported poor to no relief of pain after NALP. A closer look at this patient population reveals that patients with hormone-dependent tumors experienced better pain relief than did those with non–hormone-dependent tumors.[7] Furthermore, it appears that investigators who injected larger volumes of alcohol (4 to 6 mL) or who repeated NALP when the first procedure was not successful obtained better results, in terms of pain relief. In spite of the inherent limitations of analyzing data from multiple studies, it is obvious that NALP is an effective treatment for certain patients suffering from cancer pain.[7, 10, 17, 18]

Complications

Complications directly related to NALP are summarized in Table 66–2. Virtually all patients who undergo NALP complain of a bilateral frontal headache, which resolves spontaneously within 24 to 48 hours.[10] Diabetes insipidus develops in approximately 40% of patients who undergo the procedure. Approximately 35% of patients experience transient temperature increases up to 1.5° C after

NALP.[10, 16] These temperature aberrations are attributed to disturbance of the temperature-regulating mechanism of the hypothalamus.[10] About 20% of patients experience an increase in pulmonary secretions and mild orthopnea that, clinically, resembles congestive heart failure.[10] This problem is self-limited if careful attention is paid to the patient's fluid status. It has been postulated that this phenomenon is centrally mediated. Although the potential exists for serious ocular disturbances, a review of the literature suggests that transient visual disturbances, including diplopia, blurred vision, and loss of visual field, occur in fewer than 10% of patients who undergo neuroadenolysis of the pituitary gland.[4, 7, 16] Permanent visual disturbances occur much less often, with an average incidence of approximately 5%.[4, 7, 10, 16] Cerebrospinal fluid leakage, infection, and pituitary hemorrhage develop in fewer than 1% of patients reported but are some of the most devastating complications. If they are not recognized immediately and treated, death can result.[4, 7, 10]

TABLE 66–2 ***Incidence of Complications of Neuroadenolysis of the Pituitary***

Complication	Incidence %
Transient bilateral frontal headache	100
Diabetes insipidus	40
Hyperthermia	35
Increased pulmonary secretions	20
Transient visual disturbances	10
Permanent visual disturbances	5
Cerebrospinal fluid leakage	1
Pituitary hemorrhage	1
Infection	0.5

DISCUSSION

Neuroadenolysis of the pituitary gland is a safe, effective method for palliating diffuse cancer pain that does not respond to conservative treatment modalities. Its technical simplicity and relative safety make NALP an ideal procedure for cancer patients who have undergone a vast array of treatments. Although spinal administration of opioids has replaced NALP as the procedure of choice for many cancer pain syndromes, it is the belief of many cancer pain specialists that NALP is still underutilized today. With the needle-through-needle modification described, a more favorable risk-benefit ratio is expected. As Bonica[7] has stated, "NALP is one of the most, if not the most, effective ablative procedures for the relief of severe diffuse cancer pain."

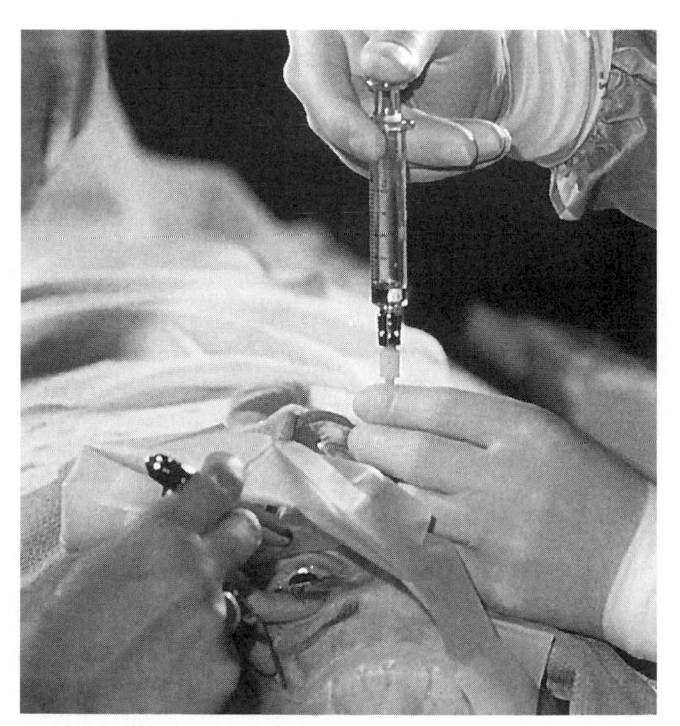

FIGURE 66–8 *The patient's eyes are exposed, and 0.2-mL aliquots of alcohol are injected as the Hinck needle is gradually withdrawn.*

REFERENCES

1. Beatson GT: On the treatment of inoperable cases of cancer of the mamma. Lancet 2:104–106, 1896.
2. Huggins C, Hodges CV: Inhibition of memory and prostate cancers by adrenalectomy. Cancer 12:131–141, 1952.
3. Luft R, Olivercrona H: Experiences with hypophysectomy. J Neurosurg 10:301–316, 1953.
4. Lipton S: Pituitary adenolysis. *In* Raj PP (ed): Practical Management of Pain, ed 2. St Louis, CV Mosby, 1992, p 908.
5. Ventifredda V, DeConno F: Moricca's operation at the National Cancer Institute of Milan. *In* Ischia S, Lipton S, Maffezzoli GF (eds): Pain Treatment. New York, Raven, 1993, pp 85–90.
6. Gianasi G: Neuroadenolysis of the pituitary of Moricca: An overview of development, mechanisms, technique, and results. Adv Pain Res Ther 7:647–648, 1984.
7. Bonica JJ: Neurolytic block and hypophysectomy. *In* Bonica J: The Management of Pain, vol 2. Philadelphia, Lea & Febiger, 1990, pp 2028–2034.
8. Corssen G, Holcomb MA, Moustapha I, et al: Alcohol induced adenolysis of the pituitary gland: A new approach to control of intractable cancer pain. Anesth Analg 56:414–421, 1977.
9. Levin AB, Katz J, Benson RC, Jones AG: Treatment of pain of diffuse metastatic cancer by stereotactic chemical hypophysectomy: Long-term results and observations on mechanisms of action. Neurosurgery 6:258–262, 1980.
10. Waldman SD, Feldstein GS: Neuroadenolysis of the pituitary: Description of a modified technique. J Pain Symptom Manage 2:45–49, 1987.
11. Yanagida H, Corssen G, Trouwborst A, Erdman W: Relief of cancer pain in man: Alcohol-induced neuroadenolysis vs. electrical stimulation of the pituitary gland. Pain 19:133–141, 1984.
12. Duthie AM: Pituitary cryoablation. Anaesthesia 38:495–497, 1983.
13. Patt RB: Neurosurgical and neuroaugmentative intervention. *In* Patt RB (ed): Cancer Pain. Philadelphia, JB Lippincott, 1993, p 489.
14. Lipton S: The injection of alcohol into the pituitary fossa (Moricca's operation). *In* Lipton S: Relief of Pain in Clinical Practice. Oxford, Blackwell Scientific, 1979, pp 179–220.
15. Levin AB, Ramirez LL: Treatment of cancer pain with hypophysectomy: Surgical and chemical. Adv Pain Res Ther 7:631–645, 1984.
16. Gianasi GC: Pituitary neuroadenolysis: An analysis of the clinical results in a group of high-risk patients. *In* Ischia S, Lipton S, Maffezzoli GF (eds): Pain Treatment. New York, Raven, 1993, pp 91–95.
17. Takeda F: Results of cancer pain relief and tumour regression by pituitary neuroadenolysis and surgical hypophysectomy. *In* Ischia S, Lipton S, Maffezzoli GF (eds): Pain Treatment. New York, Raven, 1993, pp 103–113.
18. Waldman SD: Neuroadenolysis of the pituitary. *In* Waldman SD: Atlas of Interventional Pain Management Techniques. Philadelphia, WB Saunders, 1998, pp 513–515.

CHAPTER • 67

Percutaneous Cordotomy

Steven Rosen, MD

Percutaneous cordotomy is an extraordinary technique useful primarily for cancer pain management. A radiofrequency lesion is made in the anterolateral quadrant of the spinal cord to interrupt pain transmission through the spinothalamic fibers. Good to excellent results should be achieved in close to 90% of patients, with minimal morbidity. The use of percutaneous cordotomy has declined for two reasons. First, knowledge and skill in the use of systemic and spinal narcotics are increasing. Narcotics are least effective, however, in patients with neuropathic or incident pain. Cordotomy offers such patients dramatic, sustained relief. Second, skilled practitioners are few. The technique must be performed by a practitioner skilled in percutaneous interventional work. The operator must be comfortable with the use of fluoroscopy and radiofrequency lesioning. It is to be hoped that, as interventional pain management is popularized and the number of skilled practitioners increases, percutaneous cordotomy will become a standard technique in comprehensive cancer care. When used in such a manner, percutaneous cordotomy is a gratifying procedure that helps cancer patients live out their lives free of pain and with as much dignity as possible.

HISTORICAL CONSIDERATIONS

The development of cordotomy mirrors progress in medicine. *Cordotomy* refers to creating a lesion in the spinothalamic tracts, by either a surgical scalpel or a radiofrequency generator. The first surgical cordotomy was reported by Spiller and Martin[1] in 1912. It had been noted that patients with pathologic lesions in the anterolateral quadrants of the spinal cord developed contralateral loss of pain and temperature discrimination yet retained the sensation of light touch. Spiller and Martin[1] performed their cordotomy in the midthoracic spine to relieve lower limb pain. Only high cervical cordotomy, however, could relieve pain from below the middle cervical segments.[2, 3] Despite gratifying pain relief, it became obvious that considerable morbidity was associated with high cervical cordotomy.[4] This morbidity was attributed to the surgical resection itself and to interference with automatic respiratory function. Patients would breathe on command but developed sleep apnea. The complication was especially common after bilateral high cervical lesions. Severinghaus and Mitchell[5] called this complication *Ondine's curse*, a reference to the water nymph Ondine, who, having been jilted by her husband, took away his automatic respiratory functions so that he had to remember to breathe. When he fell asleep, he died. The rate of mortality from high cervical cordotomy was cited as 4% to 25%.[6, 7]

The first percutaneous cordotomies were described by Millan and colleagues[6] in 1963, who placed a radioisotope-tipped probe near the anterolateral quadrant of the cord at C1–C2. The lesions were inconsistent, however, and radioisotope-tipped needles were not generally available. In 1965, Millan and associates[8] described percutaneous cordotomy using direct current. Lesions took 10 to 30 min to take effect, as compared with as long as 2 to 3 months after radioisotope-tipped needles were removed. Percutaneous radiofrequency cordotomy was first described by Rosomoff and associates[9] in 1965. With minor modifications, theirs is the technique used today. Lesions were reproducible and could be performed in less than a minute. The technique was relatively simple and allowed patients to enjoy pain relief who might not have been acceptable surgical risks for the more extensive open operation.

It was hoped that respiratory mortality would be less with the percutaneous approach, but this turned out not to be the case. To minimize the risk of respiratory trespass. Lin and coworkers[10, 11] developed the anterior approach. Needles were placed through either the C5–C6 or C6–C7 disc and then into the anterolateral quadrant of the cord, which is below the exit of the respiratory fibers with the phrenic nerve. It was difficult to realign poorly positioned needles embedded in disc material, however, and today the anterior approach is rarely used. Crue and associates[12] and Hitchcock[13] developed a posterior approach. The probe was placed through the posterior columns and then into the final position in the anterolateral quadrant. The high lateral cervical approach at C1–C2 is relatively simple to perform, is easy to conceptualize, and has withstood the test of time.

Since 1965, modifications have been directed toward improving target visualization. For stereotactic surgery, the target must be identified both radiologically and physiologically. After the target has been identified, it must then be destroyed in a precise and reproducible manner.

In percutaneous cordotomy, the target is the anterolateral quadrant of the spinal cord. The dentate ligament separates the anterior from the posterior quadrant. Identification of the dentate ligament greatly aids electrode placement. Millan and colleagues[6] and Rosomoff and associates[9] simply injected air to outline the anterior surface of the cord. The electrode was placed just below the anterior surface, and incremental lesions were made until either contralateral analgesia was obtained or motor weakness occurred. Onofrio[14] used an emulsion of Pantopaque (iophendylate) in air to outline both the anterior surface of the cord and the dentate ligament. This step significantly reduced the time needed to search for the anterolateral quadrant. Computed tomography (CT)–guided placement of electrodes has been described by Kanpolat.[15, 16] More precise lesioning may decrease postoperative complications by increasing the selectivity of the procedure. Gildenberg and coworkers[17] emphasized impedance monitoring to identify penetration of the spinal cord. Physiologic identification of the spinothalamic fibers was emphasized by Taren and associates.[18] Different areas of the spinal cord exhibit characteristic responses to motor and sensory stimulation.[19, 20] Evoked potentials were recorded from the anterolateral quadrant in 1983 by Campbell and Lipton.[21] Impedance monitoring to detect the subarachnoid space has also been described.[22]

After the target is identified, it must be destroyed in a precise and reproducible manner. Principles of radiofrequency lesioning have been reviewed by Cosman and colleagues.[23] A comprehensive review of radiofrequency techniques is now available.[24] A significant development has been the thermocoupled electrode.[25] Cordotomy lesions had been performed by gradually increasing the current and lesioning time while carefully observing for pain relief and monitoring for neurologic deficits. The thermocoupled electrode allows direct temperature monitoring to guide lesion making. The tissue temperature, not the current, causes neural destruction, and it could now be precisely controlled. The active tip of the Levin thermocoupled electrode was 2 mm in length and 0.5 mm in diameter, ensuring easy placement through a 20-gauge spinal needle. The resulting 4-mm oval-shaped lesion is ideal to adequately denervate the anterolateral quadrant of the cord.

The latest efforts have been devoted to defining the role of percutaneous cordotomy in comprehensive pain care. Tasker and associates[26] have described the role of cordotomy in patients with noncancer pain of spinal cord origin. Ischia and associates published several excellent articles detailing the risks and benefits of percutaneous cordotomy in cancer patients. They have described results of cordotomy for pain of vertebral body lesions[27] and that of Pancoast's tumor and upper thoracic lesions.[28] They also reported on the complementary roles of cordotomy and subarachnoid neurolysis in patients with pelvic malignancy.[29] Ischia and colleagues[30] have discussed the benefits and the respiratory risks involved in bilateral lesioning.

Histologic correlation with clinical results after cordotomy has been used to define the functional neuroanatomy of the spine. Nathan and Smith[31, 32] and Lahuerta and coworkers[33] used histologic evidence to identify respiratory pathways in the spinal cord. In a similar manner, the location of the sympathetic fibers[34] and the pathways involved in voiding and defecation[35] have been ascertained. Histologic evidence has shown that lesions 5 mm deep to the surface that destroy about 20% of the hemicord give optimal analgesia.[36] A fascinating phenomenon is the development of reference of sensation after cordotomy.[37] Mirror-image pain may develop or noxious sensations may be referred to the side of the body opposite to the cordotomy target. New subsidiary pain pathways have been postulated.[38] This observation has led to new theories about the roles of inhibitory pain pathways. Further research will continue to expand our knowledge of the intricacy of nerve transmission in humans.

INDICATIONS AND CONTRAINDICATIONS

Percutaneous cervical cordotomy is best used for unilateral cancer pain below the shoulder in patients with life expectancy less than 1 year. A lesion is created in the spinothalamic tract. Complications develop from extension of the lesion to adjoining tracts or to development of a zone of edema that temporarily interferes with transmission by adjacent fibers. In this section, the indications and contraindications to percutaneous cordotomy are reviewed, as well as published results.

It cannot be emphasized enough that pain-relieving procedures are part of comprehensive cancer care and cannot be viewed in isolation. Cancer is a complex, multifactorial disease, and it is unlikely that one procedure, no matter how well performed, will result in sustained lifelong pain relief. A percutaneous cordotomy is just one part of a comprehensive treatment plan that includes surgery, radiation therapy, medications, pain-relieving procedures, and psychological support. Review of the literature is disappointing, because few attempts have been made to define indications or to stratify results according to location of disease and type of pain. As spinal narcotic techniques have evolved, the role of cordotomy has decreased, but we can hope that it will soon be better defined.

From January 1990 to December 1998, 54 percutaneous cordotomies were performed by the author. The patients all had experienced failure of aggressive medical pain therapy. During the same interval, 58 subarachnoid pumps and 31 permanently tunneled epidural catheters were implanted in cancer patients. Depending on the study, as many as 30% of cancer patients are candidates for pain-relieving procedures or surgeries. Some of these patients can benefit from invasive but opioid-sparing techniques such as percutaneous cordotomy. More than 100 celiac ablations, hypogastric ablations, and spinal neurolyses were performed.

Indications

As mentioned, the best indication for cordotomy is unilateral cancer pain below the shoulder. Percutaneous cordotomy is generally performed at C1–C2. At this level, the spinothalamic tract is in the anterolateral quadrant of the cord. Pain fibers enter the cord through the dorsal horn and then may ascend several levels before crossing over and taking their final position in the spinothalamic tract. A lesion at C1–C2 is almost guaranteed to produce analgesia below C4 or C5, the levels that innervate the shoulder. An open surgical cordotomy at T1–T2 does not produce analgesia in the upper extremity but does produce it in the lower chest, abdomen, and lower extremity. It does not affect respiratory fibers, because they have already exited the spinal cord via the phrenic nerve. As will become clearer later, this point is important in the consideration of bilateral lesioning.

A percutaneous cordotomy is especially useful for neuropathic or incident pain. Although neuropathic pain exhibits some narcotic responsiveness,[39] brachial or sacral plexopathy generally responds poorly to medical pain therapy. Better responses can be obtained with spinal narcotic techniques, especially when local anesthetics and/or clonidine[40–43] are added. Even with these measures, however, pain relief may well be unsatisfactory or barely acceptable. Patients with brachial plexopathy from Pancoast's tumor or sacral plexopathy from pelvic malignant disease are excellent candidates for cordotomy.

Incident pain is when the patient is comfortable at rest but develops severe pain with weight bearing. Examples are pelvic, hip, femur, and humeral lesions or fractures. Incident pain may also arise from a vertebral body fracture. If affected patients are not candidates for surgical stabilization, they may be good candidates for cordotomy. Patients with incident pain who are comfortable while standing with analgesics invariably are oversedated at rest. Incident pain is extraordinarily difficult to treat with medical management. It is remarkable to see a patient with a hip fracture walk pain free after a cordotomy.

The ideal indications for cordotomy are incident pain and neuropathic pain of the lower extremity. In my series, 26 of 54 patients had incident pain and another 15 had neuropathic pain of the lower extremity. Six patients underwent cordotomy for upper extremity pain secondary to Pancoast's tumor. Seven had cordotomies for cancer-related chest wall pain. Patients with incident pain and lower extremity plexopathies are the most difficult to treat with medical or procedural interventions and are excellent candidates for percutaneous cordotomy.

Neuropathic pain must be distinguished from deafferentation pain, which would not be relieved by cordotomy. Examples of deafferentation pain are postherpetic neuralgia, thalamic pain, and many cases of pain secondary to spinal cord lesions or reflex sympathetic dystrophy. The pain is usually described as dysesthetic or causalgic. Patients complain of burning pain and show hyperpathia and allodynia. Deafferentation pain is related to the loss of afferent sensory input and usually occurs in the setting of at least partial sensory loss in the affected distribution. In a cancer patient, pain would be caused not by tumor pressing on a nerve but from actual damage to the nerve itself. Deafferentation pain is uncommon in terminal cancer patients but considerably more common in patients with noncancer, or "benign," pain. Deafferentation pain accounts for the relatively poor results of cordotomy in noncancer patients and is probably responsible for the great majority of postcordotomy dysesthesias.

Tasker and associates[26] have elucidated the role of percutaneous cordotomy in patients with spinal cord lesions. Destructive surgery, predominantly cordotomy, was most effective in patients with intermittent or evoked pain. Cordotomy was marginally effective in patients with steady pain, which was usually causalgic or dysesthetic. Again, the point is that quality and origin of pain are crucial in determining whether cordotomy is indicated, especially in a patient with noncancer pain.

The benefit of cordotomy tends to decrease with time. Although nerve regeneration has not been demonstrated, cordotomies can wear off over time. Pain can recur years later, and lesioning can sometimes be repeated, with renewed long-term benefit.[44,45] In 1974, Rosomoff[46] reported on 1279 cordotomies performed in 789 patients. Immediately after cordotomy, more than 90% of patients were pain free. By the end of 1 year, almost 40% of patients no longer had absolute pain relief. Sixteen percent of patients developed postcordotomy dysesthesia of varying degrees. Nagaro[47] classified pain recurrence as deafferentation pain or pain secondary to recovery of nerve function. Deafferentation could be secondary to increasing tumor-related peripheral nerve injury or destruction of second-order neurons by the cordotomy. Because of pain recurrence and the development of postcordotomy dysesthesias, cordotomies are not generally recommended for patients whose life expectancy is longer than 1 year. Thus, the procedure is mostly limited to terminal cancer patients. As the indications for the technique become better defined, more longer-term survivors and noncancer patients will be candidates for this powerful pain-relieving technique. At this time, patients with relatively long life expectancy should be preferentially considered for neuroaugmentation or a spinal narcotic infusion.

Because cancer is a systemic disease, unmasking of contralateral pain after a successful cordotomy is common. Most cancer pain can be satisfactorily treated with medications, and it is likely that newly unmasked pain will be relieved with analgesics alone and will be easier to treat than the pain relieved by the cordotomy. Macaluso and colleagues[48] reported the results of cordotomies in 20 patients with lumbosacral, pelvic, and lower extremity pain. Contralateral pain was unmasked in 18 patients and responded to opioids in 15, to intrathecal phenol in 1, and to contralateral cordotomy in 2. In my practice, contralateral pain was unmasked postoperatively in 5 patients, and 30 of 54 patients developed contralateral pain before death. Twenty-seven of these patients were treated with medical management. Two patients required bilateral cordotomies, and one required local anesthetic and narcotic infusion through a tunneled epidural catheter.

Contraindications

The major contraindication to cordotomy is preexisting respiratory dysfunction; this condition is discussed more fully in the section on Complications. In short, the automatic respiratory fibers course through the reticulospinal tract. The reticulospinal tract is adjacent to the spinothalamic tract. In fact, reticulospinal fibers may mingle with those of the spinothalamic tract. It is easy to see how lesions in the spinothalamic tract could interfere with automatic respiratory function. Voluntary respiratory control fibers are in the corticospinal tract located in the posterior quadrant of the cord and, so, are unlikely to be affected by a percutaneous cordotomy. Many respiratory fibers exit the cord via the phrenic nerve, which contains fibers from C3, C4, and C5. Therefore, a C1–C2 cordotomy can cause ipsilateral respiratory dysfunction along with contralateral pain relief. Cordotomy decreases the forced expiratory volume (FEV_1) by an average of 20%,[49] but it is impossible to predict beforehand who will and who will not be affected.

When does respiratory function become a concern? A patient with a lung tumor and ipsilateral pain may well depend on the function of the contralateral lung to stay alive. This would be the side on which respiratory function is affected by the contralateral cordotomy. What parameters can be used to predict the safety of the procedural intervention? At this time, no good guidelines are available. I obtain pulmonary function tests and a sniff test to check diaphragm function. An estimate is also made of the relative pulmonary function of each lung. An FEV_1 above 1.2 L would allow a small margin of safety, even after a 20% drop. As a rough guideline, a patient who is able to lie supine without difficulty is probably a good candidate for a cordotomy. This is obviously a practical screening test, because patients who could not perform this maneuver would in any case not be able to cooperate sufficiently during the procedure itself to ensure a successful outcome.

Respiratory function is an even more serious issue when bilateral cordotomy is contemplated. Bilateral procedures should be staged at least several weeks apart to allow cord edema from the first lesion to dissipate. Clearly, bilateral lesions of the reticulospinal tract have disastrous consequences. As I describe in the discussion of clinical anatomy in the next section, the spinothalamic fibers from the cervical segments are closest to the reticulospinal fibers. If the first cordotomy produces cervical analgesia, it is likely that the reticulospinal fibers were damaged. The patient is, therefore, at increased risk from contralateral cordotomy. If the second cordotomy also damages the automatic respiratory fibers, the patient is very likely to develop sleep apnea syndrome and possibly respiratory death.

In the patient considered for bilateral cordotomy when the first cordotomy produces a high level of cervical analgesia, the surgeon has three options. Tasker[50] suggests tailoring the lesion. The spinothalamic fibers serving the lumbar dermatomes are relatively far from the reticulospinal tract. Stimulation should preferentially be sought from the lumbar segments, so that the resulting lesion would be less likely to include the automatic respiratory fibers. A second option is cordotomy at or below C6. The percutaneous anterior approach is theoretically possible but in practice difficult to perform. If a contralateral cordotomy is necessary, the best option would be an open surgical procedure in the lower cervical or upper thoracic region. Of course, this would not be appropriate for the patient who needs bilateral analgesia extending to the cervical dermatomes.

At this time, there are two indications for open surgical cordotomy. The first is the situation just described. The second is unavailability of the expertise or equipment needed to perform percutaneous cordotomy. If bilateral cervical analgesia is needed, a spinal narcotic technique would be more appropriate.

There is risk of urinary retention and sexual dysfunction after unilateral cordotomy, and that risk increases significantly with bilateral lesioning. Although the risks and benefits of cordotomy should clearly be discussed in detail, it is unlikely that the need for permanent catheterization or risk of sexual dysfunction would contraindicate the procedure in a terminally ill patient with severe pain that is unresponsive to conventional pain therapy.

RESULTS

During the last decade, much work has been devoted to defining the role of cordotomy in comprehensive cancer pain. The most important work has been published by Ischia's group. They have analyzed the results of unilateral percutaneous cervical cordotomies in patients with Pancoast's tumor or thoracic malignant pain.[28] Ninety-two percent of their patients obtained excellent results, as evidenced by analgesia to pinprick in the middle cervical dermatomes. Forty-four percent of patients with Pancoast's syndrome were pain-free until death as a result of the cordotomy alone. Only 22% of patients with thoracic pain were pain-free as a result of the cordotomy alone, owing to a 70% incidence of mirror pain in this group (mirror pain is discussed fully in the section on Pitfalls). Cordotomy plus aggressive medical pain therapy, however, afforded complete pain control in 75% of patients with Pancoast's syndrome and in 86% of those with thoracic pain. Nagaro[51] and Orlandini[52] compared percutaneous cordotomy with subarachnoid phenol in patients with chest pain secondary to cancer. Subarachnoid phenol gave excellent but short-term relief. Cordotomy resulted in excellent long-term relief at the expense of generalized weakness, mirror pain, and temporary hemiparesis.

Ischia and associates[27] studied the role of unilateral cordotomy in the treatment of patients with vertebral metastatic lesions. The pain was either unilateral or bilateral. Seventy-one percent of patients obtained substantial benefit from the combination of cordotomy and appropriately used analgesics. This group also compared the roles of cordotomy and subarachnoid neurolytic block in patients with pelvic cancer.[29] The issue is important because the sacral segments tend to be missed by cordotomy, either because they are farthest from the lesion or because of the higher incidence of deafferentation pain in patients with rectal lesions. Ischia and associates[29] were able to obtain excellent relief using cordotomy for predominantly unilateral pain, subarachnoid phenol for perineal pain, and pharmacologic therapy in all cases.

Ischia's group also reported the results of bilateral percutaneous cordotomies.[31] The electrode was positioned just anterior to the dentate ligament, so that the lesion was more likely to affect the lumbar segments and less likely to damage the reticulospinal tract. Bilateral lesions were created in one session. There were no respiratory deaths in the 36 patients treated, 60% of whom substantially benefited from the procedure. Sanders[53] recently reported on patients after unilateral and then staged bilateral cordotomies. Excellent relief was noted for the unilateral procedure. Bilateral lesioning gave only 50% total pain relief at the expense of a high incidence of urinary retention and mirror-image pain.

Other authors have reported series of cancer pain patients who have undergone cordotomy. Meglio and Cioni[54] performed 53 cordotomies; excellent surgical results were noted in 63% of patients 15 weeks postoperatively. Eleven of these patients had Pancoast's syndrome, and 31 had lower extremity pain secondary to pelvic or abdominal cancer. Lahuerta and associates[55] reported on 100 cordotomies, 95% of which were performed in cancer patients. Complete pain relief was obtained in 64% of patients, and partial relief in 23%. Only one of the five patients with nonmalignant pain obtained complete relief via cordotomy. Macaluso and colleagues[48] performed 20 cordotomies for lumbosacral, pelvic, and lower extremity pain of malignant origin. Their patients' opioid requirements were reduced by 80% at 4 weeks, and the opioid reduction generally lasted up to 12 weeks. Amano and coworkers[56] described the results of 281 cordotomies. Unilateral cordotomy gave good or excellent results in 82% of patients. The rate was 95% for bilateral lesions. Jackson[57] recently described results in patients with mesothelioma after the procedure: 83% were able to decrease opioid dosage by at least half.

White and Sweet[58] compared the results of large series of open and percutaneous cordotomies in a 1979 study and found that results with the two were comparable. Eighty-five percent of patients obtained good initial analgesia after either open or percutaneous procedures. Mortality and morbidity rates, however, were lower with the percutaneous technique (see section on Complications).

Summary

Percutaneous cordotomy is an excellent technique for cancer pain management. The best indication is unilateral pain below the shoulder in a patient with a life expectancy of less than 1 year. The major contraindication to a percutaneous cordotomy is preexisting respiratory dysfunction on the side opposite the one to be rendered analgesic. Because cancer is a systemic disease, it is unlikely that cordotomy alone will ensure complete pain relief. The rate of good to excellent results of cordotomy should approach 90% when the procedure is combined with aggressive pharmacologic and other appropriate procedural therapies.

CLINICALLY RELEVANT ANATOMY

During percutaneous cordotomy, a lesion is created in the spinothalamic tract. This tract is located in the anterolateral quadrant of the spinal cord. Results and side effects depend on the size and location of the lesion. Thorough knowledge of the applied anatomy is essential to guide electrode placement and radiofrequency lesioning. The clinically relevant anatomy at C1–C2 is described here, because virtually all procedures are performed at this level.

The lateral approach to C1–C2 is optimal. Because of anterior migration of the interarticular facets, there are no bony obstacles to the anterolateral quadrant. The C1–C2 level has the largest intervertebral opening. Also, vertebral artery injury is unlikely there, because the vertebral artery generally lies well anterior to the cord. The artery enters the dura mater at the atlantooccipital space, so a lateral approach would be riskier at C0–C1. Variations in the course of the vertebral artery have been documented by Katoh and associates.[59] The vertebral artery is anterior to the cord in 95% of cases at C1–C2. In 5% of cases, however, the artery passes over the middle to posterior third of the cord. Vertebral artery injury is possible.

The other vascular structure of interest is the anterior spinal artery (Fig. 67–1), which is generally located in the anterior commissure. Perese and Fracasso[60] report almost 50% incidence of bilateral anterior spinal arteries in the cervical region. A more laterally placed anterior spinal artery could be affected by the radiofrequency lesion, and thrombosis with cord infarction is theoretically a complication.

In addition to the vascular structures, the C2 nerve root must be considered. It exits the spinal canal at the C1–C2 level and continues as the greater occipital nerve. There is a high likelihood that the cordotomy needle could impinge on the C2 nerve root, and C2 paresthesias could occur during the performance of percutaneous cordotomy. Greater occipital nerve headaches can last up to a week postoperatively. The last reason to perform cordotomy at C1–C2 has already been mentioned. Because of variable crossover of spinothalamic fibers, only high lateral cordotomies reliably produce analgesia up to C5, so that pain from brachial plexopathies may be relieved.

Figure 67–2 shows a cross section of the spinal cord at the C1–C2 level. Correlation of histologic staining after open and percutaneous lesions with the resulting sensory and motor deficits has allowed functional identification of spinal cord tracts.

The spinothalamic tract contains ascending fibers that transmit pain and temperature sensation. These neurons ascend from the dorsal root ganglion and cross through the anterior commissure to the contralateral anterolateral quadrant. The crossover[61] may be delayed by several segments, so that only a high cervical lesion reliably gives pain relief below the C5 level. These neurons terminate at various levels in the brain. That spinothalamic fibers terminate in the nucleus ventralis posterolateralis of the thalamus was demonstrated by dissection in monkeys.[62] In

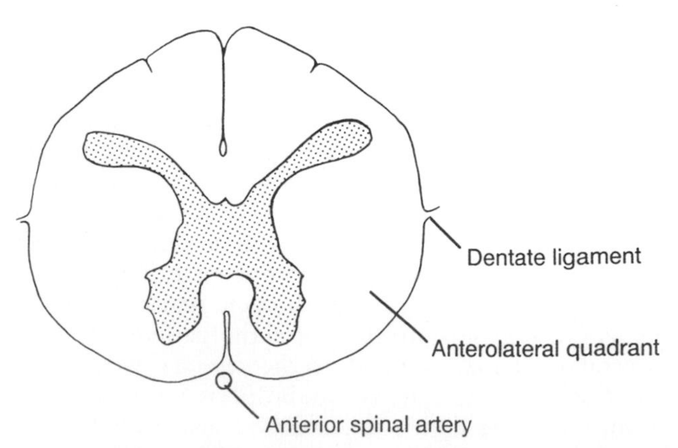

FIGURE 67–1 Axial section of the spinal cord at C1–C2 shows the anterior spinal artery, dentate ligament, and anterolateral quadrant.

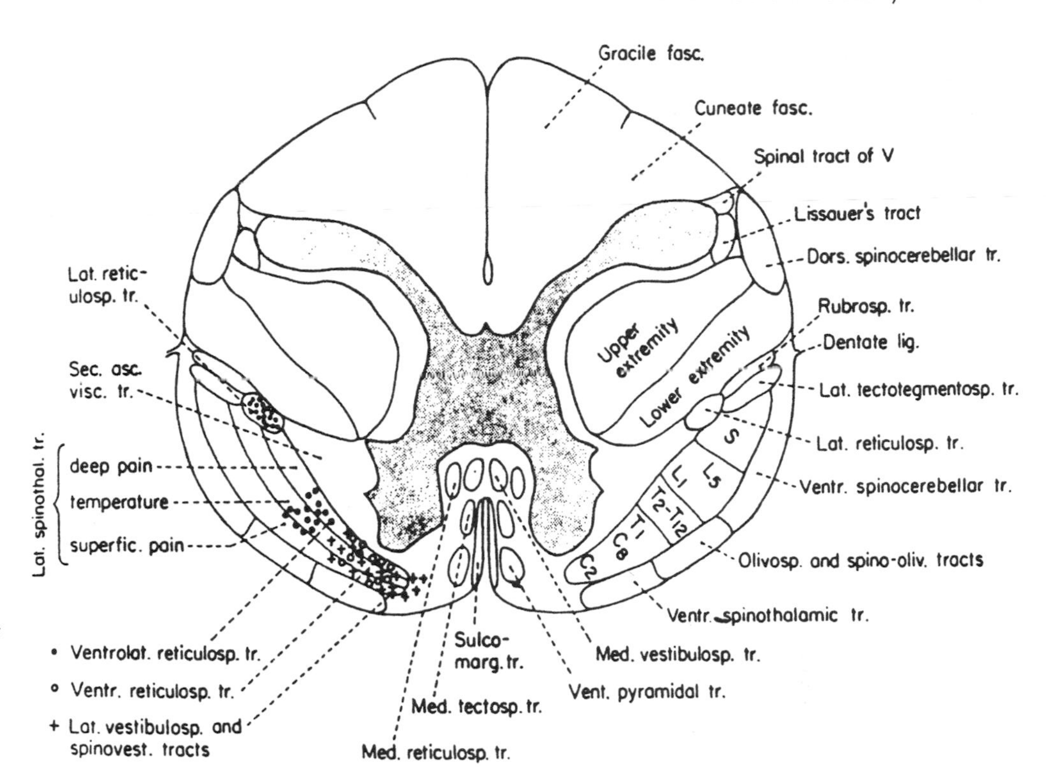

FIGURE 67–2 Axial section of the spinal cord at C1–C2. (From Taren JA, Davis R, Crosby EC: Target physiologic corroboration in stereotaxic cervical cordotomy. J Neurosurg 30:569, 1969.)

humans the same anatomic configuration was demonstrated by DiPiero and colleagues[63] using positron emission tomography (PET).[63] These researchers also found that patients with cancer pain had decreased blood flow to the contralateral thalamus that normalized after percutaneous cordotomy.

The spinothalamic tracts are organized in a somatotropic manner (see Fig. 67–2). Fibers transmitting impulses from cervical levels are more anterior, and those from the lumbar and sacral segment are more posterior. This arrangement has clinical implications, which are discussed later. Some authors stratify the spinothalamic fibers: the more superficial fibers over transmit superficial pain and deeper fibers transmit temperature and deep pain.[18] The spinothalamic tract relays pain and temperature from the periphery to the contralateral thalamus. Contralateral stimulation to deep pinprick is not felt after cordotomy in the great majority of cases.[64] Similarly, deep somatic sensations such as pressure are reduced by anterolateral cordotomy and are best correlated with cancer pain relief. Visceral pain is relieved by anterolateral cordotomy.[65] Nathan[66] studied tactile sensitivity in postcordotomy patients and reported the following results: senses of position, movement, and vibration were normal after cordotomy; graphesthesia was unaltered; light touch was unaffected; itching sensations were removed by cordotomy, but tickle sensation was unaffected. White and Sweet[65] wrote that patients who have undergone cordotomy "will be able to detect a mosquito when he alights, although they will not be able to feel him bite nor be annoyed by the subsequent itch." Temperature discrimination is generally lost after cordotomy, so patients must learn to pick up hot or cold objects with the hand in which temperature discrimination is intact. Friehs[67] reports that pain and temperature may be conducted by adjacent but separate pathways. He has noted different dermatomal levels for pain as opposed to temperature sensations after cordotomy. Usually pain and temperature discrimination are both lost. To summarize, White and Sweet[65] write, "The patient walking barefoot in the dark can tell whether he is walking on a stone or wooden floor, on a carpet or on linoleum. He must only beware that he does not step on a tack and in particular that he does not burn himself."

Figure 67–3 shows the respiratory pathways as outlined by Hitchcock and Leece.[68] Nathan[31] first worked out the location of the descending respiratory tracts. He realized that lesions of the anterolateral quadrant interfered with automatic respiration but lesions of the corticospinal tract had no effect. Fibers of the automatic respiratory tract have been found to be intermingled with reticulospinal fibers.[33] There is also somatotropic division of fibers: those controlling automatic diaphragmatic function are more anterior and those controlling intercostal and abdominal musculature are more posterior. The voluntary respiratory fibers are in the corticospinal tract. The concept of at least two

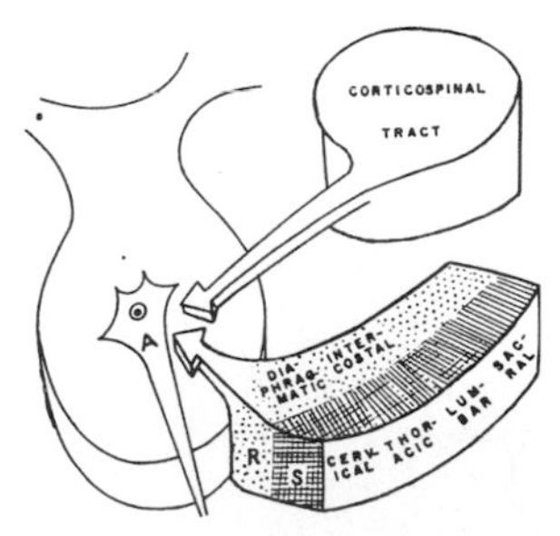

FIGURE 67–3 Somatotropic division of spinothalamic (S) and reticulospinal (R) tracts. A = axon. (From Hitchcock E, Leece B: Somatic representation of the respiratory pathways in the cervical cord of man. J Neurosurg 27:320, 1967.)

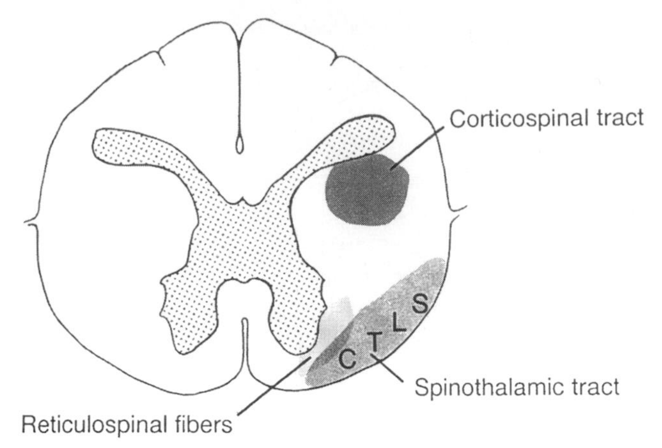

FIGURE 67–4 Interrelationship of spinothalamic and reticulospinal fibers.

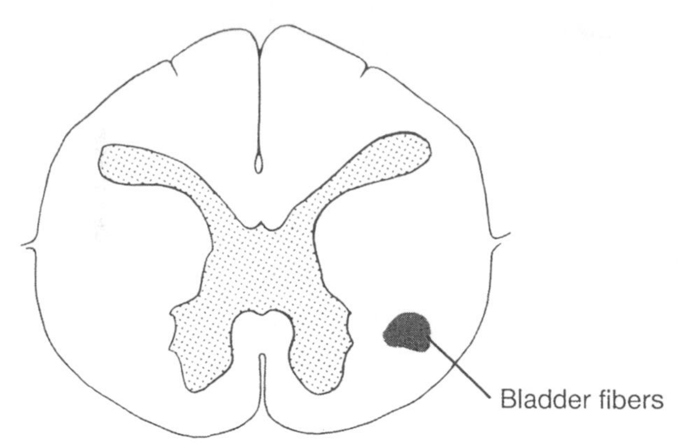

FIGURE 67–6 Location of fibers involved in micturition.

distinctive respiratory tracts, one automatic and one voluntary, explains why patients have died in their sleep after high bilateral cervical cordotomy.

The corticospinal tract lies posterior to the dentate ligament. Therefore, it is posterior to the spinothalamic and spinoreticular fibers. This tract contains fibers involving motor control. It descends uncrossed, unlike spinothalamic fibers. A lesion in the corticospinal tract produces ipsilateral weakness; a lesion in the spinothalamic tract results in contralateral loss of pain and temperature discrimination.

The concept of somatotropy in the reticulospinal and spinothalamic tracts explains why high cervical lesions are more likely to result in respiratory dysfunction. The spinoreticular fibers serving automatic diaphragmatic respirations are adjacent to, and in many cases intertwined with, the spinothalamic fibers that transmit pain and temperature sensation from the cervical segments (Fig. 67–4). Therefore, lesions involving cervical pain transmission are likely also to result in ipsilateral automatic respiratory dysfunction. This condition is of minimal importance when contralateral lung function is acceptable. Clearly, bilateral lesions are more dangerous. This concept also explains why a lesion centered in the lumbar or sacral pain fibers would be more likely to result in ipsilateral paresis secondary to cord edema affecting the nearby corticospinal tract.

The location of sympathetic preganglionic fibers has been described by Nathan and Smith.[34] These fibers lie close to the posterior portion of the anterior horn (Fig. 67–5). Transient Horner's syndrome develops after many percutaneous cordotomies. Unilateral cordotomies, however, do not upset vasomotor function, because crossing and mixing of sympathetic fibers probably starts no higher than T1.

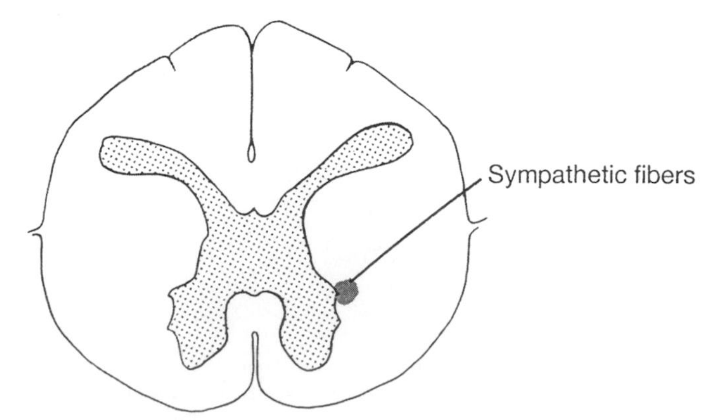

FIGURE 67–5 Location of sympathetic fibers.

Nathan and Smith[36] have also worked out the location of pathways implicated in voiding and defection. These fibers are situated lateral to the lateral horn of the gray matter (Fig. 67–6). Bilateral damage to these fibers leads to impairment of these functions. Transient impairment of bladder function can occur after percutaneous cordotomy. Such impairment is more likely in patients with preexisting disease or with bilateral lesions.

The dentate ligament is the external landmark that separates the anterior from the posterior tract (Fig. 67–7). This is an important landmark for surgical and percutaneous cordotomies, and much effort has been devoted to visualizing it during the procedure.[14,69,70] The spinothalamic tract is anterior to the dentate ligament, whereas the corticospinal tract lies posterior. As Sweet[71] has pointed out, however, the position of the dentate ligament varies, so before a lesion can be safely made, physiologic corroboration is needed to confirm that the electrode is actually in the spinothalamic tract.

Summary

Percutaneous cordotomy is an elegant demonstration of the correlation between neuroanatomy and clinical outcome. A lesion is made in the spinothalamic tract. Pain and temperature discrimination are interrupted on the contralateral side. This tract is somatotropically organized. Fibers from the cervical region are interrelated with those in the reticulospinal tract that serve automatic diaphragm functions. Those that transmit lumbar information are adjacent to the corticospinal tract. Fibers that transmit sympathetic and bladder function are also in the anterolateral quadrant of the cord. Pain relief and side effects correlate with the size and location of the lesion.

CLINICAL PEARLS AND TRICKS OF THE TRADE

The percutaneous cordotomy is described next. With rare exceptions, percutaneous cordotomy should be performed

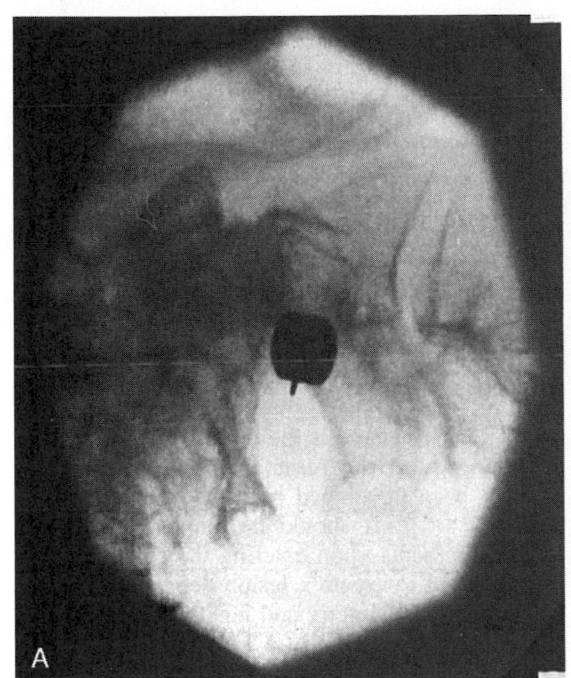

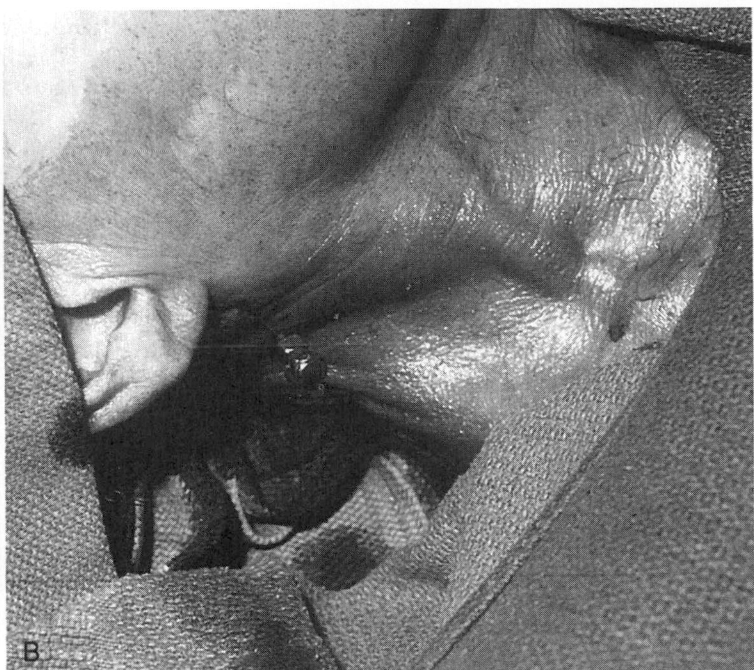

FIGURE 67–7 A, *Fluoroscopic view of initial needle placement into subarachnoid space.* B, *Photograph of needle shown in* A. *(Also in color; see Color Plates.)*

with the patient minimally sedated. The physician should conduct a thorough physical examination beforehand so that changes during and after the cordotomy may be appreciated. Mullan[72] has emphasized that considerable time should be invested in the preoperative visit. As in all radiofrequency procedures, patient cooperation is essential. Overdependence on anesthetic drugs is no substitute for adequate patient preparation.

Preoperative Preparation

Certain points must be emphasized during the preoperative interview. Patients should understand that the procedure can take as long as 1 hour and that they will have to remain supine during the procedure. As the spinal needle is inserted, the C2 nerve root can be irritated, resulting in occipital and scalp pain until the local anesthetic takes effect. Needle puncture of the dura can be uncomfortable and difficult to anesthetize. Electrical stimulation and radiofrequency lesioning are generally tolerated well. Postoperatively, patients may develop a spinal headache. Greater occipital nerve headaches can last as long as a week. Patients may need intermittent bladder catheterization, especially during the first several days. Ipsilateral paresis may develop, and the patient may need a walker, possibly for several weeks. Mirror pain develops in 10% of patients and is more common when the cordotomy is performed to relieve thoracic pain.

Over the longer term, patients will lose temperature discrimination as they gain pain relief. They must be cautioned to pick up hot or cold objects first with the hand whose temperature discrimination is intact. Sexual stimulation and function may be decreased by the cordotomy. Patients must understand that, depending on the course of the disease, contralateral pain may develop and that lifelong pain relief is unlikely.

If narcotic dosage can be reduced and mental faculties improve, patients may begin to focus on issues of death and dying. Postoperative depression can occur, so appropriate support for the patient and family should be provided for before the pain-relieving procedure. The patient must have confidence that, no matter what the postoperative course, the pain management team will continue to optimize symptom control as long as necessary.

OPERATIVE TECHNIQUE

Percutaneous cordotomy should be performed with intravenous sedation. The patient should be maximally sedated during insertion of the spinal needle from skin to the dura and during the lesioning. The patient must be alert during electrophysiologic testing. There are many variations of the operative technique, but they all follow the same general theme.[45, 73, 74] Different techniques have been developed to visualize the cord and the dentate ligament.[14, 69, 70] It should be emphasized that the impedance measurements on entering the cord and the amperage needed to create a lesion depend on several factors,[75] including the diameter and length of the active tip and the tissue conductivity. I use a Levin cordotomy electrode[25] with a Radionics lesion generator. Other excellent electrode[22, 76] and radiofrequency generators are available (Owl Instruments, Willowdale, Ontario, Canada, and Stryker-Leibinger, Dallas, Tex.).

As in many precision percutaneous techniques, proper patient positioning is essential. The patient is supine with the neck slightly flexed to enlarge the C1–C2 opening.

The fluoroscope C arm is positioned so that a true lateral view is obtained; this is essential to minimize errors from parallax and to best identify the proper radiologic targets. After the best image is visualized, the head is fixed in position. The technique is to reposition the needle continuously until the fixed target is identified.

After the patient is prepared, local anesthetic is infiltrated. It should not be injected too deep, lest the epidural or subarachnoid space inadvertently be anesthetized. A 20-gauge spinal needle is now inserted toward the apex of the C1–C2 space. Paresthesia is generally noted as the needle contracts the C2 nerve root. One milliliter of 2% lidocaine is sufficient to anesthetize the nerve root. Because this is a large nerve, it takes several minutes for the anesthetic to become effective. The spinal needle is advanced to the epidural space and then through the dura and into the cerebrospinal fluid (Fig. 67–7). Cerebrospinal fluid flow can be slow, and the surgeon should not insert the needle too aggressively. This spinal needle should be inserted anterior to the dentate ligament, so that the anterior border of the cord and the dentate ligament will be outlined by falling contrast emulsion (see later). The depth at which the dura is punctured should be noted. If any doubt exists as to correct needle position, it may be checked with an anteroposterior projection, which should show the needle medial to the midfacet line and lateral to the odontoid.

At this point, contrast emulsion is prepared. It is used to outline the important landmarks—the anterior surface of the spinal cord, the dentate ligament, and the posterior dura. The spinothalamic tract is located between the anterior border of the dura and the dentate ligament. The best emulsion is a combination of oil-based contrast agent, such as iophendylate (Pantopaque), and air. However, Pantopaque is no longer available. Alternative techniques[69,70] may not outline the dentate ligament as effectively. An excellent emulsion consists of 3 mL of Ethiodol (ethiodized oil) mixed with 7 mL of preservative-free saline and 10 mL of air. Ethiodol is iodine based, so allergic reactions can occur. The emulsion is mixed vigorously for 3 min. Excess air is evacuated. One milliliter of the emulsion is injected through a syringe with an eccentric nipple located in the dependent position.

The contrast emulsion should outline the anterior border of the cord, the dentate ligament, and the posterior dura (Fig. 67–8). If it does not, the emulsion may have been incompletely mixed, or the needle could have been posterior to the dentate ligament. Multiple lines of contrast emulsion indicate that a true lateral view was not obtained. A dual-screen C-arm fluoroscope with memory capability is recommended because the contrast emulsion can quickly pulsate away. The image should be saved for use as a reference.

The first needle is now removed, and a second is inserted at right angles to the correct area of the cord between the anterior border and the dentate ligament. This step should be performed accurately and efficiently before the contrast pulsates away. The depth of the subarachnoid space was noted during the placement of the first needle. After the needle enters the spinal fluid, the thermocoupled probe is inserted (Fig. 67–9).

Impedance measurements depend on which electrode system is being used. When the Levin cordotomy electrode is in the cerebrospinal fluid, the impedance nears 200 Ω. It rises above 1000 Ω as the probe enters the cord. At 1000 to 1500 Ω, the probe is deep enough to begin electrical stimulation.

Stimulation is first performed at 50 Hz. Spinothalamic tract stimulation generally produces contralateral thermic sensations, which patients have described variously as heat, cold, and blowing wind. These sensations occur at less than 0.4 V. If thermic stimulation occurs in the upper extremity, the patient usually obtains analgesia over the entire half of the body below C5. Thermic stimulation in the lower extremity tends to produce analgesia only over the extremity. Occasionally, pain or paresthesia is produced over a particular area of the body. If this area overlaps the painful area, lesioning is likely to have a good result. Otherwise, the probe should be repositioned until either thermic stimulation to the upper extremity is obtained or the pain or paresthesias cover the appropriate area.

Electrical stimulation is then performed at 2 Hz. If the electrode is in the spinothalamic tract, no motor stimulation occurs with less than 1 V. If ipsilateral stimulation is noted below the neck at both 2 Hz and 50 Hz, the electrode is probably in the corticospinal tract and should be repositioned anterior to the dentate ligament. Patients occasionally note ipsilateral sensations from the neck in addition to contralateral sensory stimulation. Such sensations imply that the probe is near the anterior horn cells. Similarly, stimulation of ipsilateral cervical musculature at 2 Hz and below 1 V also indicates that the probe is near the anterior horn. This does not contraindicate lesioning if contralateral sensory stimulation is obtained below 0.4 volt. If, however, stimulation is produced only in the neck, caution should be exercised, because the electrode may be too near the anterior horn cells and a lesion made here might be ineffective. High stimulation thresholds may be noted from scarring secondary to previous cervical radiation or a previous cordotomy. Stimulation parameters are summarized in Table 67–1. Electrophysiologic monitoring[77] by somatosensory evoked potentials has not been shown to improve outcome or decrease complications.

A lesion is created only after proper stimulation is obtained. Like any other radiofrequency techniques, the procedure should be abandoned if proper stimulation cannot be achieved. (This happened in 1 of my 54 cases.) Lesioning causes a mild headache that disappears after several seconds. Lesioning may be performed by either of two techniques. One utilizes a constant current, and lesioning time is increased incrementally until either analgesia to pinprick is demonstrated or side effects occur. I use a thermocoupled electrode. Lesions are made at not more than 98° C for 15-sec intervals. After each lesion, analgesia to pinprick and loss of thermal discrimination are tested for on the contralateral side. Lesion times can be increased up to 30 sec. If boiling or cavitation occurs, the voltage jumps, and the lesioning should be terminated immediately. Otherwise, an uncontrolled lesion will have been created.

Before the needle is withdrawn, it is prudent to deposit steroids directly onto the C2 nerve root sleeve. The needle is withdrawn just lateral to the midfacet line, and 0.5 mL of contrast dye is injected to outline the C2 root sleeve. Then, 20 mg of either triamcinolone or methylprednisolone acetate can be deposited to decrease the frequency and severity of any resulting C2 headache.

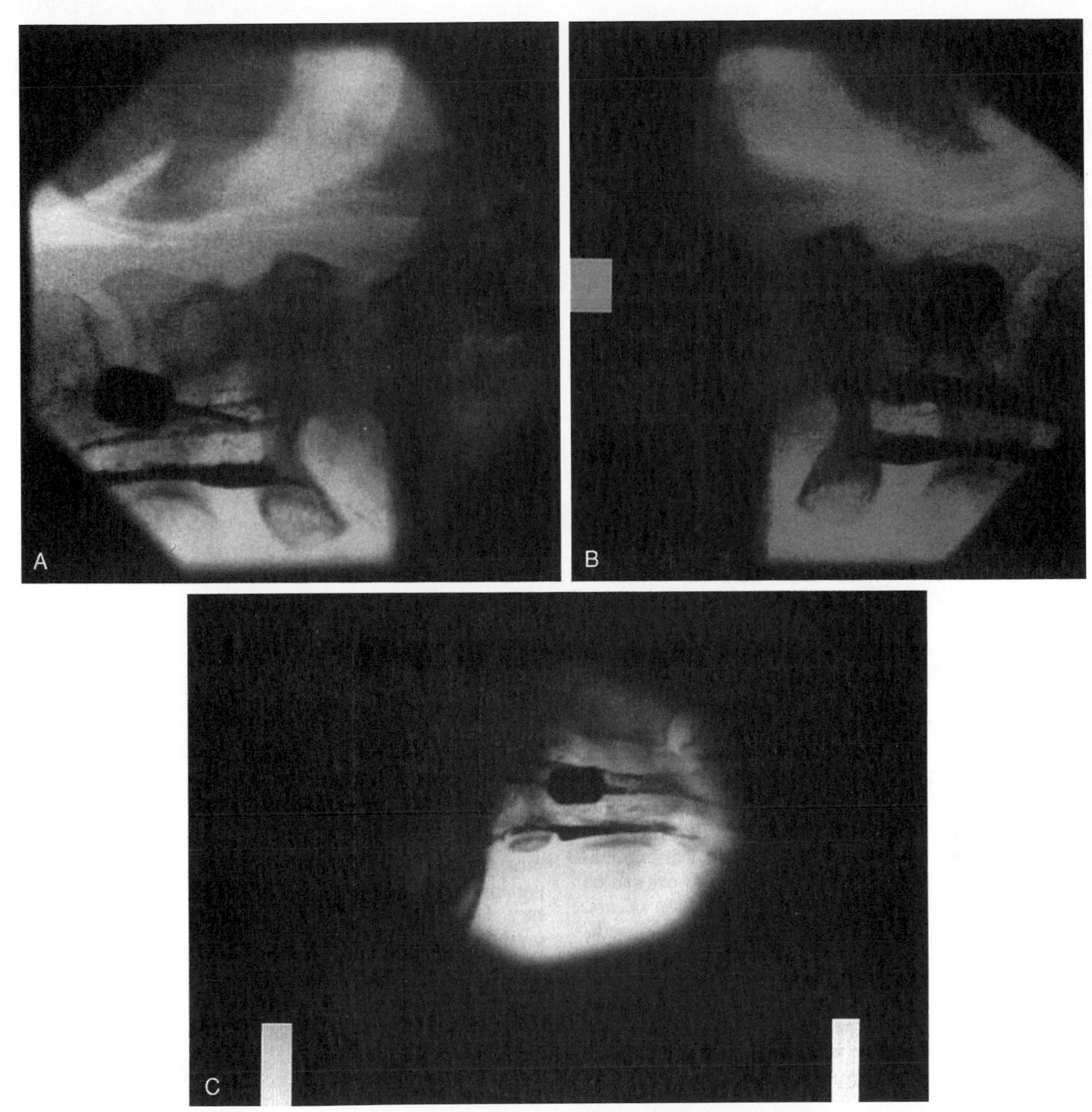

FIGURE 67–8 Three views of contrast emulsions, all outlining the anterior border of the cord, dentate ligament, and posterior border of the cord.

Kanpolat describes CT-guided cordotomy.[16] The advantage may be ease in tailoring the lesions to the painful area. There is good correlation between CT and actual cord measurements.[78] Another advantage is fewer attempts at needle positioning in difficult cases, as the anterolateral quadrant of the spinal cord can be visualized in all cases. The longer duration of the procedure is a drawback.

POSTOPERATIVE COURSE

The postoperative course after percutaneous cordotomy is generally benign. Initially patients are given high doses of steroids, which are tapered over the next week. This regimen decreases cord edema and the risk of complications. If a spinal headache occurs, bed rest is encouraged for at least 1 day. Mild analgesics are all that is necessary for discomfort at the needle insertion site. The patient should be monitored for urine output. Occasionally, bladder catheterization is necessary; this is more likely for patients with a history of prostatism or bladder dysfunction. Approximately 10% of patients develop ipsilateral paresis, which is temporary. Occasionally, patients are discharged with a walker until their motor strength returns to baseline.

Patients should be weaned from narcotics. If their pain was unilateral, they should be given 25% of preoperative doses to prevent withdrawal symptoms. When the dose is reduced, contralateral pain may be unmasked. It must be

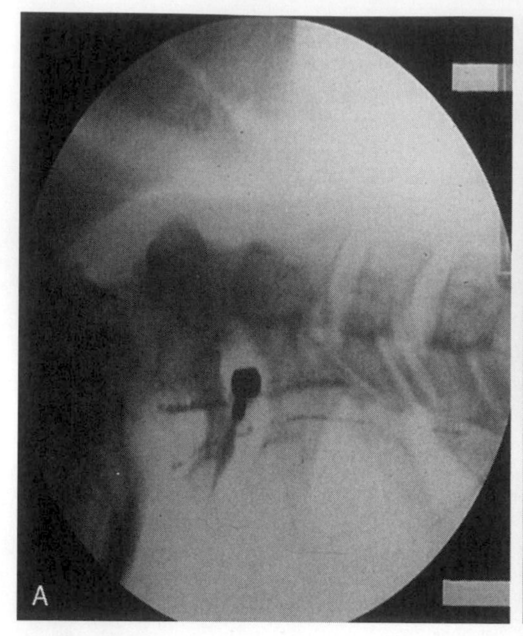

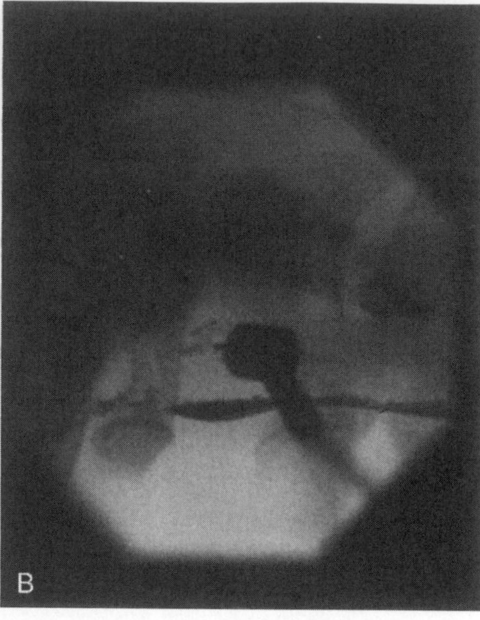

FIGURE 67–9 Two views of the thermocoupled electrode inserted into the anterolateral quadrant. Note that the contrast emulsion has dissipated.

differentiated from mirror pain, which is discussed later. If contralateral pain is discovered, radiation therapy, chemotherapy, or surgery may be appropriate in addition to medical or procedural pain treatments.

A patient whose preoperative respiratory status was suspect should be monitored for 3 days for signs of respiratory decompensation. By day 3, cord edema is decreasing, along with the risk of complications. If respiratory status is problematic, I recommend intensive care monitoring with frequent checks of respiration and serial blood gas measurements to check for evidence of carbon dioxide retention. The patients' and families' wishes concerning intubation and ventilatory support should have been discussed before the cordotomy. One of my patients died from respiratory failure after bilateral staged cordotomy while being monitored in an intensive care setting.

Summary

Visualization of the bony landmarks is critical to accurate cordotomy, and time spent positioning the patient and C-arm fluoroscopic device before the procedure is time well spent. Visualization of the dentate ligament and anterior surface of the cord helps to guide the needle toward the spinothalamic tract. Impedance values and thresholds for electrical simulation depend on the electrode being used. If the patient is adequately prepared and the technique is executed meticulously, gratifying results will be achieved.

PITFALLS

Recurrence of pain is a common problem after cordotomy. The several mechanisms for recurrence are discussed here. Treatment options depend on the mechanism of the recurrent pain.

Inadequate Lesioning

Short-term pain relief before recurrence is probably secondary to an inadequate lesion. A misplaced lesion can cause cord edema that temporarily interferes with pain transmission through the spinothalamic tract. As cord edema resolves, normal transmission returns and pain recurs. Tasker[45] repeated 2.6% of cordotomy lesions within a few weeks because of fading or falling levels of analgesia; most of the second procedures gave satisfactory results. Lahuerta[36] showed that approximately 20% of the hemicord must be destroyed to produce the most satisfactory pain relief (Fig. 67–10). Naguro[79] showed oval-shaped lesions in the anterolateral cord correlating with pain relief. Ischia and colleagues[28] emphasized that results definitely

TABLE 67–1 **Stimulation Parameters at C1–C2**

Location of Electrode	Results of Stimulation	
	At 50 Hz	*At 2 Hz*
Spinothalamic tract	Contralateral thermic stimulation at <0.4 V	No motor stimulation at <1 V
Corticospinal tract	Ipsilateral paresthesias and tetanization below neck	Ipsilateral motor stimulation below neck at <1 V
Anterior horn	Ipsilateral paresthesias and tetanization in neck	Ipsilateral motor stimulation in neck

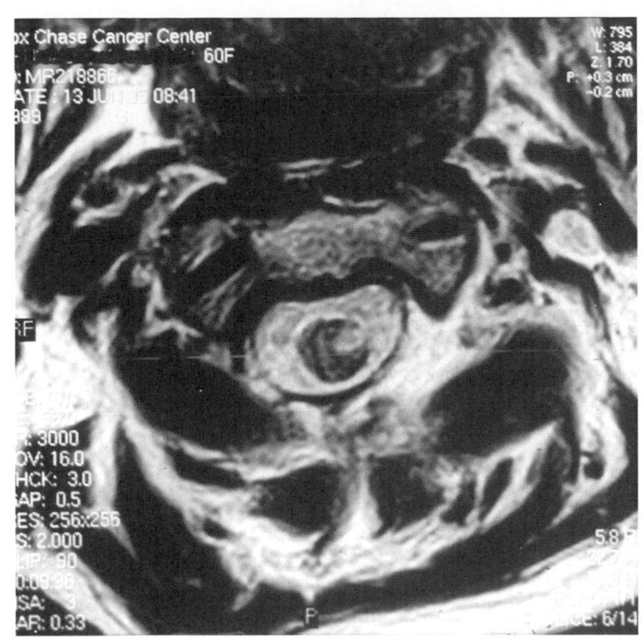

FIGURE 67–10 Postoperative MRI shows lesion in the anterolateral cord.

vary according to the ability of the surgeon, and Gybels and Sweet[74] warn, "This is not an easy procedure." It should be performed by someone skilled in the use of fluoroscopy and radiofrequency lesioning. A major source of difficulty is working from views of C1–C2 that are not true lateral views. I optimize the view of the "cathedral window" at C1–C2 before fixing both the fluoroscope and the patient's head in position. Only then is the patient prepared and draped. If a true lateral view is not obtained, multiple contrast lines can appear, so that identification of the anterolateral quadrant becomes problematic. In these cases the size of the C1–C2 opening is not optimal. Even if only the nearest dentate ligament is outlined, parallax errors confound identification of the true size and location of the anterolateral quadrant. To obviate frustration that occurs when contrast dye rapidly pulsates away from the operative site, a dual-screen fluoroscope with memory is essential. Again, it cannot be overemphasized that this procedure should be performed only by an operator skilled in precision percutaneous techniques.

New and Unmasked Pain

Unfortunately, pain can recur even after a successful lesion.[80] A common cause is unmasking of contralateral pain as narcotic doses are tapered postoperatively. Macaluso and associates[28] reported unmasked contralateral pain in 18 of 20 patients treated by cordotomy for pain from lumbosacral or pelvic cancer. This complication occurred in 5 of my 54 patients during the first postoperative week; 25 other patients developed contralateral pain before death. The great majority of cancer patients obtain satisfactory pain control with oral medications. Only a minority of such patients need invasive procedures to relieve new or unmasked pain.

I cannot overemphasize that pain-relieving procedures are but part of an overall cancer pain treatment program. Cancer is a dynamic, progressive disease, and it is likely that bilateral pain will eventually develop whether opposite or above the areas rendered analgesic by the cordotomy. Any new pain should be treated according to standard cancer pain protocols. If possible, therapy should be directed toward the underlying disease. If this is not possible, palliative radiation or surgery should be considered, complemented by adequate analgesics and pain-relieving procedures.

Complete lifelong pain relief after cordotomy is the exception rather than the rule. Tasker[45] reported that only 33.7% of his patients were totally pain-free at the latest follow-up. Forty percent developed pain opposite the side of original pain, owing either to undiagnosed or new disease or to the development of mirror pain (discussed later). Of their patients with pelvic malignant disease, Ischia and colleagues[29] reported that 36% obtained complete pain relief from cordotomy alone. Another 40% obtained relief when narcotic and nonnarcotic analgesics were added to therapy. Similar results were observed in patients with cervicothoracic pain.[28] Seventy-five percent of patients with Pancoast's tumor obtained complete pain control through cordotomy and analgesics, and 86% of those with thoracic pain obtained excellent relief. Fewer than one third of these patients, however, obtained complete relief with the procedural intervention alone. Similar results have been noted after celiac plexus ablation.[81] Only 10% to 24% of patients obtain lifelong pain relief from this block. Pain recurs as the block wears off or as tumor extends outward from the celiac plexus.

Postcordotomy Dysesthesias

When postcordotomy dysesthesia occurs it is difficult to treat. They probably constitute previously undiagnosed deafferentation pain or new deafferentation pain that developed after the cordotomy. Deafferentation pain occurs in the absence of normal afferent sensory input. In a cancer patient, the cause of the pain would no longer be pressure on neural tissue from the tumor itself but, rather, the damaged neural tissue. Tasker[45] believed that almost 40% of his patients developed deafferentation pain below a level of adequate analgesia. It occurred immediately postoperatively in 6.7% of patients, indicating that the syndrome had been present preoperatively. Another 33.7% of Tasker's patients developed dysesthesia pain postoperatively that differed in character from the pain that had been present previously. It is not clear why this situation was so frequent. Nathan and Smith[82] noted only three cases of postcordotomy dysesthesia after 74 unilateral procedures and no cases after 40 bilateral procedures. Nagaro[47] described postcordotomy dysesthesias in 15.2% of 66 patients. He believed that 2 out of 10 patients had recurrence of pain secondary to recovery of pain sensitivity; 8 out of 10 had deafferentated pain; and 6 had deafferentating peripheral nerve damage caused by tumor invasion after a successful cordotomy. Two patents had diffuse dysesthesia, presumably secondary to destruction of additional second-order neurons by the cordotomy. Regardless of the exact frequency, it is clear that cordotomies should be avoided in patients with dysesthetic sensations in areas of preexisting sensory loss.

References of Sensation

Another form of pain recurrence is known as *mirror pain* or *reference of sensation.* The pain occurs in a distribution that mirrors that present before the cordotomy. *Mirror pain* is actually a misnomer, because the pain occurs both horizontally and cranially from the preoperative location. The phenomenon has also been referred to as *allachesthesia* (*allesthesia*).[65] Painful sensations are referred from the side of the body previously rendered analgesic to the contralateral side. Reference of sensation was first described in a postcordotomy patient by Ray and Wolff,[83] in 1945. Nathan[37] reported the phenomenon in 15 patients in 1956; 13 of the cases occurred after cordotomy. Another patient had a thrombosed anterior spinal artery, and one developed the syndrome after an upper limb amputation. Nathan noted reference of sensation after 17 of 61 surgical cordotomies.[84] Nagaro and colleagues[38] counted it in 7 of their 66 patients. Ischia and associates[28] noted mirror pain in 73% of patients who had thoracic pain secondary to lung cancer or metastatic disease. This high frequency in association with chest wall lesions has been noted by many operators. Mirror pain occurred after 4 of 7 cordotomies I performed for chest wall pain.

A typical case is as follows: A patient presents with right chest wall pain from lung cancer unresponsive to conventional analgesics. The right-sided pain is eliminated by the cordotomy. Three days later, however, as analgesics are tapered, the patient develops similar left-sided pain. The right side of the body below the shoulder is still analgesic to pinprick. A workup for a new cancerous lesion is negative. The new pain is bothersome but can be controlled partially with analgesics until the patient dies (which happened 2 months later).

Nathan[37] described reference of sensation in a patient who underwent cordotomy for right-sided chest pain. Forty hours postoperatively, reference of sensation developed, so that, "When a pin was applied to the analgesic right side, the patient immediately put up his hand and covered an analogous place on the left side of the chest. When asked why he did this, he replied that he did not know. . . . Eventually he said that he could hardly believe his senses but it seemed to him that he felt the pinprick applied to the right side of the chest as if it were the left."[37] Bowsher[85] noted that naloxone increases the severity of the referred pain, indicating that the newly opened fibers were opioidergic.

If reference of pain occurs, bilateral lesioning eliminates it. Pain tends to decrease as cordotomy-induced analgesia turns to hypalgesia. Nagaro and associates[86] have theorized that subsidiary pathways connect dorsal horns both longitudinally and laterally, which in turn connect to the intact spinothalamic tract. Usually, the subsidiary pathways are inhibited by a feedback loop involving the spinothalamic tracts. Reference of pain results as release of feedback inhibition allows transmission through the intact spinothalamic tract.

For example, consider a patient whose left leg pain is relieved by a right-sided cordotomy. Reference of sensation develops, and the pain is referred to the right leg. Noxious stimuli are transmitted from the left leg through the right spinothalamic tract but are blocked by the cordotomy at C1–C2. The loss of feedback inhibition allows the signal to cross through subsidiary pathways to the intact left spinothalamic tract. The brain perceives the signal as emanating from the right side of the body. Nagaro and associates[86] described referral of left groin and thigh pain to the right chest after a right C1–C2 cordotomy. The chest pain was eliminated by an epidural block below T10, proving that the new pain was in fact referred from the originally painful region. In another article, Nagaro and associates[87] reported having relieved referred pain with thoracic intrathecal phenol applied to the side of the original cancer pain.

Summary

Recurrence of pain can be due to technical errors in the performance of the procedure. Pain may recur, however, even after successful cordotomy, sometimes because of unmasking of pain during tapering of narcotics. It can be also due to spread of new tumor ipsilateral to the lesion or above the area rendered analgesic by cordotomy. Postcordotomy pain can be either a deafferentation phenomenon or secondary to reference of sensation. Treatment options depend on proper characterization of the recurrent pain.

COMPLICATIONS

Mortality after percutaneous cordotomy is due either to rapid unexpected progression of the underlying disease or to respiratory decompensation. Morbidity includes ipsilateral paresis and urinary retention. Horner's syndrome can occur but is usually temporary. Sexual sensitivity decreases after cordotomy. Postcordotomy dysesthesias are discussed in an earlier section. Other than progression of disease and postcordotomy dysesthesias, the mortality and morbidity after percutaneous cordotomy are due entirely to the size and location of the lesion created in the anterolateral quadrant.

Respiratory Complications

Respiratory complications were first noted in the 1930s,[4] soon after the introduction of high cervical cordotomy. It was thought that the smaller, more accurate lesions made by the percutaneous technique would decrease the incidence of respiratory embarrassment, but this turned out not to be the case.

As discussed previously, the reticulospinal tract controls involuntary function of the intercostal, abdominal, and diaphragmatic muscles and is just behind or intermingled with the spinothalamic tract. The location of the reticulospinal fibers was first diagrammed by Hitchcock and Leece.[68] Lahuerta and colleagues[33] studied histologic sections at C1–C2 taken from patients who died of respiratory complications after cordotomy. They showed that all cases involved the region of the anterolateral funiculus, which contains spinothalamic fibers from the second to the fifth thoracic dermatomes. They postulated that this region may be the afferent pathway that transmits signals from the periphery to the brain stem respiratory centers. Much effort has been devoted to differentiating the afferent spinoreticular tract from the efferent reticulospinal tract. From a practical point of view, it is clear that involuntary control of respiration is transmitted through the anterolateral quadrant, and Ischia and colleagues[28] remark that bilateral cervical lesions cannot be made without "running the risk of killing the patient." Tasker[50] has emphasized "tailoring" the lesion, and Ischia and colleagues[30] have performed one-stage bilateral cervical cordotomy, taking care to align the electrode with the dentate ligament or at most 1 mm anterior to it, to avoid lesioning the anterior part of the anterolateral quadrant.

Belmusto and associates[88] were the first to note an intraoperative reduction in tidal volume immediately after section of the cord. This occurred in every case when the lesion was deep enough to produce pain relief. Nathan[31] observed similar changes and noted that respiratory movements on the affected side were not eliminated. Rosomoff and coworkers[89] observed that unilateral cordotomy resulted in little change in vital capacity but a significant reduction in tidal volume and a compensatory increase in respiratory rate. Bilateral cordotomy resulted in a significant reduction in minute ventilation. In patients with high levels of analgesia, the increase in respiratory rate was insufficient to compensate for the reduction in tidal volume. In patients who developed respiratory embarrassment, the most consistent alteration was a reduction in carbon dioxide sensitivity.

Krieger and Rosomoff[90] found that respiratory dysfunction could begin as late as 6 days after cordotomy. Subjective signs of respiratory dysfunction appeared before clinical impairment could be demonstrated. Characteristically, patients manifested the subjective sensation of panic, and respirations were interrupted with frequent sighing. Signs were similar to those of an anxiety reaction. Afterward, patients demonstrated the classic syndrome: They would hypoventilate when awake but became apneic when asleep. When awakened, they would resume breathing, but hypoventilation persisted. The most common syndrome showed a decrease in carbon dioxide response and vital capacity. Occasionally, patients manifested no change in vital capacity and an attenuated carbon dioxide response.

Lema and Hitchcock[49] measured FEV_1 after both percutaneous and open cordotomies. Eleven of 15 patients demonstrated a drop in FEV_1 after percutaneous cordotomy, the average decrease being 20%. The average decrease after open cordotomy was 25%. It was more marked with deeper incisions. Although this observation was not quantified, the authors agree that respiratory decompensation is more likely in patients who have preexisting respiratory disease or bilateral cordotomies with high cervical levels of analgesia.

Ondine's curse was named by Severinghaus and Mitchell,[5] who observed it in three patients after cordotomy. Polatty and Cooper[91] described an unfortunate patient who survived with Ondine's curse for 14 months. Nocturnal mechanical ventilation through a tracheostomy was necessary, and eventually, phrenic nerve pacemakers were implanted. Rosomoff and coworkers[89] counseled against using pharmacologic depressants in patients with postcordotomy pulmonary dysfunction. The need to titrate narcotics downward after cordotomy was emphasized by Wells and colleagues,[92] who observed respiratory depression after cordotomy in patients who took long-acting morphine preparations. Sleep apnea may disappear as postcordotomy edema subsides and reticulospinal fibers return to normal.

Patients with bilateral cordotomies are most at risk for sleep apnea. Although Ischia and associates[30] have performed bilateral cordotomies in a single session, most authors recommend staging the procedures and delaying the second cordotomy at least 2 weeks, to allow cord edema to subside. If the remaining pain is centered in the trunk or lower extremities, high open thoracic cordotomy is an option. If the pain is in the upper chest or upper extremity, contralateral cordotomy is an option if good analgesia was not obtained with the first procedure. If high levels of analgesia were achieved, performing the second cordotomy carries considerable risk.

Patients at risk for respiratory failure should be monitored in the intensive care unit. Spirometry, arterial blood gases, and vital signs should be used to guide therapy. Shortness of breath, confusion, and anxiety may herald the onset of sleep apnea. Apnea alarms may be useful. Physician, patient, and family should have a thorough discussion of the respiratory risks before the procedure. The decision to provide or withhold aggressive ventilatory support should be made at that time. The sleep apnea syndrome is generally self-limiting, and patients can be weaned off the ventilator within 2 weeks.

The incidence of postoperative respiratory failure is impossible to estimate, owing to the varying skills and experience of the operators and the lack of standardized indications for the procedure. Rosomoff and associates[93] reported a 3% incidence of major respiratory complications in 1279 cordotomies, including one death from sleep apnea.[93] Tasker[45] observed a 0.5% incidence of respiratory death and an additional 0.5% incidence of temporary respiratory failure after 380 cordotomies. Among 103 patients with cervicothoracic cancer, the incidence of respiratory failure was 4.2%; this was clearly a high-risk group.[28] White and Sweet[58] compared open and percutaneous cordotomy. Mortality after percutaneous cordotomy was 1% in 3357 cases and was primarily due to respiratory failure. The incidence was 8% after the open procedure. The difference was attributed to the longer hospitalization needed after the open procedure and to the fact that some of the patients who underwent open cordotomy would have been chosen for the percutaneous procedure after the authors had gained experience with the technique.

Paresis

As previously discussed, paresis can occur ipsilateral to the lesion, secondary to the effect of cord edema on the corticospinal tracts. Motor function should return to the preoperative level as cord edema subsides. The risk of ipsilateral hemiparesis rises if stimulation is obtained only to the contralateral lower extremity, because those fibers are closest to the corticospinal tracts. With proper electrical stimulation and a lightly sedated patient, permanent paresis should occur rarely, if at all.

Ipsilateral limb weakness was reported in 69% of patients by Lahuerta and colleagues.[55] The condition was present in only 4% of patients after 1 month. White and Sweet[58] noted transient weakness in 6.5% of patients. Tasker[45] reported transient paresis after 8% of unilateral cordotomies and 16% of bilateral procedures. Paresis persisted in 0.8% of the unilateral cordotomy group and in 1.6% of the bilateral group. Rosomoff and coworkers[93] noted a 5% incidence of temporary ipsilateral paresis; in 3% of patients the paresis proved to be permanent.

Urinary Complications

The fibers involved in micturition run near the spinothalamic fibers from the sacral segments of the body. Reported rates of permanent catheterization vary greatly, depending on surgical technique and patient selection criteria. The risk increases with bilateral lesions and in patients with preexisting bladder dysfunction, prostatism, or pelvic cancer. Tasker[45] noted deterioration of bladder function after 2.9% of unilateral procedures and after 18.8% of bilateral procedures. Catheterization was needed in 10% of patients in the series reported by Rosomoff and coworkers.[93] Two percent were left with permanent catheters, mainly for nursing convenience. Ischia and associates[28] noted permanent urinary retention in 9 of 103 patients treated with cordotomy for cervicothoracic pain, and a 7.2% catheterization rate in patients treated for neoplastic vertebral pain.[27] Urinary retention after cordotomy developed in 11.1% of the patients who underwent cordotomy for malignant pelvic disease.[29] Clearly, this group was at high risk. Palma and associates[94] reported transient bladder dysfunction in 10 of 163 patients after cordotomy.

Horner's Syndrome

Horner's syndrome may also develop after cordotomy. Referring to open procedures, Gybels and Sweet[74] state that Horner's syndrome is "almost the rule following high cervical cordotomy." After percutaneous procedures, transient self-limited Horner's syndrome can occur. Clearly, the incidence of Horner's syndrome depends on the site and location of the radiofrequency lesion. I have noted Horner's syndrome in approximately half of 29 cases, which generally disappeared within a day or so. When the sympathetic fibers are lesioned, transient hypotension can occur. This seems to be more of a problem after open cordotomies, and the risk increases with bilateral lesioning.

Sexual Dysfunction

Loss of sexual sensitivity occurs on the side rendered analgesic by cordotomy.[65] Bilateral lesions eliminate orgasm in women. Loss of erection and ejaculation can occur in males in the presence of preexisting urinary tract dysfunction or pelvic malignancy. Otherwise, libido and potency are not affected. Lahuerta and associates[64] observe that "unlike alcohol, cordotomy takes away (some of) the pleasure but not the performance."

Summary

The major risk of percutaneous cordotomy is respiratory decompensation. A sleep apnea syndrome may develop. The risk is difficult to estimate but increases with preexisting pulmonary disease and bilateral lesions producing high levels of cervical analgesia. Less serious complications include ipsilateral paresis and urinary retention. Transient Horner's syndrome may also occur. The lesser complications are generally transient. Sexual sensitivity may decrease. The risk of urinary retention increases in patients with preexisting urinary tract disease, pelvic disease, or bilateral cordotomy.

FUTURE DIRECTIONS

The use of cordotomy has declined. It is hoped that publications such as this one will stimulate interest in precision percutaneous techniques and reverse this trend. Although aggressive narcotic-based cancer pain management is an immense improvement over what was available 10 to 15 years ago, many patients are living out their lives with mediocre pain relief and significant medication side effects. This large group of unfortunate patients could benefit immensely from techniques such as percutaneous cordotomy. It bears repeating that cordotomy is complementary to other pain control techniques. Cordotomy is most valuable for patients with neuropathic or incident pain. Literature on the treatment of neuropathic pain is accumulating. New publications describe subcutaneous lidocaine,[95] systemic local anesthetics,[96] intravenous narcotics,[39] and local anesthetic epidural[41] and subarachnoid[42] infusions. Epidural and intrathecal clonidine[43, 97] may be useful for opioid-resistant neuropathic pain; ziconotide[43] may also be specific to neuropathic pain. Many patients with neuropathic pain would be excellent cordotomy candidates, were the procedure available to them.

There are too few outcome studies of interventional pain management. Ischia and colleagues have published excellent studies describing the risks, benefits, and outcomes of percutaneous cordotomy in selected cancer patients, but much work still needs to be done. Most of the studies of percutaneous cordotomy were published before use of spinal narcotics was widespread, and no studies have yet prospectively compared spinal narcotic and local anesthetic infusions with percutaneous cordotomy for cancer patients with neuropathic or incident pain. Similarly, with the exception of Tasker's[26] article on cordotomy for pain of spinal cord origin, there is no good information on how cordotomy fits into the management of pain not related to cancer.[26]

CONCLUSION

Percutaneous cordotomy is useful principally for cancer patients with unilateral pain below the shoulder and life expectancy of less than 1 year. No other procedure available to the interventional pain management specialist offers such dramatic, immediate, and long-term benefits. The goal will be to integrate percutaneous cordotomy into comprehensive pain care so that the maximum number of patients may benefit from this extraordinary technique.

REFERENCES

1. Spiller WG, Martin E: The treatment of persistent pain of organic origin in the lower part of the body by division of the anterolateral column of the spinal cord. JAMA 58:1489, 1912.
2. Foerster O: Uber die Vorderseiten Strangdurchschneidung. Arch Psychiatr Nerv Krankh 81:707, 1927.
3. Stookey B: Chordotomy of the second cervical segment for relief from pain due to recurrent carcinoma of the breast. Arch Neurol 26:443, 1931.
4. Peet M, Kahn EA, Allen SS: Bilateral cervical chordotomy for relief of pain in chronic infectious arthritis. JAMA 100:488, 1933.
5. Severinghaus JW, Mitchell RA: Ondine's curse: Failure of respiratory center automaticity while awake. Clin Res 10:122, 1992.
6. Millan S, Harper PV, Hekmatpanah J, et al: Percutaneous interruption of spinal pain tracts by means of a strontium needle. J Neurosurg 20:931, 1963.
7. Belmusto L, Owens G: Surgical control of pain in the elderly patient with cancer. Am J Surg 103:709, 1962.
8. Millan S, Hekmatpanah J, Dobben G, et al: Percutaneous, intramedullary cordotomy utilizing the unipolar anodal electrolytic lesion. J Neurosurg 22:548, 1965.
9. Rosomoff H, Carroll F, Brown F, et al: Percutaneous radiofrequency cervical cordotomy: Technique. J Neurosurg 23:639, 1965.
10. Lin PM, Gildenberg PL, Polakoff PP: An anterior approach to percutaneous lower cervical cordotomy. J Neurosurg 25:533, 1966.
11. Gildenberg PL, Lin PM, Polakoff PP, et al: Anterior percutaneous cervical cordotomy: Determination of target point and calculation of angle of insertion. J Neurosurg 28:173, 1968.
12. Crue EL, Todd EM, Carregal EJA: Posterior approach for high cervical percutaneous radiofrequency cordotomy. Contemp Neurol 30:41, 1968.
13. Hitchcock E: Stereotaxic spinal surgery: A preliminary report. J Neurosurg 31:386, 1969.
14. Onofrio EM: Cervical spinal cord and dentate delineation in percutaneous radiofrequency cordotomy at the level of the first to second cervical vertebrae. Surg Gynecol Obstet 133:30, 1971.
15. Kanpolat Y, Akyar S, Caglar S, et al: CT-guided percutaneous selective cordotomy. Acta Neurochir (Wien) 123:92, 1993.
16. Kanpolat Y, Caglar S, Akyar S, Temiz C: CT-guided procedures for intractable pain in malignancy. Acta Neurochir Suppl (Wien) 64:88–91, 1995.
17. Gildenberg PL, Zanes C, Flitter M, et al: Impedance-measuring device for detection of penetration of the spinal cord in anterior percutaneous cervical cordotomy (Technical note). J Neurosurg 30:87, 1969.
18. Taren JA, Davis R, Crosby EC: Target physiologic corroboration in stereotaxic cervical cordotomy. J Neurosurg 30:569, 1969.
19. Tasker RR, Organ LW: Percutaneous cordotomy: Physiological identification of target site. Contemp Neurol 35:110, 1973.
20. Tasker RR, Organ LW, Smith KC: Physiological guidelines for the localization of lesions by percutaneous cordotomy. Acta Neurochir Suppl (Wien) 21:111, 1974.
21. Campbell JA, Lipton S: Somatosensory evoked potentials recorded from within the anterolateral quadrant of the human spinal cord. Adv Pain Res Ther 5:23, 1983.
22. Myerson BA, von Holst H: Extramedullary impedance monitoring and stimulation of the spinal cord surface in percutaneous cordotomy. Acta Neurochir (Wien) 107:63, 1990.
23. Cosman ER, Nashold BS, Bedenbaugh P: Stereotactic radiofrequency lesion making. Appl Neurophysiol 46:160, 1983.
24. Kline MT: Stereotactic Radiofrequency Lesions as Part of the Management of Pain. Orlando, Fla, Paul M. Deutsch, 1992.
25. Levin AB, Cosman ER: Thermocouple-monitored cordotomy electrode (Technical note). J Neurosurg 53:266, 1980.
26. Tasker RR, DeCarvalho GTC, Dolan EJ: Intractable pain of spinal cord origin: Clinical features and implications for surgery. J Neurosurg 77:373, 1992.
27. Ischia S, Luzzani A, Ischia A, et al: Role of unilateral percutaneous cervical cordotomy in the treatment of neoplastic vertebral pain. Pain 19:123, 1984.
28. Ischia S, Ischia A, Luzzani A, et al: Results up to death in the treatment of persistent cervicothoracic (Pancoast) and thoracic malignant pain by unilateral percutaneous cervical cordotomy. Pain 21:339, 1985.
29. Ischia S, Luzzani A, Ischia A, et al: Subarachnoid neurolytic block (L5–S1) and unilateral percutaneous cervical cordotomy in the treatment of pain secondary to pelvic malignant disease. Pain 20:139, 1984.
30. Ischia S, Luzzani A, Ischia A, et al: Bilateral percutaneous cervical cordotomy: Immediate and long-term results in 36 patients with neoplastic disease. J Neurol Neurosurg Psychiatry 20:129, 1984.
31. Nathan PW: The descending respiratory pathway in man. J Neurol Neurosurg Psychiatry 26:487, 1963.
32. Nathan PW, Smith MC: Clinicoanatomical correlation in anterolateral cordotomy. Adv Pain Res Ther 3:71, 1979.
33. Lahuerta J, Buxton P, Lipton S, et al: The location and function of respiratory fibers in the second cervical spinal cord segment: Respiratory dysfunction syndrome after cervical cordotomy. J Neurol Neurosurg Psychiatry 55:1142, 1992.
34. Nathan PW, Smith MC: The location of descending fibres to sympathetic preganglionic vasomotor and sudomotor neurons in men. J Neurol Neurosurg Psychiatry 50:1253, 1987.
35. Nathan PW, Smith MC: The centrifugal pathway for micturition within the spinal cord. J Neurol Neurosurg Psychiatry 21:177, 1958.
36. Lahuerta J, Bowsher D, Lipton S, Buxton P: Percutaneous cervical cordotomy: A review of 181 operations on 146 patients with a study on the location of "pain fibers" in the C-2 spinal cord segment of 29 cases. J Neurosurg 80(6):975, 1994.
37. Nathan PW: Reference of sensation at the spinal level. J Neurol Neurosurg Psychiatry 19:88, 1956.
38. Nagaro T, Amakawa K, Kimura S, et al: Reference of pain following percutaneous cervical cordotomy. Pain 53:205, 1993.
39. Portenoy RK, Foley KM, Inturrisi CE: The nature of opioid responsiveness and its implications for neuropathic pain: New hypotheses derived from studies of opioid infusions. Pain 43:273, 1990.
40. Hogan Q, Haddox JD, Abram S, et al: Epidural opiates and local anesthetics for the management of cancer pain. Pain 46:271, 1991.
41. DuPen S, Kharasch ED, Williams A, et al: Chronic epidural bupivacaine-opioid infusion in intractable cancer pain. Pain 49: 293, 1992.
42. Van Dangen RIM, Crul BJP, DeBock M: Long-term intrathecal infusion of morphine and morphine/bupivacaine mixtures in the treatment of cancer pain: A retrospective analysis of 51 cases. Pain 55:119, 1993.
43. Hassenbush SJ, et al: Alternative intrathecal agents for the treatment of pain. Neuromodulation 2(2):85–91, 1999.
44. Lipton S: Percutaneous cervical cordotomy. Acta Anaesthesiol Belg 1:81, 1981.
45. Tasker RR: Percutaneous cordotomy: The lateral high cervical technique. *In* Schmidek HH, Sweet WH (eds): Operative Neurosurgical Techniques: Indications, Methods, and Results, ed 2. New York, Grune & Stratton, 1988, p 1191.
46. Rosomoff HL: Percutaneous radiofrequency cervical cordotomy for intractable pain. Adv Neurol 4:683, 1974.
47. Nagaro T, et al: Classification of post-cordotomy dysesthesia. Masui 43(9):1356–1361, 1994.
48. Macaluso C, Foley KM, Arbit E: Cordotomy for lumbosacral, pelvic and lower extremity pain of malignant origin: Safety and efficacy. Neurology 38:51, 1988.
49. Lema JA, Hitchcock E: Respiratory changes after stereotactic high cervical cord lesions for pain. Appl Neurophysiol 49:62, 1986.
50. Tasker RR: Percutaneous cordotomy: Neurosurgical and neuroaugmentative intervention. *In* Cancer Pain. Philadelphia, JB Lippincott, 1993, p 482.
51. Nagaro T, et al: Percutaneous cervical cordotomy and subarachnoid phenol block using fluoroscopy in pain control of costopleural syndrome. Pain 58:325–330, 1994.
52. Orlandini G: Evaluation of life expectancy in selection of patients undergoing percutaneous cervical cordotomy or subarachnoid phenol block for pain control of costopleural syndrome. Pain 61(3):492–493, 1995.

53. Sanders M, Zuurniond W: Safety of unilateral and bilateral percutaneous cordotomy in 80 terminally ill cancer patients. J Clin Oncol 13(6):1509–1512, 1955.
54. Meglio M, Cioni B: The role of percutaneous cordotomy in the treatment of chronic cancer pain. Acta Neurochir (Wien) 59:111, 1981.
55. Lahuerta J, Lipton S, Wells J: Percutaneous cervical cordotomy: Results and complications in a recent series of 100 patients. Ann R Coll Surg Engl 67:41, 1985.
56. Amano K, Kawamura H, Tanikawa T, et al: Bilateral versus unilateral percutaneous high cervical cordotomy as a surgical method of pain relief. Acta Neurochir Suppl (Wien) 52:143, 1991.
57. Jackson MB, Pounder D, Price C, et al: Percutaneous cervical cordotomy for the control of pain in patients with pleural mesothelioma. Thorax 54 (3):238–241, 1999.
58. White JC, Sweet WH: Anterolateral cordotomy: Open versus closed: Comparison of end results. Adv Pain Res Ther 3:47–48, 1979.
59. Katoh Y, Itoh T, Tsuji H, et al: Complications of lateral C1–C2 puncture myelography. Spine 15:1085, 1990.
60. Perese IM, Fracasso JB: Anatomical considerations in surgery of the spinal cord: A study of vessels and measurements of the cord. J Neurosurg 16:314, 1959.
61. Sweet WH, Poletti CE: Operations in the brain stem and spinal canal, with an appendix on open cordotomy. *In* Wall PD, Melzack R (eds): Textbook of Pain, ed 2. Edinburgh, Churchill Livingstone, 1984, p 624.
62. Mehler WR, Feferman ME, Nauta WJH: Ascending axon degeneration following anterolateral cordotomy: An experimental study in the monkey. Brain 83:718, 1960.
63. DiPiero V, Jones AKP, Iannotti F, et al: Chronic pain: A PET study of the central effects of percutaneous high cervical cordotomy. Pain 46:9, 1991.
64. Lahuerta J, Bowsher D, Campbell J, et al: Clinical and instrumental evaluation of sensory function before and after percutaneous anterolateral cordotomy at cervical level in man. Pain 4:23, 1990.
65. White JC, Sweet WH: Pain and the Neurosurgeon: A Forty-Year Experience. Springfield, Ill, Charles C Thomas, 1983.
66. Nathan PW: Touch and surgical division of the anterior quadrant of the spinal cord. J Neurosurg 53:935, 1990.
67. Friehs GM, Schrottner O, Pendl G: Evidence for segregated pain and temperature conduction within the spinothalamic tract. J Neurosurg 83(1):8–12, 1995.
68. Hitchcock E, Leece B: Somatotopic representation of the respiratory pathways in the cervical cord of men. J Neurosurg 27:320, 1967.
69. Krol G, Arbit E: Percutaneous lateral cervical cordotomy: Target localization with water-soluble contrast medium. J Neurosurg 79:390, 1993.
70. Lipton S: Neurolytic blocks around the head. *In* Raez GB (ed): Techniques of Neurolysis. Boston, Kluwer Academic, 1989.
71. Sweet WH: Recent observations pertinent to improving anterolateral cordotomy. Clin Neurosurg 23:80, 1975.
72. Millan S: Percutaneous cordotomy. J Neurosurg 35:360, 1971.
73. Rosomoff HL: Percutaneous spinothalamic cordotomy. *In* Wilkens RH, Rengachary SS (eds): Neurosurgery. Pain. New York, McGraw-Hill, 1985, p 2446.
74. Gybels JM, Sweet WH: Percutaneous anterolateral cordotomy. *In* Gildenberg PL (ed): Neurosurgical Treatment of Persistent Pain. Basel, Karger, 1989, p 173.
75. Fox JL: Experimental relationship of radiofrequency electrical current and lesion size for application to percutaneous cordotomy. J Neurosurg 33:415, 1970.
76. Kanpolat Y, Cosman ER: Special radiofrequency electrode system for computed tomography–guided pain-relieving procedures. Neurosurgery 38(3):602–603, 1996.
77. Zileli M, Coskun E, Yegul I, Oyar M: Electrophysiological monitoring during CT-guided percutaneous cordotomy. Acta Neurochir Suppl (Wien) 64:92–96, 1995.
78. Kanpolat Y, Akyar S, Caglar S: Diametral measurements of the upper spinal cord for stereotactic pain procedures: Experimental and clinical. Surg Neurol 43(5):478–483, 1995.
79. Nagaro T, et al: The histological changes in the spinal cord following percutaneous cervical cordotomy (PCC) and correlation of these changes with the efficacy of PCC. Masui 44(3):325–330, 1995.
80. Mooij JJA, Bosch DA, Beks JWF: The cause of failure in high cervical percutaneous cordotomy: An analysis. Acta Neurochir (Wien) 72:1, 1984.
81. Ischia S, Ischia A, Polati E, et al: Three posterior percutaneous celiac plexus block techniques. Anesthesiology 76:534, 1992.
82. Nathan PW, Smith MC: Dysesthesie après cordotomie. Med Hyg 42:1788, 1984.
83. Ray BS, Wolff SG: Studies on pain, "spread of pain," evidence on site of spread within the neuraxis of effects of painful stimulation. Arch Neurol Psychiatry 53:257, 1945.
84. Nathan PW: Results of anterolateral cordotomy for pain in cancer. J Neurol Neurosurg Psychiatry 26:353, 1963.
85. Bowsher D: Contralateral mirror-image pain following anterolateral cordotomy. Pain 88:63, 1988.
86. Nagaro T, Amakawa K, Arai T, et al: Ipsilateral referral of pain following cordotomy. Pain 55:275, 1993.
87. Nagaro T, Kimura S, Arai T: A mechanism of new pain following cordotomy: Reference of sensation. Pain 30:89, 1987.
88. Belmusto L, Brown E, Owens G: Clinical observations on respiratory and vasomotor disturbance as related to cervical cordotomies. J Neurosurg 20:225, 1963.
89. Rosomoff HL, Krieger AJ, Kuperman AS: Effects of percutaneous cervical cordotomy on pulmonary function. J Neurosurg 31:620, 1969.
90. Krieger AJ, Rosomoff HL: Sleep-induced apnea. Part I: A respiratory and autonomic dysfunction syndrome following bilateral percutaneous cervical cordotomy. J Neurosurg 39:168, 1974.
91. Polatty RC, Cooper KR: Respiratory failure after percutaneous cordotomy. South Med J 79:897, 1986.
92. Wells CJ, Lipton S, Lahuerta J: Respiratory depression after percutaneous cervical anterolateral cordotomy in patients on slow-release oral morphine. Lancet 1:739, 1984.
93. Rosomoff HL, Papo I, Loeser J, et al: Neurosurgical operations on the spinal cord. *In* Bonica JJ (ed): Management of Pain. Philadelphia, 1990.
94. Palma A, Holzer J, Cuadra O, et al: Lateral percutaneous spinothalamic tractotomy. Acta Neurochir (Wien) 93:100, 1988.
95. Brose WG, Cousins MJ: Subcutaneous lidocaine for treatment of neuropathic cancer pain. Pain 45:145, 1991.
96. Glazer S, Portenoy RK: Systemic local anesthetics in pain control. J Pain Symptom Manage 6:30–39, 1991.
97. Eisenreich J, et al: Epidural clonidine analgesia for intractable cancer pain. Pain 61:391–399, 1995.

CHAPTER • 68

Percutaneous Laser Discectomy

Sunil K. Singh, MD

Laser for treatment of lumbar disc disease is a very attractive, even seductive, technology. It is one of the best minimally invasive spine techniques and has many advantages: (1) single-step insertion of a thin needle; (2) easy access to the often difficult to reach L5–S1 disc space; (3) nuclear ablation beyond what can be suctioned or physically removed; (4) a brief outpatient procedure; (5) absence of epidural scar and postoperative pain syndromes. Despite the potential benefits, however, few of these advantages have been realized in clinical practice. Laser remains a rarely used tool for treatment of disc disease except in a few specialized centers.

THEORY

The mechanism of action of all percutaneous methods used to treat lumbar disc disease, especially that of lasers, is not obvious. A small amount of tissue is excised from the center or nuclear part of the disc, and this in turn is believed to exert an effect on a noncontiguous portion of nucleus that is protruding through annulus fibrosus and abutting an exiting nerve root. First described by Hijikata[1] in relation to the percutaneous discectomy method, the central cavity created by laser is believed to allow the nuclear protrusion to move back within the disc. A small change in disc nucleus volume can exert disproportionately large changes on the disc. Yunezawa and coworkers[2] first demonstrated significant alterations in intradiscal pressure in response to vertical load after Nd : YAG laser treatment. Their study also reported the equivalency of laser to aggressive manual curettage. Choy and Altman[3] reported greater than 50% reduction of intradiscal pressure in response to load following 1000 J of Nd : YAG laser energy. Prodoehl and associates[4] reported similar results using 1200 J from the Ho : YAG laser. There is no specimen to weigh after laser discectomy; therefore the amount of disc removed can only be approximated. By calculating the geometry of the laser tract, Choy[5] estimated that 1000 J of Nd : YAG laser energy vaporized 98.52 mg of disc. Lane and coworkers,[6] who used 1200 J each of CO_2, argon, and Ho : YAG laser energy to compare effectiveness of all, reported that Ho : YAG was superior in ablating 2.4 g of disc tissue. By comparison, an automated percutaneous discectomy clinical trial reported removal of 2 to 7 g of disc tissue with a suction cutting device. Quigley's group[7] compared an automated device, Nd : YAG, and Ho : YAG laser and clearly showed the automated device to be superior for removing the greatest mass of tissue.

LASER PHYSICS AND LASER-TISSUE INTERACTION

Laser is an acronym for *l*ight *a*mplification by *s*timulated *e*mission of *r*adiation. Stimulation of a crystal or gas with an electric current or flash lamp energizes the molecules of crystal or gas, which release photons of light. A fully reflective concave mirror can direct the light back into the crystal or gas medium toward a partially reflective concave mirror at the opposite end of the crystal or of a resonating chamber containing the gas. The light developed in this manner passes back and forth between the two mirrors until it is intense enough to pass through the partially reflective mirror as a laser beam. This laser beam is coherent, collimated, and monochromatic; its wavelength depends on the nature of the crystal or gas. The laser beam can be focused on a small spot of high energy density, creating an efficient and precise tool to heat, and ultimately to vaporize, tissue, usually by boiling the water within. For example, CO_2 gas produces laser light in the far infrared (wavelength 10.65 μm), whereas a crystal of Nd : YAG (yttrium, aluminum, and garnet crystal doped with neodymium) produces laser light in the near infrared (wavelength 1.06 μm). The effect of laser light on human tissue depends on the optical properties of the tissue and the interaction of tissue and laser. If, for example, water in tissue absorbs laser light effectively, light energy is converted quickly to heat and tissue is vaporized along with water in the tissue. Ideally, this should occur at or very near the surface of the tissue, so that little or no heat is disseminated into or through the tissue. Conversely, when water in tissue absorbs laser poorly, the energy is disseminated through the tissue and converted to heat over a larger volume, causing thermal injury. Laser light in the visible and near infrared portions of the electromagnetic spectrum easily passes through water and passes poorly through nonpigmented tissues. Its effect in intervertebral disc tissue, therefore, is less complete than that in mid and far infrared. It is possible to inject pigment into tissue so that near infrared and visible light can be absorbed more quickly, producing vaporization of the tissue with much less thermal injury. Laser light requires a mechanism whereby laser can be conveniently delivered to the tissue. Visible light and near and mid infrared lasers can be passed through a silicon fiber with minimal loss of energy, but far infrared CO_2 lasers require a free-beam or rigid wave-guide delivery system. Far infrared CO_2 lasers (better absorbed by tissues), therefore cannot easily be used in laser discectomy. A free beam is difficult to direct into the disc, and hollow, rigid wave-guide requires a constant purge jet of CO_2 gas, which has the potential to produce extrathecal emphysema.

Laser is used commonly for the purpose of precise destruction; therefore, matching the laser's wavelength to tissue absorption maximizes the efficiency of the ablative process and minimizes the thermal spread and collateral damage. For laser discectomy, the target tissue is the nucleus pulposus, the main constituent of which is water.[8] In clinical practice, it is hard to gauge the influences of the diverse absorption properties on the efficacy and safety of laser discectomy performed with any one of these lasers. Although poor tissue absorption necessitates greater energies and subsequently creates more tissue heating, laser power usually is not a limiting factor in any particular process, and heat can be dissipated by slowing the rate of energy application and increasing the length and frequency of pauses.

LASERS IN DISC DISEASE

Nd : YAG Lasers

Ascher[9] and Choy and colleagues[10] performed the first Nd : YAG laser discectomy about 15 years ago. Their procedure consisted of fluoroscopically guided insertion of a needle into the disc space to be treated and threading of a thin laser fiber through the needle into the disc space. Activation of laser with delivery of about 1200 J of energy (in short bursts to avoid heating the adjacent tissues) into the disc cavitated the nucleus and ablated a small amount of tissue. The products of vaporization (steam and carbon particles) were allowed to escape through the spinal needle surrounding the laser fiber. At the end of the procedure, the needle site was covered with a Band-Aid and the patient was discharged. These investigators postulated that removal of even a small volume of tissue from the disc resulted in a large drop in intradiscal pressure. They thought it might be the mechanism responsible for prompt and marked pain relief in patients who were treated for sciatica secondary to degenerative disc protrusion and contained herniations. They suggested that the procedure would not be useful for patients with unconfined herniations or sequestered disc fragments outside the disc space loose in the spinal canal. Ascher,[9] Choy,[10] and others have performed this procedure in more than 1000 patients. Long-term pain relief has been reported in 70% to 80% of patients by these authors. The procedure is appealing in that it is done on an outpatient basis with conscious sedation. Percutaneous laser disc decompression with a 1.06 Nd : YAG laser has been approved by the U.S. Food and Drug Administration (FDA). Generally, it is thought that laser discectomy is equivalent to other percutaneous discectomy procedures, such as chemonucleolysis and automated percutaneous lumbar discectomy (APLD) using a reciprocating suction cutter.

KTP Lasers

The crystal of potassium, titanyl, and phosphate (KTP) produces laser light that is lime green. This laser employs fiberoptics and is easily directed into disc space through a spinal needle. It was first used for laser discectomy by Davis[11] who reported results essentially similar to those described by Ascher,[9] Choy,[10] and others. The procedure was found to be safe and effective in their early experience, and KTP laser was subsequently approved by the FDA for use in this application. Manufacturers have subsequently developed side-firing probes, which make it possible to point laser energy in almost any direction, minimizing the possibility of injury to structures anterior to the spinal column such as the aorta, vena cava, and iliac vessels.

Ho : YAG Lasers

Holmium YAG (Ho : YAG) laser has wavelength in mid infrared and is absorbed well by water. It is fiberoptic. An effective dose of energy can be introduced into the disc via fibers introduced percutaneously through a needle or catheter. Ho : YAG laser is a pulsed laser, in contrast to the continuous-wave, near infrared lasers, and therefore has the theoretical advantage of producing minimal amounts of heat in adjacent tissues. With a pulse width of about 250 microseconds at 10 Hz and 1.6 J per pulse, virtually no temperature rise is noted in adjacent tissues. When 1200 J of Ho : YAG laser energy was introduced into the disc through a 400 μm fiber with the same parameters, it consistently produced a 2-cm by 1.5-cm by 1-cm defect in the nucleus pulposus. The defect can be precisely localized in the disc by fluoroscopic needle guidance. The defect should be in the posterior quadrant just anterior to the site of herniation. Early experience revealed the procedure to be safe and effective (like Nd : YAG and KTP lasers), enough so to justify FDA approval for marketing of this application.

INDICATIONS FOR LASER DISCECTOMY

Selection of patients depends on two kinds of criteria, clinical and radiographic.

- Clinical indications (identical to those for microdiscectomy)
  - Radicular symptoms
  - Concordant signs
  - Positive straight leg raise
  - Failure of supervised trial of conservative treatment
- Radiologic indications
  - Presence of disc herniation at appropriate level

Must exclude stenosis, or facet hypertrophy and disc fragment

Exclusion criteria for laser discectomy are these:

- Progressive neurologic deficit
- Previous surgery at same disc level (relative contraindication)
- Workers compensation cases (relative contraindication)

TECHNIQUE

Entry into Disc

All percutaneous methods rely on the posterolateral approach to the disc as described by Day.[12] Local anesthetic supplemented with light sedation is used to avoid inadvertent root injury.

Site of Procedure

The injection procedure can be performed in an operating room or in a special procedure room of a radiology department, provided the necessary equipment, anesthesia, emergency cart, and trained personnel are available.

Positioning

The prone or lateral decubitus position is satisfactory if the patient can be properly positioned and stabilized to afford a lateral approach to the disc space. Radiation exposure of the patient in a typical procedure is equivalent to that of a five-view lumbosacral spine series.

Needle Placement

After sterile skin preparation, as for any surgical procedure, the area is draped. The disc space is identified with the help of a C-arm fluoroscope. Disc margins are made clear by craniocaudal movement of the fluro tube. At this time the fluro tube is rotated obliquely to bring the superior articular process to the midline. An 18-gauge 7-in needle is introduced immediately anterior to the superior articular process and superior to the transverse process via a triangular safe zone. The needle is advanced in 1- to 2-cm increments in a "stop and look and go" process, to allow a change of course if it is not properly directed. Progress is viewed in anteroposterior and lateral projections with the C-arm fluoroscope, which must be of sufficient strength and quality to give a clear view of the area. The needle tip should be at the center of the disc upon completion. In most cases, the entry points in the skin for treating either the L4–L5 or the L5–S1 disc space are at the level of the iliac crest (very close to each other). The rubbery texture of the annulus is easily felt with the tip of the 18-gauge needle. Fluoroscopy precautions include the wearing of lead aprons by all personnel in the procedure and operating rooms. Lead gloves and avoiding exposing the operator's hands also reduces radiation exposure.

Laser Application

Once the needle has reached the annulus, it is advanced through the annulus and into the nucleus pulposus for a distance of about 1 cm. The fiber is then marked to prevent penetration of the tip more than 1 cm beyond the end of the needle. Owing to differences in absorption, energy requirements and rates of application also differ among lasers. Choy and Ascher[13] reported using an Nd : YAG laser as 20-W continuous energy delivered in 1-sec pulses with 1-sec pauses until 1000 to 1850 J was delivered. Davis uses KTP laser as 10- to 15-W continuous energy in 0.5-sec pulses with 0.5-sec pauses for a few minutes. The commercial KTP laser is designed to deliver up to 1250 J before it shuts down automatically and allows another 300 J to be administered before it issues a warning. Sherk and colleagues[14] use the Ho:YAG laser in the pulsed mode at 10 Hz.

RESULTS

The most extensive experience in the literature is published by Choy and Ascher[13] with Nd : YAG. They followed 333 patients for a mean duration of 26 months. The success rate was 78.4% (as measured by a good or fair response) according to MacNab.[15]

Siebert[16] reported on his first 100 patients treated with Nd : YAG. The success rate was 78% at mean follow-up of 17 months. Davis[11] reported an 85% success rate with the KTP laser, *success rate* being defined as minimal discomfort and the ability to return to gainful employment (follow-up duration was not specified). Yeung[17] reported preliminary assessment of more than 1000 patients whose lumbar herniated discs were treated with KTP laser. The reported success rate (good or excellent results) was 84%. No specifics were supplied. Ho : YAG laser was used by Sherk and coworkers[14] in a comparison of laser discectomy with conservative treatment. No differences were noted between treated and control groups. They concluded that laser discectomy is a safe procedure that appears to be effective in relieving symptoms in some patients. I use Ho : YAG laser, and my successful results are about 80% (comparable to other investigators').

COMPLICATIONS

Discitis is the only documented complication of laser discectomy. Choy's group[13] in 1993 tabulated the world experience with laser discectomy. Choy reported two cases of discitis.

CONCLUSION

Laser discectomy is a minimally invasive procedure that has been used to treat about 10,000 patients worldwide. Various laser wavelengths have been used but no consensus exists about which is most efficacious. Good candidates have a classic clinical syndrome and neuroimaging evidence of a contained herniation. Published results are in the range of 75% to 80% success.

REFERENCES

1. Hijikata S: Percutaneous nucleotomy. A new concept technique and 12 years experience. Clin Orthop 238:9–23, 1989.
2. Yunezawa T, et al: System and procedure of percutaneous intradiscal laser nucleotomy. Spine 15:1175–1185, 1990.
3. Choy DSJ, Altman P: Fall of intradiscal pressure with laser ablation. *In* Sherk HH (ed): Spine: State of the Art Reviews. Laser Discectomy. Philadelphia, Hanley & Belfus. 1993.
4. Prodoehl JA, et al: Effects of lasers on intervertebral disc pressures. *In* Sherk HH (ed): Spine: State of the Art Reviews. Laser Discectomy. Philadelphia, Hanley & Belfus, 1993.
5. Choy DSJ: Problem of the L5–S1 disc solved by needle entry with an extrathecal approach. J Clin Laser Med Surg 12:321–324, 1994.
6. Lane GS, et al: An experimental comparison of CO_2, argon and Nd:YAG laser ablation of intervertebral discs. *In* Sherk HH (ed): Spine: State of the Art Reviews. Laser Discectomy. Philadelphia, Hanley & Belfus, 1993, pp 1–9.
7. Quigley MR, et al: Laser discectomy: Comparison of automated suction, Ho:YAG laser and Nd:YAG laser systems. Spine 19:319–322, 1994.
8. Quigley MR, et al: Laser discectomy: A review. Spine 19:53–56, 1994.
9. Ascher PW: Status quo and new horizons of laser therapy in neurosurgery. Lasers Surg Med 5:499, 1985.
10. Choy DJS, et al: Percutaneous laser nucleolysis of lumbar disc. N Engl J Med 317:771–772, 1987.
11. Davis JK: Early experience with laser disc decompression. J Fla Med Assoc 79:37–39, 1992.
12. Day PL: Lateral approach for lumbar discogram and chemonucleolysis. Clin Orthop 67:90–93, 1969.
13. Choy DSJ, Ascher PW: Percutaneous laser disc decompression. Spine 17:949–956, 1992.
14. Sherk HH, et al: Results of percutaneous lumbar discectomy with lasers. *In* Sherk HH (ed): Spine: State of the Art Reviews. Laser Discectomy. Philadelphia, Hanley & Belfus 1993, pp 141–150.
15. MacNab I: Negative disc exploration: An analysis of the causes of nerve root involvement in sixty-eight patients. J Bone Joint Surg 53A:891–903, 1971.
16. Siebert W: Percutaneous laser disc decompression: The European experience. *In* Sherk HH (ed): Spine: State of the Art Reviews. Laser Discectomy. Philadelphia, Hanley & Belfus, 1993, pp 103–133.
17. Yeung AT: Consideration for the use of KTP laser for disc decompression and ablation. *In* Sherk HH (ed): Spine: State of the Art Reviews. Laser Discectomy. Philadelphia, Hanley & Belfus, 1993, pp 67–93.

CHAPTER • 69

Intradiscal Electrothermal Annuloplasty

Steven D. Waldman, MD, JD •
Steven M. Siwek, MD •
Katherine A. Waldman, OTR, MBA

Intradiscal electrothermal annuloplasty (IDA) is another step in the continuum of care for patients suffering from lumbar discogenic pain. It is a reasonable option for a discrete subset of patients—those whose pain is secondary to either an internally disrupted lumbar disc or a disc with very limited herniation and has not responded to conservative therapy, including medication management, physical therapy, epidural steroid injections, and bed rest. IDA is not indicated for back or radicular pain secondary to spinal stenosis or to significant disc herniation with nerve root compression. In this chapter we review the current status of this new treatment modality, emphasizing patient selection issues and the fine points of technique for IDA that will help the pain management specialist to improve outcomes.

THE PATHOPHYSIOLOGY OF LUMBAR DISC DISRUPTION

The exact mechanisms by which the intervertebral disc serves as a nociceptive generator have yet to be completely elucidated. It is known, however, that the lumbar intervertebral disc contains nociceptive fibers and is capable of generating pain. The nociceptive fibers are most numerous in the posterolateral portion of the disc. Pain impulses from these fibers are transmitted to the spinal cord via the dorsal root ganglion. Mechanoreceptors also present in the disc may also contribute to afferent impulses via the dorsal root ganglia. It should be noted that structures surrounding the disc such as the posterior longitudinal ligament also play an important role in the genesis of back and radicular pain.

The nociceptive fibers in the disc and surrounding structures (such as the posterior longitudinal ligament) may be stimulated by mechanical or chemical agents. Substance P release has also been implicated in the genesis of back and radicular pain secondary to the disrupted lumbar disc, as has the reinnervation of the damaged portion of the disc with small unmyelinated nociceptive fibers. Current thinking suggests that it is the interplay of all of these factors that leads to chronic stimulation of the dorsal root ganglia and resultant chronic pain. Plasticity at the spinal cord level may also contribute to the development of chronic pain in response to this continued barrage of afferent nociception from the dorsal root ganglia. Further research is required to clarify exactly how the disrupted lumbar disc causes the clinical constellation of symptoms that pain management specialists currently attribute to discogenic disease.

THE TREATMENT OF DISCOGENIC PAIN WITH HEAT

IDA is thought to ameliorate discogenic pain by three mechanisms: (1) thermal destruction of annular nociceptive nerve fibers; (2) thermal injury to collagen fibers of the annulus with subsequent healing; and (3) potential reduction in disc volume and intradiscal pressure from thermal destruction of disc tissue. To produce these effects, a heat source capable of controlled heating must be accurately placed near the nociceptive source to produce thermal injury. Several modalities for heat delivery have been developed, including the radiofrequency needle, the fiberoptic laser, and the navigable thermal catheter. Each modality has its advantages and disadvantages (Table 69–1). In this chapter we focus primarily on the clinical applications of the navigable thermal catheter, because it appears to be the most amenable to and practical for use by interventional pain management specialists.

PATIENT SELECTION

The Targeted History and Physical Examination

As with all other interventional pain management modalities, proper patient selection is mandatory to improve the

TABLE 69–1 ***Advantages and Disadvantages of Intradiscal Thermal Delivery Systems***

System	Advantages	Disadvantages
Laser Fiberoptic		
Energy source: laser	Good access to the lesion	Expense
Delivery method: straight or side-firing fiberoptic catheter	Excellent decompression effect for radiculopathy	Poor temperature control
Radiofrequency Electrode		
Energy source: radiofrequency	Easy intradiscal placement	Does not heat disc tissues well (low water content)
Delivery method: straight electrode	Cost effectiveness	Poor decompressive effect
	Safety	Small treatment area
	Minimal invasiveness	Cannot easily reach posterior disc
Intradiscal Electrothermal Catheter		
Energy source: electroresistive coil	Easy intradiscal placement	Poor decompressive effect
Delivery method: navigable catheter	Broad target zone	Cannot reach collapsed discs
	Cost effectiveness	Poor results for radicular pain
	Safety	
	Minimal invasiveness	

chances of good outcomes and to avoid side effects and complications. All patients being considered for IDA must give a detailed history and have a physical examination by the pain management specialist. Specific areas of history to be investigated include the success and failure of previous treatment modalities, the location of the pain, the presence of bowel or bladder symptoms or other neurologic deficits, and the patient's pattern of using opioids and other controlled substances, alcohol, and illicit drugs. Special attention to the neurologic examination is crucial to identifying occult preexisting neurologic deficits lest they later be attributed to the IDA procedure itself. A general assessment of the patient's level of deconditioning is also useful to help in designing a postprocedure back rehabilitation program. Coagulopathy and anticoagulant therapy are absolute contraindications to IDA, as is infection of the disc or surrounding tissues.

Previous Treatment

As a general rule, patients with chronic back or leg pain who are being considered for a trial of IDA should have experienced failure of aggressive conservative pain management. Medication management with the nonsteroidal anti-inflammatory agents, simple analgesics, and skeletal muscle relaxants, combined with bed rest, physical modalities (including heat and cold), epidural steroid injections, and a back rehabilitation program, should be used before a trial of IDA is run. Long-term opioid therapy for chronic pain remains controversial and may be a significant impediment to the overall success of IDA, since in most cases preexisting back pain intensifies for a time after IDA. For this reason, a very careful behavioral assessment is warranted before a trial when long-term opioid use has resulted in drug tolerance. The findings may help to avoid postprocedure opioid overdosing and pathologic drug-seeking behaviors.

Spinal Imaging and Testing

Patients who are being considered for IDA should undergo magnetic resonance imaging (MRI) of the lumbar spine to provide the pain management specialist with a baseline assessment of the status of the discs, vertebral bodies, and surrounding tissues. MRI also helps to identify discitis, which is often missed on clinical examination alone. Plain radiographs and computed tomographic scanning of the suspected spinal segments will delineate bone abnormalities not readily seen on MRI. Radionuclide bone scanning helps to identify tumor, infection, or impending vertebral compression fracture not demonstrated by other imaging modalities. Provocative discography, performed either at the time of IDA or before, as a separate diagnostic maneuver, is most useful in identifying which discs are causing the patient's pain. Infection is an absolute contraindication to IDA. When there is any suspicion of infection, erythrocyte sedimentation rate, complete blood count, gallium scanning, and culture of material from the suspect disc should be performed before proceeding with IDA.

Conditions Amenable to Treatment with IDA

Only certain pathologic conditions of the intervertebral disc are amenable to IDA. Primary indications for IDA include an internally disrupted disc with annular fissuring and discs with very limited and contained nuclear herniation. Other types of discogenic disease that may respond to IDA include painful postoperative discs, painful discs located above a previous fusion, and early degenerative disc disease with good preservation of disc space integrity. Discography to identify if in fact the suspected disc is responsible for the patient's pain is strongly advised when considering IDA to treat these secondary indications.

NAVIGABLE THERMAL CATHETER TECHNIQUE

Overview of Hardware

The prototype of the navigable thermal catheter for intradiscal use is the SpineCATH System (Oratec Interventions, Inc., Menlo Park, Calif.). A similar product manufactured by Radionics, Inc., is currently in clinical trials. The SpineCATH features a navigable radiopaque tip to allow positioning of the distal heating portion of the catheter close to the posterior disc. The catheter's 18-gauge diameter allows relatively easy percutaneous introduction via a 17-gauge introducer. Unfortunately, at the present time the SpinCATH System can be used only with its own special radiofrequency generator.

Patient Preparation and Positioning

The patient is placed on the fluoroscopic table in either the prone or the lateral position, the choice being based on the experience of the pain management specialist and the comfort of the patient. The lateral position has the advantage of easier access to the patient's airway should problems occur. The prone position has the advantage of being easier to implement and more consistent. If it is chosen, positioning the patient in a partially oblique position by placing a radiolucent foam wedge under the asymptomatic side may aid in identifying anatomic landmarks. After correct positioning is obtained, the skin is prepared with antiseptic solution and sterile drapes are placed.

Introducer Needle Placement

The fluoroscope is then utilized to identify the inferior end plate of the affected spinal level. For the lower spinal interspaces, this requires angling the fluoroscopic beam with a 25- to 35-degree cephalocaudal trajectory. The beam is then rotated to identify the superior articular process and to align it approximately in the middle of the inferior end plate. The skin overlying a point just lateral to the middle of the superior articular process is marked with a sterile marker to indicate the entry point of the introducer. At this point, the skin and subcutaneous tissues are anesthetized with 1.0% preservative-free lidocaine. A 3.5-in 25-gauge needle is introduced through the anesthetized area in a trajectory just anterior to the mid-point of the superior articular surface, keeping it parallel to the end plates. To avoid persistent paresthesia, the patient should be warned to report any paresthesia, as that would indicate that the needle has impinged on a nerve root. One per cent lidocaine is injected through the needle as it is introduced along this trajectory, to provide adequate anesthesia for the catheter introducer.

With the 25-gauge needle left in place to provide a radiopaque marker, the 17-gauge 6-in introducer needle is advanced just parallel to the 25-gauge needle. Under fluoroscopic guidance, the introducer needle tip should be placed just in front of the superior articular process with the needle bevel facing the posterior wall of the disc. Again, the patient should be warned to report any paresthesia. The introducer needle is advanced under fluoroscopic guidance into the annulus of the disc, which offers significant resistance to the needle and has a "gritty" feel. There will be a sudden loss of resistance as the introducer needle enters the softer annulus of the disc. The placement of the introducer needle relative to the nuclear cavity is confirmed by obtaining fluoroscopic views in all planes.

Catheter Placement

After satisfactory placement of the introducer needle within the nuclear cavity of the affected disc is confirmed, the bevel of the introducer is placed toward the posterior wall of the disc and the stylet is removed. The white marker on the tip and handle of the SpineCATH is identified and aligned with the bevel marker on the introducer to aim the curved catheter tip toward the posterior disc. The catheter is then gently advanced through the introducer needle. The first bold marker on the catheter indicates that the catheter tip has reached the bevel of the needle. Under fluoroscopic guidance, the catheter is then gently advanced to position the heating portion of the catheter close to the posterior disc. Ideally, the catheter tip should extend beyond the midline of the posterior disc (Fig. 69–1). Using small rotational movements while gently advancing the catheter helps to optimize needle placement. To ensure that the entire heating portion of the catheter is outside the introducer needle the second bold mark on the catheter *must* lie beyond the introducer needle hub. Before heating, the pain management specialist should also confirm by biplanar fluoroscopy that no portion of the catheter is outside the annulus of the disc. Forceful movements of the catheter are to be discouraged, to avoid catheter kinking or breakage. If it should become kinked, manipulation of the catheter must cease immediately. If the kinked catheter is in proper position against the posterior disc, the operator may proceed with the heating sequence. Otherwise, the introducer needle and catheter are withdrawn as a unit under fluoroscopic guidance. If any significant resistance is felt, the operator must stop withdrawing the needle and catheter immediately and determine the relative positions of both units by fluoroscopy before making further attempts at withdrawal.

Heating Sequence

Successful IDA requires heating the nociceptive tissues at a temperature high enough for the time necessary to produce thermal injury without causing thermal injury to surrounding structures and excessive pain for the patient. The heating protocol described next is recommended by a number of pain management specialists with experience in IDA,

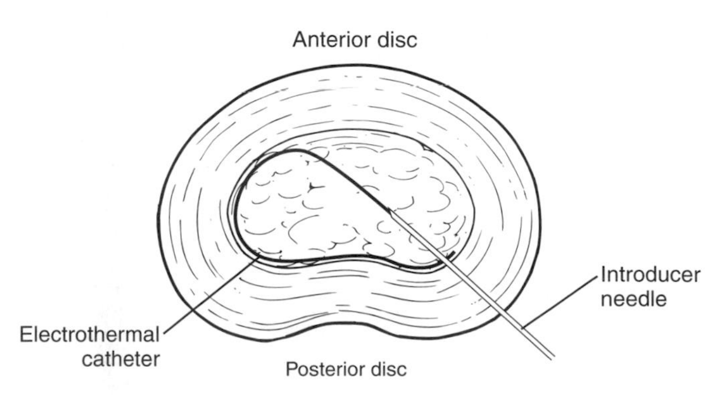

FIGURE 69–1 Proper placement of intradiscal catheter against posterior disc.

although other heating protocols have been used safely and successfully.

After proper catheter placement, the catheter is heated from 37° C (the patient's body temperature) to 65° C. After the temperature has remained at 65° C for 1 min and the patient has not complained of excessive pain, the temperature is increased by 1° C every 30 sec until it is between 80° and 90° C. The heating sequence takes approximately 15 min, during which time the patient is constantly monitored for onset of new radicular symptoms or severe back pain. Clinical experience has shown that more rapid heating sequences often produce extraordinary pain. Clinical experience and microscopic analysis of heated discs have also shown that a certain amount of heat is required to provide long-term pain relief. Temperatures less than 76° C often result in poor long-term pain relief. After the heating sequence is completed, the introducer needle and catheter are removed as a unit. Some pain management specialists prefer to carefully remove the catheter while leaving the introducer needle in place and administering intradiscal antibiotics or steroids via the needle before removing it. Sterile dressings are placed over the entry sites, and the patient is observed until vital signs and neurologic status are stable.

Postprocedure Care

The majority of patients experience exacerbation of their preprocedure back or radicular pain immediately after IDA. The patient and family should be warned of this before the procedure to reduce the fear that something has gone wrong. The postprocedure pain flare generally lasts 3 to 7 days and the patient will require additional analgesics, muscle relaxants, and, above all, reassurance. Occasionally, transcutaneous nerve stimulation and a lumbar support with rigid stays may be beneficial if movement-induced pain and spasm are problems. Patients who have received long-term opioid therapy may be particularly hard to manage during the early postprocedure period, and the pain management specialist should be prepared to hospitalize such patients to prevent medication overuse and its attendant problems and risks.

After the immediate postprocedure period, patients may expect to begin to experience pain relief gradually over a period of 4 to 6 weeks. Again, preprocedure communication with patient and family helps them to understand and accept the gradual improvement associated with IDA therapy. After 8 to 12 weeks, all patients who have undergone IDA should begin a careful back rehabilitation program under the direct supervision of a physiatrist or pain management specialist familiar with postoperative spine rehabilitation. Overaggressive therapy often results in increased pain and functional disability and is to be avoided. Return to work after IDA is based on the patient's rate of recovery. Sedentary workers usually return to work within 10 to 14 days and those who perform heavy lifting within 60 to 90 days, as recovery allows.

COMPLICATIONS

Acute complications of IDA are related to needle-induced trauma to neural structures or the vasculature. Incorrect needle placement can also result in trauma to retroperitoneal structures, including the kidneys. The incidence of such complications can be greatly reduced by giving close attention to the functional anatomy and placing the needle with biplanar fluoroscopic guidance. Thermal injuries due to improper catheter placement can also be avoided with careful attention to technique. Heating should be discontinued whenever a patient experiences new or severe back or radicular pain. Late complications of IDA are related to infection. Discitis is hard to diagnose clinically but must always be included in the differential diagnosis of persistent or excessive postprocedure pain. Failure to rapidly diagnose infection can result in life-threatening sequelae, including epidural abscess and meningitis.

CONCLUSION

Intradiscal electrothermal annuloplasty is a new and useful tool for the treatment of a variety of discogenic diseases. As with other interventional pain management techniques, proper patient selection and careful attention to the technical aspects of the procedure are crucial if optimal results are to be achieved and side effects and complications avoided. Additional experience with IDA allows the pain management specialist to further refine both patient selection and technique and improve outcomes.

SUGGESTED READING

Bogduk N: The lumbar disc and low back pain. Neurosurg Clin North Am 2:791–806, 1991.

Houpt JC, Conner ES: Experimental study of temperature distributions and thermal transport during radiofrequency current therapy of the intervertebral disc. Spine 21:1808–1831, 1996.

Intradiscal Electro Thermal Therapy Training Course Syllabus. Menlo Park, Calif., Oratec Interventions, 1999, pp 1–57.

Nakamura S: The afferent pathways of discogenic low back pain. J Bone Joint Surg 78:606–612, 1996.

Schwarzer AC: The prevalence and clinical features of internal disc disruption in patients with chronic back pain. Spine 20:1878–1883, 1995.

VanKleef M, Barendse GA: Percutaneous intradiscal radiofrequency thermocoagulation in chronic nonspecific low back pain. Pain Clinic 3:259–268, 1996.

CHAPTER • 70

Percutaneous Vertebroplasty

Sunil K. Singh, MD

Percutaneous vertebroplasty with polymethylmethacrylate (PMMA) cement is used to increase the fragility of the diseased vertebral bodies. Treatment can be curative or palliative. Depriester and coworkers have been performing percutaneous vertebroplasty since 1984.[1] Initially, the major indication was aggressive spinal hemangioma, but with experience two more indications (osteoporotic vertebral crush fracture and spinal tumors) were found.[1–3]

TREATABLE LESIONS

Percutaneous vertebroplasty is indicated for any disease—painful or not—that weakens the vertebral body. Percutaneous vertebroplasty has two objectives: analgesia and stabilization (solidification). There are three pathologic indications: osteoporotic vertebral crush fracture, malignant spinal tumors, and vertebral hemangioma.

Osteoporotic Vertebral Fracture

Osteoporosis is complicated by vertebral fracture, which may occur spontaneously or after minor trauma. The most common vertebral fracture site is the thoracolumbar junction. These fractures are commonly seen in postmenopausal women aged 60 years or older. The vertebral fractures are often very painful and are managed by immobilization, analgesic drugs, epidural steroid injections, and specific treatment of osteoporosis. Immobilization increases demineralization. In spite of long-term medical treatment, some patients have severe, persistent, incapacitating pain. Medical treatment of osteoporosis consists of prevention of fracture and use of antiresorptive agents (estrogen and calcitonin). Initial symptoms tend to disappear in 4 to 6 weeks. Repeated vertebral fractures are common and cause significant morbidity. Later consequences of vertebral fracture are loss of height, kyphosis, and chronic back pain. In these cases, vertebroplasty alleviates symptoms and reduces the duration of immobilization.[1–5]

Depriester and Deramond described their experience treating many patients between 49 to 86 years of age by this method.[6] In 75% of cases, the thoracolumbar junction was treated and in 35%, two vertebrae. Four patients were treated at three levels. All patients had severe pain despite medical treatment and immobilization. Vertebroplasty was performed 3 weeks to 5 months after onset of symptoms. Results were excellent in all cases: quick and complete relief of pain. Patients were capable of standing up and walking 24 to 48 hours after the procedure. The effects were long lasting and at follow-up results were excellent. No complications were reported. In some cases, pain increased immediately after the vertebroplasty, but it was relieved with antiinflammatory agents.[1, 3] Collapse of adjacent vertebrae in contact with the injected one is a potential risk. It was observed in one patient treated with vertebroplasty.

When a patient has only early collapse and back pain, vertebroplasty may be performed to avoid the onset or aggravation of kyphosis and secondary collapse. Vertebroplasty must be accompanied with medical treatment of osteoporosis and an orthopedic corset to stabilize the spine.[1, 3]

Spinal Tumors

Many malignant spinal tumors, such as metastases, lymphomas, and myelomas can be treated. Such tumors are often painful. Pharmacotherapy, radiotherapy, chemotherapy, and embolization can be employed, but these are often associated with failure and complications.[6]

For previously untreated painful vertebral metastasis radiotherapy is useful in 70% of cases to alleviate spinal pain, but the effect may take 2 to 6 weeks to develop.[7] Radiotherapy does not prevent vertebral crush, because of tumor necrosis and secondary spine deformity. Vertebroplasty produces analgesia by solidifying the osteolytic lesion. It is only a palliative treatment. Vertebroplasty results in quick (1–3 days) disappearance of pain, vertebral consolidation, and spinal stability.[3, 8] Results are better (significant relief of pain and return to activities of normal living in more than 70% of patients) when spinal pain is the major symptom.[6]

Patients most suitable for vertebroplasty are those suffering from an osteolytic lesion of the vertebral body without rupture of the posterior wall, with or without vertebral collapse, and with severe pain. Unfortunately, patients often have extensive osteolytic lesions with vertebral collapse and osteolysis of the posterior wall. In these cases, vertebroplasty can be performed if there is no epidural invasion by tumor. It is important to inject both osteolytic and nonosteolytic parts of vertebral body with PMMA. Two punctures via the transpedicular approach are necessary when a pedicle is possibly destroyed.

Vertebroplasty is a palliative (not curative) treatment. Vertebroplasty should be performed before radiotherapy, because the analgesic effect is immediate after vertebroplasty and delayed after radiotherapy.[9] No modification of the radiotherapy protocol is needed after PMMA injection.[10]

For persons with neurologic symptoms, vertebroplasty can be an adjunct to surgery. It can precede or follow surgery to bring about consolidation of tumor level, limiting orthopedic devices and avoiding surgical anterior corpectomy. Corpectomy is a major surgical procedure when there are many metastases or when patient's health is poor. In cases with rupture of the posterior wall and extension into the spinal canal, cement injection must be performed very carefully to avoid extravertebral cementing.[6]

If an osteolytic lesion is present in the posterior arch or if there is significant extravertebral extension, vertebroplasty is not performed. Other substances (alcohol, Ethibloc) can be injected into the tumor to produce sclerosis.[3, 11] The excellent analgesic effect of vertebroplasty encourages the treatment of metastatic lesions outside the spine (especially hip metastases) via a percutaneous approach.[3, 12]

Vertebral Hemangioma

Vertebral hemangiomas are common, benign lesions (incidence about 10%).[13] These (usually) asymptomatic lesions have a characteristic radiologic appearance, including vertical thick trabeculations on plain films, decreased density on computed tomography (CT) and hyperintensity on T1-weighted images (because of abundant fat in the lesion). Rarely, vertebral hemangiomas are aggressive by clinical or radiologic criteria. Radiologic criteria for aggressiveness are lesion growth, bone destruction, vertebral collapse, absence of fat in the vertebral body (isointense or hypointense on T1WI MRI), and an active vascular component demonstrated after contrast injection by hyperintensity on T1WI MRI. Aggressive lesions are most often seen in thoracic region (Fig. 70–1).[13] Clinical criteria of aggressiveness are severe spinal pain or neurologic signs related to compression of the nerve root or spinal cord. Clinically aggressive spinal hemangiomas are frequently aggressive on radiologic examination, especially when there are neurologic signs.[6]

Vertebroplasty is indicated for radiologically or clinically aggressive spinal hemangioma. It has the following objectives: produce analgesia; assist in radiculomedullary decompression; spinal stabilization to avoid secondary deformity; arrest pseudotumoral vascular malformation.[6]

Severe focal spinal pain with vertebral body hemangioma and without radiologic evidence of aggressiveness is treated with vertebroplasty, with 90% success. When neurologic signs (with or without spinal pain) and a radiologically aggressive hemangioma are observed, vertebroplasty is the first step. Care must be taken to avoid injecting the epidural component with PMMA. Surgery is performed as a second step, when necessary. Surgical excision of the hemangioma is easy and bloodless.[6]

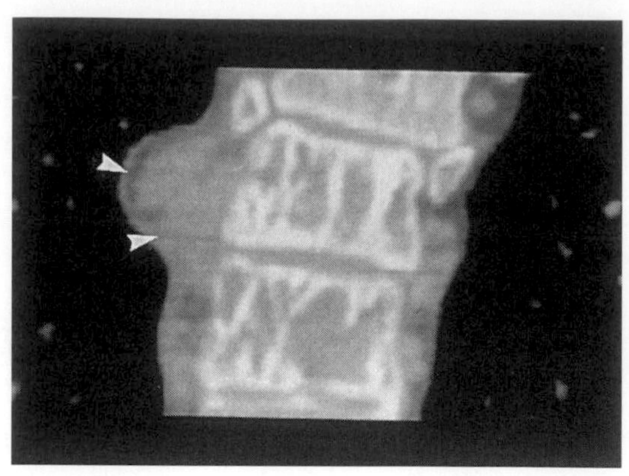

FIGURE 70–1 A CT-guided right posterolateral approach with a 10-gauge needle. (From Depriester C, et al: Percutaneous vertebroplasty: Indications, techniques, and complications. In *Connors JJ, Wojak JC [eds]: Interventional Neuroradiology: Strategies and Practical Techniques. Philadelphia, WB Saunders, 1999.)*

In the experience of Depriester, Deramond, and colleagues, vertebroplasty never aggravated the patient's clinical status.[6] In patients with progressive neurologic findings, they described rapid improvement in neurologic status after vertebroplasty because of diminution of pulsatility of the hemangioma or disappearance of the vascular shunt. They suggested the following guidelines, based on their 10 years of experience:

1. For acute or subacute cord compression, percutaneous vertebroplasty followed by decompressive laminectomy.
2. For patients with only severe spinal pain and radiologically aggressive vertebral hemangioma with an epidural component, percutaneous vertebroplasty without subsequent surgery.

MATERIALS AND DEVICES

1. Needle (MD Technologies: 1-800-338-0440)
   DBMNJ1104-11 G–4 in
   DBMNJ1106-11 G–6 in
   DBMNJ1304-11 G–4 in
2. Polymethylmethacrylate (PMMA cement)
   Howmedica Simplex
   Codman Cranioplastic Kit (Johnson & Johnson: 1-800-255-2500)
3. Barium (opacifying agent)
   Sterile barium sulfate (6-g packets) (Bryant Corporation: 1-781-935-0004)
   Unsterile barium sulfate (25-lb buckets) EZ–EM Corporation

4. Syringes
   1-mL Luer-Lok syringes (100/box)
   (1) Becton-Dickinson #309628 (Owen and Minor: 1-800-969-2742)
   (2) MSS011 (Merit Medical: 1-800-626-3748)

PREPROCEDURE PHASE

Patient Selection

The response to vertebroplasty is best when the patient has (1) one fracture that is not very compressed; (2) fracture less than 12 months old; (3) fracture older than 12 months but that is still hot on bone scan or has recently become more compressed. Patients with multiple fractures, severely compressed fractures, and old fractures certainly can benefit, but they probably do less well than the patients just described. The patient should be in significant pain and suffer lifestyle alterations because of pain from the fracture to be considered for vertebroplasty.

Before the procedure, every patient should have a detailed physical examination, MRI of the affected vertebra, and a radionuclide bone scan. Palpation of the spinous process of the affected vertebral body should elicit the pain that the patient attributes to the fracture. Bone scan confirms that the fracture is still active and, in cases of multiple fractures, helps to determine which fractures should be treated first. MRI helps to confirm that the patient's pain is not secondary to disc herniation, spinal stenosis, or infection. MRI also helps to plan the procedure, especially if the vertebral body is severely compressed.

Vertebroplasty is generally best performed in the midthoracic, lower thoracic, or lumbar spine. It is technically difficult to treat vertebral bodies above T5 (depending on patient size and anatomy). Patients whose previous spinal surgery was unsuccessful generally do not seem to respond as well to vertebroplasty. Young age is a relative contraindication to vertebroplasty because the long-term safety of the procedure is still unknown.

Informed Consent

Consent is obtained in front of the patient's family. I explain that the concept of replacing a diseased vertebral body with PMMA has been used since 1984. The procedure was developed in the United States by Jansen and Dion at the University of Virginia. I show a model of the spine and identify its parts. I explain that back pain can come from many different sources—compression fracture, disc herniation, spinal stenosis, or facet arthritis. I inform them that vertebroplasty will help the pain from compression fracture but will not do anything for pain of other causes in the spine.

I explain the following risks: infection, bleeding, contrast reaction, rib or pedicle fracture, exacerbation of pain (from leakage of PMMA to epidural or foraminal veins), paralysis. I assure the patient that these complications are unlikely to happen and that osteomyelitis and paralysis have not been reported. I emphasize that the procedure should be performed only if the patient is in significant pain and is willing to take a small risk to get relief. Some patients refuse the procedure at this point, but in my experience these are the ones with less pain, who do not need (and would not benefit from) the procedure anyway.

PROCEDURE

Anesthesia

M.A.C. Conscious sedation and local anesthesia are usually satisfactory.

Bone Trocar Placement

The patient's record is reviewed, including plain films, bone scan, and magnetic resonance images to decide which vertebra will be injected. The patient is placed in the prone position. Strict sterile technique is necessary. The patient's skin is prepared with Betadine and then draped. Anteroposterior (AP) and lateral scout films are taken. To obtain a good lateral view (in the thoracic region), it is first necessary to align the posterior ribs. Next oblique or cant the tube if necessary to ensure that the pedicles are exactly superimposed. With the flurotube in AP position, find the obliquity that projects the pedicle over the upper, outer third of the vertebral body. This point is marked with a hemostat and the skin punctured with a 27-gauge needle and infiltrated with lidocaine/bupivacaine. On a lateral projection it is determined that the needle is pointing in the proper direction to traverse the pedicle and end up in a good position near the center of the vertebral body. The AP and lateral views are used to adjust the needle as necessary until the proper path is confirmed. If the shorter needle has not reached the bone, a 22-gauge spinal needle is bounced up and down on the pedicle, infiltrating with generous amount of local anesthetic, which is also deposited in the needle tract on the way out.

With good local anesthesia, the procedure is very rarely painful. For large pedicles (lumbar, lower thoracic) I use an 11-gauge trocar and for smaller pedicles (midthoracic) a 13-gauge trocar. I advance the trocar down to pedicle and with a back-and-forth twisting motion get purchase in the bone. I start with the tip of the trocar in the upper outer third of the pedicle in most patients and direct the trocar into the vertebral body, verifying on AP and lateral views that the trocar is heading in the proper direction (Fig. 70–2). I adjust as necessary by using the beveled stylet to direct the trocar gently up or down. I do not twist the trocar too hard up or down because the pedicle could fracture. I place the tip of the trocar in the anterior third of the vertebral body when possible. The spine supports most weight on the anterior half of each vertebral body, so I attempt to fill in anteriorly as best I can. This position is generally away from large veins and offers the option of pulling the trocar back to fill the posterior portion of the vertebral body toward the end of the PMMA application.

Vertebral Body and Epidural Venography

Venography reveals the location of vertebral body veins and, so, indicates what PMMA will look like as it begins

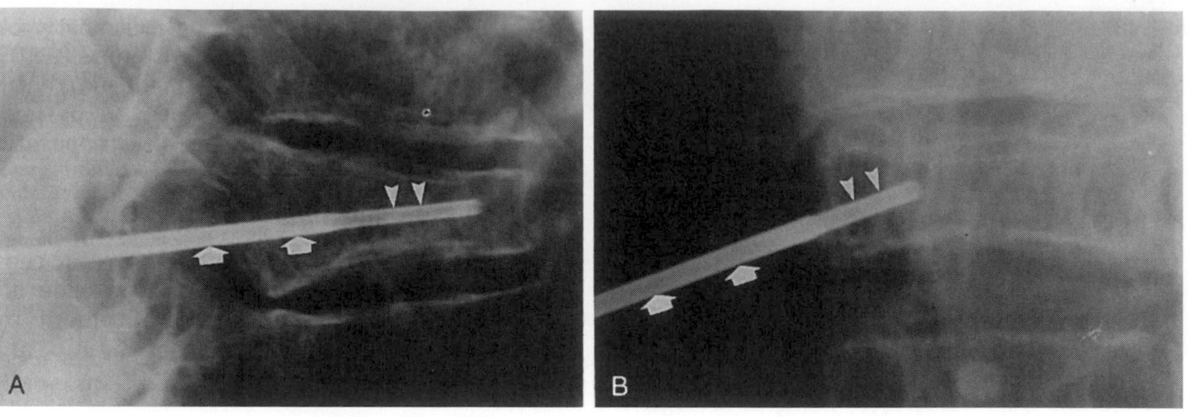

FIGURE 70–2 A, *Sagittal and* B, *frontal views of the posterolateral approach with a 10-gauge needle* (arrows) *and a 15-gauge biopsy needle* (arrowheads). *(From Depriester C, et al: Percutaneous vertebroplasty: Indications, techniques, and complications.* In *Connors JJ, Wojak JC [eds]: Interventional Neuroradiology: Strategies and Practical Techniques. Philadelphia, WB Saunders, 1999.)*

to enter the veins. Everyone does not recommend venography, but I believe it is very useful. I consider contrast allergy the only contraindication. A venogram image is placed on one of the monitors and is a useful reference if there is a question of venous filling. Venography also offers a chance to judge how much resistance will be felt when PMMA is injected into the vertebral body. In general, if it is difficult to inject contrast, it will be difficult to inject PMMA. The converse is usually true as well. PMMA viscosity can be adjusted so that it is either easy or difficult to inject. The trocar in preloaded with saline using a long spinal needle to avoid injecting a large amount of air into the vertebral body (a vascular space). Contrast is injected very slowly as the operator notes the amount of resistance to injection. When the trocar is in a good place, bone marrow will show a fine reticular blush before the paravertebral and epidural veins fill (Fig. 70–3). Venography also reveals whether the end plates and posterior wall of the vertebral body are intact.

Contrast usually leaks out of the fracture in the vertebral body. Contrast injection does not show a definite path for PMMA, because contrast is much less viscous than PMMA. It has a greater tendency to leak out of any fracture in the vertebral body, but PMMA does not always follow the same path. If contrast leaks from the vertebral body, PMMA may also, but PMMA injection can still be successful. In such cases, the viscosity of PMMA is altered to help to keep it in the vertebral body. If venography reveals that the trocar is in the middle of a large vertebral body vein, it should be pushed forward a few millimeters to avoid injecting directly into the vein. Pulling the trocar back does not work as well, since a large tract will remain that allows PMMA to enter the vein. Advancing the trocar usually seals the hole in the vein, allowing PMMA to flow into the vertebral body. Occasionally, contrast does not exit the vertebral body into the veins but instead stains the vertebral body or extravasates into the disc space. In this case, contrast injection should stop, since too much contrast in the vertebral body obscures the PMMA as it is being injected. If contrast stains the vertebral body, 20 to 30 mL of saline is injected to rinse contrast out of vertebral body.

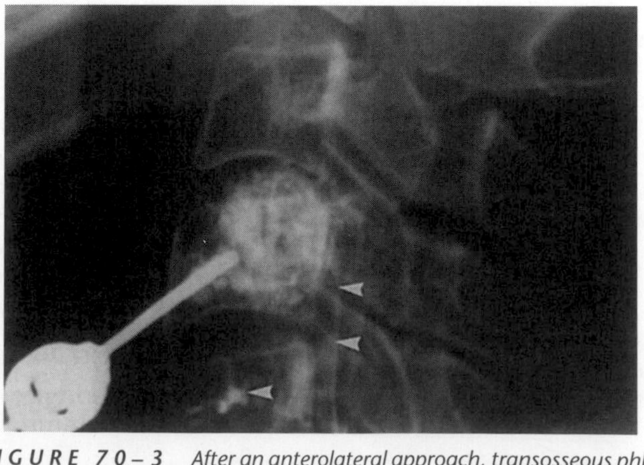

FIGURE 70–3 *After an anterolateral approach, transosseous phlebography shows the draining veins* (arrowheads). *(From Depriester C, et al: Percutaneous vertebroplasty: Indications, techniques, and complications.* In *Connors JJ, Wojak JC [eds]: Interventional Neuroradiology: Strategies and Practical Techniques. Philadelphia, WB Saunders, 1999.)*

Mixing PMMA

These instructions are for use of the Surgical Simplex kit (Howmedica). A sterile specimen cup (with measurement markers) used to hold surgical specimens is needed. One packet of PMMA from the kit is emptied into a bowl. About a third of the powder is put into the specimen cup (Simplex PMMA powder has 4 g of barium, the opacifying agent); then 3 g of sterile barium sulfate (half of the 6 g of sterile barium in the vial) is added. PMMA and barium are mixed with a sterile tongue depressor. The ampule of liquid monomer is opened, and 7 cc of liquid monomer added to the mixture of powder polymer and opacifying agent. All ingredients are mixed thoroughly with a sterile tongue depressor for about 1 min. The mixture should be about the consistency of thin pancake batter after mixing. If needed, more liquid monomer is added. (I put a 60-mL syringe without plunger on top of the liquid ampule to reduce volatile organic in the room.) Once the material is mixed, the cup is tipped to one side to pool the cement, which is sucked up slowly with a 10-mL syringe. The air is expelled from the syringe; about 8 to 9 mL of cement material remains. About 10 1-mL syringes are at hand with plungers out, ready to be backloaded with cement. About 0.4 mL of cement from the 10-mL syringe is injected into the back of each 1-mL syringe and the plungers are quickly replaced as each is filled. A filled 1-mL syringe is used to begin injecting. (Cement at the tip of the syringe polymerizes faster than unexposed cement.)

PMMA Injection

Before PMMA is injected, all remaining contrast is rinsed out of the trocar with saline. This step is necessary because any contrast remaining in the trocar would be confused with PMMA when it is injected. If venography shows very rapid venous filling or demonstrates a large vein near the needle tip or if contrast extravasates from end plates into the disc space, mixed PMMA should be relatively viscous. Cement should be thinner if the vertebral body is sclerotic or the patient has good bone density or if contrast during venography can be injected only with difficulty. If significant venous filling begins to occur, the operator should wait a minute or two, to allow the PMMA to harden a bit. More viscous cement is less likely than a thinner mixture to leak out of the veins. Another strategy is to pull the trocar back or to push it forward and inject in a different location. Because a new site will not have been investigated with venography and could harbor a large vein, cement is injected with caution. If PMMA extrudes into the disc, the same strategy is employed as when PMMA enters a vein: the operator waits for PMMA to harden or repositions the needle. Usually this seals the end plate fracture and allows the rest of the vertebral body to fill. Often it is difficult to inject PMMA into the vertebral body. A smaller quantity (0.2 mL) can be used or the trocar withdrawn a couple of millimeters. Often, this extra bit of room allows PMMA to flow into the vertebral body. PMMA is injected slowly, even if injection is easy and the vertebral body is filling properly. With faster injection, venous filling is more likely. Injection continues until the vertebral body is well filled, but is always stopped before PMMA leaks posteriorly into the epidural area or significantly fills a vein. It is almost always necessary to inject both sides of a vertebral body via a bipedicular approach. Occasionally (i.e., in the thoracic spine), it is possible to fill a vertebral body satisfactorily with a single-pedicle approach. If there is doubt about where PMMA is going, injecting must stop. The degree of pain relief is not an indicator of the degree of PMMA filling. Although the goal is to fill the vertebral body as completely as possible, good pain relief is possible with a modest filling (Fig. 70–4).

POSTPROCEDURE ORDERS

The patient remains at bed rest for few hours (mainly to allow neuroleptic anesthesia to wear off; PMMA hardens in a few minutes). Medications for postoperative pain are used as needed, and a muscle relaxant or valium if the patient has significant muscle spasm. Sitting and standing up are allowed the morning after the procedure. In most cases, postoperative pain and muscle spasm are not severe and resolve in a few days. Preprocedure narcotic doses are progressively tapered. Follow-up by phone is in order after a week, or earlier if the patient has a problem.

All patients are examined 6 weeks after vertebroplasty and plain films are obtained to examine the result. The same examination is performed 6 months later and annually thereafter.[6]

If a patient who had been doing better suddenly becomes worse, a new compression fracture may have developed. In these cases, I order a new bone scan or MRI to evaluate for a new fracture. The possibility of osteomyelitis should be kept in mind, and it is one reason that I am quick to evaluate with MRI if the patient feels worse.

COMPLICATIONS

Fortunately, complications are rare. If the patient complains of chest pain after the procedure, rib fracture must

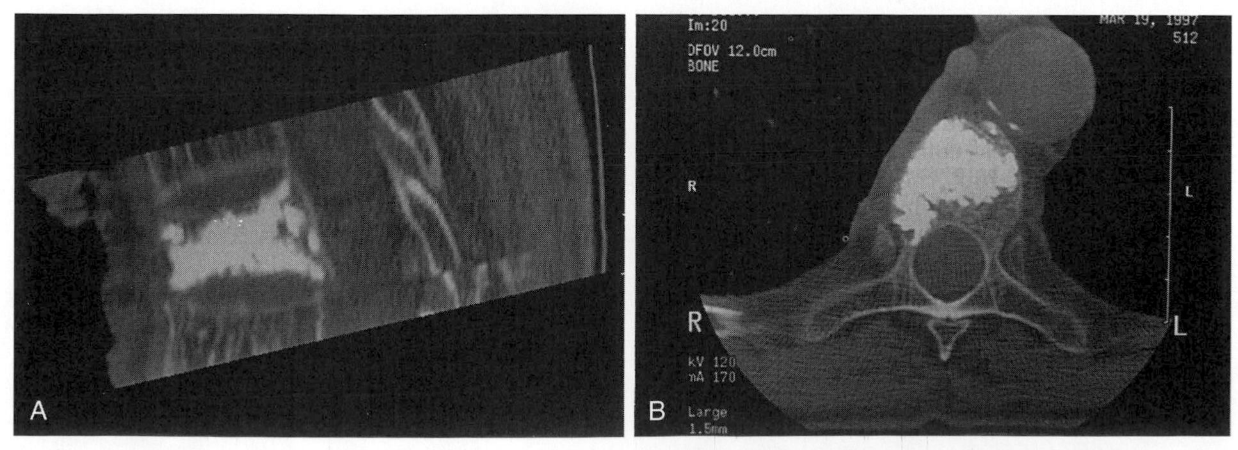

FIGURE 70–4 *Sagittal,* A, *and axial,* B, *views demonstrate a satisfactory injection in the vertebra without extravertebral leakage. (From Depriester C, et al: Percutaneous vertebroplasty: Indications, techniques, and complications.* In *Connors JJ, Wojak JC [eds]: Interventional Neuroradiology: Strategies and Practical Techniques. Philadelphia, WB Saunders, 1999.)*

be ruled out with a rib series and pulmonary embolus with a ventilation-perfusion scan. Severe back pain can be a sign of a fractured pedicle or transverse process, both easily seen on computed tomography.[14]

New radicular pain can be caused by migration of PMMA into the epidural venous plexus. Computed tomography demonstrates this very easily. The levels above and below the treated disc are viewed to look for migration into adjacent levels. Nerve root blocks may be effective, or laminectomy may be necessary. Paralysis has been reported but is very uncommon. Precautions should be taken when injecting above L1, with attention to the posterior vertebral body wall and ensuring that PMMA is not allowed to flow into the epidural venous plexus.[14]

CONCLUSION

Vertebroplasty appears to be a promising pain management technique that is useful in the treatment of certain painful conditions. Additional experience with these techniques is needed to refine patient selection criteria and the procedure itself.

REFERENCES

1. Depriester C, Deramond H, et al: Percutaneous vertebroplasty with acrylic cement in the treatment of osteoporotic vertebral crush fracture. Neuroradiology 33:149–152, 1991.
2. Deramond H, et al: Percutaneous vertebroplasty with methylmethacrylate: Technique, method, results (Abstract). Radiology 177:352, 1990.
3. Deramond H, Depriester C, et al: Percutaneous vertebroplasty. *In* Wilson D (ed): Interventional Radiology of the Musculoskeletal System. London, Edward Arnold, 1995, pp 133–142.
4. Heiss JD, et al: Brief report: Relief of spinal cord compression from vertebral hemangioma by intralesional injection of absolute alcohol. N Engl J Med 331:508–511, 1994.
5. Bascoulergue Y, et al: Percutaneous injection of methylmethacrylate in the vertebral body for the treatment of various diseases. Percutaneous vertebroplasty (Abstract). Radiology 169:372, 1988.
6. Depriester C, et al: Percutaneous vertebroplasty: Indication, technique and complications. *In* Connors J (ed): Interventional Neuroradiology. Philadelphia, WB Saunders, 1999, pp 346–357.
7. Shepherd S: Radiotherapy and management of metastatic bone pain. Clin Radiol 39:547–550, 1988.
8. Weil A, et al: Spinal metastases: Indication for and results of percutaneous injection of acrylic surgical cement. Radiology 199:241–247, 1996.
9. Garmatis CJ, et al: The effectiveness of radiation therapy in the treatment of bone metastases from breast cancer. Radiology 126:235–237, 1978.
10. Murray JA, et al: Irradiation of polymethylmethacrylate. J Bone Joint Surg 56A:311–312, 1974.
11. Cotton A, et al: Percutaneous vertebroplasty for osteolytic metastases and myeloma: Effects of the percentage of lesion filling and the leakage of methylmethacrylate at clinical follow-up. Radiology 200:525–530, 1996.
12. Cotton A, et al: Malignant acetabular osteolysis: Percutaneous injection of acrylic bone cement. Radiology 197:307–310, 1995.
13. Fox MW, et al: The natural history and management of symptomatic and asymptomatic vertebral hemangioma. J Neurosurg 78:36–45, 1993.
14. Jansen M, et al: Percutaneous polymethylmethacrylate vertebroplasty in the treatment of osteoporotic vertebral body compression fracture: Technical aspects. AJNR 18:1897–1904, 1997.

CHAPTER • 71

Chymopapain Chemonucleolysis

Sunil K. Singh, MD

Mixter and Barr introduced laminectomy for removal of disc herniation in 1934.[1] Barr wrote,[2] "Some of the people here think that open surgery for disc lesions will probably be a thing of past. This seems incredible, but I suspect that it may be true. We ought to be able to absorb some of this collagen tissue, which is there, biochemically. I will be surprised if some of us here do not see the day when disc surgery is abolished or nearly so. . . . Discs are 90% water. Why should we have to bail them out with surgical instruments?"

In 1941, Jansen isolated the enzyme chymopapain from crude papain, a proteolytic enzyme from papaya latex.[3] In 1956, Thomas demonstrated selective affinity of chymopapain for chondromucoprotein.[4] This prompted Lynan Smith to conduct experimental and clinical research with chymopapain. In 1963, Smith reported dissolution of nucleus pulposus without effect on surrounding tissues. Smith reported on human clinical trials in 1964.[5] He coined the term *chemonucleolysis* to describe dissolution of nucleus pulposus with intradiscal injection of chymopapain, which catalyzes rapid hydrolysis of the chondromucoprotein portion of nucleus pulposus. By 1975, 17,000 patients were treated experimentally with chymopapain in the United States with 72% good results. In 1980, seven U.S. centers conducted a double-blind study whose findings showed statistically significant success for chymopapain as compared with placebo.[6] In 1982, the U.S. Food and Drug Administration (FDA) approved intradiscal injection of chymopapain for managing herniated nucleus pulposus with sciatica. A double-blind study by Fraser in Australia showed the same successful results.[7] Another double-blind study published in *Spine* in 1988 demonstrated similar successful results.[8]

In 1983, 6214 orthopedic and neurologic surgeons participated in 1-day training sessions consisting of lectures and radiographically controlled mannequins to demonstrate proper needle placement via a lateral approach (introduced by Brown). Although trainers emphasized repeatedly that chymopapain should be injected by the lateral approach and under no circumstances by a posterior (Lindblom) or posterolateral (Erlacher) approach, many inexperienced surgeons ignored this warning and major complications resulted. It became clear that 1 day of training was insufficient to achieve competence. Acute transverse myelitis was a major complication reported by Smith Laboratories to the FDA. Subsequent review showed that only one patient demonstrated definite evidence of acute transverse myelitis, in retrospect an incidental finding.[9, 10] In a double-blind study, Gogan and Fraser reported that a patient developed acute transverse myelitis after saline injection.[11] Because of these problems chymopapain chemonucleolysis (CNL) procedures dropped dramatically in the United States. During the same period and since, the use of chymopapain increased in Europe and elsewhere. At the American Association of Neurological Surgeons (AANS) meeting in 1986, Professor Mario Brock of Germany said that the major problem in the United States was the inadequacy of 1-day training. In Europe, he said, such training is not allowed.

Laminectomy can result in failed back syndrome and other complications. In the United States, there are more than 2000 pain clinics, the majority of whose patients suffer the sequelae of failed back operations. Major complications of CNL due to technical errors occurred before 1987. Anaphylaxis is no longer a problem with CNL because of routine use of immunoassays (Chymofast chymopapain sensitivity test), and possibly because of the administration of histamine H1 and H2 blockers.

Of all percutaneous intradiscal procedures, only chymopapain has been approved as acceptable by the Guideline Panel for the Agency for Health Care Policy and Research[12]: "The Panel found evidence that percutaneous discectomy is significantly less efficacious than chymopapain in treating patients with lumbar disc herniation."

INDICATIONS

Patient Selection

A history of sciatica and evidence of lumbar disc herniation on physical examination of the lumbar spine is the keystone. Magnetic resonance imaging (MRI), myelography, computed tomography (CT), discography, and electromyelography (EMG) are only confirmatory of examination findings. Chymopapain is indicated for unremitting sciatica resulting from herniation of the nucleus pulposus that has not responded to conservative treatment. McCulloch found that patients with two symptoms, two signs, and one positive diagnostic test for herniated nucleus pulposus are more likely than others to respond to chymopapain chemonucleolysis. Using this "Rule of Five" (Table 71–1), *symptoms* should include leg pain dominant over back pain, specific neurologic symptoms such as paresthesia in the leg or foot; *signs* such as straight-leg raising limited to 50% of normal with or without crossover pain and with or without a positive bow-string sign, and at least two neurologic abnormalities, such as reflex abnormality, wasting, weakness, or sensory loss; and myelographic, CT, or MRI confirmation.[13, 14]

Any profound acute or progressive neurologic change, particularly cauda equina syndrome, is a contraindication to chymopapain, and surgical decompression is the treatment of choice.[15] Age limits for chymopapain CNL have become less defined. The majority of studies were done in the 18- to 60-year age group because of concern about possible effects on juvenile discs and a belief that, in patients older than 60 years, the degenerative process would deplete proteoglycan in the nucleus pulposus. Today there is evidence that adolescent herniated discs respond well to chymopapain. CNL may be appropriate also for elderly patients, particularly some in their 80s who have hydrated discs on MRI. In one long-term study of patients aged 60 to 80 years who were treated with chymopapain, Benoist[16] found that results were just as good in this group as among younger patients provided no spinal canal stenosis was associated. This study showed results similar to those of a European multicenter study that compared results in different age groups.[17] Sutton reported a study of CNL with patients younger than 19 and found the results to be comparable to those for an age-matched cohort previously subjected to open discectomy. The surgery group had a higher recurrence rate—25% as compared with 8% for those treated by CNL.[18, 19] In one more recent study on adolescents, Wilson and Mulholland reported a long-term success rate of 83%.[20]

TABLE 71–1 **Criteria for Patient Selection for Chemonucleolysis**

Sciatica or buttock pain should predominate over back pain.
Pattern of pain and paresthesia in lower limb should be in a nerve root distribution.
Nerve root tension sign should be present:
  Reduction of straight-leg raising on the affected side by typical leg pain.
  Reproduction of typical leg pain by straight-leg raising on opposite side (crossed straight-leg raising).
  Radiating leg pain when pressure is applied to the tibial nerve in popliteal fossa (bow-string sign).
  Positive femoral stretch sign.
If signs of nerve root dysfunction are present (wasting, weakness, sensory loss, reflex change), they should indicate involvement of a single nerve root.
Neuroimaging (CT, MRI, myelography) confirmation of diagnosis.
  Disc herniation that is not sequestered and where there is nerve root.
  Compromise at a level congruent with clinical signs.

TABLE 71–2 **Contraindications to Chemonucleolysis**

Absolute
  Allergy to chymopapain
  Cauda equina syndrome
  Pregnancy
  Normal CT/MRI/discogram
Relative
  Severe, uncontrolled diabetes with peripheral neuropathy
  Severe spondylolisthesis
  Old infection of disc or vertebra
  Unsuccessful surgery at symptomatic level
  Emotional instability
  Medicolegal cases
  Language barrier

CONTRAINDICATIONS

A major contraindication to CNL is chymopapain allergy (Table 71–2). A second injection of chymopapain is generally contraindicated because the initial injection may have sensitized the patient. This belief was challenged by Sutton, who performed the Chymofast test (on serum) on a series of 33 patients to determine the immunoglobulin E (IgE) titer before giving them a second injection. Only 9% had a reaction. The last 12 patients in this study were pretreated with histamine H1 and histamine H2 blockers, and they had no allergic reactions.[21]

A progressive and significant neurologic deficit such as cauda equina syndrome is a contraindication, because chymopapain response is time dependent and cauda equina syndrome is an emergency that requires prompt relief of pressure on nerve roots.

Pregnancy is a contraindication because no one has studied pregnant women. The most obvious absolute contraindication is demonstration of a normal disc on MRI, CT, or discography.

Relative contraindications include grade II or higher spondylolisthesis and an old infection of a disc or vertebra. A history of unsuccessful open discectomy at a symptomatic level is associated with fewer successful outcomes of CNL because of the presence of fibrosis. Emotional instability (major psychiatric illness) and the complicating factor of possible medicolegal action are other relative contraindications that have been associated with poor results. Patients receiving Workers Compensation have poorer results, probably because they lack the motivation to participate as necessary for a successful outcome.[22] A language or other communication barrier makes it difficult to explain the procedure thoroughly and may increase the risk of medicolegal action. Uncontrolled severe diabetes associated with neuropathy can be considered a relative contraindication.

TECHNIQUE

CNL should be done by a physician who can accurately place the needle in the disc by thinking three-dimensionally while working with only two-dimensional images. Risk of anaphylactic reaction (current prevalence 0.3%) is minimized by doing a Chymofast test and premedicating with H1 and H2 receptor blockers (diphenhydramine and cimetidine or ranitidine, respectively) 24 hours before the injection.[23] Premedication does not prevent an anaphylactic reaction but is thought to suppress the reaction somewhat so that treatment is more effective. Oral diphenhydramine or hydroxyzine, 50 mg three times a day, can serve as an H1 blocker, and ranitidine, 300 mg twice a day, as an H2 blocker.[24] Steroids are thought to stabilize cell membranes and thus reduce the release of chemical mediators for anaphylaxis. Intravenous methylprednisolone, 250 mg, can be given 1 hour before the procedure. No statistical evidence supports this position, however. Oral or intravenous hydration before injection is very important.

Anesthesia

General anesthesia is to be avoided. Awake patients can alert the physician to the early warning symptoms of impending anaphylaxis, including the burning sensation, tingling, coldness, and nausea.[25] They will also appreciate the nerve root's being touched by the needle and thus prevent neural trauma. A neuroleptic anesthetic using intravenous agents such as midazolam and fentanyl can be effectively titrated to the degree of pain experienced by the patient. General anesthesia has the advantage of allowing intubation in case of laryngospasm of anaphylaxis, but succinylcholine or tracheostomy can accommodate this complication in patients not under general anesthesia. An emergency tray to treat anaphylaxis must be ready.

Procedure

Site

The injection procedure can be performed in an operating room or in a special procedure room of a radiology department, as long as the necessary equipment, anesthesia, emergency cart, and trained personnel are available.

Positioning

The prone or lateral decubitus position is satisfactory, as long as the patient can be properly positioned and stabilized to allow a lateral approach to the disc space.[26] In a typical properly conducted procedure, radiation exposure of the patient is equivalent to that of a five-view lumbosacral spine series.

Needle Placement

After sterile skin preparation, the area is draped as for any surgical procedure. The disc space is identified with the help of a C-arm fluoroscope. Disc margins are made clear by craniocaudal movement of the fluro tube. The tube is next rotated obliquely to bring the superior articular process into the midline. An 18-gauge 7-in needle is introduced immediately anterior to the superior articular process and superior to the transverse process via the triangular safe zone. It is advanced in 1- to 2-cm increments in a "stop and look and go" fashion, to allow a change in course if necessary. Progress is viewed on anteroposterior and lateral projections of the C-arm fluoroscope, which must be of sufficient quality to provide a clear view of the area. The needle tip should be at the center of the disc upon completion. In most cases, the entry point in the skin for either the L4–L5 or the L5–S1 disc space is at the level of the iliac crest (very close to each other). The rubbery annulus is easily felt with the tip of the 18-gauge needle. A two-needle technique offers an advantage for entering the L5–S1 disc and is the preferred method at any level. To facilitate entry into the disc space, the terminal 2 cm of a 22-gauge needle is curved so that the bevel lies on the convexity. A 7-in, 22-gauge needle passed through the 3.5-in, 18-gauge needle allows greater accuracy in needle placement. A 22-gauge bent needle will allow a curved path from the side of the bevel. This technique often saves the repositioning of 18-gauge needle. With the two-needle technique, it is possible in almost all cases to place the tip of the 22-gauge needle within nucleus and thus avoid annular injection.[27] Fluoroscopy precautions include lead aprons for all personnel in the procedure or operating room. Lead gloves and avoiding exposure of the operator's hands also reduce radiation exposure.

Confirmation of Proper Needle Placement

Discography should be routinely used to confirm needle placement. Intrathecal spread of contrast material should alert the physician to terminate the procedure. Edwards demonstrated a much higher success rate with CNL when contrast material injected immediately before chymopapain had outlined the disc herniation, as compared with those cases when contrast material was confined within nucleus or inner annulus.[28] In addition, demonstration of epidural leakage of contrast alerts the physician to inject chymopapain more slowly to produce greater binding of enzyme to the nucleus. Epidural leakage is not a contraindication to chymopapain injection. For discography, water-soluble non-ionizing contrast agents are least irritating. Another method for confirming needle placement is discometry. Discometry involves determining the resistance in injecting water or saline instead of contrast agent.[29] Injection of water into the nucleus pulposus or leaking disc gives less resistance than an annular injection. A normal disc can hold as much as 2 mL of fluid with considerable resistance.

Drug Reconstitution and Injection Technique

Chymopapain is reconstituted with sterile water (free of bacteriostatic agents and preservatives that might inactivate the enzyme) and drawn into separate syringes for testing and injection, to avoid deactivation of the enzyme by reflux. Alcohol used on the vial stopper should evaporate before a needle is inserted because alcohol contamination will neutralize chymopapain.[30] The average dose of chymopapain is 2000 units. Some physicians use 200 units as a test dose to determine sensitivity. After 10 min, remaining chymopapain is injected slowly over a 4-min period. The needle is kept in place for 5 min before it is withdrawn. Since the reaction does not appear to be dose-related, a test dose seems to be of doubtful value. Some studies suggest that 1000 units may be sufficient and that it seems to reduce much of the postoperative muscle spasm and back pain, but others found no reduction in postinjection pain. If a low dose is used, it is appropriate to use 1000 units in 2 mL volume for dispersion.[31] Enzyme should be injected slowly and with the least possible force, to avoid unnecessary intradiscal pressure and, theoretically, production of cauda equina syndrome by sudden disc extrusion. The needle stylet is replaced and the needle is withdrawn. Abdel-Salam and colleagues recommend paradiscal injection of local anesthetic after chymopapain injection to reduce the incidence of back muscle spasm. Since 95% of allergic reactions such as anaphylactic shock occur within 15 min, observation in the operating or procedure room should continue for this time before the patient is transported to the recovery room, unless it is nearby and fully equipped for resuscitation.[32] The patient is observed for about 1 hour in the recovery room, then in ambulatory surgery unit for about 6 hours, and is then discharged.

Postprocedure Care

Instructions are given for getting out of bed without straining the back, gradual ambulation as tolerated, and other patient education. Any movement that is painful should be avoided. Sitting is poorly tolerlated and should be avoided initially. Sciatica or radiating pain is often relieved promptly by CNL, but back pain after the procedure is frequent (prevalence 20% to 40%). Back pain is managed with ice packs, heating pads, analgesics, muscle relaxants, nonsteroidal antiinflammatory drugs, and corset-type support. Walking and sidestroke swimming are started almost immediately, and exercise is gradually increased in duration and intensity. Patients are encouraged to return to work as soon as possible. They can return to light or sedentary work in 1 to 2 weeks and, with proper reconditioning, to medium to heavy work in 6 weeks, depending on pain relief and the pre-injection condition of the muscles.

COMPLICATIONS

The vast majority of complications (87%) occurred before the end of 1984, during the first 2 years of general use of chymopapain CNL in the United States, and none have been reported since July 1987.[33]

Immune Mediated

The most common serious complication of chymopapain CNL is an allergic reaction, specifically, anaphylactic shock. Its reported prevalence was about 1%. With routine serum IgE testing (Chymofast test), the incidence has dropped to about 0.3%. Reports continue to show a sex ratio of 10 women to 1 man and of 3 black women to 1 white woman. IgE testing is 99% accurate. A postmarketing survey by Boots (USA) Company for 1987 to 1988 shows an overall rate of anaphylaxis of 0.18%.[23] Use of H1 and H2 blocking agents (which do not influence the incidence of anaphyalxis) has rendered all reactions more amenable to treatment. The drug of choice for anaphylactic reactions is epinephrine, 0.5 to 1.0 mL of a 1 : 10,000 solution, given intravenously or intramuscularly. Epinephrine is approximately 200 times stronger than ephedrine. Oxygen (100%) and infusion of crystalloids and colloids are used to combat hypovolemic shock. Dopamine may be used if sustained adrenergic support is needed. Dopamine, 5 μg/kg/min, increases cardiac output and improves renal blood flow. Less dangerous allergic reactions include rash and urticaria; they respond to antihistamines and may require oral or injectable steroids.

Neurologic

Reported neurologic complications were due to improper intrathecal injection of chymopapain. Acute transverse myelitis identified in one patient who had had CNL about 3 weeks earlier could not conclusively be attributed to enzyme; it may have been only an unfortunate coincidence. In five other patients, acute transverse myelitis was suspected, but on subsequent investigation none was found to be due to chymopapain. Since April 15, 1984, more than 135,000 chymopapain injections have been given in the United States, and no new cases of acute transverse myelitis have been reported.[10]

Discitis

The term *discitis* has commonly been associated with CNL because of the exacerbation of back pain that frequently follows the procedure. Radiographic evidence of discitis after CNL has been reported in 1% of patients[29] and has generally been regarded as the result of a chemical or an aseptic process. The bactericidal effect of chymopapain has been the main explanation for the low incidence of bacterial discitis after CNL.[29] The incidence of discitis can be greatly reduced by observing strict aseptic technnique and giving a preoperative antibiotic such as intravenous cephazolin.[34]

FAILED CHEMONUCLEOLYSIS

When sciatica remains unrelieved after 6 weeks or disabling back pain persists beyond 3 months, CNL has failed. A persistent disc herniation, a free fragment, and nerve root canal stenosis are common causes of persistent sciatica. Discogenic back pain, facet arthritis, and discitis are possible causes of continued disabling back pain. Persistent sciatica requires further clinical evaluation, including assessment of any alteration in the pattern of pain and of changes in nerve root tension or neurologic signs. Before open surgery is undertaken, it is wise to reinvestigate the patient with MRI, CT, or CT myelography. Results of laminectomy for failed CNL are quite satisfactory.[35, 36] Brock and colleagues concluded in a study that previous unsuccessful CNL has no influence on either short-term or long-term results of subsequent microsurgery.[35] Disc fragment excision alone is required for a persistent herniation or a free fragment of disc tissue. Nerve root canal decompression is necessary for root canal stenosis. Discogenic back pain with restricted mobility is occasionally severe enough to warrant single-level surgical stabilization, provided that adjacent discs are essentially normal on MRI or discography.

Post-CNL Laminectomy Compared with Repeat Laminectomy

In a prospective 1- to 13-year follow-up of 53 post-CNL laminectomy patients and 50 repeat discectomy patients, long-term results were better for the post-CNL laminectomy group than for those who had repeat laminectomy.[37]

LONG-TERM RESULTS

Long-term follow-up of 3120 patients of 13 investigators (aged 7 to 20 years) who underwent CNL shows successful results for 71% to 93% (average 77%).[38] A Norwegian paper reported 92% successful results after CNL.[39] Nordby and Wright's reported average was 76.2% from a review of 45 studies published between 1985 and 1993.[40] Wilson and Mulholland concluded,[41] "The recurrence rate after CNL has proved to be at least as low as that of surgical discectomy, and the durability of a successful outcome following CNL is significantly better than following surgery." Gogan and coworkers' 10-year follow-up of Fraser's 10-year double-blind study comparing CNL with placebo showed successful results in 80% of CNL patients and 35% in the saline group.[42]

REPEAT CNL

Sutton was the first surgeon to report successful results from CNL performed in Canada.[21] Since then, similar success rates have been reported by Deutman and coworkers in the Netherlands.[43] Repeat chymopapain injection is not approved by the FDA at present, but with the availability of IgE chymopapain test and pre-CNL preparation of patients with H1 and H2 blockers, there is no reason to withhold this valuable procedure from patients who had good long-term results from their initial laminectomy and have either a recurrent herniated disc or a herniated disc on the opposite side (at the same level or another).

CERVICAL CHEMONUCLEOLYSIS

During the past decade, reports from Europe have claimed favorable results for cervical CNL in a few small series of patients.[44-46] More recently, Krause and colleagues reported results for 190 patients with cervical radiculopathy from cervical disc herniation treated by CNL.[47] The majority of patients had symptoms between 6 weeks to 3 months, and the majority of lesions occurred at C6–C7 (120 cases) or C5–C6 (57 cases). The mean age of patients was 42 years and most were men. The procedure was carried out through a right-sided anterolateral approach. Very slow injection of 0.7 to 0.8 mL (1500 units) of Chymodiactin was preceded by discography. Successful outcomes were reported for 86% of patients within 1 week of the procedure. Results were observed far sooner than with lumbar CNL, as reflected by a relatively rapid reduction of disc herniation in 80% of cases subsequently assessed by CT. Complications reported included a case of discitis attributed to a gastrointestinal organism. Only 5% of patients required operation for failure, and the authors concluded that there was no justification for the restrictions on use of chymodiactin in the cervical spine that had been imposed by the manufacturer. Castresana and colleagues conducted a prospective study to evaluate the effectiveness of chymopapain injection for cervical disc herniation and to establish the effectiveness of treatment by MRI follow-up. The study group consisted of 87 patients with cervical radiculopathy from cervical disc herniation treated by CNL.[48] In most cases, symptoms disappeared within hours or the first few days after injection. There were no incidents or complications. Two patients reported itching in the feet. Lower neck pain was a frequent finding after chymopapain injection. Three procedures were failures, and those patients were treated with surgery at the injected level 1 month to 1 year later. Sixty-eight patients were examined by MRI 2 weeks to 51 months after chymopapain injection to determine its effect on disc herniation. In 51 cases (70.8%), herniation disappeared altogether and in 9 cases (12.5%) almost completely. In 7 cases (9.7%) herniation was significantly reduced, and in 5 (6.9%) no significant change in disc morphology was observed. Of those 5 patients, 2 achieved a satisfactory result and only one required fusion. The investigators reported, "Effectiveness of chemonucleolysis in dissolving the soft disc component and decompressing the nerve root is evidenced by the rapid disappearance of symptoms experienced by 90% patients and total recovery from sensory and motor deficits in most cases, also confirmed by other authors. The total lack of complications with cervical chymopapain nucleolysis makes it especially attractive as compared with conventional surgery. MRI follow-up examination of injected discs confirms the enzyme's rapid lytic action on the soft component, removing or significantly reducing 83% of soft cervical disc herniations." I achieved similar results (80%–90%) among about 50 patients 1 have treated in the past 3 years.

ALTERNATIVE ENZYMES

Collagenase demonstrated a wide range of safety in all tissues except through intrathecal injection. No allergy was demonstrated in guinea pig studies. An initial group of 52 patients had a 78% success rate and no systemic or local toxic effects, but the phase III investigation was aborted in 1984 when operative findings in Germany revealed involvement of end plates, bone, ligament, and epidural fat. It was determined that collagenase used in German studies was more potent than that used in the United States. Pain relief is slow with collagenase, which usually takes effect within 3 to 6 weeks. The major action of collagenase is on collagen, whereas chymopapain has no effect on collagen.

Chondroitinase ABC is an enzyme from the bacterium *Proteus vulgaris* that has lytic action on the nucleus pulposus comparable to that of chymopapain. Investigation is under way in Japan and the United States.

Cathepsin G (obtained from human neutrophil leukocytes), *chymotrypsin* (purified from human pancreatic juices), and *cathepsin B* (purified from human liver) have been injected into rabbit discs, and all are effective in removing the nucleus pulposus. The potency of cathepsin G and chymotrypsin is in the range of chymopapain's, whereas cathepsin B is about half as effective. Chymotrypsin has been used for some years in one type of cataract surgery, to digest zonules of lens. No antigenic response has been noted in humans during these procedures.[49]

SUMMARY

Chymopapain injection is a safe and effective procedure when performed properly. Results are similar to those of surgical discectomy in relieving radiculitis from herniated nucleus pulposus. The most important advantage of CNL over laminectomy is that it does not produce scar tissue, a serious complication that can occur after laminectomy. The advantage of CNL over percutaneous discectomy is that chymopapain may be injected into noncontained extruded discs as long as the fragment is contiguous with the disc interspace. CNL may be performed as an outpatient procedure in a radiology suite, to obviate the occasional risk of complications from general anesthesia and the tremendous operating room costs. CNL is substantially less expensive than laminectomy in short-term and long-term results. Most poor results are related to ill-advised patient selection or technical error. Chymopapain is not neurotoxic. It is an allergenic foreign protein and can cause anaphylaxis, which can be reduced or modified by a Chymofast test and preinjection use of H1 and H2 blockers. The rates of death, infection, and neurologic complications are significantly lower with CNL than with laminectomy. The choice of CNL as an alternative to laminectomy should be offered to every patient who meets the criteria for surgery. Research is in progress to find a chemonucleolytic enzyme that is safer and more effective.

REFERENCES

1. Mixter WJ, Barr JS: Rupture of the intervertebral disc with involvement of the spinal canal. N Engl J Med 211:210–215, 1934.
2. Barr JS: Lumbar disc lesions in retrospect and prospect. Clin Orthop 129:4–8, 1977.
3. Jansen EF, Balls AK: Chymopapain: A new crystalline proteinase from papaya latex. J Biol Chem 137:459–460, 1941.
4. Thomas L: Reversible collapse of rabbit ears intravenous papain and prevention of recovery by cortisone. J Exp Med 104:245–252, 1956.
5. Smith L: Enzyme dissolution of the nucleus pulposus in humans. JAMA 187:137–140, 1964.
6. Javid MJ, Nordby EJ, et al: Safety and efficacy of chymopapain in herniated nucleus pulposus with sciatica. Results of a randomized double-blind study. JAMA 249:2489–2494, 1983.
7. Fraser RD: Chymopapain for the treatment of intervertebral disc herniation. The final report of a double blind study. Spine 8:815–818, 1984.
8. Dabezies DJ, Langford K, et al: Safety and efficacy of chymopapain in the treatment of sciatica due to herniated nucleus pulposus. Results of randomized double-blind study. Spine 13:561–565, 1988.
9. Eguro H: Transverse myelitis following chemonucleolysis. Report of a case. J Bone Joint Surg 65A:328–330, 1983.
10. Nordby EJ, Wright PH: Safety of chemonucleolysis. Adverse effects reported in the USA 1982–1991. Clin Orthop 293:123–134, 1993.
11. Gogan WJ, Fraser RD: Chymopapain. A 10-year double blind study. Spine 7:388–394, 1992.
12. US Department of Health and Human Services: Acute low back pain problems in adults. The Guideline Panel for the Agency for Health Care Policy and Research in the United States, 1994.
13. McCulloch JA: Chemonucleolysis. J Bone Joint Surg 59:45–52, 1977.
14. McCulloch JA: Chemonucleolysis. Experience with 2000 cases. Clin Orthop 146:128–135, 1980.
15. Nordby EJ: Diagnosis and patient selection. *In* Brown JE, Nordby EJ (eds): Chemonucleolysis. Thorofare, NJ, Slack, 1985, pp 45–60.
16. Benoist M: Lumbar discal herniation in the elderly: Long-term results of chymopapain chemonucleolysis. Eur Spine J 2:149–152, 1993.
17. Benoist M, Mulholland R: Chemonucleolysis: Results of a European survey. Acta Orthop Belg 49:32–47, 1983.
18. Sutton CJ Jr: Current concepts in chemonucleolysis. International Congress and Symposium Series. J R Soc Med 72:205–211, 1985.
19. Sutton CJ Jr: Chemonucleolysis in the management of herniated lumbar discs in the adolescent. Presented at International Intradiscal Therapy Society meeting, Fort Lauderdale, FL, March 10, 1988.
20. Wilson LF, Mulholland RC: Adolescent disc protrusions: A long-term follow-up of chymopapain therapy. Eur Spine J 1(3):156–162, 1991.
21. Sutton CJ Jr: Repeat chemonucleolysis. Clin Orthop 206:45–49, 1986.
22. Greenough CG, Fraser RD: The effects of compensation on recovery from low-back injury. Spine 14:947–955, 1989.
23. Periodic adverse drug experience to the FDA on Chymodiactin (1987): The Boots (USA) Company, Inc., Lincolnshire, Illinois.
24. Philbin DM, Moss J: The use of H1 and H2 histamine antagonists with morphine anaesthesia: A double-blind study. Anaesthesiology 55:292–296, 1981.
25. Hall BB, McCulloch JA: Anaphylactic reactions following the intradiscal injection of chymopapain under local anaesthesia. J Bone Joint Surg 65A: 1212–1219, 1983.
26. Shields CB, Arpin EJ: Prone position chemonucleolysis. *In* Brown JE, Nordby EJ, Smith L (eds): Chemonucleolysis. Thorofare, NJ, Slack, 1985, pp 119–127.
27. McCulloch JA, Waddell G: Lateral lumbar discography. Br J Radiol 51:498–502, 1978.
28. Edwards WC: CT discography: Prognostic value in the selection of patients for chemonucleolysis. Spine 12:792–795, 1987.
29. McCulloch JA: Discometry. *In* McCulloch JA, Macnab I (eds): Sciatica and chymopapain. Baltimore, Waverly, 1983.
30. Chung BU: Bent-tip single needle technique. *In* Brown JE, Nordby EJ (eds): Chemonucleolysis. Thorofare, NJ, Slack, 1985, pp 143–165.
31. Kiester PD, et al: Is the effect of chymopapain on disc proteoglycans dose related? North American Spine Society paper, Quebec City, Canada. June 30, 1989.
32. Abdel-Salam A, et al: A new paradiscal injection technique for the relief of back spasm after chemonucleolysis. Br J Rheumatol 31:491–493, 1992.
33. Nordby EJ, Fraser RD: Chemonucleolysis. The Adult Spine: Principles and Practice, 1989–2008, 1997.
34. Osti OL, Fraser RD: Discitis after discography. The role of prophylactic antibiotics. J Bone Joint Surg 72B:271–274, 1990.
35. Brock M, et al: The results of lumbar disc surgery following unsuccessful chemonucleolysis. Acta Neurochir 112:65–70, 1991.
36. Deburge A, et al: Surgical findings and results of surgery after failure of chemonucleolysis. Spine 10:812–815, 1985.
37. Javid MJ, et al: Long-term follow up of postchymopapain laminectomy patients versus repeat laminectomy patients. Presented at the International Intradiscal Therapy Society Meeting, La Jolla, CA, March 14–15, 1995.
38. Nordby EJ: Editorial comment: Long-term results in chemonucleolysis. Clin Orthop 206:2–3, 1986.
39. Brautaset NJ, et al: Lumbale skiveprolapser behandlet med kymopapain. Tidsskr Nor Laegeforen 112:2335–2339, 1992.
40. Nordby EJ, Wright PH: Efficacy of chymopapain in chemonucleolysis: A review. Spine 19:3578–3583, 1994.

41. Wilson LF, Mulholland RC: The long-term results of chemonucleolysis. *In* Wittenberg RH, Steffan R (eds): Chemonucleolysis and Related Intradiscal Therapies. New York, Thieme, 1995, pp 69–75.
42. Gogan WJ, Fraser RD: Chymopapain. A 10-year double blind study. Spine 7:388–394, 1992.
43. Deutman RD, et al: Repeat chemonucleolysis. Presented at the Eighth Annual Meeting International Intradiscal Society Meeting, La Jolla, CA, March 15–19, 1995.
44. Bonafe A: Chymopapain cervical chemonucleolysis. Preliminary results in 15 cases. *In* Bonneville J-F (ed): Focus on Chemonucleolysis. Berlin, Springer-Verlag, 1986, 126–132.
45. Castresana FG, et al: Cervical chemonucleolysis. Presentation of three cases. Early results. International Intradiscal Therapy Society meeting, Orlando, FL, March 10, 1989.
46. Lazorthes Y, et al: Chemonucleolysis of cervical disks: Preliminary results in 15 cases of root compression. *In* Sutton JC (ed): Current Concepts in Chemonucleolysis, J R Soc Med 72:217–233, 1985.
47. Krause D, et al: Cervical nucleolysis: Indications, technique, results. 190 patients. J Neuroradiol 20:42, 1993.
48. Castresana FG, et al: Cervical chymopapain nucleolysis. Percutaneous spine techniques. Neurosurg Clin North Am :1–16, 1996.
49. Javid MJ, et al: Current status of chymopapain in herniated nucleus pulposus. Neurosurg Q 62:662–666, 1985.

INDEX

Note: Page numbers in *italics* indicate illustrations; those followed by t refer to tables.